PROSTHETIC AND BIOPROSTHETIC HEART VALVES

Collected Reprints (1966-2019)

By

William C. Roberts, MD

and

Colleagues

ISBN: 979-8-88862-142-4
Printed in the United States of America on acid-free paper.

Table of Contents

*Articles are numbered based on WCR's CV.

Bacterial Endocarditis Involving Prosthetic Mitral Valves

Clinical and Pathologic Observations

WILLIAM C. ROBERTS, MD, AND ANDREW G. MORROW, MD, BETHESDA, MD

The clinical and necropsy findings are described in two patients who developed staphylococcal endocarditis following replacement of the mitral valve with Starr-Edwards prostheses. In each, death resulted from large thrombi which formed on the prostheses, causing them to become both stenotic and incompetent. The character and extent of the infection in the mitral annulus would have made secondary operative intervention fruitless.

BACTERIAL or fungal endocarditis is an infrequent but dreaded complication of cardiac valve replacement. At the National Heart Institute, more than 150 patients have undergone mitral valve replacement with Starr-Edwards prostheses. None of these patients developed endocarditis as an immediate consequence of the operation, but fatal infections have occurred in two patients in the late postoperative period. Previous reports concerning endocarditis in patients with prosthetic valves [1-3] generally have emphasized the clinical features of the disease, and have suggested prophylactic measures to prevent its occurrence.[4] The present report focuses attention on the pathologic features of this cardiac infection, as demonstrated by the findings in the two patients who developed infective endocarditis after mitral valve replacement.

Accepted for publication April 22, 1966.

From the Clinic of Surgery, National Heart Institute, National Institutes of Health, Bethesda, Md.

Reprint requests to Laboratory of Pathology, Clinic of Surgery, National Heart Institute, National Institutes of Health, Bethesda, Md 20014 (Dr. Roberts).

Report of Cases

CASE 1 (06-11-64).—A man 47 years of age had his calcified stenotic mitral valve replaced with a Starr-Edwards prosthesis on April 29, 1965. On the day before, the day of, and on each of the seven days after the cardiac operation he received erythromycin ethylsuccinate (1.0 gm intramuscularly), streptomycin (1.0 gm intramuscularly) and sodium methicillin (12 gm intramuscularly). This prophylactic regimen was utilized because the patient had had allergic manifestations when he had been given penicillin on other occasions. The patient's postoperative course was uneventful, but some weeks after discharge he developed a superficial ulcer on his left lower leg. On July 21, at his local hospital, a split-thickness skin graft was applied to the ulcerated area. No local or systemic antibiotics were administered before or immediately after the procedure. Eight hours following the grafting operation, the patient had a chill, vomited, and became disoriented. On the following day he was semicomatose, incontinent of urine and feces, his temperature was 105.8 F. (41 C); later that day signs of left hemiparesis became evident. Chloramphenicol, streptomycin, and kanamycin sulfate were then administered, and a blood culture obtained two days later remained sterile. On August 5, penicillin (15 million units intravenously) and methicillin (4 gm intravenously) daily were substituted for the other antibiotics. On August 15, all antibiotics were discontinued, since no improvement had occurred, and three blood cultures obtained on August 19 grew *Staphylococcus aureus*, coagulase positive. The patient died on August 20.

The heart (A65-186) was returned to us for examination. The orifice of the prosthetic mitral valve was occluded by a large vegetation (Fig 1) which, on microscopic examination, contained numerous clumps of gram-positive cocci. The infected thrombotic material also was present on the ventricular aspect of the prosthesis, attached to both the Teflon and metallic rings and to the base of each of the four metallic struts (Fig 2). About

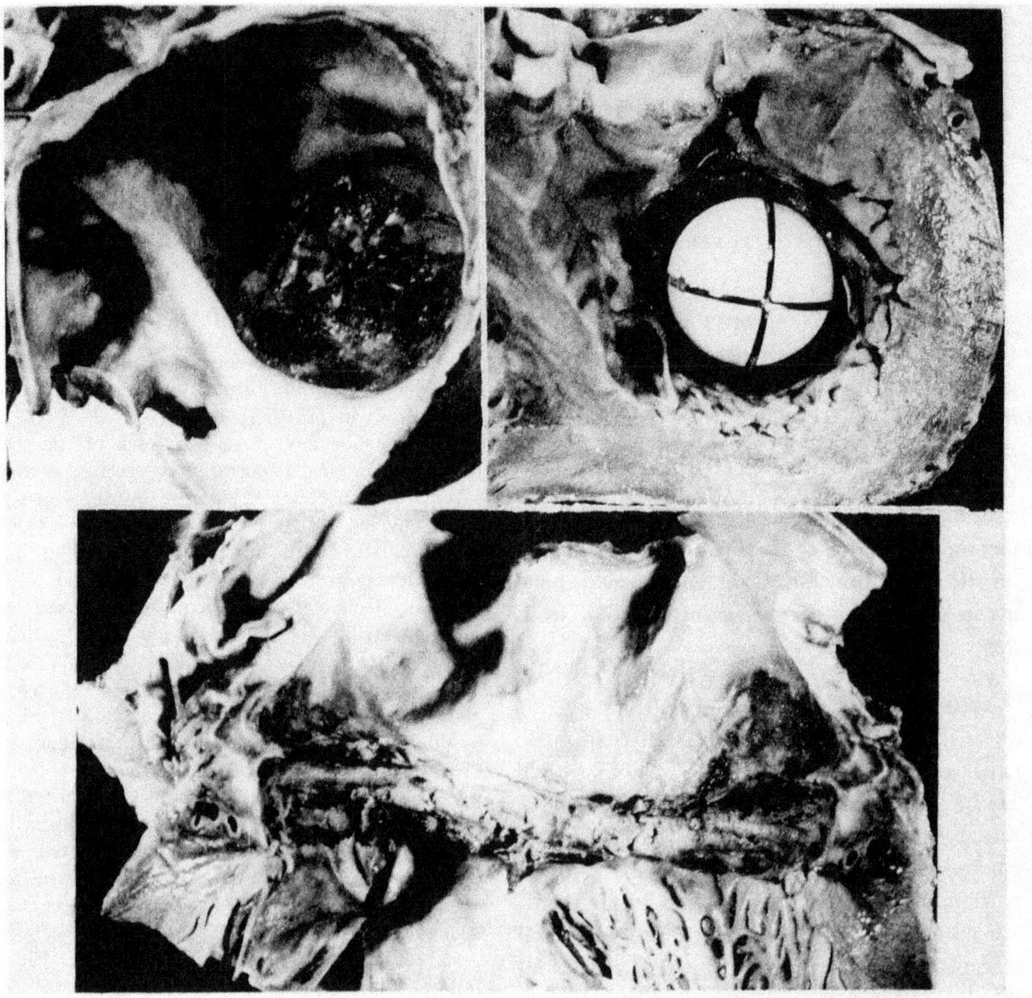

Fig 1.—Heart of patient 1. *Top left,* Opened left atrium, showing the prosthetic mitral orifice completely obscured by a large thrombus. *Top right,* Opened left ventricular cavity disclosing vegetative material about the metallic base of the prosthesis. *Bottom,* Opened left atrium, mitral annulus, and left ventricle. The entire mitral annulus is necrotic. Acute necrotizing inflammation also is present in the adjacent myocardium, and in the atrioventricular sulcus surrounding the coronary vessels.

30% of the circumference of the Teflon fixation ring of the prosthesis was not attached to the mitral annulus, but since the unattached portion of the fixation ring was covered by infected thrombus, which also was adherent to the left atrial wall, no peribasilar communications were present. Following removal of the prosthesis, the entire mitral annulus was found to be necrotic, and the inflammatory process also was present in the subepicardial tissue of the artrioventricular sulcus, and in the adjacent myocardium (Fig 3). Histologic sections of the myocardial walls disclosed acute and subacute abscesses and infarcts. Many intramural coronary arteries contained infected emboli, and had acutely inflamed walls (Fig 4). Focal infarcts also were present in the spleen (240 gm), kidneys and brain.

CASE 2 (05-68-27).—A 46-year-old man had a stenotic and incompetent mitral valve replaced with a Starr-Edwards prosthesis on July 23, 1964. Cardiac catheterization eight months later (March 1965) disclosed that the left atrial pressure and cardiac output had returned to normal, and he was asymptomatic. He continued to be well until Nov 5, 1965, when he suddenly fainted, and during the next 24 hours he vomited several times, became listless and anorexic. On November 19 he noted fever (102 F [39.9 C]), and consulted his physician who administered an antibiotic, which was probably erythromycin. He was readmitted to the National Heart Institute on November 24 and was lethargic and disoriented. His temperature rose daily to 102 F (39.9 C). On auscultation the sounds of the prosthetic mitral valve were normal, and no murmur suggesting mitral regurgitation was audible. Dental examination revealed his teeth to be in excellent condition, except for two small cavities. The white blood cell count was 41,000/cu mm, and the hematocrit, 41%. On November 28 cultures of blood drawn during the previous four days grew *Staphylococcus albus,* and daily doses of penicillin (100 million units intravenously) and streptomycin (2 gm intramuscularly) were initiated. The patient became hypotensive, evidenced progressively decreasing cardiac output, and died on Nov 30, 1965.

At autopsy (A65-221), the orifice of the prosthetic mitral valve was almost totally occluded by a thrombus, and thrombus was also present on the ventricular aspect of the mitral prosthesis (Fig 5). Cultures of left ventricular blood at autopsy were sterile, but cultures of the thrombus on the valve grew *S albus.* The movement of the ball in the cage of the Starr-Edwards prosthesis was severely limited by the mass of infected thrombus, and the ball was neither able to extend to the apex of the cage nor to seat completely (Fig 6). The entire mitral annulus was necrotic, and the inflammatory process was present in the adjacent myocardium, and in the subepicardial fat of the atrioventricular sulcus (Fig 7). A histologic section of the mitral annulus is shown in Fig 3. Gram-positive organisms in clumps were identified in the mitral vegetations. Several organizing microinfarcts were present in the left ventricular wall near its base, but no acute microinfarcts, abscesses, or coronary arterial emboli were found. Multiple cerebral and splenic infarcts were present.

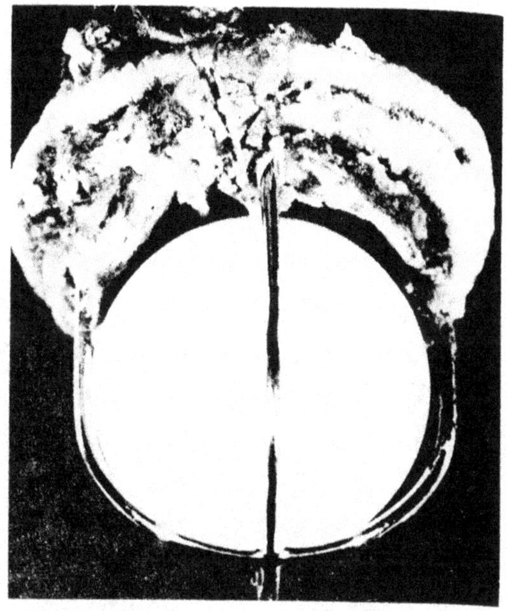

Fig 2.—The Starr-Edwards mitral valve removed from the heart of patient 1. The infected thrombus restricts the motion of the ball, and prevents it from seating completely. As a result, the prosthetic valve is both stenotic and incompetent.

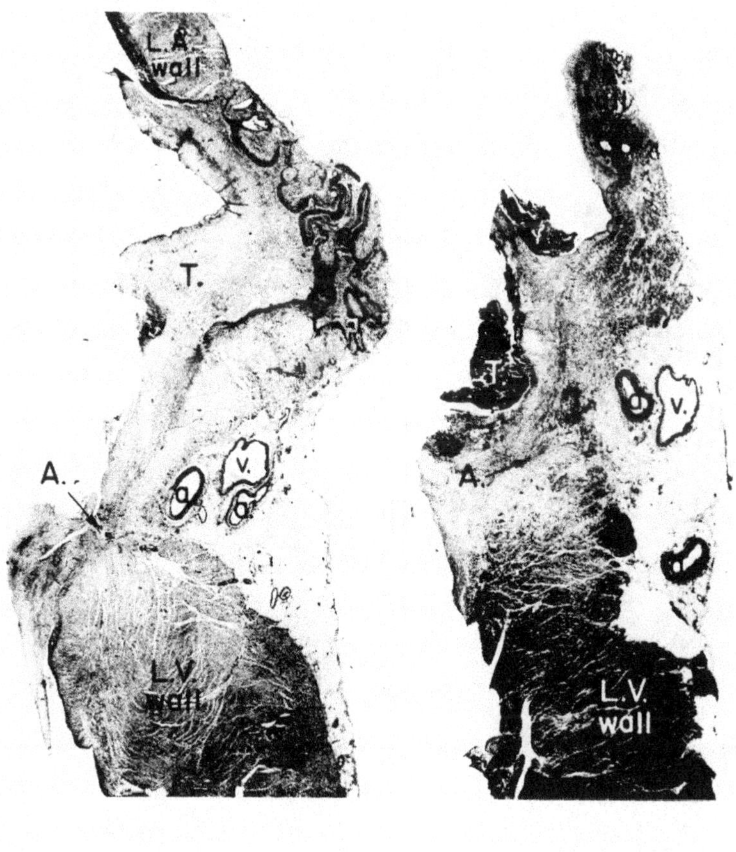

Fig 3.—Section of left atrial (*L.A.*) and left ventricular (*L.V.*) walls and mitral annulus (*A., arrow*) in patients 1 (at left) and 2 (at right). The infected thrombus (*T.*) covers a considerable portion of the left atrial endocardium, and extends into the adjacent myocardium and into the atrioventricular sulcus. (*a.*) indicates coronary artery and (*v.*) coronary sinus (hematoxylin and eosin; × 3, reduced about 15%).

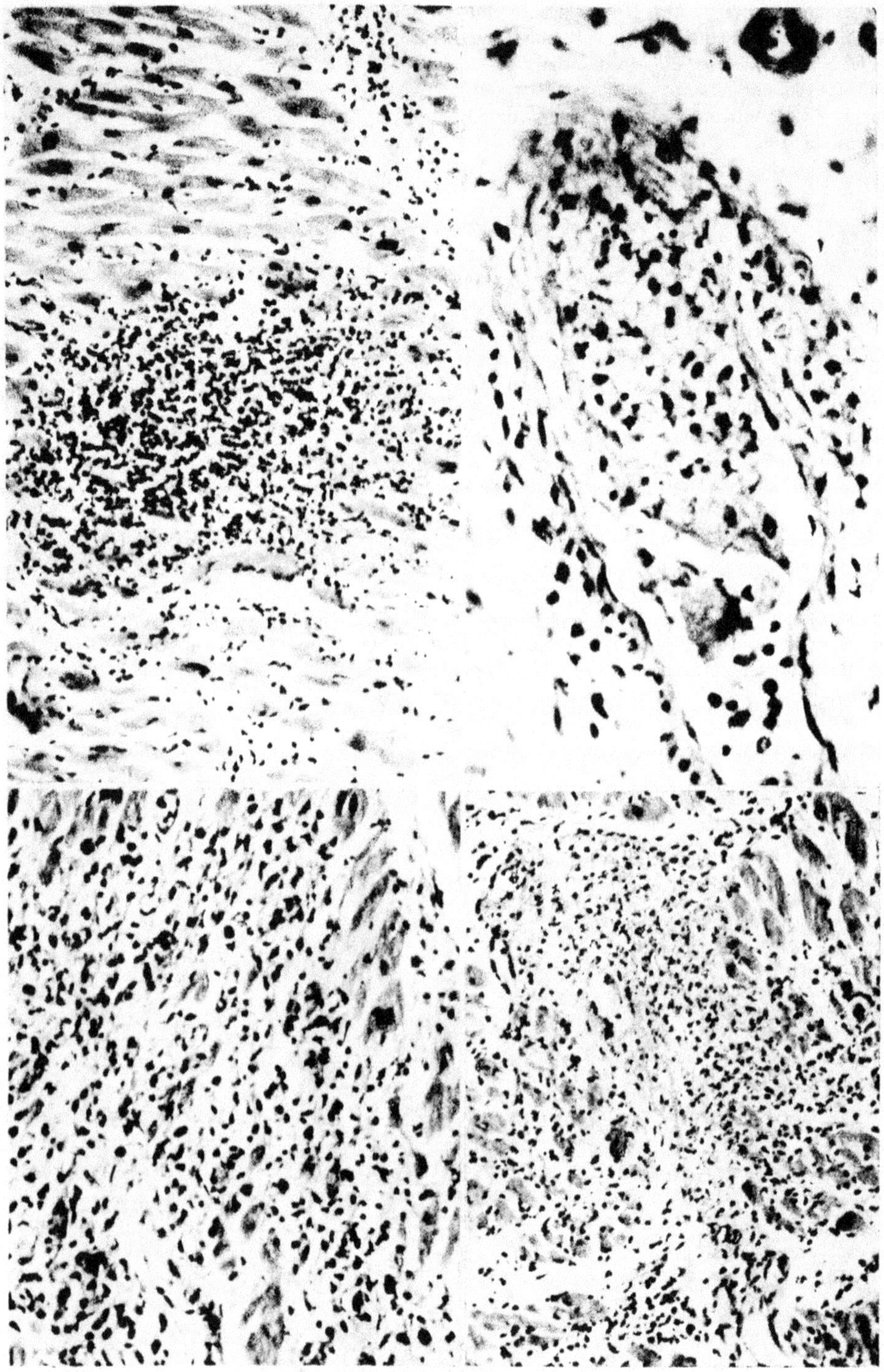

Fig 4.—Lesions in the left ventricular wall in patient 1. *Top left,* Acute abscess (hematoxylin and eosin, × 160). *Top right,* Intramural coronary artery containing infected embolus. The inflamed embolus appears to burrow into the vessel wall producing an acute arteritis (hematoxylin and eosin, × 400). *Bottom left,* Organizing abscess. Other areas disclosed both acute and healed microinfarcts. The lesion illustrated probably represents a transitional stage between acute abscess or acute infarct, and healed microinfarct (hematoxylin and eosin, × 186). *Bottom right,* Acute vasculitis probably resulting from an infected embolus penetrating its wall (hematoxylin and eosin, × 186).

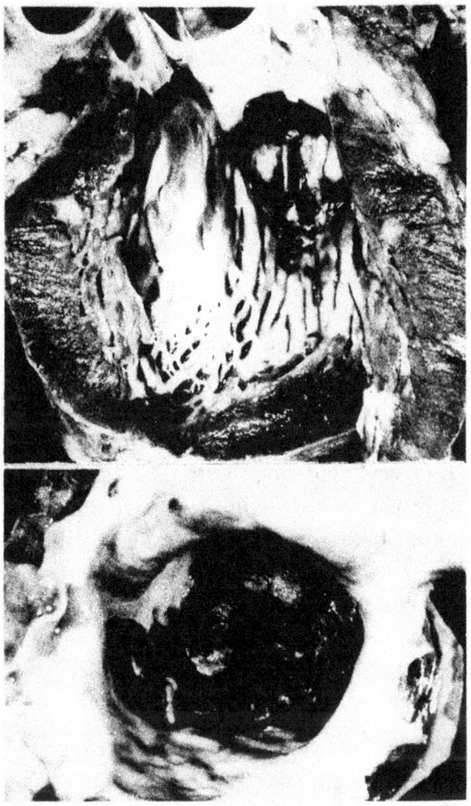

Fig 5.—Opened left ventricle and aortic valve (*top*) and opened left atrium (*bottom*) in patient 2. The infected thrombus is located on both the atrial and ventricular aspects of the Starr-Edwards mitral prosthesis, and from the atrial aspect the prosthetic orifice is seen to be obliterated. The thickened left ventricular endocardium appears to result primarily from healing of the stumps of the amputated papillary muscles.

Comment

The courses of the two patients described above, and the reported experiences of others,[1-3] indicate that infection at the site of a prosthetic cardiac valve is almost always fatal, and that death usually occurs within a month following the onset of signs and symptoms. Death from endocarditis at the site of a prosthetic aortic valve is usually related to detachment of the valve from the aortic annulus, with resulting severe aortic regurgitation and cardiac failure.[4] In the present two patients, the infected thrombi or vegetations on the mitral prostheses interfered with the motion of the ball in the cage and death resulted from obstruction to flow and to valvular incompetence.[5] Although the fixation ring of the mitral prosthesis was partially detached from the mitral annulus in each of the two patients described, a regurgitant leak between the prosthetic ring and the mitral annulus did not occur since the areas of disruption were covered by thrombi.

Staphylococcus is the organism most often responsible for endocarditis in patients with prosthetic valves. It is well recognized that staphylococci produce an acute destructive endocarditis,[6] and this fact is again emphasized by the two patients described herein. Not only did the infectious process involve the mitral ring in each patient, but it ex-

Fig 6.—The mitral prosthesis removed from the heart of patient 2. The movement of the ball in the cage is severely restricted by the mass of the infected thrombus. Several sutures had torn away from the necrotic annulus. The valve is seen from both its anterior and posterior aspects.

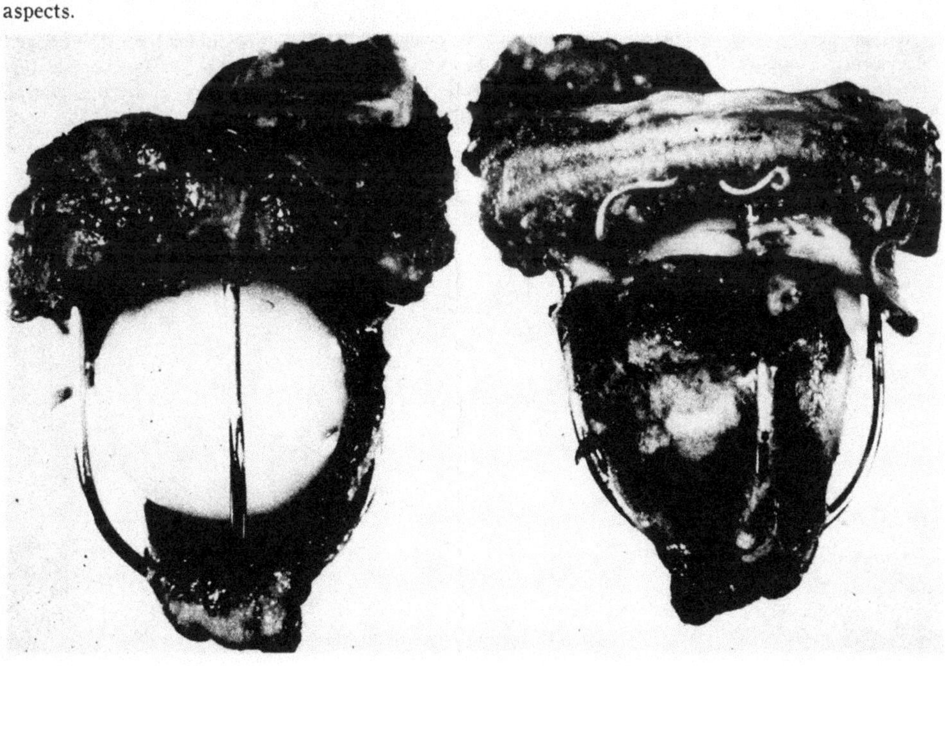

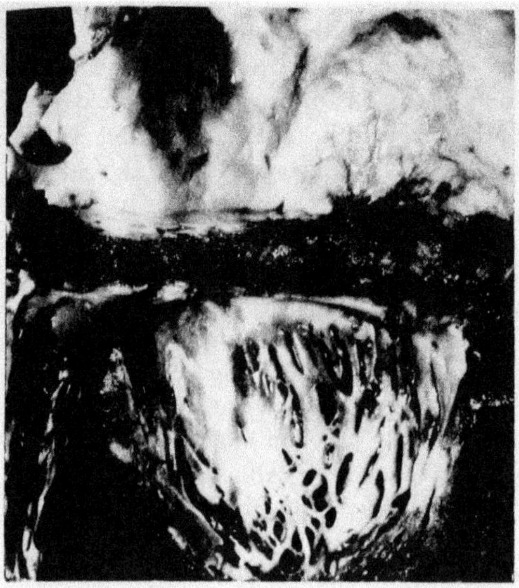

Fig 7.—Opened left atrium, mitral annulus, and left ventricle in patient *2* following removal of the mitral prosthesis. The entire mitral ring is necrotic.

tended into the adjacent myocardium, and into the subepicardial adipose tissue of the left atrioventricular sulcus. The extent of the infection and the character of the tissue of the mitral annulus in these patients clearly indicate that an attempt at secondary operative intervention would have been fruitless. Consequently, since presently available antibiotics are rarely effective in eradicating infection at the site of a prosthetic cardiac valve the infection must be prevented. In patient 1, the infection could, perhaps, have been prevented by prophylactic antibiotics administered before and immediately after the skin grafting operation, but no source of infection was evident in patient 2. The value of prophylactic penicillin in patients with rheumatic heart disease who undergo dental procedures is well established, but the necessity of even more vigorous prophylactic regimens in patients with prosthetic cardiac valves who undergo similar procedures has only recently been emphasized.[4]

Generic and Trade Names of Drugs

Sodium methicillin—*Dimocillin-RT*, *Staphcillin*.
Kanamycin sulfate—*Kantrex*.
Chloramphenicol—*Chloromycetin*.
Erythromycin ethylsuccinate—*Erythrocin Ethyl Succinate*, *Pediamycin*.

REFERENCES

1. Amoury, R.A.; Bowman, F.O.; and Malm, J.R.: Endocarditis Associated With Intracardiac Prostheses: Diagnosis, Management and Prophylaxsis, *J Thorac Cardiov Surg* **51**:36, 1966.
2. Stein, P.D.; Harken, D.E.; and Dexter, L.: The Nature and Prevention of Prosthetic Valve Endocarditis, *Amer Heart J* **71**:393, 1966.
3. Herr, R., et al: Special Problems Following Valve Replacement: Embolus, Leak, Infection, Red Cell Damage, *Ann Thorac Surg* **1**:403, 1965.
4. Cohn, L.H., et al: Bacterial Endocarditis Following Aortic Valve Replacement: Clinical and Pathologic Correlations, *Circulation* **33**:209, 1966.
5. Roberts, W.C., and Morrow, A.G.: The Mechanisms of Acute Left Atrial Thrombosis After Mitral Valve Replacement: Pathologic Findings Indicating Obstruction to Left Atrial Emptying, *Amer J Cardiol*, to be published.
6. Sheldon, W.H., and Golden, A.: Abscesses of the Valve Rings of the Heart: A Frequent but Not Well Recognized Complication of Acute Bacterial Endocarditis, *Circulation* **4**:1, 1951.

Late Postoperative Pathological Findings After Cardiac Valve Replacement

By William C. Roberts, M.D., and Andrew G. Morrow, M.D.

A NUMBER of previous reports from this and other clinics have described the use of Starr-Edwards prostheses in the operative management of acquired mitral and aortic valve disease. In general, these studies have assessed the effectiveness of the prosthetic valves in terms of immediate and late mortality and also by comparisons of pre- and postoperative clinical, radiographic, electrocardiographic, and hemodynamic examinations. However, less attention has been directed to the pathological anatomy of hearts in which Starr-Edwards valves have functioned for long periods of time. At the National Heart Institute, the hearts of 20 patients who died at late postoperative intervals after mitral and/or aortic valve replacement have been examined. The results of these examinations and correlations with appropriate antemortem clinical data are presented in this report.

Clinical and Pathological Observations

Starr-Edwards valves have been utilized in this clinic for replacement of one or more cardiac valves in 280 patients with congenital or acquired heart disease. Of these 280 patients 82 have died, and 78 were studied at necropsy. Of the latter number 58 patients died within one month of operation and 20 from one and one-third to 28 months after operation (average ten months). Pertinent clinical and pathological data concerning these 20 patients are summarized in table 1. The mitral valve had been replaced in six patients, the aortic in 12, and both mitral and aortic valves in two.

From the Clinic of Surgery, National Heart Institute, National Institutes of Health, Bethesda, Maryland.

Causes of Death

Five patients died of infection: staphylococcal endocarditis occurred at the site of the valvular prosthesis in four,[1, 2] and pulmonary nocardiosis secondary to dexamethasone therapy for serum hepatitis was the cause of death in the fifth.[3] Two patients (nos. 3 and 19) died of ventriculoatrial regurgitation around prosthetic mitral valves. One patient (no. 6) developed progressive thrombosis on the ventricular aspect of a mitral prosthesis; it became severely stenotic, and she died of congestive failure. Two patients who had Marfan's syndrome had replacement of the aortic valve and the ascending aorta; one died of associated mitral regurgitation and the other of renal failure caused by an associated aneurysm in the descending thoracic aorta. One patient with a prosthetic mitral valve had an intracerebral hemorrhage secondary to warfarin-produced hypoprothrombinemia.

The nine remaining patients died suddenly and unexpectedly; one had had a mitral replacement and eight aortic replacements. Three of the patients with prosthetic aortic valves and the one with the mitral prosthesis had had acute myocardial infarctions documented before operation; in the three with aortic valves, left ventricular aneurysms were evident at necropsy. The infarcts and aneurysms in two patients (nos. 7 and 16) followed acute bacterial endocarditis involving the aortic valve and were apparently the result of coronary arterial emboli. In the third patient (no. 12), myocardial infarction and aneurysm resulted from extensive coronary arterial atherosclerosis. Four of the nine patients who died suddenly complained of chest pain immediately before death, but necropsy showed changes of acute myocardial infarction in only one (no. 15). Eight of these nine patients had severe coronary arterial narrowing, and extensive myocardial scarring was present in each of them. The patient with the mitral prosthesis who died suddenly had had complete heart block before operation, and a pacemaker had been implanted at the time of valve replacement. The pacemaker was functioning after death, but a fatal Adams-Stokes attack could have resulted from failure of the heart to respond to the stimulation.

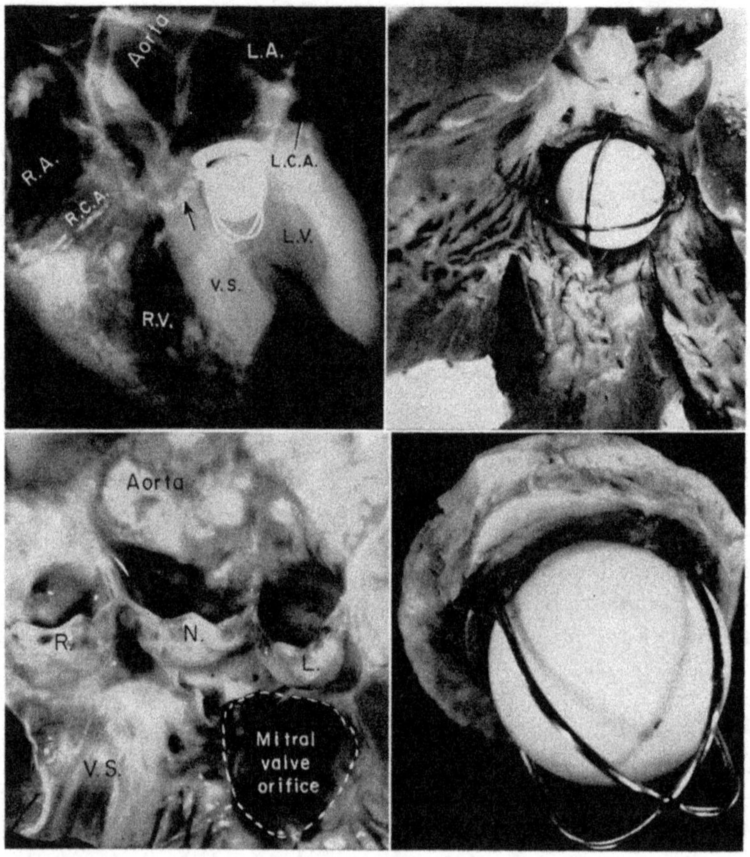

Figure 1

Heart of patient 1. This 53-year-old woman with mitral stenosis and regurgitation and mild aortic and tricuspid regurgitation underwent mitral replacement seven months earlier. Complete heart block, the result of calcium destroying the bundle of His, appeared four years before death, and a pacemaker had been inserted at the time of valve replacement. She died suddenly at home. Top left: Radiograph of the heart, showing the position of the ball during ventricular systole. The ball is unable to seat completely because of thrombus. The arrow designates a mass of calcium in the area of the bundle of His. Calcium deposits are also present in the right (R.C.A.) and left (L.C.A.) coronary arteries, and complete focal luminal occlusions of these vessels were present. R.A. = right atrium; R.V. = right ventricle; L.A. = left atrium; L.V. = left ventricle; V.S. = ventricular septum. Top right: Opened left ventricle and aortic valve showing thrombus on the mitral prosthesis. There is considerable endocardial thickening of the left ventricle. Bottom left: Close-up of opened aorta, aortic valve, and left ventricular outflow tract. This patient's aortic regurgitation resulted from mild fibrous contraction of each of the three cusps (R. = right; N. = noncoronary; L. = left). The mitral annulus is designated by the dashed line. Bottom right: Excised mitral prosthesis, showing thrombus on the metallic ring and bases of two struts. This thrombus prevented the ball from seating completely and resulted in mitral regurgitation, although regurgitation was not detected clinically.

Table 1

*Clinical and Pathological Data in Twenty Patients Who Died After Valve Replacement with Starr-Edwards Prostheses**

Pt.	Age / Sex	Preop lesions	Valve replaced	Anti-coagulants post-operatively	Interval operation to death (months)	Cause of death	Thrombus on prosthesis	Peribasilar fistula	Coronary artery disease	Associated disease
1	53 / F	MS, MI, TI	Mitral	Warfarin	7	Sudden	++	0	Gr. 5/5	Healed myocardial infarct; complete heart block and pacemaker; angina pectoris
2	65 / F	MS	Mitral	Warfarin	8	Cerebral hemorrhage	0	0	Gr. 3/5	0
3	29 / M	MS, MI, TI	Mitral	Warfarin	9	Congestive heart failure	++	+	0	0
4	46 / M	MS, MI, TI	Mitral	0	4	Staphylococcal endocarditis	++	0	0	0
5	48 / M	MS, MI, TI	Mitral	Warfarin	17	Staphylococcal endocarditis	++	0	Gr. 4/5	0
6	15 / F	Congenital MI	Mitral	Warfarin	12	Congestive heart failure	++	0	0	Cerebral embolus postop; congenital fibroelastosis, left ventricle
7	26 / M	AI	Aortic	0	3	Sudden	+	0	Gr. 5/5	Healed myocardial infarct; left ventricular aneurysm
8	55 / M	AS	Aortic	0	1¾	Staphylococcal endocarditis	0	+	Gr. 5/5	Healed myocardial infarct
9	48 / M	AS, AI	Aortic	0	4	Sudden	0	0	Gr. 4/5	Angina pectoris only after operation
10	51 / M	AS, AI	Aortic	0	12	Staphylococcal endocarditis	++	+	Gr. 2/5	0
11	21 / M	AI, MI	Aortic	0	7½	Died 2 wk after mitral replacement	+ (aortic)	+ (aortic)	Gr. 3/5	Marfan's syndrome
12	60 / F	AS	Aortic	0	20	Sudden	+	0	Gr. 5/5	Healed myocardial infarct; left ventricular aneurysm; angina pectoris
13	51 / M	AS	Aortic	0	1 1/3	Sudden	+	0	Gr. 3/5	Angina pectoris
14	41 / M	AI	Aortic	0	2½	Thrombosed aneurysm in descending thoracic aorta	+	0	Gr. 2/5	Marfan's syndrome
15	50 / M	AS, AI	Aortic	0	24	Sudden; acute myocardial infarct	++	+	Gr. 4/5	Angina pectoris

16	24/M	AS	Aortic	0	9	Sudden	++	0	0	Healed myocardial infarct; left ventricular aneurysm; arthrogryposis multiplex congenita
17	27/M	AI	Aortic	0	13	Sudden	+	0	0	0
18	41/M	AS	Aortic	0	28	Sudden	+	0	Gr. 2/5	Extensive subendocardial fibrosis, left ventricle
19	47/M	AI, MI	Aortic, mitral	Warfarin	6½	Congestive heart failure	+ (mitral)	+ (mitral)	Gr. 1/5	0
20	45/M	MS, MI, AI	Aortic, mitral	Warfarin	10	Pulmonary nocardiosis	++ (mitral)	+ (mitral)	Gr. 2/5	Chronic hepatic disease

*Key to abbreviations:
MS and MI = mitral stenosis and mitral regurgitation.
AS and AI = aortic stenosis and aortic regurgitation
TI = tricuspid regurgitation.
Thrombus + = present but not functionally significant.
Thrombus ++ = present and functionally significant.

Grading of coronary arterial narrowing:
Gr. 1/5 = up to 25% occlusion of lumen.
Gr. 2/5 = 26 to 50% occlusion.
Gr. 3/5 = 51 to 75%.
Gr. 4/5 = 76 to 99%.
Gr. 5/5 = complete occlusion.

Prosthetic Valve Thrombi

Thrombi were found on the prosthetic valves at necropsy in 17 of the 20 patients (figs. 1 to 6). Seven of the 17 had been receiving warfarin. Three of the 17 patients with thrombi were among those who died of bacterial (staphylococcal) endocarditis. Only one of the remaining 14 patients with thrombus on their valves had had evidence of systemic emboli during life or at necropsy. In seven of the 14 patients, the thrombus had rendered the prosthesis incompetent, stenotic, or both, but in the others valve function was not impaired. Of the nine patients who died suddenly, eight had thrombus on their prostheses. The thrombi were usually located at the junction of the struts and the metallic rings and extended up the struts for variable distances. In patient 15, who also had a small peribasilar leak, the extensive thrombus on the struts prevented random motion of the ball, which became grooved by the struts. In addition to its being discolored and grooved (fig. 6), the weight of the prosthetic ball in this patient was 9.1% greater than when it had been inserted 24 months earlier.[4] Rarely, a thrombus was attached only to the metallic ring of the prosthesis. In no patient was thrombus located only at the apex of the cage of the prosthesis. Histological study of several of the thrombi disclosed that they consisted predominantly of fibrin; no bacteria or fungi were seen.

Fistulae Around Prosthetic Valve Rings

As noted, mitral peribasilar communications were considered to be responsible for death in two patients, and in three additional patients, excluding those with staphylococcal endocarditis, such communications were also present (fig. 7). Two were around prosthetic mitral valves and one at the base of an aortic valve. The presence of these accessory communications was established before death in the patient with the aortic prosthesis (no. 15) but in only one of the four patients with mitral prostheses.

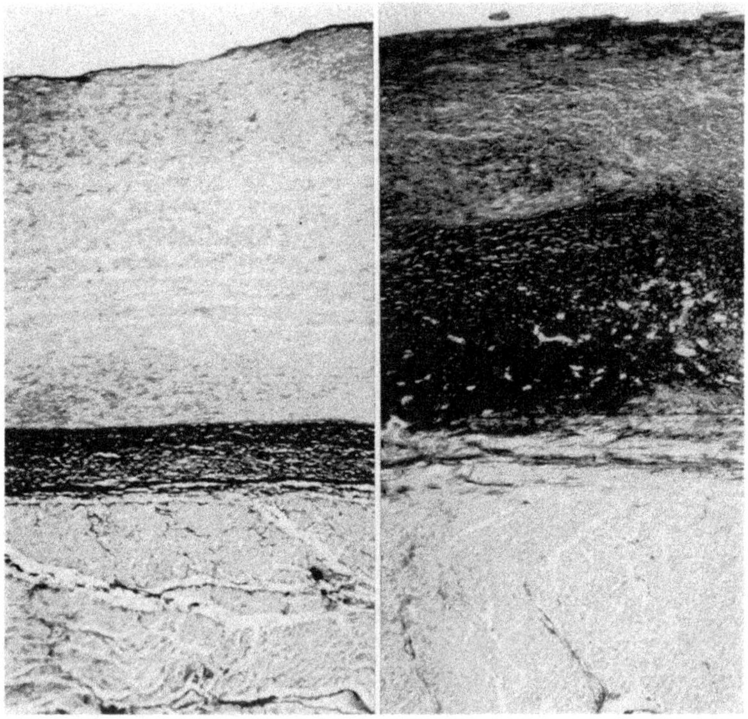

Figure 2

Photomicrographs of left atrial wall (left) and left ventricle (right) in patient 1. Elastic fibers stain black. There is marked thickening of the endocardium of the left atrium, and this fibrous reaction is free of elastic fibrils. In contrast, there is also marked endocardial thickening of the left ventricle, but this connective tissue contains numerous elastic fibers. The left atrial and left ventricular endocardial thickening illustrated was observed in nearly all patients who had undergone mitral replacement but was unusually severe in this patient. Elastic tissue stains; each ×32.

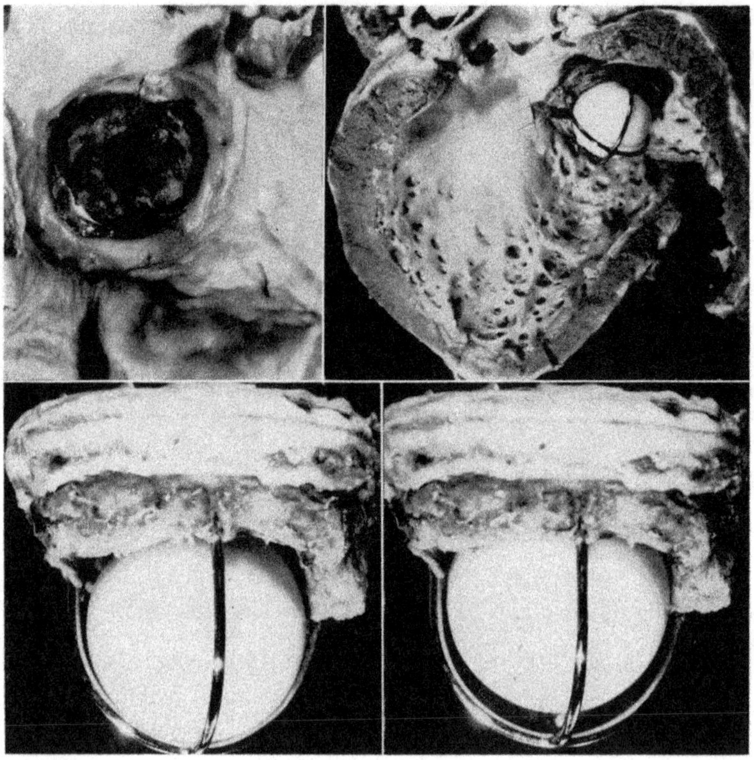

Figure 3

Heart and prosthesis in patient 6. This 15-year-old girl had congenital mitral regurgitation and endocardial fibroelastosis of the left ventricle. Seven days after replacement of the mitral valve with a 4-M Starr-Edwards prosthesis, she had a cerebral embolus. At catheterization nine and one-half months after operation, the cardiac index had returned to normal (3.2 L/min/m²), but the mean left atrial and left ventricular end-diastolic pressures were increased to 20 and 18 mm Hg, respectively; no pressure gradient was present across the valve. Two and one-half months after this catheterization, she developed severe heart failure and died. At autopsy the prosthesis was found to have been made severely stenotic and slightly incompetent by a large thrombus. Top left: The left atrium is opened, showing the thrombus partially occluding the prosthetic mitral orifice. Fibrous tissue has completely covered the Teflon fixation ring and the sutures. Top right: Opened left ventricle and aortic valve showing the ventricular aspect of the mitral prosthesis. There is diffuse endocardial fibroelastosis of the left ventricle. Bottom left: Excised mitral prosthesis showing massive thrombosis. The ball is in the position it would assume during ventricular diastole. Bottom right: The ball is now seated, a position it would assume during ventricular systole. The movement of the ball is extremely limited. Histological sections of the thrombus revealed that it consisted mainly of fibrin and that it contained no bacteria or fungi.

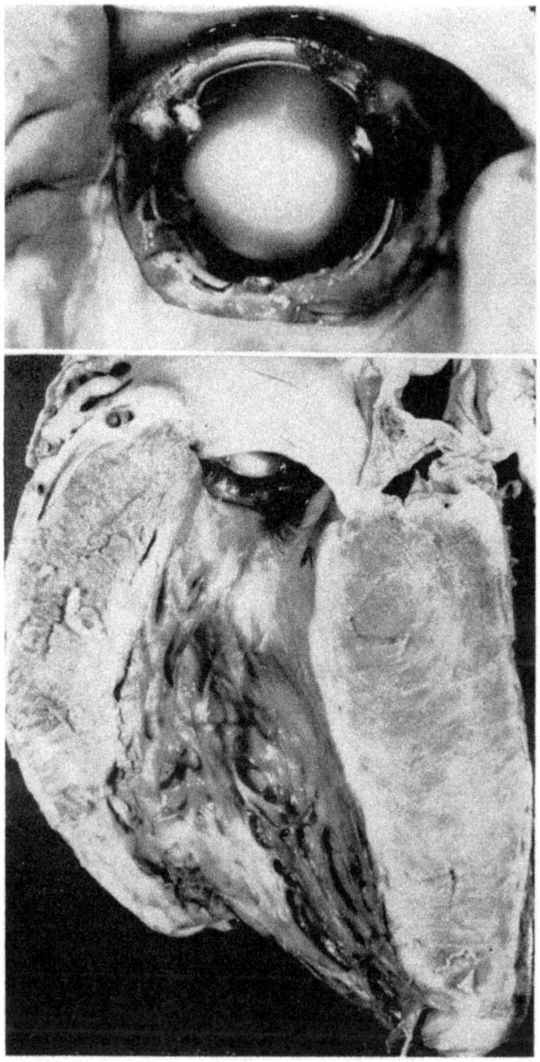

Figure 4

Aortic prosthesis of patient 7 from below showing adherent thrombus (top) and bisected left ventricle showing an aneurysm (bottom). This 26-year-old man was found dead in bed three months after valve replacement. The left ventricular infarct and aneurysm were secondary to a coronary arterial embolus which occurred at the time of aortic valve bacterial endocarditis two years before operation. The cause of the sudden death was not determined.

Intimal Thickening of the Aortic Root and Proximal Coronary Arteries

In each of the 14 patients with prosthetic aortic valves, there was intimal thickening in the aortic root, including the area of the coronary arterial ostia (figs. 8 to 10). This thickening was produced by the deposition of fibrous tissue, which was devoid of foam cells, on the internal elastic membrane of the proximal portion of the ascending aorta. The degree of intimal proliferation varied from minimal in patient 13, who died 40 days after valve replacement, to extremely severe in patients 9 and 12, who died four and 20 months, respectively, after valve replacement. In patient 9, not only was the intima of the aortic root thickened, but there was severe intimal thickening in the proximal 1-cm segments of the right and left coronary arteries. Also, the coronary vessels distal to this point were widely patent (fig. 9). In this patient coronary arterial perfusion cannulae could not be inserted into the ostia at the time of necropsy, although such cannulae had been utilized without difficulty at the time of valve replacement four months earlier. This man, who was 48 years old, had not had chest pain before operation, but two months postoperatively he developed angina pectoris and thereafter had numerous anginal attacks until death. The other patients demonstrated similar although less severe alterations in the aortic root and proximal coronary arteries. In patient 12, who had a ventricular aneurysm, the coronary ostia were so small that the coronary arteries could not be cannulated at the time of operation. In this patient intimal thickening involved not only the ascending aorta and proximal coronary arteries, but also the entire coronary bed, and the changes were clearly attributable to arteriosclerosis.

Associated Myocardial and Endocardial Lesions (Figs. 1 to 3)

Although only five patients had had clinical evidence of myocardial infarction preoperatively, all of the 20 were found at necropsy to have foci of interstitial and replacement fibrosis in the left ventricle. In each of the eight patients in whom the mitral valve was replaced, the stumps of the amputated papillary muscles were covered by fibrous tissue, and in six of them, the fibrous process extended to involve other areas of left ventricular endocardium as well. One of these patients (no. 6) had been considered preoperatively to have rheumatic mitral regurgitation.

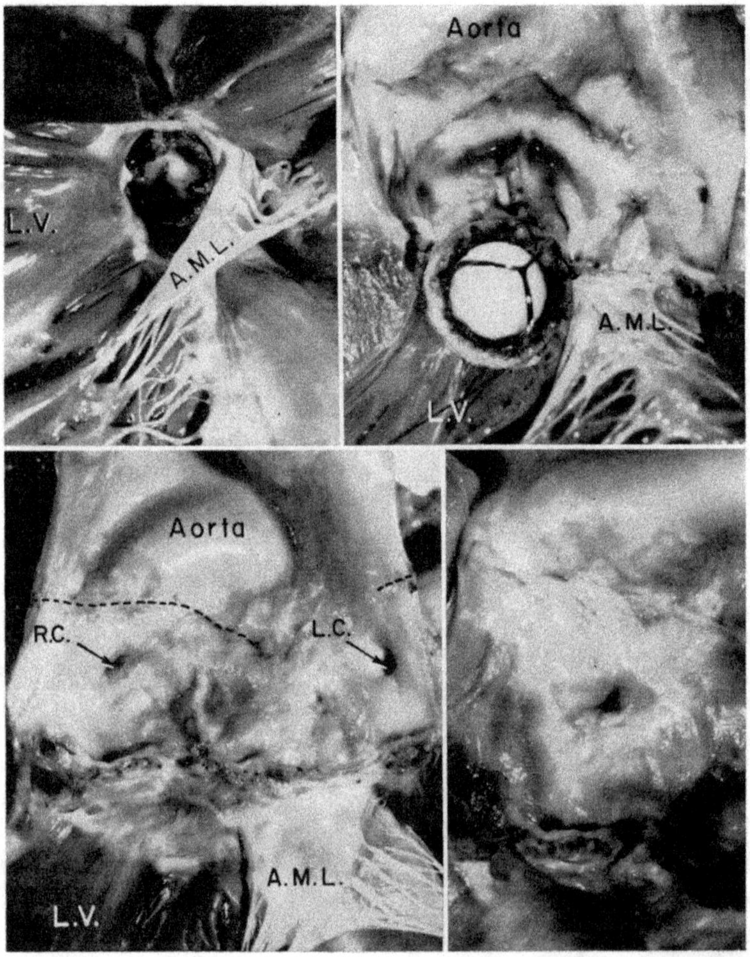

Figure 5

The heart of patient 15 who died of acute myocardial infarction 24 months after valve replacement for calcific aortic stenosis. He had been well postoperatively until one day before death when he experienced precordial pain. Motion of the ball was severely limited by thrombus on the metallic ring and on the struts. Top left: Valve as seen from the left ventricle (L.V.), showing the thrombus. A.M.L. = anterior mitral leaflet. Top right: Opened aorta, aortic valve ring, and left ventricle (L.V.). A wooden stick designates a peribasilar communication. Bottom left: The right (R.C.) and left (L.C.) coronary ostia are indicated. There is considerable intimal thickening in the aortic root. The healed aortotomy incision is shown by the dashed line. It is apparent that intimal proliferation extends some distance from the aortotomy incision. Bottom right: Ostium of right coronary artery; it is narrowed by fibrous intimal proliferation.

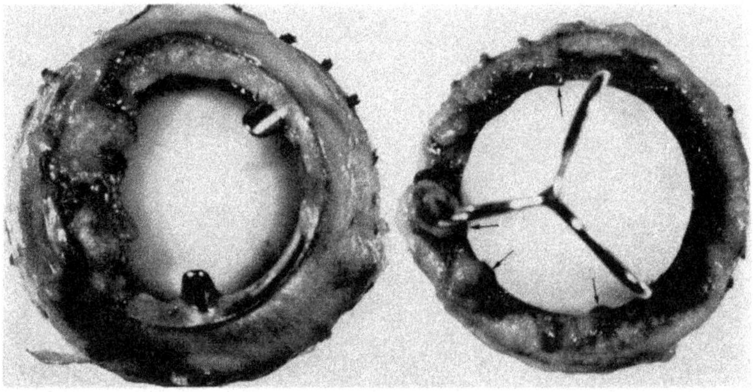

Figure 6

Excised aortic prosthesis (size 9A) in patient 15. Left: As seen from the left ventricular aspect. Right: As seen from the aortic aspect. Several grooves (arrows) are evident in the ball, which was unable to move randomly because of thrombus on the struts and because of increases in its volume (4%) and weight (9%).

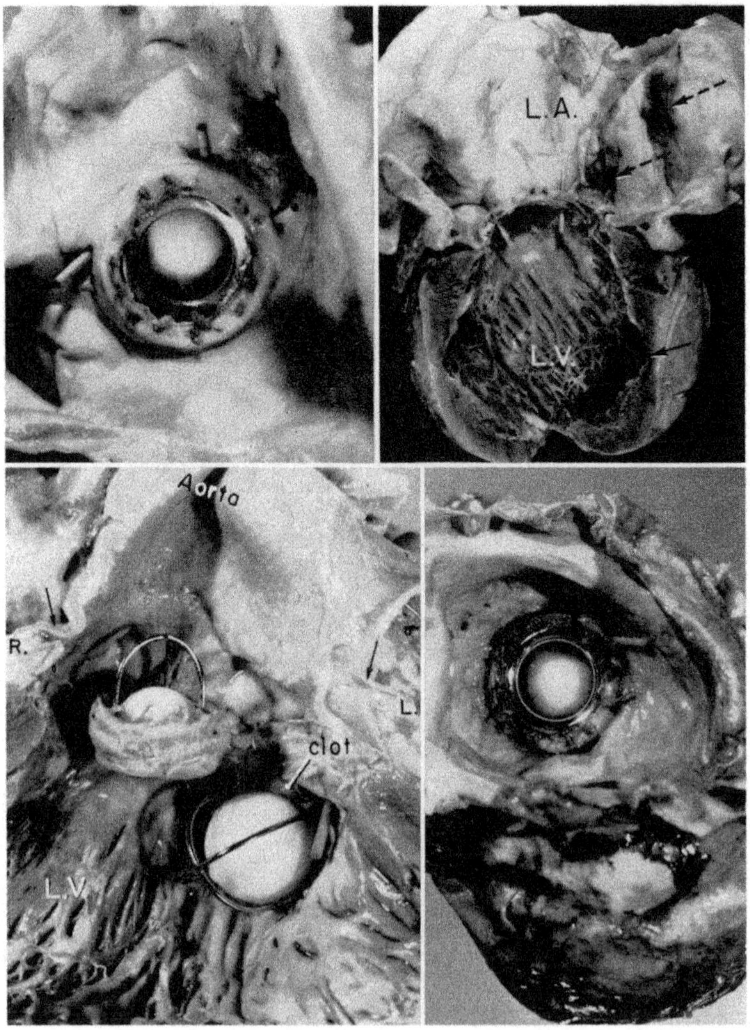

Figure 7

Two of the 20 patients underwent replacement of both mitral and aortic valves. Each developed thrombi on and fistulae around the mitral prostheses. The two upper photographs are the heart of patient 19, who died of severe cardiac failure six and one-half months after valvular replacement. At autopsy the cause of the failure was found to be regurgitation at three sites about the mitral fixation ring. Top left: Mitral prosthesis from left atrial aspect. Small wooden sticks are placed in the peribasilar fistulae. Thrombus was present on the ventricular aspect of the prosthesis, but it did not appear to interfere with movement of the ball. Top right: Opened left atrium (L.A.), mitral ring, and left ventricle (L.V.) in the same patient. Sticks again demonstrate the sites of the peribasilar communications. The dashed arrows depict mural thrombi, and the solid arrow shows the sites where the papillary muscles had been removed. The wall of the left ventricle is thinned in these areas. Bottom left: Heart in patient 20. This man died ten months after valve replacement of pulmonary nocardiosis secondary to chronic steroid therapy for serum hepatitis. At necropsy, the ostia of the coronary arteries (R. and L.) were somewhat narrowed. Thrombus was present on the mitral prosthesis. The single peribasilar communication, which was not detected clinically, is better illustrated in the bottom right view, which shows the opened left atrium.

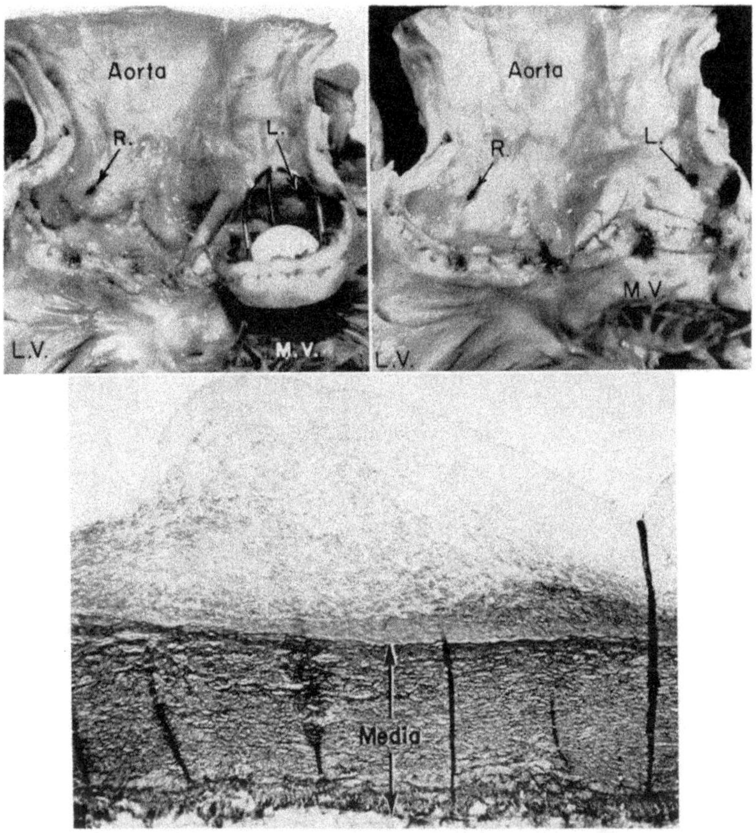

Figure 8

Aortic root region in patient 9. This 48-year-old man, who had no chest pain before valve replacement for aortic stenosis, developed angina pectoris two months postoperatively and died during an anginal attack. At operation, four months before death, both coronary arteries were cannulated without difficulty, but at autopsy cannulae could not be inserted. The upper photographs show the opened aorta, aortic annulus, and left ventricular (L.V.) outflow tract. There is considerable intimal proliferation in the aorta, and the ostia of both right (R.) and left (L.) coronary arteries are narrowed by this process. M.V. = anterior leaflet of mitral valve. The lower photograph shows a section of aortic wall about 1 cm above the level of the coronary ostia. There is marked intimal proliferation, and in certain areas the intima is thicker than the aortic media. The superimposed connective tissue contains few elastic fibrils. Elastic tissue stain, ×25.

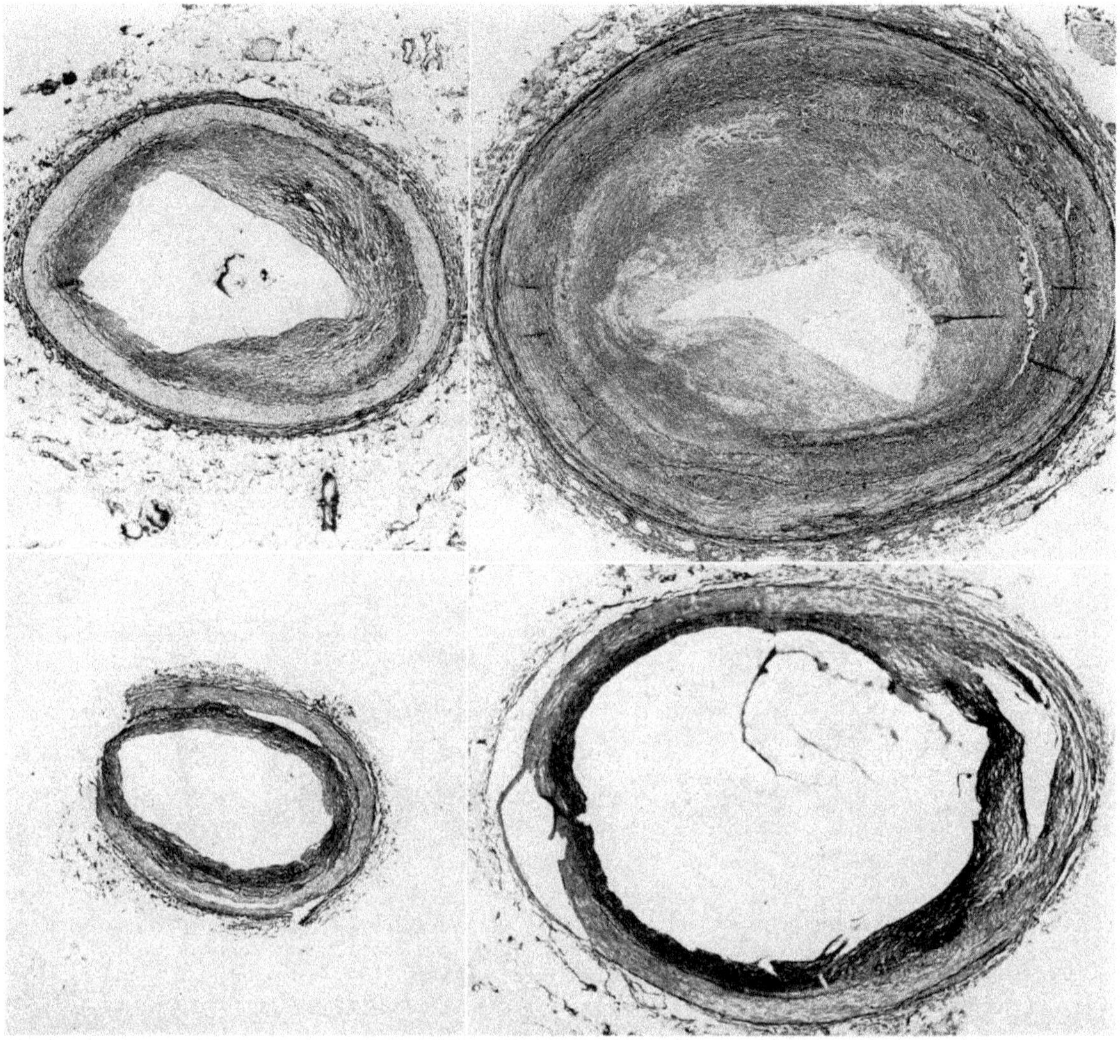

Figure 9

Photomicrographs of sections of the coronary arteries of patient 9. Top left: Right coronary artery at its origin showing considerable intimal proliferation. This vessel is somewhat hypoplastic. Bottom left: Right coronary artery 1.5 cm from its origin. At this point, and distally, the lumen is widely patent. Top right: Left coronary artery at its origin. There is severe luminal narrowing, the result of intimal proliferation. Bottom right: Left coronary artery immediately proximal to its bifurcation into anterior descending and left circumflex branches; both branches were widely patent. Elastic tissue stains; all × 20.

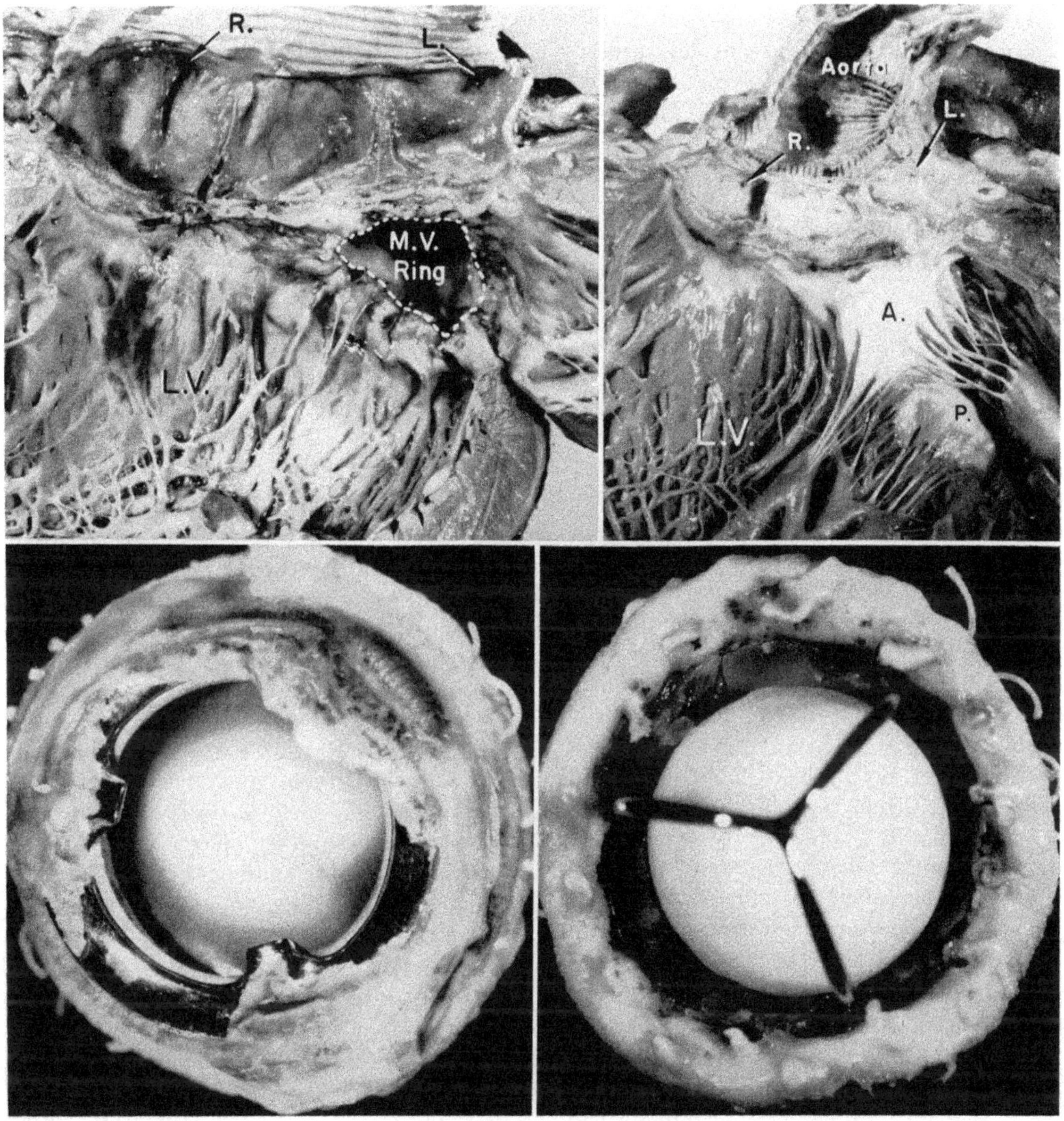

Figure 10

Two of the 20 patients included in this study died of complications of the Marfan syndrome, and their opened aortae, aortic valve rings, and left ventricles are shown in the upper photographs. In each patient the ascending aorta as well as the aortic valve was replaced. Top left: Patient 11, a 21-year-old man, underwent aortic valve replacement seven and one-half months before death. At postoperative catheterization six and one-half months later he was found to have severe mitral regurgitation, and two weeks before death the mitral valve was replaced with a Starr-Edwards prosthesis. At the second operation the aortic prosthesis was found to be incompetent and to contain a thrombus; several sutures were placed to obliterate the peribasilar communication. The intima of the aortic root is thickened, and the coronary ostia (arrows) are narrowed. The proximity of the aortic graft to the ostia may, however, have played a role in narrowing them. The mitral valve (M.V.) ring is calcified. The proximal 1 cm of the coronary arteries in this patient were narrowed. Top right: Patient 14, a 41-year-old man, underwent replacement of the aortic valve and ascending aorta two and one-half months

At necropsy, however, examination of the left ventricle indicated that the valvular regurgitation had resulted from severe congenital endocardial fibroelastosis (fig. 3). The endocardium of the left atrium also was extensively thickened, although focally, in all the patients in whom the mitral valve had been replaced. The endocardium of the left ventricle also showed localized scarring in three patients with prosthetic aortic valves, but each of them had had a myocardial infarction preoperatively.

Discussion

It is well appreciated that thrombus formation on the prosthesis is one of the more important late complications of cardiac valve replacement. Thrombosis may be even more prevalent than previously appreciated since it was evident in 17 of the 20 patients studied. Only one of these patients with noninfected thrombus had clinical or anatomical evidence of systemic embolization, and the episode in this patient occurred several days after operation. Obviously, thrombus may occur on a prosthetic cardiac valve without interfering with valve function, and this was the case in seven of the 14 patients with noninfected thrombi. In the other seven there was convincing anatomical evidence that the thrombus rendered the prostheses stenotic, incompetent, or both, but in three the degree of valvular imcompetency produced was minimal. It is difficult from this study to draw conclusions regarding the efficacy of anticoagulants in patients with prosthetic cardiac valves. Five of the 14 patients with noninfected thrombi had been receiving warfarin, and two of the three patients who did not have thrombi were not on anticoagulants.

The cause of the thickening of the intima of the aortic root and of the proximal coronary arteries is of considerable interest. In each of the 14 patients with prosthetic aortic valves, some degree of fibrous proliferation was found in these areas, and it was clear from necropsy examination that the healing of the aortic incision was not the responsible factor since intimal thickening also was present at some distance from it. It also appears unlikely that the changes in the coronary ostia and proximal coronary arteries were related to the insertion of coronary arterial cannulae at the time of valve replacement. In all of these patients smooth, ball-tipped metal cannulae, held by hand, were utilized to perfuse the left coronary artery. In none was damage to the ostium observed at the time of operation, and in no patient was a purse-string suture placed about the coronary ostium. In only one of these 14 patients was ostial narrowing evident at the time of aortic valve replacement, and it would appear that these changes occurred in the postoperative period. It is unlikely that any functional disturbances are produced by intimal thickening in the ascending aorta itself. On the other hand, when this process involves the ostia and proximal coronary arteries, the effects may be compared to those of syphilitic aortitis. The flow of blood through a normal aortic valve and ascending aorta is laminar, but when a ball-valve prosthesis is present, flow in these areas is grossly turbulent.[5] The anatomical indicator of localized turbulent flow is intimal proliferation,[6] and the present findings suggest that the intimal fibrosis observed in these patients may be a previously unrecognized consequence of aortic valve replacement.

References

1. Cohn, L. H., Roberts, W. C., Rockoff, S. D., and Morrow, A. G.: Bacterial endocarditis

before he died of the nephrotic syndrome, secondary to an obstructing aneurysm in the descending thoracic aorta. The ostium of the right (R.) coronary artery is very small. This narrowing again may have been related to the proximity of the aortic suture line. L. = ostium of left coronary artery; L.V. = left ventricle; A. = anterior mitral leaflet; P. = posterior mitral leaflet. Bottom left and bottom right: Aortic valve prosthesis in patient 14. Some of the thrombus was removed inadvertently at necropsy. Probably no hemodynamically significant lesion resulted from the presence of this thrombus.

following aortic valve replacement: Clinical and pathological correlations. Circulation **33:** 209, 1966.

2. ROBERTS, W. C., AND MORROW, A. G.: Bacterial endocarditis involving prosthetic mitral valves: Clinical and pathologic observations. Arch Path (Chicago) **82:** 164, 1966.
3. ROBERTS, W. C., BERARD, C. W., AND BRAUNWALD, N. S.: Pulmonary abscess following steroid therapy for serum hepatitis. To be published in Dis Chest.
4. STARR, A., PIERIE, W. R., RAIBLE, D. A., EDWARDS, M. L., SIPOSS, G. G., AND HANCOCK, W. D.: Cardiac valve replacement: Experience with the durability of silicone rubber. Circulation **33** and **34** (suppl. I): I-115, 1966.
5. TEMPLE, L. J., SERAFIN, R., CALVERT, N. G., AND DRABBLE, J. M.: Principles of fluid mechanics applied to some situation in the human circulation and particularly to the testing of valves in a pulse duplicator. Thorax **19:** 261, 1964.
6. EDWARDS, J. E., AND BURCHELL, H. B.: Endocardial and intimal lesions (jet impact) as possible sites of origin of murmurs. Circulation **18:** 946, 1958.

Causes of early postoperative death following cardiac valve replacement

Clinico-pathologic correlations in 64 patients studied at necropsy

William C. Roberts, M.D., and Andrew G. Morrow, M.D., Bethesda, Md.

Since the introduction of prosthetic cardiac valves, a number of reports from this and other clinics have described the clinical and hemodynamic results of their application in patients with valvular heart disease. Less attention has been given, however, to the anatomic study of hearts in which prosthetic valves have functioned for varying periods of time. Recently, we described the pathologic findings in the hearts of patients who died in the late postoperative period following valve replacement with Starr-Edwards prostheses.[1] The present report focuses attention on the cardiac findings at necropsy in 64 subjects who died in the early postoperative period following single or multiple valve replacement. The relationship between the anatomic findings and the principal cause or causes of death is described and illustrated, and particular attention is given to potentially avoidable technical problems that may be associated with the use of the prostheses.

Patients studied

Among the patients with either congenital or acquired heart disease who have had replacement of one or more cardiac valves with Starr-Edwards prostheses at the National Heart Institute, 110 have died. Ninety-three of these subjects were studied at necropsy: 64 died within 1 month of operation, and 29 after longer intervals, up to 56 months following operation. The ages of the 64 patients who died within 1 month of operation ranged from 14 to 65 years (average was 44 years); 33 were women, and 31 were men. Twenty-three of the 64 patients were over 50 years of age, and 6 were under 20 years of age. Preoperatively, 42 patients were in Functional Class III, and the other 22 in Functional Class IV (New York Heart Association Classification). The mitral valve only had been replaced in 28 patients, the aortic only in 27, both mitral and aortic valves in 6, both mitral and tricuspid valves in 1, and the tricuspid alone in 2. Fourteen patients died in the operating room, and 18 others within 48 hours of operation; 49 of the total group of 64 patients died within the first postoperative week. The principal causes of death in the 64 patients are summarized in Table I, and each is considered in greater detail below. In 36 patients, death was attributed to a single factor, in 24 subjects to 2 factors, and in 4 patients to either 3 or 4.

From the Clinic of Surgery, National Heart Institute, National Institutes of Health, Bethesda, Md. 20014.
Received for publication April 26, 1967.

Table I. *Incidence of early fatal complications in 64 patients in whom one or more cardiac valves were replaced with Starr-Edwards prostheses*

	Complication	*No. of patients*
I.	Dysfunction of the prosthetic valve	22
II.	Hemorrhage	20
III.	Acute myocardial infarction	15
IV.	Associated uncorrected valvular disease	7
V.	Cerebral emboli or cerebral hemorrhage	4
VI.	Pulmonary complications	6
VII.	Sudden death (arrhythmia)	5
VIII.	Infection	5
IX.	Occluding left atrial thrombi unassociated with dysfunctioning valvular prostheses	4
X.	Occluding right atrial thrombi	3
XI.	Dissecting aortic aneurysm	3
XII.	Uncertain cause	2
Total		96 (complications in 64 patients)

I. Dysfunction of the prosthetic valve. Mechanical interference with proper functioning of the prosthesis was a major cause of death in 22 patients. Fourteen subjects had had isolated mitral valve replacement, 3 had had isolated aortic valve replacement, and 5 had had both the mitral and aortic valves replaced. Twelve of these 22 patients died in the operating room or within 24 hours of operation.

In 12 patients in whom isolated mitral replacement was performed, and in 3 in whom both mitral and aortic valves were replaced, the 2M or 3M mitral prosthesis utilized could not be accommodated by the left ventricular cavity. In each of these 15 patients, the muscular ventricular septum protruded into the cage of the valve, the ball could not descend fully, and obstruction to left atrial emptying (prosthetic mitral stenosis) resulted[2] (see Figs. 1 and 9). Preoperatively, the mitral lesion in all but 2 of these subjects was pure or predominant mitral stenosis, and the left ventricle in each was normal or nearly normal in size.

One of the 2 patients whose mitral lesion preoperatively was pure regurgitation, but who nevertheless had obstruction to left atrial emptying, was a 14-year-old girl with associated congenital endocardial fibroelastosis. In her the left ventricular cavity was too small to accommodate the 3M mitral prosthesis utilized. The second patient, a 25-year-old man, also had congenital mitral regurgitation but, in addition, severe aortic regurgitation and mild aortic stenosis; the 4M mitral prosthesis inserted was again too large for the left ventricle, and the muscular septum protruded into the cage (Fig. 1). At necropsy, 8 of these 15 patients had thrombi which occluded the mitral orifice. In them, thrombosis appeared to be the anatomic expression of stasis of blood in the left atrium, the result of abnormally low flow across the functionally stenotic prosthesis. Four of the 8 subjects with anatomic evidence of obstruction to left atrial emptying, but without left atrial thrombosis, died in the operating room. In another patient, a small 21-year-old woman with predominant mitral regurgitation who had undergone mitral replacement, there did not appear to be any interference with the descent of the ball in the cage, but the outflow tract of the left ventricle appeared obstructed by the prosthetic ball (3M). In this patient, the cage lay in an unusually transverse position in the left ventricle, and its apex contacted the muscular ventricular septum just below the aortic valve. Left bundle branch block, which had not been present preoperatively, was recorded 12 hours postoperatively, and she died 22 hours following operation after a course typical of the low cardiac output syndrome.

In 2 patients with isolated aortic valve replacement, and in 3 patients with double valve replacement, an aortic prosthesis was utilized that was too large for the ascending aorta into which it was inserted. As a re-

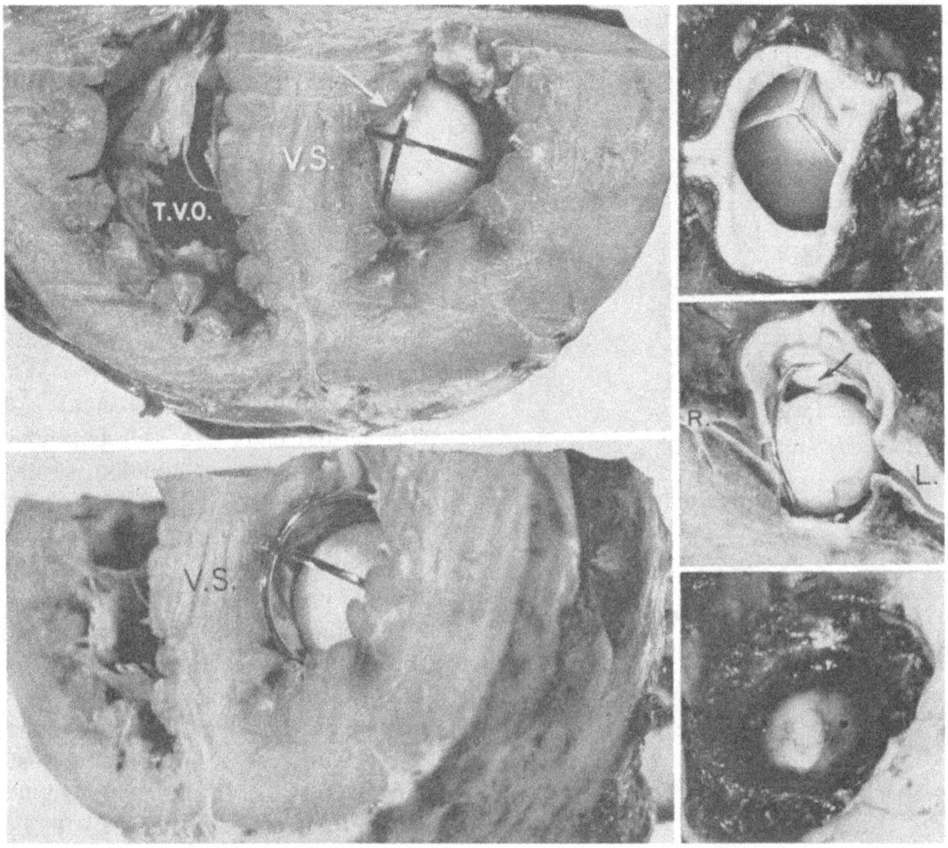

Fig. 1. Views of the heart of the patient with dysfunction of both mitral and aortic prostheses. The left photographs show the ventricular septum bulging into the mitral cage limiting the descent of the ball (*arrow*). *T.V.O.*, Tricuspid valve orifice. *Right upper* and *right middle:* Not only was the motion of the mitral ball severely limited, but also that of the aortic ball, despite the insertion of a relatively small-sized prosthesis (8A). The apex of the cage is eccentrically located as seen from above (*right upper*) and the wall of the aorta protrudes between 2 of the metallic struts, restricting the movement of the ball in the cage. In the right middle view, the anterior wall of the aorta is removed and demonstrates that the wall of the aorta inverted when the aortotomy was closed (*arrow*). The match head demonstrates the remaining narrowed valvular orifice. *R.* and *L.*, Right and left coronary arteries, respectively. *Right lower:* Thrombosed mitral orifice as viewed from the left atrium. Stasis of blood in this chamber, secondary to low flow across the obstructed prosthetic valves, appeared to have caused occlusion of the orifice.

sult, the aortic wall protruded into the cage and prevented the valve from opening fully (Fig. 1). The 2 subjects in whom isolated aortic replacement was performed had pure aortic stenosis preoperatively; the ascending aortas were noted to be small at the time of operation, and small prostheses (8A or 8AT) were utilized. The aortic lesion preoperatively in 1 patient with double valve replacement was aortic regurgitation and in the other 2 it was combined stenosis and regurgitation. Nevertheless, in each the ascending aorta was small and, again, small-sized prostheses (8A, 8A and 7A) were utilized. The patient with pure aortic regurgitation who had a dysfunctioning aortic prosthesis, but an apparently normally functioning mitral prosthesis, also had an occluding left atrial thrombus at necropsy.

Four patients died because of incompe-

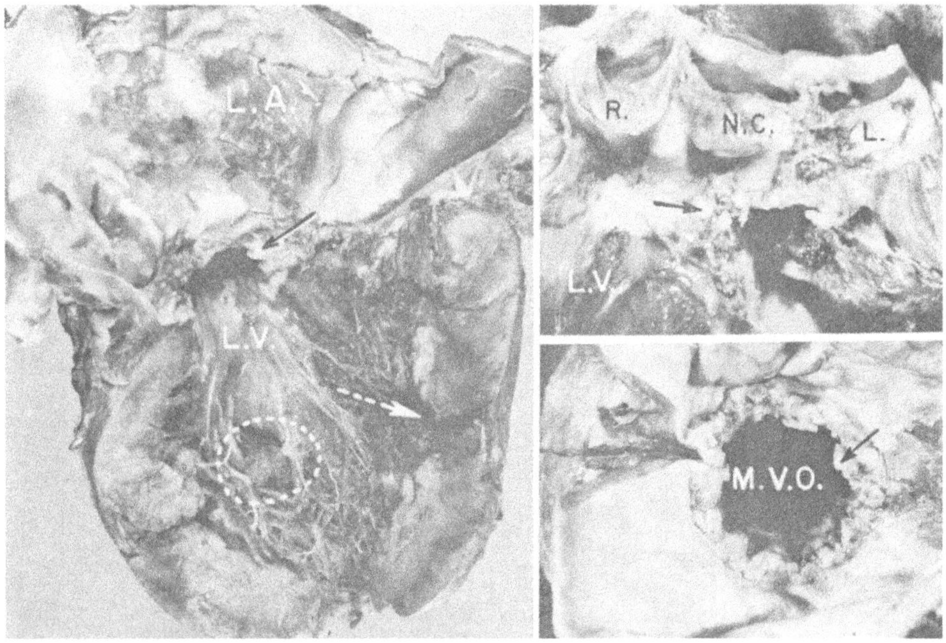

Fig. 2. Prosthetic mitral regurgitation, secondary to a calcific nodule in the annulus, which prevented complete seating of the ball. This 42-year-old man (A64-147) had a stenotic and incompetent mitral valve replaced with a 3M Starr-Edwards prosthesis, and died 5 hours postoperatively after manifesting the low cardiac output syndrome. *Left:* Opened left atrium (*L.A.*) and left ventricle (*L.V.*) and mitral annulus following removal of the prosthesis. The solid arrow points to the nodule of calcium which interfered with the seating of the ball. The dashed arrow indicates the site where the papillary muscles were amputated, and the myocardial wall is thin in this area. The dashed circle encloses a small fibroma which was an incidental necropsy finding. *Right upper:* Opened aortic valve and left ventricle. The nodule of calcium (*arrow*) is just below the noncoronary (*N.C.*) cusp. Aortic valvuloplasty also was done in this patient. *R,* Right anterior cusp. *L,* Left anterior cusp. *Right lower:* Mitral valve orifice (*M.V.O.*) from the left atrium. The arrow indicates the calcific nodule which caused the mitral prosthesis to be incompetent.

tent prostheses. In 1, who had undergone isolated mitral replacement, the ball was prevented from seating by a nodule of calcium extending into the cage between its base and apex; severe mitral regurgitation resulted (Fig. 2). In the second patient, a large nodule of calcium indented the Teflon ring of an aortic prosthesis, the ball was prevented from seating, and severe aortic regurgitation resulted (Fig. 3). In the third patient, who had undergone both mitral and aortic valve replacements, the aortic ball was prevented from seating completely because it contacted one of the metallic struts of the mitral prosthesis during ventricular diastole[3] (Fig. 4). In the final patient, regurgitation through the aortic prosthesis resulted from displacement of the Teflon ring by a diminutive aortic annulus (Fig. 5).

II. Hemorrhage. Uncontrolled bleeding was the principal cause of death in 18 patients, and a major contributing cause in 2 others. Ten patients had had isolated aortic valve replacement, 5 had combined mitral and aortic valve replacement, and 5 had mitral replacement, one accompanied by aortic valvuloplasty and another by tricuspid annuloplasty. Bleeding in 12 subjects was diffuse and from multiple sites, most commonly from adhesion secondary to previous thoracotomies. Two of these 12 patients also had calcific adhesive pericarditis, and removal of the calcific pericardium, which was necessary to open the heart, led to

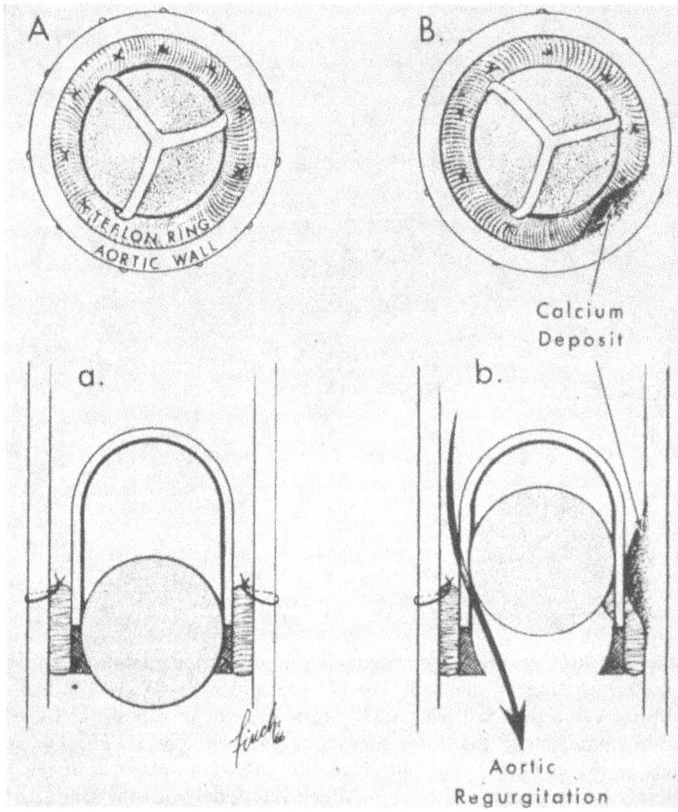

Fig. 3. Diagram which demonstrates the mechanism by which a calcific nodule in the aortic valve ring indented the Teflon ring of an aortic prosthesis, prevented the ball from seating, and resulted in fatal aortic regurgitation (*right*). Normal seating of the ball is illustrated at the *left*. The patient was a 49-year-old woman (A63-183) with severe aortic stenosis (150 mm. Hg peak systolic pressure gradient). She died in the operating room following replacement of the aortic valve with an 8A Starr-Edwards prosthesis. Severe aortic regurgitation following discontinuation of cardiopulmonary bypass led to cardiac arrest. The annulus in this patient was small, but the smallest prosthesis available at the time was utilized.

bleeding. Bleeding in one patient presumedly resulted from prolonged cardiopulmonary bypass (4 hours).

Specific sites of bleeding were identified in 8 patients. The left ventricular wall was perforated in 2 patients, in 1 during excision of a papillary muscle. In another patient, bleeding occurred from the venous cannulation site in the right ventricle. Removal of a large deposit of calcium, which had extended from the mitral leaflets through the annulus into the left ventricular myocardium, caused a separation of the left atrium from the left ventricle in another patient (Fig. 6). Three patients bled from incisions in the aorta; in one the ascending aorta was too small to accept readily a 7A prosthesis, and the incision was closed under considerable tension; in the second patient, *Serratia species* mediastinitis caused separation of the aortotomy on the twenty-third postoperative day; the third patient died from a laceration of the ascending aorta, made inadvertently when the aorta was dissected. In the eighth, massive intraperitoneal bleeding resulted from puncture of a vessel in the abdominal wall during paracentesis in the postoperative period. Two of the 19 patients with intrathoracic bleeding evidenced clinical signs of cardiac tamponade.

III. Acute myocardial infarction. Necro-

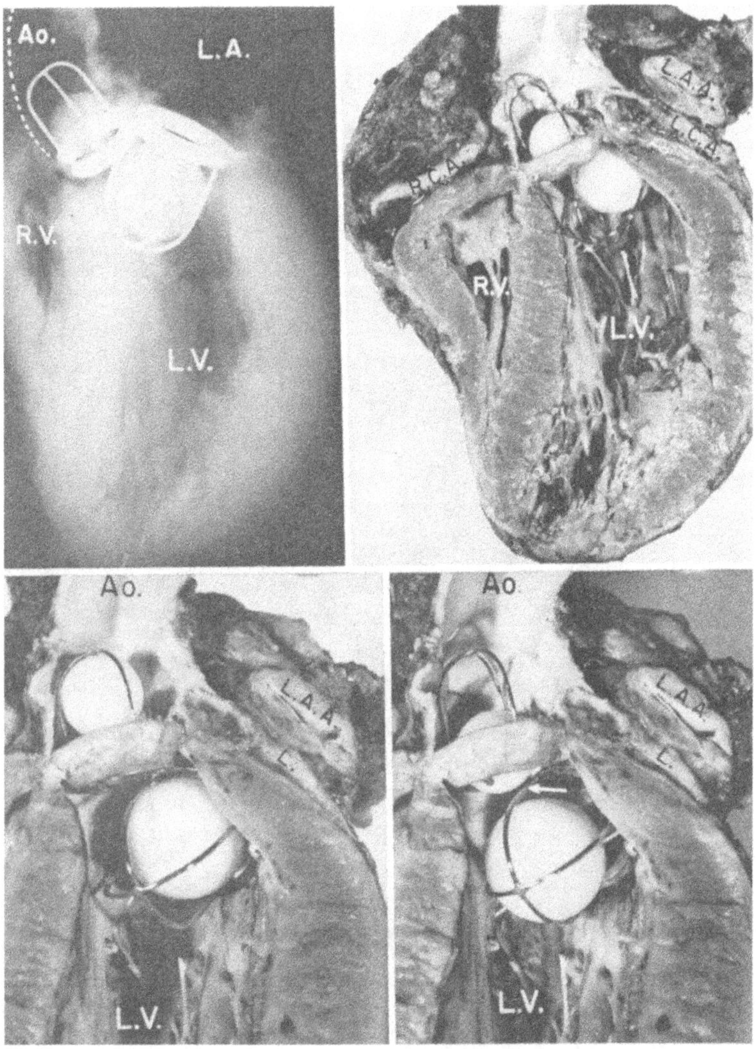

Fig. 4. Prosthetic aortic regurgitation. This 45-year-old man (A65-121) had hemodynamic and angiographic evidence of severe mitral and aortic regurgitation and both valves were replaced with Starr-Edwards prostheses. After both valves had been inserted, there was evidence of some aortic regurgitation, but this was not considered to be of significant magnitude and the aortotomy was not reopened. Postoperatively, however, a diastolic murmur was audible along the left sternal border, the blood pressure was low (90/60 mm. Hg), and there were manifestations of a reduced cardiac output. Because of the possibility of the mitral valve having become occluded by thrombus, reoperation was performed 4 days after the initial operation. After bypass was initiated the left atrium was opened. No thrombus was present, but there was massive regurgitation of blood from the aorta into the left ventricle. Refractory arrest occurred during the procedure.

At necropsy, both mitral and aortic valves were found to be securely sutured, and no peribasilar communications were present. Aortic regurgitation resulted from incomplete seating of the ball of the aortic prosthesis, which contacted one of the struts (*arrow*) of the mitral prosthesis during ventricular diastole (*lower right*). Simulated ventricular systole is shown in the *lower left* photograph. A radiograph of the intact specimen is shown in the *upper left*, and the specimen following removal of the anterior wall of the ventricles is shown in the *upper right*. The close proximity of the two prostheses to one another is apparent. The Starr-Edwards mitral prosthesis is size 5M, the largest manufactured. Had a smaller mitral prosthesis been utilized, contact of the aortic ball with the metallic strut of the Starr-Edwards valve would not have occurred. (From Roberts et al., J. Thoracic & Cardiovas. Surg. 52: 189, 1966, The C. V. Mosby Company.)

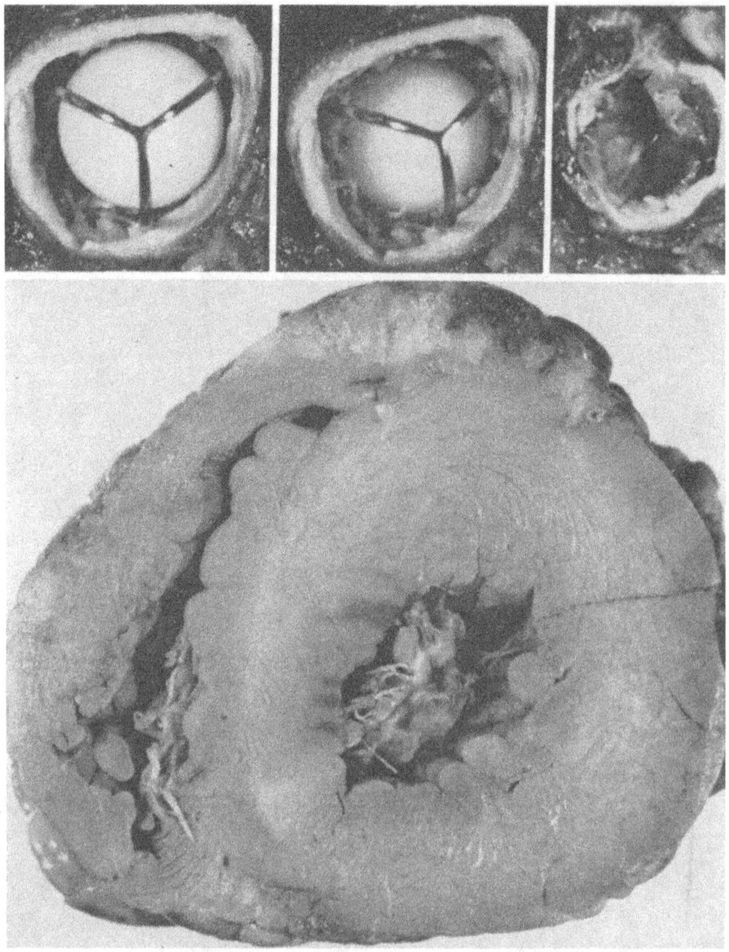

Fig. 5. Aortic valve area and transverse section of the right and left ventricles in a 65-year-old woman whose stenotic aortic valve was replaced with an 8A Starr-Edwards prosthesis (A65-190). Following discontinuance of cardiopulmonary bypass, the patient was severely hypotensive and cardiac arrest occurred 5 minutes later. At necropsy, the aortic prosthesis was found to be too small for the aortic root into which it was inserted. Although the ball could ascend completely, the area between the ball and aortic wall was small; the ball was unable to seat because its Teflon ring was pushed inward by the narrowed "annulus." *Upper left:* Position of the ball during simulated ventricular systole. *Upper middle:* Ball pushed into seated position. The ball was unable to descend freely. *Upper right:* The narrowed left ventricular outflow tract and aortic root is shown following removal of the prosthesis. *Lower:* The left ventricular wall is markedly thickened, and its cavity is filled by the mitral valvular leaflets. Even though a relatively small aortic prosthesis was utilized in this patient it was not small enough.

sis of myocardial fibers adjacent to the site where the apical left ventricular drain had been inserted was noted in all patients who died after aortic valve replacement. Also, in all patients who had had mitral replacement, there was focal acute infarction of the myocardial fibers at the stumps of the amputated papillary muscles. In addition to these expected foci of myocardial necrosis, larger and apparently functionally significant areas of acute infarction were observed in 15 patients: 10 had had mitral replacement (one with tricuspid replacement also), and 5 aortic valve replacement. In 8 of the 15

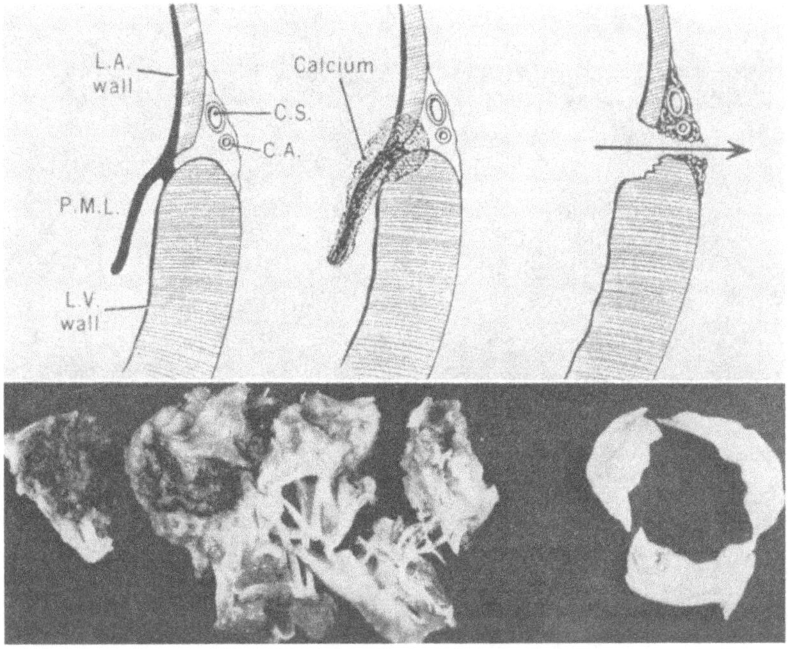

Fig. 6. Complication of extensive calcium deposition in the mitral annulus. This 44-year-old man (A66-40) underwent mitral and aortic valve replacement because of mitral stenosis and aortic regurgitation. The mitral valve is extensively calcified (*lower left*), and was removed in several pieces. The calcium had extended through the mitral annulus into the left atrioventricular sulcus, and, during removal of it, the left atrial wall was separated from the left ventricular wall (*upper middle* and *upper right*). Attempts to close the defect following valve replacement were unsuccessful and massive bleeding occurred. The area of the mitral annulus of a normal heart is shown diagrammatically in the upper left. The left atrial (*L.A.*) myocardium is not connected to the left ventricular (*L.V.*) myocardium. The posterior mitral leaflet (*P.M.L.*) is formed by the junction of endocardium from the left atrium and left ventricle. *C.S.*, Coronary sinus. *C.A.*, Coronary artery. *Lower right:* Resected aortic valve which was severely incompetent, but not calcified.

subjects, myocardial infarction could be attributed to technical factors at operation: occlusion of one or both coronary arterial ostia by aortic dissection (1 patient), by the Teflon ring of the aortic valve prosthesis (1 patient), and by the suture line of a Teflon graft which had replaced an ascending aortic aneurysm (1 patient) (Fig. 7). Massive bleeding and prolonged periods of shock preceded death in 4 patients with infarcts. In the eighth patient, the coronary sinus was lacerated and repaired.

The causes of the acute myocardial infarctions in the other 7 subjects are less clear. Before death, each of the 7 patients had had prolonged periods of inadequate cardiac output, hypotension, arrhythmia, and pulmonary congestion; in 5 of them many of the degenerated myocardial fibers were the site of acute dystrophic calcification (Figs. 8, 9, and 10). It appears that in these patients acute myocardial infarction was the anatomic expression of inadequate coronary arterial perfusion of variable cause, and/or the result of inadequate cardiac output. Two of the 7 patients, however, had dysfunctioning mitral prostheses, another had associated massive tricuspid regurgitation following tricuspid annuloplasty, and another had a large pulmonary infarct. A fifth patient had sustained cerebral air embolization, and may also have had air

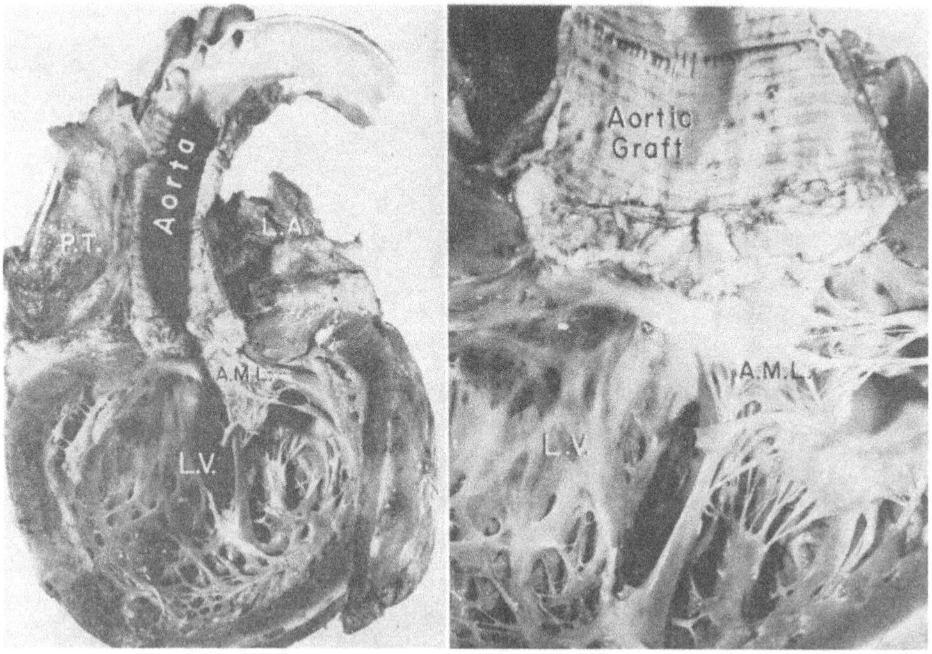

Fig. 7. Acute myocardial infarction following replacement of the aortic valve and ascending aorta. Preoperatively, this 56-year-old woman (A64-223) had massive aortic regurgitation and an aneurysm of the ascending aorta. At operation, the right coronary artery was found to be occluded, and it was divided. The aortic graft, however, partially occluded the ostium of the left coronary artery. The patient died of a large acute posterior myocardial infarct 45 hours following operation. *Left:* Opened left ventricle (*L.V.*) and aorta. *A.M.L.*, Anterior mitral leaflet. *P.T.*, Pulmonary trunk. *L.A.*, Left atrium. *Right:* Close-up view of aortic annulus and graft suture line. Neither coronary ostium is apparent.

emboli to the coronary arteries. Only the mitral valve had been replaced in each of the 7 patients, none had significant coronary arterial disease, none was elderly (ages 41 to 51 years), and in all the infarcts were multiple, primarily subendocardial, and involved both ventricular walls. Several of the patients had undergone external cardiac massage postoperatively, and the relationship of this procedure to the myocardial injury is uncertain.

In only 4 of the total group of 15 patients was acute myocardial infarction apparent electrocardiographically, but complete electrocardiograms were not uniformly obtained.

IV. Associated uncorrected valvular disease. In 7 patients, associated valvular malformations were not corrected by valve replacement, and were considered major causes of death. The associated lesion in 3 patients was tricuspid regurgitation: in all, tricuspid annuloplasties had been performed, but the repairs dehisced postoperatively, and massive tricuspid regurgitation resulted. In each of 2 other patients, mitral commissurotomy, performed in association with aortic valve replacement, resulted in severe mitral regurgitation. In 2 additional subjects, who had aortic replacement for aortic stenosis, severe and previously unrecognized mitral stenosis was found at necropsy; both were women.

V. Cerebral emboli or cerebral hemorrhage. Six patients sustained cerebral emboli at operation or in the early postoperative period. In 3 patients, who never recovered consciousness, emboli were considered the major cause of death. Calcific emboli were found in cerebral arteries in 2 of them (Fig.

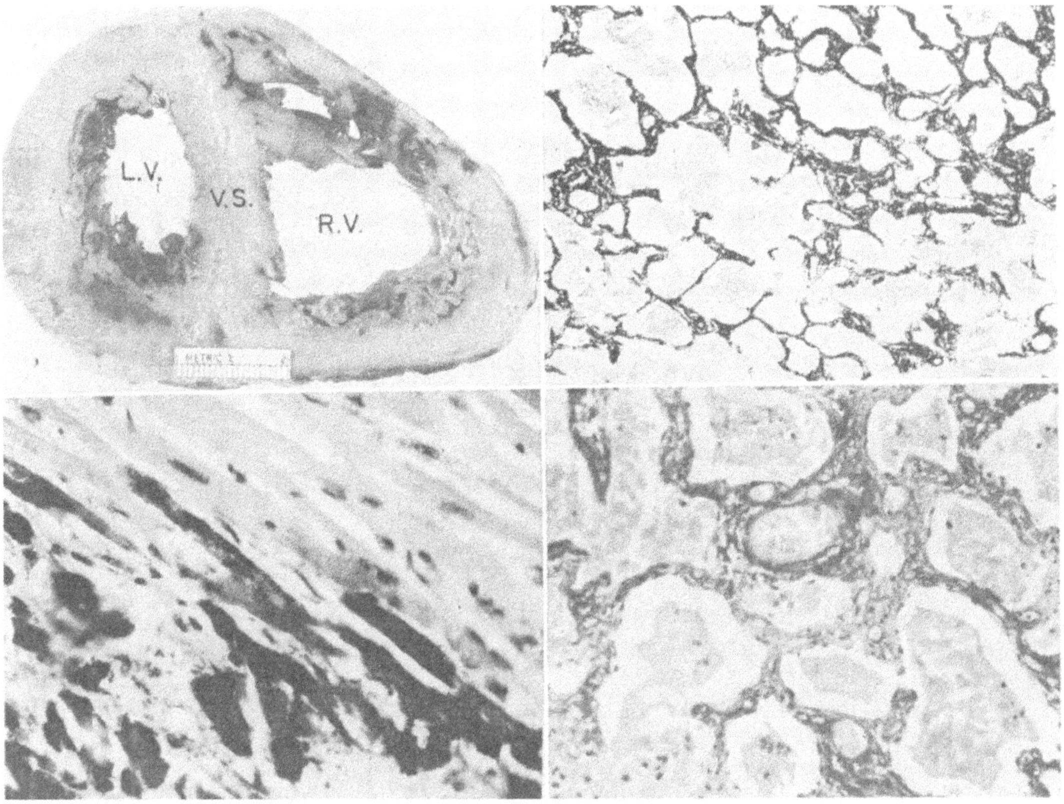

Fig. 8. Myocardial and pulmonary calcification in a patient who died after mitral and tricuspid valve replacements. *Upper left:* Transverse section of ventricles shows dark areas of myocardium in each ventricle. Sections of these areas disclosed that they were foci of severe myocardial degeneration, and that many of the necrotic myocardial fibers were calcified *(lower left;* von Kossa stain; orig. mag. ×187). *Upper right:* Section of lung stained for calcium reveals heavy deposits of calcium (which appears black) in virtually every alveolar septum (von Kossa stain; orig. mag. ×63.) *Lower right:* Close-up view of alveolar septa shows distribution of calcium deposits in them. (Hematoxylin and eosin stain; orig. mag. ×187.)

Myocardial fiber calcification was found in 4 other patients in this study, but none had pulmonary calcification as well. The above patient also had heavy deposits of calcium in the striated muscle. The cause of this calcification is uncertain, and whether or not it was present before operation or appeared only afterward is also unknown. The calcium deposition in the above-described patient was not related to abnormal blood levels of calcium, phosphorus, or magnesium. Determinations of serum calcium, phosphorus, and magnesium were made on 2 days during the week before operation and on 5 days during the postoperative period; each was normal.

10), and, in the third patient, embolism resulted from air which was not evacuated from the left atrial appendage. A fourth patient died of a massive intracerebral hemorrhage on the twenty-third day after aortic valve replacement. She was receiving therapeutic doses of Warfarin, and the hemorrhage was attributed to trauma, sustained when she fell from bed; it was considered, however, that the fall could have been precipitated by an embolus which was undetectable at autopsy. In 2 other subjects, only minor and transient neurologic deficits had been noted before death.

VI. Pulmonary complications. In 5 patients, pulmonary hemorrhage or infarction was a major cause of death. Two patients had intra-alveolar hemorrhage of such se-

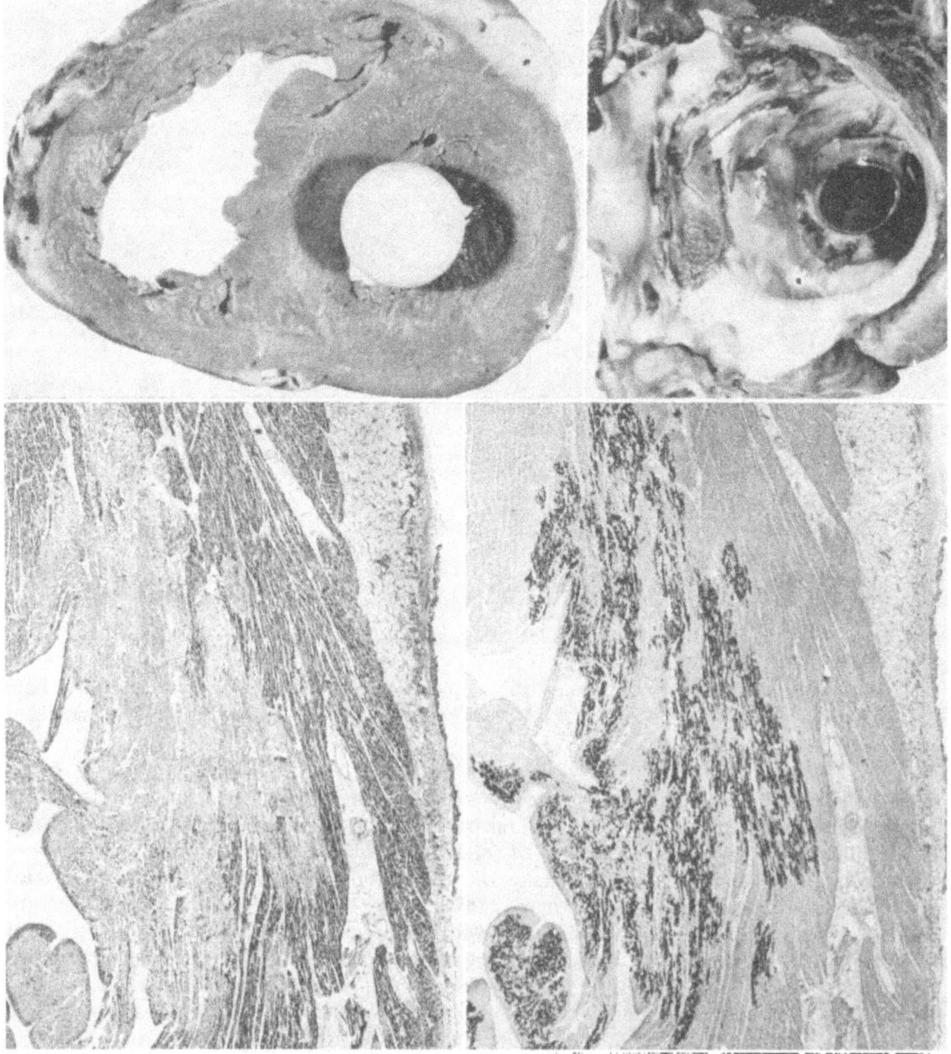

Fig. 9. Heart of a 42-year-old woman (A65-151) who had severe mitral stenosis and regurgitation, and balanced systemic and pulmonary arterial pressures. She died 5 days following replacement of the mitral valve, and the entire postoperative course demonstrated typical features of the low cardiac output syndrome. At necropsy, the mitral prosthesis was found to be too large for the left ventricular cavity, even though a small-sized prosthesis had been used. *Upper left:* Transverse section of ventricles just below the atrioventricular rings show that the prosthetic ball is very large in comparison to the left ventricular cavity. *Upper right:* Left atrium. Thrombus is present at the atriotomy suture line, but the prosthesis is free of thrombus. *Lower left:* Photomicrograph of a section of left ventricle shows large areas of myocardial fiber degeneration. (Phosphotungstic-acid hematoxylin stain; orig. mag. ×14.) *Lower right:* Same section, but now stained for calcium (black), indicates severe dystrophic calcification of the myocardium. Degenerated areas such as these almost surely interfere severely with myocardial function.

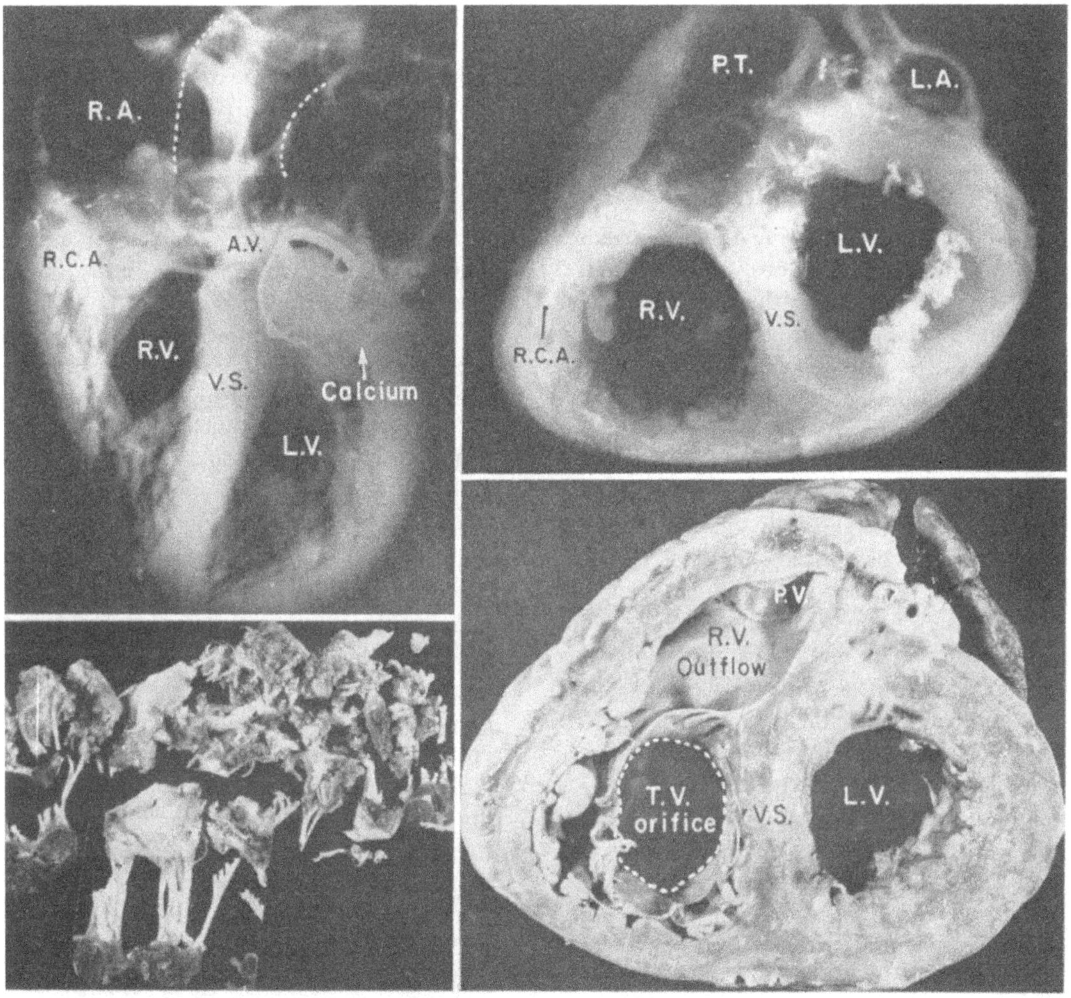

Fig. 10. Systemic emboli following replacement of an extremely calcified, stenotic, and incompetent mitral valve. This 51-year-old man (A66-150) never awakened postoperatively, and roentgenograms of the skull suggested a calcific embolus in the right middle cerebral artery; the embolus was found at necropsy 5 days following operation. The mitral valve was removed in numerous fragments (*lower left*), and presumably at least one escaped into the systemic circulation. *Upper left:* Anteroposterior radiograph of the heart. There is considerable residual calcium in the mitral annulus and adjacent left ventricular myocardium, as well as in the aortic valve (*A.V.*) and right coronary artery (*R.C.A.*). The prosthesis is size 3M. *Upper right:* Radiograph of the specimen shown in the lower right. Only the basal portions of the ventricles remain, and massive residual cardiac calcification is again evident.

verity that air exchange became impossible. In 1 of these subjects, who died 3 days following operation, the lungs had been over-expanded at the time of operation, the result of malfunction of the respirator. Three patients had large pulmonary infarcts and in 1 of them, the infarcts became infected, ruptured, and produced empyema and pericarditis. The 5 subjects with pulmonary hemorrhage or infarction died from 3 to 12 days (average, 6 days) following operation.

VII. Sudden death (arrhythmia). Death occurred suddenly and unexpectedly in 5 patients, and in 3 there were no anatomic causes apparent at necropsy. One patient, a

16-year-old girl who preoperatively had pure aortic regurgitation, had cardiac arrest on the sixteenth postoperative day while she was preparing to be discharged; a 59-year-old man died suddenly on the twelfth postoperative day while riding in a wheel chair; and a 15-year-old girl had cardiac arrest 30 hours following mitral valve replacement, after a previously smooth course. In the latter patient, the left ventricular papillary muscles removed at operation were analyzed for catecholamines, and exceptionally low levels of epinephrine and norepinephrine were found. The fourth patient, a 45-year-old man, whose first week following aortic valve replacement was entirely uneventful, died suddenly on the eleventh postoperative day during physical therapy; at necropsy a pheochromocytoma, weighing 21 grams, was found in one adrenal gland. The fifth patient, a 59-year-old man, was found dead in bed 20 days following mitral valve replacement after a previously smooth postoperative course. At necropsy, numerous Aschoff bodies were found in the myocardium and pericardium, and, in addition, there was extensive old replacement and interstitial fibrosis of the left ventricular wall. Although there was no luminal narrowing of the extramural coronary arteries, several small intramural coronary arteries were occluded. Foreign-body type giant cells and doubly refractile material, probably talc, were present within these vessels at the sites of occlusion. These lesions are interpreted as coronary emboli resulting from a mitral commissurotomy performed 10 years earlier.

VIII. Infection. In 2 patients, infection was a major cause of death and in 3 others it was a contributory cause. One patient developed *Serratia species* mediastinitis, which led to disruption of the aortotomy. The second, a 17-year-old girl who had had several pulmonary emboli before mitral replacement, developed Klebsiella pneumonitis postoperatively, and rupture of the infected pulmonary infarcts led to empyema and infective pericarditis. In the other 3 patients, death was principally attributable to other factors, but evidence of infection was present at necropsy. One patient developed disseminated candidiasis following peritoneal dialysis for acute renal failure. The renal failure, however, was precipitated by excessive bleeding, which was the major cause of his death. A second patient, who died on the fourteenth postoperative day, had bronchopneumonia from mixed organisms, and the third had *Staphylococcus aureus* mediastinitis and pericarditis.

It is noteworthy that none of the total group of 64 patients who died within 1 month of valve replacement had infection at the site of attachment of the prosthesis.

IX. Occluding left atrial thrombi unassociated with dysfunctioning valvular prostheses. In addition to the 9 patients who developed left atrial thrombi secondary to dysfunctioning prostheses (see I), 4 other patients were found to have occluding left atrial thrombi at necropsy; in none of them was there malfunction of the mitral prosthesis. Each of the 4 had a markedly decreased cardiac output postoperatively; 2 had massive tricuspid regurgitation following disruption of tricuspid annuloplasties, a third, who also had tricuspid regurgitation, had massive pulmonary infarction. The fourth patient with left atrial thrombosis had pure mitral regurgitation preoperatively and a huge left ventricular cavity. A massive myocardial infarct on the first postoperative day impaired left ventricular function, decreased the cardiac output, produced stasis, and eventual thrombosis of the prosthesis.

X. Occluding right atrial thrombi. In each of the 3 patients in whom the tricuspid valve was replaced with a Starr-Edwards prosthesis, thrombus occluded the right atrial orifice of the prosthesis. Two patients had isolated replacement of the tricupsid valve: 1 of them also had a mitral commissurotomy, and in the second, tricuspid, mitral, and aortic valvulotomies had been performed 2 months before the tricuspid replacement. In the third patient, the mitral as well as tricuspid valve was replaced. The postoperative period in each of these 3 subjects was characterized by features typical of the low cardiac output syndrome, and thrombosis of the valves in them was considered to be the result of low flow across the tricuspid orifice with resulting stasis of blood in the right atrium. In 2 patients, a 4M Starr-Edwards prosthesis was utilized, and, in the third, a 3M prosthesis. In none was there evidence of interference with movement of the ball in the cage at necropsy. Thrombosis of the prosthesis was considered a primary cause of death in 2 of the subjects, whereas mitral regurgitation following mitral commissurotomy was considered the principal cause in the third, in whom right atrial thrombosis apparently occurred only as a terminal event.

XI. Dissecting aortic aneurysm. In 3 patients, death was directly attributable to dissecting aortic aneurysm. In 2 patients the dissection was related to insertion of a femoral arterial cannula, and each died of this complication (Fig. 11). In the third patient, dissection originated at the aortotomy, and eventually let to dissection and occlusion of the proximal coronary arteries; this patient died 2 days after aortic valve replacement.

XII. Death from uncertain cause. An adequate anatomic explanation for death was not apparent in 2 patients. One, a 34-year-old man with aortic regurgitation and ventricular septal defect, died 24 hours following aortic valve replacement and closure of the defect. His course postoperatively was typical of the low cardiac output syndrome. At necropsy, there were no recent myocardial infarcts, and the ball moved normally in the valve. His heart, however, weighed 1,250 grams, the largest we have seen. The second patient, a 64-year-old man, died in the operating room following aortic valve replacement. Ventricular fibrillation occurred following thoracotomy, but he was resuscitated. Electrocardiograms during cardiopulmonary bypass showed progressive changes of myocardial degeneration, despite perfusion of the coronary arteries. He was hypotensive when bypass was discontinued, and ventricular fibrillation occurred several minutes later. At necropsy, there were several intramural hemorrhages in the myocardium adjacent to the aortic valve, including the areas of atrioventricular node and bundle (Fig. 12).

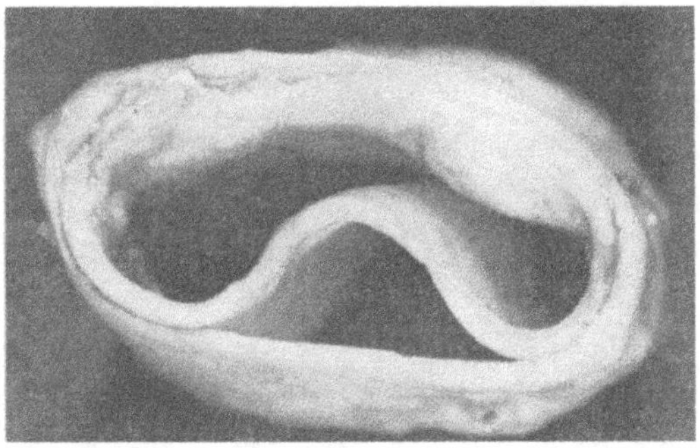

Fig. 11. Aortic dissection following femoral arterial cannulation. Two or 3 seconds following initiation of cardiopulmonary bypass in this 59-year-old woman (A63-218), the ascending aorta distended abnormally, and it was apparent that a dissection had occurred from the site of the arterial cannulation to the root of the aorta. Shown here is the aorta (about the level of the diaphragm). The dissection occurred in the outer media. Death in 3 patients was the result of traumatic aortic dissection.

Conclusions

In these 64 patients, an analysis of the causes of death in the early postoperative period discloses that more than half of the 96 fatal complications were the result of potentially avoidable errors in operative management. For example, in 17 patients the mitral prostheses utilized were too large, leading to obstruction to left atrial emptying (15 patients), obstruction to left ventricular outflow (1 patient), and aortic regurgitation (1 patient). Three aortic valves which were too large caused obstruction to outflow in two instances, and aortic regurgitation in another. Two valves were rendered incompetent by residual calcific deposits which could have been excised. Seven of the twenty deaths from bleeding were the direct result of technical misadventure, as were four of the acute myocardial infarctions. All of the deaths related to an associated and uncorrected valvular malformation could have been avoided. Thus, tricuspid annuloplasty is not to be depended upon for

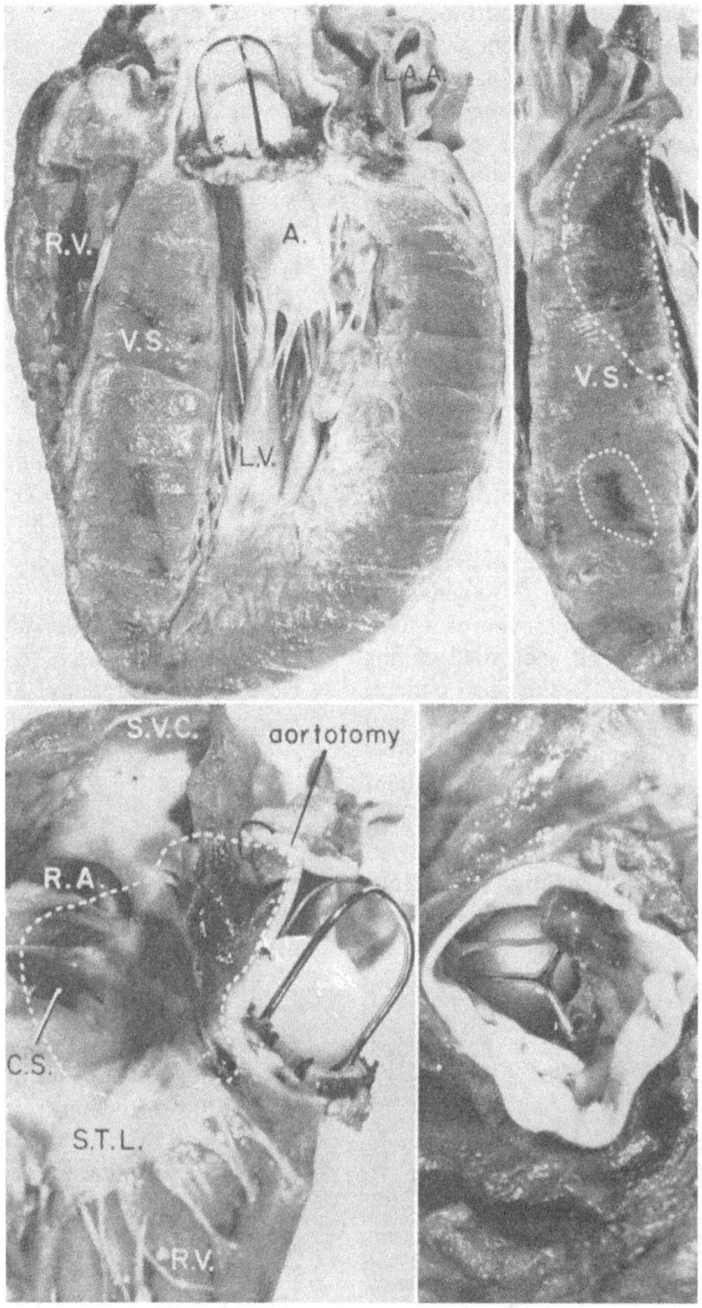

Fig. 12. Extensive interstitial myocardial hemorrhages may occur following replacement of any cardiac valve. The 19-year-old girl (A66-179), whose heart is shown, died of a pulmonary complication (massive intra-alveolar hemorrhage probably secondary to an anesthesia accident at the time of operation) 3 days following aortic valve replacement. There are numerous focal hemorrhages in the ventricular septum (*V.S.*) (*upper*), and diffuse hemorrhages in the right atrial (*R.A.*) wall adjacent to the aortic root. Extensive hemorrhage in the area between the ostium of the coronary sinus (*C.S.*) and membranous ventricular septum (*lower left*) may produce heart block, although block did not occur in this patient. *S.T.L.*, Septal tricuspid leaflet. *S.V.C.*, Superior vena cava. *Lower right:* A thrombus formed between the aortic suture line and the apex of the aortic valve prosthesis (size 9A). This patient was the only one of the 64 in whom thrombus was found on an aortic valve prosthesis.

effective relief of tricuspid regurgitation, and mitral valve replacement must be performed if doubt exists as to the effectiveness of mitral commissurotomy. The deaths of 2 patients as the result of undiagnosed mitral stenosis emphasize once more the importance of detailed preoperative assessment of mitral valve function in women who apparently have only calcific aortic stenosis. Three cases of fatal cerebral emboli, those resulting from calcific debris or air, could have been prevented by more careful attention to operative details. Two of the infections, presumably incurred at operation, must be attributed to faulty aseptic technique. Dissections of the aorta could have been avoided by more careful manipulation of the femoral cannula or by cannulation at another site. Finally, thrombosis of tricuspid prostheses has not been encountered since disc valves of low profile configuration have been used at this site.

Recognition and appreciation of the factors listed above have resulted in improved judgment and technique in valve replacement, and a lower immediate mortality. Thus, of the 98 patients in whom one or more cardiac valves were replaced in 1964, 19 died within 1 month following operation. Single or multiple valve replacements were carried out in 96 patients during 1966 and the first 2 months of 1967; 11 of these patients died within the first postoperative month. A comparison of the sizes of the mitral prostheses utilized during each of these periods is of interest. Of the 47 patients who had mitral replacement in 1964, 2M Starr-Edwards prostheses were inserted in only 7, and in 16 patients 4M prostheses were utilized. In contrast, 2M valves were used in 28 of the 56 patients who had mitral replacement during 1966 and early 1967, and in only 10 patients were 4M prostheses utilized.

One of the unexpected findings in this study was the demonstration of an anatomic cause of death in virtually all of the patients who had manifested the low cardiac output syndrome.[4] The most common cause of the syndrome was a dysfunctioning valvular prosthesis. In 7 patients with this syndrome, multiple subendocardial acute myocardial infarcts, unassociated with significant coronary arterial disease, were observed at necropsy; in 5 patients many of the necrotic myocardial fibers were calcified. Interestingly, each of the 7 patients had had mitral valve replacement, and such multiple focal infarcts were not observed in any patient who had undergone isolated aortic valve replacement.

REFERENCES

1 Roberts, W. C., and Morrow, A. G.: Late Postoperative Pathologic Findings After Cardiac Valve Replacement, Circulation (Suppl.) **35:** 48, 1967.

2 Roberts, W. C., and Morrow, A. G.: Mechanisms of Acute Left Atrial Thrombosis After Mitral Valve Replacement: Pathologic Findings Indicating Obstruction to Left Atrial Emptying, Am. J. Cardiol. **18:** 497, 1966.

3 Roberts, W. C., Lambird, P. A., Gott, V. L., and Morrow, A. G.: Fatal Aortic Regurgitation Following Replacement of the Mitral and Aortic Valves: A Mechanical Complication of Double Valve Replacement, J. Thoracic & Cardiovas. Surg. **52:** 189, 1966.

4 Morales, A. R., Fine, G., and Taber, R. E.: Cardiac Surgery and Myocardial Necrosis, Arch. Path. **83:** 71, 1967.

Anatomic Studies of Hearts Containing Caged-ball Prosthetic Valves

WILLIAM C. ROBERTS AND ANDREW G. MORROW

Clinic of Surgery, National Heart Institute, National Institutes of Health, Bethesda, Maryland

The 1960's will probably be remembered in the annals of cardiology as the era during which prosthetic replacement of cardiac valves was initiated. In September 1960, a Conference on Prosthetic Valves for Cardiac Surgery was held in Chicago, and investigators from this and other countries presented results of partial or total cardiac valve replacement in experimental animals, and in some patients (1). At the conference, Starr described the unsuccessful use of a caged-ball prosthesis in one patient, but added that "this type of valve holds much promise." Since September 1960, approximately 40,000 Starr-Edwards caged-ball prostheses have been furnished to surgeons by the Edwards Laboratories, and prosthetic valves of other design have also been employed with success.

Since 1962 Starr-Edwards valves have been utilized at the National Heart Institute in approximately 350 patients. Subsequently, 120 of them have died, and necropsies have been performed in 98. The causes of death in these subjects, and the findings in their hearts at necropsy, are summarized in the report which follows.

PATIENTS STUDIED

Of the 98 patients in whom necropsy was performed, 65 died within one month of operation (early death), and 33 at later periods up to 56 months postoperatively. The cardiac valves which were replaced in all of these patients are listed in Table I. All patients were in functional classes III or IV before operation. Of the 65 subjects who died within a month of operation, 32 were women and 33 were men, and their ages ranged from 14 to 65 years (average 44). Of the 33 patients who died later, 7 were women and 26 were men, and their ages ranged from 15 to 69 years (average 44).

ANALYSIS OF THE EARLY POSTOPERATIVE DEATHS

The types and incidence of fatal complications in the 65 patients who died within one month of operation are listed in Table II; they have been discussed more fully in a previous publication (2). Sixteen subjects died in the operating room, 18 others within 48 hours of operation, and a total of 50 had died within a week of operation.

Mechanical interference to proper functioning of the prosthesis was a major cause of death in 22 patients. In 21 of them the prosthesis utilized was too large for either the left ventricle or ascending aorta into which it was inserted, and motion of the caged ball was limited. In each of 16 patients in whom mitral replacement was carried out, the muscular ventricular septum protruded into the cage of the valve, the ball could not open fully, and obstruction to left atrial

[1] Presented at the Topics in Clinical Medicine, postgraduate course in internal medicine, conducted by Philip A. Tumulty, M.D., sponsored by the Department of Medicine, The Johns Hopkins University School of Medicine and Hospital.

TABLE I

Necropies following Starr-Edwards Valve Replacement

Valve Replaced	Early Death	Late Death	Total
Mitral	28	8	36
Aortic	28	17	45
Mitral and Aortic	6	7	12
Tricuspid	2	0	2
Tricuspid and Mitral	1	1	2
	—	—	—
	65	33	98

TABLE II

Incidence of Fatal Complications in the Early Postoperative Period in 65 Patients Following Starr-Edwards Valve Replacement

Complication	No. Patients
I. Prosthetic dysfunction	22
II. Hemorrhagic diathesis	20
III. Acute myocardial infarct	15
IV. Associated uncorrected or undiagnosed valvular disease	7
V. Intracranial lesions (emboli)	4
VI. Pulmonary complications	6
VII. Sudden death (arrhythmia)	5
VIII. Infection	5
IX. Occluding LA thrombi unassociated with dysfunctioning valvular prostheses	4
X. Occluding RA thrombi	3
XI. Dissecting aortic aneurysm	3
XII. Uncertain cause	2
	—
Total	97 complications in 65 patients

emptying (prosthetic mitral stenosis) resulted (Figs 1–4). Preoperatively the mitral lesion in 14 of the 16 patients was pure or predominant mitral stenosis, and the left ventricle in each was normal or nearly normal in size. The majority of these subjects had a 3M Starr-Edwards prosthesis inserted, and a valve of this size is too large to function properly in a normal-sized left ventricular cavity. At necropsy, eight of these 16 patients had thrombi which occluded the mitral orifices (3). In them, thrombosis appears to have been the anatomic expression of stasis of blood in the left atrium, the result of abnormally low flow across the functionally stenotic prosthesis. Four of the eight subjects with prosthetic mitral stenosis without left atrial thrombosis died in the operating room.

In five patients in whom the aortic valve was replaced (four also had mitral replacement) the aortic prosthesis utilized was too large for the ascending aorta, despite the insertion of small-sized (8A) prostheses in each of them (Figs 4 and 5). The aortic wall protruded into the cage and prevented the valve from opening fully.

Three patients died from incompetent prostheses. In two, the ball was pre-

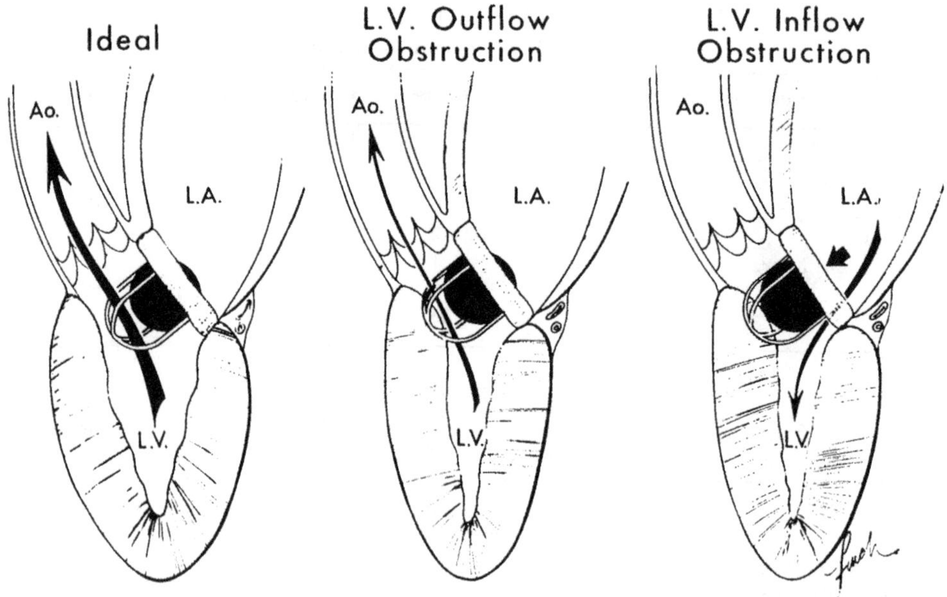

FIG 1. Diagram demonstrating the machanism of dysfunction of a Starr-Edwards mitral prosthesis. On the left is shown the *ideal* position of this prosthesis: the apex of the cage does not contact the ventricular septum, and the ball descends freely and seats completely. In one of the patients studied by us, there appeared to be obstruction to left ventricular (L.V.) outflow as demonstrated in the middle diagram, but this complication is unusual following mitral replacement. More frequently, the burrowing of the cage of the mitral prosthesis into the ventricular septum prevents descent of the ball, producing prosthetic mitral stenosis or left ventricular inflow obstruction. This complication has occurred mainly in patients who preoperatively had pure or predominant mitral stenosis without significant aortic valvular disease. With this lesion, the left ventricular cavity is of normal size, or smaller than normal, and its posterior wall is shorter than normal (21). The shortening of the posterior wall causes the mitral prosthesis to lie transversely in the left ventricular cavity, and the more transverse it lies the greater the chance of its contracting the ventricular septum. In contrast, in patients with pure mitral regurgitation, the apex of the cage will not infrequenly point directly toward the apex of the left ventricle.

vented from completely seating by protruding nodules of calcium; in the third patient, who underwent double valve replacement, the aortic ball contacted one of the metallic struts of the mitral prosthesis during ventricular diastole, preventing it from seating (4).

Uncontrolled bleeding occurred in 20 patients. In 12, the bleeding was from multiple sites, most commonly from adhesions secondary to previous thoracotomies, while in eight patients specific sites of bleeding were identified. The latter were generally the result of technical misadventures, and lacerations of the wall of the heart or aorta occurred in seven subjects.

Acute myocardial infarction was the third most frequent fatal complication, and it occurred in 16 patients. In nine the infarcts were large, usually single, and clearly secondary to associated conditions, most often hemorrhage; in the other seven, the infarcts were multiple, primarily subendocardial, associated in five subjects with dystrophic calcification, and their etiology is less clear. Before death each of these seven patients had prolonged periods of inadequate cardiac output, hypotension, arrhythmia, and pulmonary congestion. Whether the infarcts in them were simply the anatomic expressions of inadequate coro-

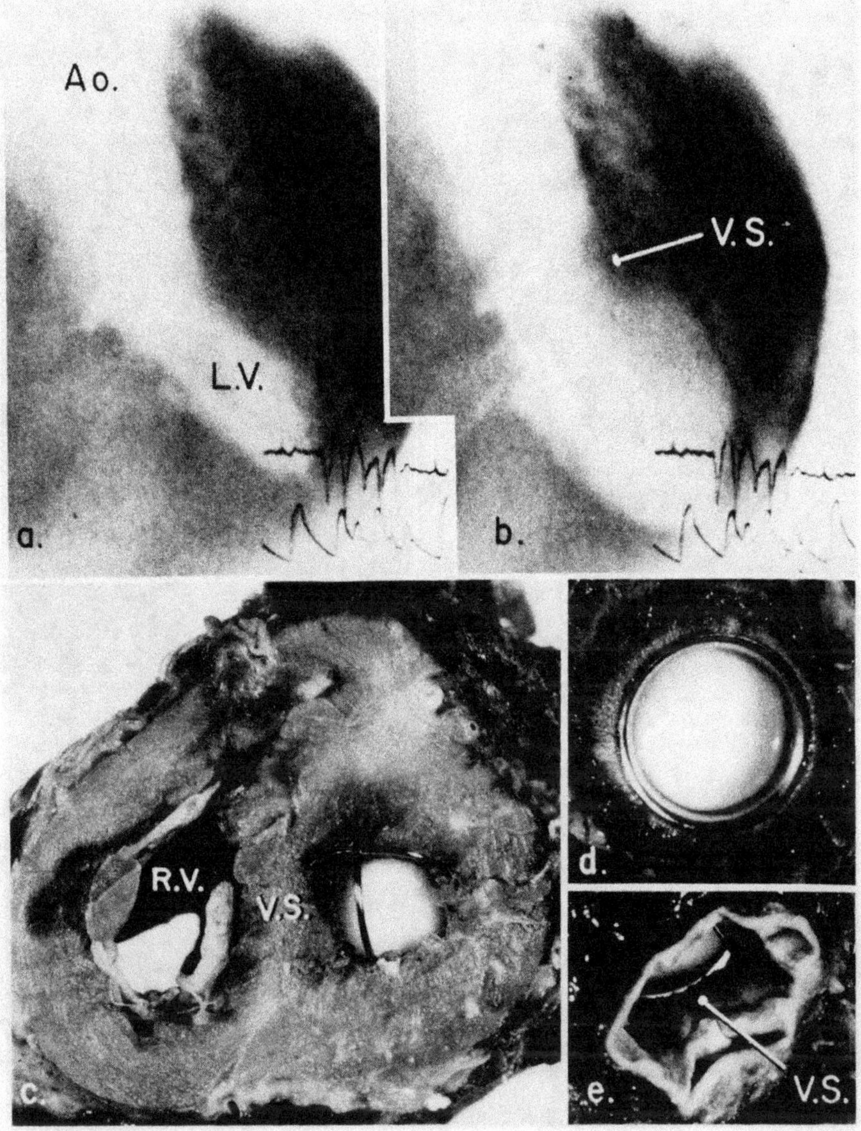

Fig 2. Cineangiocardiogram exposed in the right anterior oblique projection (*a.* and *b.*) and the heart (*c.*, *d.*, and *e.*) of a cachetic, Class IV, 57-year-old man (A56-170) with severe mitral stenosis. He had a small left ventricular cavity which was evident preoperatively on the cineangiocardiagram. *a.*, angiocardiographic appearance of the left ventricular cavity at peak systole. *b.*, at end-diastole. The diameter of the left ventricular outflow tract, even during diastole, is smaller than the diameter of the ascending aorta. In both angiocardiographic frames, the electrocardiogram and brachial arterial pressure pulse recorded simultaneously also are shown. The systolic and diastolic appearance of the ventricle is that during the first normal cycle following ventricular extrasystoles. Valve replacement was performed, but after insertion of the prosthesis, death resulted from bleeding from the cannulation site in the right ventricle. The autopsy appearance of the left ventricular cavity and the size 3M prosthesis are shown in *c*. Protrusion of the ventricular septum into the mitral cage almost totally blocked motion of the ball. In this patient, there also appeared to be obstruction to left ventricular emptying. With the mitral ball in the closed position simulating ventricular systole (*d.*), the photograph in *e.* was taken. Following excision of the three aortic valve cusps, the mitral ball is seen almost to contact the muscular ventricular septum and to obstruct the outflow tract. (Reproduced with permission from the American Journal of Cardiology, **18:** 497, 1966, reference 3).

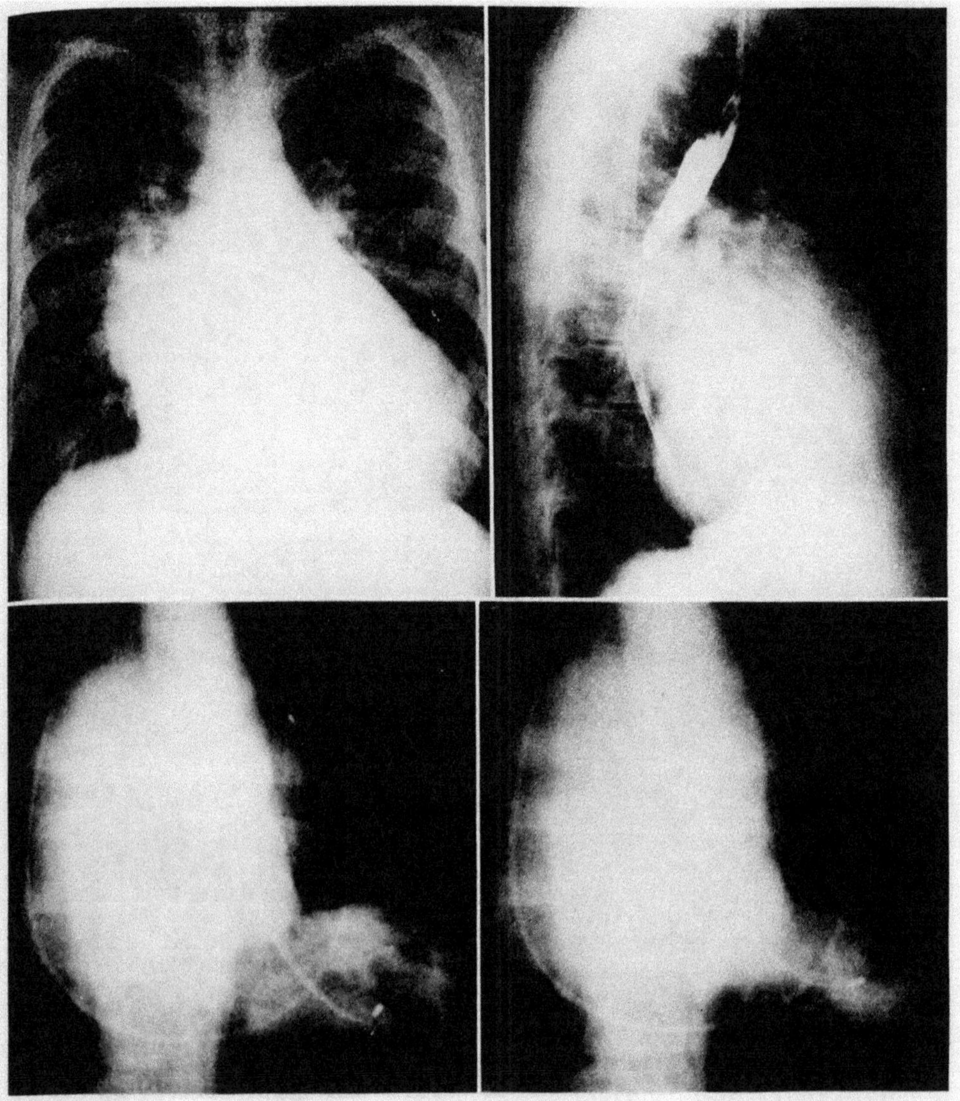

FIG. 3. Chest roentgenograms (*upper*), and left ventricular angiocardiograms (*lower*) in a 25-year-old man (A65-133) with congenital mitral and aortic regurgitation, and slight (18 mm Hg peak systolic pressure gradient) aortic stenosis. Although the cardiac silhouette is huge, the enlargement is due primarily to myocardial hypertrophy rather than to cavity dilatation (see Fig 4). The aortic valve was congenitally bicuspid. The size of the left ventricular cavity during diastole (*lower left*) and systole (*lower right*) are shown.

nary arterial perfusion, of variable cause, could not be determined. Interestingly, in each of the seven subjects only the mitral valve had been replaced, none had significant coronary arterial disease, and none were old (ages 41 to 51 years). In only four of the 16 patients was acute myocardial infarction apparent electrocardiographically after operation.

The other fatal complications (listed in Table II) were less frequent than those discussed above. *Associated uncorrected valvular disease* was the major cause of death in seven patients. The associated lesion in three subjects was tricuspid regurgitation: tricuspid annuloplasties had been performed in all, but

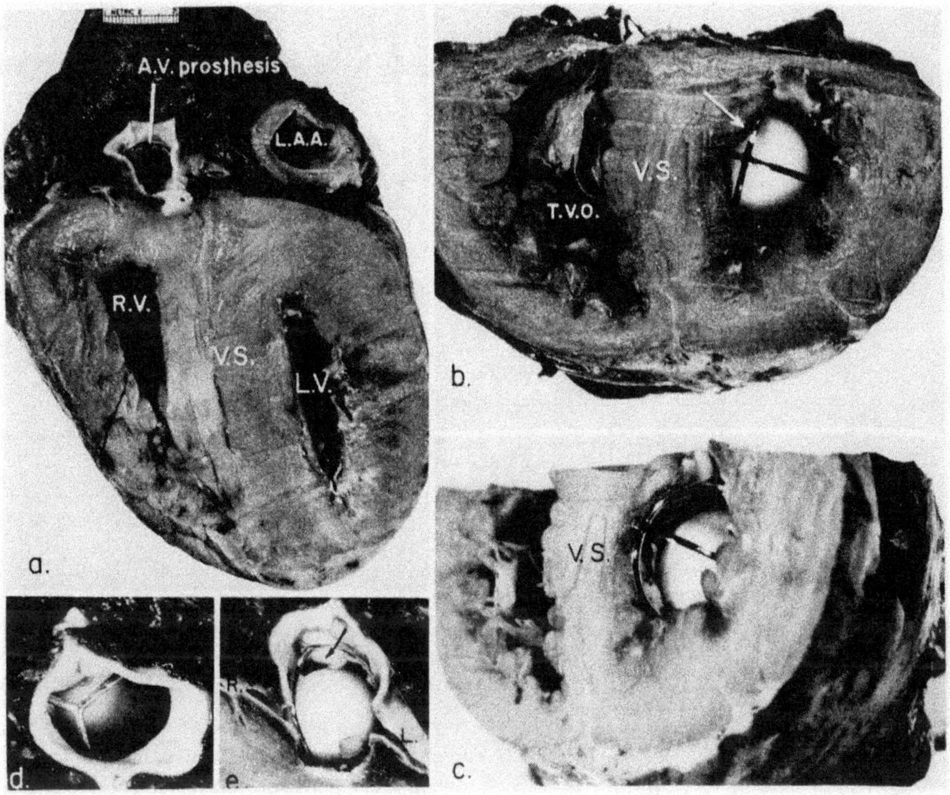

FIG 4. Heart of the patient whose x-rays are shown in Figure 3. This man died 24 hours following replacement of the aortic valve with an 8A Starr-Edwards prosthesis, and the mitral valve with a 4M prosthesis. The walls of both ventricles are extremely hypertrophied, and the ventricular cavities are relatively small, despite both valve lesions being of the incompetent or volume variety. The mitral prosthesis (seen in *b.* and *c.*) is too large, and the ventricular septum bulges into the cage, severely limiting the descent of the ball with resulting prosthetic mitral stenosis. Not only was the motion of the mitral ball severely limited in this patient, but also that of the aortic ball, despite the insertion of a relatively small sized prosthesis (8A) (*d.* and *e.*). In *d.* the aortic prosthesis is seen from above. The apex of the cage is eccentrically located, and the wall of the aorta protrudes between two of the metallic struts, restricting the movement of the ball in the cage. In *e.* the anterior wall of he aorta has been removed, demonstrating that the wall of the aorta inverted when the aortotomy was closed (arrow). A.V. = aortic valve; L.A.A. = left atrial appendage; R.V. = right ventricle; L.V. = left ventricle; V.S. = ventricular septum; T.V.O. = tricuspid valve orifice; R. = right and L. = left coronary artery. (Reproduced with permission from the American Journal of Cardiology, **18:** 497, 1966, reference 3).

the repairs dehisced postoperatively, and massive tricuspid regurgitation resulted. In each of two other patients mitral commissurotomy, performed in association with aortic valve replacement, resulted in severe mitral regurgitation. In two additional subjects who had aortic replacement for aortic stenosis, severe and previously unrecognized mitral stenosis was found at necropsy. *Pulmonary complications* consisted of massive intra-alveolar hemorrhage in two subjects, and pulmonary infarcts in three others. Each of the latter also had pulmonary infarcts preoperatively. Although *arrhythmias* occurred in a number of patients, in only five could they be listed as the major cause of death. In each of the five, death occurred suddenly and unexpectedly, and in three of them there was no anatomic explanation. The fourth was found at necropsy to have a large pheo

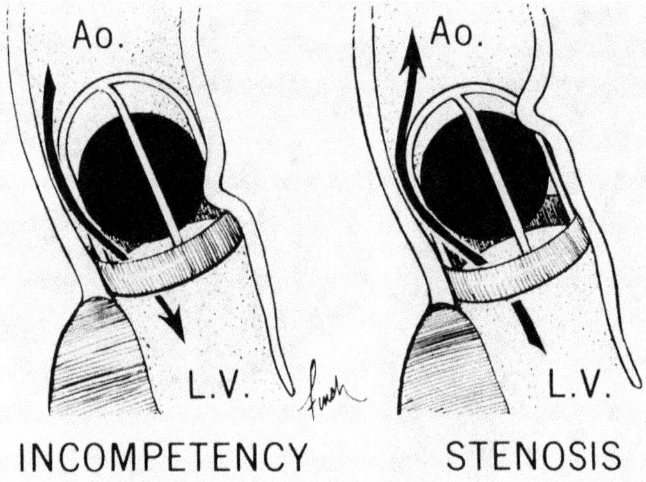

FIG. 5. Diagram demonstrating how an aortic valvular prosthesis may function improperly. If the wall of the aorta is caused to invert toward the lumen, for example by an unremoved nodule of calcium, the ball is prevented from seating completely and aortic regurgitation occurs. If the invagination of the aorta toward the lumen is more cephalad, the systolic motion of the ball may be limited, causing prosthetic stenosis.

chromocytoma of the adrenal gland, and the fifth had active rheumatic carditis, as evidenced by the presence of numerous Aschoff bodies, and multiple old microinfarcts secondary to talc emboli in numerous intramural coronary arteries. *Infection* was a major cause of death in only two patients, and a contributory cause in three others. One of the two developed a Gram-negative infection superimposed on a pulmonary infarct which ruptured and caused empyema. The second developed *serratia* specie mediastinitis, which spread to the aortotomy incision and disrupted it. Although *left atrial thrombi* were usually the result of dysfunctioning prostheses (nine patients), four patients had thrombi without anatomic evidence of valvular malfunction. Each of the four had markedly decreased cardiac output for varying reasons. *Occluding right atrial* thrombi occurred in each of the three patients in whom the tricuspid valve was replaced with a Starr-Edwards prosthesis.

COMMENTS AND CONCLUSIONS CONCERNING THE EARLY POSTOPERATIVE DEATHS

In these 65 patients, an analysis of the causes of death in the early postoperative period discloses that more than half of the 96 fatal complications were the result of potentially avoidable errors in operative management. For example, in 18 patients the mitral prostheses utilized were too large, leading to obstruction to left atrial emptying (16 patients), obstruction to left ventricular outflow (one patient), and aortic regurgitation (one patient). Three aortic valves which were too large caused obstruction to outflow in two instances, and aortic regurgitation in another. Two valves were rendered incompetent by residual calcific deposits which could have been excised. Seven of the 20 deaths from bleeding were the direct result of technical misadventure, as were five of the acute myocardial infarctions. All of the deaths related to an associated and uncorrected valvular malformation could have been avoided. Thus, tricuspid annuloplasty is not to be depended upon for effective relief of tricuspid regurgitation, and mitral valve replacement must be performed if doubt exists as to the effectiveness of mitral commissurotomy. The two patients who died as the result of undiagnosed mitral stenosis emphasize once more the importance of detailed preoperative assessment of mitral valve function in patients with a history of acute rheumatic fever or chorea who apparently have only calcific aortic stenosis. Three of the fatal cerebral emboli, those resulting from calcific debris or air, could have been prevented by more careful attention to operative details. Two of the infections, presumably incurred at operation, must be attributed to faulty aseptic technique. Dissections of the aorta could have been avoided by more careful manipulation of the femoral cannula, or by cannulation at another site. Finally, thrombosis of tricuspid prostheses has not been encountered since disc valves of low profile configuration have been used at this site.

Recognition and appreciation of the factors listed above have resulted in improved judgment and technique in valve replacement, and a lower immediate mortality. Thus, of the 98 patients in whom one or more cardiac valves were replaced in 1964, 19 died within one month following operation. Single or multiple valve replacements were carried out in 81 patients during 1966 and 10 died within the first postoperative month. A comparison of the sizes of the mitral prostheses utilized during each of these periods is of interest. Of the 47 patients who had mitral replacement in 1964, 2M Starr-Edwards prostheses were inserted in only seven, and in 16 patients 4M prostheses were utilized. In contrast, 2M valves were used in 20 of the 47 patients who had mitral replacement during 1966, and in 10 patients 4M prostheses were utilized. Only two of 34 patients in whom one or more cardiac valves were replaced in the first five months of 1967 has died, and each of them had had aortic valve replacement; of the 16 subjects in whom the mitral valve was replaced, a size 2M prosthesis was utilized in 14 of them and a 3M prosthesis in the other two.

One of the unexpected findings in this study was the demonstration of an anatomic cause of death in virtually all of the patients who had manifested the low cardiac output syndrome (5). The most common cause of the syndrome was a dysfunctioning valvular prosthesis. In seven patients with this syndrome, multiple subendocardial acute myocardial infarcts, unassociated with significant coronary arterial disease, were observed at necropsy; in five patients many of the necrotic myocardial fibers were calcified. Interestingly, each of the seven patients had had mitral valve replacement, whereas such multiple focal infarcts were not observed in any patient who had undergone isolated aortic valve replacement.

ANALYSIS OF THE LATE POSTOPERATIVE DEATHS

The pertinent clinical and pathologic data in the 33 patients who died later than one month following replacement of one or more cardiac valves with Starr-Edwards prostheses are summarized in Table III. Some observations in 20 of these subjects have been described elsewhere (6).

CAUSES OF DEATH

Staphylococcal infection developed at the sites of attachment of prosthetic cardiac valves in five patients (7–9). The pertinent clinicopathologic observations in them are summarized in Table IV. With the exception of one patient,

TABLE III

Late Deaths following Starr-Edwards Cardiac Valve Replacement

Valve Replaced	No. Patients	Survival from Operation (mo)	Thrombus on Prosthesis	Ring Leak	Anti-coagulants	Cause of Death
Mitral	8	7–56 (Av 16.6)	7*	2	7	Sudden = 1 ABE = 2 Prosthetic MR or MS = 4 Other = 1
Aortic	17	1.3–37 (Av 13.0)	13†	5†	2	Sudden = 10 ABE = 3 Other = 4
Mitral and Aortic	7	1.5–44 (Av 15.4)	6‡	2§	7	Sudden = 1 CHF = 4 Prosthetic MR = 1 Ruptured appendix = 1
Mitral and Tricuspid¶	1	9	1	0	1	Sudden = 1
41	33	1.3–56 (Av 14.4)	27	9	17	Sudden = 13 ABE = 5 Prosthetic MR or MS = 5 CHF = 4 Other = 6

* Two patients had prosthetic staphylococcal endocarditis.
† Three patients had prosthetic staphylococcal endocarditis.
‡ Mitral valve in all 4; aortic valve also in 3.
§ Mitral valve in each.
¶ Kay-Shiley tricuspid valve.
Abbreviations: ABE = acute staphylococcal endocarditis: MR = mitral regurgitation; MS = mitral stenosis; CHF = congestive heart failure.

each died within 45 days following the onset of symptoms and/or signs of infective endocarditis. In two patients operative procedures (dental extractions in one and a skin graft in one) precipitated the septicemia, but in two no precipitating cause for the infection was apparent. In each of the five patients the infective process involved the entire annulus where the prosthesis had been inserted, and extended into the adjacent myocardium and epicardium. In two of the three patients with infection at the site of a prosthetic aortic valve (Fig 6), the inflammatory process extended through the atrial septum to the area of the atrioventricular node, and caused a high degree of atrioventricular block. The extent of the infection, and the character of the tissue of the valve annuli in these patients, clearly indicates that an attempt at secondary operative intervention would have been fruitless. Consequently, since presently available antibiotics are rarely effective in eradicating infection at the site of a prosthetic cardiac valve, the infection must be prevented. The value of penicillin in patients with rheumatic heart disease who undergo dental or other operative procedures is well established, but the necessity of an even more vigorous prophylactic regi-

TABLE IV

Infective Endocarditis at the Site of Caged-ball Prostheses

Patient	Age/ Sex	Valve Replaced	Organism	Precipitating Cause	Length of Infection	Conduction Disturbance	Interval Op. to Death (mo)	Cause of Death
1) F.H. A63-176	55 M	Aortic	Staph. epidermidis	AMI	16 mo., intermittent	1° H.B. 2° H.B. 2° H.B. LBBB	Bahnson cusp-26 Muller valve-5½ S-E valve-1½	AR
2) W.L. A64-189	51 M	Aortic	Staph. epidermidis	Teeth extractions	45 days	LBBB	13½	AR
3) A.S. A65-186	47 M	Mitral	Staph. aureus	Skin graft	30 days	0	4	MS
4) T.G. A65-221	46 M	Mitral	Staph. epidermidis	Unknown	25 days	0	4	MS
5) W.B. A67-22	48 M	Aortic	Staph. epidermidis	Unknown	16 days	1° H.B. 2° H.B. Nodal	3	AR

Abbreviations: H. B. = block; LBBB = left bundle branch block, AR = "aortic" regurgitation; and MS = "mitral" stenosis.

men in patients with prosthetic cardiac valves who undergo similar procedures has only recently been emphasized (7). Death in the three patients with infected aortic valve prostheses was the result of massive aortic regurgitation secondary to partial or total detachment of the prosthesis. Death in the two subjects with infected mitral prostheses was the result of obstruction to the mitral orifice, secondary to large infected thrombi (vegetations) on the atrial aspect of the prostheses.

Infection was the cause of death in one other patient; he developed pulmonary nocardiosis secondary to dexamethasone therapy for serum hepatitis (10).

Congestive cardiac failure was the cause of death in eight patients: in three of them the failure was the result of ventriculo-atrial regurgitation around prosthetic mitral valves; in two patients the failure was secondary to progressive thrombosis of the prosthetic valves, aortic in one and mitral in the other, and the ball in each was nearly immobile; in the other three patients the cause of the cardiac failure is less certain. Each had had both mitral and aortic replacements. One of the three died shortly after receiving blood transfusions for intravascular hemolytic anemia. The other two subjects developed severe right sided, as well as left sided, cardiac failure several months following operation. At autopsy, both had extensive acquired endocardial fibroelastosis of the left ventricle, and this may have been responsible for cardiac decompensation. Two patients, who had *Marfan's syndrome,* had replacement of the aortic valve and the ascending aorta: one died of associated mitral regurgitation, and the other of renal failure caused by an associated aneurysm in the descending thoracic aorta. Two patients died of complications of *warfarin-induced hypoprothrombinemia*: one of a massive intracerebral hemorrhage, and the second of bilateral subdural hematomas. Another patient died of complications of a cerebral arterial embolus. One patient

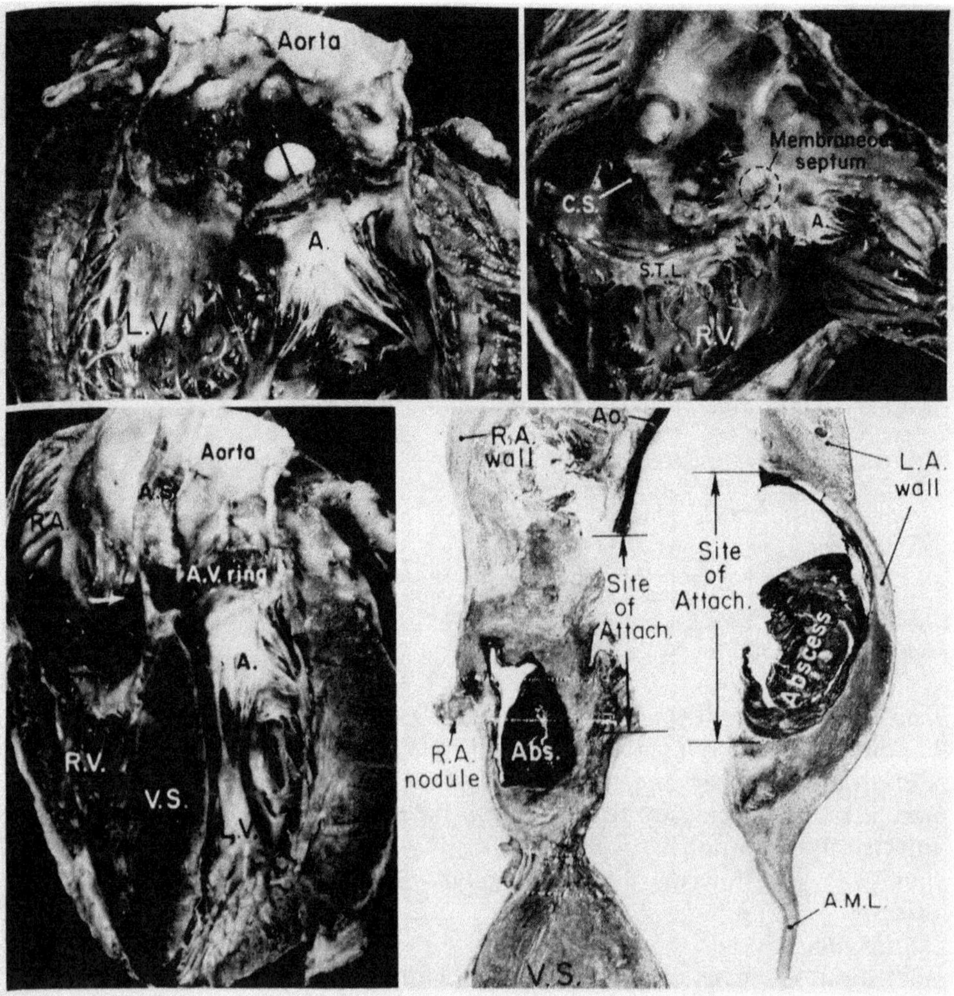

FIG. 6. *Staphylococcus epidermidis* infection at the site of an aortic valve prosthesis in a 48-year-old man, in whom valve replacement was performed three months before death (patient #5, Table IV). Preoperatively, this patient had severe aortic stenosis (86 mm Hg peak systolic pressure gradient) and regurgitation. His postoperative period was uneventful until 16 days before death when fever, chills, myalgias and weakness appeared without any apparent precipitating event. When seen at the National Heart Institute 10 days before death the blood pressure was 120/54 mm Hg, and a loud murmur typical of aortic regurgitation was audible. Blood cultures were positive, but despite extensive antibiotic therapy, the heart progressively enlarged, the valve became more detached, and he died. *Upper left:* Opened aorta, aortic valvular ring, and left ventricle (L.V.). The site of attachment of the prosthesis is necrotic and the prosthesis has prolapsed slightly into the left ventricular cavity. Approximately 40 percent of the prosthetic ring had become detached before death. A. = anterior mitral leaflet. *Upper right:* Opened right atrium, tricuspid valve, and right ventricle (R.V.). The atrial septum and membraneous ventricular septum (dashed circle) is extensively infiltrated by inflammatory necrotic material, which extends through these structures to form two infected nodules (arrows) on the right atrial endocardium. Thus, right atrial infective endocarditis was the result of the extension of this necrotizing process. The area between the ostium of the coronary sinus (C.S.) and membraneous ventricular septum is the location of the atrioventricular conduction tissue, which was destroyed by the infective process. A high degree of atrioventricular block resulted. S.T.L. = septal tricuspid leaflet; A. = anterior tricuspid leaflet. *Lower left:* The anterior wall of the heart has been removed, showing extension of the infection from the aortic valvular (A.V.) ring, through the atrial septum (A.S.), and membraneous ventricular septum (V.S.). The arrow again designates one of the right atrial (R.A.) infected nodules. *Lower middle:* Section of aortic root and adjacent structures. The infection spread from the site of attachment of the prosthesis into the right atrial wall (R.A.), atrial and membraneous ventricular septum. A cystic abscess (Abs.) also is present between the right atrial nodule and the site of attachment. Phosphotungsten acid hematoxylin stain, ×1.7. *Lower right:* Another section of aortic root and adjacent structures. This section is from another area and includes the anterior mitral leaflet (A.M.L.) and inflamed left atrial wall (L.A.). The abscess extends around the entire circumference of the aortic "ring." Hematoxylin and eosin stain, ×2.4.

died of a noncardiac condition, ruptured appendix, but at necropsy he had extensive prosthetic thrombosis.

The remaining 13 patients died *suddenly* and unexpectedly: one had had a mitral replacement, ten had aortic replacement, one both tricuspid and mitral replacement, and one had both aortic and mitral replacement. Death in two patients, occurring 29 and 37 months, respectively, following operation, was the result of dislodgement of aortic balls from their cages, with the production of sudden and massive aortic regurgitation. Necropsy in one of these patients was limited to the chest organs, so that the site to which the ball migrated in him is uncertain, but in the second subject the ball had impacted at the aortic bifurcation, as in a patient reported elsewhere (11). In two additional patients who underwent valve replacement (aortic in one; mitral and aortic in one) in this clinic and died suddenly elsewhere 28 and 36 months, respectively, following operation, the aortic balls had dislodged from their cages and migrated to the bifurcation of the abdominal aorta. The hearts of these two subjects have been unavailable for study by us and therefore these two patients are not included in our necropsy survey. Death in another patient was the result of acute myocardial infarction. The cause of death in the other 10 subjects is uncertain. Three of the patients with prosthetic aortic valves and the one patient with isolated mitral replacement had had acute myocardial infarctions documented before operation; in the three with aortic valves, left ventricular aneurysms were evident at necropsy. Five of the 13 patients who died suddenly complained of chest pain immediately before death, but necropsy showed changes of acute myocardial infarction in only the one mentioned. Nine of these 13 patients, however, had severe coronary arterial narrowing, and extensive myocardial scarring was present in each of them.

OTHER NECROPSY OBSERVATIONS IN THE 33 PATIENTS WHO DIED LATE

Prosthetic valve thrombi (Figs 7 and 8): Thrombi were found on the prosthetic valves at necropsy in 27 of the 33 patients; 14 of the 27 had been receiving warfarin, and three of the six patients without prosthetic thrombi had been receiving warfarin. Four of the 27 subjects with thrombi were among those who died of bacterial (Staphylococcal) endocarditis. Only four of the remaining 23 patients with thrombi on their valves had had evidence of systemic emboli during life. In at least 11 of these 23 patients, the thrombus had rendered the prosthesis incompetent, stenotic, or both, but in the others valve function was not impaired. Of the 13 patients who died suddenly, 11 had thrombus on their prostheses. In each the thrombi were located at the junction of the struts and metallic rings, extended up (or down for mitral) the struts for variable distances, and occasionally completely covered the metallic rings. In one patient, who also had a small peribasilar leak, the extensive thrombus on the struts prevented random motion of the ball, which became grooved by the struts. In addition to its being discolored and grooved, the weight of the prosthetic aortic ball in this patient was 9.1 percent greater than when it had been inserted 24 months earlier. In still another patient with an aortic prosthesis, which had been in place for 30 months, the silicone rubber ball was made completely immobile by thrombus, was deep yellow in color (rather than white), soft in consistency, and grooved. Histologic study of several of the thrombi disclosed that they consisted mainly of fibrin and

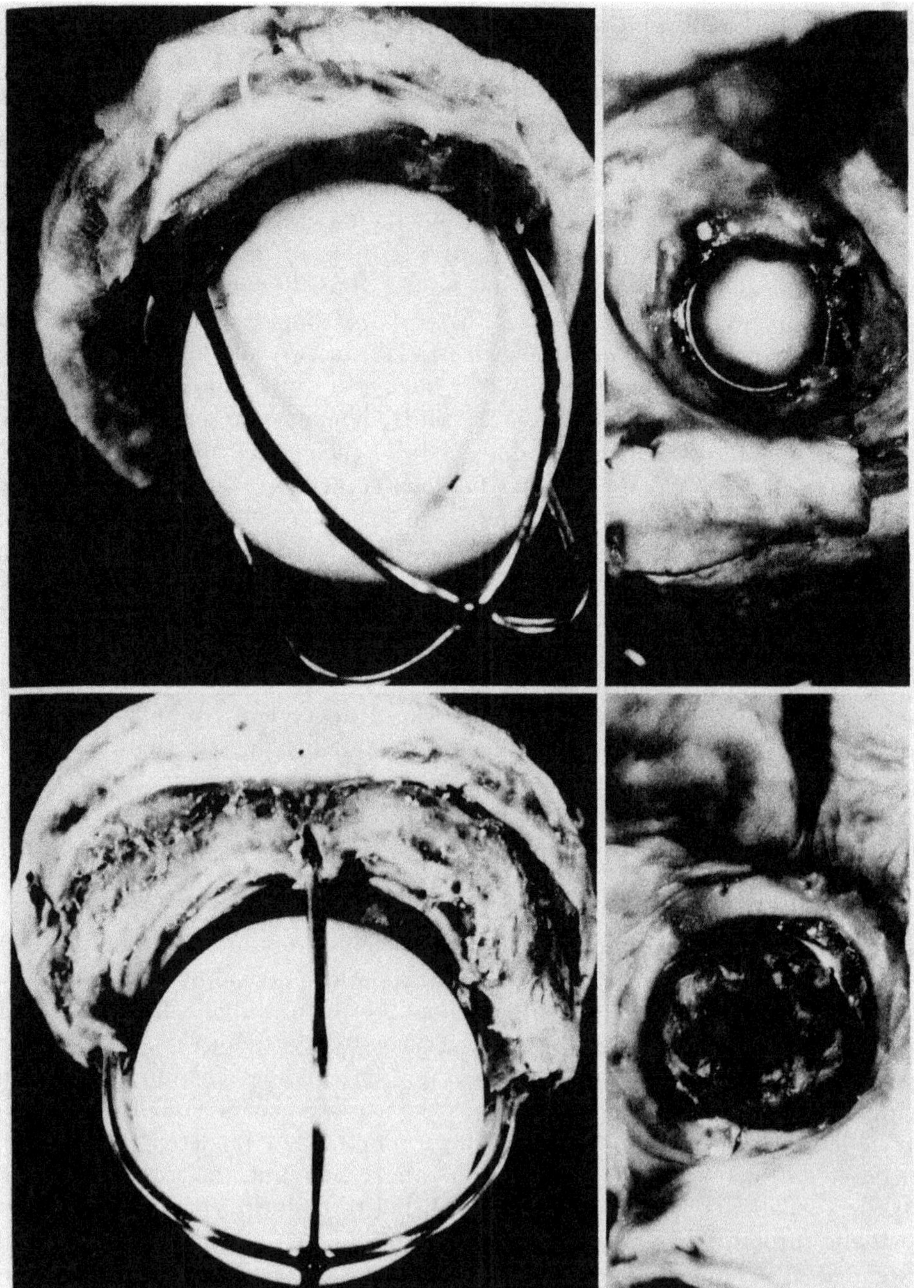

FIG. 7. Mitral valvular thrombi. *Upper:* Thrombus on this prosthesis encompasses the bases of each of the four metallic struts. The thrombus protrudes slightly into the cage and prevents the ball from seating completely. Thus, prosthetic mitral regurgitation occurred. This same prosthesis as seen from the left atrial aspect is shown in the upper right photograph. This patient was a 43-year-old woman (A65-43) who died suddenly and unexpectedly seven months following mitral replacement. *Lower:* The heavily thrombosed mitral prosthesis of a 15-year-old girl (A66-54) who had undergone mitral replacement 11 months earlier. Signs and symptoms of a cerebral embolus occurred seven days following operation, but never thereafter. She died of congestive cardiac failure, the result of prosthetic mitral stenosis. The range of motion of the prosthetic ball was only 2 mm. The same valve as viewed from the left atrium is shown in the lower right photograph. Only one other patient studied by us had this much noninfected thrombus on a cardiac valvular prosthesis.

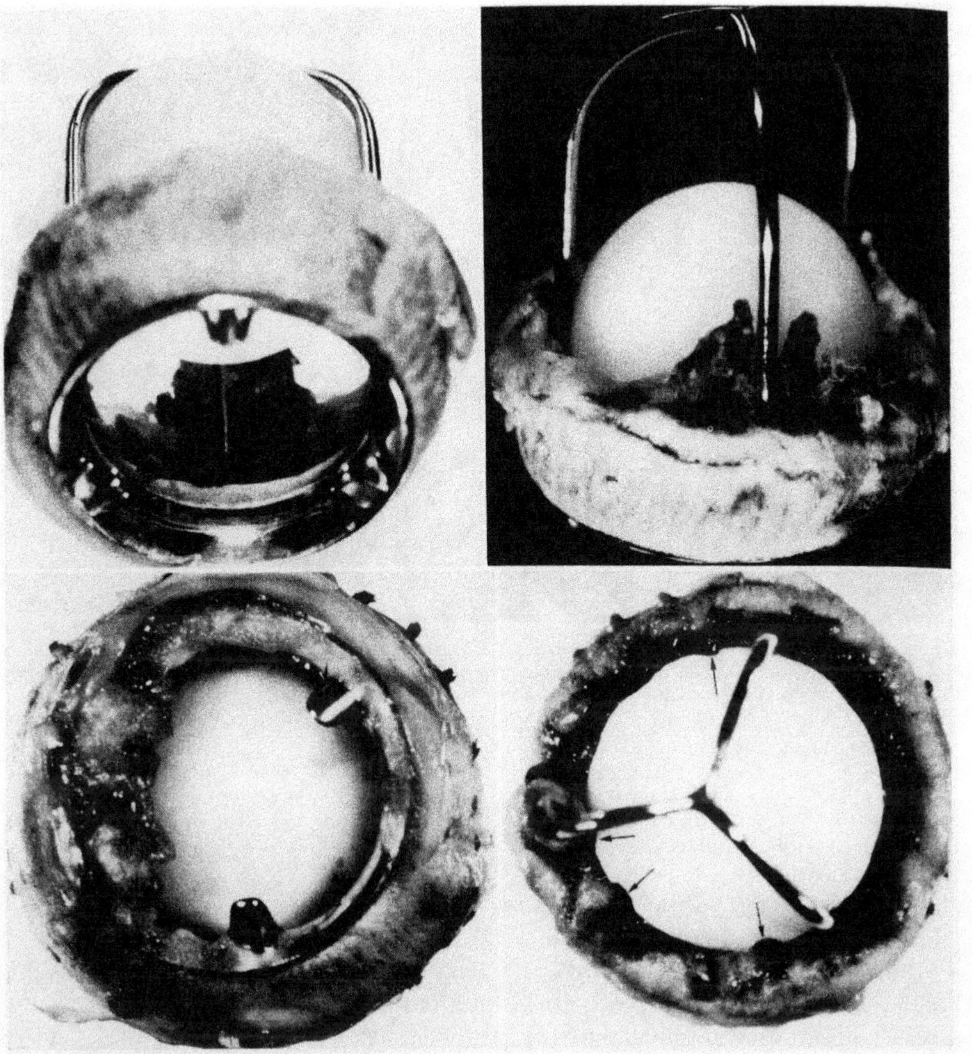

FIG 8. Aortic valvular thrombi. *Upper:* Aortic valvular prosthesis in a 24-year-old man (A65-185) who died suddenly and unexpectedly nine months following valve replacement. The preoperative clinical features of this patient were reported elsewhere (22). This small thrombus, extending up one of the three metallic struts from the metallic ring, did not interfere with movement of the prosthetic ball. *Lower:* Aortic valvular prosthesis in a 50-year-old man (A65-143) who died of an acute myocardial infarction 24 months following valve replacement. Thrombus covers portions of the metallic ring and encompasses one of the metallic struts. The small arrows point to grooves made in the ball by the metallic struts. The area for ball movement was severely limited because of ball swelling and because of strut thrombus protruding into the cage.

platelets, and were devoid of bacteria or fungi except in the five subjects with documented Staphylococcal endocarditis.

Fistulae around prosthetic valve rings (Fig 9): As noted, mitral peribasilar communications were considered to be responsible for death in three patients, and in three additional subjects, excluding those with bacterial endocarditis, such communications also were present: two were around mitral prostheses, and one, an aortic prosthesis. The presence of accessory communications was estab-

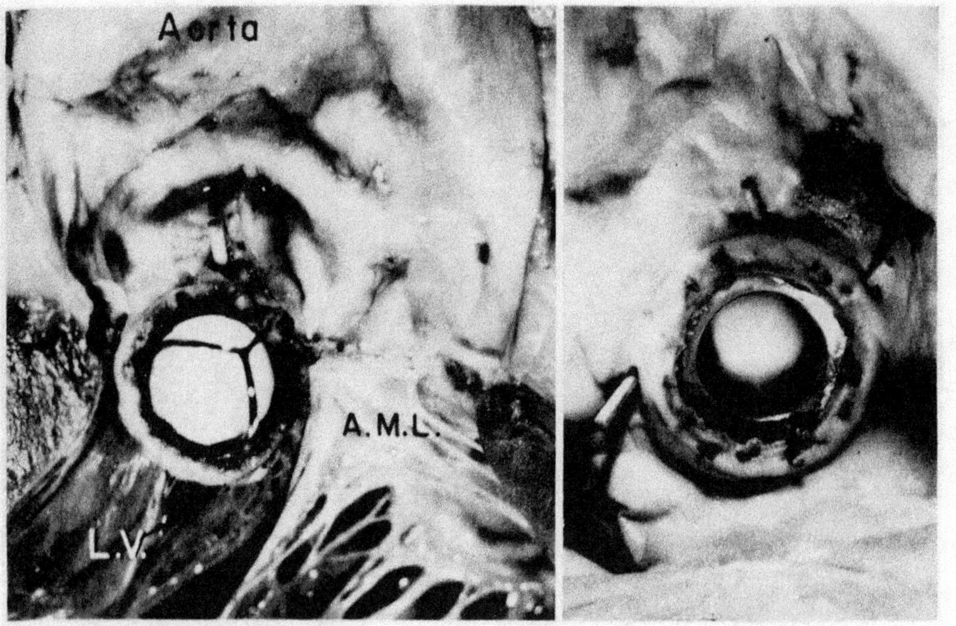

FIG. 9. Peribasilar prosthetic regurgitation. *Left:* Opened aorta, aortic valve "ring," and left ventricle (L.V.) in a 50-year-old man (A65-143) who had a precordial murmur typical of aortic regurgitation in the late postoperative period. A stick has been inserted into the fistula at the site of attachment of the prosthetic valve. A.M.L. = anterior mitral leaflet. *Right:* Mitral prosthesis as seen from the left atrium of a 47-year-old man (A64-90) who died six and one half months following mitral and aortic valve replacements. In the late postoperative period he developed severe congestive heart failure, but a murmur of mitral regurgitation was not audible. The three peribasilar fistulae, each containing a stick, readily explain the cardiac failure.

lished before death in the patient with the aortic prosthesis, but in only two of the five patients with mitral prostheses.

Rockoff and associates recently summarized the clinical, hemodynamic, and angiocardiographic features of patients studied in this clinic with left ventriculoatrial regurgitation secondary to partial detachment of a mitral ball-valve prosthesis (12). The characteristic pansystolic murmur is often absent when mitral regurgitation occurs through a peribasilar communication, and consequently left ventricular angiocardiography is the only means of precisely diagnosing this complication during life. This procedure should be performed on all patients who fail to improve following mitral valve replacement, or who exhibit abnormal cardiac dynamics at postoperative cardiac catheterization.

Intimal thickening of the aortic root and proximal coronary arteries (Figs 10 and 11): In each of the 24 patients (22 men, 2 females; ages 21–69, average, 45 yrs) with prosthetic aortic valves, there was intimal thickening in the aortic root, which included the area of the coronary arterial ostia. This thickening was produced by the deposition of fibrous tissue, which was devoid of foam cells, on the internal elastic membrane of the proximal portion of the ascending aorta. The degree of intimal proliferation varied from minimal to severe; in some patients it was diffuse and in others it was focal. In addition to the changes in the aortic root in all 24 patients, there also was intimal proliferation of varying degrees around one or both coronary arterial ostia in 16 of them: in eight this prolifera-

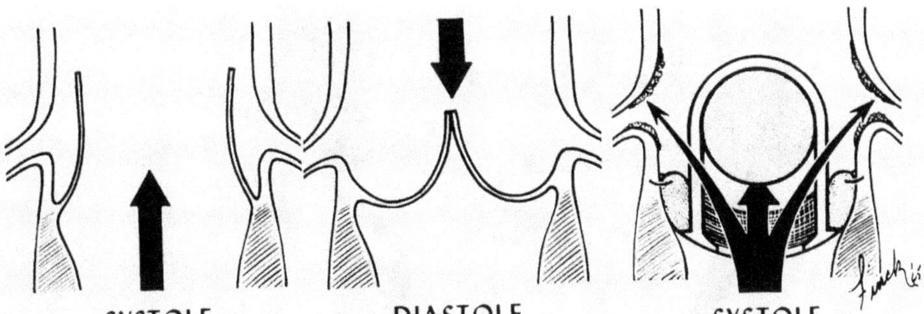

FIG 10. Diagrammatic representation of the aortic valve region in the normal heart (left and center) and following replacement with a caged-ball prosthesis. Flow of blood during systole across the normal aortic valve is laminar, and the coronary arteries fill mainly by retrograde flow during diastole. Following caged-ball prosthetic replacement, the flow of blood across the aortic valve area is no longer laminar. The force of left ventricular ejection is directed centrally, as in the normal, but the ball prevents central flow, producing severe turbulence in the area. Thus, during ventricular systole blood between the surface of the ball and the intima of the aortic root is flowing in a turbulent fashion. The anatomic indicator of turbulent flow under high pressure is intimal proliferation which has been observed in the proximal aorta of each of the 24 subjects dying in the late postoperative period following aortic valve replacement. Since the coronary ostia are no longer "guarded," so to speak, by the aortic cusps during ventricular systole and, much more importantly, since they are in the area of turbulent flow, they also are subject to intimal proliferation which has been observed in them in several subjects (see text).

tion was in the area of the right coronary ostium, but in seven there was no narrowing of it, and in one the ostium was severely narrowed. The other seven patients had narrowing of varying degrees of both coronary ostia. In three of the seven, the narrowing was mild and functionally insignificant; in the other four there was considerable narrowing of each coronary ostium and of the proximal main left and right coronary arteries as well. Two of the latter four patients, however, had had replacement of the ascending aorta by a graft at the time of valve replacement, and the proximity of the suture line to the coronary ostia may have been a factor producing ostial narrowing. The third patient had severe narrowing, not only of the ostia, but of the entire coronary arterial tree, secondary to atherosclerosis. The fourth patient had severe intimal thickening in the proximal 1 cm segments of the right and left coronary arteries, but the coronary vessels distal to this point were widely patent. In this patient, coronary arterial perfusion cannulae could not be inserted into the ostia at the time of necropsy, although such cannulae had been utilized without difficulty at the time of valve replacement only four months earlier. This man, who was 48 years old, had not had chest pain before operation, but two months postoperatively he developed angina pectoris, and thereafter numerous anginal attacks. This patient also had mild anemia postoperatively, and at necropsy the presence of considerable amounts of iron in his kidneys indicated that the anemia was secondary to intravascular hemolysis (13, 14). The presence of the anemia in him may be interpreted as indicating that there was excessive turbulence of blood in the area of the valvular prosthesis.

The thickening of the intima of the aortic root appears to have occurred in these patients in the postoperative period. It was clear from necropsy examination that the healing of the aortotomy incision was not the responsible factor,

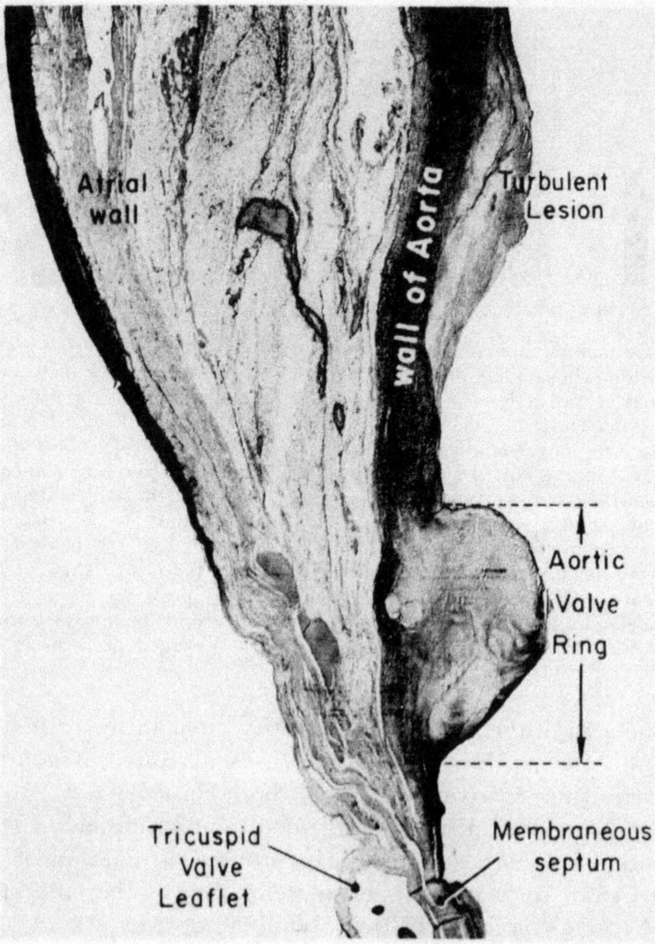

FIG. 11. Section including aortic valve "ring" where a Starr-Edwards aortic valve prosthesis had been attached 20 months earlier in this 60-year-old woman (A64-225). Above the aortic valve ring on the intimal surface of the aorta is a protrusion which is interpreted to be the result of severe turbulent flow in the aortic root beween the base and apex of the prosthetic cage as discussed in Figure 10. The membraneous ventricular septum, septal tricuspid valve leaflet, and atrial wall are designated for orientation purposes. Elastic van Gieson stain ×7.

since intimal thickening also was present at some distance from it. In only one of the 24 patients was coronary ostial narrowing evident at the time of aortic valve replacement. It is unlikely that any functional disturbances are produced by intimal thickening in the ascending aorta itself. On the other hand, when this process involves the ostia and proximal coronary arteries, the effects, when severe, may be compared to those of syphilitic aortitis. The flow of blood through a normal aortic valve and ascending aorta is laminar, but when a ball-valve prosthesis is present, flow in these areas is grossly turbulent (15). The anatomic indicator of localized turbulent flow is intimal proliferation (16). Although the changes in the coronary ostia and proximal coronary arteries were relatively unimpressive in most of the 24 patients, their average survival following valve replacement was 14 months (range 1.3–44 months). It is possible that the intimal proliferation in these areas will become more extensive with time; however, it is encouraging that no coronary ostial narrowing was observed in the longest survivor (44 months) of these 24 subjects.

Associated endocardial lesions (Figs 12 and 13): In each of the 15 patients who had mitral replacement there was some degree of left ventricular endocardial thickening at necropsy. The stumps of the amputated left ventricular papillary muscles in each of these patients were covered by fibrous tissue, but in 12 of the 15 patients the fibrous process extended to involve other areas of left ventricular endocardium as well. In one of these 12 subjects, a 14-year-old girl who had mitral regurgitation preoperatively, the endocardium of the entire left ventricle was thickened, and it was clear that in her the fibrous proliferation, which contained numerous elastic fibers, was the result of primary congenital endocardial fibroelastosis. In the other 11 patients, all of whom were middle-aged adults, with extensive though patchy left ventricular endocardial thickening, the fibrous proliferation almost certainly appeared following operation. This secondary endocardial fibroelastosis was especially severe in three and moderately severe in one of the six patients who had aortic as well as mitral valve replacement. One of the patients with double valve replacement had no endocardial fibroelastosis, but he lived only one and one half months following operation. The other five lived from 6 to 44 months following valve replacement. Left ventricular endocardial thickening did not occur in patients with isolated aortic valve replacement, unless there had been a previous myocardial infarct (three patients).

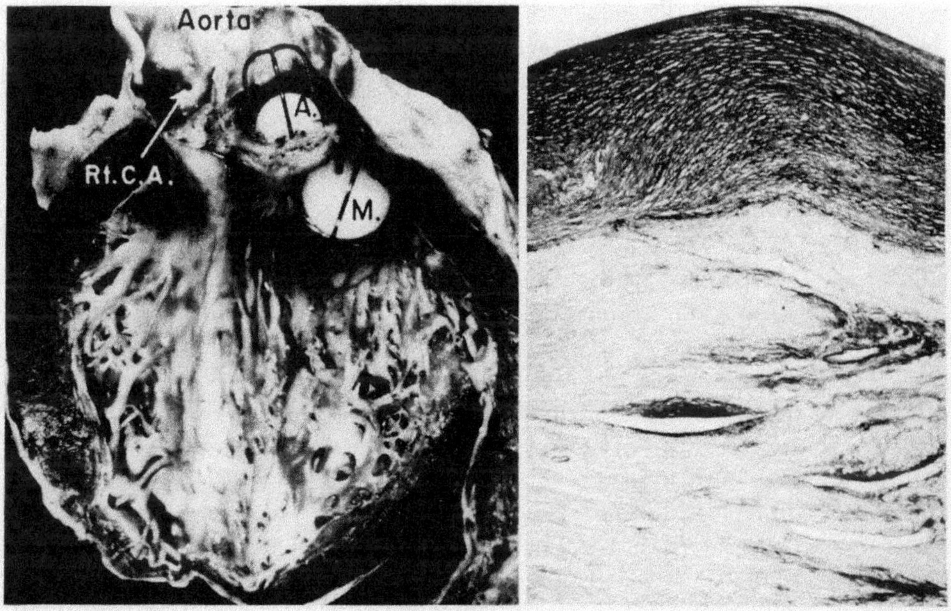

FIG 12. Secondary diffuse left ventricular endocardial fibroelastosis in a 56-year-old man (A67-50) who died 11 months following replacement of the aortic (A.) and mitral (M.) valves with Starr-Edwards prostheses. The endocardium of the left ventricular papillary muscles, partially excised at the time of operation, was not thickened, thus indicating that the endocardial thickening occurred in the postoperative period. This patient died of severe congestive cardiac failure which probably was related to the endocardial thickening. *Right:* Section demonstrating the severe thickening of the left ventricular endocardium which contains numerous elastic fibers. Elastic van Gieson stain, ×22.5.

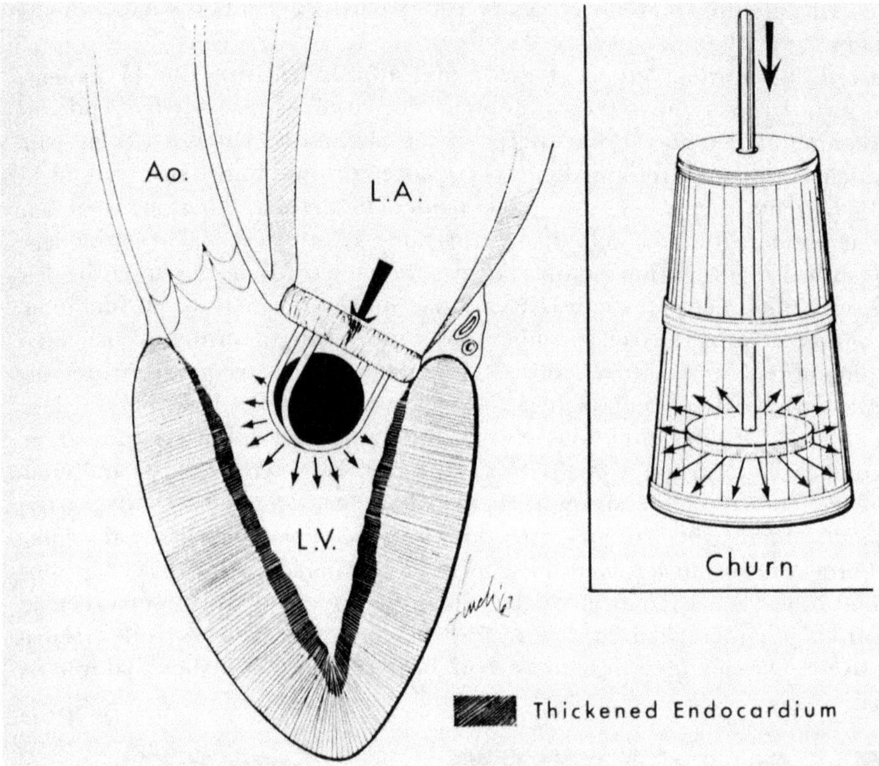

FIG. 13. Diagrammatic representation of the possible mechanism of the secondary left ventricular (L.V.) endocardial fibrosis which occurs commonly following replacement of the mitral valve with a caged-ball prosthesis. The cage and ball of the mitral prosthesis are located within the left ventricular cavity. Thus, when the ball moves, either descends or ascends, it pushes blood laterally, consequently producing turbulence. This effect may be compared to the turbulence produced by the butter churn. Again, the anatomic indicator of turbulent flow is proliferation of connective tissue on the surface in contact with that flow; in this case, endocardium. Ao. = aorta; L.A. = left atrium.

The functional consequence of extensive, focal, acquired left ventricular endocardial fibroelastosis is uncertain. This process was the only abnormal anatomic cardiac finding in two subjects who had severe unexplained progressive congestive heart failure several months following operation, and may have been the cause of the cardiac failure in them. Although the endocardial thickening which occurs over the stumps of the amputated papillary muscles is simply a healing phenomenon, the cause of the more widespread left ventricular endocardial thickening is uncertain. Turbulent flow of blood in this chamber produced by the caged ball in it may be the explanation.

The endocardium of the left atrium also was extensively thickened in all 15 patients who had mitral replacement. In contrast to the endocardial fibrosis in the left ventricle, which contained numerous elastic fibers, that which occurred in the left atrium was, with rare exception, devoid of elastic fibers. The left atrial endocardial thickening also almost certainly appeared postoperatively, and may have been precipitated by operative trauma to this chamber's wall.

Traumatic intravascular hemolysis: It is now well appreciated that intravascular hemolysis occurs in virtually all patients with malfunctioning Teflon aortic valves (13), and in a few patients with incompetent and stenotic aortic valves which have not been operated upon (14). The intravascular hemolysis in these subjects is the result of trauma to erythrocytes traversing the malfunctioning natural or artificial aortic valve. The anatomic indicator of intravascular hemolysis is renal hemosiderosis ("blue kidney" (14)); the mechanisms by which iron is deposited in the kidneys have been described elsewhere (13). The kidneys were available for examination in 17 of the 33 subjects who died in the late postoperative period. In 14 of the 17 patients histologic sections stained by the Prussian blue reaction disclosed iron in the kidneys (Table V): in nine the amounts of iron deposited in the kidneys (almost entirely in the proximal tubules) were heavy (3+ or 4+ on a 1–4+ scale), in two moderate (2+) and in three trace or minimal (1+). Of these 17 subjects, the aortic valve alone had been replaced in nine, the mitral alone in three, and both mitral and aortic in five. Three of the 12 with renal iron had accessory peribasilar communications at necropsy, and each of them had heavy deposits of iron in their kidneys. Of the three subjects with renal hemosiderosis following isolated mitral replacement, one had a large peribasilar leak, a second had a huge prosthetic thrombus, and the third, who had only trace amounts of renal iron, had acute staphylococcal infection at the site of the prosthesis. Two of the subjects with heavy renal deposits of iron had had malfunctioning Teflon aortic valve prostheses which were replaced with Starr-Edwards prostheses three and 12 months, respectively, before death.

Although the deposits of iron in the kidneys at times produce striking anatomic lesions, no significant renal damage or impairment of renal function appears to occur as a result of this deposition (13, 14). The bone marrow is usually able to compensate for the increased red blood cell destruction, and significant anemia is uncommon. The hematocrit values in the late postoperative period were available in 11 of the 14 patients with renal hemosiderosis: in seven the hematocrit was normal ($\geqq$ 40%), and in four it was low (34% in one, and 37% in each of three). The patient with a hematocrit of 34%, however, had infectious endocarditis, which probably was responsible for the anemia in him.

Degeneration of the prosthetic ball (ball variance) (Figs 14 and 15): At the time of insertion, the prosthetic balls are white, firm, smooth, and glistening. Variation from these normal features have not been observed in any of the mitral prosthetic balls (poppets) examined by us in the late postoperative period.

TABLE V

Renal Hemosiderosis in Patients Dying in the Late Post-Operative Period following Cardiac Valve Replacement with Starr-Edwards Prosthesis

Valve Replaced	No. Pts.	Renal Iron		
		Heavy or Moderate	Trace	None
Aortic	9*	5	2	2
Aortic and Mitral	3*	2		1
Mitral	3*	2	1	
Totals	15	9	3	3

* 1 patient had peribasilar communications.

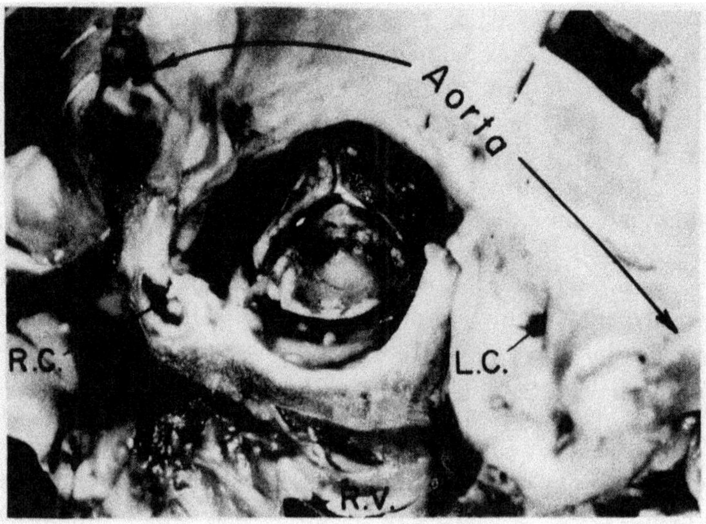

FIG. 14. Aortic ball variance. Shown here is an immobile aortic ball which is swollen, rather soft in consistency and yellow in color. It had been inserted 30 months earlier and, postoperatively, this 50-year-old man (A67-107) had at least four systemic emboli and during his last two months, severe intractable cardiac failure. The ball was impacted in the cage and almost certainly was both stenotic and incompetent. Some type of ball variance probably occurs late following all aortic valve replacements, but this degree of ball variance is extreme and unusual. R.V. = right ventricle; R.C. = ostium, right coronary artery; and L.C. = ostium, left coronary artery.

Alteration has occurred, however, in the aortic valve balls which have functioned for long periods. For some time it has been recognized that the silicone rubber aortic balls take up lipid materials (17). Starr, Hancock and others have shown that the prostheses in individuals in whom lipids are absorbed into the aortic ball, frequently are tight fitting or have perivalvular leaks (17, 18). The increase in blood velocity and turbulence which occurs under these conditions appears to be the principle mechanism involved in the uptake of lipids (18). The lipids apparently make the silicone rubber less resistant to abrasion and damage. The most frequent abnormality observed in these aortic balls is surface dullness with loss of the glistening white appearance of the ball. This degree of ball variance appears to be an early indication of ball degeneration, and has been seen in several of the aortic prosthetic balls examined by us. Discoloration per se, however, appears to be of no functional significance. Alteration in size of the ball, on the other hand, is of considerable physiologic significance. In each of the two patients mentioned previously, in whom the aortic ball embolized, it may be assumed that the ball either became smaller or broke apart (19). In two other subjects vertical grooves, corresponding to the struts, were present in the aortic balls (Figs 8 and 14). In each, the balls were virtually immobile, the result probably of both swelling of the balls (20) and of impingement on their movement by thrombus surrounding the metallic struts. In one of these two patients the ball was deep yellow in color and soft in consistency (Fig 14).

Dislodgement of an aortic ball from its cage may be suspected in any individual following caged ball aortic valve replacement, who suddenly develops chest or abdominal pain, rhythm disturbance or syncope, or shock and on auscultation demonstrates a murmur of aortic regurgitation and absent opening and

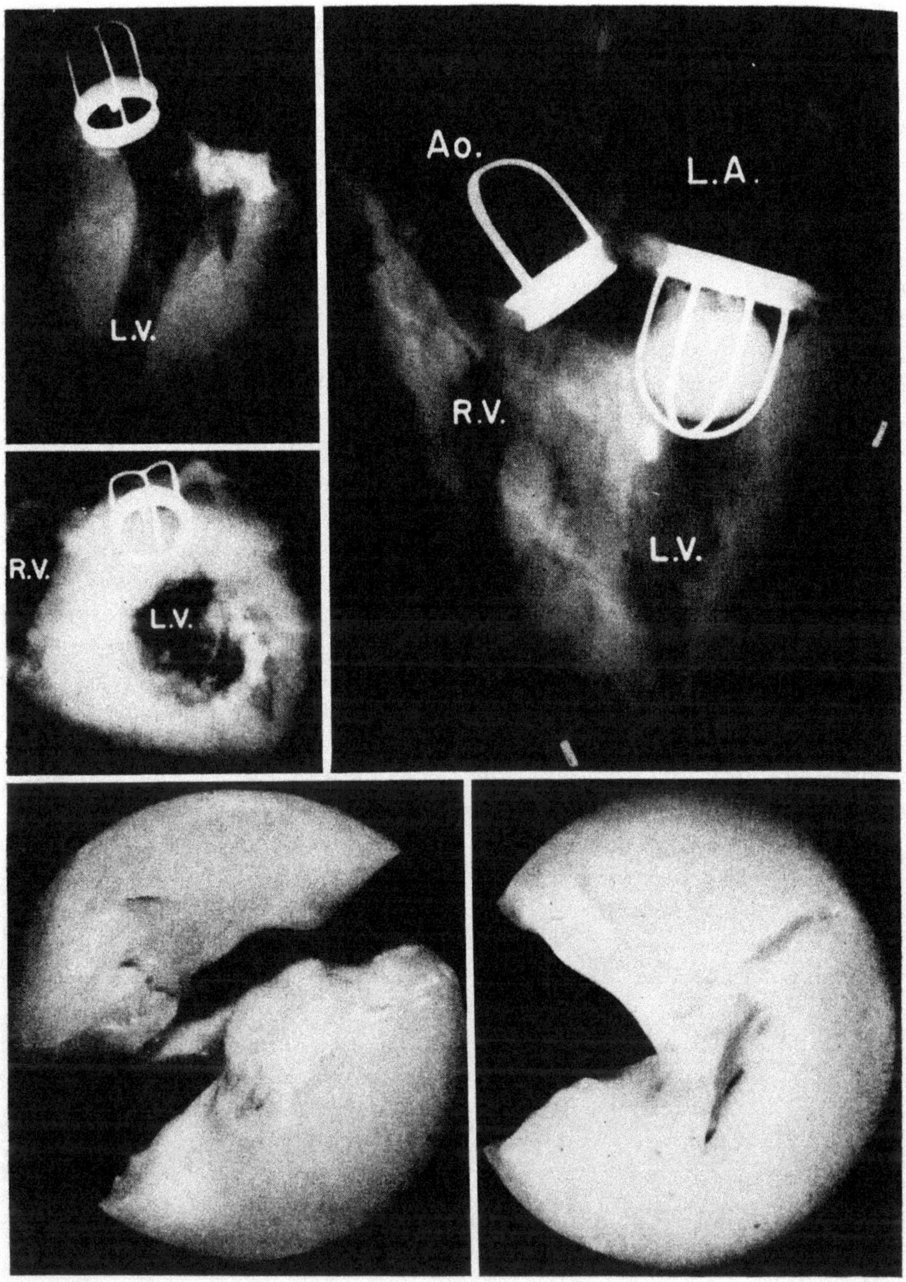

FIG 15. Another extreme of ball variance is marked atrophy and/or splitting of the aortic ball. *Upper and middle left:* Roentgenograms of the heart of a 56-year-old man (A67-85) who died suddenly and unexpectedly 37 months following aortic valve replacement. The radiographs show the prosthetic aortic cage, but the ball is missing, having dislodged and embolized to the abdominal aorta. The calcium is in the mitral valve. L.V. = left ventricle; R.V. = right ventricle. *Upper right:* Roentgenogram of the heart of a 52-year-old woman (A67-142) who died suddenly and unexpectedly 29 months following replacement of both mitral and aortic valves with Starr-Edwards prostheses. Again, the aortic ball is absent having dislodged to the abdominal aorta. Ao. = aorta; L.A. = left atrium. *Lower:* The aortic ball, seen from two views, from another patient, L.M., and it too had dislodged from the aortic valve prosthetic cage and was found at operation in the abdominal aorta. This patient suddenly and unexpectedly collapsed 28 months following aortic valve replacement, and died about one hour later. The severe splitting of the ball allowed it to be dislodged.

closing prosthetic clicks. Since the ball generally migrates to the aortic bifurcation, the arterial pulses in the legs may be expected to be absent. Since aortic ball dislodgement usually causes death within hours, emergency operation is necessary. There is not time for cardiac catheterization or angiocardiography before reoperation. Median sternotomy would appear to be the ideal initial incision, but the abdominal wall should also be prepared for possible extension of the thoracic incision. With initiation of femoral arterial inflow, the ball, lodged at the aortic bifurcation, may be forced to the thoracic aortotomy. If the ball is not returned by the force of the femoral arterial infusion, it may have never ascended the aorta, but may have fallen into the left ventricular cavity. A new ball must be inserted into the aortic cage. The cage itself does not need to be replaced unless a large portion of the prosthetic ring is detached, or unless the prosthesis is improperly situated. Certainly thrombus, if present, should be removed from the prosthetic struts or ring. If the old ball is not returned to the thoracic aortotomy by the force of the femoral arterial bypass pressure, and if it is not present in the left ventricle, exploration of the abdominal aorta is indicated. One of the subjects who underwent aortic valve replacement in this clinic suddenly collapsed 28 months later while attending church. This individual on arrival at another hospital several minutes later was found to have absent femoral pulses, a diagnosis of embolus to the aortic bifurcation was made, and laparotomy was performed. On exploration of the abdominal aorta, the aortic prosthetic ball, which was nearly split in half (Fig 15), was found rather than a clot. Cardiac arrest prevented further operative intervention, but the chances of survival would appear to have been greater had initial thoracotomy been performed and a new ball inserted into the prosthetic cage.

CONCLUSIONS

Prosthetic cardiac valve replacement has brought new life to many patients during this decade. The initial technical problems involved in the insertion have, for the most part, been eliminated, and the immediate operative mortality now is low. What period of survival may be expected for these individuals, however, remains in doubt. Prosthetic thrombosis continues to be a major problem which has been altered little by anticoagulant therapy. Regurgitation around prosthetic valves is becoming less frequent as more experience is being gained in their insertion. Degeneration of the aortic prosthetic ball is becoming a major problem. If the ball swells, its movement becomes limited; if the ball becomes smaller, it may embolize. The use of a metal ball may lessen the problem of ball variance, and the covering of the metallic struts may lessen the tendency for thrombus to develop on them. Infection at the site of the prostheses remains an ever dangerous problem, particularly since a precipitating cause for the infection is often not apparent. The cause of sudden death, usually following aortic valve replacement, continues to be the most frequent mode of exitus, and only occasionally is an anatomic explanation apparent.

Thus, cardiac valve replacement had added a new and temporarily effective therapy for patients with severe valvular cardiac disease. Valve replacement at this time, however, should be reserved for the patient who is severely limited (functional class III or IV) by his valvular disease.

ADDENDUM

Since this manuscript was submitted for publication, autopsies have been performed on four additional patients who died in the late postoperative period following replacement of one or more cardiac valves with Starr-Edwards prostheses. One patient died of a noncardiac complication (barroom brawl), but the other three died of results of degeneration of the aortic prosthetic ball. One died 47 months postoperatively of prosthetic aortic stenosis secondary to severe swelling of the ball which was yellow, grooved, softened, and immobile. The other two patients died of dislodgement of balls from aortic valve cages with migration to the abdominal aorta. Each of these two patients died suddenly and unexpectedly 32 and 36 months, respectively, following aortic valve replacement. The aortic ball in each was fractured, discolored, and grooved.

Thus, we have now studied the hearts of four patients, and the dislodged ball only in another patient, who died of embolization of the prosthetic aortic ball. The length of survival following operation in these five subjects ranged from 28 to 37 months (average = 32 mo). One of these five patients had a peribasilar aorto-left ventricular communication. Trauma to erythrocytes traversing the prosthetic aortic valve was severe in at least three of these subjects since large quantities (3+ and 4+) of stainable iron were present in their kidneys. The kidneys were not available for examination in the other two patients. In three of these five subjects size 8AT prostheses had been utilized, in one size 9A, and in one size 10A. Fracturing with embolization or swelling with impaction of the aortic prosthetic silicone rubber ball may prove to be the major late complication following replacement of the aortic valve with Starr-Edwards prostheses.

REFERENCES

1. Merendino, K. A., Morrow, A. G., Lillehei, C. W. and Muller, W. H., Jr., Editors: *Prosthetic Valves for Cardiac Surgery*. Charles C Thomas, Springfield, Ill., 1961, p. 586.
2. Roberts, W. C. and Morrow, A. G.: Causes of early postoperative death following cardiac valve replacement: Clinico-pathologic correlations in 64 patients studied at necropsy. J. Thorac. Cardiov. Surg., **54**: ——, 1967.
3. Roberts, W. C. and Morrow, A. G.: Mechanisms of acute left atrial thrombosis after mitral valve replacement. Pathologic findings indicating obstruction to left atrial emptying. Amer. J. Cardiol., **18**: 497, 1966.
4. Roberts, W. C., Lambird, P. A., Gott, V. L. and Morrow, A. G.: Fatal aortic regurgitation following replacement of the mitral and aortic valves. A mechanical complication of double valve replacement. J. Thorac Cardiov. Surg., **52**: 189, 1966.
5. Morales, A. R., Fine, G. and Taber, R. E.: Cardiac surgery and myocardial necrosis. Arch. Path., **83**: 71, 1967.
6. Roberts, W. C. and Morrow, A. G.: Late postoperative pathologic findings after cardiac valve replacement. Circulation, **35**(Suppl. 1): 48, 1967.
7. Cohn, L. H., Roberts, W. C., Rockoff, S. D. and Morrow, A. G.: Bacterial endocarditis following aortic valve replacement. Clinical and pathologic correlations. Circulation, **33**: 209, 1966.
8. Roberts, W. C. and Morrow, A. G.: Bacterial endocarditis involving prosthetic mitral valves. Clinical and pathologic observations. Arch. Path., **82**: 164, 1966.
9. Archard, H. O. and Roberts, W. C.: Bacterial endocarditis after dental procedures in patients with aortic valve prostheses. J. Amer. Dent. Ass., **72**: 648, 1966.
10. Roberts, W. C., Berard, C. W. and Braunwald, N. S.: Roentgenogram of the month. Dis. Chest, **51**: 439, 1966.
11. Ablaza, S. G. G., Blanco, G., Maranhao, V. and Goldberg, H.: Fatal extrusion of ball from Starr-Edwards aortic valve prosthesis. J. Thorac Cardiov. Surg., **50**: 401, 1965.
12. Rockoff, S. D., Ross, J., Jr., Oldham, N. H., Jr., Mason, D. T., Morrow, A. G. and Braunwald, E.: Ventriculo-atrial regurgitation following prosthetic replacement of the mitral valve. Angiocardiographic and hemodynamic findings. Amer. J. Cardiol., **17**: 817, 1966.

13. ROBERTS, W. C. AND MORROW, A. G.: Renal hemosiderosis in patients with prosthetic aortic valves. Circulation, **33:** 390, 1966.
14. ROBERTS, W. C.: Renal hemosiderosis (blue kidney) in patients with valvular heart disease. Amer. J. Path., **48:** 409, 1966.
15. TEMPLE, L. J., SERAFIN, R., CALVERT, N. G. AND DRABBLE, J. M.: Principles of fluid mechanics applied to some situations in the human circulation and particularly to the testing of valves in a pulse duplicator. Thorax, **19:** 261, 1964.
16. EDWARDS, J. E. AND BURCHELL, H. B.: Endocardial and intimal lesions (jet impact) as possible sites of origin of murmurs. Circulation, **18:** 946, 1958.
17. STARR, A., PIERIE, W. R., RAIBLE, D. A., EDWARDS, M. L., SIPOSS, G. G. AND HANCOCK, W. D.: Cardiac valve replacement: Experience with the durability of silicone rubber. Circulation, **33**(Suppl.): 115, 1966.
18. HANCOCK, W. D.: Edwards Laboratories, Inc., Santa Ana, California, Personal Communication, May 26, 1967.
19. NEWMAN, M. M. HOFFMAN, M. S. AND GESINK, M. H.: Mechanical failure of Starr-Edwards aortic prosthesis due to ball fracture. J. Thorac. Cardiov. Surg., **53:** 398, 1967.
20. LAFORET, E. G.: Death due to swelling of ball component of aortic ball-valve prosthesis. New Eng. J. Med., **276:** 1025, 1967.
21. KIRCH, E.: Alterations in size and shape of individual regions of heart in valvular disease. Verh. Deutsch. Ges. Inn. Med., Kong., **41:** 324, 1929.
22. FRIEDMAN, W. F., MASON, D. T. AND BRAUNWALD, E.: Arthrogryposis multiplex congenita associated with congenital aortic stenosis. J. Pediat., **67:** 682, 1965.

Secondary Left Ventricular Endocardial Fibroelastosis Following Mitral Valve Replacement

Cause of Cardiac Failure in the Late Postoperative Period

By William C. Roberts, M.D., and Andrew G. Morrow, M.D.

ANALYSES of late death among patients in whom one or more cardiac valves have been replaced with caged-ball prostheses have disclosed that such patients either die suddenly and unexpectedly, usually without previous indication of significant cardiac dysfunction, or that they die after a period of progressively more severe congestive cardiac failure.[1] Sudden death is uncommon after mitral replacement but is the most frequent mode of late death after aortic replacement. Sudden death may be the result of arrhythmia or asystole, dislodgment of the ball from an aortic prosthetic cage, or acute myocardial infarction from any cause. Late death following a period of cardiac failure occurs if the movement of the prosthetic ball is restricted by infected or noninfected thrombus or by swelling of the ball, leading to stenosis of the prosthesis or regurgitation through it. Regurgitation through a peribasilar communication may also lead to cardiac failure and death, as may associated uncorrected valvular or myocardial disease. Another important but hitherto unemphasized cause of heart failure after valve replacement is extensive secondary endocardial fibroelastosis of the left ventricle. A description of this lesion, observed at necropsy in patients who died after cardiac valve replacement, and speculations concerning its pathogenesis and significance constitute the report that follows.

From the Clinic of Surgery, National Heart Institute, National Institutes of Health, Bethesda, Maryland.

Patients Studied

Among the patients who have undergone replacement of one or more cardiac valves with Starr-Edwards prostheses at this Institute between 1961 and 1967, approximately 120 have died. Of the 103 in whom necropsy was performed, 66 died within one month of operation (early death) and 37 at later periods up to 56 months (average 16.6 months) after operation (late death). The ages of the 37 patients who died later ranged from 15 to 69 years (average 44). The cardiac valves which had been excised at the time of operation and the hearts of the 103 necropsied patients were examined.

Results

None of the patients who died within a month of operation had endocardial fibrosis of the left ventricle. Likewise, in the 20 patients who died in the late postoperative period after isolated aortic valve replacement, endocardial fibrosis was observed only in a localized area at the left ventricular apex where the drainage cannula had been inserted at the time of operation and in three patients who had had previous myocardial infarctions. In contrast, larger areas of left ventricular endocardial thickening were observed at necropsy in each of the 16 patients who died in the late postoperative period after mitral valve replacement. The interval between operation and death in these 16 patients ranged from 1.5 to 56 months (average 15.9). Eight of the 16 subjects had isolated mitral replacement, seven had both mitral and aortic valves replaced, and one had mitral

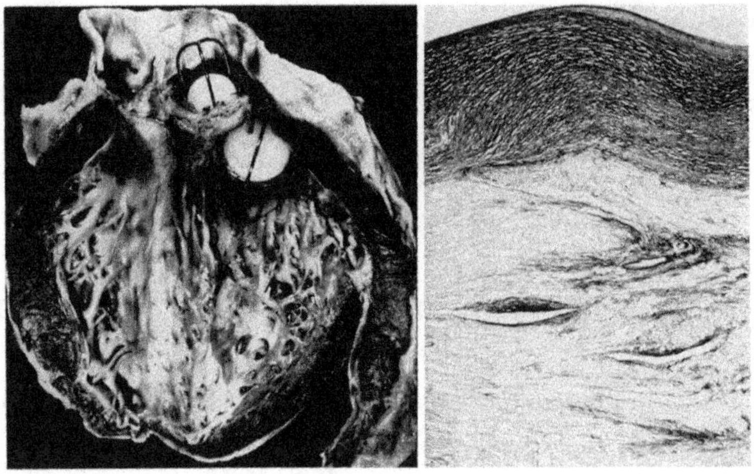

Figure 1

The opened left ventricle (left) and photomicrograph of its thickened endocardium (right) in case 1. The endocardium is diffusely thickened, and the myocardium is free of scars. Right: The thickened endocardium contains numerous elastic fibers, which stain black. Elastic van Gieson stain, ×25.

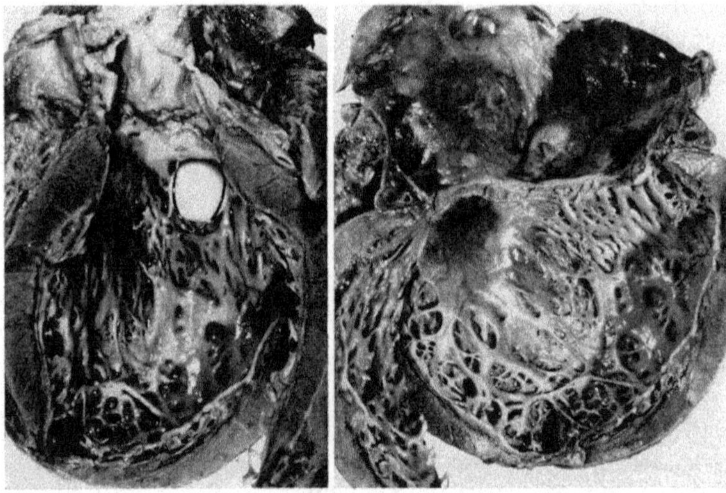

Figure 2

The opened left ventricle in case 2. Left: The ascending aorta, aortic valve "ring," and left ventricle are opened. The aortic valve prosthesis has been removed. Right: The opened left atrium, mitral annulus, and left ventricle are shown. The Starr-Edwards mitral prosthesis has now been removed. The endocardium of both left atrium and left ventricle is greatly thickened. The left ventricular myocardial wall is focally scarred in the immediate subendocardial areas.

and tricuspid prostheses. The stumps of the amputated left ventricular papillary muscles and the left ventricular apex (site of drain insertion at operation) in each of these 16 patients were covered by fibroelastic tissue, but in 13 of them, the fibrous process involved other areas of left ventricular endocardium as well. In one of the 13 subjects, a 14-year-old girl who had had evidence preoperatively of mitral regurgitation since age three, the endocardium of the entire left ventricle was diffusely and uniformly thickened, and it was clear that the fibrous proliferation, which contained numerous elastic fibers, was primary

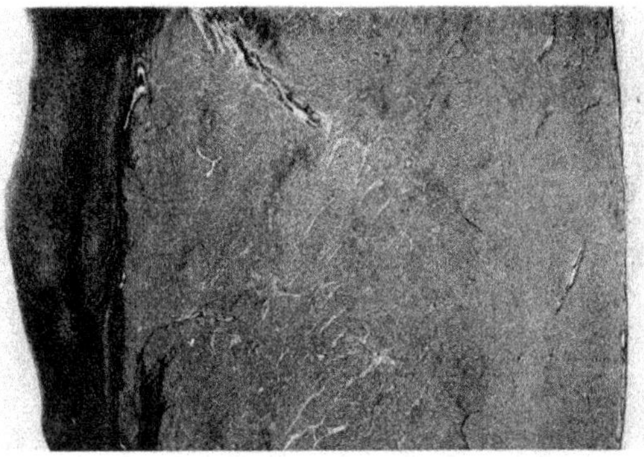

Figure 3

Photomicrograph of a section which includes the entire thickness of the left ventricular wall in case 2. The endocardium is thickened by fibroelastic tissue. The immediate subendocardial myocardium is partially replaced by dense fibrous tissue, but deeper in the myocardium no scars are present. Elastic van Gieson stain, ×9.

congenital endocardial fibroelastosis. Also, she was the only patient in whom the endocardium covering the amputated left ventricular papillary muscles was diffusely thickened. In the other 12 patients, all of whom were adults (average age 47 years; range 29 to 65), extensive though patchy left ventricular endocardial thickening was evident and almost certainly had occurred after operation. The most extensive secondary left ventricular endocardial fibrosis was observed in two patients who had had aortic as well as mitral valve replacement (figs. 1 to 3). In these patients the left ventricular endocardial thickening was believed to have been of functional significance. The clinical and pathological findings in these two patients are described in detail below. Both had severe, intractable cardiac failure several months postoperatively without other anatomical explanations. In the other 11 patients with significant, though less severe, left ventricular endocardial fibrosis (figs. 4 to 7), death was clearly attributable to other causes: mitral regurgitation through a peribasilar communication, infection at the site of the prosthesis, thrombosis of the prosthesis, dislodgment or swelling of the ball in the aortic valve prosthesis, hemorrhage secondary to warfarin-induced hypoprothrombinemia, hepatitis, or an unrelated noncardiac condition.

The endocardium of the left atrium was also extensively thickened in all 16 patients who had had mitral valve replacement. In contrast to the endocardial fibrosis in the left ventricle, which contained numerous elastic fibers, that which occurred in the left atrium was, with rare exceptions, devoid of elastic fibers. The left atrial endocardial thickening also almost certainly appeared postoperatively, probably the result of operative trauma to the wall of this chamber.

Description of Patients

Case 1

J. B., a 56-year-old man, had had rheumatic fever at age six but was asymptomatic until age 43 when he began to experience attacks of vertigo. A year later, signs and symptoms of left-sided congestive cardiac failure were apparent. A mitral commissurotomy was performed when he was 52 years old, but two years later severe cardiac failure recurred. By age 55 (February, 1966) he was in functional class IV (New York Heart Association) and had massive edema, a pulsating liver, and jaundice.

Cardiac catheterization showed a 74-mm Hg peak systolic pressure gradient between the left ventricle (195/15 mm Hg) and radial artery (121/66 mm Hg) and a 10-mm Hg mean diastolic pressure gradient between the left atrium (mean pressure 23; v wave 36 mm Hg) and left ventricle. The cardiac index was 1.7 L/min/m^2 and the A-V O_2 difference 8.2 vol%. The pressure in the pulmonary artery was 74/30 mm Hg, in the right ventricle 74/5 mm Hg, and in the right atrium the mean pressure was 5 mm Hg. Cineangiocardiograms with injections into the

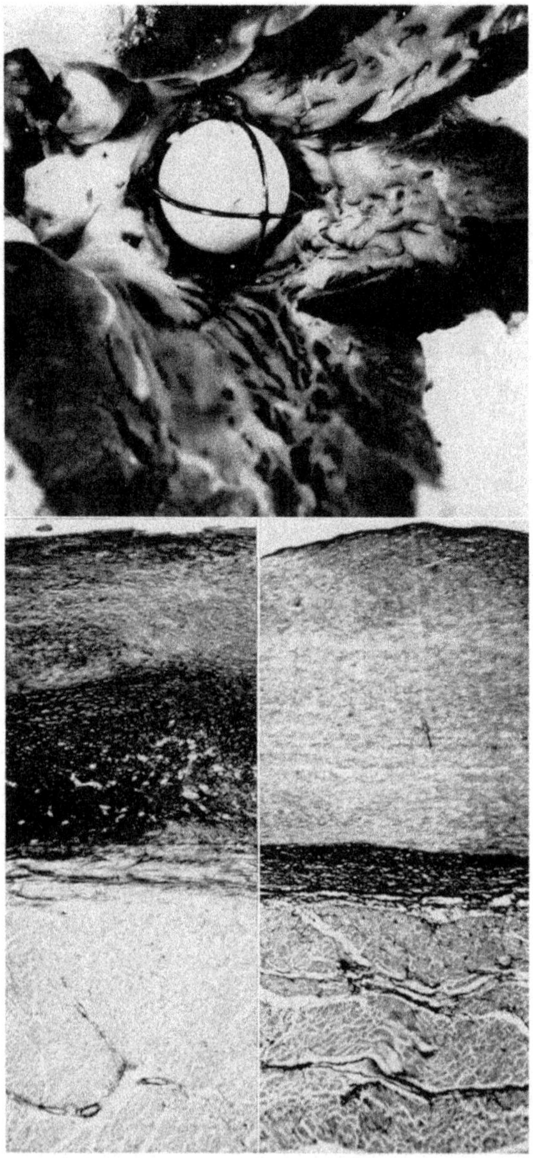

Figure 4

The opened left ventricle (upper) and photomicrographs of sections of left ventricle and left atrium (lower) in a 53-year-old woman who died suddenly and unexpectedly seven months after replacement of the mitral valve. Although the left ventricular endocardium is diffusely thickened, no clinical manifestations resulted. The mitral prosthesis contains thrombus, and its ball seats incompletely. Lower left: Sections of left ventricle showing the severely thickened endocardium. The elastic fibers stain black. Lower right: Section includes the entire thickness of the left atrial wall. The fibrous tissue superimposed on the normal endocardium, which contains elastic fibers (stained black), is devoid of elastic fibers. Elastic van Gieson stains, each ×32.

left ventricular cavity and aortic root disclosed severe mitral and aortic regurgitation. In March, 1966, the mitral valve was replaced with a 2M and the aortic valve with an 8A Starr-Edwards prosthesis. Transient renal failure occurred immediately after operation, but two months postoperatively, the patient's condition was considerably improved. Four months after operation, however, signs of congestive cardiac failure recurred, and six months postoperatively, he was severely symp-

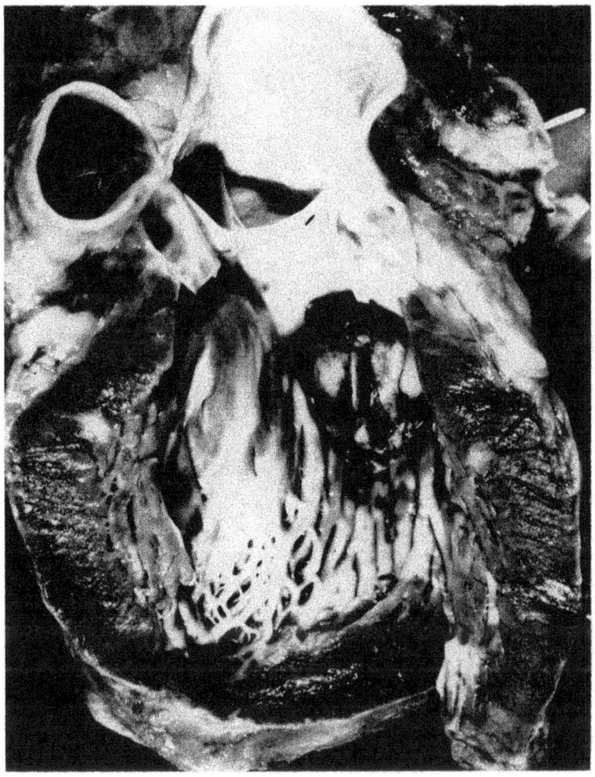

Figure 5

Opened left ventricle, aortic valve, and ascending aorta in a 46-year-old man who died of Staphylococcus albus *infection at the site of the mitral prosthesis 16 months after valve replacement. The endocardium of the left ventricle is extensively thickened. His postoperative course, however, was uneventful until signs of the infective endocarditis appeared 25 days before he died.*

tomatic and again in functional class IV. Repeat catheterization at this time showed the following pressures in mm Hg: pulmonary artery 60/35, right ventricle 60/20, right atrial mean 20, v wave 24, pulmonary arterial wedge mean 20, v wave 29, left ventricle 109/18, and brachial artery 115/70. The cardiac index was 1.8 L/min/m^2. His cardiac failure failed to improve despite extensive therapy, and he died in February, 1967, 11 months after operation.

At necropsy the heart weighed 520 g, the mitral and aortic prostheses were securely fixed, and no peribasilar communications were present. There was a small amount of antemortem thrombus on each prosthesis, but this did not interfere with proper movement and seating of the balls. The most unusual finding was extensive endocardial thickening of the left ventricle (fig. 1). There were virtually no foci of interstitial or replacement fibrosis in the left ventricular myocardium. Except for insignificant narrowing (between 25 and 50%) of the anterior descending branch, the lumens of coronary arteries were widely patent.

Case 2

J. L., a 36-year-old man who had acute rheumatic fever at age nine, was asymptomatic until age 18 when exertional dyspnea appeared. Acute rheumatic fever recurred at age 28, and at age 30 he had signs of an embolus to the left femoral artery. At age 33 an embolus to the aortic bifurcation apparently occurred, and a year later there was transient paralysis of the right hand. By now, dyspnea was so severe that he was unable to work. At age 36 (August, 1966) he was in functional class III, and cardiac catheterization was performed. The left atrial (mean 23, v wave 35) to left ventricular mean diastolic pressure gradient was 18 mm Hg, and the left ventricular (150/8) to brachial arterial (140/60) peak systolic pressure gradient was 10 mm Hg. The pulmonary arterial pressure was 40/22, right ventricle 40/9, and right atrial mean pressure 3 mm Hg. The

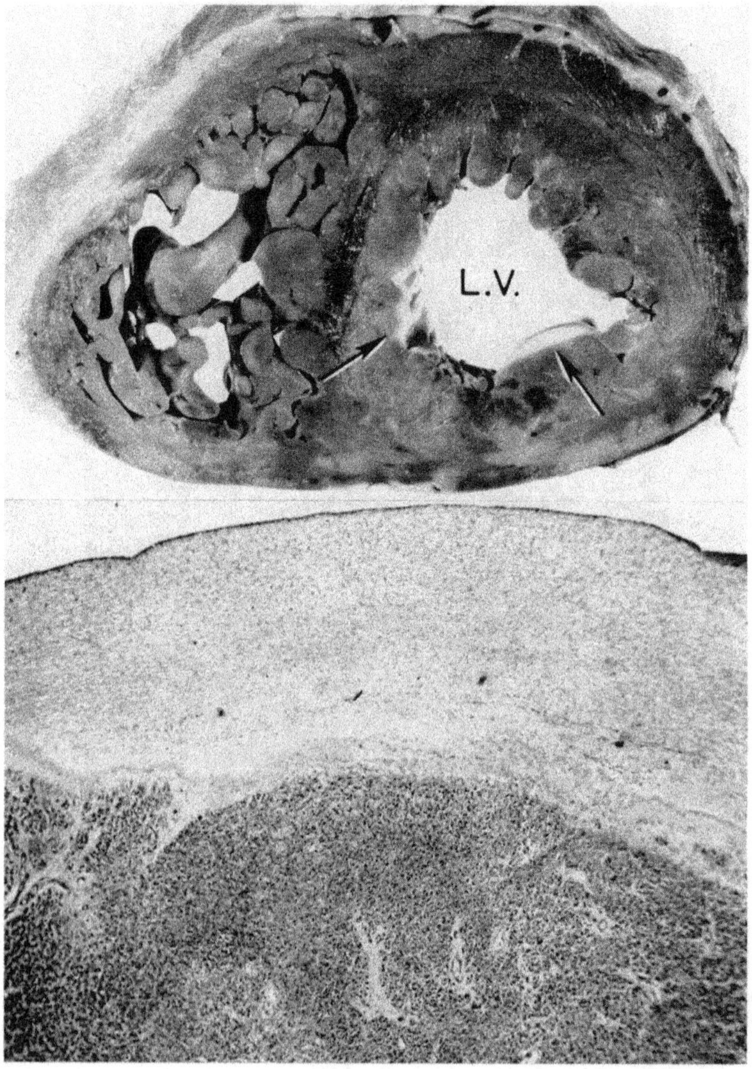

Figure 6

Transverse section of the cardiac ventricles and a photomicrograph of a section of left ventricle in a 47-year-old man who died of Staphylococcus aureus *infection at the site of a mitral prosthesis four months after mitral valve replacement. The endocardium of the left ventricle (L.V.) is focally thickened (arrows). Bottom: Section of thickened left ventricular endocardium. Hematoxylin and eosin stain, ×25. This patient was well postoperatively until one month before death when signs and symptoms of the cardiac infection appeared.*

cardiac index was 1.7 L/min/m^2. Cineangiocardiograms with injections into the left ventricle and aortic root disclosed mild mitral regurgitation and severe aortic regurgitation. In September, 1966 the aortic and mitral valves were replaced with Starr-Edwards prostheses (8A and 2M). During the first postoperative months his condition was greatly improved. Four months after operation, however, signs of congestive cardiac failure were apparent, and by six months postoperatively he was severely edematous, jaundiced from hepatic congestion and hypoxia, and was in functional class IV. Fluoroscopy disclosed that his left ventricle was severely dilated and contracted poorly. He was readmitted at this time, and severe cardiac decompensation persisted despite therapy. He died in March, 1967, seven months after valve replacement, in intractable cardiac failure.

At necropsy the heart weighed 700 g, both prostheses were securely fixed, and there were no peribasilar communications. Although antemor-

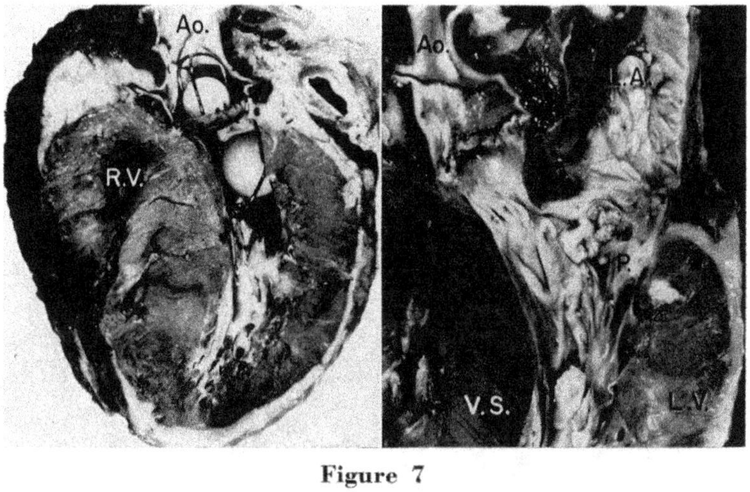

Figure 7

Heart of a 42-year-old man who had his mitral valve replaced with a Starr-Edwards prosthesis at another institution 20 months before death. Before replacement the anterior mitral leaflet was excised, but neither the papillary muscles nor the posterior mitral leaflet was removed. He was greatly improved for five months thereafter, but then signs of cardaic failure recurred. When function was class IV, one month before death, he was admitted to the National Heart Institute for the first time. Studies disclosed that the aortic valve was stenotic and incompetent and that the mitral prosthesis was incompetent. At reoperation a peribasilar mitral leak was found and closed and the aortic valve replaced. He died the next day after excessive bleeding.

At autopsy the endocardium of the left ventricle and left atrium were found to be extensively thickened without underlying myocardial fibrosis. Left: The anterior one-half of the ventricles has been removed, demonstrating the two prostheses and the thickened left ventricular endocardium. R.V. = right ventricle. Right: Closeup of the left ventricle (L.V.), aortic root (Ao.), and mitral annulus after removing the prostheses. The extensive focal thickening of the endocardium is apparent. P. = posterior mitral leaflet, L.A. = left atrium, V.S. = ventricular septum.

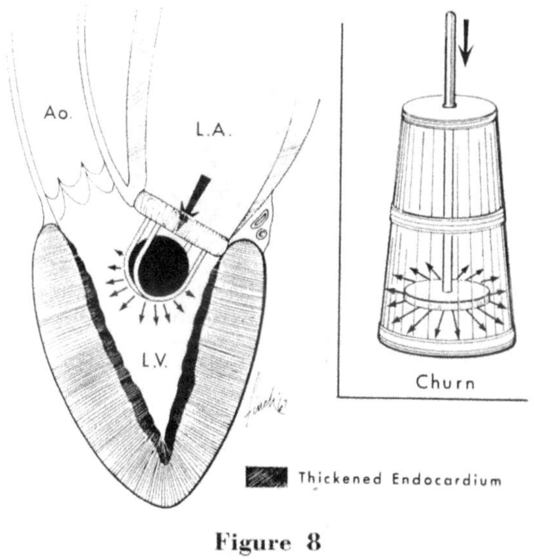

Figure 8

Diagrammatic representation of the possible mechanism of the secondary left ventricular (L.V.) endocardial fibrosis after replacement of the mitral valve with a caged-ball prosthesis. The cage and ball of the mitral prosthesis are located within the left ventricular cavity. Thus, when the ball moves, either descends or ascends, it pushes blood laterally, producing turbulence. This effect may be compared to the turbulence produced by the butter churn. The anatomical indicator of turbulent flow is proliferation of connective tissue on the surface in contact with that flow; in this case, endocardium. Ao. = aorta; L.A. = left atrium.

tem thrombi were present on each prosthesis, the clots were small and did not interfere with proper movement or seating of the balls. The endocardium of the left ventricle was diffusely thickened by fibrous tissue (fig. 2). The coronary arteries were normal, and the left ventricular myocardium, except focally in the immediate subendocardial regions, was virtually free of foci of interstitial and replacement fibrosis.

Comment

The endocardial thickening which occurs over the stumps of the amputated papillary muscles after mitral replacement may be re-

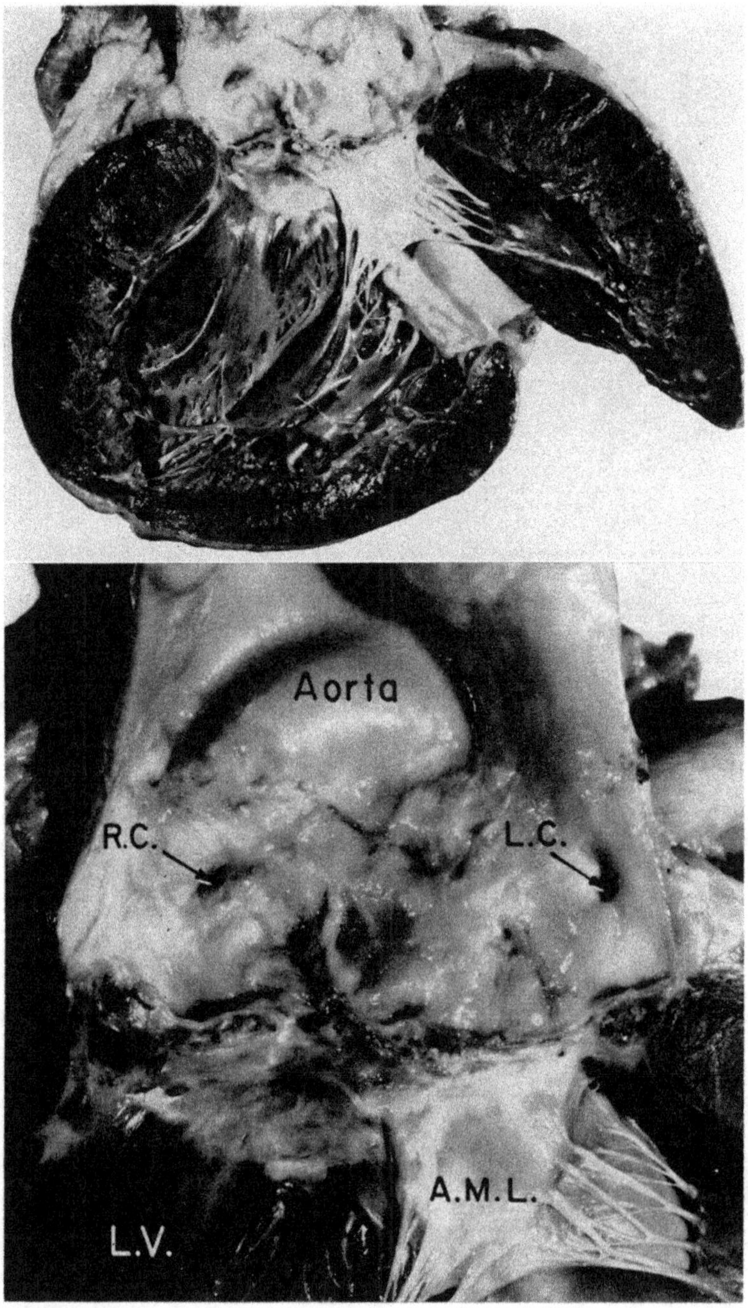

Figure 9

The left ventricle and aortic root in a 50-year-old man who died suddenly and unexpectedly of an acute myocardial infarction 24 months after aortic valve replacement. These photographs are shown for contrast with those of the hearts of patients who died late after mitral valve replacement. There is no endocardial thickening of the left ventricle (upper). In contrast, there is considerable intimal proliferation in the aortic root, and this is attributed to turbulence produced by the aortic valve prosthesis, in a manner similar to endocardial thickening of the left ventricle after mitral valve replacement. R.C. and L.C. = ostia of the right and left coronary arteries, respectively; L.V. = left ventricle; and A.M.L. = anterior mitral leaflet.

garded as simple healing. The cause of the more widespread left ventricular endocardial thickening observed in these patients is uncertain but may be the result of turbulent blood flow in this chamber. The leaflets and chordae tendineae of the natural mitral valve are within the left ventricular cavity, but these structures are thin, readily movable, and the blood flows *centrally* or between the two leaflets. In contrast, after insertion of a caged-ball mitral prosthesis, blood flows *peripherally* or around the caged ball, and the endocardial lining of the left ventricle is not protected from blood flowing across the mitral prosthesis. Also, the ball in the prosthetic mitral valve moves up and down, imparting a churning turbulence to the blood within the left ventricular cavity (fig. 8). The anatomical indicator of turbulent flow is fibrous proliferation, and in this case its site is the left ventricular endocardium. Similar fibrous proliferation occurs in the aortic root after replacement of the aortic valve with a caged-ball prosthesis (fig. 9).

Left ventricular endocardial thickening may also result from degeneration of the underlying myocardium. In an occasional patient with primary myocardial disease or long-standing active rheumatic carditis, the endocardium of the left ventricle is found at necropsy to be mildly opacified. The actual endocardial thickening in these conditions, although it may be extensive, is much less than that observed in the hearts studied after mitral valve replacement. The endocardium is constantly bathed with chamber blood, but apparently it is one of the last sites to be perfused by coronary arterial blood. Thus, diminished coronary flow from any cause could possibly cause endocardial thickening. The lesion is unusual in patients with coronary arterial disease, however, except over sites of actual, healed myocardial infarcts. In the present patients no correlation existed between the degree of coronary arterial narrowing and the presence or severity of left ventricular endocardial fibroelastosis, and neither of the two patients with the most severe endocardial thickening had significantly narrowed coronary arteries.

The rate at which endocardial thickening develops after mitral valve replacement would seem to be variable, but at least several weeks and probably several months are necessary for the changes to occur. Significant thickening was observed four months after mitral replacement in one patient, and one of the two patients in whom this lesion was most severe died of cardiac failure only six months after double valve replacement.

Summary

Secondary endocardial fibrosis of variable severity was observed in the left ventricle in 13 of 16 patients after mitral valve replacement. Similar lesions were not observed in any of 20 patients who died in the late postoperative period after isolated aortic valve replacement. The left ventricular endocardial thickening is believed to be the result of turbulent flow, produced in the left ventricle by the caged ball within it. Severe impairment of cardiac function appeared to result from the process in two of the 13 patients: each developed intractable and ultimately fatal cardiac failure several months after double valve replacement, and the extensive endocardial thickening was the only anatomical cause for failure in both patients. Thus, secondary left ventricular endocardial fibrosis appears to be another, although uncommon, cause of cardiac failure in the late postoperative period after replacement of the mitral valve with a caged-ball prosthesis.

Reference

1. Roberts, W. C., and Morrow, A. G.: Anatomic studies of hearts containing caged-ball prosthetic valves. Johns Hopkins Med J **121**: 271, 1967.

Fatal Degeneration of the Silicone Rubber Ball of the Starr-Edwards Prosthetic Aortic Valve*

William C. Roberts, M.D., F.A.C.C. *and* Andrew G. Morrow, M.D., F.A.C.C.

Bethesda, Maryland

Late complications following replacement of one or more cardiac valves with caged ball prostheses have been described by workers from this clinic and others.[1–3] Among these are: thrombosis of the prosthesis; fistulas around the base of the prosthesis; diffuse secondary left ventricular endocardial fibroelastosis after mitral valve replacement; aortic intimal proliferation with narrowing of the ostia of the coronary arteries after aortic valve replacement; bleeding secondary to warfarin-induced hypoprothrombinemia; aneurysm formation at the site of excision of left ventricular papillary muscles; and degeneration of the silicone rubber aortic ball (ball variance).[4] Since the latter complication may prove a frequent and at times fatal consequence of replacement of the aortic valve with a silicone rubber ball in a metal cage, a review of this complication appeared warranted. We therefore studied 36 necropsy subjects who died late after aortic valve replacement.

Patients Studied

From December 1961 to January 31, 1968, at the National Heart Institute, 462 patients underwent replacement of one or more cardiac valves with Starr-Edwards prostheses. Aortic valve replacement was carried out in 271 patients (52 of whom also had mitral and 2 tricuspid valve replacement). Mitral valve replacement was performed in an additional 191 patients (13 of whom also had tricuspid valve replacement). Approximately 150 of the 462 patients subsequently died. Autopsies were performed in 122 of these patients, of whom 75 died within one month of operation and 47 at later periods. Thirty-five of the 47 patients who died late had had aortic valve replacement (9 also a mitral valve replacement), and 12 patients had had isolated mitral valve replacement. The interval from operation to death in the 35 patients who died late after aortic valve replacement, with or without mitral valve replacement, ranged from 1.3 to 46 months (average 18); in the 12 patients who died late after mitral valve replacement it ranged from 3 to 56 months (average 15).

Results

Evidence of ball degeneration or variation was defined as gross alteration in ball color, shape and consistency, or the presence of surface damage (abrasion or fracture). None of the patients who died in the early postoperative period and none of the 12 patients who died late after isolated mitral valve replacement had evidence of degeneration of the silicone rubber ball. Likewise, none of the 23 autopsy subjects who died less than 24 months after aortic valve replacement had evidence of ball variation. In contrast, all of the 12 remaining patients, who died 24 months or longer after aortic valve replacement, had evidence of ball degeneration.

In 11 of the 12 patients the degree of ball variation was severe; in 6 the ball had atrophied, fractured, and become dislodged from the cage; in 5 it had swollen and become impacted within the cage (Table I; Fig. 1 to 6). In the twelfth patient, who died 28 months after aortic valve replacement, the ball was slightly discolored, but its surface was smooth and it moved

* From the Section of Pathology and the Clinic of Surgery, National Heart Institute, National Institutes of Health, Bethesda, Md. 20014.

Address for reprints: William C. Roberts, M.D., Section of Pathology, National Heart Institute, Bethesda, Md. 20014.

TABLE I
Degeneration of the Prosthetic Aortic Valve Ball

Case No.	Age & Sex	Interval from Op. to Death (mo.)	Mode of Death	Size of Aortic Prosthesis	Peribasilar Leak	Prosthetic Thrombus	State of Prosthetic Ball	Impaction of Ball in Cage	Dislodgment of Ball from Cage	Ball Migration Site
1	50M	24	Sudden	9A	Yes	++	Swollen	Yes	No	
2	50M	30	CHF	10A	No	++	Swollen	Yes	No	
3	52M	46	CHF	8A	No	+	Swollen	Yes	No	
4	37M	35	CHF	10A	No	+	Swollen	Yes	No	
5	59M	36	Sudden	10A	No	++	Swollen	Yes	No	
6	56M	37	Sudden	10A	No	0	Fractured	No	Yes	?Abd. Aorta
7	52F	29	Sudden	8AT	No	0	Fractured	No	Yes	Abd. Aorta
8	51M	37	Sudden	9A	Yes	+	Fractured	No	Yes	Abd. Aorta
9	32M	37	Sudden	8AT	No	++	Fractured	No	Yes	Abd. Aorta
10	26M	28	Sudden	8A	...	...	Fractured	No	Yes	Abd. Aorta
11	61F	32 (Av. 33.7)	Sudden	8AT	No	++	Atrophied	No	Yes	LV

+ = thrombus did not interfere with proper functioning of the prosthesis.
++ = thrombus caused prosthesis to function improperly.
Abd. = abdominal; CHF = congestive heart failure; LV = left ventricle; Op. = operation.

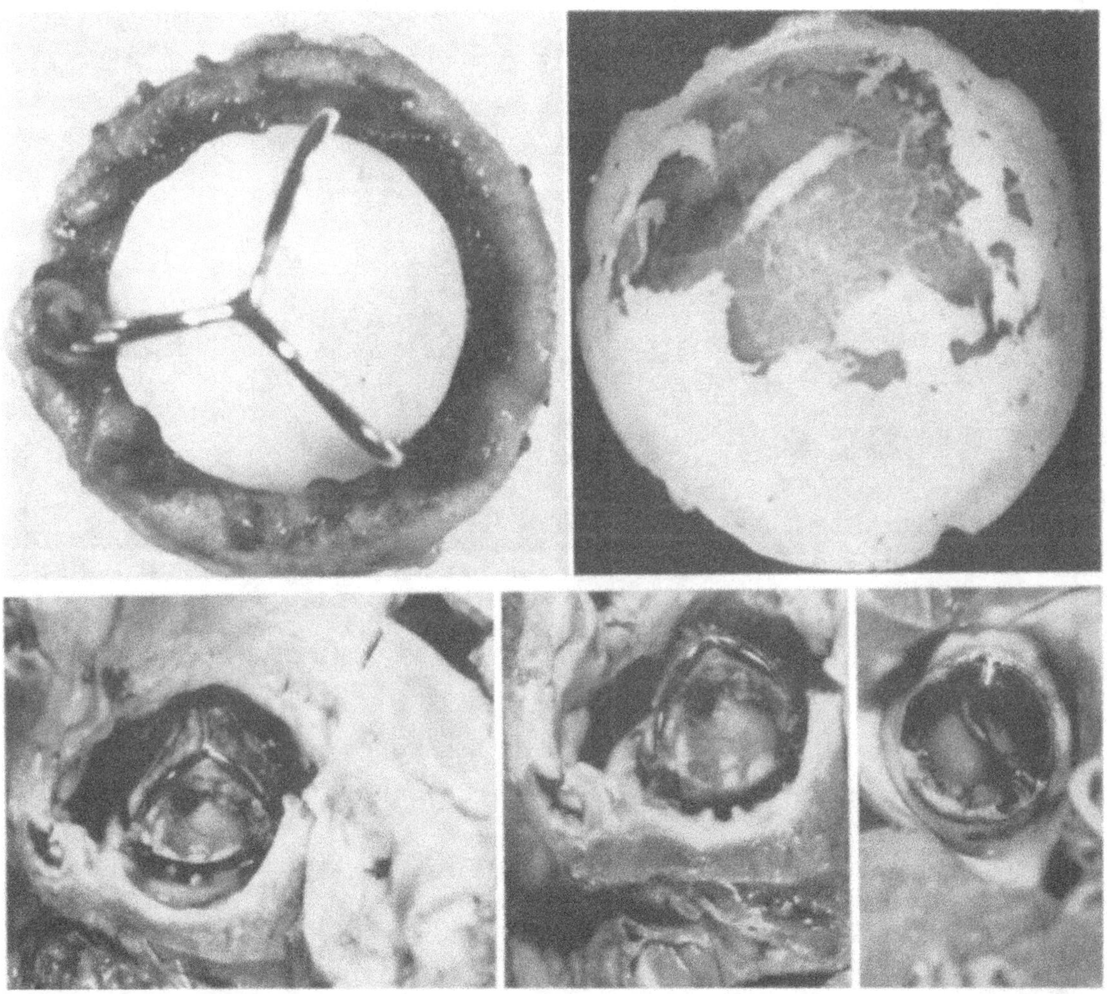

Figure 1. *Swollen, impacted silicone rubber aortic balls in 3 patients.* **Upper left,** Case 1. The valve had been implanted 24 months earlier. The ball is swollen (7 per cent increase in volume compared to its original size) and grooved and moves with difficulty in the cage. **Lower panel,** Case 2. The aortic ball is swollen, yellow, grooved and immobile. Thrombus is present between the ball and struts (**lower left** and **lower middle**) and on the metallic ring (**lower right**). **Upper right,** Case 3. The aortic ball, swollen, grooved and discolored, was impacted in the cage.

freely within the cage. Two subjects (Cases 8 and 9) with totally dislodged aortic balls almost certainly had had embolization of fragments of silicone rubber earlier, as indicated by the presence of particles of refractile material in and about large foreign body giant cells in the liver, spleen and lymph nodes (Fig. 4). They were the only patients in the group of 12 with aortic ball deterioration in whom these organs were available for examination. Of the 11 patients with either ball impaction or dislodgment, 2 had fistulas between the prosthetic ring and the natural valve annulus and 9 had antemortem thrombi on the prostheses (Fig. 2). In 4 of the 9 patients the thrombi appeared to have interfered with proper functioning of the prosthesis.

Evidence of intravascular hemolysis, as indicated by renal hemosiderosis,[5] was present in 5 of the 6 subjects with deteriorated aortic balls whose kidneys were available for examination. Deposition of iron in the cytoplasm of the proximal convoluted tubules is the anatomic indicator of intravascular hemolysis, and the amounts present were large in all 5 subjects.

Comments

Ball deterioration may prove to be a common if not invariable late consequence of replacement of the aortic valve with a silicone rubber ball in a metal cage. In each of the 12 necropsy subjects (Table I) who died 24 months or later after aortic valve replacement with a Starr-Edwards pros-

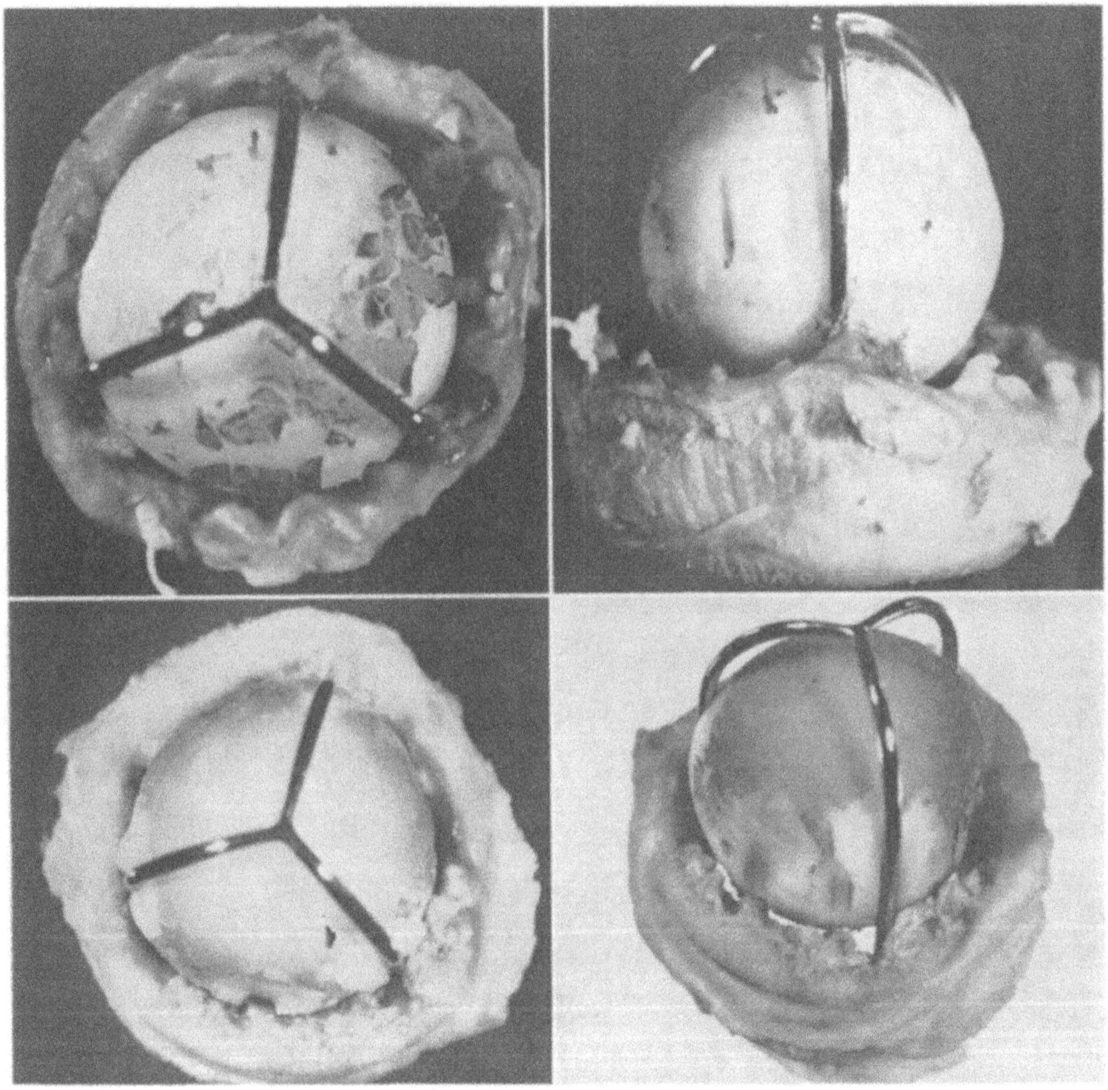

Figure 2. *Swollen, impacted and discolored aortic silicone rubber balls in 2 additional patients.* **Upper,** Case 4. The aortic ball is impacted, grooved and distorted. **Lower,** Case 5. This swollen, grooved, yellow ball was immobile.

thesis, the silicone rubber ball was degenerated, and in 11 of the 12 the deformed ball was the cause of death. Eight of the 11 died suddenly and unexpectedly without previous symptoms of cardiac dysfunction. The remaining 3 died after periods of congestive cardiac failure. The shortest interval between operation and death in the 11 patients was 24 months, and in this patient (Case 1, Table I) the aortic ball was swollen, grooved and impacted in the cage (Fig. 1). A large peribasilar communication and considerable antemortem prosthetic thrombus in this patient appear to have accelerated ball deterioration. The next earliest death (Case 10) occurred 28 months after valve replacement, and no peribasilar communication or significant thrombus was present on the prosthesis (Fig. 5). In another patient who died 28 months after valve replacement, the aortic ball showed only mild evidence of degeneration, which was not a factor in his sudden unexplained death. All 9 necropsy subjects who died later than 28 months after aortic valve replacement had severe evidence of ball degeneration, with either impaction of the ball in the cage or dislodgment from it.

Previous Reported Experience: There have been other reports of ball degeneration after replacement of the aortic valve with a Starr-Edwards (S-E) or Magovern prosthesis (silicone rubber ball). Ablaza and associates[6] described a pa-

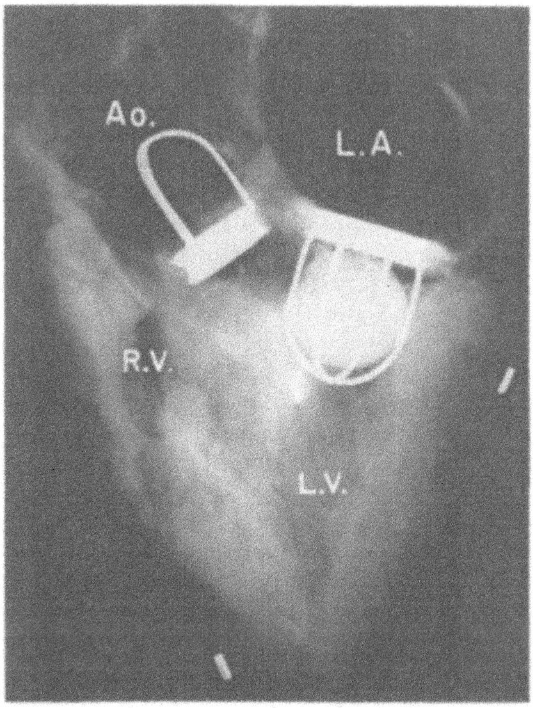

Figure 3. Case 7. *Radiograph of heart specimen revealing an absent aortic ball.* Both mitral and aortic valves had been replaced 29 months earlier. The patient died suddenly and unexpectedly, and at necropsy the aortic ball was found in the abdominal aorta. The mitral ball was normal. Ao. = aorta; L.A. = left atrium; L.V. = left ventricle; and R.V. = right ventricle.

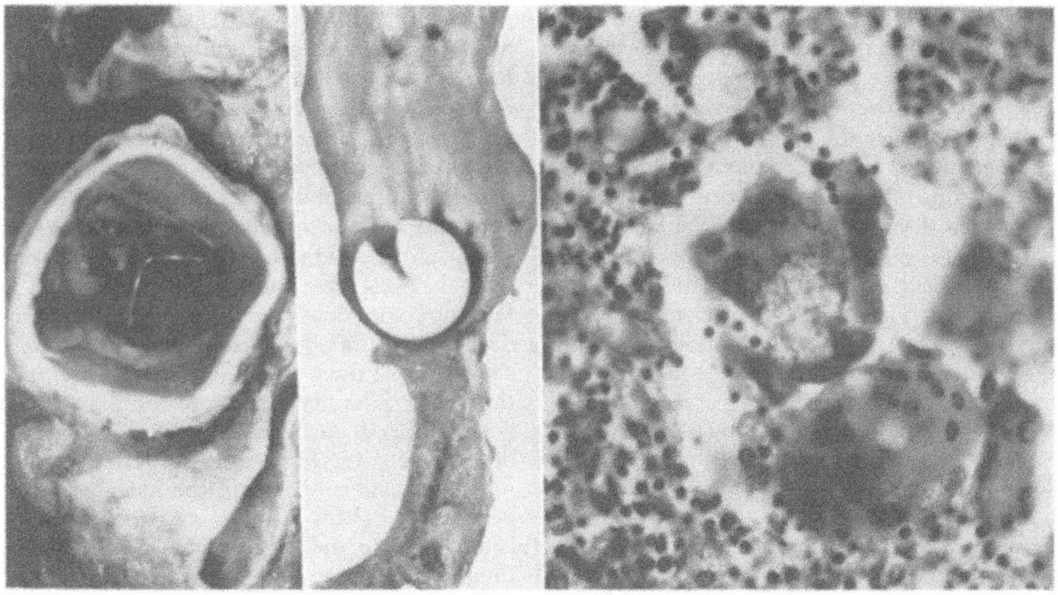

Figure 4. Case 9. *Dislodged aortic ball.* The aortic cage at autopsy was empty (**left**), and the ball was found in the abdominal aorta (**center**). The ball was white and fractured and weighed 1.809 gm. compared to 2.121 gm. at the time of insertion. **Right,** *photomicrograph of refractile material in and about giant cells.* This refractile material almost certainly represents particles of silcone rubber which had embolized earlier to the liver, spleen and lymph nodes. (Hematoxylin and eosin × 400.)

tient who died suddenly only 11 months after replacement of the aortic valve with a 9A S-E prosthesis. Starr et al.,[4] however, raised the possibility that an 8A ball had inadvertently been inserted into a 9A S-E cage in this patient. Newman and associates[7] described embolization of the silicone rubber ball 34 months after replacement of the aortic valve with an 11A S-E prosthesis. The ball was fractured and opaque. Hairston and associates[8] also described a patient in whom the aortic ball dislodged from the cage producing sudden death 34 months after valve replacement with a 9A S-E prosthesis. Magovern,[9] Logan,[10] and Laforet[11] have each reported a patient in whom the silicone rubber ball of a Magovern aortic prosthesis swelled and impacted in the cage. Logan's patient died "approximately 2½ years" and Laforet's patient 20 months after valve implantation. In April 1966 Starr summarized the findings in 17 cases of previously implanted aortic balls returned to the Edwards Laboratories from 14 institutions. These balls had functioned in patients for periods ranging from 3½ to 24 months. The patient who survived 24 months is the patient of our Case 1 (Table I). Only 4 of the 17 patients whose courses were summarized by Starr died because of ball degeneration: 3 from ball dislodgment and 1 (our Case 1) from ball impaction. In the 3 patients who died from ball expulsion the intervals between operation and death were 3½, 11 and 11 months, respectively. One of the latter patients had been reported on earlier by Ablaza et al.[6] Starr also raised the possibility that a size 8A ball had been inserted into a size 9A cage in the patient who died of ball expulsion only 3½ months after valve replacement, and this may also have occurred in both patients who died 11 months after replacement. By July 1967, 93 degenerated aortic silicone rubber balls had been returned to the Edwards Laboratories. The average period of implantation was 25 months in these subjects. The number in whom ball variance caused death by either dislodgment or impaction was not stated.

More recently Herr and associates[12] described variance of the silicone rubber ball of the Starr-Edwards prosthesis in 26 patients. In 13 ball degeneration was found at autopsy, and the interval from aortic valve replacement to death ranged from 15 to 42 months (average 28). Death in 8 patients was not related to deterioration of the poppet, but in each of the 5 remaining subjects death was sudden and due to swelling of the ball with impaction in the cage. In the other 13 patients evidence of variance of the aortic ball was discovered at reoperation. The interval between valve implantation and reoperation ranged from 18 to 49 months (average 37). Preoperatively, the diagnosis of ball variance in these 13 patients was based on change in the aortic opening sound, which instead of having a sharp clicking quality, was soft or muffled or had disappeared. Phonocardiography confirmed these auscultatory observations. Interestingly, 6 of the 13 patients reoperated upon were asymptomatic. In none of the 26 patients with aortic ball variance described by Herr et al. had the ball become dislodged from the cage.

Mitral Ball Variance: Degeneration of the silicone rubber ball of the Starr-Edwards *mitral* prosthesis has been described to our knowledge in only 1 patient.[13] This patient, who had both mitral and aortic valves replaced with Starr-Edwards prostheses 47 months earlier, was reoperated upon because of clinical evidence of aortic ball variance. At operation not only did the aortic ball show evidence of degeneration, but the mitral ball was yellow in color. Therefore, the mitral ball was also removed and on analysis at the Edwards Laboratories was found to have increased in weight by 4 per cent and in dimension by 2 to 3.4 per cent. There was no evidence, however, that the degenerated mitral ball was functioning improperly. Cooley and associates[14] mentioned swelling and sticking of the silicone rubber ball in 1 patient who had an SCDK-Cutter mitral prosthesis inserted several months earlier. In this type of prosthesis the ball contacts the struts, not a metal ring, under high pressure and velocity. In addition we have observed severe degeneration of the silicone rubber in a Hufnagel discoid mitral as well as Hufnagel discoid aortic valve in a submitted heart from a 23 year old man. The mitral and aortic discoid prostheses had been implanted 33 months before death. In contrast to the severe degeneration of the silicone rubber portion of each of these discs the polypropylene portion of the discs was intact. Thus, it appears that silicone rubber in a mitral ball or disc may also degenerate. However, at least in the case of the mitral silicone rubber ball, the incidence of degeneration at this point is extremely small in comparison to the high incidence of degeneration of the silicone rubber prosthetic aortic ball. This difference is further emphasized by the fact that the number of Starr-Edwards mitral prostheses and aortic prostheses supplied to surgeons is approximately equal.[15] Differences

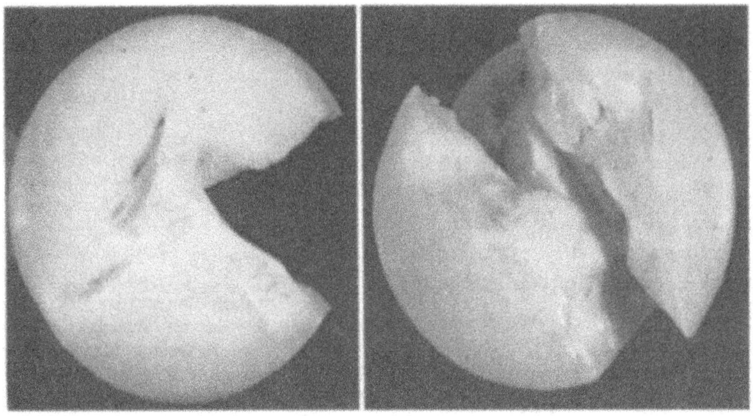

Figure 5. Case 10. *Fractured, disolodged aortic ball.* The ball was found in the abdominal aorta.

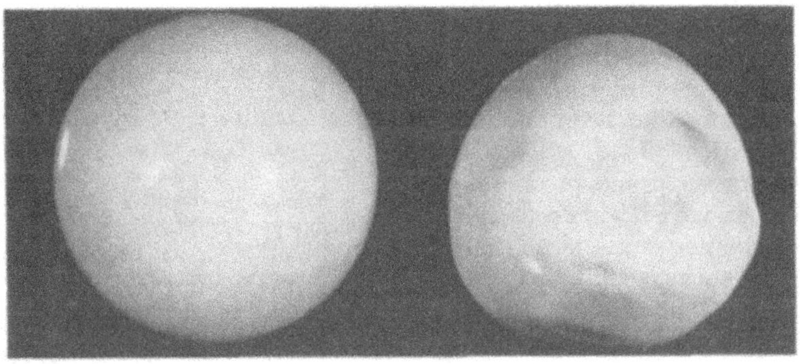

Figure 6. Case 11. *Dislodged aortic ball* (**right**). The ball, found in the left ventricle, was severely atrophied. At **left** a normal-sized ball is shown for comparison.

in aortic and mitral valvular blood velocities are probably the explanation. Typically, the orifice diameters of aortic prostheses are smaller than those of mitral prostheses, and the time of ventricular systole is approximately half that of ventricular diastole for a patient at rest. The velocity of flow through the orifice of the average aortic prosthesis is at least three times greater than the velocity through the orifice of the average mitral prosthesis. Also, the aortic ball contacts both the valve ring and the apex of the cage under high pressure, whereas the mitral ball contacts only the ring under high pressure, since the ball passes to the apex of the cage during ventricular diastole. The cause of the degeneration of the silicone rubber aortic ball is uncertain. All variant balls examined by the Edwards Laboratories have contained lipids, which apparently make the silicone rubber susceptible to wear. These lipids are extractable, and the rubber returns to a near normal state afterward.

Clinical Implications: The therapeutic implication of degeneration of the silicone rubber prosthetic ball is obvious. In such case the ball, or the entire valve, needs to be replaced, but the most appropriate time for reoperation is presently uncertain. One of the frightening features of ball degeneration is its clinical silence until sudden catastrophe occurs. Eight of the 11 patients described herein died suddenly and unexpectedly after long periods of being asymptomatic. Herr and associates,[12] as mentioned earlier, have relied on auscultation and phonocardiography as the best clinical indicators of ball degeneration. Thus, even if the patient is asymptomatic and the aortic opening click is absent or muffled, or if the character or intensity of the opening sound is variable from beat to beat, they advocate reoperation with replacement of the ball or the entire prosthesis. In none of the 11 patients described herein were phonocardiograms recorded. However, the phonocardiograms of patients with prosthetic valves are now being assessed at the National Heart Institute by power spectrum analysis, and it is hoped that this method may provide more precise information on the development of ball variance and the need for replacement of the poppet or valve.

The introduction of the hollow metal (stellite 21) ball in a prosthesis with fabric-covered struts and orifice offers hope that ball degeneration will be eliminated. This newer prosthesis, introduced in 1967, has yet to be tested adequately, however, and no conclusions concerning its superiority are justified at this time.

Summary

Fatal degeneration of silicone rubber balls of Starr-Edwards prosthetic aortic valves is described in 11 of 271 patients who underwent aortic valve replacement. Among 35 autopsy subjects, none of the 23 who died less than 24 months after operation had evidence of ball degeneration, whereas severe degeneration was present in 11 of 12 patients who died more than 24 months after operation. In 6 patients the ball had atrophied, fractured and become dislodged from the cage, and in 5 it had swollen and become impacted within the cage.

Degeneration of the silicone rubber ball may be an inevitable late complication of replacement of the aortic valve with a Starr-Edwards prosthesis. Therefore, reoperation and replacement of these degenerated aortic balls will be necessary in many patients. The ideal time for reoperation, however, is not yet determined. Whether the use of a hollow metal ball will prevent this complication remains to be seen.

Addendum

Since this manuscript was submitted a 41 year old man, who had had his aortic valve replaced with an 11A, model 1000, Starr-Edwards prosthesis 65 months earlier, died after mitral valve replacement. At the second operation the aortic silicone rubber ball was found to be discolored, but its surface was smooth; it did not appear swollen or atrophied, and it moved normally. Thus, despite a 65 month implantation period the aortic silicone rubber ball was only mildly degenerated, and it functioned normally. Nevertheless, it was replaced for precautionary reasons.

References

1. Roberts, W. C. and Morrow, A. G. Late postoperative pathologic findings after cardiac valve replacement. *Circulation*, 35 (Suppl. i): 48, 1967.
2. Roberts, W. C. and Morrow, A. G. Anatomic studies of hearts containing caged-ball prosthetic valves. *Johns Hopkins M. J.*, 121: 271, 1967.
3. Roberts, W. C. and Morrow, A. G. Secondary left ventricular endocardial fibroelastosis following mitral valve replacement: cause of cardiac failure in the late postoperative period. *Circulation*, 35 (Suppl. ii): 101, 1968.
4. Starr, A., Pierie, W. R., Raible, D. A., Edwards, M. L., Siposs, G. G. and Hancock, W. D. Cardiac valve replacement: Experience with the durability of silicone rubber. *Circulation*, 33 (Suppl i): 115, 1966.
5. Roberts, W. C. and Morrow, A. G. Renal hemosiderosis in patients with prosthetic aortic valves. *Circulation*, 33: 390, 1966.
6. Ablaza, S. G. G., Blanco, G., Maranhao, V. and Goldberg, H. Fatal extrusion of the ball from a Starr-Edwards aortic valve prosthesis: Report of a case. *J. Thoracic & Cardiovas. Surg.*, 50: 401, 1967.
7. Newman, M. M., Hoffman, M. S. and Gesink, M. H. Mechanical failure of Starr-Edwards aortic prosthesis due to ball fracture. *J. Thoracic & Cardiovas. Surg.*, 53: 398, 1967.
8. Hairston, P., Summerall, C. P. and Muller, W. H. Jr. Embolization of silastic ball from Starr-Edwards prosthesis: Case report and comments. *Ann. Surg.*, 166: 817 1967.
9. Magovern, G. J. Discussion of Magovern, G. J., Kent, E. M. and Cushing, W. B. Sutureless mitral valve replacement. *Ann. Thoracic Surg.*, 2: 474, 1966.
10. Logan, W. D., Jr. In Ref. 9, p. 474.
11. Laforet, E. G. Death due to swelling of ball component of aortic ball-valve prosthesis. *New England J. Med.*, 276: 1025, 1967.
12. Herr, R. H., Kloster, F. E., Yukiyasu, S. and Starr, A. Diagnosis and management of "ball variance" following aortic valve replacement. *Circulation*, 35 (Suppl. ii): 141, 1968.
13. Chappel, P. E., Edwards Laboratories, Inc. Personal communication, May 1, 1968.
14. Cooley, D. A., Bloodwell, R. D., Beall, A. C., Jr., Gill, S. E. and Hallman, G. L. Total cardiac valve replacement using SCDK-Cutter prosthesis: Experience with 250 consecutive patients. *Ann. Surg.*, 164: 428, 1966.
15. Robinson, D. K., Edwards Laboratories, Inc. Personal communication, October 2, 1967.

Compression of anomalous left circumflex coronary arteries by prosthetic valve fixation rings

William C. Roberts, M.D., and Andrew G. Morrow, M.D., Bethesda, Md.

Damage to a coronary artery is a rare but recognized complication of cardiac valve replacement. Thus, the ostium of a coronary artery may be occluded by the fixation ring of an aortic valve prosthesis, or the proximal portion of the artery may be lacerated or dissected during cannulation.[1,2] The left circumflex coronary artery, located in the atrioventricular sulcus in close proximity to the mitral annulus, may be damaged during mitral valve replacement.[3] A more unusual complication of valve replacement has recently been observed in 2 patients with severe valvular heart disease in whom the left circumflex coronary artery arose from the right coronary artery. In each patient the anomalous coronary artery was compressed by the fixation rings of mitral and/or aortic valvular prostheses; in 1 patient, obstruction of the vessel led to fatal myocardial infarction. A brief description of the clinical and necropsy findings in these 2 patients is the subject of this report.

Descriptions of patients

CASE 1. W. R. (06-83-61), a 45-year-old man, was severely incapacitated, and severe mitral and aortic regurgitation were demonstrated at preoperative hemodynamic and angiographic assessments. At operation, the ascending aorta and aortic "annulus" were both relatively small, and the aortic valve was replaced with a size 8A Starr-Edwards prosthesis. The incompetent mitral valve was replaced with a 3M Starr-Edwards prosthesis. During the entire postoperative period the patient evidenced signs of inadequate cardiac output, and administration of isoproterenol was required to maintain an adequate systemic arterial pressure. Urine output initially was adequate, but oliguria appeared and the blood urea nitrogen rose to 200 mg. per 100 ml. Progressive hypoxia was treated by tracheostomy and assisted resuscitation; circulatory depression persisted and the patient died on the tenth postoperative day.

At autopsy (A68-22), the heart weighed 1,040 grams; the left ventricle and left atrium were greatly dilated. No thrombus was present on either prosthetic valve, but the aortic valve appeared large in proportion to size of the aorta into which it had been inserted. The left circumflex coronary artery arose from the right coronary artery immediately after its origin from the aorta. The left circumflex branch passed behind the aorta in the groove between both prosthetic valve rings (Fig. 1). The rings of the prostheses compressed the anomalous left circumflex branch, probably totally obstructing its lumen. After the left circumflex branch passed behind the aorta and pulmonary trunk it coursed normally in the left atrioventricular sulcus. The lateral wall of the left ventricle was focally hemorrhagic and acutely infarcted (Fig. 1).

CASE 2. M. G. (01-72-82), a 53-year-old woman, developed signs of cardiac dysfunction at the age of 37 years. When she had been studied at the age of 47, the pulmonary arterial pressure was 90/36, right ventricle 90/12, right atrial mean pressure 10 and v wave 13, and left atrial mean pressure 20 and v wave 50 mm. Hg;

From the Section of Pathology and the Clinic of Surgery, National Heart Institute, National Institutes of Health, Bethesda, Md. 20014.

Received for publication Oct. 7, 1968.

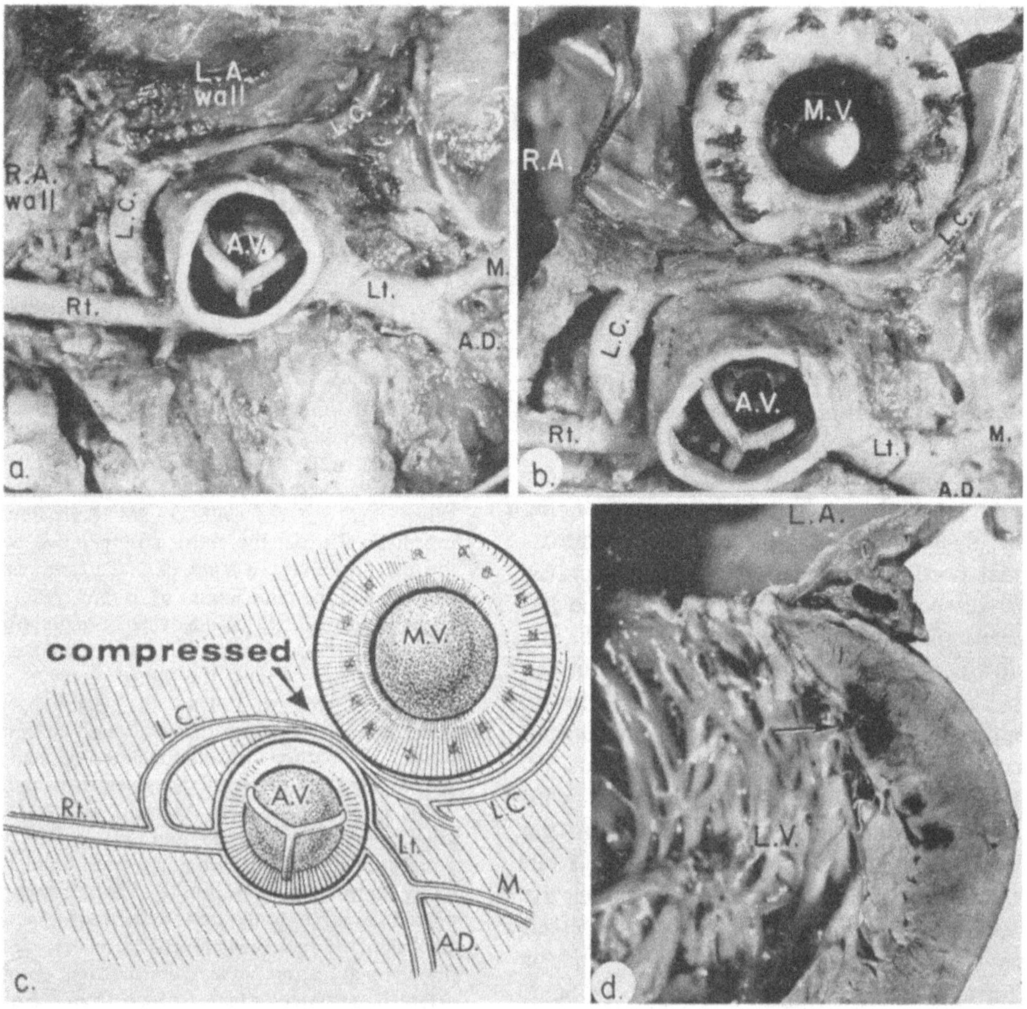

Fig. 1. Patient 1. *a,* Aortic root viewed from above shows the Starr-Edwards aortic valve *(A.V.)* prosthesis and the origins of the coronary arteries. The left circumflex *(L.C.)* arises from the right *(Rt.)* coronary artery immediately after the latter's origin from the aorta. The left circumflex coronary artery passes posteriorly, between the aortic root and base of the left atrium *(L.A.).* Its course thereafter is normal. The origin and distribution of the left *(Lt.)* coronary artery and its branches, anterior descending *(A.D.)* and marginal *(M.),* are normal. *R.A.,* Right atrium. *b,* The wall of the left atrium has now been excised, better demonstrating compression of the left circumflex coronary artery between the fixation rings of the mitral and aortic prostheses, shown diagrammatically in *c. d,* Cut surface of lateral walls of left atrium *(L.A.)* and left ventricle *(L.V.)* demonstrates focal hemorrhagic infarction *(arrow)* of the ventricular wall.

simultaneous left ventricular and brachial arterial pressures were 125/10 and 125/70 mm. Hg, respectively, and the left atrial and left ventricular mean diastolic pressure gradient was 8 mm. Hg. At operation, the mitral valve was replaced with a 4M Starr-Edwards prosthesis. The early course after operation was uneventful, but review of electrocardiograms 3 years postoperatively showed evidence of anterior myocardial infarction in the past and an intraventricular conduction defect, neither of which had been present before operation. At cardiac catheterization, 4½ years after mitral valve replacement, the pulmonary arterial pressure was 44/21 mm. Hg, the pulmonary arterial wedge mean pressure was 17 with v waves 20, and simultaneous left ventricular and brachial arterial pressures were 152/20 and 130/70 mm. Hg, respectively. A sudden cerebrovascular accident occurred 5⅔ years after valve replacement, and she died.

At autopsy (A68-141), the heart weighed 800 grams, and thrombus was present on the prosthetic valve. The left circumflex coronary artery arose from the right coronary artery, and passed behind the aorta in the groove between the prosthetic mitral ring and the base of the aorta (Fig. 2). The lumen of this artery was compressed by the prosthetic valve ring but sections of the vessel showed that it was patent (Fig. 3). The left circumflex coronary artery thereafter coursed normally in the left atrioventricular sulcus. Extensive scarring was present in the lateral wall of the left ventricle and in the free wall beneath the anterolateral papillary muscle (Fig. 3).

Comment

Origin of the left circumflex coronary artery from the right coronary artery is noted in about 0.3 per cent of autopsied subjects.[4] It originates just after the origin of the right coronary artery, and courses posteriorly around and between the root of the aorta and the left atrial wall, nearly at the level of the mitral annulus. Normally, the aortic and mitral annuli are pliable structures, but when either or both valves are replaced with caged-ball prostheses the valve rings become rigid. Consequently, if both mitral and aortic valves are replaced with rigid ring-type prostheses, and if the left circumflex coronary artery arises anomalously, the lumen of this vessel can be compressed between the two prosthetic annuli. In Patient 1, the anomalous left circumflex coronary artery was almost certainly occluded in this manner, as evidenced by the acute infarct of the lateral free wall of the left ventricle, the area normally supplied by the left circumflex coronary artery. In Patient 2, the mitral valve only was replaced, but the anomalous left circumflex coronary was nevertheless caught between the rigid mitral prosthetic annulus and the aortic root, which, of course, was distended by systemic arterial pressure. Although the anomalous coronary artery in this patient was not occluded, its lumen was much smaller than normal and the lateral and anterior walls of the left ventricle were focally scarred.

Antemortem diagnosis of anomalous origin of the left circumflex coronary artery from the right coronary artery was not accomplished in either patient. Even had the anomaly been appreciated at operation, it is unlikely that correction of the anomaly would have been warranted. External compression of the anomalous left circumflex coronary arteries may have been lessened or prevented in each patient, however, by use of smaller-sized mitral prostheses.

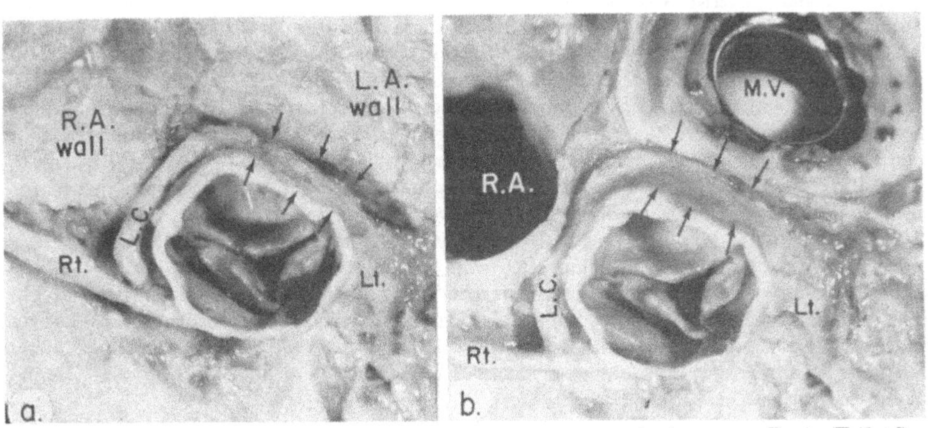

Fig. 2. Aortic root in Patient 2. *a,* The left circumflex *(L.C.)* coronary artery arises anomalously from the right *(Rt.)* coronary artery and is narrowed between the fixation ring of the mitral prosthesis and the base of the aorta. The site of compression of the anomalously arising vessel is shown by the *arrows. b,* The atrial walls have now been excised, demonstrating the mitral valve *(M.V.)* prosthesis. *R.A.,* Right atrium. *Lt.,* Left main coronary artery.

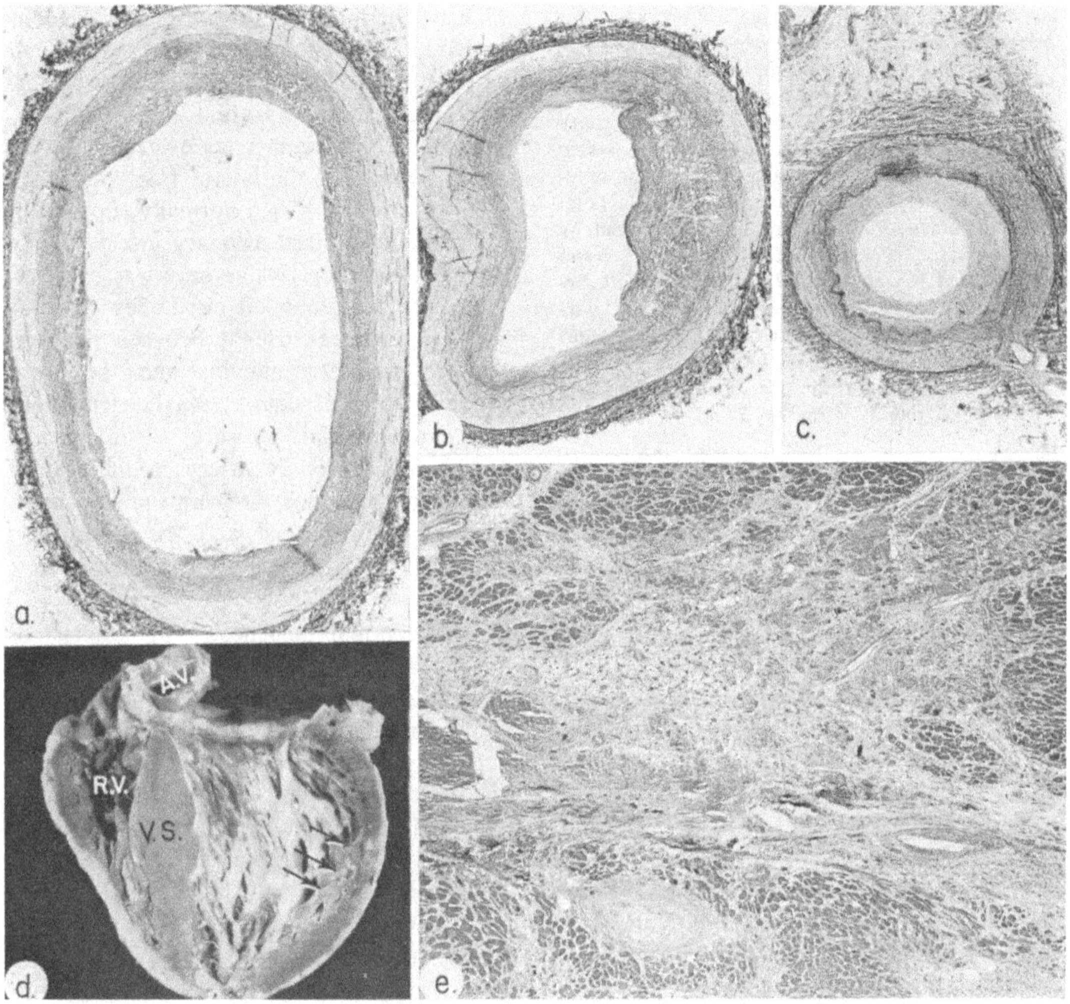

Fig. 3. Coronary arteries and cardiac ventricles in Patient 2. *a,* Cross-section of right main coronary artery 2 cm. from its origin from the aorta is shown for comparison with *b* and *c. b,* Left circumflex coronary artery 1 cm. after its origin from the right coronary artery. *c,* Left circumflex coronary artery more distal to *b* at the site of its being squeezed between the mitral prosthetic ring and the aortic root (see Fig. 2, between the *arrows*). The photomicrographs shown in *a, b,* and *c* were each taken at the same magnification (× 22) and demonstrate the degree of narrowing of the anomalously arising left circumflex coronary artery. The narrowing of this vessel clearly resulted from external compression to it by the fixation ring of the mitral prosthesis. Elastic van Gieson stains were used in the sections in each of the 3 photomicrographs. *d,* Posterior one half of the cardiac ventricles demonstrates thinning and fibrosis *(arrows)* of the left ventricular free wall at a site normally supplied by the left circumflex coronary artery. The left ventricular endocardial thickening is a late anatomic observation after replacement of the mitral valve with a Starr-Edwards prosthesis.[5] *R.V.,* Right ventricle. *V.S.,* Ventricular septum. *A.V.,* Aortic valve cusp. *e,* Section of portion of lateral wall of left ventricle shows extensive myocardial replacement and interstitial fibrosis. (Hematoxylin and eosin stain; × 16.)

REFERENCES

1 Roberts, W. C., and Morrow, A. G.: Causes of Early Postoperative Death Following Cardiac Valve Replacement. Clinico-pathologic Correlations in 64 Patients Studied at Necropsy, J. THORACIC & CARDIOVAS. SURG. **54:** 422, 1967.

2 Roberts, W. C., and Morrow, A. G.: Anatomic Studies of Hearts Containing Caged-Ball Prosthetic Valves, Johns Hopkins M. J. **121:** 271, 1967.

3 Danielson, G. K., Cooper, E., and Tweeddale, D. N.: Circumflex Coronary Artery Injury During Mitral Valve Replacement, Ann. Thoracic Surg. **4:** *53, 1967.*

4 White, N. K., and Edwards, J. E.: Anomalies of the Coronary Arteries; Report of Four Cases, Arch. Path. **45:** 766, 1948.

5 Roberts, W. C., and Morrow, A. G.: Secondary Left Ventricular Endocardial Fibroelastosis Following Mitral Valve Replacement. Cause of Cardiac Failure in the Late Postoperative Period, Suppl. to Circulation *37* and *38:* II-101, 1968.

Chronic Intravascular Hemolysis (Renal Hemosiderosis) after Incomplete Prosthetic Closure of a Ventricular Septal Defect and Noncalcific Aortic Regurgitation

THOMAS J. LIDDY, M.D., AND WILLIAM C. ROBERTS, M.D.

Pathologic Anatomy Branch, National Cancer Institute and Section of Pathology, National Heart and Lung Institute, National Institutes of Health, Bethesda, Maryland 20014

ABSTRACT

Liddy, Thomas J., and Roberts, William C.: Chronic intravascular hemolysis (renal hemosiderosis) after incomplete prosthetic closure of a ventricular septal defect and noncalcific aortic regurgitation. Amer. J. Clin. Path. 53: 839–842, 1970. Clinical and pathologic features of the case of an 11-year-old boy who underwent operative repair of tetralogy of Fallot nine months before death are described. Aortic regurgitation was produced inadvertently at operation during an unsuccessful patch closure of the ventricular septal defect. Postoperatively, the child developed severe cardiac failure and mild anemia. During a second operation seven days before death, aortic blood, which regurgitated through the aortic valve, was observed to contact the nonendothelialized ventricular septal patch, which only partially closed the septal defect. Erythrocytes were traumatized by the jet of blood contacting the nonendothelialized patch, liberating free hemoglobin, which was filtered by glomeruli and reabsorbed by renal tubules (renal hemosiderosis). Intravascular hemolysis after patch closure of ventricular septal defect has not been described previously.

CHRONIC INTRAVASCULAR HEMOLYSIS occurs occasionally in patients with severe calcific aortic valvular stenosis and regurgitation.[4] After replacement of aortic valves with a caged-ball or Teflon-leaflet prosthesis, however, intravascular hemolysis invariably occurs,[3, 5, 7] but it usually is not clinically significant. Chronic intravascular hemolysis also occurs occasionally in patients with partial atrioventricular canals after prosthetic closure of the atrial septal defects, with or without repair of the cleft anterior mitral leaflets.[6, 8, 10] The hemolysis in these patients has been attributed to contact of erythrocytes regurgitated from the left ventricle at high velocity and pressure against the prosthetic atrial septal patch. A review of the literature disclosed that intravascular hemolysis after operative closure of ventricular septal defect with prosthetic material has not been described. However, intravascular hemolysis did develop in a patient studied by us, in whom aortic valvular regurgitation was produced inadvertently while a ventricular septal defect was being closed incompletely. Clinical and autopsy findings in this patient are described.

Received April 10, 1969; accepted for publication May 27, 1969.

Dr. Liddy's present address is: St. Barnabas Medical Center, Livingston, N. J. 07039.

Requests for reprints should be directed to Dr. Roberts.

Report of a Case

An 11-year-old boy had undergone repair of tetralogy of Fallot eight months before admission to the National Heart Institute.

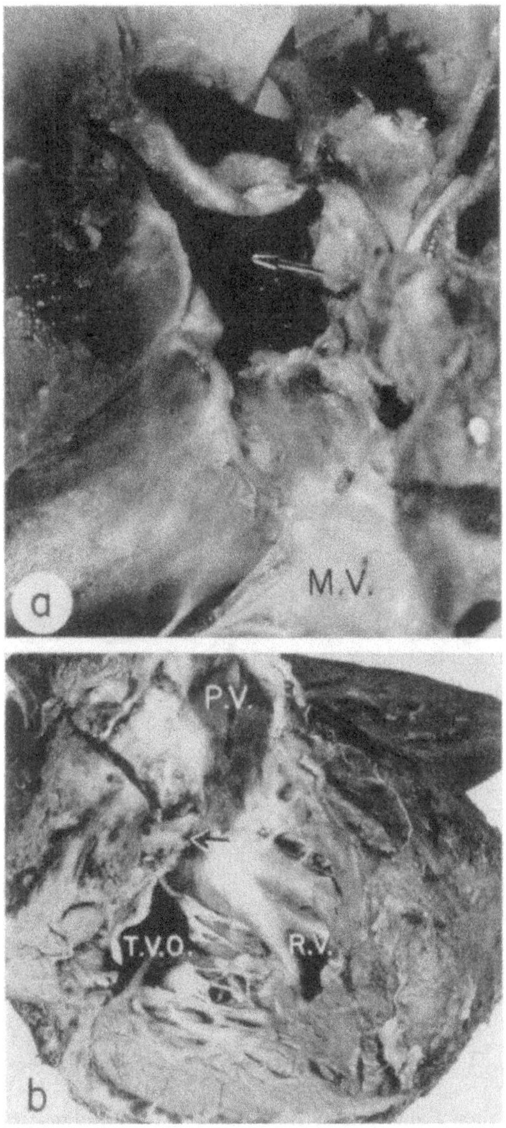

FIG. 1. Opened heart of the patient. *a* (upper), the aortic root, aortic valvular cusps, Ivalon patch (*arrow*), anterior leaflet of the mitral valve (*M.V.*), and the ventricular septum. The patch closing the ventricular septal defect is not covered by endothelium. The perforations in the noncoronary cusp are not seen in this view. *b* (lower), the right ventricle (*R.V.*), tricuspid valvular orifice (*T.V.O.*), ventricular septal patch (*arrow*), and site of the surgically removed pulmonic valvular cusps (*P.V.*).

The ventricular septal defect allegedly had been closed by an Ivalon patch and the valvular and infundibular pulmonic stenosis was thought to be alleviated. During closure of the septal defect, a suture had caught an aortic valvular cusp and aortic regurgitation occurred. Severe right-sided congestive failure, evident immediately after operation, became progressively more severe. Catheterization a month after operation disclosed a residual large left-to-right shunt at the ventricular level.

When admitted to the National Heart Institute for the first time eight months later (a month before death), the patient was severely ill (class IV). A grade 5/6 ejection-type systolic murmur was audible over the entire precordium and a grade 4/6 decrescendo diastolic blowing murmur was heard along the left sternal border. The hematocrit was 37%, hemoglobin 11.3 Gm. per 100 ml., platelet count 59,000 per cu. mm., and leukocyte count 6,000 per cu. mm. Serum iron was 86 μg. and the total iron-binding capacity, 330 μg. The direct Coombs' test proved negative. Total serum bilirubin was 2.7 mg. per 100 ml. and blood urea nitrogen, 10 mg. per 100 ml. Urine was normal. Repeat cardiac catheterization disclosed a left-to-right shunt (1.5 to 1) at the ventricular level and elevated right ventricular (60/20 mm. Hg) and right atrial pressures (mean, 17; *a* wave, 23; *v* wave, 23 mm. Hg). The femoral arterial pressure was 110/48 mm. Hg. At reoperation (seven days before death), two perforations, each about 0.5 cm. in diameter, were found in the noncoronary aortic valvular cusp. The aortic valvular cusps were fibrotic, smooth, and free of calcific deposits; the two perforations, which were responsible for the severe aortic regurgitation, were closed by sutures. It was apparent that the regurgitant stream was in direct line with the ventricular septal patch, which was not covered by endothelium. The residual shunt resulted from partial detachment of the ventricular septal patch; the detached portion was reapproximated to the margin of the defect by sutures. Postoperatively,

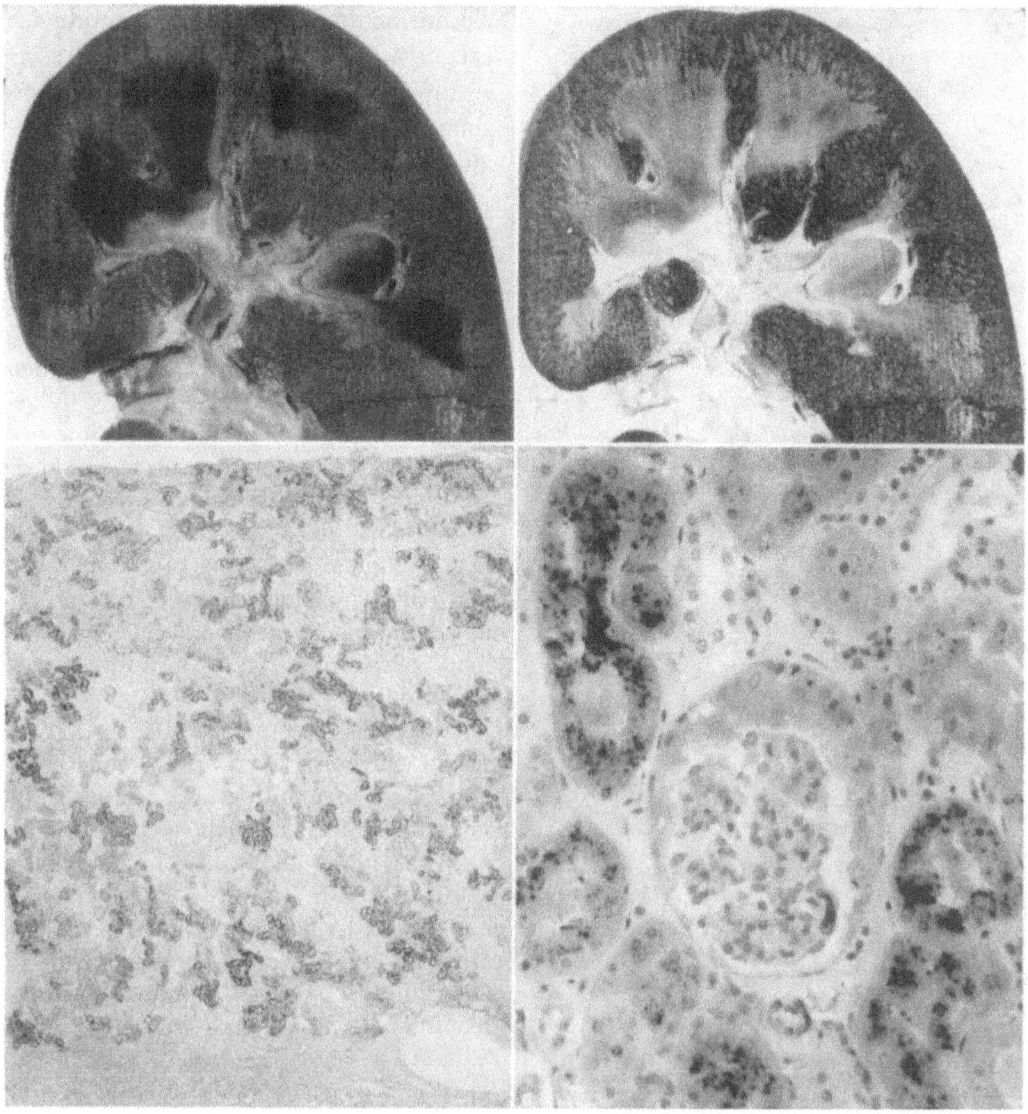

FIG. 2. Kidney. Upper left, cut section. Upper right, same kidney after soaking in Prussian blue solution for 2 min. The cortex stained dark blue, indicating heavy deposits of iron, whereas the medulla did not stain. Lower left, photomicrograph of a section of kidney stained by the Prussian blue method. The dark-stained tubules indicate deposits of iron. The medulla (*bottom*) is free of iron deposits. × 20. Lower right, close-up showing that the iron deposits are situated predominantly in the cytoplasm of the proximal convoluted tubules, although some iron-positive material is present in Bowman's space and in the lumen of the proximal tubules. × 230.

the patient had prolonged periods of hypotension, grand mal seizures, and hyperbilirubinemia (1·7 mg. per 100 ml.), and died.

At autopsy, the ventricular septal defect and the aortic valvular perforations were well closed (Fig. 1). The erythroid elements in the bone marrow were hyperplastic and large deposits of iron were present in the cytoplasm of the proximal convoluted tubules of the kidney (Fig. 2). No stainable iron was present in the liver or spleen.

Comments

The intravascular hemolysis almost certainly resulted from damage to erythrocytes which contacted the nonendothelialized ventricular septal patch. Blood which regurgitated from the aorta through the perforated aortic valvular cusp and ejected from the left ventricle through the residual ventricular septal defect had direct contact with the prosthetic patch. Although few clinical tests for hemolysis were performed, there is unequivocal anatomic evidence, *i.e.*, renal hemosiderosis, that chronic intravascular hemolysis had occurred. Chronic intravascular hemolysis is the only condition which causes severe renal hemosiderosis without associated deposits of iron in the liver or spleen.[2] Acute hemolysis (resulting from cardiopulmonary bypass, for example) may cause glomerular filtration of hemoglobin, but hemosiderin in these patients is present only in the tubular lumens and in Bowman's spaces.[5] Prolonged periods of intravascular hemolysis are necessary before stainable iron can be detected in the cells of the proximal convoluted tubules. The amount of intravascular hemolysis required to produce severe renal hemosiderosis is not precisely known, but the extracorpuscular hemoglobin, at least initially, must exceed 100 to 140 mg. per 100 ml. plasma for hemoglobin to filter through renal glomeruli.[1] Prolonged intravascular hemolysis, however, depletes the serum haptoglobin, and this threshold falls accordingly.[9] The hemolysis in the patient described was well compensated, since he was only mildly anemic. The pronounced erythroid hyperplasia of the bone marrow in the presence of normal arterial oxygen saturation, however, indicates an active stimulus to erythropoiesis.

References

1. Lathem, W.: The renal excretion of hemoglobin: Regulatory mechanisms and the differential excretion of free and protein-bound hemoglobin. J. Clin. Invest. **38**: 652–658, 1959.
2. Leonardi, P., and Ruol, A.: Renal hemosiderosis in the hemolytic anemias: Diagnosis by means of renal biopsy. Blood **16**: 1029–1038, 1960.
3. Pirofsky, B., Sutherland, D. W., Starr, A., and Griswold, H. E.: Hemolytic anemia complicating aortic-valve surgery. An autoimmune syndrome. New Eng. J. Med. **272**: 235–239, 1965.
4. Roberts, W. C.: Renal hemosiderosis (blue kidney) in patients with valvular heart disease. Amer. J. Path. **48**: 409–419, 1966.
5. Roberts, W. C., and Morrow, A. G.: Renal hemosiderosis in patients with prosthetic aortic valves. Circulation **33**: 390–398, 1966.
6. Sayed, H. M., Dacie, J. V., Handley, D. A., Lewis, S. M., and Cleland, W. P.: Haemolytic anaemia of mechanical origin after open heart surgery. Thorax **16**: 356–360, 1961.
7. Sears, D. A., and Crosby, W. H.: Intravascular hemolysis due to intracardiac prosthetic devices. Diurnal variations related to activity. Amer. J. Med. **39**: 341–354, 1965.
8. Sigler, A. T., Forman, E. N., Zinkham, W. H., and Neill, C. A.: Severe intravascular hemolysis following surgical repair of endocardial cushion defects. Amer. J. Med. **35**: 467–480, 1963.
9. Veneziale, C. M., McGuckin, W. F., Hermans, P. E., and Mankin, H. T.: Hypohaptoglobinemia and valvular heart disease: Association with hemolysis after insertion of valvular prostheses and in cases in which operation had not been performed. Mayo Clin. Proc. **41**: 657–662, 1966.
10. Verdon, T. A., Jr., Forrester, R. H., and Crosby, W. H.: Hemolytic anemia after open-heart repair of ostium-primum defects. New Eng. J. Med. 269: 444–446, 1963.

Lethal Ball Variance in the Starr-Edwards Prosthetic *Mitral* Valve

William C. Roberts, MD; Gilbert E. Levinson, MD; and Andrew G. Morrow, MD, Bethesda, Md

Lethal degeneration of a silicone rubber ball of a Starr-Edwards *mitral* prosthesis implanted for 78 months occurred. Variance of mitral silicone rubber poppets requires longer periods of implantation than required for degeneration of aortic poppets. Syncope or near syncope and congestive cardiac-failure appearing more than four years after mitral replacement with a silicone rubber poppet suggests ball variance. Alterations in intensity of the opening sound of the mitral prosthesis in the absence of arrhythmias further suggests this diagnosis.

Degeneration or variance of the silicone rubber poppet is now a well-recognized late complication of aortic valve replacement with a caged-ball prosthesis.[1,2] Constant trauma of the ball against the metallic struts and valve base by the high pressures of both systole and diastole is considered of importance in causing degeneration. In contrast to its common occurrence in the aortic position, degeneration of a silicone rubber poppet of a *mitral* caged-ball prosthesis thus far has been rare. Recently, however, severe degeneration of the silicone rubber ball was observed in a woman who had had isolated mitral valve replacement at the National Heart and Lung Institute with a Starr-Edwards prosthesis 78 months before death. Observations in this patient are described in this report.

Patient Summary

A 41-year-old woman who died on Nov 17, 1969, underwent mitral valve replacement with a 3M Starr-Edwards prosthesis on May 21, 1963. The immediate postoperative course was uneventful and the patient was considerably improved. A grade 1-2/6 apical systolic murmur was heard initially 18 months after operation and persisted thereafter. The murmur was described as pansystolic by some and as ejection type by others. In addition, a grade 1-2/6 diastolic blowing murmur along the left sternal border was audible during the three years before death. Sudden transient unilateral hemiplegia occurred three years after operation, despite warfarin sodium therapy. Five years postoperatively dermal petechiae and menometrorrhagia appeared leading to iron deficiency anemia. Six years postoperatively hysterectomy was performed. Overt congestive cardiac-failure and hemolytic anemia (direct Coombs' test positive) occurred in the early postoperative period. The opening and closing sounds of the mitral prosthesis appeared normal. Six months later, or two months before death, the patient had returned to near normal status. The blood hematocrit reading and reticulocyte count were normal and easy fatiguability was the patient's only symptom. A month later epigastric discomfort appeared and 26 days later, or four days before death, hematemesis (600 ml) occurred and anemia (hematocrit value, 32%) reappeared. The prothrombin time was 130 seconds (control, 12) and the hypoprothrombinemia was attributed to documented excessive salicylate ingestion. No recurrence of bleeding occurred (vitamin K therapy) but her condition steadily worsened. Alteration in the intensity of the opening sound of the prosthesis was detected by auscultation during this hospi-

Received for publication April 3, 1970; accepted May 20.

From the Section of Pathology and the Clinic of Surgery, National Heart and Lung Institute, Bethesda, Md, and the Division of Cardiovascular Diseases, Department of Medicine, New Jersey College of Medicine and Dentistry, Newark.

Reprint requests to Section of Pathology, National Heart and Lung Institute, Bethesda, Md 20014 (Dr. Roberts).

talization. Tachycardia, fever, pallor, and a right upper lobe pulmonary infiltrate appeared, and the patient was found dead in bed.

At autopsy, the pulmonary infiltrate was typical of lobar pneumonia. The viscera was congested. The silicone rubber ball of the mitral prosthesis showed evidence of severe degeneration (Figure). It was uniformly yellow, fractured at two sites, and swollen in an oblong manner. Neither a peribasilar left ventricular atrial communication nor antemortem prosthetic thrombus was present.

Comment

It is disappointing indeed to observe degeneration of the silicone rubber ball of the Starr-Edwards mitral prosthesis in the patient described. The degeneration of the poppet in this patient may well prove not to be an isolated occurrence but an indication of other such events to come. When degeneration of the silicone poppet of the Starr-Edwards prosthetic aortic valve was first observed, investigators attributed ball variance to associated peribasilar aortic left ventricular leaks, to antemortem thrombus on the prosthesis, to elevated blood lipid levels, or to chronic alcoholism. Rapidly, however, it became apparent that the silicone rubber in the aortic prosthetic cage could not withstand the trauma of contact against the metallic struts and ring under systemic pressure, whether or not associated lesions, particularly peribasilar leaks, were present.

At the National Heart and Lung Institute we have examined the silicone rubber poppets in 68 patients who died after one month (range 1.3 to 78 months [average, 20]) of replacement of one or more cardiac valves with Starr-Edwards prostheses. Degeneration of the prosthetic poppet was not observed in any of the 43 patients who died less than 24 months after valve replacement. Of the 25 patients who died 24 months or longer after valve replacement, 17 patients had had only the aortic valve replaced, four had had only the mitral valve replaced, and four had had both mitral and aortic valves replaced. Of the 21 aortic valve poppets examined, 17 showed degeneration. In ten patients the balls were discolored, swollen, grooved, and impacted in the cage, and caused prosthetic stenosis (implantation period 24 to 67 months [average, 45 months]). In six patients the balls were fractured or atrophied, and had dislodged from the cage causing fatal aortic regurgitation (implantation period 28 to 37 months [average, 33 months]); interestingly, all six of the patients in whom the ball dislodged underwent valve replacement in 1965, and all six died in 1967. In the 17th patient the aortic ball was discolored but not grooved, swollen, or fractured and it functioned normally for 65 months. Of the remaining four aortic poppets examined no gross ball degeneration was present (implantation period, 27 to 45 months [average, 36 months]). Of the eight mitral poppets examined, seven were normal (implantation period, 28 to 68 months [average, 43 months]) and only in the patient described herein did the ball show severe degeneration.

Degeneration of silicone rubber poppets of caged ball mitral prostheses has occurred in at least nine other patients: four in SCDK-Cutter[3-5] and five in Starr-Edwards[6] type prostheses. Sanderson et al[4] described swelling, softening, and "light canary-yellow" discoloration of the silicone rubber poppet of a Cutter mitral prosthesis inserted 37 months earlier. Chemical analysis of the ball revealed cholesterol and triglyceride deposits. Changes in the intensity and timing of the opening and closing clicks of the prosthesis were noted before reoperation in this patient who was in "moderate" congestive cardiac-failure. Leatherman et al[3] described two patients who had mitral valve replacements with Cutter prostheses eight and ten months, respectively, before reoperation, which was performed because of the sudden appearance of syncope or presyncope in both patients. The prosthetic sounds in each patient were of variable intensity and irregular, despite sinus rhythm. At reoperation, the mitral poppet in each patient was white and swollen, and movement of the poppet in the cage was impaired. Connolly and associates[6] described swelling (16% increase from original weight and 5% increase from original dimensions), yellow discoloration, and grooving of the silicone rubber ball of a mitral Starr-Edwards prosthesis (model 6000) implanted 50 months earlier. Muffling and finally disappearance of the opening sound of the prosthesis, along with acute pulmonary edema, suggested the diagnosis of mitral ball variance in their patient. At reoperation the swollen poppet moved only with difficulty and then only for a short distance within the cage, "obviously causing severe obstruction." In addition to the mitral poppet in the patient described by Connolly et al, P. E. Chappell, Jr. (written communication, January 1970) described four other Starr-Edwards mitral valve poppets (all of the model 6000 series) returned to the laboratory because of ball variance. The period of implantation in the four patients varied from 50 to 67 months. All four poppets were discolored and each showed slight loss of weight. One showed minor surface damage, and

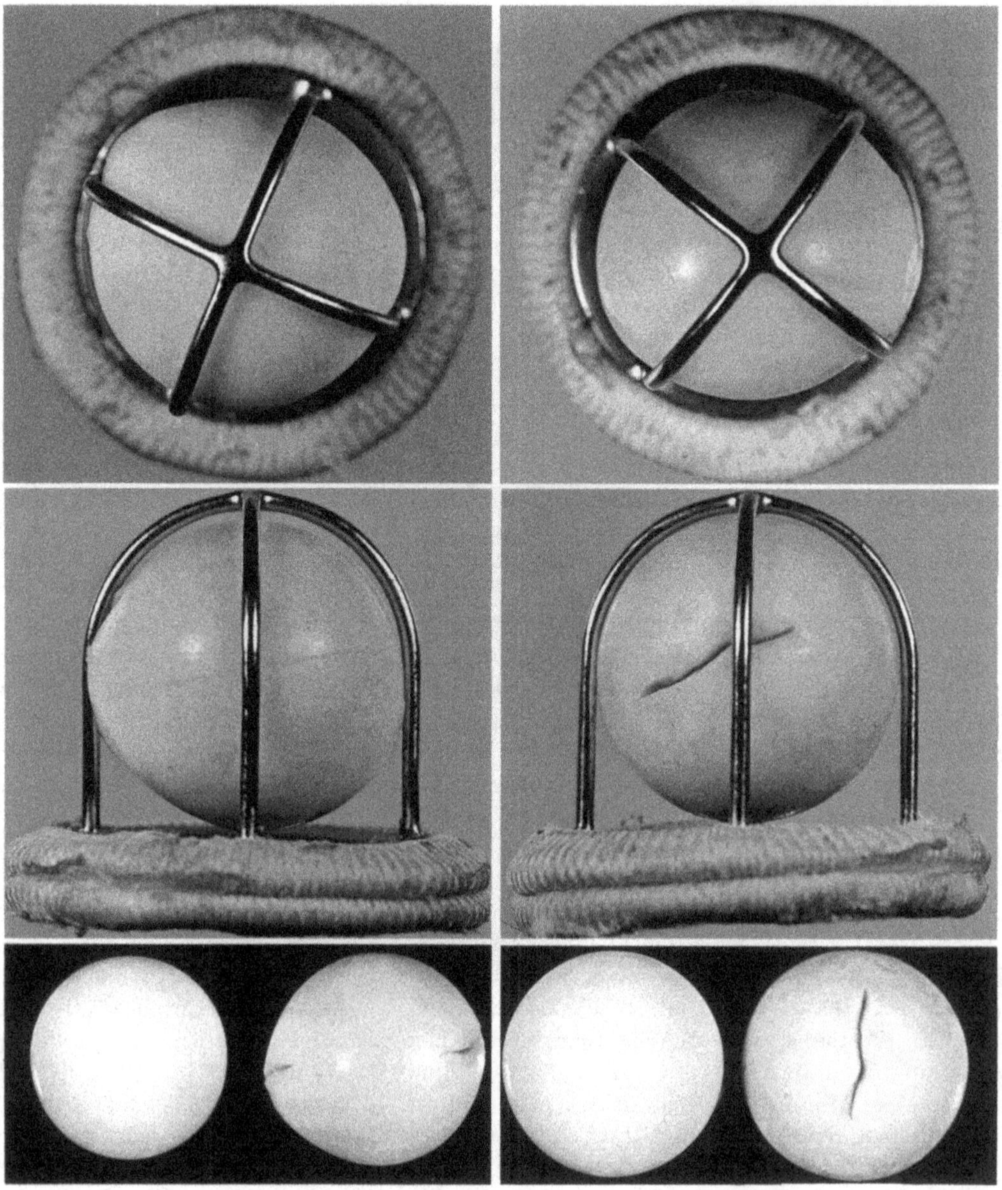

Prosthetic mitral valve in patient described. Top, Two views of prosthesis from above. When ball is in position shown on the left it is immobile. Middle, Two views from side. On the left ball is immobile. Bottom, White poppet is a normal 3M Starr-Edwards ball for comparison with yellow, fractured, swollen, and deformed poppet of present patient, also size 3M originally. Two fractures are visible on view on left, and the length of one fracture is visible in view on right.

one was split. No prosthetic dysfunction occurred in any of the four patients. With the probable exception of the fractured poppet and of the swollen ball in the patient described by Connolly et al, none of the other seven mitral poppets mentioned were degenerated to the degree present in the present patient. The poppet in her was oblong, and when its longest diameter was at a right angle to the metallic struts of the cage, movement of the ball could occur only with manual pressure. When the long diameter of the ball was parallel with the struts, however, the ball moved well when the cage was tilted back and forth; soon the poppet's axis would change, and then it could neither extend fully to the apex of the cage nor seat completely. It seems likely, therefore, that valve function was normal with some beats and abnormal with others. It is probable that death occurred when the ball was made immobile for a brief period in the cage. In addition to the variance of the caged mitral silicone rubber ball, we have observed severe degeneration of the silicone rubber in a Hufnagel discoid mitral as well as Hufnagel discoid aortic prosthesis in a heart from a 23-year-old man operated on elsewhere. The prostheses had been implanted 33 months earlier. In contrast to the severe degeneration of the silicone rubber portion of each of these disks, the polypropylene portions of the disks were intact.

It is clear that the incidence of degeneration of the silicone rubber of mitral prostheses is low at this time, compared to the incidence of degeneration of the silicone rubber in the aortic valve position. This difference is further emphasized by the fact that the total number of Starr-Edwards mitral prostheses and aortic prostheses supplied to surgeons is approximately equal (30,000 of each type). Differences in aortic and mitral valvular blood velocities are probably the explanation. Typically, the orifice diameters of aortic prostheses are smaller than those of mitral prostheses, and the time of ventricular systole is approximately half that of ventricular diastole for a patient at rest. The velocity of flow through the orifice of the average aortic prosthesis is at least three times greater than the velocity through the orifice of the average mitral prosthesis. Also, the aortic ball contacts both the valve ring and the apex of the cage under high pressure, whereas the mitral ball contacts only the ring under high pressure (except in the Cutter prosthesis) since the ball passes to the apex of the cage during ventricular diastole.

The period of implantation necessary to produce significant mitral poppet degeneration is unknown at present. In our patient the period was 78 months, but much shorter periods have been observed. Peribasilar leaks or prosthetic thrombus may shorten this period. The presence or absence of peribasilar leaks was not mentioned in the nine other patients described with variant mitral balls. The shortest implantation period in which severe aortic poppet degeneration was observed was 24 months. This patient also had a peribasilar communication.[1]

Clinical features of *aortic* ball variance are variable, but this diagnosis must be suspected in any patient in whom a prosthesis containing silicone rubber has been in place 24 months or longer. When the aortic ball swells, congestive cardiac-failure usually ensues and alterations of prosthetic sounds are often apparent. Dislodgement of the aortic ball from the cage has not been preceded by symptoms of cardiac dysfunction in the six patients studied by us. The clinical features resulting from severe degeneration of the silicone rubber *mitral* poppet also are variable, and consist of syncope or near syncope, congestive heart-failure, and alterations in prosthetic sounds. Sanderson et al[4] in their patient with a variant mitral Cutter ball showed that the interval between aortic closure and mitral opening sound varied from 0.10 to 0.62 seconds (normal, 0.07 to 0.15 seconds), and the opening sound disappeared in the patient described by Connolly et al[6] and varied in our patient. Mitral ball degeneration should thus be considered in any patient doing poorly four or more years after mitral replacement, and reoperation may be necessary in many of these patients. It is hoped that the hollow metal ball in Starr-Edwards prostheses of current design will not degenerate. This newer prosthesis, introduced in 1967, had yet to be tested adequately, however, and no conclusions concerning its superiority are yet justified.

References

1. Roberts WC, Morrow AG: Fatal degeneration of the silicone rubber ball of the Starr-Edwards prosthetic aortic valve. *Amer J Cardiol* 22:614-620, 1968.
2. Hylen JC, et al: Aortic ball variance: Diagnosis and treatment. *Ann Intern Med* 72:1-8, 1970.
3. Leatherman LL, et al: Malfunction of mitral ball-valve prosthesis due to swollen poppet. *J Thorac Cardiovasc Surg* 53:398-400, 1967.
4. Sanderson RG, Hall AD, Thomas AN: The clinical diagnosis of ball variance in a mitral valve prosthesis. *Ann Thorac Surg* 6:473-475, 1968.
5. Beall AC Jr, et al: Prosthetic replacement of cardiac valves: Five and one-half years' experience. *Amer J Cardiol* 23:250-257, 1969.
6. Connolly DC, Harrison CE Jr, Ellis FH: Ball variance in a Starr-Edwards prosthetic mitral valve causing acute pulmonary edema (diagnosis by auscultation before onset of symptoms). *Mayo Clin Proc* 45:20-24, 1970.

Hemodynamic confirmation of obstruction to left ventricular inflow by a caged-ball prosthetic mitral valve

Case report

Richard L. Shepherd, D. Luke Glancy, Edward B. Stinson, and William C. Roberts, Bethesda, Md.

It is now generally recognized that insertion of a large caged-ball mitral prosthesis into a relatively small-sized left ventricular cavity may lead to obstruction of the left ventricular inflow or outflow or both.[1-4] Recently, routine postoperative cardiac catheterization was performed on a patient who had undergone double valve replacement for combined mitral and aortic stenosis 6½ months earlier. A significant pressure gradient between the left atrium and left ventricle was documented at catheterization, and its mechanism was later established by necropsy. Pertinent clinical and anatomic features of the mitral obstruction by the mitral prosthesis in this patient are presented in this report.

Case report

L. K., a 58-year-old man, was evaluated at the National Heart and Lung Institute in July, 1971, because of a 1 year history of progressive fatigue, orthopnea, frequent paroxysms of nocturnal dyspnea, and one episode of pulmonary edema.

From the Cardiology Branch, Clinic of Surgery, and Section of Pathology, National Heart and Lung Institute, Bethesda, Md. 20014.

Received for publication July 19, 1972.

Address for reprints: Richard L. Shepherd, M.D., Cardiology Branch, National Heart and Lung Institute, Bldg. 10, 7B-15, Bethesda, Md. 20014.

Physical examination revealed a markedly prolonged carotid upstroke, an aortic ejection murmur, a diastolic blowing murmur along the left sternal margin, and a diastolic rumble at the apex. The electrocardiogram indicated left ventricular hypertrophy with "strain." Chest roentgenograms showed left ventricular and left atrial enlargement and dilatation of the ascending aorta. Fluoroscopy revealed extensive calcific deposits on the aortic valve. Cardiac catheterization data are summarized in Table I.

On July 29, 1971, the aortic valve was replaced with a 9A, Model 2320 Starr-Edwards prosthesis, and the mitral valve was exchanged for a 4M, Model 6320 Starr-Edwards prosthesis. The immediate postoperative period was complicated by mild low-output syndrome treated with isoproterenol. The patient was discharged on Aug. 15, 1971, on a regimen of digoxin, furosemide, and warfarin. In November he voluntarily discontinued warfarin, and 2 weeks later he suddenly developed transient right-sided hemiparesis and dizziness; warfarin therapy was reinstituted. At the time of readmission to the National Heart and Lung Institute in February, 1972, the patient was nearly asymptomatic. Neurologic examination revealed normal findings. The prosthetic valve sounds were crisp, and no murmurs were heard. Postoperative cardiac catheterization data are shown in Table I. Five days after catheterization he died suddenly while still in the hospital.

At necropsy, the heart was enlarged (total weight 450 grams), but neither ventricle was dilated. Each of the four struts of the mitral prosthetic cage were in contact with endocardium of left ventricle, and the mitral poppet was pre-

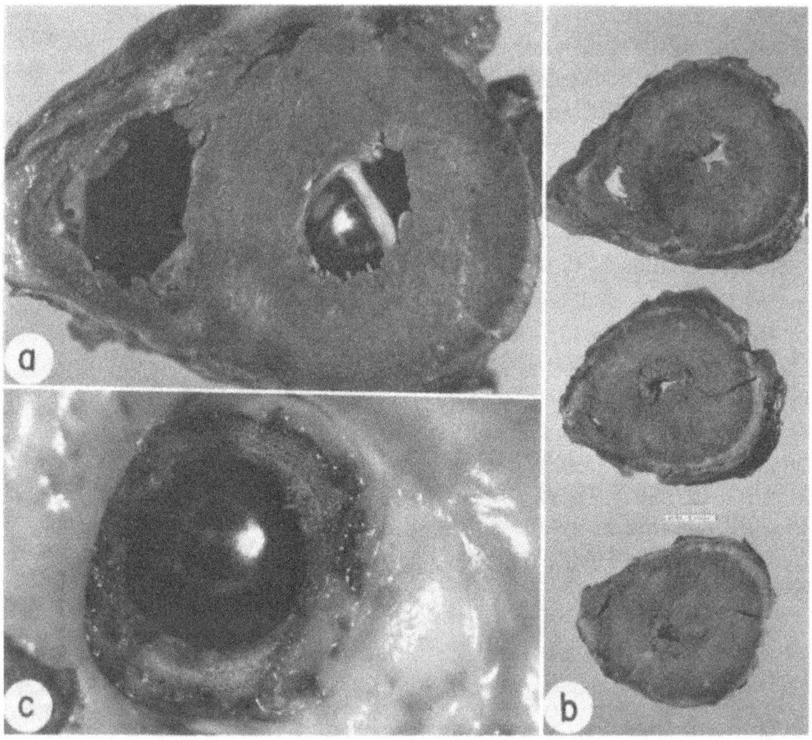

Fig. 1. *a,* Transverse section of the ventricles shows that the Starr-Edwards mitral prosthesis fills the entire left ventricular cavity at this level. The poppet was prevented from descending completely by the ventricular septum which bulged into the cage. The cloth-covered struts, which are visible in this view, are completely covered by collagen. The left ventricular wall is hypertrophied. Other transverse sections caudal to this one are shown in *b.* The left ventricular cavity is extremely small. *c,* View of mitral prosthesis from left atrium. The entire "floor" of this chamber is occupied by the prosthesis.

vented from descending fully by ventricular septum which protruded into the cage (Fig. 1). Collagen deposits covering the struts of the mitral prosthesis were thin and did not inhibit free movement of the poppet. No thrombus was present in the primary orifice or on the struts of the mitral prosthesis. There was no thrombus on the aortic prosthesis, and the aortic poppet moved freely. The left ventricle showed no foci of fibrosis or necrosis. There was no evidence of a recent systemic or pulmonary embolus.

Comments

The patient described above died 6½ months after aortic and mitral valve replacement for severe aortic stenosis and mild-to-moderate mitral stenosis. In retrospect, it would appear that the 4M Starr-Edwards mitral prosthesis was too large for this patient's normal-sized left ventricular cavity; the obstruction associated with the prosthesis was more severe than that caused by the excised mitral valve.

Table I. *Catheterization data**

Parameter	*July 5, 1971 (24 days before operation)*	*Feb. 7, 1972 (6½ months after operation)*
Pulmonary artery (mm. Hg)	38/18 (26)	34/16 (22)
Pulmonary artery wedge (mm. Hg)	(16)	(14)
Left ventricle (mm. Hg)	205/30	125/6
Left brachial artery (mm. Hg)	102/55 (70)	125/70 (90)
Left ventricle-pulmonary artery wedge (mm. Hg)†	7	11
Cardiac output (L./min.)	3.48	4.87
Aortic valve area (sq. cm.)	0.32	
Mitral valve area (sq. cm.)	1.96	1.59

*Figures in parentheses are mean values.
†Mean diastolic gradient.

The cause of sudden death 5 days after cardiac catheterization is uncertain, but it is highly probable that stenosis of the prosthetic mitral valve was a contributing cause. Necropsy showed that the prosthetic obstruction was due to protrusion of the interventricular septum into the cage of the mitral prosthesis, which prevented free descent of the poppet. It has been postulated[5] that a caged-ball mitral valve prosthesis may be too large for the left ventricle into which it is inserted, but hemodynamic and anatomic confirmation of this concept has previously been lacking. More severe forms of prosthetic dysfunction probably result in low-output syndrome and early postoperative death, and the increased mortality rate which has been reported in patients with small left ventricles[6] may be due in part to dysfunction of the prosthesis.

REFERENCES

1 Morrow, A. G., Clark, W. D., Harrison, D. C., and Braunwald, E.: Prosthetic Replacement of the Mitral Valve: Operative Methods and the Results of Preoperative and Postoperative Hemodynamic Assessments, Circulation **29:** 2, 1964 (Suppl.).

2 Morrow, A. G., Oldham, H. N., Elkins, R. C., and Braunwald, E.: Prosthetic Replacement of the Mitral Valve. Preoperative and Postoperative Clinical and Hemodynamic Assessment in 100 Patients, Circulation **35:** 962, 1967.

3 Glancy, D. L., O'Brien, K. P., Reiss, R. L., Epstein, S. E., and Morrow, A. G.: Hemodynamic Studies in Patients With 2M and 3M Starr-Edwards Prostheses: Evidence of Obstruction to Left Atrial Emptying, Circulation **29, 30:** 113, 1969 (Suppl. I).

4 Reis, R. L., Glancy, D. L., O'Brien, K. P., Epstein, S. E., and Morrow, A. G.: Clinical and Hemodynamic Assessments of Fabric-Covered Starr-Edwards Prosthetic Valves, J. Thorac. Cardiovasc. Surg. **59:** 84, 1970.

5 Roberts, W. C., and Morrow, A. G.: Mechanisms of Acute Left Atrial Thrombosis After Mitral Valve Replacement: Pathologic Findings Indicating Obstruction to Left Atrial Emptying, Am. J. Cardiol. **18:** 497, 1966.

6 Terzaki, A. K., Cokkinos, D. V., Leachman, R. D., Meade, J. B., Hallman, G. L., and Cooley, D. A.: Combined Mitral and Aortic Valve Disease, Am. J. Cardiol. **25:** 588, 1970.

Structural alterations in tissue cardiac valves implanted in patients and in calves

John W. Yarbrough, M.D., William C. Roberts, M.D., and Robert L. Reis, M.D.,** Bethesda, Md.*

Heterograft cardiac valves are supplied in a wide range of sizes and are prepared before implantation. Fresh, beta-propiolactone–treated, gamma-irradiated, freeze-dried, frozen, and formalin-fixed valves all have been utilized in patients.[1] Although initial hemodynamic results were good and thromboembolic complications were minimal, these valves have not been durable.[2-4] Because it forms strong cross linkages of collagen while allowing flexibility of tissue and because its bonds are not biodegradable, glutaraldehyde is now being used as a preservative for heterograft valves.[1] Reports of heterograft valves previously fixed with glutaraldehyde have been encouraging.[5] This paper describes anatomic findings in glutaraldehyde-fixed porcine aortic heterograft valves in 6 patients and in 1 calf. In addition, structural alterations in other types of tissue valves implanted in 4 patients and in 6 calves are described for comparison.

From the Clinic of Surgery and Section of Pathology, National Heart and Lung Institute, National Institutes of Health, Bethesda, Md. 20014.

Received for publication Sept. 6, 1972.

Address for reprints: Dr. William C. Roberts, Section of Pathology, National Heart and Lung Institute, National Institutes of Health, Bethesda, Md. 20014.

*Present address: Department of Surgery, Duke University Medical Center, Durham, N. C.

**Present address: Department of Surgery, University of Kansas Medical Center, Kansas City, Kan.

Material

Seventeen tissue valves, implanted for 7 to 240 days (mean 93), were examined at necropsy: Ten had been implanted in patients and seven in Holstein calves (Table I). Except for the three formalin-fixed valves, all had been placed on Reis-Hancock flexible stents.[6] Fourteen had been implanted at the National Heart and Lung Institute, whereas the three formalin-fixed porcine heterograft valves were implanted into human subjects elsewhere and later were submitted by Hancock Laboratories for histologic studies. The ten porcine heterografts were prepared before implantation by Hancock Laboratories, and the other seven heterotopic tissue valves were prepared at the National Heart and Lung Institute at the time of implantation by the method described previously.[6, 7] The tissue valves were implanted into the mitral position in all 7 calves. Of the 10 human subjects, 6 had mitral valve replacement, 3 had aortic replacement, and 1 had tricuspid replacement.

At necropsy, the previously implanted valves were fixed in either 10 per cent buffered formalin or 3 per cent glutaraldehyde. After fixation, sections were taken from one or more leaflets of each valve, processed, cut, stained, and examined histologically. One section from each cusp

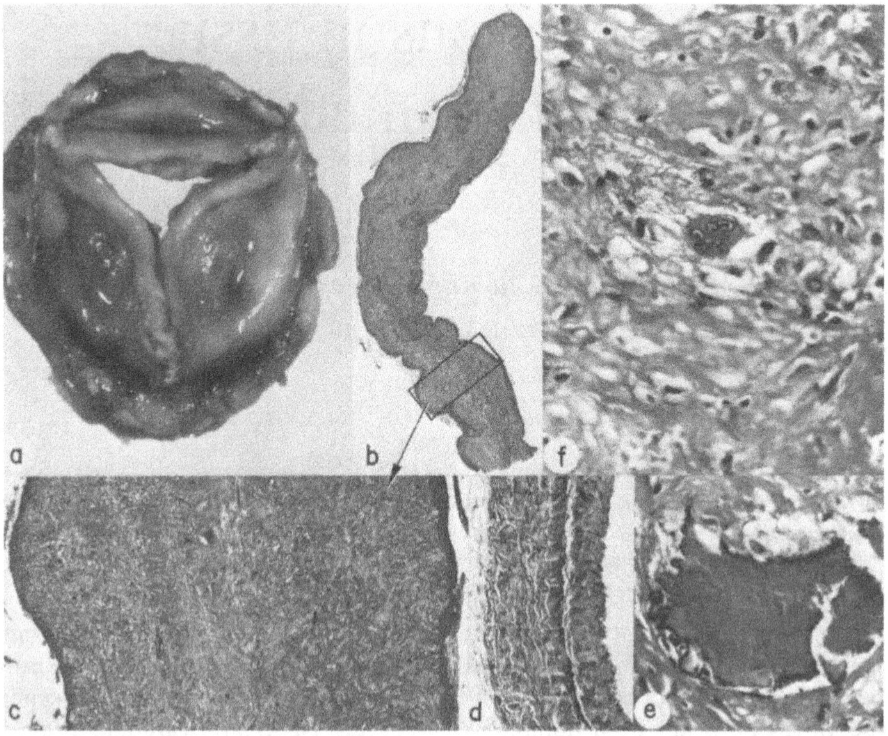

Fig. 1. Fresh autogenous pericardial valve implanted in the mitral position in a 50-year-old woman 39 days before death. There was no evidence of dysfunction of this tissue valve during the postoperative period. *a*, View of pericardial valve from above. The cusps are thickened and one is retracted. The valve orifice was competent when water was injected under pressure into the left ventricle at necropsy. *b*, Photomicrograph of section through one cusp. The surfaces of the cusp are lined by fibrin. The cusp is about four times thicker than normal. *c*, Close-up view of the area shown in *brackets* in *b*. This implanted parietal pericardium may be compared to its thickness at the time of implantation, a portion of which is shown in *d*. Both *c* and *d* were taken at the same magnification. The thickening of the implanted pericardium is due mainly to proliferation of fibrous tissue, which probably resulted from organization of the surface fibrin. *e*, Deposit of calcium in the implanted valve. *f*, Close-up of portion of implanted valve shows a multinucleated cell. Its significance is uncertain. (Hematoxylin and eosin stains. Original magnifications: *b*, ×11; *c* and *d*, ×70; *e* and *f*, ×400.)

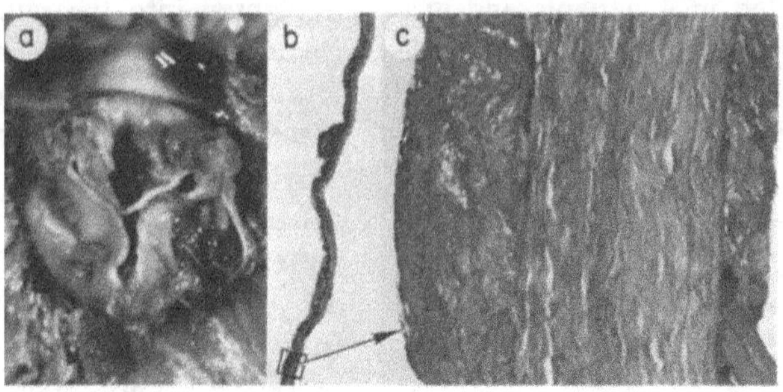

Fig. 2. Fresh autogenous pericardial valve implanted in the mitral position in a calf 7 days before death. The pericardial valve appeared to function normally during the entire postoperative period, and, at necropsy, injection of water into the left ventricle under pressure indicated that the valve was competent. *a*, Pericardial valve as viewed from left ventricle. The leaflets are mildly thickened. *b*, Low-power photomicrograph of section of one cusp. *c*, Blow-up of area in *brackets* shown in *b*. The cusp is nearly twice normal thickness. The thickening is due to fibrin-platelet thrombus on its surface. The margins of the original parietal pericardium are clearly visible. (Hematoxylin and eosin stains. Original magnifications: *b*, ×6; *c*, ×160.)

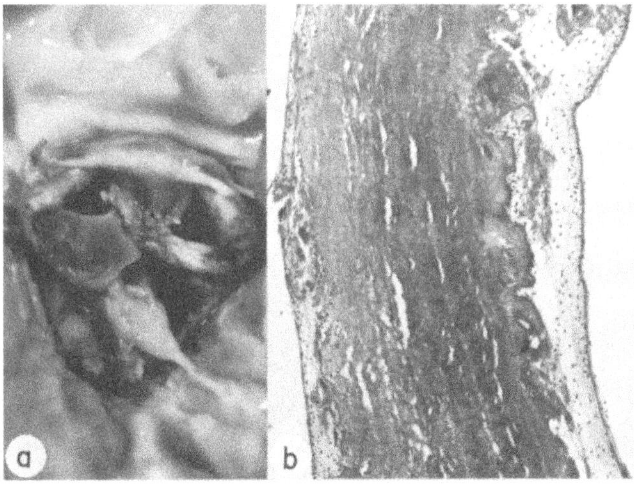

Fig. 3. Fresh autogenous parietal pericardium valve implanted in a calf 82 days before its death. The calf did poorly postoperatively, and signs of mitral regurgitation and infective endocarditis were evident at least 1 month before death. *a,* Tissue valve as viewed from left ventricle. The cusps are torn and perforated. There are no signs of infection at the site of attachment of the rigid frame to the natural mitral annulus. *b,* Section of portion of one cusp. The entire valve is necrotic and edematous. A few polymorphonuclear leukocytes are visible. No stainable colonies of organisms were observed, but the calf was being given antibiotics during the entire postoperative period. (Hematoxylin and eosin stain. Original magnification: *b,* ×100.)

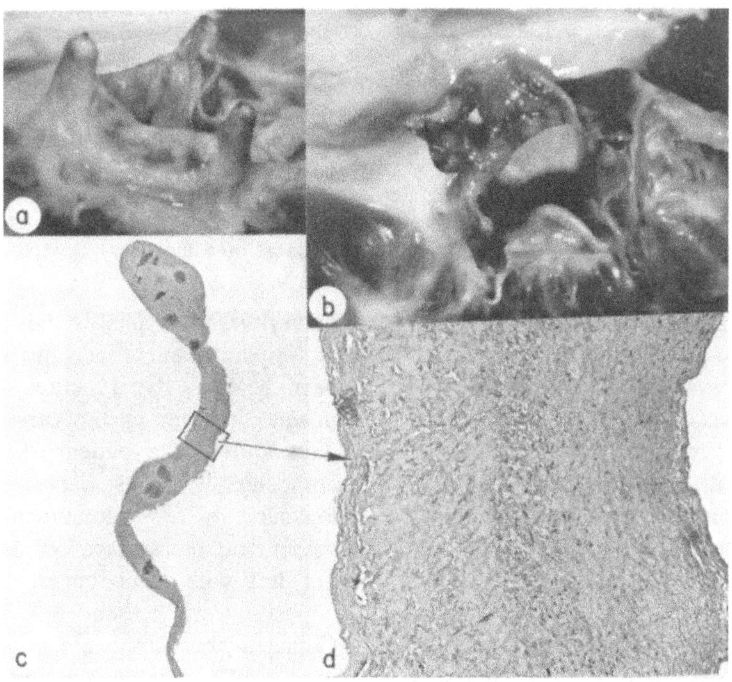

Fig. 4. Fresh autogenous pericardial valve implanted into the mitral position of a calf 116 days before its death. *a,* The cusps are diffusely thickened and retracted. *b,* One cusp tore and prolapsed into the left atrium. *c,* Photomicrograph of one of the nonprolapsed cusps shows the diffuse thickening. A close-up of the area in *brackets* is shown in *d.* There is considerable fibrous thickening of the implanted parietal pericardium. No colonies of organisms were seen on histologic study of the prolapsed cusp. (Hematoxylin and eosin stain. Original magnifications: *c,* ×8; *d,* ×100.)

Table I. *Tissue valves evaluated*

Type of valve	Patients	Days	Calves	Days
	Subjects and duration of implantation			
Fresh autogenous pericardium	1	39	3	7-116
Fresh autogenous fascia lata	0	-	1	80
Glutaraldehyde-fixed human fascia lata	0	-	2	48, 56
Formalin-fixed porcine aortic valve	3	80-240	0	-
Glutaraldehyde-fixed porcine aortic valve	6	14-180	1	110
Totals	10	14-240	7	7-116

Table II. *Severity of morphologic changes in implanted tissue valves*

Type of valve	No. of subjects	Gross	Microscopic
		Changes after implantation (0-4+)	
Fresh autogenous pericardium	4	++++	++++
Fresh autogenous fascia lata	1	+++	++++
Glutaraldehyde-fixed human fascia lata	2	++++	++++
Formalin-fixed porcine aortic valve	3	++++	++++
Glutaraldehyde-fixed porcine aortic valve	7	+	+
Total	17		

was stained with hematoxylin and eosin, Verhoeff–van Gieson, methenamine silver, and periodic acid–Schiff.

Results

The four fresh autogenous pericardial valves were thickened and retracted by 30 days after implantation (Figs. 1 to 4) (Table II). Two valves implanted in calves were perforated and detached from the commissures. Grossly, each appeared infected, but microscopically no stainable organisms were found in the leaflets. All

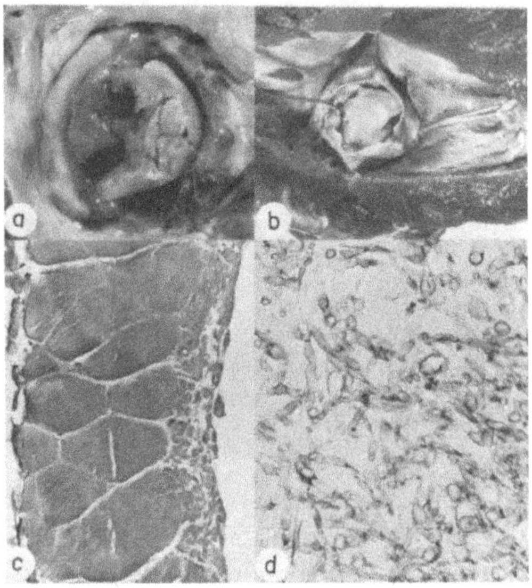

Fig. 5. Fresh autogenous fascia lata valve implanted into the mitral position of a calf 80 days before its death. Initially he did well postoperatively but later developed overt congestive cardiac failure. A diastolic rumble that suggested mitral stenosis became audible. At necropsy, the mitral orifice was partially obstructed by a large fungal mass attached primarily to the rigid-frame portion of the tissue valve. *a,* View of tissue valve from left atrium shows the large fungal mass. *b,* View of valve from left ventricle again shows the fungal mass obstructing the orifice. *c,* Photomicrograph of a section of one cusp. The fascia lata is necrotic, devoid of cells, and not thickened. *d,* Candida species in the fungal mass. (Hematoxylin and eosin stain [*c*] and methenamine silver stain [*d*]. Original magnifications: *c,* ×160; *d,* ×400.)

valves were less pliable than they had been at implantation. Since no murmurs had been heard, valve function was considered normal in both of the calves that lived 7 days and in the patient. The valves were competent when tested post mortem. Histologically, a few mononuclear cells were present on the surfaces of each valve cusp but not within the cusps. Minute calcific deposits were present in all valve cusps. Collagen fibers appeared intact in the valve implanted in the patient but were necrotic in each of the 3 calves. Fibrous tissue was present in each valve cusp, except in the valve implanted 7 days before death. Fibrin deposits were present on all valves. The thickening of the valve in the patient was primarily due to fibrous tissue, almost sure-

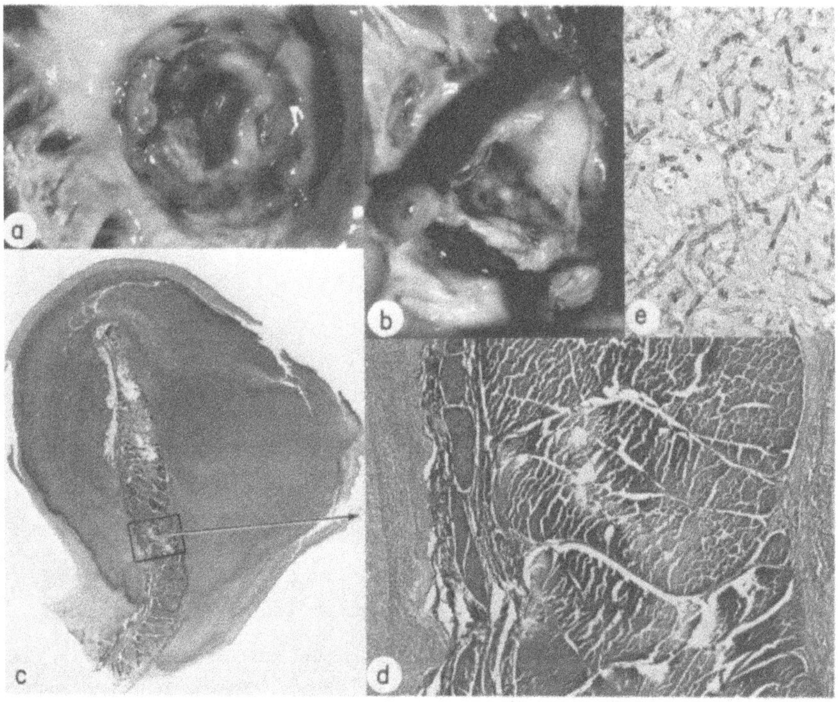

Fig. 6. Glutaraldehyde-fixed human fascia lata valve implanted in the mitral position in a calf 56 days before its death. The calf did poorly from the time of implantation and died of severe congestive cardiac failure. The orifice of the valve became obstructed by a large fungal mass (*a, b,* and *c*). *a,* View of stenotic valve from left atrium. *b,* View from left ventricle. *c,* Photomicrograph shows fungal ball totally encapsulating the fascia lata cusp. *d,* Close-up view shows necrosis of the fascia lata with total absence of cells. *e,* Candida species identified in the obstructing mass. (Hematoxylin and eosin stains [*c* and *d*] and methenamine silver stain [*e*]. Original magnifications: *c,* ×5; *d,* ×40; *e,* ×400.)

ly the result of organization of fibrin. Vascular channels, located primarily at the base of the leaflet, were present in the valve of the human subject.

The one fresh autogenous fascia lata valve (Fig. 5) implanted in a calf for 80 days was made stenotic by a large mycotic thrombus which occluded the orifice. This mass was attached to the sewing ring and to the atrial surface of the cusps. Candida species were found in the occluding mass. A few focal fibrin deposits were present on the leaflets, but generally the cusps were not thickened. However, the leaflets were necrotic.

The two glutaraldehyde-fixed human fascia lata valves (Figs. 6 and 7) were examined 48 and 56 days, respectively, after implantation in calves. Both were stenotic, rigid, focally but extensively calcified, and necrotic. Focal fibrin deposits were present on the implanted valves in both calves. The valvular stenosis in 1 calf was worsened by a large mycotic thrombus which was attached to two of the three cusps; it contained Candida species. No cellular infiltrates were present in the leaflets.

Each of the three formalin-fixed porcine aortic valves (Figs. 8 to 10) was retrieved from a patient because of valve failure either due to detachment of a cusp from a commissure or to perforation or tearing of a cusp. Histologically, the leaflets in all 3 patients were necrotic and mildly thickened. The cusps were devoid of inflammatory cells except at their bases, where mononuclear cells were present. The adjacent aorta also was necrotic, and its intima was thickened

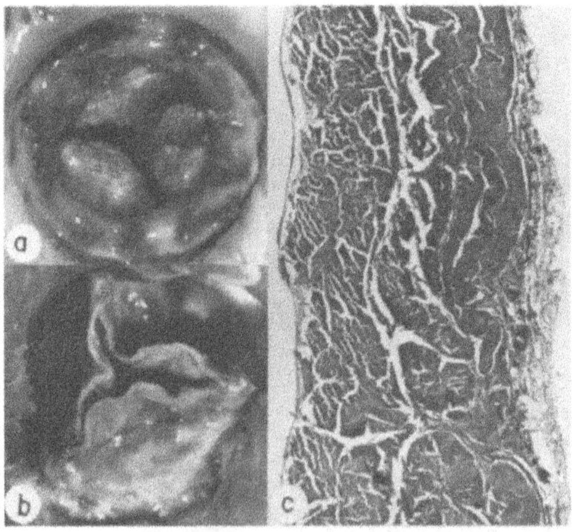

Fig. 7. Glutaraldehyde-fixed human fascia lata valve implanted in the mitral position of a calf 48 days before its death. The calf did poorly from the beginning of the postoperative period and died of progressive congestive cardiac failure. The valve cusps were not freely pliable at the time of insertion, and at necropsy the cusps were rigid. *a*, View of valve from left atrium. *b*, View from left ventricle. *c*, Photomicrograph of portion of one cusp. The fascia in this area is necrotic and free of cells. In other areas, fibrous tissue covered the ventricular surfaces. In most areas the cusps were extensively calcified. The rigidity of the cusps at necropsy could be attributed primarily to the presence of the calcific deposits. (Hematoxylin and eosin stain. Original magnification: *c*, ×65.)

by a loose fibrous tissue that contained multinucleated cells. No calcific deposits were present.

The seven porcine valves fixed in stabilized glutaraldehyde* (Figs. 11 to 16) appeared normal grossly. The leaflets were thin, translucent, and freely mobile. Valve function appeared normal in each. However, one of the seven valves contained a large thrombus in one of the three sinuses (Fig. 15). Microscopically, the cusps contained elongated cells, similar to those seen in a control valve (Fig. 17). Small foci of necrosis were noted in three of the seven implanted valves (Figs. 12, 14, and 16). The sinus surfaces of the cusps of three valves were covered by mesothelial-like cells arranged more or less perpendicular to

*Supplied by Hancock Laboratories, Inc., Orange, Calif.

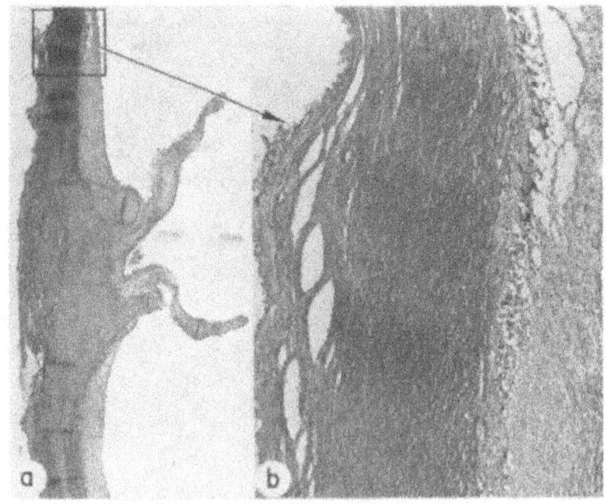

Fig. 8. Formalin-fixed porcine aortic valve implanted in a patient 90 days before his death. *a*, Section includes commissure, two aortic valve cusps, and adjacent aorta. The cusps at their bases contain mononuclear cells, and the adjacent intima of the aorta is thickened. *b*, Close-up of area in *brackets* shown in *a*. The media of the entire aorta is necrotic, the intima is thickened, and giant cells are present at the junction of the media and intima. (Hematoxylin and eosin stains. Original magnifications: *a*, ×20; *b*, ×100.)

the cuspal surfaces (Fig. 12). These cells occasionally grouped together to form giant cells. Deposits of fibrin were superimposed on the lining cells. No lining cells, fibrin, or fibrous tissue were present on the upstream surfaces of the cusps except at their bases adjacent to the myocardium. No calcium was found in the cusps.

Discussion

Although the numbers of patients (10) and calves (7) involved in the present study were small, the results of morphologic examination of the seventeen tissue valves are quite clear. Whether in human subjects or in calves, the parietal pericardial and fascia lata valves appear to be poor substitutes for natural valves. The fresh pericardial mitral valve in the patient was four times thicker than it had been when inserted only 39 days before death. Similar thickening and focal calcification of pericardial valves have been observed by others.[8, 9] The thickening appeared to result from deposition of successive layers of fibrin which were transformed into fibrous tissue. In each of the 2 calves

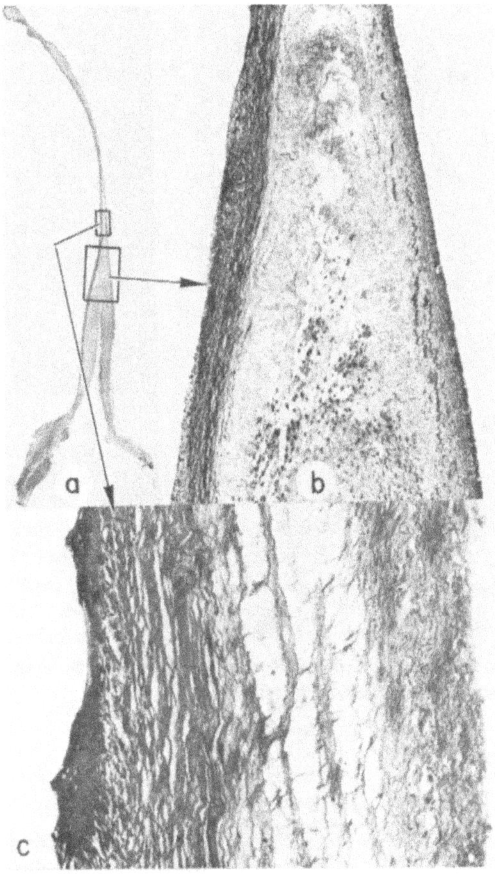

Fig. 9. Formalin-fixed porcine aortic valve implanted in a patient 150 days before his death. *a,* Low-power photomicrograph of one cusp. It is quite edematous. *b,* Close-up of area shown in *brackets* in *a.* Mononuclear cells infiltrate the core of the cusps, and that portion near the margins is totally necrotic. The core portion of the cusp is severely edematous. *c,* Close-up view of another area in *brackets* shown in *a.* The cusp in this area is totally necrotic, devoid of cells, and covered on one surface by a fibrin thrombus. (Hematoxylin and eosin stains. Original magnifications: *a,* ×5; *b,* ×63; *c,* ×250.)

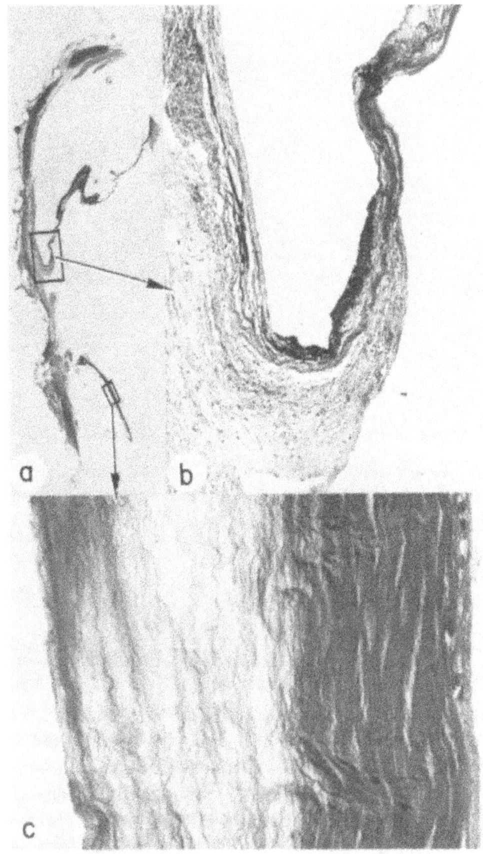

Fig. 10. Formalin-fixed porcine aortic valve implanted in a patient 240 days before his death. *a,* Section includes portions of aorta and of two cusps. A close-up of one area in *brackets* is shown in *b.* Fibrin thrombus is present on the aortic surface of this cusp near its attachment to the aorta. Inflammatory cells also are present in the cusp at this point. *c,* Close-up of another area in *brackets.* Here the cusp is totally necrotic and devoid of cells. (Hematoxylin and eosin stains. Original magnifications: *a,* ×5; *b,* ×63; *c,* ×310.)

that survived over 7 days with fresh pericardial valves, portions of the cusps became detached and both valves were necrotic. It is probable that infective endocarditis caused the major portion of the destruction in each of these animals, but that was not proved.

All three fascia lata valves, whether implanted when fresh or after glutaraldehyde fixation, became rigid, their orifices stenotic, and the tissue necrotic. The rigidity was due to deposition of fibrous tissue and extensive calcific deposits on the surfaces of the fascia lata cusps. The stenosis was produced by the rigidity of the cusps and by the presence of large mycotic thrombi obstructing the orifices (in 2 of the 3 calves). The cause of the latter in each was Candida species infection. Thus, the tissue valves were sites of infection in 4 of the 7 calves: The cusps were extensively damaged, and the valves were made purely incompetent in each of the 2 animals with pericardial valves; however, in the 2 with fascia lata valves, the

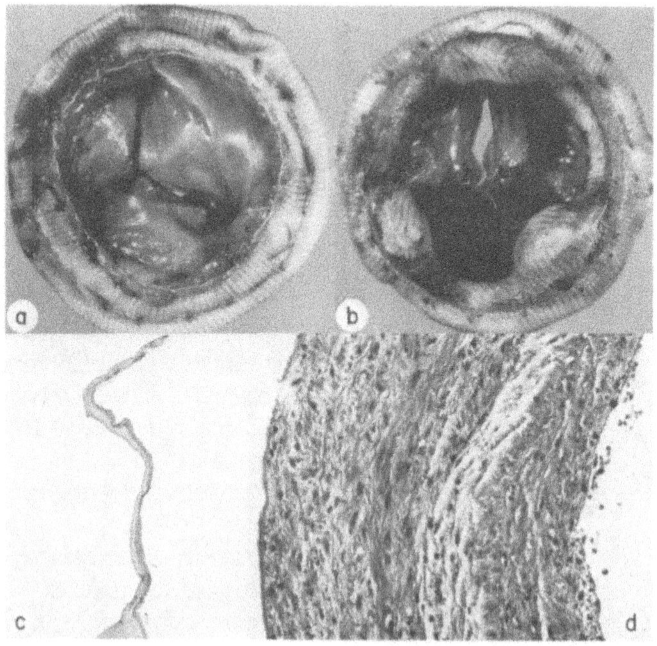

Fig. 11. Glutaraldehyde-fixed porcine aortic valve implanted in the mitral position of a 44-year-old man 14 days before his death. Preoperatively he had severe mitral stenosis. His postoperative course was so smooth that he was discharged 12 days after operation. He collapsed suddenly at home 2 days later and died immediately. *a,* View of valve from left atrium. *b,* View from left ventricle. The cusps are freely movable and devoid of thrombus. *c,* Photomicrograph of section through one cusp. *d,* Close-up view shows many cells and no necrosis. These leaflets appear well preserved. (Hematoxylin and eosin stains. Original magnifications: *c,* ×10; *d,* ×290.)

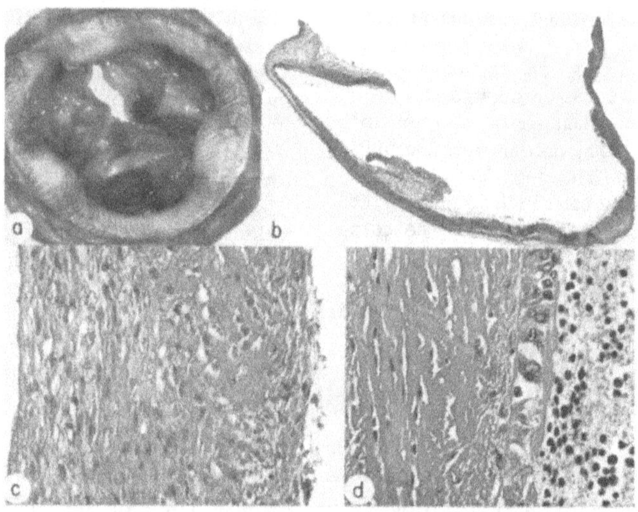

Fig. 12. Glutaraldehyde-fixed porcine aortic valve implanted into tricuspid valve position in a 50-year-old woman 39 days before her death. There was no evidence of dysfunction of this valve in the postoperative period. *a,* View of valve as it appeared from right ventricle. The cusps are freely mobile. *b,* Photomicrograph of section of one cusp. The cusps are focally but minimally thickened. A small thrombus adheres to one surface. *c,* Close-up view through one area of cusp shows near normal appearance. *d,* Close-up view of another area of the same cusp. Here the surface of the cusp is covered by mesothelial-like cells. (Hematoxylin and eosin stains. Original magnifications: *b,* ×20; *c* and *d,* ×400.)

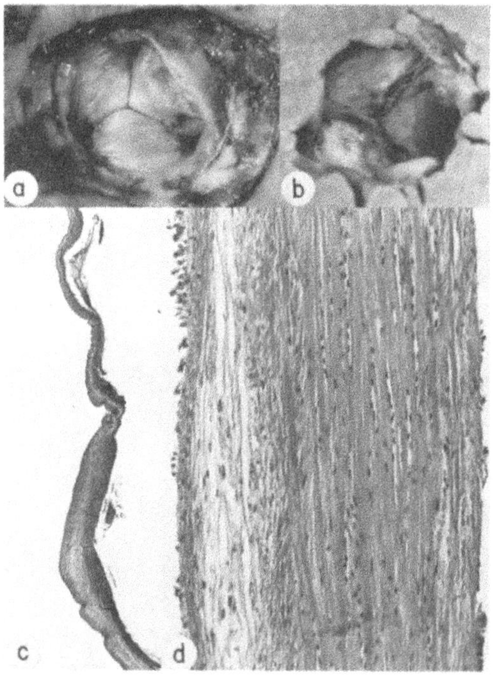

Fig. 13. Glutaraldehyde-fixed porcine aortic valve implanted in the mitral position in a 60-year-old man for pure mitral regurgitation. He died 50 days after the valve replacement, having been unconscious for 45 days. This implanted valve appeared to have functioned normally during the entire postoperative period. *a*, Implanted valve as viewed from left atrium. *b*, Same valve as viewed from left ventricle. The orifice is competent and the leaflets are freely mobile. *c*, Some portions of the leaflets are thickened. A close-up view of a portion of one cusp is shown in *d*. The valve appears well preserved. (Hematoxylin and eosin stains. Original magnifications: *c*, ×11; *d*, ×160.)

infective process formed larger mycotic masses which caused the orifices to be stenotic. Although infection involving a Starr-Edwards caged-ball prosthesis occurs at the site of attachment of the prosthetic valve to the natural valve annulus,[10, 11] the infection in the four tissue valves involved only the cusps. No infection was present beneath the prosthetic rings. The tissue valve may be particularly susceptible to infection by Candida species.[12]

The most rigid of all the tissue valves utilized in this study were the glutaraldehyde-fixed fascia lata valves. These valves were stiff at the time of implantation. They were utilized in 7 calves, but 5 of the animals died of acute pulmonary edema (probably from stenosis of the fascia lata valves) shortly after implantation. These 5 were not included in this study. The 2 included in this study lived 48 and 52 days, respectively, but each animal was in severe congestive cardiac failure during the entire postoperative period. The fresh fascia lata valve utilized in 1 calf in this study was quite mobile at the time of implantation, but it too was stiff and nonmobile when examined 80 days after implantation. McEnany and associates[13] recently reviewed their results with autologous fascia lata mitral valves in 72 patients. In the 53 operative survivors, 60 per cent were dysfunctioning to varying degrees up to 2 years. These authors concluded that fascial valves were poor substitutes for the natural valves when used in the mitral position. This valve has become altered after insertion in the aortic position also.[12, 14]

The porcine aortic valve appears to be a good substitute tissue valve if fixed in glutaraldehyde but a poor substitute if fixed in formalin. Each of the three formalin-fixed porcine valves evaluated in this study partially tore from its attachment between 90 and 150 days after implantation, causing severe valvular regurgitation in each. In contrast to the pericardial and fascia lata valves, the formalin-fixed porcine valves remained freely mobile. However, they appeared necrotic on histologic examination.

The glutaraldehyde-fixed porcine valves may well prove to be good substitute tissue valves. None of the 6 patients in this study who had these valves had evidence of valvular dysfunction postoperatively. Furthermore, these valves now have been implanted in 64 other patients by one of us (R. L. R.), and there has been no clinical evidence of valve dysfunction in any after a 20 month follow-up period. Examination of the glutaraldehyde-fixed porcine aortic valves utilized in the 6 patients and in 1 calf in this study showed that only minimal thickening occurred, and most areas of the cusps appeared well preserved by light microscopy. The cusps in all 7 subjects

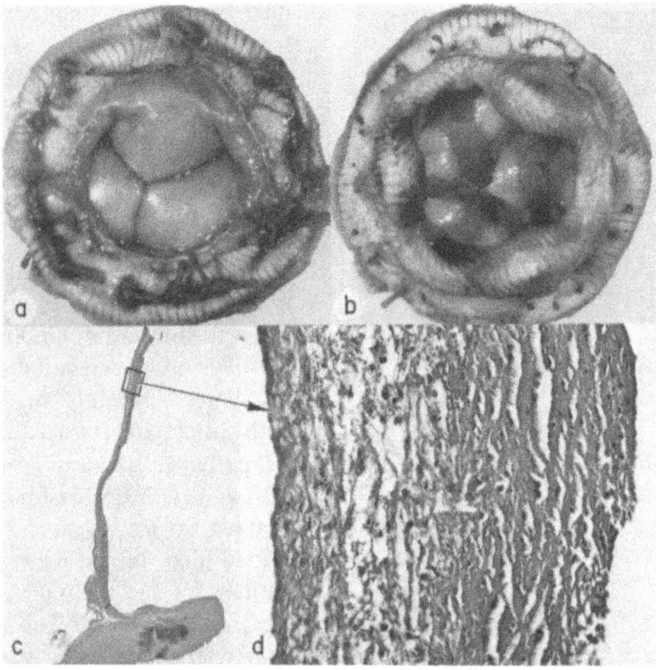

Fig. 14. Glutaraldehyde-fixed porcine aortic valve implanted in the mitral position in a 55-year-old woman for severe mitral stenosis 130 days before her death. This patient appeared to die from parenchymal pulmonary disease. There was no evidence that the implanted valve functioned abnormally at any time during the postoperative period. *a*, Implanted valve as viewed from left atrium. *b*, Valve as viewed from left ventricle. *c*, Photomicrograph of section of one cusp of the implanted valve. The cusps are not thickened and are freely mobile. *d*, Close-up of an area of the cusp. The cells are well preserved, but the cusp is probably focally edematous. (Hematoxylin and eosin stains. Original magnifications: *c*, ×11; *d*, ×370.)

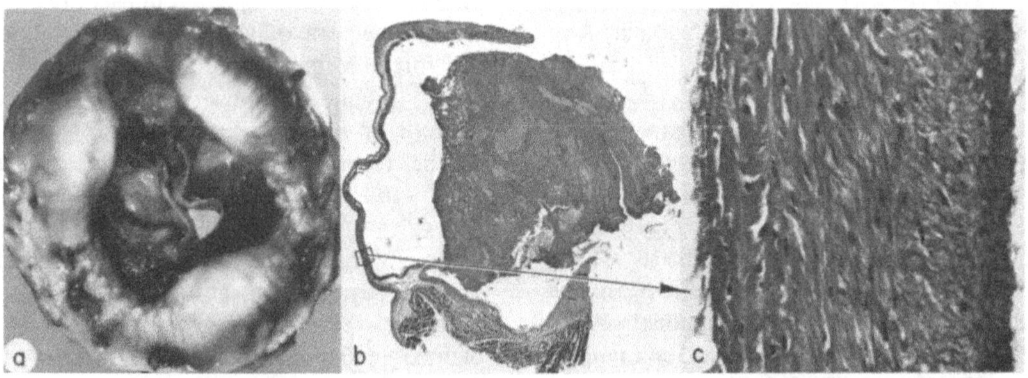

Fig. 15. Glutaraldehyde-fixed porcine aortic valve implanted in the aortic position for pure aortic regurgitation in a 51-year-old man 150 days before his death. This patient was asymptomatic postoperatively. He was found dead in bed at home. The cause of the sudden unexpected death is unclear. *a*, At necropsy, a thrombus filled one of the three sinuses of the implanted aortic valve. One week before he died, a 35 mm. Hg peak systolic pressure gradient was found between the left ventricle and brachial artery. The sinus thrombus may have accounted for the pressure gradient. *b*, Photomicrograph of section through implanted valve cusp and sinus thrombus. The distal portion of the cusp is mildly thickened. *c*, Close-up view of portion of cusp. The valve appears well preserved. (Hematoxylin and eosin stains. Original magnifications: *a* and *b*, ×11; *c*, ×400.)

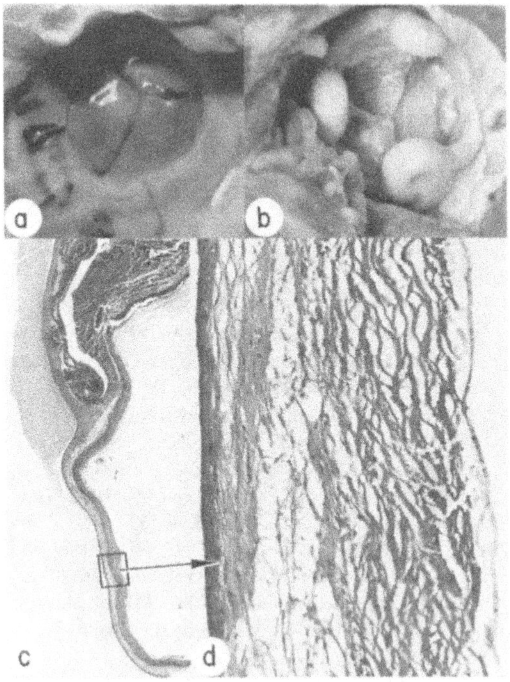

Fig. 16. Glutaraldehyde-fixed porcine aortic valve implanted into the mitral position of a calf 110 days before death. The valve functioned normally during the entire postoperative period. *a*, Implanted valve as viewed from left atrium. *b*, Valve as viewed from left ventricle. *c*, Photomicrograph of section through one cusp. *d*, Close-up view of portion of cusp. The valve cusps were freely mobile. The valve appears quite edematous and contains fewer cells than normally. (Hematoxylin and eosin stains. Original magnifications: *c*, ×10; *d*, ×160.)

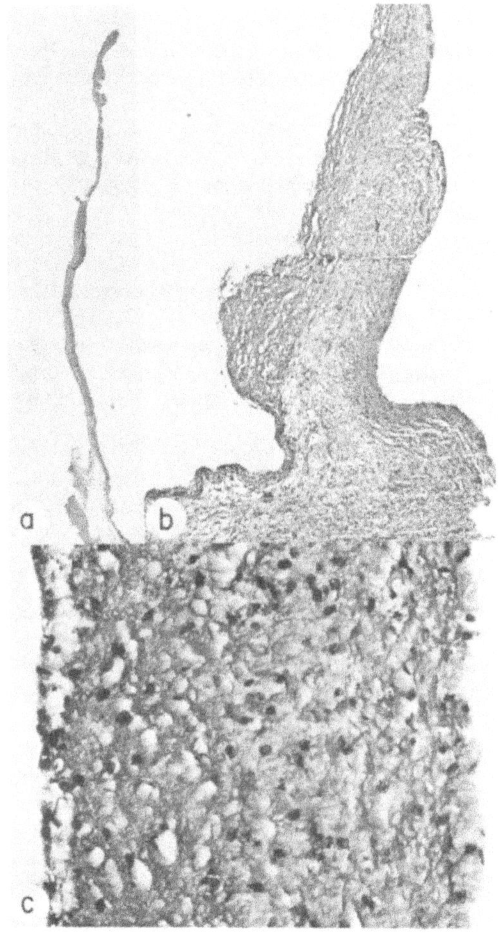

Fig. 17. Section of a control porcine aortic valve fixed in stabilized glutaraldehyde but never implanted. *a*, Portion of a cusp straightened out. *b*, Higher-power view of base of another cusp. *c*, Close-up view of portion of one cusp. Compared to this and other control valves the glutaraldehyde fixed porcine valves showed the collagen fibers in the cusps to be aligned in a radial fashion. The collagen in the control valve, as shown here, has a more disorganized appearance. Although they did elongate, the nuclei of the glutaraldehyde-fixed valves were better maintained than the more spherical nuclei of the control valves as shown here. (Hematoxylin and eosin stains. Original magnifications: *a*, ×8; *b*, ×63; *c*, ×400.)

were freely mobile and competent at necropsy. Death in the 6 patients was due to factors unrelated to the tissue valve.

Summary

Morphologic observations have been presented on tissue valves implanted in 10 patients and in 7 calves for periods ranging from 7 to 240 days. It appears that fresh autogenous pericardium, fresh autogenous or glutaraldehyde-fixed human fascia lata, and formalin-fixed porcine aortic valves are unacceptable substitutes for the natural cardiac valves when prepared by these methods. In contrast, the relatively minimal histologic changes in the glutaraldehyde-fixed porcine aortic valves and the lack of signs of dysfunction for up to 20 months after implantation offer encouragement that this tissue valve will prove to be a good valve substitute.

REFERENCES

1 Gerbode, F., editor: Proceedings of the First International Workshop on Tissue Valves, October 4-5, 1969, Ann. Surg. **172:** 1, 1970.

2 O'Brien, M. F.: Heterograft Aortic Valves for Human Use: Valve Bank, Techniques of Measurement, and Implantation, J. THORAC. CARDIOVASC. SURG. **53:** 392, 1967.

3 Ionescu, M. I., Mashhour, Y. A. S., and Uboler, G. H.: Reconstructed Heterograft Aortic Valves for Human Use, Thorax **23:** 221, 1968.

4 Buch, W. C., Kosek, J. C., and Angell, W. W.: Deterioration of Formalin-Treated Aortic Valve Heterografts, J. THORAC. CARDIOVASC. SURG. **60:** 673, 1970.

5 Carpentier, A., Lemaigre, G., Robert, L., Carpentier, S., and Dubost, C.: Biological Factors Affecting Long-Term Results of Valvular Heterografts, J. THORAC. CARDIOVASC. SURG. **58:** 467, 1969.

6 Reis, R. L., Hancock, W. D., Yarbrough, J. W., Glancy, D. L., and Morrow, A. G.: The Flexible Stent: A New Concept in the Fabrication of Tissue Valve Prostheses, J. THORAC. CARDIOVASC. SURG. **62:** 683, 1971.

7 Kaiser, G. A., Hancock, W. D., Lukban, S. B., and Litwak, R. S.: Clinical Use of a New Design Stented Xenograft Heart Valve Prosthesis, Surg. Forum **20:** 137, 1969.

8 Suzuki, A., Mackrell, J., and Kay, E. B.: Mitral Valve Replacement With Transplant Valves, J. THORAC. CARDIOVASC. SURG. **60:** 13, 1970.

9 Björk, V. O., and Hultquist, G.: Teflon and Pericardial Aortic Valve Prostheses, J. THORAC. CARDIOVASC. SURG. **47:** 693, 1964.

10 Cohn, L. H., Roberts, W. C., Rockoff, S. D., and Morrow, A. G.: Bacterial Endocarditis Following Aortic Valve Replacement: Clinical and Pathologic Correlations, Circulation **33:** 209, 1966.

11 Roberts, W. C., and Morrow, A. G.: Bacterial Endocarditis Involving Prosthetic Mitral Valves: Clinical and Pathologic Observations, Arch. Pathol. **82:** 164, 1966.

12 Hudson, R. E. B.: Pathology of Heart Valve Grafting, *in* Ionescu, M. I., Ross, D. N., and Wooler, G. H., editors: Biological Tissue in Heart Valve Replacement, London, 1972, Butterworth & Co., Ltd., pp. 835-886.

13 McEnany, M. T., Ross, D. N., and Yates, A. K.: Valve Failure in Seventy-Two Frame-Supported Autologous Fascia Lata Mitral Valves: Two-Year Follow-Up, J. THORAC. CARDIOVASC. SURG. **63:** 199, 1972.

14 Silver, M. D., and Trimble, A. S.: Structure of Autologous Fascia Lata Heart Valve Prostheses, Arch. Pathol. **93:** 109, 1972.

Pathologic Anatomy of Cardiac Valve Replacement: A Study of 224 Necropsy Patients

William C. Roberts, Bernadine H. Bulkley, and Andrew G. Morrow

DURING THE PAST 12 YR numerous reports have described the use of prostheses of various types to replace malfunctioning cardiac valves. Most valvular prostheses have been evaluated in terms of clinical and hemodynamic improvement, and less attention has been given to alterations observed at necropsy. This report focuses attention on findings at necropsy in 224 patients who died after replacement of one or more cardiac valves at the National Heart and Lung Institute from 1963 through October 1972.

PATIENTS STUDIED

The 224 patients were divided into two groups: (1) 128 patients dying within 2 mo of operation (early deaths), and (2) 96 patients dying at later periods up to 116 mo (late deaths). Not included among the 224 patients were three who died during operation before valve replacement could be carried out: One had cardiac arrest during thoracotomy and two had acute dissection of the entire aorta with compression-occlusion of the coronary arteries immediately after cardiopulmonary bypass was instituted. The cardiac valves replaced in the 224 patients are listed in Table 1.* All patients were in functional classes III or IV (New York Heart Association Classification) before operation. The ages and sexes of the patients are summarized in Table 2. Of the 224 patients, 141 (63%) were males and 83 (37%) were females; their ages ranged from 4–69 yr (average 46). The functional valve lesions necessitating valve replacement are summarized in Table

---

From the Section of Pathology and the Clinic of Surgery, National Heart and Lung Institute, National Institutes of Health, Bethesda, Md.

William C. Roberts, M.D.: *Chief, Section of Pathology, National Heart and Lung Institute, National Institutes of Health, Bethesda, Md.; Associate Professor of Pathology and Medicine (Cardiology), Georgetown University School of Medicine, Washington, D.C.* Bernadine H. Bulkley, M.D.: *Staff Associate, Section of Pathology, National Heart and Lung Institute, National Institutes of Health, Bethesda, Md.* Andrew G. Morrow, M.D.: *Chief, Clinic of Surgery, National Heart and Lung Institute, National Institutes of Health, Bethesda, Md.*

Reprint requests should be addressed to William C. Roberts, M.D., Building 10A, Room 3E-30, National Heart and Lung Institute, National Institutes of Health, Bethesda, Md. 20014.

*Tables 1–23 are compiled in the appendix at the end of this paper, pp. 575–585.

3. All 224 patients had undergone cardiac catheterization preoperatively. Of 281 valves replaced, stenosis of some degree occurred in 194 valves (69%), and the remaining 87 valves (31%) were purely incompetent. There was no correlation between the functional valve lesion and the incidence of early or late death. Most stenotic valves also were incompetent, and in some the predominant hemodynamic lesion was regurgitation rather than stenosis. All purely regurgitant valves had no pressure gradients across them.

The *etiology of the valvular lesions* was variable. Most patients undergoing isolated aortic valve replacement for either stenosis or pure regurgitation had nonrheumatic lesions:[1-3] Congenitally malformed valves, particularly the bicuspid condition, was the most common cause of isolated aortic stenosis. Of 29 patients undergoing valve replacement for isolated pure aortic regurgitation, the etiology was rheumatic in ten (each also had anatomic disease of the mitral valve), "cystic medial necrosis" of aorta in four (three had the Marfan syndrome), healed infective endocarditis in five (on congenitally malformed valves in three and on previously normally formed valves in two), congenitally bicuspid valve (never the site of infection) in one, prolapsed aortic cusp associated with ventricular septal defect in three, unknown in three, and syphilis, arteriosclerosis, and ankylosing spondylitis, one each. Combined mitral and aortic disease and combined mitral, aortic, and tricuspid disease was nearly always rheumatic in origin. Mitral stenosis was of rheumatic origin in all subjects. Sixteen of 17 patients in whom the tricuspid valve was replaced also had mitral stenosis; the seventeenth had tricuspid valve was replaced also had mitral stenosis; the seventeenth had tricuspid valve replacement only after he was unable to come off cardiac bypass after aortic valve replacement. Of the 24 patients undergoing replacement for isolated pure mitral regurgitation, the etiology was rheumatic or probably rheumatic in 12, congenital endocardial fibroelastosis in two, ruptured chordae tendineae on previously normal valves (secondary to healed infective endocarditis,[4]) in five, floppy mitral valve in one, cleft mitral valve associated with ostium primum defect in one, papillary muscle fibrosis secondary to coronary heart disease in one, hypertrophic (asymmetric) cardiomyopathy in one, and unknown in one. Both patients with primary muscle disease, hypertrophic cardiomyopathy or papillary muscle dysfunction, died early.

The 281 prosthetic valves used in the 224 patients are shown in Table 4. The sizes of the 250 Starr-Edwards prostheses employed are summarized in Table 5. There was no correlation between the size of the prosthetic valve utilized and the incidence of early or late death. In addition to one or more valve replacements in the 224 patients, valve annuloplasty or commissurotomy also was performed in 13 patients, 12 of whom died early. Four other patients, each of whom had pure aortic regurgitation had their ascending aortas replaced with grafts: Two died early and two died late; three had aortic "cystic medial necrosis," and the fourth had syphilis.

Accurate[5] weights of the hearts in the 224 patients are summarized in Table 6. No significant difference was noted between the weights of hearts of those patients dying early and those dying late when corresponding sexes and similarly replaced valves were compared.

Significant extramural coronary arterial luminal narrowing occurred in 36 (16%) of the 224 patients (Table 7). At least one of the three major extramural coronary arteries (right, anterior descending and left circumflex) was narrowed > 75% by old plaques in each of the 36 patients. The per cent of patients with this degree of narrowing in both early and late death groups were similar: 15% in the former and 18% in the latter. The average age of these 36 patients was 52 yr; 30 were men and six were women. Only one was < 40 yr of age, and he was a 26-yr-old man who had coronary arterial narrowing secondary to an embolus dislodged from vegetations on the aortic valve; the embolus subsequently organized. Only 10 of the 36 patients with severe coronary arterial luminal narrowing by old lesions had healed transmural infarcts; nine others had subendocardial free wall scars.

Embolic material was found in *intramural coronary arteries* on histologic sections* in 12 of 128 patients (9%) dying early and in 9 of 96 patients (9%) dying late after valve replacement. The embolic material consisted of *calcium* in seven patients, *foreign particle* (refractile anisotropic material), probably silicone,[6] in seven, *fibrin-platelets* in five, both calcium and foreign particle in one, and *bone marrow* in one. Excision of the cardiac valves *intact* at operation may lower the frequency of calcific emboli.[7] The most common site of emboli to intramural coronary arteries was left ventricular papillary muscle. The myocardium adjacent to the occluded artery often was focally necrotic or fibrotic.

Aschoff bodies were observed on histologic section in only two of the 224 patients. Each died early and each had anatomic disease of both mitral and aortic valves.

Various findings in patients dying early are illustrated in Figs. 1–19 and in those dying late, in Figs. 20–40.

ANALYSIS OF THE EARLY POSTOPERATIVE DEATHS

The intervals between operation and death (prosthetic valve implantation periods) in the 128 patients dying within 2 mo of operation are summarized in Table 8. Seventy-eight patients (61%) died within 1 wk, and 93 of the 128 patients (72%), within 2 wk of operation. The prime causes of death (one principal cause per patient) are shown in Table 9. The per cent of patients dying from *prosthetic dysfunction* was 28%. In the early experience with cardiac valve replacement with rigid frame prostheses, relatively large-sized prostheses were employed, and not infrequently the prostheses utilized were too large for either the left ventricle or aortic root into which they were inserted[8–12] (Figs. 1–4). The motion of the poppets in these circumstances was limited. Beginning about 1965, efforts were made to use smaller protheses, and the mortality rate, particularly after mitral replacement, dropped. With the introduction of Starr-Edwards prostheses with fully cloth-covered struts and bases in 1967, (models 6300 and 2300), it became apparent[13,14] that the smaller mitral and aortic prostheses were inherently stenotic, and that stenosis probably worsened as tissue grew into the cloth bordering the orifice and also into the struts. By late 1968 the manufacturer had widened the orifice areas of these prostheses (models 6310 and 2310). Prosthetic

*A total of 1310 histologic sections of myocardium were reexamined in the 224 patients. This averaged 5.9 sections of heart in each patient. In most patients at least one section from the wall of each cardiac chamber was examined; in all patients at least one section of left ventricular wall was studied.

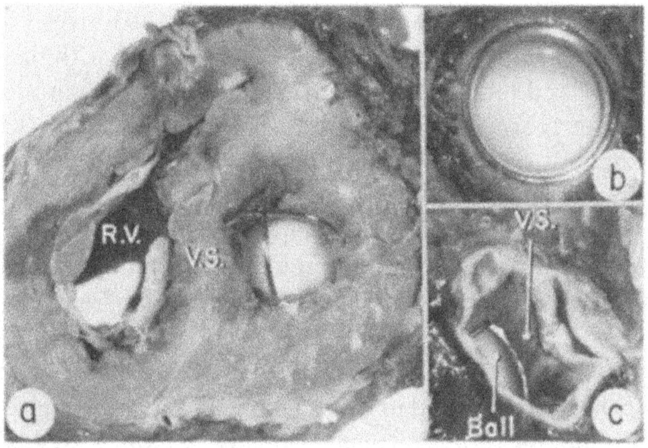

Fig. 1. Prosthetic dysfunction. Heart (weight = 360 g) of a cachectic, functionally class IV, 57-yr-old man with severe mitral stenosis preoperatively. Following replacement of mitral valve with size 3M Starr-Edwards prosthesis, patient was unable to come off cardiopulmonary bypass and died in operating room. At autopsy (A65-170), the mitral prosthesis was shown after transverse sectioning of ventricles (A) to be too large for left ventricular cavity. Ventricular septum (V.S.) protruded into mitral cage almost totally blocking motion of ball. In this patient there also appeared to be obstruction to left ventricular emptying. With the mitral ball in the closed position simulating ventricular systole (B), the photograph in C was taken. Following excision of the three aortic valve cusps, the mitral ball is seen almost to contact the muscular ventricular septum and obstruct the outflow tract. (By permission.[12])

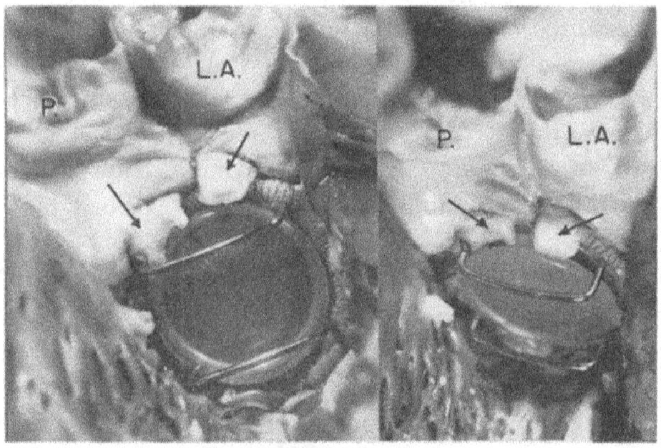

Fig. 2. Prosthetic dysfunction. Opened left ventricle and aortic valve in a 51-yr-old woman in whom the stenotic mitral valve was replaced with Kay-Shiley disc prosthesis. Her 3-day postoperative period was characterized by features of low cardiac output syndrome. At necropsy (A70-200), two fragments (arrows) of unexcised anterior mitral leaflet prevented complet‹ seating of disc during ventricular systole. Regurgitation, therefore, must have occurred, and this mechanical interference appears to be prime explanation for low cardiac output syndrome postoperatively. P. and L.A., posterior (non-coronary) and left anterior aortic valve cusps.

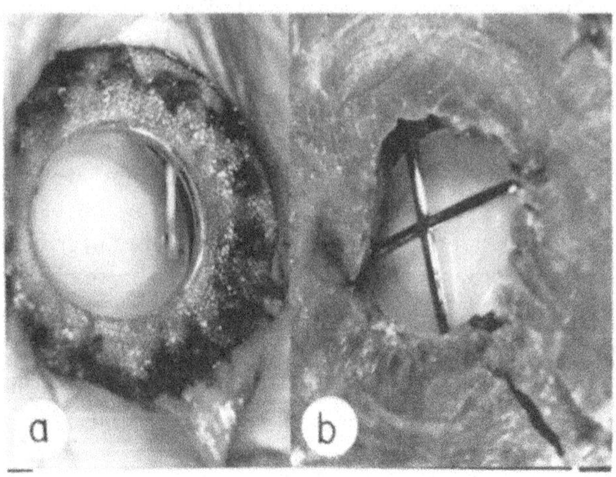

Fig. 3. Prosthetic dysfunction. Starr-Edwards mitral prostheses (model 6520, size 3M) implanted in this 38-yr-old man (A72-47) 48 hr before death. (A) Mitral valve as viewed from left atrium. A small chorda tendinea not excised at operation protrudes between disc and metallic base, causing incomplete closure. (B) Same valve viewed from left ventricle. Margins of the disc contact endocardium of left ventricle at most points. Death in this patient appears to be related to the prosthesis being too large for the left ventricle, causing obstruction to left atrial emptying.

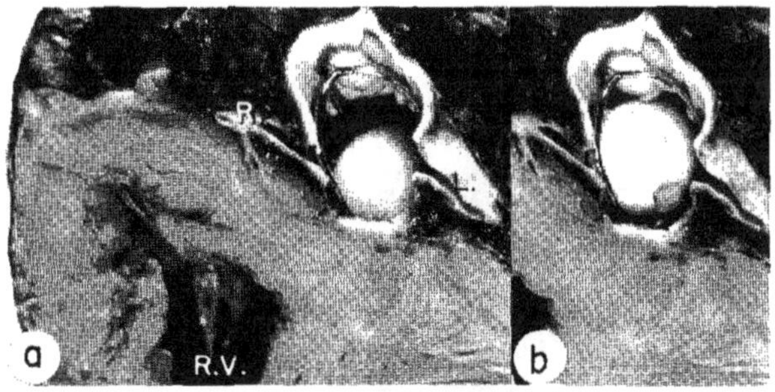

Fig. 4. Prosthetic dysfunction. Opened aortic valve in a 25-yr-old man (A65-133) with congenitally malformed mitral and aortic valves, causing severe mitral and aortic regurgitation and slight aortic stenosis. The aortic prosthesis, even though it is a small-sized one (8A Starr-Edwards), is too large for the aortic root. During simulated ventricular diastole (A) ball is seated, but during simulated ventricular systole (B) ball is prevented from ascending completely to apex of cage by wall of the aorta, which protrudes between two metallic struts, restricting ball movement in cage. A match head projects from the residual prosthetic orifice. R.V., right ventricle; R. and L., right and left coronary arteries.

dysfunction reappeared dramatically in mid-1970, however, when the manufacturer decreased the third-strut clearances (between the surface of the prosthetic aortic balls and the inner margins of the cloth-covered struts) from 0.040–0.070 to 0.008–0.020 inches (Figs. 5–8). Five deaths listed under "prosthetic dysfunction" in Table 9 resulted from this manufacturing error, which was corrected in late 1970. The current Starr-Edwards aortic valve (model 2320) has a third-strut clearance of 0.050–0.060 inches, except at its base, which has a smaller clearance. The cloth on this newer model also has been altered; polypropylene has been added to the Teflon on the struts and on the sewing ring. It is hoped that the polypropylene will decrease the frequency of strut cloth wear. The current Starr-Edwards mitral prosthesis (model 6320) has a uniform radial cage-to-ball clearance of 0.017–0.021 inches, and this clearance is maintained constant from base to dome. Polypropylene also has been added to its Teflon cloth. The metal struts have now been united at the domes of both new prostheses; in previous models the struts were held together at their domes only by cloth.

It is hazardous to implant a large-sized prosthesis into a relatively small-sized

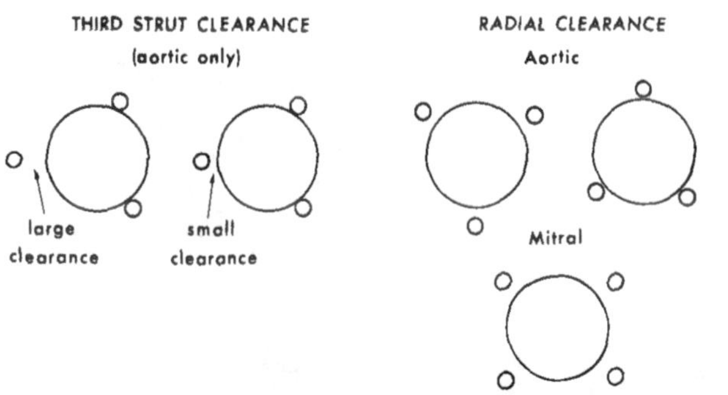

Fig. 5. Diagram to illustrate the concepts of third strut and radial clearance of caged-ball prostheses. With development of cloth-covered aortic prostheses, it was believed that large ball-to-cage third-strut clearance (distance between the surface of the prosthetic aortic ball and inner margin of strut) of earlier models would allow excessive lateral motion of ball and lead to cloth wear and chattering of metal ball within cage. Hence, to "guide" the poppet, the third-strut clearance of the model 2310 aortic prosthesis was decreased from 0.04–0.07 to 0.008–0.02 in. Growth of tissue over the cloth of the strut reduced third-strut clearance even further, causing the ball to stick in the mid-portion of the cage. In the model 2320, third-strut clearance was increased to 0.05–0.06 in, except at the base, where close-clearance was initially retained. Radial-cage-to-ball clearance of mitral valve also was decreased in some model 6310 cloth-covered prostheses, but current model 6320 has uniform radial-cage-to-ball clearance of 0.017–0.021 in.

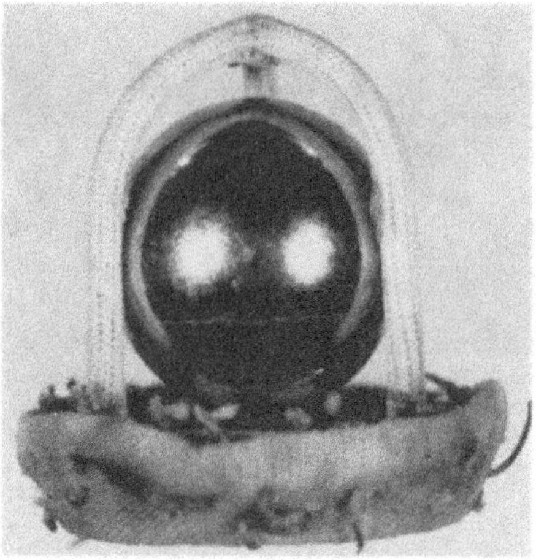

Fig. 6. Prosthetic dysfunction from close-clearance Starr-Edwards aortic prostheses, Aortic prosthesis (size 10A) in which the ball stuck in the mid-portion of cage. This 45-yr-old man died suddenly five days postoperatively. At necropsy (A70-227), ball was immobile as shown and a small thrombus was present on inner aspects of each of the three struts about midway between base and apex. The clearance between the surface of the ball and one strut when ball was pushed against the other two struts (so-called third-strut clearance) was only 4 mils when this prosthesis was manufactured.

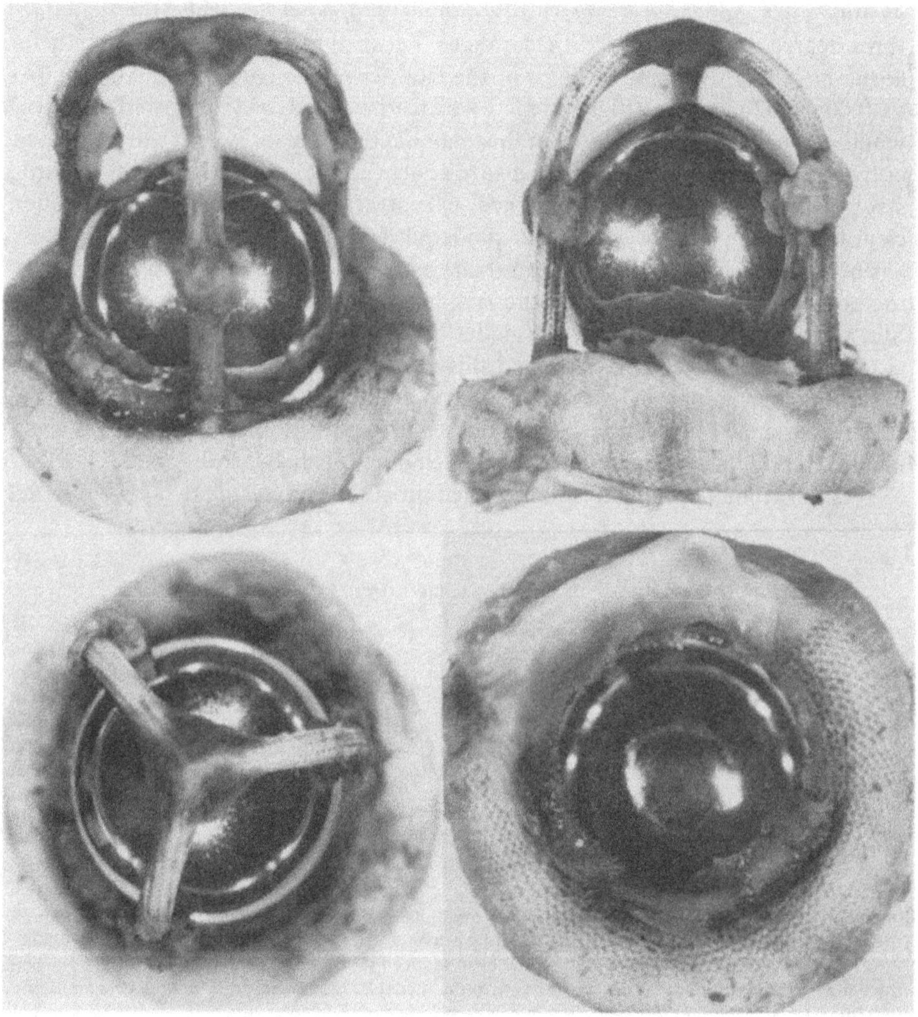

Fig. 7. Prosthetic stenosis due to thrombi on close-clearance Starr-Edwards aortic valve. This 29-yr-old man (A71-197) died suddenly 12 mo after replacement with a close-clearance Starr-Edwards cloth-covered aortic prosthesis (site 11A, Model 2310). Thrombi formed near junctions of the vertical and curved portions of strut, causing ball to stick in mid-position. He developed these prosthetic thrombi and renal embolism despite warfarin therapy.

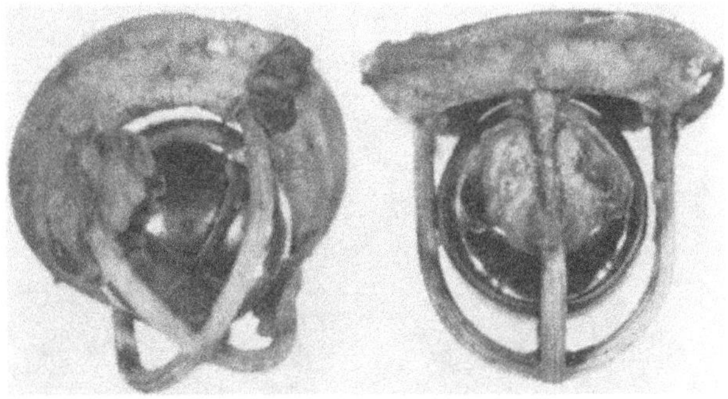

Fig. 8. Mitral prosthesis (size 3M) that developed thrombi on three of the four struts, causing immobility of the ball. This 56-yr-old man (A70-244) died 20 days postoperatively as a result of the ball's sticking. The exact clearance between the surface of the ball and the inner margins of the struts in this four-strut prosthesis is uncertain, but it is reduced. *Thrombi on mid-struts* unassociated with thrombi on bases of prostheses occur, in our experience, only in the close-clearance prosthesis manufactured in 1970.

left ventricle or ascending aorta. In 28 (Table 9) patients who died early, death was attributed at necropsy to prosthetic dysfunction because of disproportion between the size of the prosthesis and the size of the left ventricle (20 patients) or ascending aorta (eight patients) into which the prosthesis had been inserted. The 20 dysfunctioning mitral prostheses represent 24% of the 83 patients dying early after mitral replacement with rigid-framed prostheses. In 12 of the 20 patients, a 3M- or 4M-sized Starr-Edwards prosthesis had been utilized to replace a stenotic mitral valve. (The 3M Starr-Edwards prosthesis is too large for a normal-sized left ventricular cavity, and because this cavity is often of normal size in patients with isolated mitral stenosis, this prosthesis may be too large in this circumstance.) Disproportion between size of cavity and size of prosthesis was a less frequent cause of death among patients with aortic valve prostheses, representing 12% of 65 early deaths. Small-sized (7A, 8A or 2M) Starr-Edwards prostheses were used, however, in eight patients, and Kay-Shiley prostheses in two patients with prosthetic stenosis. Thus, it appears that some left ventricles and aortas are simply not large enough for rigid-framed prostheses. Central orifice prostheses are presently preferred in these selected patients.

Table 10 lists what was considered the principal cause of death in each patient. Nearly all patients dying several days or more after operation had evidence of "hepatic failure," "renal failure," or "pulmonary insufficiency." These manifestations do not represent failure of the particular organ, however, but are manifestations of that organ's inadequate arterial perfusion because of cardiac pump failure from known or unknown causes. With the exception of a few patients dying suddenly, presumably from arrhythmias, most patients dying early from the causes listed in Table 10 had evidence of *inadequate cardiac output* sometime in the postoperative period. Inadequate arterial perfusion to the lungs is usually manifested by *alveolar hemorrhage,*[15] (Fig. 19) and acute pneumonia is often superimposed. Inadequate arterial perfusion of the *liver* leads to *centrolobular hemorrhage, with or without necrosis* (Fig. 19), an anatomic picture identical to acute hepatic venous congestion. Inadequate arterial perfusion of the *kidneys* usually does not lead to histologically visible anatomic renal changes, probably because oliguria or anuria is not prolonged. True *hemoglobinuric nephrosis* (tubular necrosis) was infrequent. Inadequate perfusion of bowel may cause mucosal and submucosal hemorrhages (Fig. 19). Focal *left ventricular subendocardial and papillary muscle necrosis* (Fig. 19) occurred in many patients

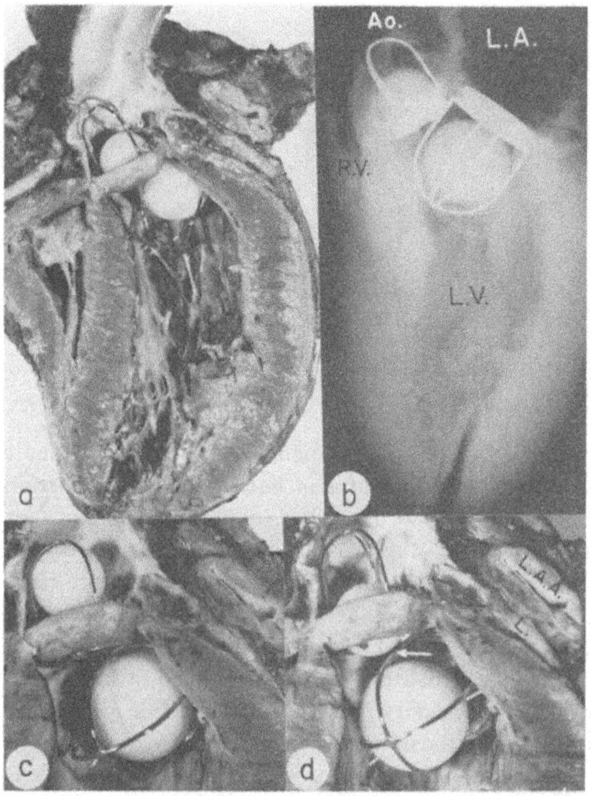

Fig. 9. Prosthetic dysfunction from contact of two prostheses. This 45-yr-old man underwent mitral and aortic valve replacement with Starr-Edwards prostheses for severe mitral and aortic regurgitation. After both valves had been inserted, there was evidence of regurgitation through or around the aortic prosthesis. A blowing diastolic murmur was audible along left sternal border postoperatively. Four days after the initial operation, thoracotomy was performed because of possibility of atrial thrombosis. No thrombus was found after left atriotomy, but there was massive regurgitation of blood from aorta into left ventricle. Refractory cardiac arrest occurred during procedure. Necropsy (A65-121) disclosed that both prostheses were securely sutured, and no peribasilar communications were present. The aortic regurgitation resulted from incomplete seating of the ball of the aortic prosthesis, which contacted one of the metallic struts of the mitral prosthesis during ventricular diastole. (A) Longitudinal section of the cardiac ventricles and aorta; (B) radiograph of the heart, again demonstrating the close proximity of the two prostheses to one another; (C and D) close-up views of the left ventricular outflow tract during simulated ventricular systole (C) and diastole (D). Arrow points to metallic strut of mitral cage, which contacted the aortic ball during ventricular diastole. Pressure in the aorta at beginning of ventricular diastole not only returned ball toward its seating position but, almost certainly, also caused movement of entire aortic prosthesis toward the left ventricle. Consequently, the aortic ball was prevented from seating by the mitral strut and aortic regurgitation resulted. Ao., aorta; R.V., right ventricle; L.V., left ventricle; L.A., left atrium; L.A.A., left atrial appendage; and L., left coronary artery. (By permission.[11])

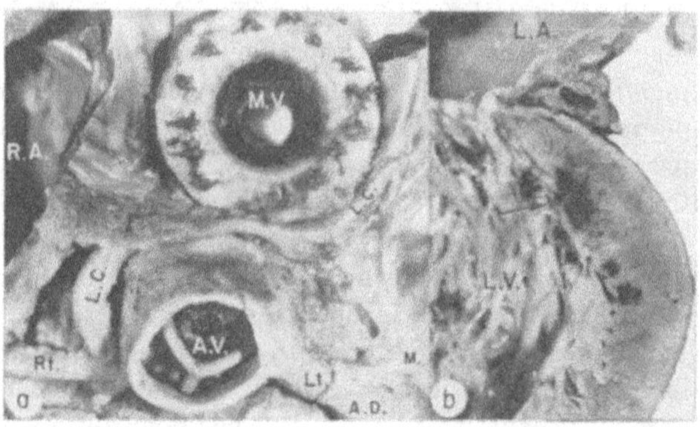

Fig. 10. Prosthetic dysfunction from compression of anomalous left circumflex (L.C.) coronary artery by rings of mitral (size 3M) (M.V.) and aortic (size 8A) (A.V.) Starr-Edwards prostheses. This 45-yr-old man with severe mitral and aortic regurgitation underwent double valve replacement 10 days before death. The entire postoperative period was characterized by features of low cardiac output syndrome. At necropsy (A68-22), the left circumflex (L.C.) coronary artery was found to arise from first portion of the right (Rt.) coronary artery and to course in groove between aortic root and base of the left atrium (L.A.) (A). This anomalously arising artery was compressed between rings of the two rigid-frame caged-ball prostheses. As a result, the lumen of the left circumflex coronary artery was occluded by this external compression leading to necrosis of the lateral wall of the left ventricle (L.V.) (B). R.A., right atrium; Lt., left main coronary artery; A.D., anterior descending coronary artery; and M., marginal coronary artery. (By permission.[9])

with the low cardiac output syndrome (Table 11). This necrosis may be simply the anatomic consequence of poor myocardial oxygenation, the result of inadequate coronary perfusion, although others[16–18] consider it the cause of the low cardiac output syndrome. Subendocardial and papillary muscle necrosis, in our view, is infrequently the cause of the low cardiac output syndrome, because it was seen as frequently in subjects having known anatomic causes of death, e.g., prosthetic dysfunction or bleeding, or associated uncorrected valve disease, etc. (see Table 8 or 10) as in those without an anatomic cause of death.

Focal myocardial necrosis of the stumps of the amputated left ventricular or right ventricular papillary muscles is to be expected after mitral and tricuspid valve replacements, respectively. The only exceptions occurred in patients dying very early (usually in the operating room) or who survived long enough for healing to occur. Also, nearly all patients had a drain inserted into the left ventricular cavity from its apex at operation. Consequently, nearly all patients dying early had transmural necrosis at the apex of the left ventricle, or, if they died late, transmural fibrosis, at this site. Necrosis or fibrosis at the left ventricular apex, therefore, was not included in the tabulations shown in Table 11. *Contraction bands*[19] appear to be the earliest lesion of myocardial necrosis in these patients. Calcification of individual necrotic myocardial fibers (Fig. 17) occurred in 12 patients. The cause of this *myocardial dystrophic calcification* is uncertain, but it probably results from myocardial ischemia because a similar lesion

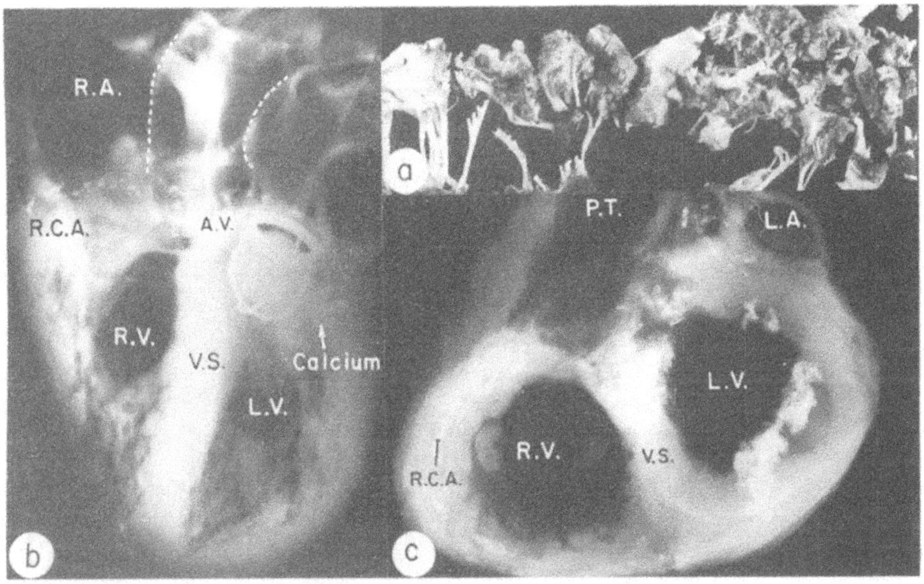

Fig. 11. Cerebral embolus after replacement of an extremely calcified, stenotic, and incompetent mitral valve, a complication of removing too little cardiac calcium. This 51-yr-old man (A66-150) never awakened postoperatively, and roentgenograms of the skull suggested a calcific embolus in the right middle cerebral artery; the embolus was found at necropsy 5 days after operation. Mitral valve was excised in numerous fragments (A), and presumably at least one escaped into the systemic circulation. (B) Radiograph shows considerable residual calcium in the mitral anulus and adjacent left ventricular myocardium, as well as in the aortic valve (A.V.) and right coronary artery (R.C.A.). The prosthesis is size 3M. (C) Radiograph of cephalad portions of cardiac ventricles and of both atria and great vessels. Amount of mitral calcific deposits remaining is very large. (By permission.[8])

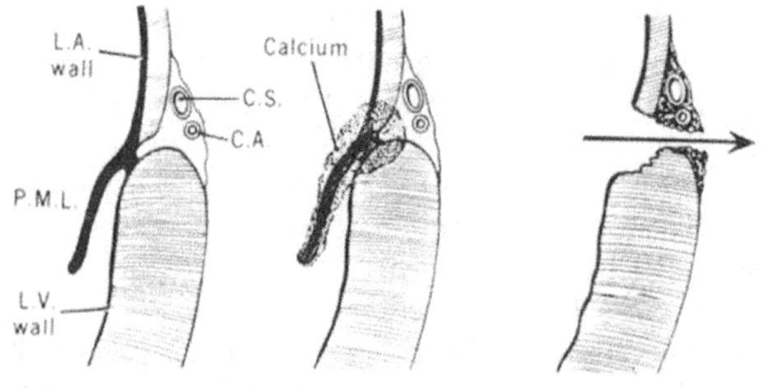

Fig. 12. Rupture of the heart at the left atrioventricular sulcus, a complication of removing too much mitral valvular calcium. If mitral leaflet calcium extends into the anulus, the surgeon will be unable to remove the deposit completely. If all mitral anular calcium is removed, as attempted in one patient, the left atrial wall may be separated from the left ventricular wall with massive bleeding. This diagram also depicts how the left atrial (L.A.) myocardium normally is totally separated from the left ventricular (L.V.) wall. The posterior mitral leaflet (P.M.L.) is formed by the junction of endocardium from the left atrium and left ventricle. C.S., coronary sinus; C.A., coronary artery.

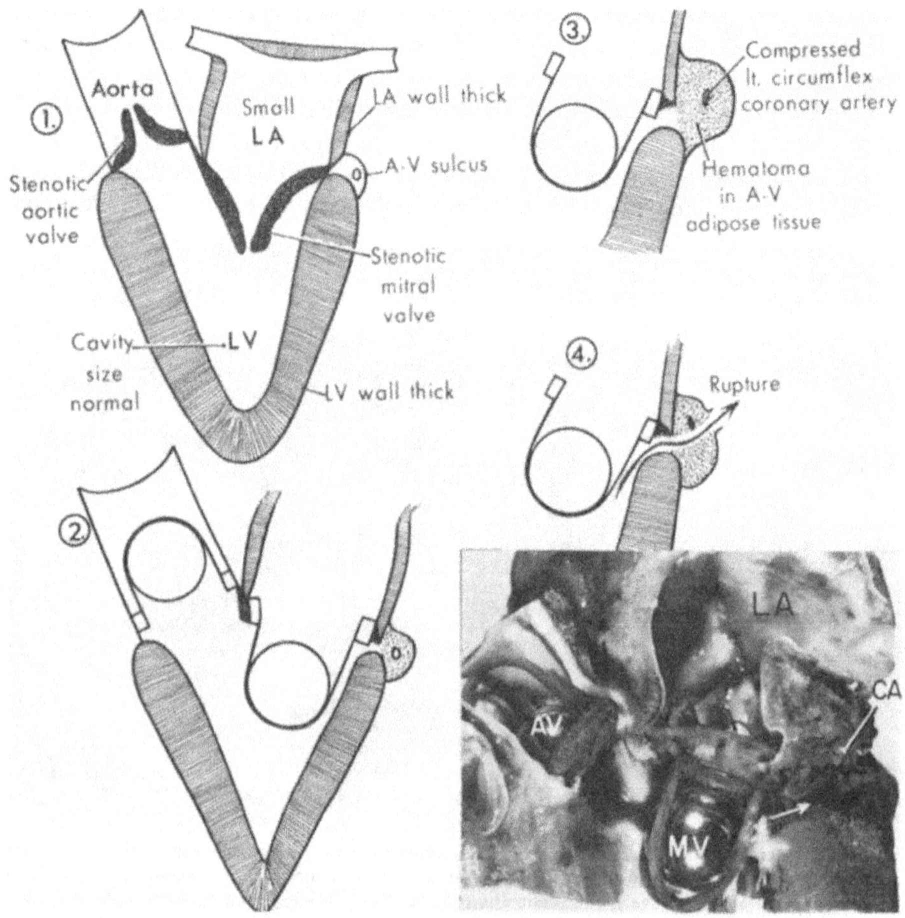

Fig. 13. Rupture of left atrioventricular (AV) sulcus during excision of mitral valve in a 57-yr-old woman (A72-1?4) with combined mitral and aortic stenosis. She died of "low cardiac output syndrome" 2 days after replacement of both valves (9A and 2M Starr-Edwards prostheses). The normal size of the left atrium prevented good exposure of the mitral valve from the interatrial groove incision and a portion of anulus was excised during excision of the valve leading to disruption of the left AV sulcus.

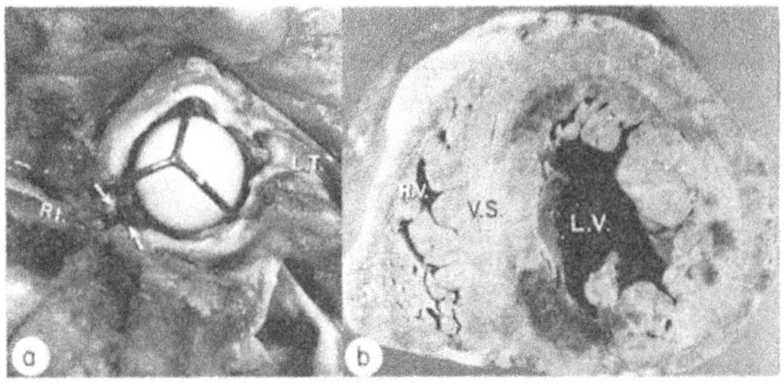

Fig. 14. Thrombotic occlusion of the proximal right coronary artery after replacement of mitral (size 2M) and aortic (size 8A) valves with Starr-Edwards prostheses. This patient's entire 6-day postoperative period was characterized by features of the low *cardiac output syndrome*. At necropsy (A67-207), a thrombus (between the arrows) was present in the mouth of the right (Rt.) coronary artery, having extended cephalad from the base of the prosthetic aortic valve (A). Several foci of necrosis were present in the left ventricular (L.V.) wall, and the largest one was in the posteroseptal wall (B). Many necrotic myocardial fibers were calcified (see Fig. 17). Lt., left coronary artery; R.V., right ventricle; and V.S., ventricular septum.

can be produced in myocardium of dogs by anoxia.[20] Determinations postoperatively of serum calcium, phosphorus, and magnesium in four of these 12 patients were normal.

Intramyocardial hemorrhage (Fig. 18) occurred in all patients dying within 7 days of operation. Intramyocardial hemorrhage occurred adjacent to all incisions in the walls of cardiac chambers. In all subjects in whom the atrium was entered via a dissection into the interatrial groove, bleeding of considerable extent occurred in the atrial septum. The extravasated blood not infrequently extended caudally into the area of the atrioventricular (AV) node or bundle or both. Extravasated blood usually occurred in the area of the AV node or bundle after aortic valve replacement because of the proximity of the valve and the conduction

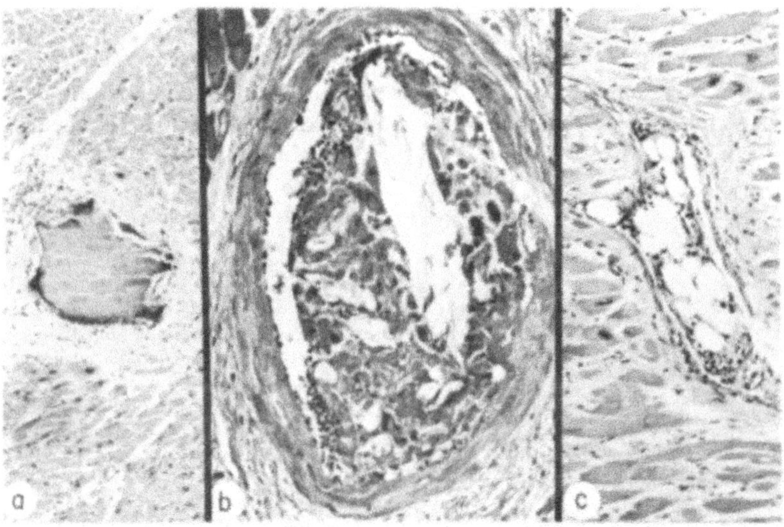

Fig. 15. Emboli to intramural coronary arteries. The emboli were of various types and probably most occurred at or shortly after valve replacement. (A) Calcific embolus in 60-yr-old woman (A64-225) in whom a heavily calcified, bicuspid, stenotic, aortic valve was replaced 20 mo earlier. (B) Foreign particle embolus in a 46-yr-old man (A69-33) in whom a heavily calcified predominantly incompetent mitral valve was excised 6 days before death. (C) Bone marrow embolus in a 41-yr-old man (A65-102) who underwent aortic valve replacement 7 days before death because of pure aortic regurgitation. Hematoxylin and eosin stains. (A) × 99, (B) × 250, (C) × 160.

tissue. Petechiae occurred also on endocardium and epicardium of nearly all patients dying early. Epicardial, myocardial, and endocardial hemorrhages were more frequent and extensive after cardiac massage.

ANALYSIS OF THE LATE POSTOPERATIVE DEATHS

The pertinent clinical and pathologic data in the 96 patients dying later than 2 mo after valve replacement are summarized in Tables 12 and 13.[21,22]

Causes of Death

These are listed (one principal cause per patient) in Table 13. *Forty patients died suddenly* and unexpectedly without preceding periods of congestive cardiac failure postoperatively. The aortic valve had been replaced in 30 of the 40 patients (six also had had mitral replacement), nine had had isolated mitral replacement, and one had had both mitral and tricuspid valves replaced. Either swelling and impaction (seven patients) or dislodgment (six patients) of aortic silicone rubber balls caused death in 13 patients. Five patients had coronary arterial emboli. No recent anatomic cardiac lesion was observed in the remaining 22 patients: Two of them, however, had severely narrowed coronary arterial ostia, and six others had severe (>75%) luminal narrowing by old plaques of one or more of the three major coronary arteries; two others had cloth-covered prosthetic aortic valves known to be moderately stenotic (50 mm Hg peak systolic pressure gradients), and one had a porcine valve known to be stenotic (35 mm Hg peak systolic gradient). The coronary arteries were free of luminal narrowing in the remaining 11 patients, but three had transmural left ventricular scars with aneurysm formation at sites of excision of left ventricular papillary muscles.

Forty-two patients died after periods of congestive cardiac failure. Five were not improved by operation, and their deaths are attributed to underlying cardiac disease. The other 37 patients were improved by operation, but heart failure

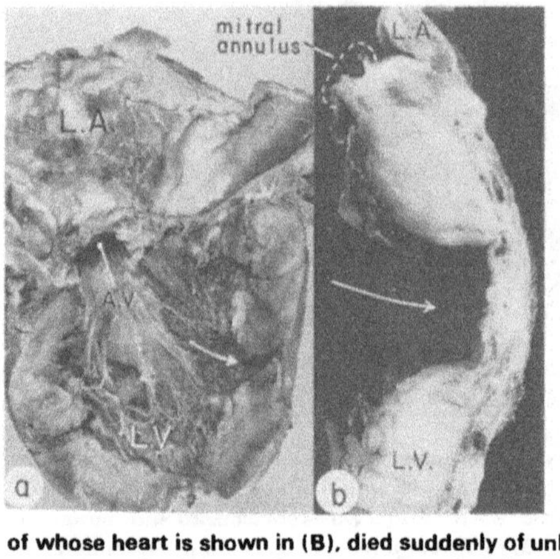

Fig. 16. Rupture and aneurysm formation at site of excision of left ventricular papillary muscles during or after mitral valve replacement. When the left ventricular papillary muscles are excised at operation, these structures are grasped with a clamp and pulled toward the left atrium. If they are pulled too vigorously before excision, a portion of the left ventricular free wall beneath the papillary muscles may also be excised. In both (A) and (B) too much left ventricular (L.V.) free wall beneath the papillary muscles (arrows) was excised, producing probable functional aneurysms in each. The 42-yr-old man (A64-147) whose heart is illustrated in (A) died 5 hr after mitral replacement. He had clinical features of the low cardiac output syndrome. The 58-yr-old woman (A68-14), a portion of whose heart is shown in (B), died suddenly of unknown cause 3 mo after mitral replacement. This is a gross longitudinal section of left atrial (L.A.) wall, mitral anulus, and left ventricular wall. Left ventricular wall beneath excised papillary muscle consisted entirely of fibrous tissue. A.V., aortic valve.

reappeared and progressed in each. Problems with the prosthetic valve accounted for death in 22 of the 37 patients: swelling with impaction of the aortic (seven patients) or mitral (one patient) silicone rubber poppets; infection at the site of attachment of the prosthesis (five patients); parabasilar prosthetic leaks (three); extensive secondary endocardial fibrosis of the left ventricle (two); prosthetic thrombosis (three); and obstruction of the prosthetic orifice due to faulty design and to overgrowth of tissue (one). In only four patients could death

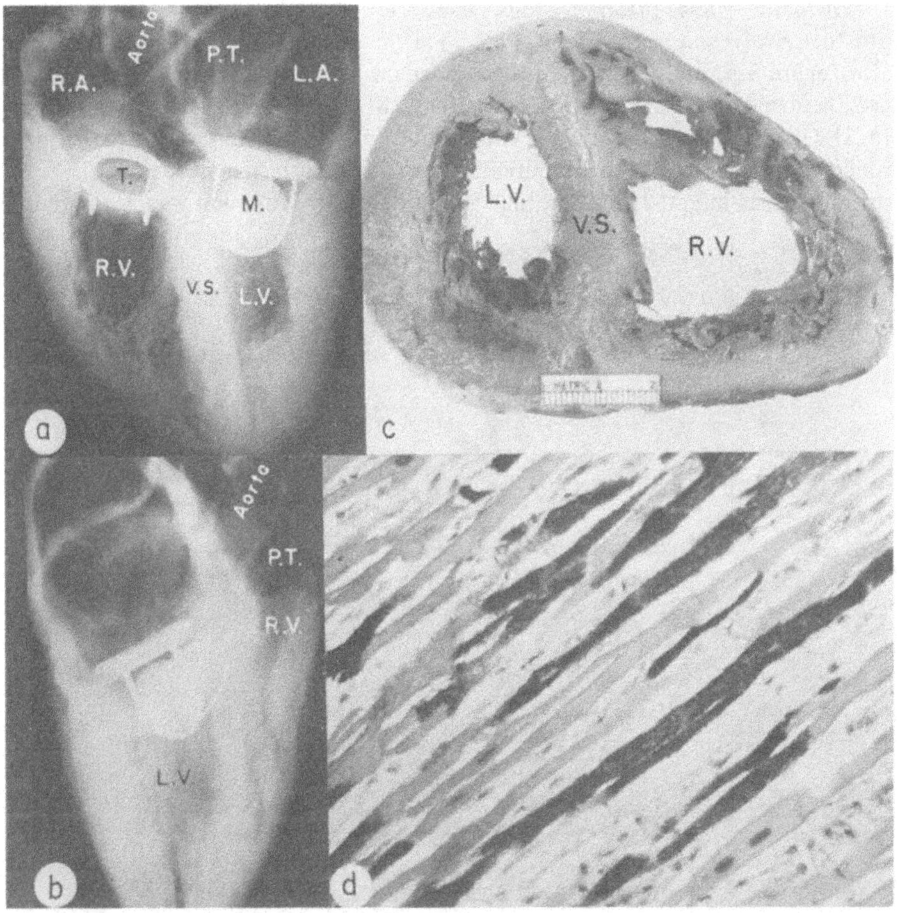

Fig. 17. Dystrophic calcification in cardiac and skeletal (pharyngeal) muscle fibers and in lung in a 46-yr-old woman who died 20 days after replacement of the mitral valve with a Starr-Edwards prosthesis (M.) and of the tricuspid valve with a Kay-Shiley prosthesis (T.). This patient's entire postoperative period was characterized by the low cardiac output syndrome. Radiographs of the excised heart at necropsy (A66-146) disclosed focal calcific deposits in the walls of both left (L.V.) and right (R.V.) ventricles (A and B). R.A., right atrium; L.A., left atrium; P.T., pulmonary trunk; and V.S., ventricular septum. A transverse section of cardiac ventricles (C) shows focal lesions in walls of both chambers. *Since the patient was severely jaundiced these myocardial lesions had a greenish color.* Histologic section of several myocardial lesions disclosed that they consisted of necrotic myocardial fibers, many of which contained calcific deposits (D). Hematoxylin and eosin stain. × 200. The cause of the focal calcific deposits in individual myocardial and skeletal muscle fibers and in alveolar septal walls and pulmonary arteries in the above patient is unknown. Determinations of serum calcium, phosphorus, and magnesium were made on 2 days during the week before operation and 5 days after operation; each was normal.

be attributed to myocardial fibrosis, in four others to associated uncorrected valve disease, and in seven the cause was never determined.

None of the remaining 14 patients had evidence of congestive cardiac failure postoperatively. They died of noncardiac causes (six patients), central nervous system catastrophies (seven patients), or hepatitis (one patient).[23]

Necropsy Observations

Prosthetic valve thrombi (Figs. 6–8, 14, 22). Thrombi were found on prosthetic valves at necropsy in 71 (80%) of the 96 patients dying later than 2 mo after operation, and 49 of them had received warfarin (Table 12). Of the 118 prosthetic valves utilized in these 96 patients, 81 (69%) had antemortum thrombi. In 21 (30%) of the 71 patients with thrombi, the thrombus appeared to have rendered the prosthesis incompetent, stenotic, or both, but in four of them the thrombus was infected. In the other 50 patients valve function was not impaired

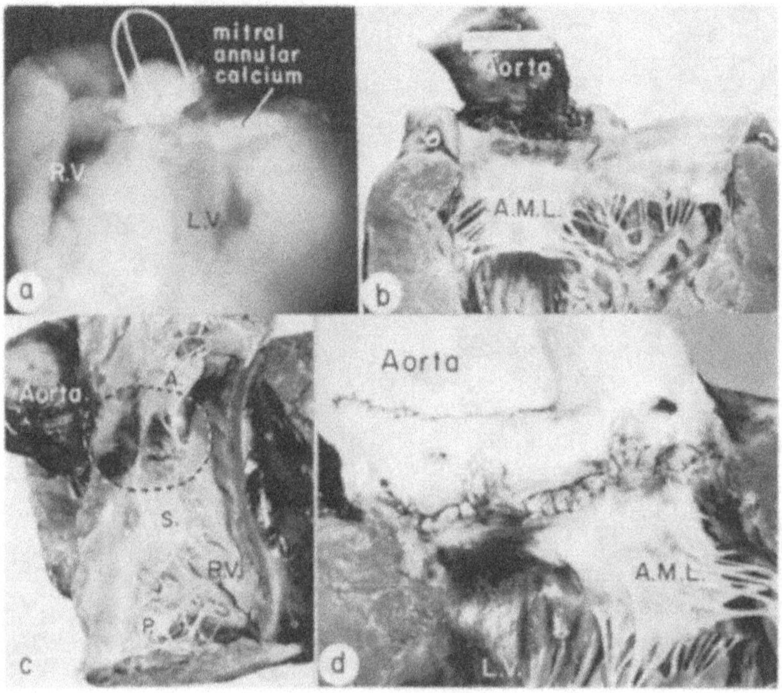

Fig. 18. Extensive myocardial and endocardial hemorrhages after aortic valve replacement. This 64-yr-old man had his stenotic aortic valve replaced with a size 9A Starr-Edwards prosthesis. During cardiopulmonary bypass he had progressive myocardial deterioration evidenced on electrocardiogram even though the coronary arteries were being perfused. Immediately after coming off cardiopulmonary bypass, the heart rate slowed and nodal rhythm was present. Ventricular fibrillation occurred several minutes later and he died. At necropsy (A66-109), radiograph of the specimen (A) disclosed extensive calcification of the mitral anulus, although the mitral leaflets and chordae tendineae were normal (B). The interstitial myocardium adjacent to the aortic root contained numerous extravasated erythrocytes. Their presence in the area of the atrioventricular node (C) (broken circle) and bundle (D), both of which are hemorrhagic, may have accounted for the severe bradycardia. Subendocardial hemorrhages in the left ventricular (L.V.) outflow tract are apparent. Entire membraneous ventricular septum is hemorrhagic. R.V., right ventricle; A.M.L., anterior mitral leaflet; and A., S., and P., anterior, septal and posterior tricuspid leaflets.

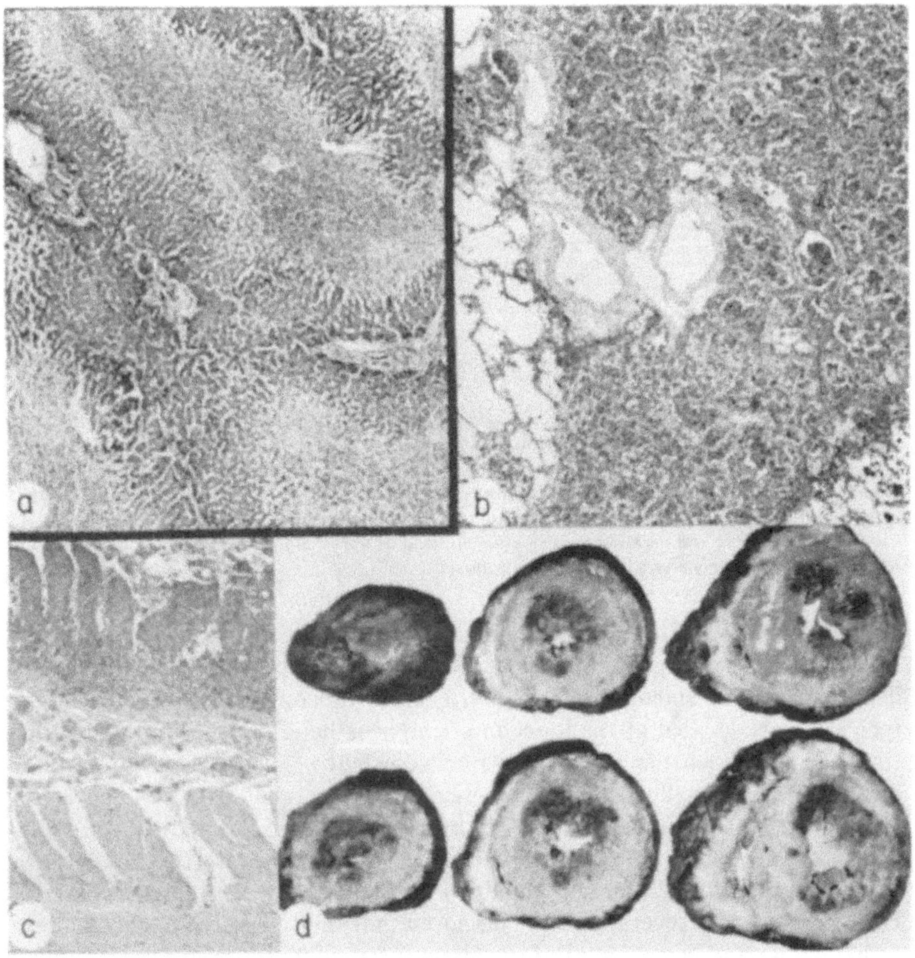

Fig. 19. Lesions in liver (A), lung (B), bowel (C), and heart (D) resulting from inadequate oxygenation of these organs after cardiac valve replacement. These lesions are the pathologic consequences of the low cardiac output syndrome. Inadequate arterial perfusion of the liver leads to centrolobular hemorrhage and necrosis (A), a lesion identical to that resulting from passive venous congestion of the liver. This 30-yr-old woman (A69-33) died 2 days after mitral valve replacement. The liver weighed 1640 g. (B) Pulmonary alveolar hemorrhage ("shock lung") in the same patient (A69-33). This lesion was more common than alveolar edema following valve replacement.[15] (C) Hemorrhage into the bowel mucosa occuring in a 31-yr-old man (A69-53) who died 6 days after mitral valve replacement. (D) Transverse sections of cardiac ventricles in a 57-yr-old woman (A72-124) who died 2 days after aortic and mitral valve replacement. Several foci of subendocardial necrosis are present in left ventricle. These foci of myocardial necrosis are considered consequences not causes of low cardiac output syndrome. Hematoxylin and eosin stains. × 40 (A, B and C).

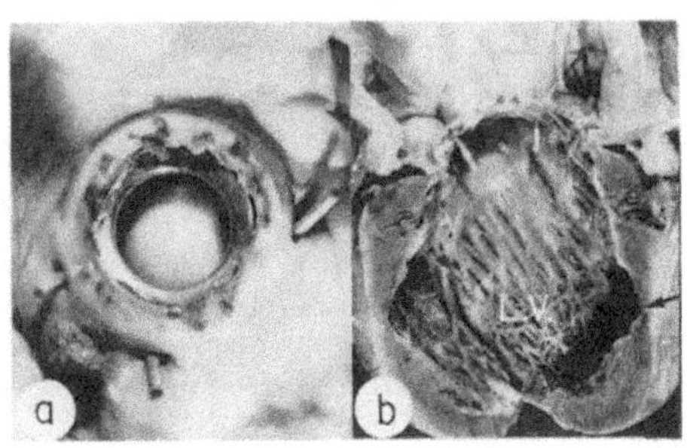

Fig. 20. *Prosthetic peribasilar communications.* (A) Mitral prosthesis implanted 6 mo earlier in a 47-yr-old man (A64-90). Small wooden sticks are inserted into each of the three peribasilar leaks. Small communications as shown here apparently may cause severe regurgitation during life. (B) Opened left atrium, mitral anulus and left ventricle (L.V.) in the same patient. Wooden sticks again designate the sites of the peribasilar leaks. Excessive left ventricular muscle (arrow) was excised when the papillary muscles were removed at the time of mitral replacement. This excessive removal of left ventricular wall probably resulted in a functional aneurysm during life. This patient died of severe congestive cardiac failure, but a murmur of mitral regurgitation was not audible postoperatively.

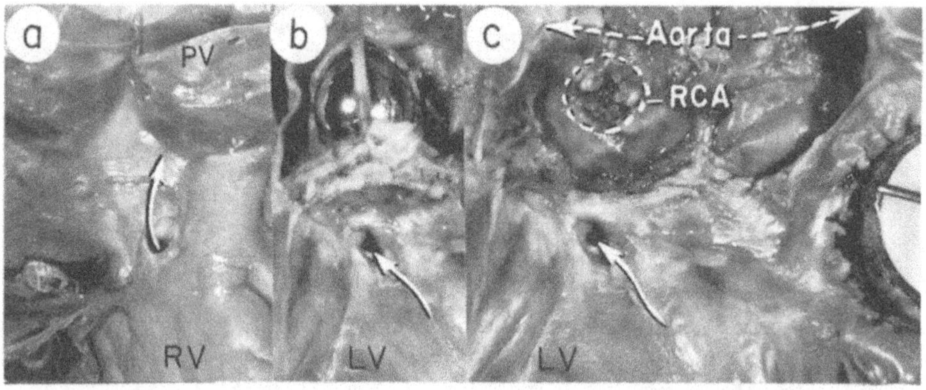

Fig. 21. Operatively induced ventricular septal defect during aortic valve replacement with Starr-Edwards prosthesis (size 10A, 2320) implanted 52 mo earlier in a 62-yr-old man (A72-36) who died of associated uncorrected valve disease. His aortic valve prosthesis apparently had functioned well. (A) Opened right ventricular (RV) outflow tract and pulmonic valve (PV) showing defect (arrow). (B) View of left ventricular (LV) outflow tract showing defect (arrow) just below base of aortic prosthesis. (C) View of left ventricle and ascending aorta after removal of aortic prostheses. Complete occlusion of ostium of right coronary artery (RCA) also was present.

by the thrombus. Although 71 patients had prosthetic thrombi at necropsy, only 16 (23% of those with thrombi; 18% of the total of 96 patients) had clinical evidence of systemic embolism during life. The thrombi on noncloth-covered struts typically were located at the junction of the prosthetic struts with the metallic rings, extending up the aortic struts and down the mitral struts for variable distances, occasionally completely covering the metallic rings. In the close-clearance aortic prostheses, however, thrombi formed in the mid-portion of the struts, sparing both apex and base (Figs. 6–8). In nonclose-clearance cloth-covered struts, thrombi formed initially at the apices, not at the bases (Fig. 22). Histologic study of several thrombi disclosed that they consisted mainly of fibrin and platelets and were devoid of bacteria or fungi, except in the subjects with documented septicemia.

Fistulae around prosthetic valve rings (Fig. 20). Peribasilar communications occurred in 11 patients (11%) (excluding those with infective endocarditis). Five

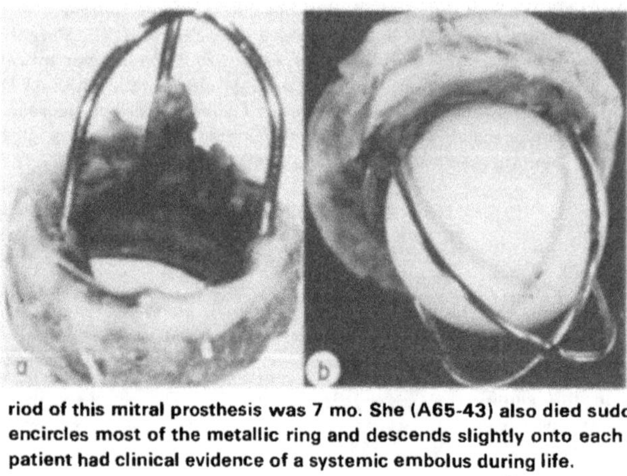

Fig. 22. Prosthetic thrombus on Starr-Edwards aortic (A) and mitral (B) prostheses. (A) This prosthesis had been implanted for 37 mo. The patient (A67-176) died suddenly and unexpectedly from dislodgement of the ball from the aortic cage (see Fig. 24C). Thrombus encircles the inner lining of the prosthetic ring and the caudal half of one of the three metallic struts. (B) The implantation period of this mitral prosthesis was 7 mo. She (A65-43) also died suddenly and unexpectedly. Thrombus encircles most of the metallic ring and descends slightly onto each of the four metallic struts. Neither patient had clinical evidence of a systemic embolus during life.

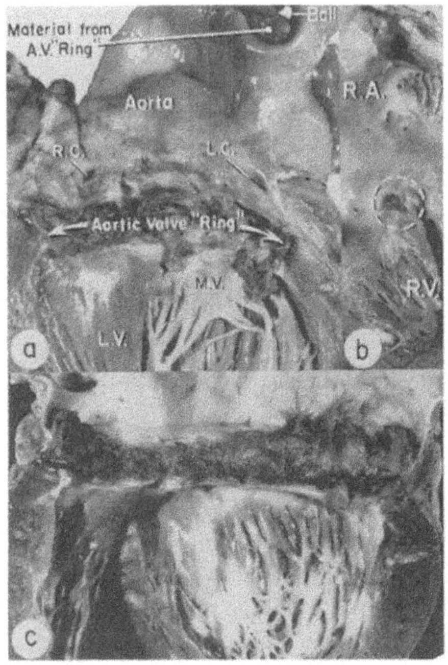

Fig. 23. Infection at the site of attachment of aortic (A and B) and mitral (C) prostheses. (A) Patient A64-189 (see Table 14). Opened left ventricle (L.V.), aortic valve (A.V.) "ring" and ascending aorta. The infection in this patient totally dislodged the aortic Starr-Edwards prosthesis, which migrated to the tranverse aorta. The prosthetic ball is visible. R.C., right coronary ostium; L.C., left coronary ostium; and M.V., anterior mitral valve leaflet. (B) Opened right atrium (R.A.), tricuspid valve, and right ventricle (R.V.) in same patient. Circled lesion is a ring abscess, having extended through from the necrotic prosthetic "ring." (C) Opened left atrium, mitral anulus, and left ventricle in patient A65-221 (see Table 14). The anulus is totally necrotic. The necrotizing nature of infections at sites of attachment of prosthetic valves appears to preclude successful reoperation once infection is established.

had isolated aortic valve replacement; three had isolated mitral replacement, but reoperation in two closed the peribasilar communications; and in three, both mitral and aortic valves had been replaced. In the three patients with two valves, fistulae were present around mitral rings only. The presence of an accessory communication was established before death in each of the 4 patients with periaortic ring leaks, but in only two of the five patients with paramitral ring leaks.[24] The mitral peribasilar communications were considered the cause of death in two patients (Table 13). The frequency of peribasilar prosthetic fistulae appears to be decreasing.

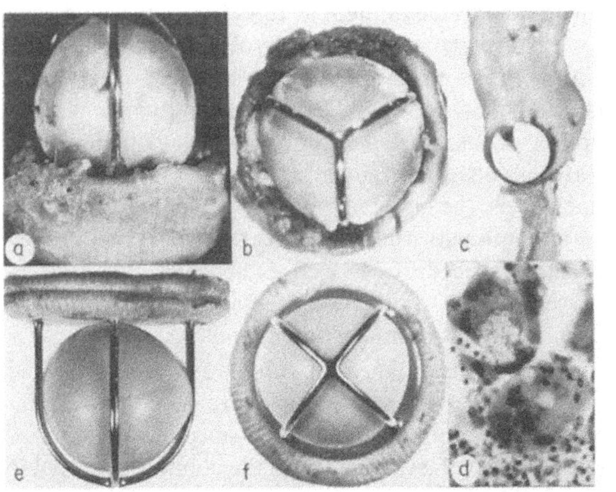

Fig. 24. Degeneration of silicone rubber poppets of Starr-Edwards prostheses. (A and B) Swollen, grooved, yellow, impacted aortic valve poppets implanted for 60 mo. (C) This fractured poppet suddenly dislodged from the aortic valve cage and migrated to the abdominal aorta. He died suddenly (A67-176). Particles of probably silicone rubber within giant cells were found in the liver, spleen, and in several lymph nodes in this patient (D) suggesting that small fragments of silicone rubber dislodged periodically for some time before total ball dislodgement occurred. (E and F) Swollen, deformed, yellow, impacted mitral poppet, which had been implanted 78 mo earlier. This patient died as a result of the swelling of this ball.

In addition to peribasilar leaks, defects in the cardiac septa below valve annuli may develop. Such was the case in the patient described in Fig. 21. He had a small ventricular septal defect created at the time of operation.

Infection at the site of attachment of a prosthetic cardiac valve (Fig. 23). Pertinent clinicopathologic observations in the eight patients who died of this complication are summarized in Table 14.[25,26] Three died within 2 mo of valve replacement, two precipitated by operative wound infections, and the third had infection before operation. The other five patients developed valve infection later, after periods of time sufficient to allow healing of the operative wounds. Precipitating events were clear in three of them and unknown in two. *Staphylococcus epidermidis* was the offending bacterium in five patients, *Staphylococcus aureus* in one, *Proteus mirabilis* in one, and *Serratia marcescens* in one. The intervals from the onset of symptoms or signs consistent with infective endocarditis to death ranged from 16–90 days. Five patients developed conduction disturbances, heart block or bundle-branch block during the period of cardiac infection. Death in four of the five patients with infected aortic prostheses resulted from partial or complete detachment of the prosthesis with production of massive aortic regurgitation, heart failure, and death. Prosthetic detachment, which was partial, occurred in only one of the three patients with infection at sites of attachment of mitral prostheses. All three patients with infected mitral prostheses developed large infected left atrial thrombi, which partially obstructed the mitral orifices.

Infection at sites of attachment of rigid-frame prosthetic valves, particularly in the case of the aortic prostheses, tends to extend deeply into adjacent structures. In four of the five patients with infected aortic prostheses, the inflammatory process extended through the atrial septum to the area of the atrioventricular node and caused a high degree of atrioventricular block. Although prosthetic infective endocarditis cured by antibiotics has been reported, considerable doubt exists as to whether the patients described actually had infection on or at the site of attachment of the prosthesis, or whether they had septicemia without endocarditis; the latter appears more likely. The extent of the infection and the character of the tissue beneath the prosthetic anuli in our patients clearly indicate that an attempt at secondary operative intervention in them at this late stage would have been fruitless. If reoperation has a place in the therapy of prosthetic infective endocarditis, the operative intervention must come early, because once the infection beneath the prosthetic ring is well established, the outcome is fatal regardless of the mode of therapy. Thus, since neither presently available antibiotics or operative methods are effective in eradicating infection at sites of attachment of prosthetic cardiac valves, the infection must be prevented. The value of administering penicillin to patients with rheumatic heart disease before they undergo dental or other operative procedures is well established, but an even more vigorous prophylactic regimen is probably necessary in patients with prosthetic cardiac valves who must undergo similar procedures.

Degeneration (variance) of the silicone rubber prosthetic ball (Fig. 24). Of the 118 prosthetic valves used in the 96 patients who died late, 87 contained silicone rubber poppets, 23 had hollow metal balls, and 4 had silicone rubber discs. Four other patients had porcine aortic valves. Damage to the poppets occurred in none of the patients in whom metal balls or discs were used, but the implantation periods were relatively short (range, 3–52 mo; average, 16) in these 23 patients.

Of the 87 silicone rubber poppets, 45 had been implanted for periods <24 mo, and all appeared normal at necropsy. Of the 42 silicone rubber poppets implanted for 24 mo or longer, 20 were normal, and 22 showed evidence of degeneration or variation consisting of gross alteration in ball color, shape, consistency, volume, and/or surface damage, abrasion, or fracture (Table 15). Only five of the 17

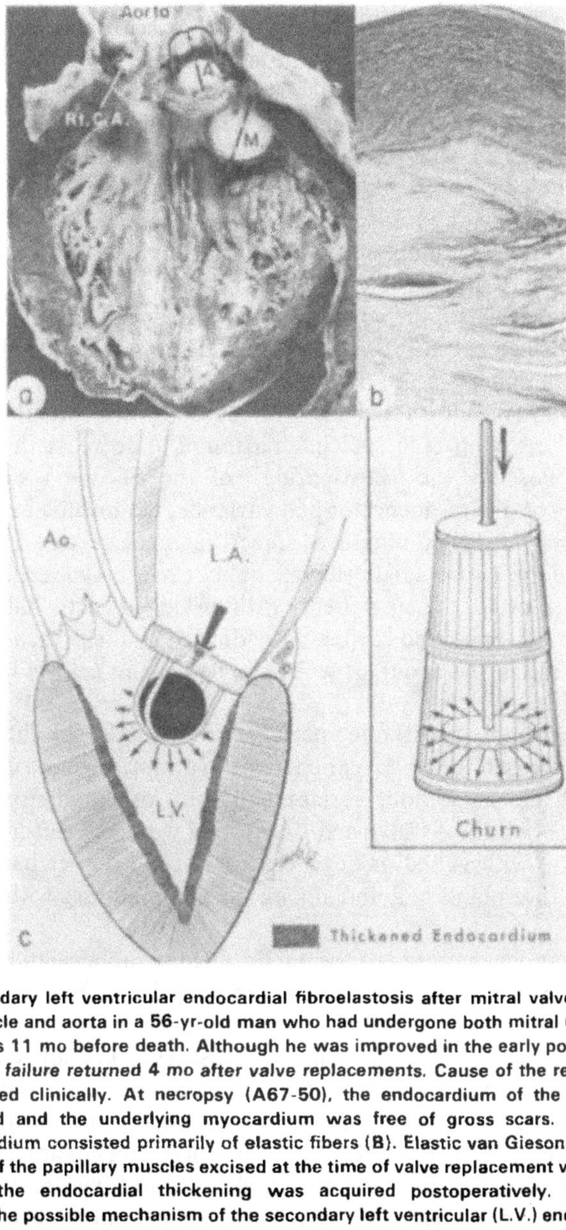

Fig. 25. **Secondary left ventricular endocardial fibroelastosis after mitral valve replacement. (A) Opened left ventricle and aorta in a 56-yr-old man who had undergone both mitral (M.) and aortic (A.) valve replacements 11 mo before death. Although he was improved in the early postoperative period, *congestive cardiac failure returned 4 mo after valve replacements.* Cause of the recurrence of failure was not determined clinically. At necropsy (A67-50), the endocardium of the left ventricle was diffusely thickened and the underlying myocardium was free of gross scars. Histologically, the thickened endocardium consisted primarily of elastic fibers (B). Elastic van Gieson stain. × 25. Since the endocardium of the papillary muscles excised at the time of valve replacement were not thickened, it is clear that the endocardial thickening was acquired postoperatively. (C) Diagrammatic representation of the possible mechanism of the secondary left ventricular (L.V.) endocardial fibroelastosis after replacement of the mitral valve with a caged-ball prosthesis. The cage and ball of the mitral prosthesis are located within the left ventricular cavity. Thus, when the ball moves, either descends or ascends, it pushes blood laterally, producing turbulence. This effect may be compared to the turbulence produced by the butter churn. The anatomic indicator of turbulent flow is proliferation of connective tissue on the surface in contact with that flow; in this case, endocardium. Ao., aorta; L.A., left atrium. (By permission.[31])**

mitral silicone rubber balls implanted for <24 mo showed evidence of degeneration: In three the poppets were discolored but functioned normally; in two the poppets were discolored, swollen and impacted.[27] All five had been implanted for 78 mo or more, and had an average implantation time of nearly twice that of the normal poppets (100 and 58 mo, respectively). Of the 25 silicone rubber aortic poppets implanted for 24 mo or longer, 17 showed evidence of degeneration: In ten the poppets were swollen (usually about 10% increase in volume compared to the poppet volume at the time of implantation), grooved, and impacted in the cage; in six the balls had fractured and embolized from the cage (in five patients the dislodged poppets were found in the aortic bifurcation; in one it had fallen back into the left ventricular cavity).[28] In 16 patients ball variance was the cause of death. The seventeenth variant aortic poppet showed only mild discoloration, and this change did not cause the prosthesis to function abnormally. The average implantation periods for the eight normal and 17 abnormal poppets were similar, 45 and 41 mo, respectively.

All six patients in whom the aortic ball had dislodged from the cage underwent aortic valve replacement in 1964 and all died in 1967. We have not observed silicone rubber ball embolism in any prosthetic valve implanted after 1964. Some manufacturers of silicone rubber balls for cardiac valve prostheses altered the processing of these poppets in 1965 in an attempt to decrease their propensity to absorb lipids. Possibly the "post-curing" of the silicone rubber will have a beneficial effect on the frequency of ball variance, but insufficient data presently are available on poppets manufactured since 1965 to be certain.

Not only can the entire aortic silicone rubber ball embolize, but so may portions of it.[28,29] In two of the six patients with dislodged aortic balls, fragments of silicone rubber had embolized earlier, as evidenced by the presence of particles of refractile material in and about large foreign body giant cells in liver, spleen, and lymph nodes.

The frequency of prosthetic peribasilar fistulae or thrombi was not significantly increased in the 22 patients with variant silicone rubber poppets as compared with the 20 without variant balls but also implanted for 24 mo or longer. Three peribasilar fistulae and 17 thrombi were encountered among the 22 prosthetic valves with varied or degenerated silicone rubber balls, whereas two fistulae and 16 thrombi were found among the 20 prostheses with normal silicone rubber balls.

It is clear that degeneration of the aortic silicone rubber ball is far more common at this time than is degeneration of a mitral silicone rubber ball, and, to our knowledge, variance of a tricuspid prosthetic poppet has not been reported. That the total number of Starr-Edwards mitral prostheses and aortic prostheses supplied to surgeons is approximately equal further emphasizes this difference in frequency. Differences in pressure and flow across aortic and mitral prostheses are probably the explanation. Typically, the orifice diameters of aortic prostheses are smaller than those of mitral prostheses, and the time of ventricular systole is approximately half that of ventricular diastole for a patient at rest. The velocity of flow through the orifice of the average aortic prosthesis is at least three times greater than the velocity through the orifice of the average mitral prosthesis. Also, the aortic ball contacts both the valve ring and the apex of the cage under

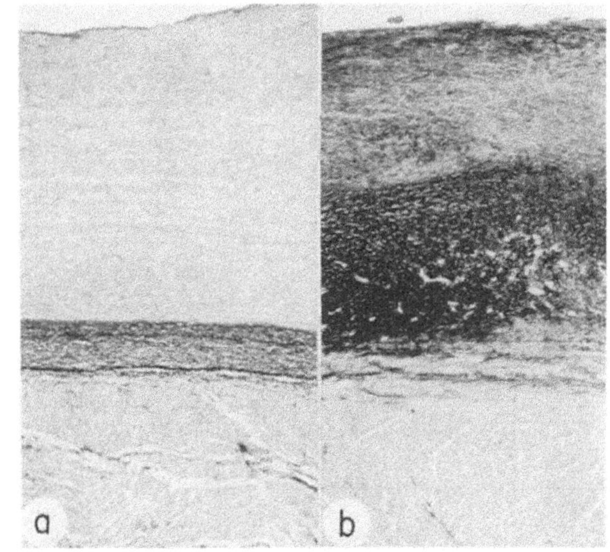

Fig. 26. Secondary endocardial fibrosis of left atrium in addition to secondary endocardial fibroelastosis of left ventricle after mitral valve replacement. Shown are sections of left atrial (A) and left ventricular walls (B), each stained for elastic fibers (Elastic van Gieson stains, each × 32), in a 53-yr-old woman (A65-43) who died suddenly and unexpectedly 7 mo after replacement of the mitral valve with a Starr-Edwards prosthesis without recurrence of symptoms of cardiac dysfunction postoperatively. Endocardial thickening of the left atrium is always found in patients dying late after mitral replacement. In contrast to that occurring in the left ventricle, however, the secondary left atrial endocardial thickening is uncertain but may be the result of local trauma at the time of operation. (By permission.[21])

high pressure, whereas the mitral ball contacts only the ring under high pressure, since the ball passes to the apex of the cage during ventricular diastole.

It is unclear why one aortic or mitral silicone rubber poppet degenerates and why another aortic or mitral poppet implanted for a similar period shows no evidence of degeneration. Table 15 showed that 17 (72%) of 25 aortic silicone rubber poppets implanted for an average of 41 mo showed degeneration, whereas 8 other

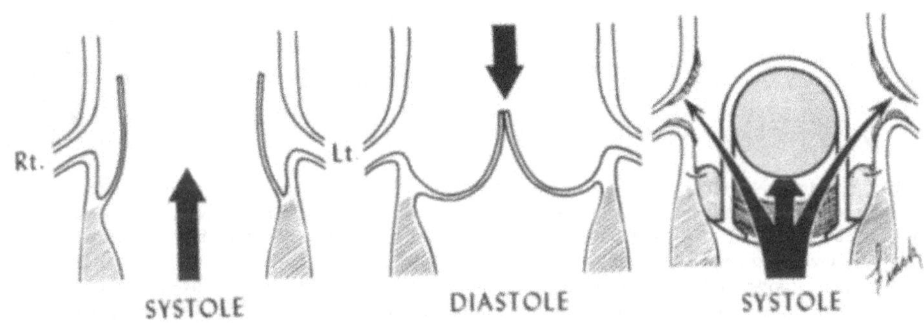

Fig. 27. Diagrammatic representation of the aortic valve region in the normal heart (left and center) and after replacement with a caged-ball prosthesis. Flow of blood during systole across the normal aortic valve is laminar, and the coronary arteries fill mainly by retrograde flow during diastole. Following caged-ball prosthetic replacement, the flow of blood across the aortic valve area is no longer laminar. The force of left ventricular ejection is directed centrally, as in the normal, but the ball prevents central flow, producing severe turbulence in the area. Thus, during ventricular systole blood between surface of the ball and intima of the aortic root is flowing in a turbulent fashion. The anatomic indicator of turbulent flow under high pressure is intimal proliferation, which has been observed in the proximal aorta of each subject dying in the late postoperative period after aortic valve replacement. Since the coronary ostia are no longer "guarded," so to speak, by the aortic cusps during ventricular systole and, much more importantly, since they are in the area of turbulent flow, they also are subject to intimal proliferation, which has been observed in them in several subjects (see text). (By permission.[10])

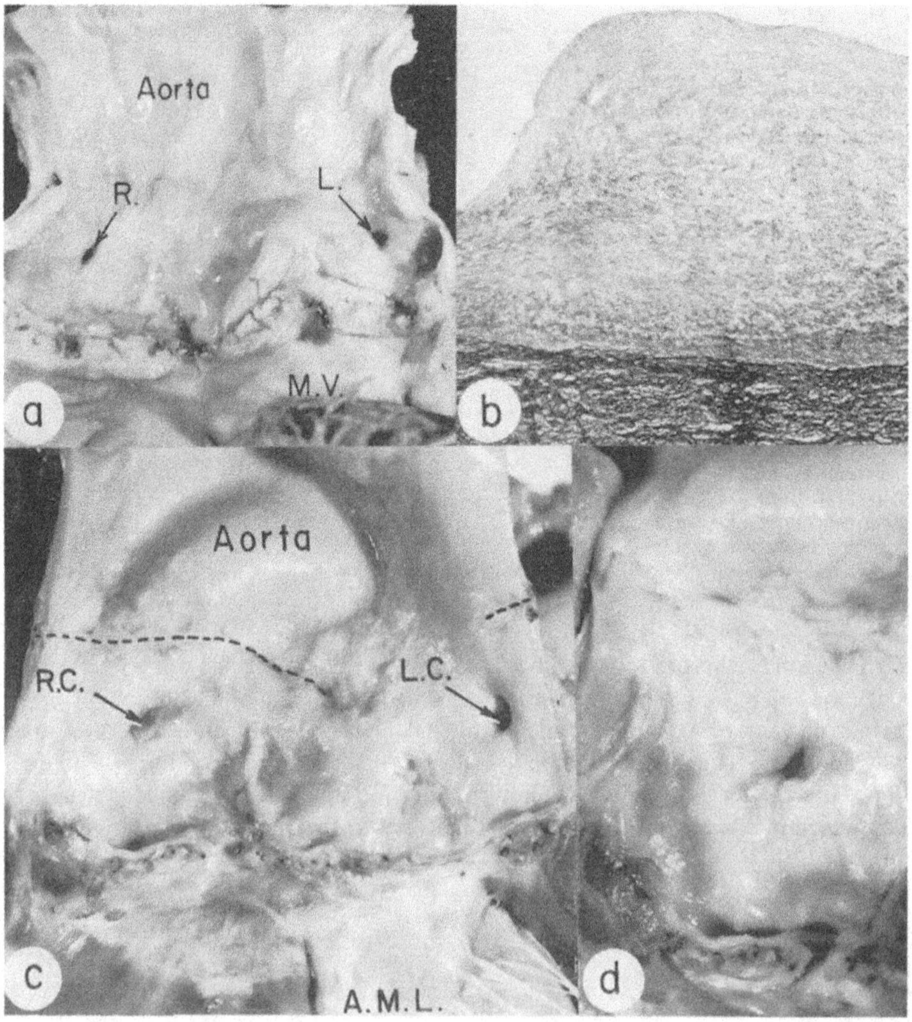

Fig. 28. Intimal proliferation in ascending aorta late after aortic valve replacement. Opened aorta and left ventricular outflow tract (A) in a 48-yr-old man who underwent aortic valve replacement with a Starr-Edwards prosthesis 4 mo earlier. Before operation he had no chest pain but 2 mo postoperatively he developed angina pectoris and died during one of the attacks. At operation, both right (R.) and left (L.) coronary arteries were cannulated without difficulty, but at necropsy (A64-163) cannulae could not be inserted. (A) Considerable intimal proliferation is apparent and both coronary ostia are small. The aortotomy incision is completely obscured by fibrous tissue. (B) Section of ascending aorta showing that the thickening is due to proliferation of fibrous tissue devoid of elastic fibers. The underlying media is normal. Elastic van Gieson stain. × 25. Sections of the coronary arteries in this patient are shown in Fig. 23. This patient had severe renal hemosiderosis, the result of trauma to erythrocytes traversing the aortic prosthesis. (C) Opened aorta and left ventricular outflow tract in a 50-yr-old man (A65-143) who died suddenly 24 mo after aortic valve replacement. Again, there is intimal proliferation in the aorta but it is focal. There is no intimal proliferation about the left coronary (L.C.) ostium as contrasted to its presence about the right (R.C.) one. The broken line designates the previous aortotomy incision. A.M.L., anterior mitral leaflet. (D) Close-up of the narrowed right coronary arterial ostium in this patient.

aortic poppets implanted for an average of 45 mo showed no degeneration. Could it be that the trauma to the poppet produced by the force of left ventricular ejection was greater in the patients with variant aortic balls? A possible quantification of this trauma might be obtained by determining the amount of intravascular hemolysis caused by the turbulent flow of blood across the valvular prosthesis. The anatomic indicator of intravascular hemolysis is renal hemosiderosis.[29,30] Although the per cent of patients with renal hemosiderosis was similar, the amount of iron present in the kidneys of the patients with degenerated silicone rubber poppets was greater than in those without degeneration but with similarly long implantation periods. Kidneys were available for examination in 17 patients in whom Starr-Edwards prostheses with silicone poppets had been im-

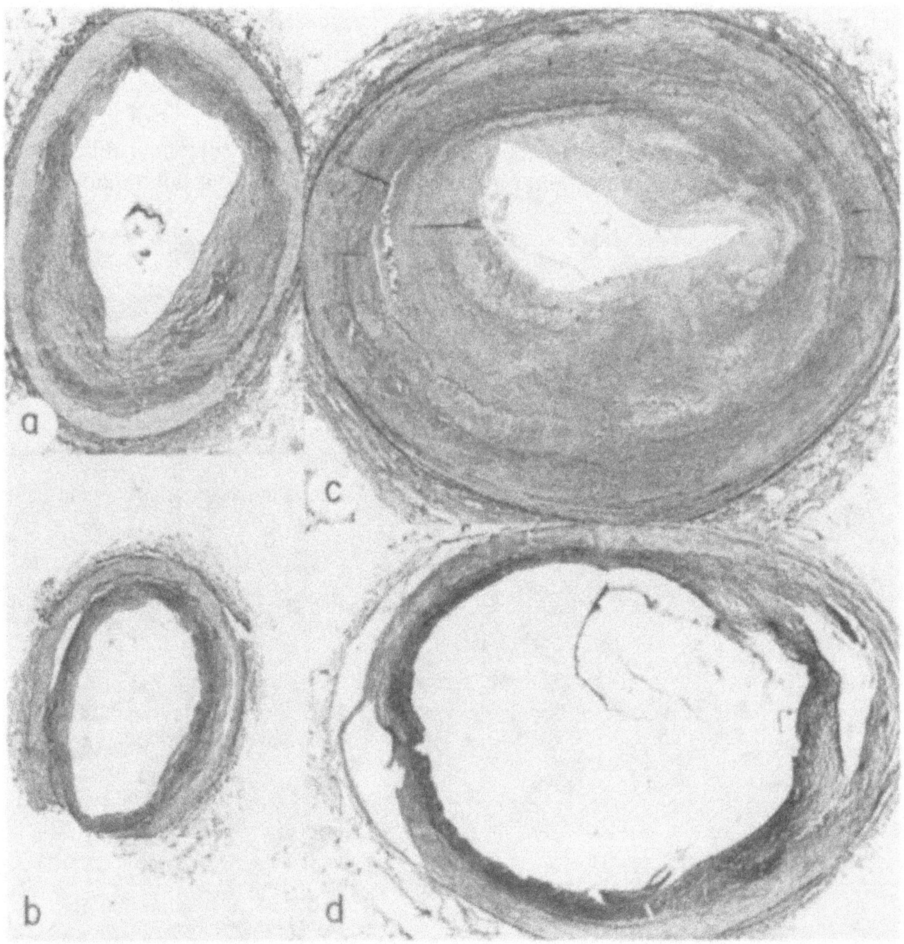

Fig. 29. Photomicrographs of the coronary arteries in the patient whose aortic root is illustrated in Fig. 22 A and B. (A) Right coronary artery at its ostium showing considerable intimal proliferation. This artery is hypoplastic. (B) Right coronary artery 1.5 cm from its ostium. At this point, and distally, the lumen is widely patent. (C) Left coronary artery at its ostium. The lumen is severely narrowed, the result of intimal proliferation. (D) Left coronary artery immediately proximal to its bifurcation into anterior descending and left circumflex branches; both branches were widely patent. Elastic van Gieson stains, all × 20. (By permission.[21])

planted for 24 mo or longer. Thirteen of the seventeen had iron deposits (Prussian blue stains) in the cytoplasm of proximal renal tubular cells: Of the ten with ball variance eight had renal iron deposits; of the seven with normal poppets, five had renal hemosiderosis. Among the aortics without ring leak, however, none of two without ball variance had renal hemosiderosis, and seven of nine *with* ball variance had renal hemosiderosis.

Clinical features of *aortic* ball variance are variable, but this diagnosis must be suspected in any patient in whom a prosthesis containing a silicone rubber poppet has been in place 24 mo or longer. When the aortic ball swells, death may occur suddenly, or may be preceded by congestive cardiac failure. Alterations of prosthetic sounds are often apparent. Dislodgement of the aortic ball from the cage was not preceded by symptoms of cardiac dysfunction in any of our six patients. The clinical features resulting from severe degeneration of the silicone rubber *mitral* poppet also are variable, and consist of syncope or near syncope, congestive heart failure, and alterations in prosthetic sounds. Aortic ball degeneration should be considered in any patient doing poorly 2 yr or more after aortic valve replacement with a prostheses containing a silicone rubber ball. Mitral poppet degeneration should be considered in any patient doing poorly 5 yr

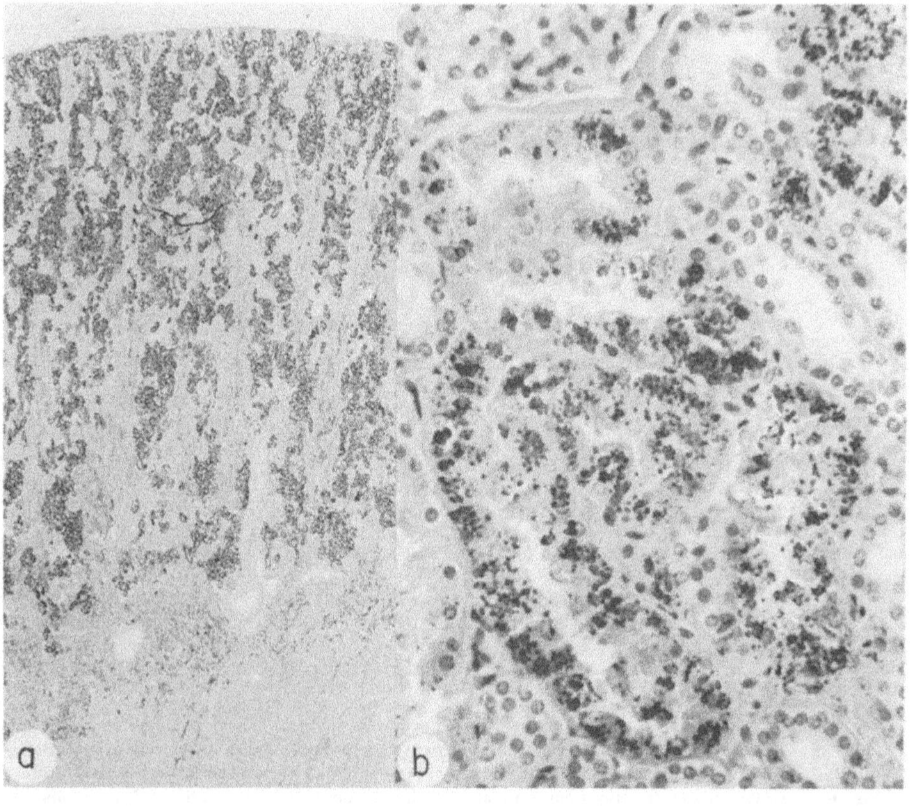

Fig. 30. Renal hemosiderosis late after aortic valve replacement (A64-10). (A) Section of kidney stained for iron (Prussian blue) disclosing numerous deposits of iron in renal tubules. × 16. (B) Close-up view showing deposits of iron in the cytoplasm of the proximal tubules. Hematoxylin and eosin stains. × 290.

or more after mitral valve replacement with a prosthesis containing a silicone rubber poppet. It is hoped that the hollow metal ball made of Stellite 21 alloy (Table 16) in Starr-Edwards prostheses of current design will not degenerate. This newer prosthesis, introduced in 1967, as yet has shown no evidence of wear.

Secondary left ventricular endocardial fibroelastosis after mitral valve replacement (Figs. 25 and 26). In each of the 49 patients who died late after mitral replacement, some degree of left ventricular endocardial thickening was found at necropsy.[31] In each of these patients, the stumps of the amputated left ventricular papillary muscles and the left ventricular apex, the site of drain insertion at operation, were covered by fibrous tissue, but in 35 of the 49 patients the fibrous process extended to involve other areas of left ventricular endocardium as well.

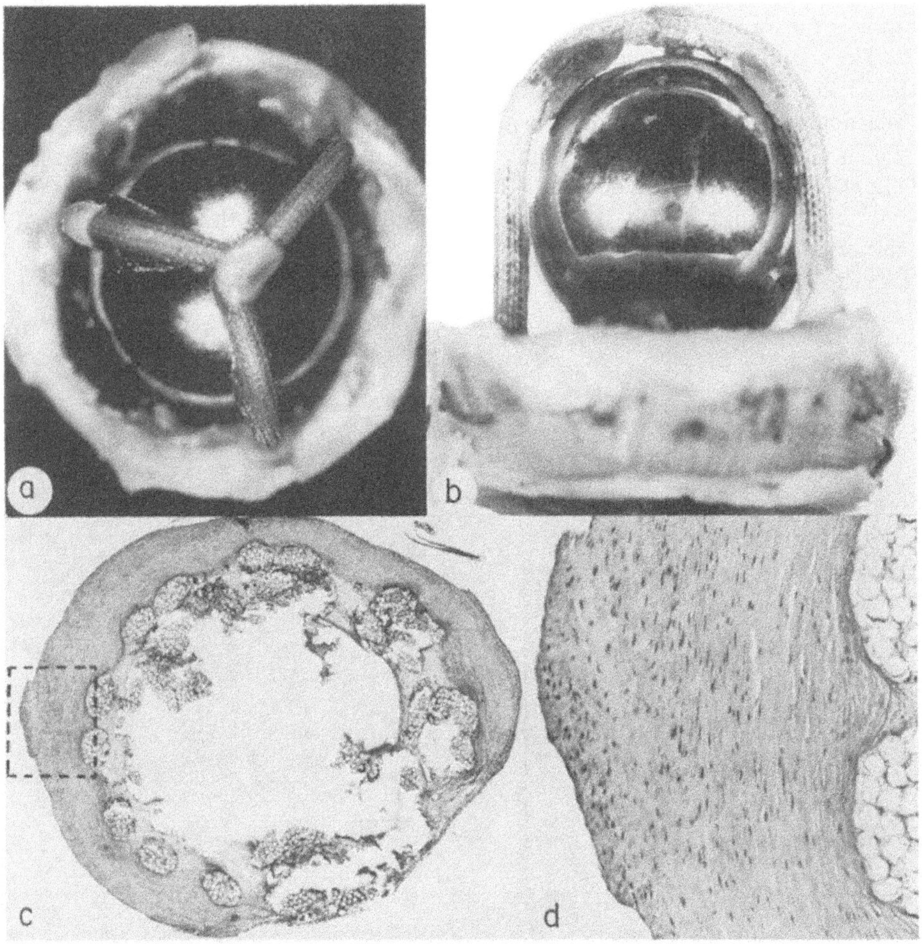

Fig. 31. Collagen deposits on cloth-covered struts of Starr-Edwards prosthesis implanted in a 53-yr-old man (A70-54) for 12 mo. (A) Prosthesis as viewed from above showing a collagen plaque at the apex of the cage. (B) Same prosthesis viewed laterally showing both collagen plaques and fibrin platelet thrombi on the Teflon-covered struts. (C) Section of collagen plaque after removal of the cloth from the metallic strut. (D) Close-up of the area shown in C, showing that fibrous tissue, containing many fibroblasts, covers the cloth. Hematoxylin and eosin stains. (C) × 34, (D) × 160.

The absence of endocardial thickening of the papillary muscles excised at the time of mitral valve replacement (except in one patient, a 15-yr-old girl who had primary endocardial fibroelastosis) and the presence of extensive left ventricular endocardial fibrous tissue containing numerous elastic fibers at necropsy indicates that the endocardial fibroelastosis was acquired postoperatively. The most extensive secondary left ventricular endocardial fibrosis was observed in two patients who had had aortic as well as mitral valve replacements. In these patients the left ventricular endocardial thickening was believed to have been of functional significance. Both had severe, intractable cardiac failure several mo postoperatively without other anatomic explanation. In the other patients with significant, although less severe, left ventricular endocardial fibrosis, death was attributable to other causes. Left ventricular endocardial thickening did not occur in patients with isolated aortic valve replacement, unless there had been a previous myocardial infarct.

The endocardium of the left atrium also was focally but extensively thickened in all 49 patients who had had mitral valve replacement. In contrast to the left ventricular endocardial fibrosis, which contained numerous elastic fibers, that which occurred in the left atrium, with rare exception, was devoid of elastic fibers. The left atrial endocardial thickening almost certainly appeared postoperatively also, probably the result of operative trauma to the interior lining of this chamber.

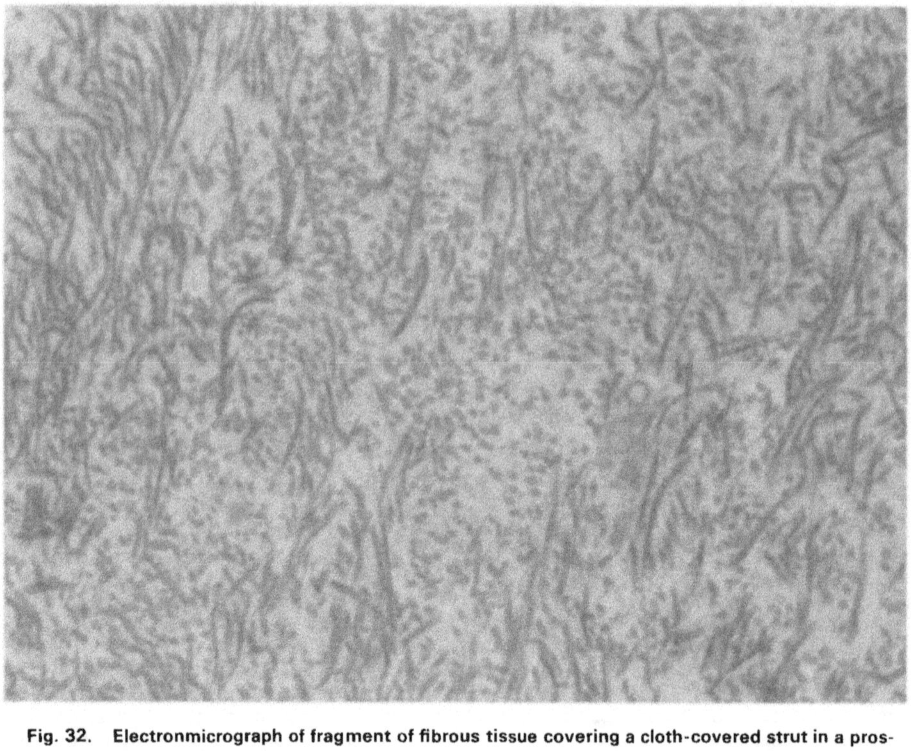

Fig. 32. Electronmicrograph of fragment of fibrous tissue covering a cloth-covered strut in a prosthesis inserted about 1 yr earlier. Tissue covering the strut consists entirely of collagen fibrils with a few fibroblasts. × 37,755. (Electronmicrograph taken by Dr. Victor J. Ferrans.)

The endocardial thickening, which occurs over the stumps of the amputated papillary muscles after mitral replacement, may be regarded as simple healing. The cause of the more widespread left ventricular endocardial thickening observed in these patients is uncertain, but it may be the result of turbulent blood flow in this chamber. The leaflets and chordae tendineae of the natural mitral valve are within the left ventricular cavity, but these structures are thin and readily movable, and the blood flows centrally, between the two leaflets. In contrast, after insertion of a caged-ball mitral prosthesis, blood flows peripherally, or around the caged ball, and the endocardial lining of the left ventricle is not protected from blood flowing across the mitral prosthesis. Also, the ball in the prosthetic mitral valve moves up and down, imparting a churning turbulence to the blood within the left ventricular cavity. The anatomic indicator of turbulent flow is fibrous proliferation, and in this case its site is the left ventricular endocardium. Similar fibrous proliferation occurs in the aortic root after replacement of the aortic valve with a caged-ball prosthesis.

Intimal thickening of the aortic root and proximal coronary arteries after aortic valve replacement (Figs. 27–29). In each of the 66 patients with prosthetic aortic valves, there was intimal thickening in the aortic root. This thickening appears to have been produced by the deposition of fibrous tissue, devoid of foam cells, on the internal elastic membrane of the proximal portion of the ascending aorta. The degree of intimal proliferation varied from minimal to severe; in some patients it was diffuse, and in others, focal.

In addition to the changes in the aortic root in all 66 patients, 37 also had intimal proliferation, with or without actual narrowing, of one or both coronary arterial ostia or proximal coronary arteries. One of the difficulties encountered in evaluating coronary ostial narrowing in these patients was inherent differences in the sizes of the ostia. In most subjects with aortic valvular disease, the left coronary arterial ostium is larger than the right; often the difference is striking. Thus, if the right coronary ostium is smaller than the left one, postoperative narrowing can be assumed to have occurred only if there is extensive intimal proliferation about the origin of the vessel. In 18 patients, there was intimal proliferation about the right ostium; it caused severe narrowing in 4 patients. The other 19 patients had narrowing of varying degree of both coronary ostia. In 14 of the latter 19 subjects, the narrowing was mild and functionally insignificant, and in the other 5, there was considerable narrowing of each ostium and of the proximal main left and right coronary arteries as well. Two of the latter 5 patients, however, had had replacement of the ascending aorta by a graft at the time of valve replacement, and the proximity of the suture line to the coronary ostia may have been a factor in the production of ostial narrowing. The third patient had severe narrowing, not only of the ostia but of the entire coronary arterial tree, secondary to atherosclerosis. The fourth patient had severe intimal thickening in the proximal 1-cm segments of the right and left coronary arteries, but the coronary vessels distal to this point were widely patent. In this patient, coronary arterial perfusion cannulae could not be inserted into the ostia at the time of necropsy, although such cannulae had been utilized without difficulty at the time of valve replacement only 4 mo earlier. This man, who was 48 yr old, had not had chest pain before operation, but 2 mo postoperatively began to have angina pectoris and thereafter had numerous anginal attacks. This patient also had mild anemia postoperatively, and at necropsy the presence of large amounts of iron in his kidneys indicated that the anemia was secondary to intravascular hemolysis. The presence of the anemia in this patient may be interpreted as indicating an excessive turbulence of blood in the area of the valvular prostheses. The fifth patient died suddenly; both coronary arterial ostia were severely narrowed.

The thickening of the intima of the aortic root appears to have occurred in these patients during the postoperative period. It was clear from necropsy examination that the healing of the aortotomy incision was not the responsible factor, since intimal thickening also was present at some distance from it. In only 2 of the 66 patients was coronary ostial narrowing evident at the time of aortic valve replacement. It is unlikely that any functional disturbances are produced by intimal thickening in the ascending aorta itself. When this process involves the ostia and proximal coronary arteries, however, the effects, when severe, may be compared to those of syphilitic aortitis.

The flow of blood through a normal aortic valve and ascending aorta is laminar, but when a ball-valve prosthesis is present, flow in these areas is grossly turbulent. The anatomic indicator of localized turbulent flow is intimal proliferation.

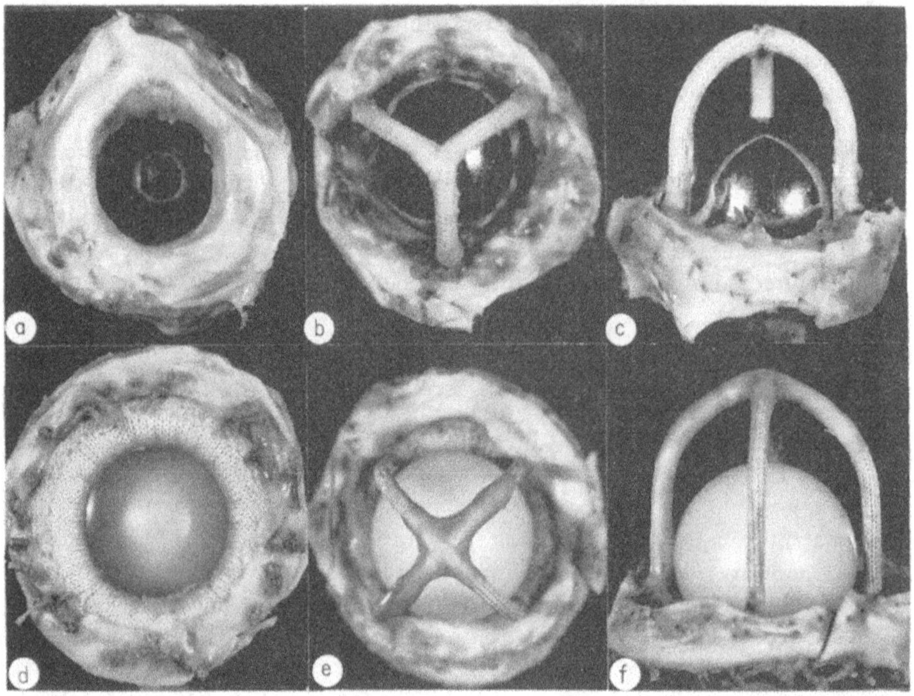

Fig. 33. Starr-Edwards prostheses. (A, B, and C) Aortic prosthesis (size 9A, model 2300). (D, E, and F) Mitral prosthesis (size 3M, model 6300). Each was implanted for 44 mo in a 58-yr-old man (A71-162). He died 8 hr after the onset of severe chest pain. Note the heavy deposition of fibrous tissue (collagen) on the ventricular aspect of the aortic prosthesis (A) and the relatively light deposition on the atrial aspect of the mitral prosthesis (D). Furthermore, the deposits of collagen on the aortic struts are thin and the Teflon is easily visible (B and C). In contrast, heavy deposits of collagen are present at the apices of each of the four struts of the mitral prosthesis (E) and on the vertical portions of two of the four struts of the mitral prosthesis (F).

Although the changes in the coronary ostia and proximal coronary arteries were relatively unimpressive in most of the 66 patients, their average survival time after valve replacement was relatively short. It is possible that intimal proliferation in these areas will become more extensive with time.

Traumatic intravascular hemolysis (Fig. 30). It is now well appreciated that intravascular hemolysis occurred in virtually all patients with malfunctioning flexible Teflon aortic valves,[29] and in a few patients with incompetent and stenotic aortic valves that have not been operated upon.[30] The intravascular hemolysis in these subjects is the result of trauma to erythrocytes traversing the malfunctioning natural or artificial aortic valve. The anatomic indicator of intravascular hemolysis is renal hemosiderosis, the so-called blue kidney. The mechanisms by which iron is deposited in the kidneys have been described elsewhere.[29]

The kidneys were available for examination in 51 of the 96 subjects dying late (Table 17). In 36 (71%) of the 51 patients, histologic sections stained by the Prussian blue reaction, disclosed iron in the kidneys. The amount of iron deposited in the kidneys, almost all of it in the cytoplasm of the proximal tubules, was heavy in 27 patients and in 9 it was minimal or mild. The valves replaced in the patients with renal hemosiderosis are shown in Table 17. Eight patients with peribasilar fistulae (not caused by infective endocarditis) had kidneys available for examination, and all eight had renal hemosiderosis. All but one of the eight had aortic prostheses. The degree of intimal proliferation in the aortic root was striking in all 28 patients with heavy deposits of renal iron after aortic replacement. As mentioned earlier, it would appear that both aortic root intimal

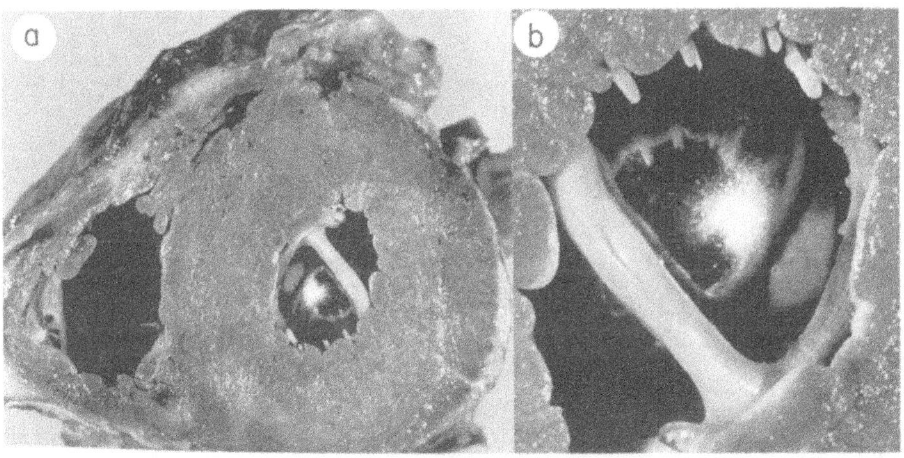

Fig. 34. Prosthetic dysfunction. Starr-Edwards cloth-covered mitral prosthesis (model 6320, size 4M) implanted in a 58-yr-old man (A72-31) 6.5 mo before death. His preoperative lesion was aortic stenosis and mitral stenosis, and left ventricular cavity was of normal size. (A) Mitral prosthesis as viewed from left ventricle. (B) Close-up of same valve. Each of the four struts of the mitral prosthesis contacts endocardium of left ventricle and the ventricular septum bulges into the mitral cage, preventing the metal poppet from descending completely to apex of cage. Cloth-covered struts show considerable collagen overgrowth. Mean diastolic pressure gradient between left atrium and left ventricle before valve replacement was 7 mm Hg, and at catheterization 6 mo postoperatively this gradient was 11 mm Hg. Thus, this case is an example of prosthetic stenosis confirmed by hemodynamic study. If a smaller sized prosthesis had been utilized, for example a 2M rather than a 4M, obstruction may not have resulted. (By permission.[40])

proliferation and renal hemosiderosis are indicators of excessive trauma to blood as it is ejected against the aortic poppet and aortic wall.

Although deposits of iron in kidneys produce striking anatomic lesions, no significant renal damage or impairment of renal function appears to occur as a result of this deposition. The bone marrow is usually able to compensate for the increased red blood cell destruction. The hematocrit values in the late postoperative period were available in 25 of the 36 patients with renal hemosiderosis: In 12 the hematocrit was normal ($\geq$ 40%) and in 13 it was low (32%–37%).

Fatal central nervous system hemorrhage associated with hypoprothrombinemia after cardiac valve replacement. Of 67 patients on warfarin dying > two months after operation, five died of complications of anticoagulation (Table 18). Three of the five had developed serum hepatitis in the early postoperative period with striking elevations of prothrombin times. The other two patients also developed severe hypoprothrombinemia, but neither had hepatitis.

Systemic emboli from prostheses were a cause of late death in ten of the 96 patients and prosthetic thrombosis the cause in one. All but two of these 11 patients had been on warfarin. Of the 29 patients not on warfarin, two died as a result of emboli. Thus, *the hazards of long-term anticoagulants may outweigh their clinical benefit.*

Aneurysm formation at sites of excised left ventricular papillary muscles after mitral valve replacement (Figs. 16 and 20). In three patients who had had

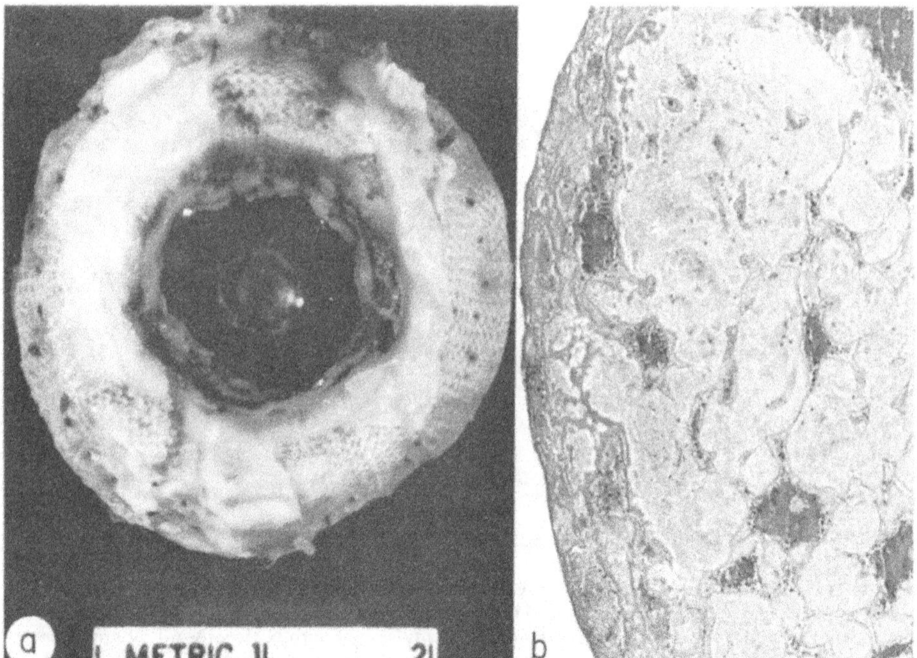

Fig. 35. Starr-Edwards aortic valve as viewed from the ventricular aspect in a 45-yr-old man (A69-281) who had valve replacement 23 mo earlier. This patient had a model 2300 prosthesis (the present one is model 2320), which was made stenotic by the manufacturer. The inlet orifice was further narrowed in this patient by a rim of fibrin-platelet thrombus (B). This patient had a 50 mm Hg peak systolic pressure gradient between left ventricle and aorta and the entire gradient appears to be at the inlet of the prosthesis. Hematoxylin and eosin stain. × 80 (B).

mitral valve replacements 3, 6, and 9 mo, respectively, before death, necropsy disclosed fibrosis of the entire left ventricular free wall beneath the site of amputation of one of the papillary muscles.[22] The thinness of the left ventricular walls at these sites indicates that functional aneurysms had been present during life. Left ventricular saccular aneurysms are almost certainly the result of excision of a portion of left ventricular free wall beneath the papillary muscles at the time of mitral valve excision. This complication may be prevented by not pulling the papillary muscle toward the left atrium at the time it is severed at operation. No known clinical consequences resulted from the left ventricular aneurysms in any of the three patients, although two died suddenly without other anatomic explanation. One patient died in the operating room from perforation of the left ventricular wall at the site of excision of one of the papillary muscles.

Calcification of mitral anulus. A previously undescribed late complication of valve replacement with rigid-framed caged-ball prostheses is calcification at the site of attachment of the prosthesis. Six (Table 19) patients dying 44–116 mo (average, 88) after mitral replacement for pure regurgitation had calcific deposits in prosthetic anuli. None of the six had valvular or anular calcification preoperatively or at operation. The anular calcific deposits at necropsy varied from focal to diffuse. The most extensive deposits occurred in two patients in whom the implantation periods exceeded 100 mo.

The mechanism of calcification of the mitral anuli in these patients is uncertain, but it is likely that constant to-and-fro movement of rigid-framed prostheses accelerates wear of the tissues beneath the site of attachment. A danger of prosthetic ring calcification is obvious in the event of reoperation to replace a faulty prosthesis. Because prostheses appear to be held in place by su-

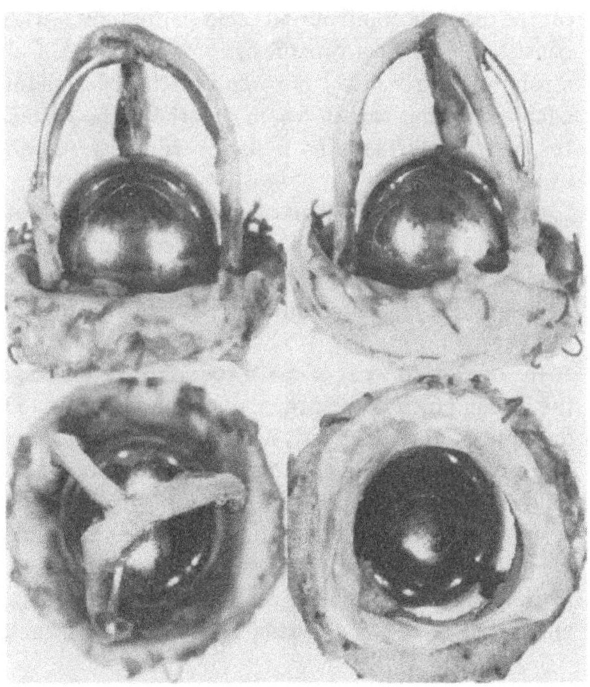

Fig. 36. Wear of cloth on struts of Starr-Edwards prosthesis (size 11A, model 2310) implanted 24 mo earlier in a 50-yr-old man who died of cancer. Upper: Lateral views of prosthesis. Lower left: Prosthesis as viewed from above. Lower right: Prosthesis as viewed from left ventricle. Collagen has covered the seat of the prosthesis but there has been little ingrowth of tissue on the cloth of the struts. Severe through-and-through wear of cloth exposed two of the three metallic struts. Although evidence of increased red cell destruction was present, the valve apparently functioned well.

tures and not by ingrowth of tissue, it is also possible that calcific deposits at prosthetic rings might tear sutures and cause peribasilar leaks.

Status of cloth-covered struts of Starr-Edwards prosthetic valves in patients dying later than 2 mo after cardiac valve replacement (Figs. 7, 31–36). Twenty-five cloth-covered prostheses implanted in 20 patients from 3–52 mo (average, 18) were examined (Table 20). Of 15 aortic prostheses, eight were model 2300, five, model 2310, and two, model 2320. Of nine mitral prostheses, four were model 6300, four, model 6310, and one, model 6320. One prosthesis implanted in the tricuspid position was model 6300. On gross examination some struts appeared free of tissue covering; however, on histologic examination, each of the 25 prostheses showed some degree of tissue growth over the cloth of the struts and bases. The initial deposit, as learned from histologic study of a number of cloth-covered prostheses in patients dying early (< 2 mo after operation), appears to be a fibrin-platelet thrombus. This material organized into dense fibrous tissue containing fibroblasts, and rarely exhibited vascular channels and mononuclear cells. Electron microscopic examination of the fibrous tissue covering the struts and bases in two patients dying late disclosed that it consisted of collagen fibrils and an occasional fibroblast[32,33] (Fig. 32). Thus, the dense fibrous tissue covering the cloth should be referred to as collagen. In several patients dying late (> 2 mo after operation), fibrin-platelet deposits were observed on the struts or bases, or both, adjacent to dense collagen.

The collagen deposits appear to form first at the apex of the cage, except in the close clearance prostheses where the deposits form on the vertical portions of the struts just before they bend to form the apex. The deposits cover some struts in their entirety; in others they are focal on one strut and grossly absent on another of the same prosthesis.

The amount of tissue growing over the struts is not proportional to the length of the implantation period, and in patients with two prostheses, it did not consistently favor a prosthesis in one position. Collagen deposition on the cloth struts was fairly heavy in some prostheses implanted for less than 6 mo, but in each of two patients in whom prostheses had been implanted for 35 and 40 mo, respectively, virtually no tissue overgrowth was observed on the struts on gross examination.

Cloth wear on the struts was observed in two of the 25 prostheses examined. Both were aortic valves: One had been implanted for 24 mo, and the other for 25 mo (Fig. 36). Fibrin platelet thrombi also were present on the struts. Two aortic valves with longer implantation periods (35 and 52 mo) were free of cloth wear and thrombi.

In addition to wear of cloth covering the struts, disruptions also may occur in the Teflon cloth in the orifice of the model 6310–6320 mitral valves. These cloth disruptions may be minor, or they may produce significant regurgitation and require reoperation. Significant cloth disruption has been observed as soon as 2 mo following valve replacement. These periorifice cloth disruptions may in part result from damage at the time of valve replacement by the prosthesis holder. Nevertheless, the use of polypropylene orifice cloth instead of Teflon is currently being evaluated. It may be less susceptible to damage from the valve holder, less apt to migrate over the stud edges, and less liable to unravel or run should a break in the yarn occur. Interestingly, disruption of orifice cloth in the composite seat of the aortic prostheses (models 2310–2320) has been far less frequent, and at this time of no clinical significance.

Although thrombo-embolism is less with cloth-covered prostheses,[34,35] compared to similar noncloth-covered prostheses, hemolysis is increased. As mentioned earlier, renal hemosiderosis is an anatomic indicator of intravascular hemolysis. Kidneys were available for histologic examination in 49 of the 92 patients dying late with rigid-framed ball valve prostheses (Table 21). Cloth-covered prostheses had been used in 14 of the 49 patients; renal iron was present in 12 patients (86%) and heavy in 10 (71%). Of the 35 patients with noncloth-covered struts, 24 (69%) had renal hemosiderosis and 18 (51%) had heavy deposits of renal iron. Excluding ten patients with peribasilar leaks (which in

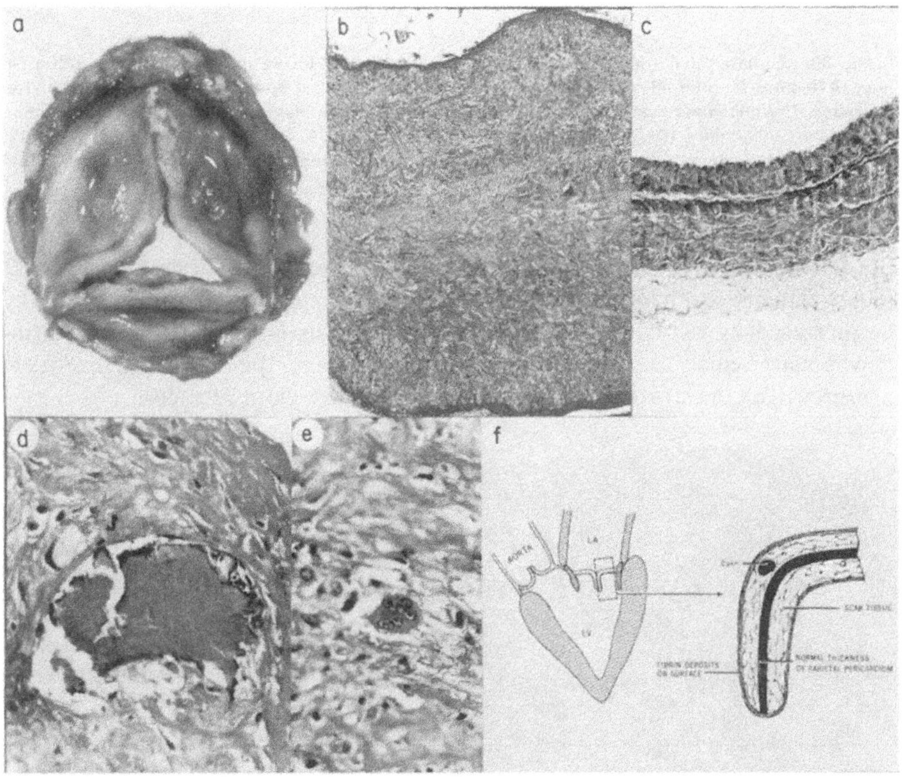

Fig. 37. Fresh autogenous pericardial valve implanted in mitral position in a 50-yr-old woman (A71-61) 39 days before death. There was no evidence of dysfunction of this tissue valve during the postoperative period. (A) View of pericardial valve from above. The "cusps" are thickened and one is retracted. The valve orifice was competent when water was injected under pressure into the left ventricle at necropsy. (B) Photomicrograph of section through one "cusp." The surfaces of the "cusp" are lined by fibrin. The cusp is about four times thicker than normal. The implanted parietal pericardium may be compared to its thickness at time of implantation, a portion of which is shown in C. Both B and C were taken at the same magnification. Thickening of the implanted pericardium is due mainly to proliferation of fibrous tissue, which probably resulted from organization of surface fibrin. (D) Deposit of calcium in the implanted valve. (E) Close-up of portion of implanted valve showing multinucleated cell of uncertain significance. (F) Schematic diagram of changes (seen in B), which occurred in the implanted autogenous pericardial valve. Hematoxylin and eosin stains. C and D, × 70. E and F, × 400.

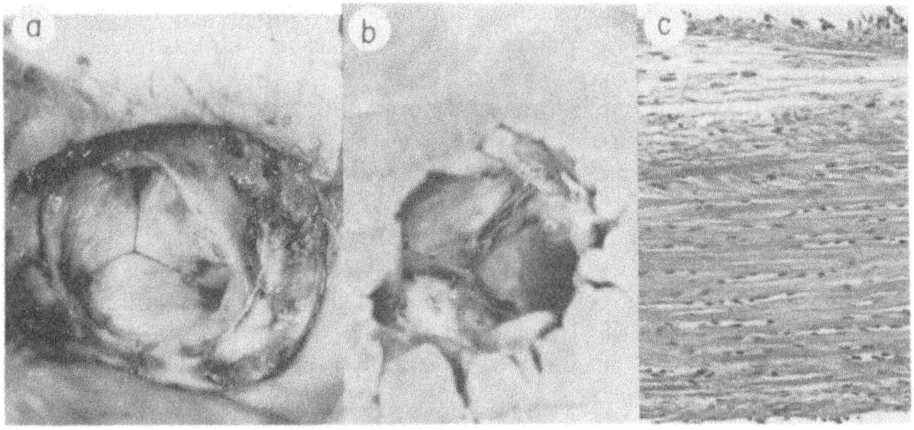

Fig. 38. Glutaraldehyde-fixed porcine aortic valve implanted in the mitral portion in a 60-yr-old man (A70–280) for pure mitral regurgitation. He died 50 days after operation but never awoke after operation. The implanted tissue valve functioned normally. (A) Implanted valve, which is competent, viewed from left atrium. (B) Same valve viewed from left ventricle. The leaflets are freely mobile. (C) Photomicrograph of a portion of one cusp. The cuspal tissue appears well preserved. Hematoxylin and eosin stain. × 160.

themselves may cause intravascular hemolysis), heavy deposits of renal iron were present in 10 of 26 (39%) patients without cloth-covered prostheses and in 9 of 13 (69%) patients with cloth-covered prostheses. Although hemolysis may initially be increased by the cloth covering of the prosthesis and lead to increased intravascular hemolysis, trauma to erythrocytes may then diminish as tissue overgrowth on the struts and bases smooths the rough cloth surfaces.

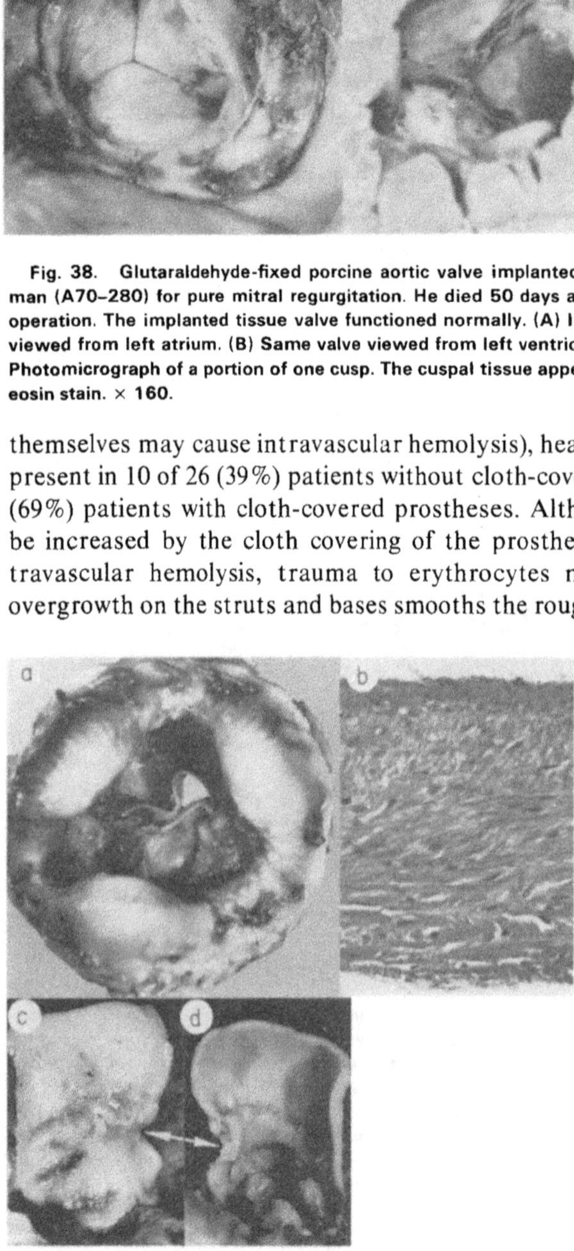

Fig. 39. Glutaraldehyde fixed porcine aortic valve implanted in aortic position in a 51-yr-old man (A71–78) 150 days before death. He died suddenly at home of uncertain cause after a previously asymptomatic postoperative course. (A) Porcine valve as viewed from above showing thrombi in two of three sinuses of Valsalva. One week before death a 35 mm Hg peak systolic pressure gradient between left ventricle and brachial artery was demonstrated, and the gradient may have been due to the thrombi causing poor leaflet mobility and to the small orifice of the tissue involved. (B) Photomicrograph of section of implanted valve cusp. The cuspal tissue appears well preserved and free of inflammation or necrosis. Hematoxylin and eosin stain. × 400. (C and D) Views of ascending aorta anteriorly (C) and of porcine valve from above (D). Arrow designates the healed aortotomy incision, which appears to cause some narrowing anatomically. Note close apposition of the struts of the porcine valve at the central orifice (suggesting inherent stenosis).

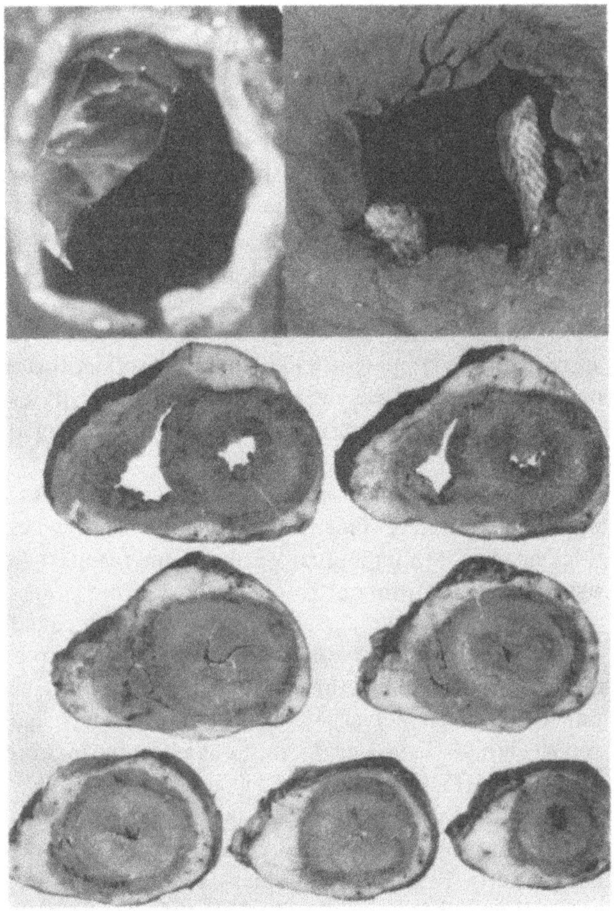

Fig. 40. Porcine aortic heterograft, fixed in stabilized glutaraldehyde, implanted in the mitral position for stenosis in a 44-yr-old man (A71–101) 14 days before death. He had a smooth early postoperative course and was discharged 12 days after operation. Two days later he died suddenly. Upper left: View from aorta showing stint of mitral prosthesis partially obstructing left ventricular outflow. Upper right: View of porcine valve from left ventricle showing two of three stints of the tissue valve frame contacting left ventricular endocardium. Left ventricular cavity is smaller than normal, and cavity obliteration in systole had been demonstrated by left ventricular cineangiography before operation. The lower photograph shows transverse cuts of the ventricles disclosing a very small left ventricular cavity.

Myocardial necrosis and fibrosis in patients dying late after cardiac valve replacement. The incidence and location of myocardial necrosis and fibrosis in these patients are summarized in Table 22. In contrast to the frequency of its occurrence in the patients who died early (Table 11), myocardial necrosis was rare in the patients dying late, occurring in only five patients, and in three of them it was limited to papillary muscle. Myocardial fibrosis, in contrast, occurred in 72 of the 96 patients: In 30 it was limited to papillary muscle; in 15 it occurred in the subendocardium of the left ventricular free wall or ventricular septum, or both, in addition to papillary muscle; and in 27 patients, it was transmural. Transmural fibrosis in three patients was located in the free walls beneath sites where left ventricular papillary muscles had been excised.

Tissue valves (Figs. 37–40). Porcine aortic valve heterografts fixed in stabilized glutaraldehyde were utilized in seven of the 224 patients (Table 23): Five were placed in the mitral position, one in the aortic, and one in the tricuspid. No patient had clinical evidence of systemic emboli and none received warfarin. Three patients died early and four died late (4–14 mo) after operation. Of the patients dying early, one never awoke postoperatively; one, who also had a parietal pericardial mitral valve, died of upper gastrointestinal bleeding; and one was unable to maintain adequate blood pressure for unknown reasons after mitral replacement. All three valves appeared to function well postoperatively. Of the four patients dying > 2 mo after valve replacement, the cause was uncertain in each: Two died of progressive congestive cardiac failure and two died suddenly. Clinically, none had evidence of valvular dysfunction, and necropsy did not provide explanations for death. In one patient dying suddenly with a porcine heterograft in the aortic position, a systolic pressure gradient of 35 mm Hg between left ventricle and brachial artery was documented 1 wk before death. At necropsy, thrombus was present within the sinuses of Valsalva of two of the three cusps. This was the only porcine valve to contain thrombus.

At necropsy, all seven porcine valves appeared in good condition: The leaflets were freely mobile, not thickened, and not calcified; the orifices were neither stenotic nor incompetent. On histologic section, the cusps were not inflammed or necrotic. Renal hemosiderosis was absent in all seven patients, and none had significant left ventricular endocardial thickening or ascending aortic intimal thickening.

The fresh autogenous pericardial valve fared less well. After only 39 days, it was approximately four times thicker than when inserted (Fig. 37). The thickening of the implanted pericardium resulted from proliferation of fibrous tissue organized from fibrin.

Tissue valves have certain advantages over caged-ball or disc prostheses: A central nonobstructive orifice causes less trauma to blood constituents and to adjacent vascular linings; thrombi are infrequent and, therefore, anticoagulants are unnecessary. Hemolysis is decreased, although significant hemolysis has been reported in fascia lata grafts that have become incompetent.[36] The long-term fate of these grafts, however, is as yet undetermined. A variety of tissue valves have been tried. Parietal pericardium is not a good valve substitute because it thickens rapidly and loses its mobility.[37,38] It also appears highly susceptible to infective endocarditis. Fascia lata is poor as a valve substitute because it is inherently too stiff and rapidly becomes even more stiff from fibrosis and calcification.[37,39]

The porcine aortic valve, when fixed in stabilized glutaraldehyde, appears to be a good valve substitute. Similar valves fixed in formalin, however, have rapidly degenerated.[37] The porcine valves in our seven patients were well preserved, and each appeared to have functioned normally, up to 14 mo after implantation in one patient. From clinical and morphologic standpoints, death in all seven appeared unrelated to the tissue valves *per se*. The porcine heterografts fixed in stabilized glutaraldehyde are promising, and deserve thorough and continuing clinical evaluation.

SUMMARY

Necropsy observations are described in 224 patients who died from 1963 through October 1972 after replacement of one or more cardiac valves by prostheses: 128 patients died within 2 mo of operation, and 96 patients at later periods up to 116 mo. Of the 281 valves replaced, Starr-Edwards prostheses were used in 250. Prosthetic dysfunction continues to be the most common cause of death (approximately 30%) in patients dying either early or late after valve replacement. It is hoped that the metal balls and cloth-covered struts will decrease the late frequency of prosthetic dysfunction, but not enough time has elapsed for this altered prosthesis to be tested adequately. Present data indicate that the frequency of clinical embolism and prosthetic thrombosis after use of the cloth-covered prostheses is less than that observed in the noncloth-covered prostheses. Cloth wear with possible dislodgement and increased intravascular hemolysis, however, remains of concern. The frequencies of peribasilar fistulae, infection at sites of attachment of prostheses, and aneurysm formation at sites of excision of left ventricular papillary muscles are decreasing. It appears that secondary left ventricular endocardial fibroelastosis after mitral replacement, aortic root and coronary ostial intimal proliferation after aortic valve replacement and calcification of valve anuli will only increase with time after valve replacement. The latter changes may prove to be major long-term problems.

It is clear after a decade of cardiac valve replacement that the ideal valve prosthesis is not yet available, or if available, not adequately tested. Thus, valve replacement at this time must be reserved for the patient severely disabled by cardiac valve disease.

APPENDIX

Table 1. Patients Studied at Necropsy After Cardiac Valve Replacement

Valve Replaced	Early Death (<2 mo)	Late Death (>2 mo)	Totals
Aortic (A)	42	47	89
Mitral (M)	52	28	80
A + M	20	18	38
Tricuspid (T)	2	0	2
T + A	1	0	1
T + M	8	2	10
T + M + A	3	1	4
Totals	128	96	224

Table 2. Age and Sex in 224 Necropsy Patients Dying After Cardiac Valve Replacement

	Early (<2 Mo) Deaths					Late (>2 Mo) Deaths				
Valve Replacement	No. Males	No. Females	Total Patients	Age Range	Average (Yr)	No. Males	No. Females	Total Patients	Age Range	Average (Yr)
Aortic (A)	29	13	42	5–65	45	44	3	47	21–69	46
Mitral (M)	25	27	52	4–63	43	11	17	28	15–65	48
A + M	12	8	20	25–27	46	16	2	18	23–63	49
Tricuspid (T)	0	2	2	42 & 57	49	0	0	0	—	—
T + A	1	0	1	20	20	0	0	0	—	—
T + M	1	7	8	32–57	45	0	2	2	49 & 51	50
T + M + A	2	1	3	33–54	45	0	1	1	52	52
Totals	70 (54%)	58 (46%)	128	4–67	(45)	71 (74%)	25 (26%)	96	15–69	(47)

Table 3. Types of Functional Valve Lesions Requiring Valve Replacement

Valve Replaced	Early Deaths: Stenosis	Early Deaths: Pure Regurgitation	Early Deaths: Totals	Late Deaths: Stenosis	Late Deaths: Pure Regurgitation	Late Deaths: Totals
Aortic (A)						
A only	26	16	42	34	13	47
A + M	12	8	20	14	4	18
A + M + T	2	1	3	1	0	1
A + T	0	1	1			
Mitral (M)						
M only	38	14	52	18	10	28
M + A	14	6	20	16	2	18
M + T	8	0	8	1	1	2
M + T + A	3	0	3	1	0	1
Tricuspid (T)						
T only	1	1	2	0	0	0
T + M	3	5	8	0	2	2
T + A	0	1	1	0	0	0
T + M + A	2	1	3	0	1	1
Totals	109	54	163	85	33	118
	(67%)	(33%)	(100%)	(72%)	(28%)	(100%)

Table 4. Prosthetic Valves Used in the 224 Necropsy Patients

Valve Replaced	Type Prosthesis: Starr-Edwards	Kay-Shiley	Magovern	Porcine Heterograft	Pericardial Valve	Totals
Aortic	127	0	4	1	0	132
Mitral	116	10	0	5	1	132
Tricuspid	7	9	0	1	0	17
Totals	250	19	4	7	1	281

Table 5. Sizes of Starr-Edwards Prostheses Employed

Valve Replaced	Valve Sizes							
Aortic	7A	8A	9A	10A	11A	12A	13A	Totals
Early deaths								
No.	3	22	17	12	7	2	1	64
(%)	(4)	(34)	(27)	(19)	(11)	(3)	(2)	(100)
Late deaths								
No.	2	17	9	15	16	2	2	63
(%)	(3)	(27)	(15)	(24)	(25)	(3)	(3)	(100)
Mitral	1M	2M	3M	4M				Totals
Early deaths								
No.	1	21	42	8				72
(%)	(1)	(29)	(59)	(11)				(100)
Late deaths								
No.		9	20	15				44
(%)		(21)	(45)	(34)				(100)
Tricuspid	2M	3M	4M					Totals
Early deaths								
No.	0	3	3					6
Late deaths								
No.	0	1	0					1
								250

Table 6. Weight (Range [Avg.]) of Hearts in Patients With Prosthetic Cardiac Valves

	Early (< 2 Mo) Deaths			Late (> 2 Mo) Deaths		
Valve Replaced	Males	Females	All	Males	Females	All
Aortic (A)	440–1250 (735)	450–800 (588)	440–1250 (694)	440–1350 (707)	330–340 (330)	330–1350 (699)
Mitral (M)	350– 850 (595)	300–600 (464)	300– 850 (517)	400– 870 (669)	370–800 (525)	370– 800 (610)
A + M	450–1090 (730)	440–550 (530)	440–1090 (657)	450– 960 (718)	420–530 (475)	420– 850 (688)
Tricuspid (T)	—	670 & 760 (715)	670 & 760 (700)	—	—	—
T + A	700 (700)		700 (700)			
T + M	390 (390)	350–680 (530)	350– 680 (530)	—	570 & 610 (590)	570 & 610 (590)
T + M + A	660 & 750 (705)	690	660 & 690 (700)	—	540	540 (540)

Table 7. Extramural Coronary Arterial Luminal Narrowing > 75% by Old Atheroscerotic Plaques in Patients With Prosthetic Cardiac Valves

	Early	Late
Aortic (A)	7 of 42	10 of 47
Mitral (M)	9 of 52	6 of 28
M + A	3 of 10	1 of 18
Tricuspid ± M ± A	0 of 14	0 of 3
	19 of 128 (15%)	17 of 96 (18%)

Table 8. Period of Time Between Valve Replacement and Death in the 128 Patients Dying Early

	Day of Death After Operation							
Valve Replaced	Zero	1–3	4–7	8–14	15–21	22–30	31–60	Totals
Aortic (A)	10	11	6	5	4	2	4	42
Mitral (M)	6	15	15	3	7	3	3	52
A + M	5	3	1	5	1	0	5	20
Tricuspid (T)	0	1	0	1	0	0	0	2
T + A	0	1	0	0	0	0	0	1
T + M	1	1	2	1	1	0	2	8
T + M + A	0	0	0	0	1	2	0	3
Totals	22*	32	24	15	14	7	14	128

*Sixteen patients died in the operating room.

Table 9. Prosthetic Stenosis* as a Cause of Early Death (<2 Mo)

	Total No. of Patients	Patients With Prosthetic Dysfunction	Prosthesis Size				
			SE	SE	SE	K-S	Magovern
Mitral Valve	83	20 (24%)	2M	3M	4M		
MS		18	4	11	1	2	0
MR		2	0	2	0	0	0
			SE	SE	SE	SE	
Aortic Valve	65	8 (12%)	7A	8A	9A	11A	
AS		2	0	1	0	0	1
AR		6	1	2	2	1	0

*Prosthetic stenosis caused by prostheses' being too big for ventricular cavity or aortic root.

Abbreviations: AS, aortic stenosis; AR, aortic regurgitation; K-S, Kay Shiley prosthesis; MR, mitral regurgitation; MS, mitral stenosis; SE, Starr-Edwards prosthesis.

Table 10. Causes of Death Early (<2 Mo) After Cardiac Valve Replacement (128 Necropsy Patients)

	Valves Replaced					
	Aortic (A)	Mitral (M)	M + A	Tricuspid (T)	T + M + A	Totals No. (%)
1. Prosthetic dysfunction	9	19	4	1	4	37(28)
Prosthesis too big for ventricular cavity or aortic root (prosthetic stenosis)	5	18	2	1	2	28
Prosthetic ball prevented from seating completely (prosthetic regurgitation)	2	0	0	0	2	4
Manufacturing error: low clearance with sticking of poppet	2	1	2	0	0	5
2. No anatomic cause	14	15	4	0	7	40(31)
Low cardiac output syndrome	7	13	3	0	7	30
Sudden (? arrhythmia)	4	2	1	0	0	7
Pump failure (in operating room)	3	0	0	0	0	3
3. Bleeding	7	2	2	0	1	12(10)
4. Technical mishap	5	3	4	0	0	12(10)
5. Central nervous system catastrophe	3	6	1	0	0	10(8)
6. Associated undiagnosed or uncorrected valve disease	1	4	1	1	0	7(5)
7. Infection	2	1	1	0	0	4(3)
At site of attachment of prosthesis	1	1	1	0	0	3
Other	1	0				1
8. Miscellaneous	1	2	3	0	0	6(5)
Totals	42	52	20	2	12	128(100)

Table 11. Myocardial Necrosis and Fibrosis in 128 Patients Dying *Early* After Cardiac Valve Replacement

	Aortic (A) (42 Patients)	Mitral (M) (52 Patients)	A + M (20 Patients)	Tricuspid ± M ± A (14 Patients)	Totals 128 Patients (%)
Myocardial necrosis, LV					
Papillary muscles only	6	26	3	7	42 (33)
Subendocardium*	6	10	3	1	20 (16)
Transmural†	4	10	4	3	21 (16)
Myocardial fibrosis, LV‡					
Papillary muscles only	4	10	0	2	16 (13)
Subendocardium*	14	5	5	2	26 (20)
Transmural†	4	3	0	1	8 (6)

*Inner half of wall of left ventricle (LV) or ventricular septum; papillary muscles usually also involved.

† Excludes patients with necrosis or fibrosis in the papillary muscle and subendocardial regions, although necrosis or fibrosis at these sites also usually are present.

‡ Replacement fibrosis only. Excludes interstitial and perivascular fibrosis, visible histologically, which occurred to varying degrees in most patients. Six patients with myocardial necrosis (four transmural) and 13 patients with myocardial fibrosis (four transmural) had luminal narrowing > 75% by old plaques of one or more of the three major extramural coronary arteries. In three patients, transmural necrosis involved only the free wall of the left ventricle at sites where excision of papillary muscles had occurred.

Table 12. Deaths Late (>2 Mo) After Cardiac Valve Replacement

			Prosthetic Thrombus				
Valve(s) Replaced	No. Patients	Implantation Periods (Mo) Range (Average)	No. Patients With Thrombi (No. Prostheses)	Patients With Thrombi on Warfarin	Thrombi Causing Dysfunction	*Clinical* Emboli	Ring* Leak
Aortic (A)	47	2.5–67 (26)	35 (35)	17	10	7	5
Mitral (M)	28	3–116 (38)	21 (21)	17	7	6	3
A + M	18	2.1–70 (20)	13 (21)	13	2	3	3
M + Tricuspid (T)	2	9 and 29 (19)	2 (4)	2	2	0	0
M + T + A	1	40	0	0	0	0	0
118 valves	96	2.1–116 (28)	71 (81)	49	21	16	11

*Patients with infective endocarditis at site of prosthesis were excluded.

Table 13. Causes of Death Late (>2 Mo) After Cardiac Valve Replacement (96 Necropsy Patients)

Cause	Valves Replaced				Totals
	Aortic (A)	Mitral (M)	M + A	Tricuspid + M	No. (%)
1. Prosthetic dysfunction	19	6	6	1	32 (33)
Degeneration, silicone rubber ball	13	2	3	0	18
Peribasilar leak	0	1	1	0	2
Prosthetic stenosis	4	0	1	1	6
Prosthetic thrombosis	0	1	0	0	1
Infective endocarditis	2	2	1	0	5
2. *Factors secondarily related to prosthesis*	6	9	5	0	20 (21)
Systemic embolism (acute)					
Myocardial infarction	2	2	1	0	5
Cerebral infarction	0	4	0	0	4
Bowel infarction	0	1	0	0	1
CNS hemorrhage from hypoprothrombinemia	2	2	1	0	5
Secondary endocardial fibrosis, LV *	0	0	2	0	2
Secondary intimal fibrosis, ascending aorta	2	0	0	0	2
Hepatitis	0	0	1	0	1
3. Sudden, cause uncertain	10	5	2	1	18 (19)
4. Underlying cardiac disease	9	6	3	1	19 (20)
Chronic CHF, cause uncertain	4	4	2	1	11
Extensive myocardial fibrosis, LV	1	0	1	0	2
Complications of Marfan Syndrome	2	0	0	0	2
Associated uncorrected valve disease	2	2	0	0	4
5. Noncardiac	3	2	2	0	7 (7)
Totals	47	28	18	3	96 (100)

Abbreviations: CHF, *congestive heart failure;* CNS, *central nervous system;* LV, *left ventricle.*

Table 14. Infection at Sites of Attachment of Starr-Edwards Prostheses

Patient	Age/Sex	Valve Replaced	Valve Infected	Interval Op→Death	Length of Infection	Precipitating Cause	Organism	Conduction Disturbance	Cause of Death
Early Deaths									
A63-176	55/M	Aortic	Aortic	45 days	45 days	Unknown	*Staphylococcus epidermidis*	1°HB, 2°HB LBBB	AR
A68-57	60/F	Mitral	Mitral	38 days	30 days	Wound infection	*Proteus mirabilis*	0	MS
A70-144	36/M	Aortic Mitral	Aortic	35 days	23 days	Wound infection	*Staphylococcus epidermidis*	0	Stroke AR
Late Deaths									
A64-189	51/M	Aortic	Aortic	13 mo	45 days	Teeth extractions	*Staphylococcus epidermidis*	LBBB	AR
A65-186	47/M	Mitral	Mitral	4 mo	30 days	Skin graft	*Staphylococcus aureus*	0	MS
A65-221	46/M	Mitral	Mitral	4 mo	25 days	Unknown	*Staphylococcus epidermidis*	0	MS
A67-22	48/M	Aortic	Aortic	3 mo	16 days	Unknown	*Staphylococcus epidermidis*	$1°HB_N$ 2°HB, Nodal	AR
A68-33	57/M	Aortic Mitral	Aortic	7 mo	90 days	Wound infection	*Serratia marcescens*	1°HB LBBB	AR

Abbreviations: AR, aortic regurgitation; 1° HB, *PR* interval > 0.20 sec; 2° HB, second degree heart block; LBBB, left bundle branch block; MS, mitral stenosis.

Table 15. Status of Silicone Rubber Poppets Implanted 24 Mo or Longer

Valve	Total	Normal	Abnormal	Discolored but Functioned Normally	Discolored, Swollen and Impacted	Discolored, Fractured, Dislodged
Aortic						
No. Poppets	25	8	17	1	10	6
Implantation						
period (mo)		27–70	24–67	65	24–67	28–37
Range (average)		(45)	(41)		(43)	(33)
Mitral						
No. Poppets	17	12	5	3	2	0
Implantation						
period (mo)		28–116	78–114	105–114	78 and 94	0
Range (average)		(58)	(100)	(100)	(86)	
Totals	42	20	22	4	12	6

Table 16. Composition of Stellite 21

Chemical Element	Nominal Composition	Atomic Number	Atomic Weight
Cobalt (Co)	58%–69%	27	58.94
Chromium (Cr)	25%–30%	24	52.01
Molybdenum (Mo)	4.5%–6.5%	42	95.95
Nickel (Ni)	1.5%–3.5%	28	58.69
Iron (Fe)	Up to 2%	26	55.85
Carbon (C)	0.2%–0.4%	6	12.01

Table 17. Renal Hemosiderosis in Patients Dying Later After Cardiac Valve Replacement

Valve	No. Patients	Renal Iron			
		Absent	Present	3+ or 4+	1+ or 2+
Aortic	30	8	22	17	5
Aortic + mitral	8	2	6	5	1
Mitral	12	5	7	5	2
Mitral + tricuspid	1	0	1	0	1
Totals	51	15	36	27	9
		(29%)	(71%)		

Table 18. Fatal CNS Hemorrhage Associated With Hypoprothrombinemia After Cardiac Valve Replacement

Patient	Age/Sex	Interval (Mo) Op → Death	Hepatitis	Warfarin
S63-2617	23/M	2	+	+
A69-27	53/M	3	+	+
A69-292	44/F	4	+	+
A65-81	65/F	8	0	+
A67-29	69/M	14	0	+

Table 19. Calcification of Anulus After Mitral Valve Replacement

Patient	Age/Sex	Pre-op Mitral Lesion	Calcium MV Pre-op	Prosthetic Implantation Period (mos)	Calcium Prosthetic Anulus	Peribasilar Ring Leak
A67-118	47/M	Pure MR	0	44	+	0
A72-30	63/M	Pure MR	0	70	+	+
A70-123	49/F	Pure MR	0	79	+	0
A72-107	49/F	Pure MR	0	105	+	0
A72-44	45/F	Pure MR	0	111	+	0
A72-88	29/F	Pure MR	0	116	+	0

Abbreviations: MR, mitral regurgitation; MV, mitral valve.

Table 20. Necropsy Study of Cloth-covered Starr-Edwards Prostheses Implanted > 2 Mo (25 Prostheses in 20 Patients)

	No. Patients	Implantation Period Range (Average) (Mo)	Valve Model Numbers					
			2300/2310/2320			6300/6310/6320		
Aortic (A)	11	3–52 (23)	5	5	1	—	—	—
Mitral (M)	5	3–7 (5)	—	—	—	1	4	0
A + M	3	3–44 (18)	2	0	1	2	0	1
A + M + T	1	40	1	0	0	2	0	0
Totals	20	3–52 (18)	8	5	2	5	4	1

Table 21. Renal Hemosiderosis: Cloth-covered vs. Noncloth-covered Struts

	Rigid-framed Prosthesis in Patients Dying Late	
	Cloth-covered Struts	Noncloth-covered Struts
No. patients	14	35
No. aortics	10 (72%)	28 (80%)
No. with renal iron	12 (86%)	24 (69%)
No. with heavy deposits	10 (71%)	18 (51%)

Table 22. Myocardial Necrosis and Fibrosis in 96 Patients Dying Late After Cardiac Valve Replacement

	Aortic (A) 47 Patients	Mitral (M) 28 Patients	A + M 18 Patients	Tricuspid + Mitral 3 Patients	Totals 96 Patients (%)
Myocardial necrosis, LV					
Papillary muscles only	1	0	0	2	3(3)
Subendocardium*	0	0	1	0	1(1)
Transmural†	0	1	0	0	1(1)
Myocardial fibrosis, LV‡					
Papillary muscles only	14	5	7	4	30(31)
Subendocardium*	8	2	4	1	15(16)
Transmural†	14	10	3	0	27(28)

*Inner half of LV (left ventricular) free wall or ventricular septum. Papillary muscle also usually involved.

† Excludes patients with papillary muscle and subendocardial necrosis or fibrosis, although necrosis or fibrosis at these sites also was present in most of these patients.

‡ Replacement fibrosis only. Excludes interstitial and perivascular fibrosis, visible histologically, which occurred to varying degrees in most patients.

Table 23. Porcine Aortic Valve Heterografts

Patient	Age	Sex	Valve Replaced	Valve Size (mm)	Implantation Period (mo)	Cause of Death	Thrombus on Prosthesis	Renal Iron
Early (<2 mo)								
A70-280	60	M	MV	34	1.7	CNS catastrophe	0	0
A71-61	50	F	TV†	30	1.3	Bleeding	0	0
A71-101	44	M	MV	29	0.5	Unknown*	0	0
Late (>2 mo)								
A71-78	51	M	AV	25	5	Sudden	+	0
A71-113	55	F	MV	25	4	Unknown*	0	0
A71-181	64	F	MV	29	6	Unknown*	0	0
A72-190	50	F	MV	29	14	Sudden	0	0

* Inadequate cardiac output of uncertain etiology

† Mitral valve also replaced with tissue valve made of parietal pericardium.

Abbreviations: MV, mitral valve; TV, tricuspid valve; AV, aortic valve; CNS, central nervous system.

REFERENCES

1. Roberts WC: The structure of the aortic valve in clinically isolated aortic stenosis. An autopsy study of 162 patients over 15 years of age. Circulation 42:91, 1970

2. —: The congenitally bicuspid aortic valve. A study of 85 autopsy cases. Am J Cardiol 26:72, 1970

3. —: Anatomically isolated aortic valvular disease. The case against its being of rheumatic etiology. Am J Med 49:151, 1970

4. —, Braunwald E, Morrow AG: Acute severe mitral regurgitation secondary to ruptured chordae tendineae. Clinical hemodynamic and pathologic considerations. Circulation 33:58, 1966

5. —: Examining the precordium and the heart. Chest 57:567, 1970

6. Helmsworth JA, Gall EA, Perrin EV, et al: Occurrence of emboli during perfusion with an oxygenator pump. Surgery 53:177, 1963

7. Roberts WC, Morrow AG: Cardiac valves and the surgical pathologist. Arch Pathol 82:309, 1966

8. —, —: Causes of early postoperative death following cardiac valve replacement. J Thorac Cardiovasc Surg 54:422, 1967

9. —, —: Compression of anomalous left circumflex coronary arteries by prosthetic valve fixation rings. J Thorac Cardiovasc Surg 57:834, 1969

10. —, —: Anatomic studies of hearts containing caged-ball prosthetic valves. Johns Hopkins Med J 121:271, 1967

11. —, Lambird PA, Gott VL et al: Fatal aortic regurgitation following replacement of the mitral and aortic valves. A mechanical complication of double valve replacement. J Thorac Cardiovasc Surg 52:189, 1966

12. —, Morrow AG: Mechanisms of acute left atrial thrombosis after mitral valve replacement. Am J Cardiol 18:497, 1966

13. Glancy DL, O'Brien KP, Reis RL, et al: Hemodynamic studies in patients with 2M and 3M Starr-Edwards prostheses: Evidence of obstruction to the left atrial emptying. Circulation 39 and 40 (Suppl. I): I/113, 1969

14. Reis RL, Glancy DL, O'Brien K, et al: Clinical and hemodynamic assessments of fabric-covered Starr-Edwards prosthetic valves. J Thorac Cardiovasc Surg 59:84, 1970

15. Buja LM, Freed TA, Berman MA, et al: Pulmonary alveolar hemorrhage. A common finding in patients with severe cardiac disease. Am J Cardiol 27:168, 1971

16. Taber RE, Morales AR, Fine G: Myocardial necrosis and the postoperative low-cardiac-output syndrome. Ann Thorac Surg 4:12, 1967

17. Morales AR, Fine G, Taber RE: Cardiac surgery and myocardial necrosis. Arch Pathol 83:71, 1967

18. Niles NR, Sandilands JR: Pathology of heart valve replacement surgery: Autopsies of 62 patients with Starr-Edwards prostheses. Dis Chest 56:373, 1969

19. Reichenbach DD, Benditt EP: Myofibrillar degeneration. A response of the myocardial cell to injury. Arch Pathol 85:189, 1968

20. Buja LM, Levitsky S, Ferrans VJ, et al: Acute and chronic effects of normothermic anoxia on canine hearts: Light and electron microscopic evaluation. Circulation 43 and 44 (Suppl. I): I/44, 1971

21. Roberts WC, Morrow AG: Late postoperative pathological findings after cardiac valve replacement. Circulation 35 and 36 (Suppl. I): I/48, 1967

22. —, —: Later postoperative pathologic findings following cardiac valve replacement with Starr-Edwards prostheses, in Brewer LA III (ed): Prosthetic Heart Valves. Springfield, Ill, Thomas, 1969

23. —, Berard CW, Braunwald NS: Roentgenogram of the month. Dis Chest 51:439, 1967

24. Rockoff SD, Ross J Jr, Oldham NN Jr, et al: Ventriculo-atrial regurgitation following prosthetic replacement of the mitral valve. Angiocardiographic and hemodynamic findings. Am J Cardiol 17:817, 1966

25. Cohn LH, Roberts WC, Rockoff SD, et al: Bacterial endocarditis following aortic valve replacement. Clinical and pathologic correlations. Circulation 33:209, 1966

26. Roberts WC, Morrow AG: Bacterial endocarditis involving prosthetic mitral valves. Clinical and pathologic observation. Arch Pathol 82:164, 1966

27. —, Levinson GE, Morrow AG: Lethal ball variance in the Starr-Edwards prosthetic *mitral* valve. Arch Intern Med 126:517, 1970

28. —, Morrow AG: Fatal degeneration of the silicone rubber ball of the Starr-Edwards prosthetic aortic valve. Am J Cardiol 22:614, 1968

29. —, —: Renal hemosiderosis in patients with prosthetic aortic valves. Circulation 33:390, 1966

30. —: Renal hemosiderosis (blue kidney) in patients with valvular heart disease. Am J Path 38:409, 1966

31. —, Morrow AG: Secondary left ventricular endocardial fibroelastosis following mitral valve replacement. Cause of cardiac failure in the late postoperative period. Circulation 37 and 38 (Suppl. II): II/101, 1968

32. —, Reis RL, Ferrans VJ, et al: Anatomic studies on cloth-covered Starr-Edwards prosthetic valves implanted for longer than two months (abstract). Am J Cardiol 29:287, 1972

33. Winter TQ, Reis RL, Glancy DL, et al: Current status of the Starr-Edwards cloth-covered prosthetic cardiac valves. Circulation 45 and 46 (Suppl I):I/14, 1972

34. Isom OW, Williams CD, Falk EA, and et al: Long-term evaluation of cloth-covered metallic ball prostheses. J Thorac Cardiovasc Surg 64:354, 1972

35. Hodam R, Anderson R, Starr A, et al: Further evaluation of the composite seat cloth-covered aortic prosthesis. Ann Thorac Surg 12:621, 1971

36. Dave KS, Madan CK, Pakrashi BC, et al: Chronic hemolysis following fascia lata and Starr-Edwards aortic valve replacement. Circulation 46:240, 1972

37. Yarbrough JW, Roberts WC, Reis RL: Structural alterations in tissue cardiac valves implanted in humans and calves. J Thorac Cardiovasc Surg, in press

38. Suzuki A, Mackrell J, Kay EB: Mitral valve replacement with transplant valves. J Thorac Cardiovasc Surg 60:13, 1970

39. McEnany MT, Ross DN, Yates AK: Valve failure in seventy-two frame-supported autologous fascia lata mitral valves. Two-year follow-up. J Thorac Cardiovasc Surg 63:199, 1972

40. Shepherd RL, Glancy DL, Stinson EB, et al: Hemodynamic confirmation of obstruction to left ventricular inflow by a caged-ball prosthetic mitral valve. J Thorac Cardiovasc Surg 65:252, 1973

Results of Valve Replacement for Severe Mitral Regurgitation Due to Papillary Muscle Rupture or Fibrosis

D. LUKE GLANCY, MD, FACC
EDWARD B. STINSON, MD
RICHARD L. SHEPHERD, MD
SAMUEL B. ITSCOITZ, MD
WILLIAM C. ROBERTS, MD, FACC
STEPHEN E. EPSTEIN, MD
ANDREW G. MORROW, MD, FACC

Bethesda, Maryland

Late results of mitral valve replacement for papillary muscle rupture (four patients) or fibrosis without rupture (five patients) are described for the first time. Patients underwent operation 3 months to more than 13 years (median 14 months) after the onset of severe mitral regurgitation. Preoperatively all had holosystolic murmurs, atrial and ventricular gallops, cardiomegaly and cardiac failure. Three had class III and six had class IV functional capacity (New York Heart Association Classification). Atrial fibrillation developed in the three patients who had mitral regurgitation for more than 3 years. Left atrial mean pressure (average 27 mm Hg) and *V* waves (average 46 mm Hg) were greatly increased in all but one patient, and cardiac index (average 2.0 liters/min per m^2) was reduced in all but one. No finding distinguished patients with rupture from those without rupture. The left ventricular angiogram was the best preoperative guide to postoperative results. Of five patients with poor left ventricular contractions, four died (one suddenly 2 days postoperatively and three with cardiac failure, two 6 months and one 62 months postoperatively); 4 months after operation one is limited by the residua of a cerebral embolus. None of the three studied postoperatively showed hemodynamic improvement. In contrast, of four patients with fair or good left ventricular contractions preoperatively, three have class I or II functional capacity 23, 60, 64 months, respectively, after operation, and one died suddenly 41 months after operation. All three studied postoperatively showed marked hemodynamic improvement.

The early results of operation for mitral regurgitation due to papillary muscle rupture or dysfunction without rupture have been described,[1-22] but the late results have not. Four patients we[1] have previously described were followed up for 5 years after mitral valve replacement for papillary muscle rupture. During this interval we studied and operated upon an additional five patients who had severe mitral regurgitation due to papillary muscle fibrosis and dysfunction without rupture. This report describes the clinical, hemodynamic and anatomic features in the nine patients, compares these features in patients with and without papillary muscle rupture and assesses the effects of operation and the factors influencing the late postoperative results.

From the Cardiology Branch, Section of Pathology, and Clinic of Surgery, National Heart and Lung Institute, Bethesda, Md. 20014. Accepted February 28, 1973.

Address for reprints: D. Luke Glancy, MD, Section of Cardiology, Department of Medicine, Louisiana State University Medical Center, 1542 Tulane Ave., New Orleans, La. 70112.

Results

Preoperative Clinical Features

All nine patients were men aged 49 to 69 years (average 57 years) at the time of operation (Table I). Seven had been hospitalized with clinical features of acute myocardial infarction 3 to 65 months be-

TABLE I

Preoperative Clinical Features, Operative Findings, Postoperative Follow-Up

Case no.	Age at Operation (yr)	Months from Infarct to Operation (mo)	AP	Edema	NYHA Functional Class	Cardiac Rhythm	ECG	Chest X-ray C/T	Chest X-ray LA Enlargement	Involved Papillary Muscle	Prosthesis Model	Prosthesis Size	Follow-up (mo)	Current Status
							Papillary Muscle Rupture							
1	59	15	0	+	IV	Sinus	AMI	0.56	2+/4+	Anterior	S-E6120	2M	62	Died of CHF
2	51	3	0	+	IV	Sinus	IMI	0.54	1+/4+	Posterior	S-E6120	2M	41	Died suddenly
3	69	13	0	+	IV	Sinus	IMI	0.62	2+/4+	Posterior	S-E6120	2M	64	Early class II
4	59	14	+	0	IV	Sinus	SEI	0.50	0	Anterior	S-E6120	2M	60	Class II (PAF → III)
							Papillary Muscle Fibrosis Without Rupture							
5	49	6	0	0	III	Sinus	AMI	0.55	1+/4+	Posterior	S-E6120	2M	6	Died of CHF
6	57	?	0	+	III	AF	IMI	0.65	3+/4+	Both	S-E6300	3M	6	CHF, died suddenly
7	51	42	+	+	IV	AF	IMI	0.75	3+/4+	Both	S-E6310	3M	0	Died postop day 2
8	65	8	+	+	III	Sinus	SEI	0.56	1+/4+	Posterior	Kay-Shiley	#4	23	Class I
9	53	65	0	+	IV	AF	IMI	0.63	3+/4+	Posterior	S-E6520	3M	4	Limited by stroke

AF = atrial fibrillation; AMI = anterior myocardial infarct; AP = angina pectoris; CHF = congestive heart failure; C/T = cardiothoracic ratio; ECG = electrocardiogram; IMI = inferior myocardial infarct; LA = left atrial; NYHA = New York Heart Association; PAF = paroxysmal atrial fibrillation; postop = postoperative; S-E = Starr-Edwards; SEI = subendocardial ischemia or infarct.

fore operation, and in each a cardiac murmur had been noted before discharge. Two patients had not been hospitalized for myocardial infarction. One of the two patients (Case 7) experienced pain in the right jaw during exertion 42 months before operation, but the pain had been replaced by dyspnea when he presented to a hospital several months later with congestive failure and the electrocardiographic findings of remote inferior wall infarction. The second patient (Case 6) had never had precordial pain. He was known to have had a cardiac murmur for 13 years; 4 years before operation atrial fibrillation and heart failure developed. His electrocardiogram suggested old inferior wall infarction. All patients experienced severe dyspnea, fatigue and orthopnea before operation, and seven also had right-sided failure with marked peripheral edema. Only three of the nine patients had angina pectoris, and in one (Case 8) it appeared for the first time after myocardial infarction. In no patient was angina the limiting symptom. Three patients had class III functional capacity (New York Heart Association classification) at the time of operation, and the other six, including all four with papillary muscle rupture, had class IV functional capacity.

At the time of operation, six patients had sinus rhythm and three, each with papillary muscle dysfunction and mitral regurgitation for at least 3 years, had atrial fibrillation. Seven patients were examined during sinus rhythm, and each had an atrial (S_4) gallop. All nine patients had a ventricular (S_3) gallop and a holosystolic apical murmur (Fig. 1).

The electrocardiogram showed inferior wall infarction in five patients, and anterior wall infarction in two. The electrocardiogram was of no help in determining whether a papillary muscle was ruptured and was only partially accurate in predicting which muscle was involved. All five whose electrocardiogram showed an inferior wall infarction had involvement of the posterior papillary muscle, but two also had involvement of the anterior muscle. The electrocardiographic patterns of anterior wall infarction and of subendocardial ischemia were each associated with involvement of the anterior muscle in one patient and of the posterior muscle in another.

All patients had generalized cardiomegaly with a cardiothoracic ratio of 0.5 or more on the posteroanterior chest roentgenogram (Table I); in four patients this ratio exceeded 0.6. In one patient left atrial size appeared to be normal on roentgenograms taken in the four standard views after barium swallow. The other eight patients had various degrees of left atrial enlargement. Cardiothoracic ratio and left atrial size were greatest in the three patients who had papillary muscle fibrosis without rupture, long-standing mitral regurgitation and atrial fibrillation. No patient had a giant left atrium.

Preoperative Hemodynamic Findings

All patients underwent preoperative cardiac catheterization (Table II, Fig. 2). Despite digitalis and diuretic therapy, pulmonary arterial pressure was in-

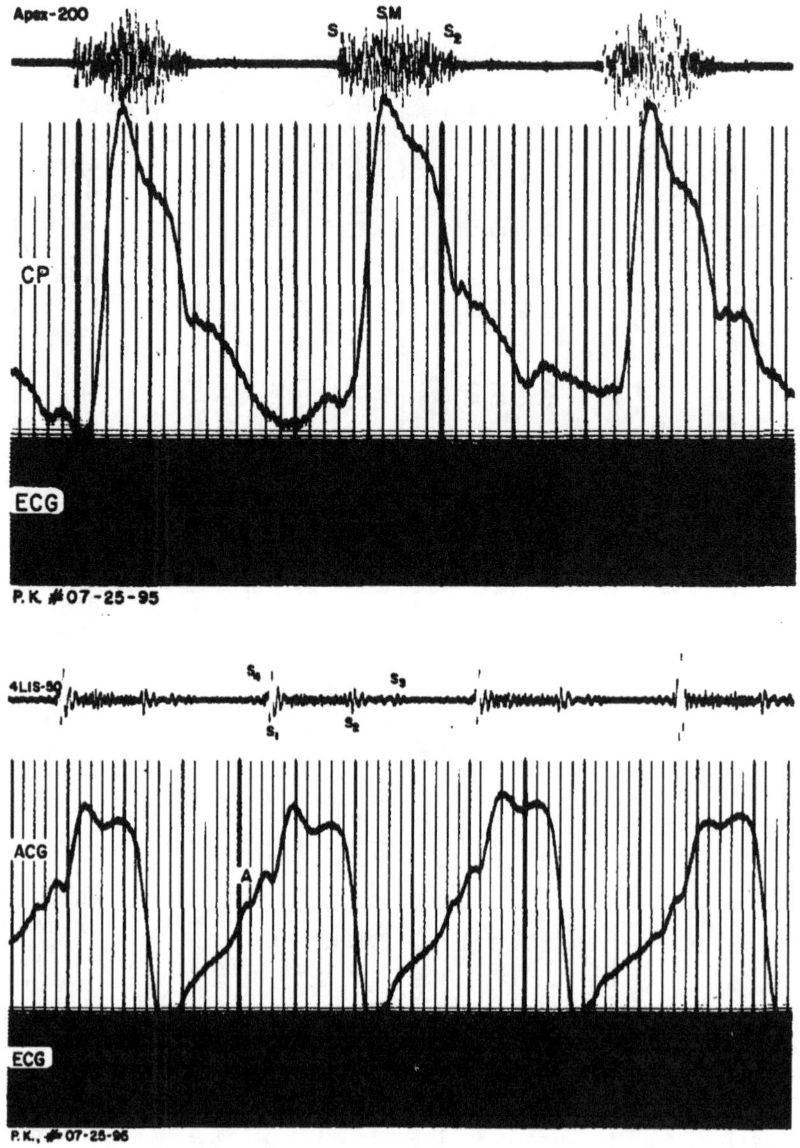

FIGURE 1. Case 4. Phonocardiograms. The systolic murmur (SM) begins with the first heart sound (S_2) and extends to the second sound (S_2). Third (S_3) and fourth (S_4) heart sounds are present, and a large *A* wave is seen on the apex cardiogram (ACG). CP = carotid pulse tracing; 4 LIS = fourth left intercostal space.

creased in all patients, and the levels of right ventricular end-diastolic and right atrial mean pressure were above the upper limits of normal in six. Eight patients had increased left atrial or pulmonary arterial wedge mean pressure and unusually large *V* waves (40 to 62 mm Hg) (Fig. 3). In one patient (Case 4), left atrial *V* wave and mean pressures were at the upper limits of normal. The left ventricular end-diastolic pressure level was abnormally high in eight of the nine patients, and the cardiac index was low in six of the seven patients in whom it was measured.

Mitral regurgitation was judged by selective left ventricular angiogram to be severe in all nine patients. Regurgitant volume was not quantified, but appeared to be equally large in patients with and without papillary muscle rupture. Prolapse of a mitral valve leaflet into the left atrium was seen only in Patient 7, who had papillary muscle fibrosis without rupture and a prolapsing posterior leaflet. Generalized or focal abnormalities, or both, of left ventricular contraction were recognized in all but one patient (Case 8). Contractions were judged to be fair or good in four patients (Fig. 4), three of whom had ruptured papillary muscles, and poor in five patients, four of whom had papillary muscle dysfunction without rupture. Coronary arteriograms were not obtained.

Operative Findings and Early Results

Rupture involved a single head of the anterior papillary muscle in two patients and a single head of the posterior muscle in the other two (Table I). In the patient (Case 2) with the shortest interval (3 months) between infarction and operation, necrotic myocardial fibers were observed in the ruptured papillary muscle head. In the other three patients, the ruptured papillary muscle head was composed of fibrous tissue with only a few viable subendocardial fibers. In three of the five patients without rupture, the posterior papillary muscle was fibrotic (Fig. 5), and in the

TABLE II

Hemodynamic Data

	Pressures (mm Hg)												Quality of LV Contractions on Angiogram
	RA mean		RV S/ED		PA S/ED (mean)		PAW or LA V wave (mean)		LV S/ED		Cardiac Index (liters/min/per m²)		
Case no.	Pre	Post	Pre	Post	Pre	Post	Pre	Post	Pre	Post	Pre	Post	
						Papillary Muscle Rupture							
1	4	7	60/6	62/10	60/30(37)	62/31(42)	49(29)	44(32)	75/19	93/28	1.9	2.0	Poor
2	14	1	60/13	28/3	60/28(40)	28/8(16)	42(28)	14(7)	74/17	...	1.7	1.5	Fair
3	10	2	80/16	42/3	80/33(52)	42/17(27)	42(28)	17(11)	110/10	...	1.2	2.9	Good
4	0	...	37/5	...	37/13(27)	...	17(12)	...	97/13	...	2.3	...	Fair
						Papillary Muscle Fibrosis Without Rupture							
5	13	15	72/15	73/15	72/42(53)	73/35(47)	..(27)	42(29)	90/30	90/36	1.7	2.4	Poor
6	2	...	32/3	...	32/12(22)	...	40(20)	...	85/16	...	3.2	...	Poor
7	21	...	112/20	62/10	112/50(80)	62/35(45)	52(33)	44(36)	120/19	74/24	...	...	Poor
8	15	8	95/19	67/11	95/40(60)	67/32(47)	60(35)	37(22)	125/20	225/14	...	3.0	Good
9	10	...	88/16	...	88/35(54)	...	62(30)	...	120/18	...	2.2	...	Poor

LA = left atrial; LV = left ventricular; PA = pulmonary arterial; PAW = pulmonary arterial wedge; Pre = preoperative; Post = postoperative; RA = right atrial; RV = right ventricular; S/ED = systolic/end-diastolic.
Figures in parentheses indicate mean pressures.

other two, both papillary muscles were scarred. The excised mitral valve was replaced by a Starr-Edwards caged-ball prosthesis in seven cases, and by a disc-type prosthesis in Cases 8 and 9 (Table I).

Patient 7 had signs of low cardiac output and died on the second postoperative day of intractable ventricular arrhythmias. Autopsy revealed severe triple vessel coronary artery disease, marked cardiomegaly (heart weight 750 g) and left ventricular dilatation, an extensive old posteroinferior infarct, thrombi in the right atrial appendage and recent pulmonary emboli with infarcts.

Patient 9 had had atrial fibrillation for 4 months before operation, but reversion to sinus rhythm occurred at the end of the procedure. Two weeks after operation he had a cerebral embolus, despite continued anticoagulation with warfarin, and was found to have atrial fibrillation again. His condition has steadily improved, but he remains limited by right hemiparesis and expressive aphasia. The condition of the other seven patients improved dramatically in the early postoperative period.

Postoperative Hemodynamic Findings

Six patients underwent postoperative cardiac catheterization (Table II, Fig. 2). The studies were usually performed 6 months after operation, but in Case 7 the data shown were obtained on the operat-

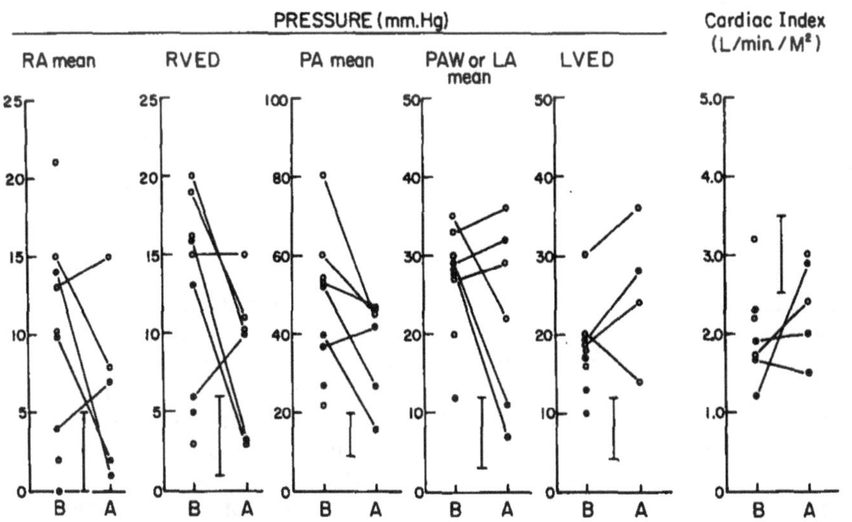

FIGURE 2. Intracardiac pressures and cardiac index before (B) and after (A) mitral valve replacement in patients with papillary muscle rupture **(solid circles)** and papillary muscle fibrosis without rupture **(open circles)**. Each **vertical bar** indicates the range of normal values. LA = left atrial; LVED = left ventricular end-diastolic; PA = pulmonary arterial; PAW = pulmonary arterial wedge: RA = right atrial; RVED = right ventricular end-diastolic.

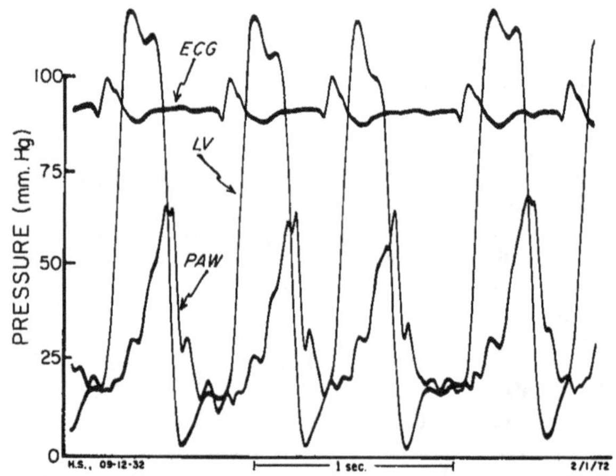

FIGURE 3. Case 9. Pulmonary arterial wedge (PAW) and left ventricular (LV) pressure tracings. The pulmonary arterial wedge *V* waves are huge, and left ventricular end-diastolic pressure is increased.

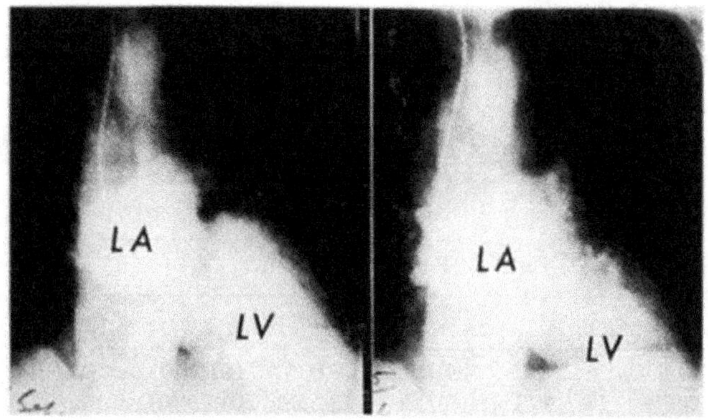

FIGURE 4. Case 3. Left ventricular angiograms exposed in diastole **(left)** and systole **(right)**. There is marked regurgitation of contrast material from left ventricle (LV) to left atrium (LA). Overall left ventricular contraction was judged to be good despite poor motion of the inferior wall.

ing table after valve replacement. Of the three patients with ruptured papillary muscles, the two whose preoperative angiograms revealed fair or good left ventricular contractions (Cases 2 and 3) showed striking hemodynamic improvement postoperatively; the patient with poor contractions had essentially unchanged hemodynamics postoperatively (Case 1). Of the three patients with papillary muscle dysfunction, two had a poorly contracting left ventricle preoperatively, and their hemodynamic status was not improved by operation. Patient 8 had good contractions before operation, and his postoperative hemodynamic status was improved although the left atrial pressure remained increased, because of a large (11 mm Hg) mean diastolic gradient across a small Kay-Shiley prosthesis. He also has had systemic arterial hypertension since operation.

Late Results of Operation

Of the eight patients who survived the early postoperative period, four have subsequently died. Patient 5 died of progressive congestive failure 6 months after operation. Patient 6 also continued to have signs and symptoms of cardiac failure, but his death, 6 months after operation, was sudden and presumably due to an arrhythmia. The condition of Patient 2 was greatly improved after operation both symptomatically and hemodynamically. Aside from several episodes of atrial fibrillation, he did well until 39 months after operation when he was hospitalized for a prolonged episode of chest pain and paroxysmal atrial tachycardia with heart block. He died suddenly 2 months after leaving the hospital and 41 months after operation. Again, death presumably was due to an arrhythmia. Necropsy revealed old complete occlusion of the right coronary artery, an old aneurysm of the inferior wall of the left ventricle and a normal mitral valve prosthesis. After operation Patient 1 had a marked decrease in symptoms but showed no hemodynamic improvement. Symptoms of congestive failure gradually recurred, but with use of digitalis and diuretic agents and with careful attention to sodium intake for 5 years his functional capacity remained in late class II or early class III and he had no angina pectoris although he had symptoms of dyspnea and fatigue. For several months before death his failure grew worse, and 6 weeks before death he had a cerebral embolus. Although he gradually recovered from the stroke, his cardiac status steadily deteriorated and he died with shock 62 months after operation.

Four patients are alive 64, 60, 23 and 4 months, respectively, after operation (Table I). Patient 3 is now 74 years old and has early class II functional capacity. He can walk a mile slowly, but experiences dyspnea if he walks rapidly. Patient 4 usually has late class II functional capacity, but has paroxysms of atrial fibrillation that cause his symptoms of dyspnea and fatigue to increase to class III severity. Patient 8 was completely asymptomatic, but 20 months after operation therapy with warfarin was temporarily discontinued in anticipation of dental extractions. Five days later he presented with pulmonary edema with faint prosthetic valve sounds and an apical grade 2/6 blowing holosystolic murmur. He underwent emergency operation. The disc of his Kay-Shiley mitral prosthesis was virtually immobilized by old and new thrombi. The prosthesis was replaced with a porcine aortic valve mounted on a flexible stent,[23] and 3 months after operation the patient is again asymptomatic. Four months postoperatively Patient 9 remains limited by hemiparesis, as described earlier.

Neither the intracardiac pressure measurements nor the cardiac output determinations could be used preoperatively to predict postoperative survival or hemodynamic results. Patients who had papillary muscle fibrosis without rupture, especially those with long-standing mitral regurgitation, an enlarged heart and atrial fibrillation, seemed to have a less favorable course after valve replacement than the patients with papillary muscle rupture. However, the

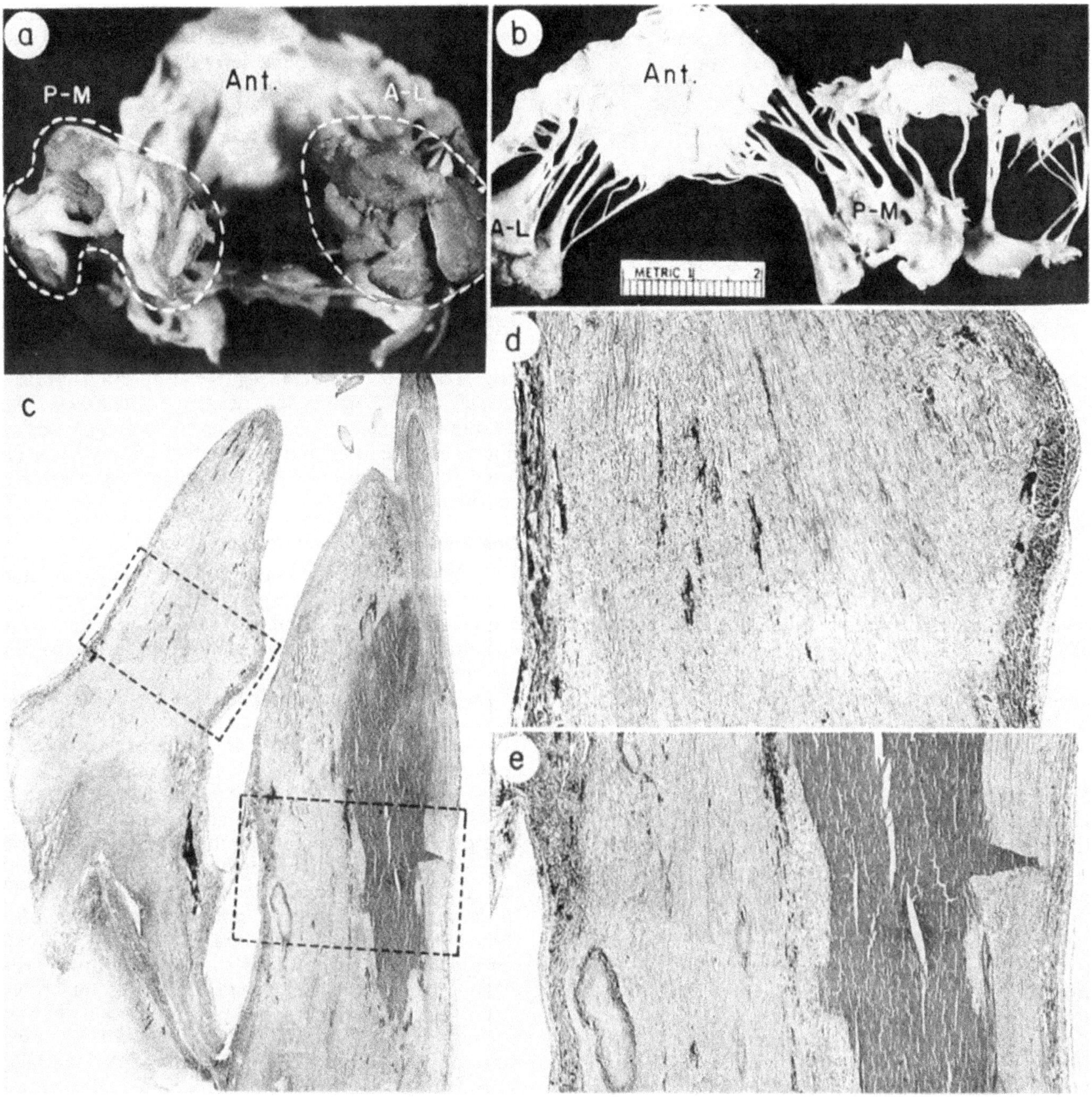

FIGURE 5. Case 5. Excised mitral valve **(a,b)** and photomicrographs **(c,d,e)** of portions of posteromedial (P-M) left ventricular papillary muscle in a patient who had papillary muscle necrosis *without* rupture during acute myocardial infarction 6 months before valve replacement. This patient was the only one among the five without rupture who had myocardial necrosis in the excised papillary muscle. **a,** intact mitral valve showing extensive necrosis and fibrosis of the posteromedial papillary muscle. The anterolateral muscle (A-L) is normal. **b** opened valve showing atrial aspects of the leaflets. **c** section of each of two trunks of the posteromedial muscle showing only fibrous scarring in one (close-up in **d**) and both fibrosis and necrosis in the other (close-up in **e**). Only the myocardial fibers in the most peripheral portions of the muscles are preserved. (These peripheral fibers probably are oxygenated directly by blood from the left ventricular cavity and not by blood from the coronary arteries, which supply the remainder of the papillary muscle.) Hematoxylin-eosin ×8.5 **(c)**, ×25 **(d)**, and ×20 **(e)** all reduced by 10 percent. Ant. = anterior mitral leaflet.

preoperative left ventriculogram was clearly the best predictor of operative results (Table III). Patients with poor left ventricular contractions had no hemodynamic improvement and had a low rate of long-term survival, whereas the opposite was true for patients with fair or good left ventricular contractions.

Discussion

Clinical Features

Mitral regurgitation and coronary artery disease frequently coexist. Although the two conditions are often unrelated, as in patients with both coronary

TABLE III

Quality of Left Ventricular Contractions as Determined by Angiogram vs. Postoperative Results

LV Contractions	Total Patients (no.)	Patients Who Died (no.)	Patients Who Survived (no.)
Poor	5	4* (2 days, 6 mo, 6 mo, 62 mo)	1 (4 mo)
Fair–good	4	1† (41 mo)	3† (23 mo, 60 mo, 64 mo)

* In the three patients in this group who underwent postoperative catheterization studies, the findings demonstrated unimproved hemodynamic status.

† The patient who died and two of the three survivors underwent postoperative catheterization studies. The findings in all three cases demonstrated improved hemodynamic status.

Figures in parentheses indicate time after operation.

atherosclerosis and rheumatic mitral valve disease, mitral regurgitation is commonly caused by coronary disease and papillary muscle infarction. When one or more heads of an infarcted papillary muscle rupture, severe mitral regurgitation invariably results and is often rapidly fatal.[16] If the remainder of the left ventricular myocardium has not been too severely damaged, the patient may survive the acute infarction to be left with chronic severe mitral regurgitation. This was the case in our first four patients.

Burch et al.[24] have drawn attention to mitral regurgitation occurring as the result of papillary muscle dysfunction without actual rupture. Mild mitral regurgitation due to papillary muscle dysfunction appears to be a common disorder, occurring in up to 55 percent of patients with acute myocardial infarction[25] and in 15 to 25 percent of patients with severe chronic ischemic heart disease.[26-28] Severe regurgitation is unusual but, when it occurs, the findings are similar to those in patients with papillary muscle rupture. The murmur is usually first heard during hospitalization for acute infarction. If the patient survives, he subsequently presents with chronic mitral regurgitation and symptoms of congestive failure rather than with angina pectoris. The cardiac rhythm is sinus during the first few years of mitral regurgitation, but atrial fibrillation eventually supervenes. A ventricular gallop is invariably heard, and an atrial gallop also is heard when the patient has sinus rhythm.

In patients with mild mitral regurgitation due to papillary muscle dysfunction, holosystolic,[25] ejection[24,25] and late[25,29,30] systolic murmurs have been described, but when mitral regurgitation is severe, the murmur is always holosystolic. It often is harsher than the blowing murmur of rheumatic mitral regurgitation and may be crescendo-decrescendo in character (Fig. 1). The electrocardiographic pattern is most often that of old inferior wall infarction, but patterns of anterior wall infarction or subendocardial ischemia also are seen. If severe mitral regurgitation has been present for 3 months or more, generalized cardiomegaly with left atrial enlargement is the rule and, in patients surviving several years, the heart is as large as in many patients with rheumatic mitral regurgitation. The longer duration of mitral regurgitation probably accounts for the larger size of the heart in our patients without papillary muscle rupture than in those with rupture. With occasional exceptions, as in Case 4, and regardless of left atrial size, cardiac catheterization reveals marked left atrial hypertension with large *V* waves. Angiocardiograms demonstrate severe mitral regurgitation with focal or generalized impairment, or both, of left ventricular contraction, but prolapse of a mitral leaflet into the left atrium can be recognized only occasionally. Thus, severe mitral regurgitation due to infarction of a papillary muscle usually has characteristic features that distinguish it from mitral regurgitation due to other causes, but we know of no way to determine preoperatively whether the papillary muscle is ruptured.

Operative Findings and Results

Repair of the mitral apparatus has been attempted in patients with mitral regurgitation due to papillary muscle infarction,[2,3] but the results have not been encouraging. Valve replacement appears to be the operation of choice under most circumstances. Although eight of our nine patients survived the first postoperative month (a survival rate approximating that of all patients undergoing isolated mitral valve replacement at the National Heart and Lung Institute[23,31,32]), only 23 (61 percent) of 38 patients previously reported on[4-22] survived the early postoperative period. Thus, operative mortality rates for valve replacement are probably higher in patients with mitral regurgitation due to coronary disease than in those with other types of mitral regurgitation. Although the number of patients in our study is small our results also suggest that the long-term prognosis after mitral valve replacement is less favorable in patients with papillary muscle infarction than in patients with other types of isolated mitral valve disease. As assessed by the life-table method, 50 percent of the first 100 patients undergoing mitral valve replacement at the National Heart and Lung Institute were alive 8 1/2 years postoperatively,[33] and results were better in patients with predominant regurgitation than in those with predominant stenosis. In our study, 50 percent of patients were dead within 5 years. Patients in our study were older and more severely ill than most patients undergoing valve replacement for rheumatic mitral regurgitation. In addition, they had various degrees of left ventricular impairment due to coronary artery disease and myocardial infarction. These factors undoubtedly are responsible for the less favorable long-term results in our study. Nevertheless, the results are at least as good as the results in patients undergoing double valve replacement for mitral and aortic disease, for in this group 50 percent of patients were dead in slightly less than 3 years.[34]

Both in our series and in that reported from the Massachusetts General Hospital,[20] operative results were somewhat better in patients with papillary muscle rupture than in those with dysfunction without rupture, but in our series we were unable to determine preoperatively whether the papillary muscle was ruptured. This is not a serious disadvantage because the preoperative left ventricular cineangiogram appears to be an even better predictor of operative results. Thus, patients with fair or good left ventricular contractions and gross mitral regurgitation usually show clinical and hemodynamic improvement, but patients with poor left ventricular contractions, especially those with only moderate mitral regurgitation, usually do not.

Operative indications: None of our patients and few of those reported on by others[15,17,19,22] were operated upon within a month of myocardial infarction and the onset of mitral regurgitation. Although some patients are alive who might not have survived without operation, valve replacement under these circumstances seems to carry a high risk. Moreover, the onset of left ventricular failure in a patient with acute infarction and severe mitral regurgitation is not necessarily indicative of progressive deterioration and death. For example, in one patient referred to us for valve replacement because of severe mitral regurgitation and several episodes of pulmonary edema, cardiac failure began to decrease 3 weeks after infarction. Five years later this patient is receiving no cardiac medications, experiences no symptoms, has a normal-sized heart and a soft, short apical systolic murmur. Thus, we believe that the indications for valve replacement in patients with chronic severe mitral regurgitation are the same whether or not the cause is papillary muscle infarction, but the indications for valve replacement during acute infarction need to be defined further.

Role of aortocoronary bypass: The role of concomitant aortocoronary bypass in patients undergoing mitral valve operations for chronic regurgitation due to papillary muscle infarction also needs to be established. Both enthusiastic[35] and discouraging[36] reports of combined operations have appeared. Although the operation might prevent or delay arrhythmic deaths or future infarction, our experience[37] suggests that left ventricular performance is more often adversely affected than improved by bypass operation, a finding of particular relevance in a group of patients whose major problem after mitral valve replacement often is chronic left ventricular failure.

Acknowledgment

We thank Dr. James Bacos, Washington Hospital Center, who performed the preoperative cardiac catheterizations in Cases 8 and 9 and generously allowed us to use the data.

References

1. **Morrow AG, Cohen LS, Roberts WC, et al:** Severe mitral regurgitation following acute myocardial infarction and ruptured papillary muscle. Hemodynamic findings and results of operative treatment in four patients. Circulation 37: suppl II:124–132, 1968
2. **Adicoff A, Alexander CS, Ferguson JN, et al:** Surgical repair of ruptured papillary muscle complicating posterior myocardial infarction. Amer J Cardiol 11:246–252, 1963
3. **Horlick L, Merriman JE, Robinson CLN:** Case of mitral insufficiency following myocardial infarction with rupture of a papillary muscle: improvement following re-attachment of the papillary muscle and plication of the mitral valve. Canad Med Ass J 94:192–195, 1966
4. **Holloway DH Jr, Whalen RE, McIntosh HD:** Systolic murmur developing after myocardial ischemia or infarction. JAMA 191:888–892, 1965
5. **De La Torre A, Linhart JW, Bartley TD:** Mitral valve replacement in a patient with mitral regurgitation secondary to rupture of a papillary muscle. Ann Intern Med 67:387–392, 1967
6. **Shelburne JC, Rubinstein D, Gorlin R:** A re-appraisal of papillary muscle dysfunction. Correlative clinical and angiographic study. Amer J Med 46:862–871, 1969
7. **Bartle SH, Hermann HJ:** Acute mitral regurgitation in man: hemodynamic evidence and observations indicating an early role for the pericardium. Circulation 36:839–851, 1967
8. **Spencer FC, Reppert EH, Stertzer SH:** Surgical treatment of mitral insufficiency secondary to coronary artery disease. Arch Surg (Chicago) 95:853–861, 1967
9. **Bashour RA:** Mitral regurgitation following myocardial infarction: the syndrome of papillary mitral regurgitation. Dis Chest 48:113–122, 1965
10. **Fluck DC, Taubman JO, Cleland WP, et al:** Acute mitral incompetence after acute myocardial infarction, with successful early treatment by mitral valve prosthesis. Lancet 2:1052–1054, 1966
11. **Klughaupt M, Flamm MD, Hancock EW, et al:** Nonrheumatic mitral insufficiency. Determination of operability and prognosis. Circulation 39:307–316, 1969
12. **Berman DA, Grismer JT:** Postmyocardial infarction syndrome followed by left ventricular aneurysm with papillary muscle dysfunction. Amer J Cardiol 25:349–352, 1970
13. **Ronan JA Jr, Steelman RB, De Leon AC Jr, et al:** The clinical diagnosis of acute severe mitral insufficiency. Amer J Cardiol 27:284–290, 1971
14. **Lee KS, Johnson T, Karnegis JN, et al:** Clinical pathologic conference. Amer Heart J 79:258–264, 1970
15. **Schimert G, Lajos TZ, Greene DG, et al:** Surgery for postinfarction complications (abstr). Circulation 38: suppl VI:VI–174, 1968
16. **De Busk RF, Harrison DC:** The clinical spectrum of papillary muscle disease. New Eng J Med 281:1458–1467, 1969
17. **De Busk RF, Kleiger RE, Ebnother CL, et al:** Successful early operation for papillary muscle rupture. Chest 58:175–178, 1970
18. **Austen WG, Sanders CA, Averill JH, et al:** Ruptured papillary muscle: report of a case with successful mitral valve replacement. Circulation 32:597–601, 1965
19. **Austen WG, Sokol DM, De Sanctis RW, et al:** Surgical treatment of papillary muscle rupture complicating myocardial infarction. New Eng J Med 278:1137–1141, 1968
20. Case records of the Massachusetts General Hospital. Case 22–1969. New Eng J Med 280:1228–1236, 1969
21. Case records of the Massachusetts General Hospital. Case 6–1970. New Eng J Med 282:327–335, 1970
22. Case records of the Massachusetts General Hospital. Case 26–1970. New Eng J Med 282:1421–1429, 1970
23. **Reis RL, Hancock WD, Yarbrough JW, et al:** The flexible stent: a new concept in the fabrication of tissue heart valve prostheses. J Thorac Cardiovasc Surg 62:683–689, 1971

24. **Burch GE, De Pasquale NP, Phillips JH:** The syndrome of papillary muscle dysfunction. Amer Heart J 75:399–415, 1968
25. **Heikkila J:** Mitral incompetence complicating acute myocardial infarction. Brit Heart J 29:162–169, 1967
26. **Hamilton GW, Murray JA, Kennedy JW:** Quantitative angiocardiography in ischemic heart disease. The spectrum of abnormal left ventricular function and the role of abnormally contracting segments. Circulation 45:1065–1080, 1972
27. **Rackley CE, Dear HD, Baxley WA, et al:** Left ventricular chamber volume, mass and function in severe coronary artery disease. Circulation 41:605–613, 1970
28. **Glancy DL:** Unpublished data
29. **Steelman RB, White RS, Hill JC, et al:** Midsystolic clicks in arteriosclerotic heart disease: a new facet in the clinical syndrome of papillary muscle dysfunction. Circulation 44:503–515, 1971
30. **Cheng TO:** Late systolic murmur in coronary artery disease. Chest 61:346–356, 1972
31. **Morrow AG, Oldham NH, Elkins RC, et al:** Prosthetic replacement of the mitral valve: preoperative and postoperative clinical and hemodynamic assessments in 100 patients. Circulation 35:962–979, 1967
32. **Winter TQ, Reis RL, Glancy DL, et al:** Current status of the Starr-Edwards cloth-covered prosthetic cardiac valves. Circulation 45: suppl I: 14–24, 1972
33. **Levine FH, Copeland JC, Morrow AG:** Prosthetic replacement of the mitral valve. Continuing assessments in the 100 patients operated upon during 1961–1965. Submitted for publication
34. **Melvin DB, Tecklenberg PL, Hollingsworth JF, et al:** Computer-based analysis of preoperative and postoperative prognostic factors in 100 patients with combined aortic and mitral valve replacement. Circulation; in press
35. **Cheng TO, Bashour T, Adkins, PC:** Acute severe mitral regurgitation from papillary muscle dysfunction in acute myocardial infarction. Successful early surgical treatment by combined mitral valve replacement and aortocoronary saphenous vein bypass graft. Circulation 46:491–497, 1972
36. **Spencer FC, Green GE, Tice DA, et al:** Coronary artery bypass graft for congestive heart failure: a report of experiences with 40 patients. J Thorac Cardiovasc Surg 62:529–542, 1971
37. **Itscoitz SB, Shepherd RL, Glancy DL, et al:** Deterioration of myocardial function following aortocoronary bypass operation (abstr). Clin Res 21:427, 1973

Calcification of prosthetic valve anuli: A late complication of cardiac valve replacement

Bernadine H. Bulkley, M.D.
Andrew G. Morrow, M.D.
William C. Roberts, M.D.
Bethesda, Maryland

The known late complications of cardiac valve replacement include thrombosis, infection, peribasilar valvar leaks, endocardial fibrosis, embolism, and degeneration of materials of the prostheses.[1] Another late complication, previously undescribed, is calcification at the sites of attachment of prostheses. This report describes this complication in eight necropsy patients.

Patients and results

Cardiac findings were reviewed in 96 necropsy patients who died more than 2 months after replacement of one or more cardiac valves with rigid-framed prostheses (usually Starr-Edwards prostheses). Seventy-two patients with calcific deposits in the excised valves were eliminated: 66 of them had had stenotic valves and six had had purely incompetent valves. The remaining 24 patients, all of whom had had purely incompetent, non-calcified valves (aortic in 13, mitral in 13) form the basis of this report. Isolated mitral replacement had been performed in 11, isolated aortic in 11, and both mitral and aortic in two. The prosthetic implantation periods in the 24 patients ranged from 3 to 116 months (average 32) (Table I). Of the 13 patients with aortic prostheses, two had calcific deposits at the sites of attachment of the prostheses; their valve implantation periods were 12 and 70 months, respectively. Of the 13 patients with mitral prostheses, seven had anular calcific deposits, and the implantation periods in six were 70 months or longer; the implantation periods in the six patients without calcific deposits ranged from 3 to 12 months (average seven months). The average ages of the seven patients with (48 years) were similar to those of the six patients without (47 years) prosthetic anular calcium.

The extent of prosthetic anular calcific deposits, graded 1^+ to 4^+ (Fig. 1), varied in the eight patients, but in all the deposits were located on and between sutures. The sutures utilized in all patients were fabricated of braided Dacron covered with a film of Teflon. The

From the Section of Pathology and the Clinic of Surgery, National Heart and Lung Institute, National Institutes of Health, Bethesda, Md.

Received for publication April 23, 1973.

Reprint requests to: Dr. William C. Roberts, Section of Pathology, National Heart and Lung Institute, Bethesda, Md. 20014.

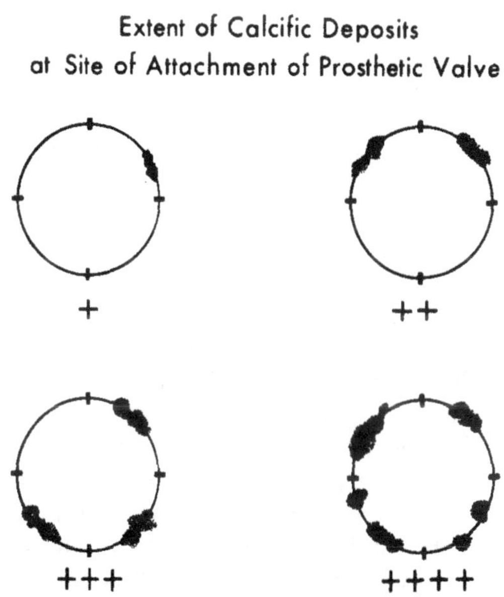

Fig. 1. Extent of calcific deposits at site of attachment of prosthetic valve. Scale of grading extent of periprosthetic anular calcium. With 1^+, calcium is located in only 1 quadrant; with 4^+ in all 4 quadrants.

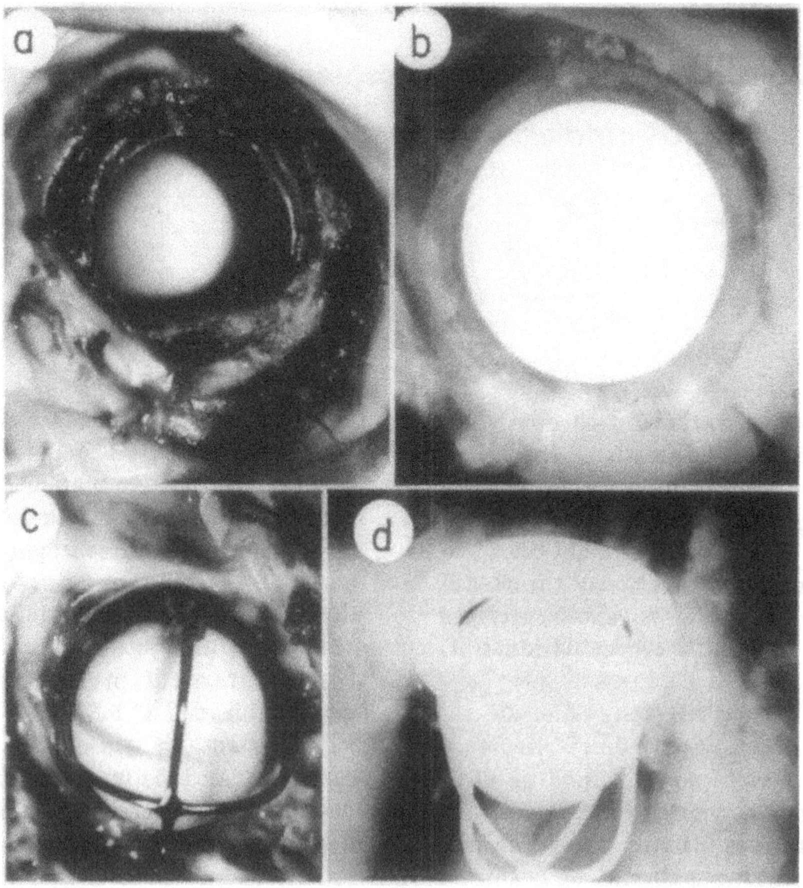

Fig. 2, a through **d**.Calcification of the Starr-Edwards prosthetic mitral anulus in a 49-year-old woman (A70-123) who underwent replacement 6½ years earlier. The prosthesis viewed from left atrium **(a)** and **(b)** and from left ventricle **(c)** and **(d)**. The radiographs show calcific deposits, not visible grossly, in the mitral anulus. The calcific deposits are located primarily in and around sutures.

deposits in several patients are illustrated in Figs. 2 to 5.

Comments

Calcification of prosthetic anuli is a late complication of cardiac valve replacement. Of 26 previously non-calcified, purely incompetent valves excised 3 to 116 months (average 76) earlier, calcific deposits developed around prosthetic anuli in nine. Of the seven valves (one aortic, six mitrals) in place for six years or more, all had prosthetic anular calcific deposits. Of the 13 patients with prosthetic mitral valves, only one of seven with implantation periods of less than 70 months contained anular calcium, but all six patients with implantation periods of more than 70 months contained anular calcium. Of the 13 patients who had undergone aortic valve replacement, only one had been in place for as long as 70 months, and it contained prosthetic anular calcium. Of the 12 patients with prosthetic aortic valves in place for less than 70 months, one had anular calcific deposits.

Calcification of the mitral anulus is frequently seen in elderly persons, commonly in association with calcification of aortic valve cusps and coronary arteries, and it is believed to be a consequence of the wear-and-tear of aging.[2] Calcification in the mitral anular area may be accelerated, however, by conditions which elevate left ventricular pressure (systemic hypertension, left ventricular outflow obstruction),[3,4] presumably because they increase wear-and-tear on the mitral valve. Similarly, constant to-and-fro motion of rigid-framed prostheses may increase wear at the sites of attachment and accelerate the appearance of dystrophic calcification.

Because its amount increases with time, calcific deposits in prosthetic rings probably will

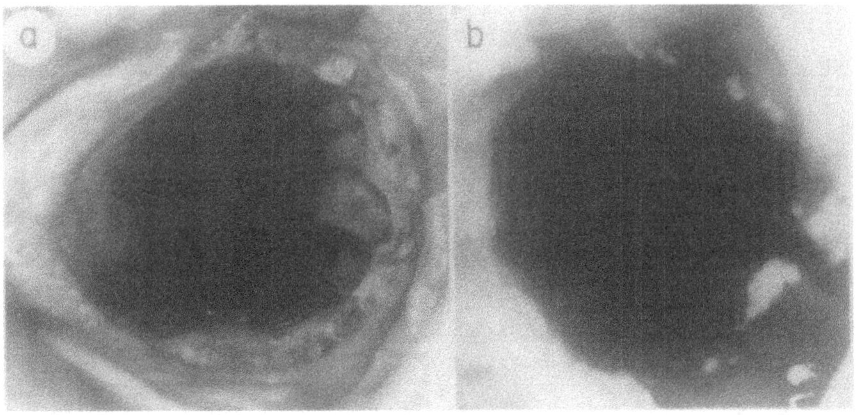

Fig. 3, a and **b.** Calcification of mitral anulus in a 49-year-old woman (A72-107) who died suddenly nine years after mitral valve replacement with a Starr-Edwards prosthesis. At necropsy, the prosthesis showed no sign of dysfunction. Shown is the mitral anulus **(a)**, viewed from left atrium after the prosthesis was removed, and a roentgenogram **(b)** showing calcific deposits.

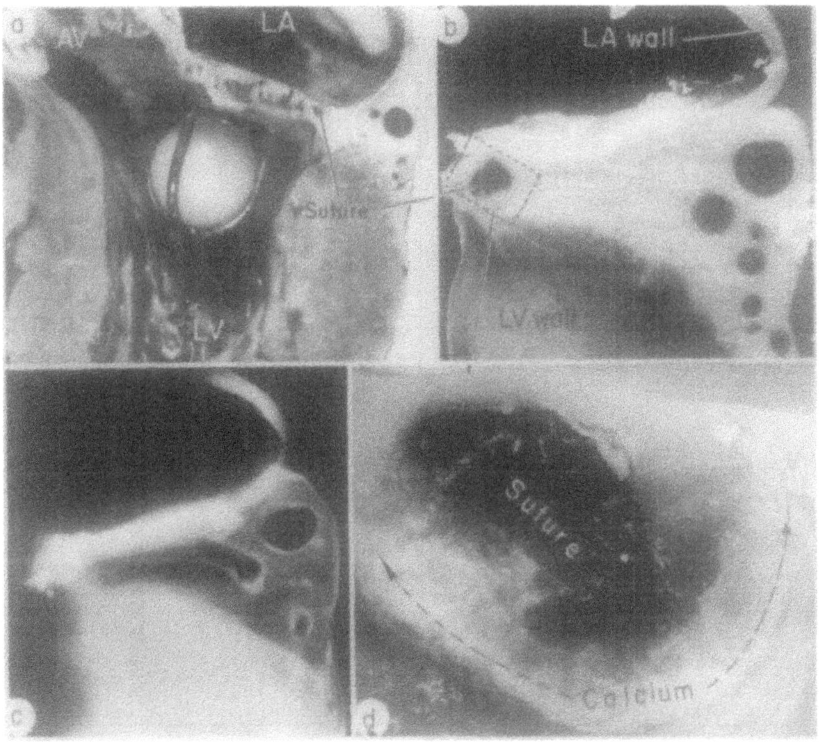

Fig. 4, a through **d.** Calcification of mitral anulus in a 45-year-old woman (A72-44) who died nine years after mitral valve replacement. Shown **(a)** is the left atrium (*LA*), left ventricle (*LV*), and the mitral prostheses. Calcific deposits in the prosthetic anuli are seen on the radiograph **(b)**. The prosthesis is held in place by sutures **(c)** and not by ingrown tissue. Closer view of the suture **(d)** shows its encasement in a ring of calcium.

become more common. In none of our patients was prosthetic anular calcium visible by roentgenography during life, but in none was the implantation period longer than 10 years. Possibly, with longer periods, the deposits might reach a degree visible by radiograph during life. Calcific deposits in anuli might cause suture rupture and peribasilar leaks. Ring calcification may be a hazard to reoperation to replace faulty prostheses.

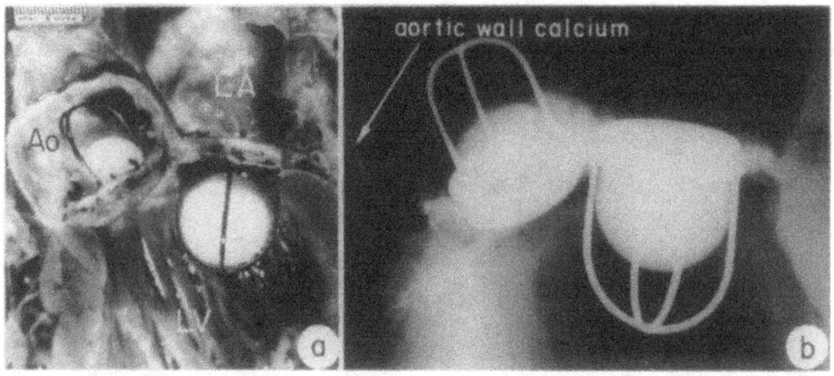

Fig. 5, a and **b.** Calcification of mitral and aortic prosthetic anuli in a 63-year-old man (A72-30) who had undergone double valve replacements with Starr-Edwards prostheses (size 4M and 11A) 70 months earlier. A transverse section through the left heart shows left atrium (*LA*), left ventricle (*LV*), and aorta (*Ao*). A small peribasilar left ventricular-left atrial communication was present around the prosthetic mitral ring involving less than 10 per cent of the circumference of the mitral anulus. Roentgenogram (**b**) demonstrates calcific deposits both in aortic and mitral prosthetic rings and in the aortotomy site. The other patient with double valve replacement had calcific deposits in the mitral but not in the aortic prosthetic anulus.

Table I. Occurrence of prosthetic ring calcification in patients dying late after replacement of non-calcified purely incompetent valves with rigid-framed prostheses

Mitral					*Aortic*				
Patient	*Age (yr.)*	*Sex*	*Prosthetic implantation period (mos.)*	*Calcium prosthetic anulus (0-4+)*	*Patient*	*Age (yr.)*	*Sex*	*Prosthetic implantation period (mos.)*	*Calcium prosthetic anulus (0-4+)*
A69-62	65	M	3	0	A63-170	26	M	3	0
A69-292	44	F	4	0	A71-78	51	M	5	0
A71-32	55	M	7	0	A67-197	52	M	8	0
A68-197	52	M	8	0	A68-89	33	M	8	0
A67-119	49	F	9	0	A70-226	49	M	11	0
A66-54	15	F	12	0	A71-197	29	M	12	++
A67-118*	47	M	44	++	A66-6	27	M	13	0
A72-30*	63	M	70	+++	A67-7	53	M	14	0
A70-123	49	F	79	+++	A67-107	50	M	30	0
A70-10	57	F	80	++	A71-138	30	M	35	0
A72-107	49	F	105	++++	A67-118*	47	M	44	0
A72-44	45	F	111	++++	A72-36	62	M	52	0
A72-88	29	F	116	+++	A72-30*	63	M	70	+++

*Aortic and mitral valves replaced.

Summary

A previously undescribed late complication of cardiac valve replacement is calcification at the site of attachment of prostheses. Of 24 patients in whom purely incompetent, non-calcified mitral or aortic valves were replaced with rigid-framed prostheses 3 to 116 months earlier, nine (seven mitral, two aortic) of 26 valves had prosthetic anular calcific deposits. Of the eight prostheses in place for 70 months or longer all contained anular calcific deposits; only one of the 18 valves in place for less than 70 months had periprosthetic calcific deposits. The extent of prosthetic calcium also increased with time. The mechanism of formation of prosthetic anular calcium is uncertain, but accelerated wear of the tissues beneath the prostheses due to the constant to-and-fro motion of the rigid frames may be a factor. Possible complications of prosthetic anular calcific deposits include suture rupture, peribasilar leak, and increased hazard to reoperation.

REFERENCES

1. Roberts, W. C., Bulkley, B. H., and Morrow, A. G.: The pathologic anatomy of cardiac valve replacement. A study of 224 necropsy patients, Progr. Cardiovas. Dis. **15**:539, 1973.
2. Roberts, W. C., and Perloff, J. K.: Mitral valvular disease. A clinicopathologic survey of the conditions causing the mitral valve to function abnormally, Ann. Intern. Med. **77**:939, 1972.
3. Roberts, W. C., Perloff, J. K., and Constantino, T.: Severe valvular aortic stenosis in patients over 65 years of age, Am. J. Cardiol. **27**: 497, 1971.
4. Ewy, G. A., Marcus, F. I., Bohajalian, O., Burke, H. L., and Roberts, W. C.: Muscular subaortic stenosis, Am. J. Cardiol. **22**:126, 1968.

Prosthetic Aortic Stenosis

A Method to Prevent Its Occurrence by Measurement of Aortic Size from Preoperative Aortogram

By RONALD P. SENINGEN, M.D., BERNADINE H. BULKLEY, M.D., AND WILLIAM C. ROBERTS, M.D.

SUMMARY

A cause of early death after aortic valve replacement with a caged-ball prosthesis is obstruction to left ventricular outflow because the prosthesis is too large for the aortic root. Of 68 patients dying within two months of aortic valve replacement, death in ten, each of whom had had intractable low cardiac output after operation, was attributed at necropsy to prosthetic aortic stenosis, despite the use of small sized (8A Starr-Edwards) prostheses in seven of them. The diameters of the aorta at the sinotubular junction, determined from the preoperative cineangiograms, in the seven patients with prosthetic stenosis were < 30 mm in all. Poppet clearances, defined as the differences between poppet and aortic root diameters, ranged from 4 to 12 mm (avg. 9). In contrast, the diameters of the aortas at the sinotubular junctions in eight control patients (unobstructed prosthetic aortic valves and early death from other causes) were > 30 in all but one, and the poppet clearances ranged from 12 to 19 mm (avg. 15). Thus, prosthetic aortic stenosis is likely to develop after aortic valve replacement with rigid-framed caged ball valves if the preoperative aortograms disclose aortic diameters at the sinotubular junctions to be < 30 mm. In such patients, either the aorta must be widened for a caged-ball prosthesis or a central flow valve must be used.

Additional Indexing Words:

Aortic valve   Cardiac valve replacement   Cardiac operation

WHENEVER THE MITRAL or aortic valve is replaced with a caged-ball prosthesis, some degree of stenosis is nearly always produced by the prosthesis.[1-5] The obstruction is usually relatively mild, but on occasion the degree of stenosis is considerable.[1-5] Anatomic features of fatal prosthetic mitral and prosthetic aortic stenosis have been described[6-10] but fatal prosthetic stenosis has not been documented hemodynamically in the early postoperative period. If the prosthetic stenosis is extremely severe, cardiac function may not be restored in the operating room after valve replacement. Also, cardiac catheterization is infrequently performed during the first few days after operation. As a consequence, diagnosis of fatal prosthetic obstruction has been made almost exclusively[11] at necropsy.

To help predict and perhaps prevent its occurrence, the sizes of the aortic roots measured by preoperative angiogram were compared to the sizes of the implanted prosthetic aortic poppets in patients with necropsy-diagnosed prosthetic aortic obstruction, and these measurements were compared to those in necropsy patients with replaced aortic valves but without prosthetic obstruction.

From the Department of Diagnostic Radiology, Clinical Center, and the Section of Pathology, National Heart and Lung Institute, National Institutes of Health, Bethesda, Maryland 20014.

Received October 16, 1973; revision accepted for publication January 3, 1974.

Address for reprints: William C. Roberts, M.D., Chief, Section of Pathology, National Heart and Lung Institute, National Institutes of Health, Bethesda, Maryland 20014.

Patients Studied and Methods

Of 68 patients dying within two months of aortic valve replacement, death in ten was attributed at necropsy to prosthetic stenosis. Of the 10, seven who had preoperative aortic cineangiograms form the basis of this report (tables 1 and 2). Preoperatively, 5 patients had pure aortic regurgitation and 2 had aortic stenosis. Death occurred in the operating room in 1 patient, and in 6, from 1 to 8 days (avg. 4) after valve replacement. Size 8A to 11A (avg. 8.6) Starr-Edwards prostheses were used. In each of the latter 6 patients, death was attributed to the low cardiac output syndrome.* At necropsy, the prosthesis in each appeared to be too large for the aorta. At least 2 of the 3 struts of the cage came into contact with the wall of aorta which protruded into the cage and prevented adequate movement of the poppet (figs. 1 and 2).

*All patients had at one time direct systemic systolic pressures of < 90 mm Hg. Each also had evidence of underperfusion of at least one organ system: brain (disorientation or seizures); bowel (pain or bleeding); kidney (oliguria); lung (alveolar infiltrates = alveolar hemorrhage [shock lung]); liver (hyperbilirubinemia); and skin (peripheral cyanosis or coldness). The hypotension and organ-perfusion inadequacy responded poorly or not at all to therapy, including vasopressors. These signs of low organ perfusion were confirmed by necropsy examination in all patients.

Table 1
Data in Patients Studied

Patient	Sex/Age (years)	MVR	LV-SA PSG (mm Hg)	LA-LV MDG (mm Hg)	AR (0-4)	MR (0-4)	Interval Operation to Death (days)	Size/Model No. SE Prosthesis	Diameter (mm) of Poppet	Diameter (mm) of aorta at S-T Junction	Clearance (mm)
WITH PROSTHETIC STENOSIS											
1. A67-207	F/51	+	51	12	4+	2+	7	8A 1200	15	20	5
2. A72-235	F/45	+	0	11	2+	0	1	8A 2300	15	23	8
3. A65-133	M/25	+	18	0	2+	3+	1	8A 1000	15	23	8
4. A68-3	M/29	+	0	0	4+	1+	3	11A 2300	18	26	8
5. A73-39	F/55	+	0	17	3+	0	OR	8A 2320	15	26	11
6. A68-67	F/37	+	0	10	4+	0	2	8A 2300	15	27	12
7. A67-311	M/42	0	0	0	4+	2+	8	9A 1200	17	29	12
WITHOUT PROSTHETIC STENOSIS											
8. A73-9	M/59	0	0	7	4+	2+	50	11A 2320	18	30	12
9. A71-149	F/52	0	0	0	4+	1+	44	8A 2320	15	28	13
10. A71-63	F/54	+	0	0	3+	3+	13	9A 2310	16	30	14
11. A72-124	F/57	+	35	5	3+	1+	2	9A 2320	16	30	14
12. A71-94	M/41	+	28	18	2+	3+	56	9A 2310	16	30	14
13. A67-88	M/33	0	160	0	0	0	OR	8A 1200	15	30	15
14. A66-40	M/45	+	0	19	3+	0	OR	8A 1200	15	33	18
15. A64-107	M/36	+	0	7	3+	2+	OR	8A 1000	15	34	19

Abbreviations: AR = aortic regurgitation; LA = left atrium; LV = left ventricle; MDG = mean diastolic gradient; MR = mitral regurgitation; MVR = mitral valve replacement; PSG = peak systolic gradient; SA = systemic artery; SE = Starr Edwards; S-T = sinotubular.

Of the remaining 58 necropsy patients who died < 2 months after aortic valve replacement, 8 were selected as controls on the basis of their having measurable aortic root cineangiograms (i.e., grids present on the frames), similar preoperative lesions and similar sized prostheses (Starr-Edwards) as those in the 7 patients with prosthetic stenosis. Preoperatively, 5 patients had pure aortic regurgitation, and 3 had aortic stenosis. Death occurred in the operating room in 3 patients and from 2 to 56 days (avg. 33) after valve replacement in the other 5 patients. Size 8A to 11A prostheses (avg. 8.7) were utilized. Death was due to technical mishaps in 4 patients, unexplained low cardiac output in 2, unexplained sudden death in 1, and non-cardiac causes in 1. At necropsy, the aortic poppets moved freely in the cages and never did more than 1 of the 3 struts of the prosthesis contact the aortic wall (fig. 3).

The hearts in the 7 patients with prosthetic stenosis weighed 310 to 1040 g (avg. 670), and those in the 8 controls, 500 to 1100 g (avg. 630). None of the 15 patients had had the Marfan or Marfan-like syndrome, and none had had a portion of ascending aorta resected.

Cineaortogram Evaluation

The diameters of the aortic roots were measured from preoperative cineaortograms, corrected for geometric magnification, in all 15 patients. The internal diameter of each aorta was measured at the sinotubular junction (the most proximal portions of the tubular aortas or the most cephalad extensions of the sinuses of Valsalva), and at a level 2 cm above the sinotubular junction (fig. 4). Both measurements were taken from the same cine frame at maximal systolic aortic distention. These measurements were performed without prior knowledge of the clinical or necropsy findings. The diameters of the aortic prosthetic poppets (supplied by Edwards' Laboratories) were compared to the diameters of the aortas and the differences (maximal clearances) were recorded (tables 1 and 2).

Table 2
Prosthetic Aortic Stenosis

	No. Patients	Diameter (mm) of aorta at S-T junction	Diameter (mm) of aorta 2 cm above S-T junction	Size of prosthesis (Starr-Edwards)	Diameter (mm) of poppets utilized	Maximal clearances (mm)
I. Stenotic prosthetic aortic valve	7	20-29 (25)	29-39 (33)	8A-11A (8.6)	15-18 (16)	4-12 (9)
II. Non-stenotic prosthetic aortic valve (controls)	8	28-34 (31)	29-39 (36)	8A-11A (8.7)	15-18 (16)	12-19 (15)

Comments

Malfunction of an implanted prosthesis is a common cause of death in the early postoperative period after cardiac valve replacement.[6-10] Of 133 patients dying early (< 2 mo) after replacement of one or more cardiac valves with caged ball prostheses (mainly Starr-Edwards), 34% died from prosthetic dysfunction.[10] Of the 68 necropsy patients with aortic prostheses, death in 10 resulted because the prosthesis was too large for the aorta into which it had been inserted. All 10 patients with prosthetic aortic stenosis had evidence of inadequate cardiac output postoperatively. Prosthetic stenosis in all 10 patients was diagnosed only at necropsy.

Studies in the patients with prosthetic stenosis demonstrated that measurement of aortic size from preoperative aortograms can predict those patients who are at high risk of developing prosthetic aortic stenosis. The critical diameter of the ascending aorta at the sinotubular junction is about 30 mm. This measurement was < 30 mm (avg. 25) in each of the 7 patients with fatal prosthetic aortic stenosis but in only 1 of the 8 control patients with normally functioning aortic prostheses of similar size (avg. 31).

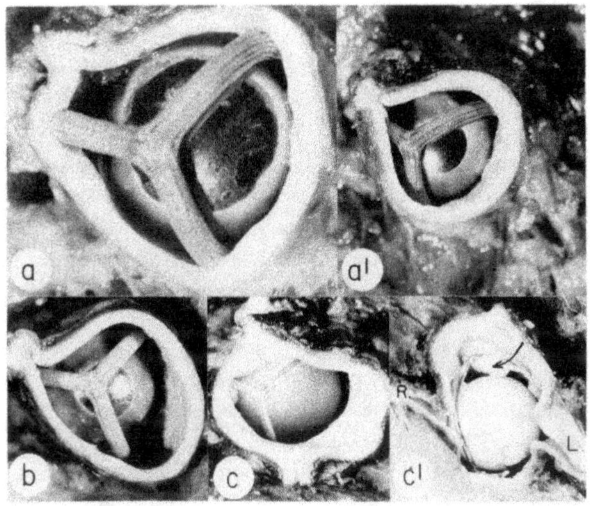

Figure 1

Prosthetic aortic stenosis. Shown here are photographs of rigid-framed caged-ball aortic prostheses in patients #2 (a, a¹), #5 (b) and #3 (c, c¹). The aortic prostheses, even though small (8A, Starr-Edwards), are too large for the aortas into which they had been placed. The struts of the cages contact the aortic walls which protrude between the struts to contact the poppets and restrict their movement. During simulated ventricular systole (c') the poppet is prevented from ascending completely to the apex of the cage by the intruding aortic wall. A match head projects from the narrowed prosthetic orifice. R. and L. = right and left coronary arteries.

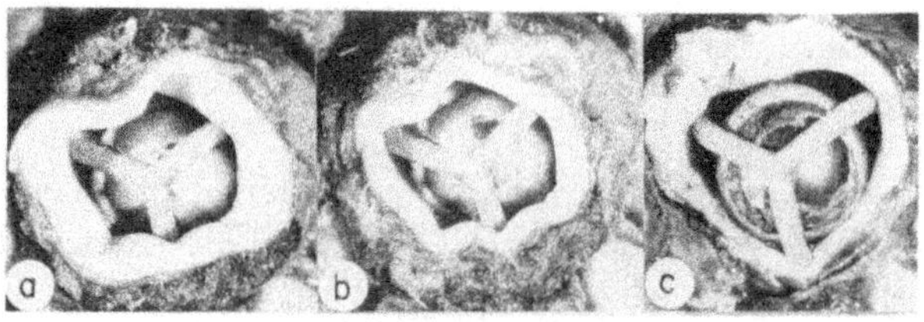

Figure 2

Prosthetic aortic stenosis in patient #4. The ascending aorta at 2 cm above (a), at 1 cm above (b), and at the sinotubular junction itself (c).

Moreover, prosthetic stenosis occurred in 5 of the 7 patients despite the use of small sized (8A) prostheses. Thus, some aortas are simply not large enough for even these small rigid-framed caged ball prostheses. Aortic diameters measured 2 cm above the sinotubular junctions did not correlate with the development of prosthetic aortic stenosis. Hence, at operation the aorta above the sinuses of Valsalva may appear of adequate size to readily accommodate a rigid-framed prosthesis, but at the same time, the size of aorta at the sinotubular junction may be too small to accept the prosthesis.

Thus, measurement of the diameter of aorta from the preoperative cineaortogram at the level of the sinotubular junction can be used to predict those patients in whom prosthetic stenosis is likely to develop after aortic valve replacement with a rigid-framed caged-ball prosthesis. Those patients with aortic diameters < 30 mm are at high risk, and in such patients widening of the aorta should be considered if caged-ball prostheses are implanted or central flow type prostheses should be used. Knowledge of this measurement recently proved helpful in a patient undergoing aortic valve replacement. The diameter of aorta at the sinotubular junction measured 29 mm on the preoperative cineaortogram. After valve replacement the heart functioned poorly, prosthetic aortic stenosis was suspected, and the aortic root was widened with a patch. The heart then functioned well after discontinuation of cardiopulmonary bypass and the postoperative course was smooth.

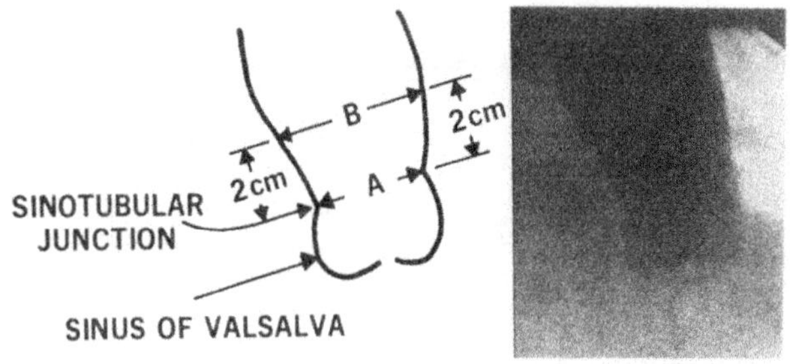

Figure 4

Cineaortogram in the right anterior oblique view with corresponding line drawing. Measurement A represents the internal aortic diameter at the junction of the sinus of Valsalva and tubular aorta (sinotubular junction); measurement B, the internal aortic diameter 2 cm above the sinotubular junction.

In addition to the measurements performed in the 15 patients described herein, the diameters of aorta at, and just above, the sinotubular junctions were measured from preoperative cineaortograms in 8 other patients, all of whom underwent cardiac catheterization about 6 months after aortic valve replacement with Starr-Edwards prostheses. The sizes of the aortic prostheses in these 8 patients, however, averaged 11.1: in 5, size 11A prostheses were used; in 2, size 12A; and in 1, size 10A. The diameters of aorta at the sinotubular junctions in these 8 patients ranged from 32 to 38 mm (avg 36), and the poppet clearances from 15 to 20 mm (avg 17). The peak systolic pressure gradients between left ventricle and systemic artery at the 6-month postoperative catheterization studies were < 25 mm Hg in each of the 8 patients. Although these patients are not comparable to our necropsy patients, these data clearly indicate that the diameters of the sinotubular junctions and the poppet clearances are considerably smaller in the patients with fatal prosthetic aortic stenosis than in the patients without significant prosthetic aortic stenosis.

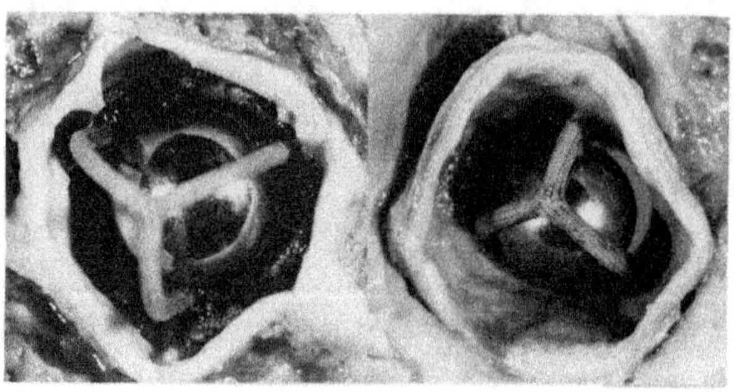

Figure 3

Two examples of non-stenotic aortic prostheses. The aortic walls do not contact the poppets or the struts of the protheses, and poppet movement is unimpeded.

References

1. Morrow AG, Oldham NH, Elkins RC, Braunwald E: Prosthetic replacement of the mitral valve: Preoperative clinical and hemodynamic assessments in 100 patients. Circulation **35**: 962, 1967
2. Kloster FE, Fauchi C, Mourdjinis A, Hodam R, Starr A, Griswold HE: Hemodynamic studies in patients with cloth-covered composite-seat Starr-Edwards valve prostheses. J Thorac Cardiovasc Surg **60**: 879, 1970

3. Glancy DL, O'Brien KP, Reis RL, Epstein SE, Morrow AG: Hemodynamic studies in patients with 2M and 3M Starr-Edwards prostheses: Evidence of obstruction to left atrial emptying. Circulation **39 & 40** (suppl I): I-113, 1969
4. Winter TQ, Reis RL, Glancy DL, Roberts WC, Epstein SE, Morrow AG: Current status of the Starr-Edwards cloth-covered prosthetic cardiac valves. Circulation **45 & 46** (suppl I): I-14, 1972
5. Hawe A, Fry RL, Ellis FH Jr: Late hemodynamic studies after mitral valve surgery. J Thorac Cardiovasc Surg **65:** 351, 1973
6. Roberts WC, Morrow AG: Mechanisms of acute left atrial thrombosis after mitral valve replacement. Pathologic findings indicating obstruction to left atrial emptying. Am J Cardiol **18:** 497, 1966
7. Roberts WC, Morrow AG: Anatomic studies of hearts containing caged-ball prosthetic valves. Johns Hopkins Med J **121:** 271, 1967
8. Roberts WC, Morrow AG: Causes of early postoperative death following cardiac valve replacement. J Thorac Cardiovasc Surg **54:** 422, 1967
9. Roberts WC, Morrow AG: Causes of death and other anatomic observations after cardiac valve replacement. Adv Cardiol **7:** 226, 1972
10. Roberts WC, Bulkley BH, Morrow AG: Pathologic anatomy of cardiac valve replacement. A study of 224 necropsy patients. Progr Cardiovasc Dis **15:** 539, 1973
11. Shepherd RL, Glancy DL, Stinson EB, Roberts WC: Hemodynamic confirmation of obstruction to left ventricular inflow by a caged-ball prosthetic mitral valve. J Thorac Cardiovasc Surg **65:** 252, 1973

Cardiac pathology after aortic valve replacement using Hufnagel trileaflet prostheses: a study of 20 necropsy patients

Michael C. Fishbein, M.D.*
William C. Roberts, M.D.
Abner Golden, M.D.
Charles A. Hufnagel, M.D.
Washington, D. C. and Bethesda, Md.

Of the various prostheses used to replace malfunctioning cardiac valves, several have had extensive clinical evaluation but only a few have been examined systematically at necropsy. In the pathology laboratory of the National Heart and Lung Institute, cardiac morphologic findings have been described in nearly 300 patients dying after valve replacement using Starr-Edwards prosthesis,[1] or tissue valves.[2] During the past eight years the hearts of 81 patients dying after cardiac replacement using trileaflet (20 patients) or disc valves (61 patients) also have been examined by us. This report describes necropsy observations in the 20 patients who died after replacement of the aortic valve with a trileaflet prosthesis consisting of three self-suspended flexible cusps made of polypropylene and covered by silicone rubber (Fig. 1).[3] No previous reports describing morphologic alterations in this particular prosthesis have appeared.

Patients studied

Clinical and pathologic findings in the 20 patients are summarized in Tables I and II. Seven patients died within two months of operation (early deaths) (Table I) and 13 patients, at later periods up to 58 months (late deaths) (average 22 months) (Table II). In 18 patients only the aortic valve was replaced; in the other two, the mitral valve also was replaced, a discoid valve[4] being utilized in each. The 20 patients ranged in age at death from 26 to 76 years; 13 were men, and seven were women. All but two patients were in functional class III or IV before valve replacement.

Of the 20 patients, 17 had stenotic and three had purely incompetent aortic valves. The aortic valves were congenitally malformed in six patients: one had a quadricuspid valve.[7] The remaining 14 patients, seven of whom also had anatomic disease of the mitral valve, had three-cuspid aortic valves. The etiology of the valve lesions in the seven patients with associated mitral disease is considered rheumatic[8]; the cause is uncertain in four and degenerative in origin[9] in three.

Significant (> 75 per cent) luminal narrowing of at least one of the three major (right, left circumflex, and left anterior descending) coronary arteries occurred in three patients (Patient No. 1, Table I; Patients Nos. 9 and 10, Table II) and was the cause of death in one. This patient (No. 9, Table II) died of an acute myocardial infarction 23 months after valve replacement. She was the only patient dying six months or longer after valve replacement without evidence of prosthetic degeneration or thrombosis.

Early deaths

Of these seven patients, three died within one week and all seven within three weeks of operation. None died on the day of operation. Extensive thrombus formation (Fig. 2) on the prostheses with obstruction to a coronary arterial ostium and myocardial necrosis caused death in four patients, two of whom also probably had some pros-

From the Departments of Pathology and Surgery, Georgetown University Medical Center, Washington, D. C., and the Section of Pathology, National Heart and Lung Institute, Bethesda, Md.

Received for publication June 17, 1974.

Reprint requests: Dr. William C. Roberts, Building 10A, Room 3E30, National Institutes of Health, Bethesda, Md. 20014.

*Present address: Department of Pathology, Harbor General Hospital, Torrance, Calif. 90509.

Table I. Clinical and necropsy data in patients dying early (< 2 months) after Hufnagel tri-leaflet aorti

Necropsy No.	Age (years)	Sex	Functional class (NYHA)	No. A-V cusps	Preoperative valve lesions				LV-SA PSG (mm. Hg)	LA-LV MDG (mm. Hg)	Date AVR (mo./year)
					AS	AR	MS	MR			
1. 69A-135	59	M	IV	3	+	+	0	0	†*	0	3/69
2. 67A-549	61	M	IV	1	+	+	0	0	20	0	10/67
3. 68A-435	43	M	IV	3	+	+	0	+	†*	0	8/68
4. 69A-345	60	F	IV	2	+	+	0	0	80	0	7/69
5. 69A-451	50	F	III	3	+	+	0	0	100	0	9/69
6. 69A-497	54	M	IV	3	+	+	+	+	35	15	9/68
7. 68A-577	51	F	III	4	0	+	0	0	0	0	11/68

Abbreviations: A = annuloplasty or valvuloplasty; AMI = acute myocardial infarction; AR = aortic regurgitation; AS = aortic stenosis; AV = aortic v
MDG = mean diastolic gradient; MR = mitral regurgitation; MS = mitral stenosis; MV = mitral valve; NYHA = New York Heart Association; O

*Cardiac catheterization not performed but valve obviously stenotic.

†Uncorrected by mitral valvuloplasty.

‡Patch inserted to widen aortic root.

Table II. Clinical and necropsy data in patients dying late (> 2 months) after Hufnagel tri-leaflet aortic

Necropsy No.	Age (years)	Sex	Functional class (NYHA)	No. A-V cusps	Preoperative valve lesions				LV-SA PSG (mm. Hg)	LA-LV MDG (mm. Hg)	Date AVR (mo./year)	A-V size inside diameter (mm.)
					AS	AR	MS	MR				
1. 68A-207	74	F	III	3	+	+	0	+	70	0	2/68	16
2. 68A-483	51	M	III	3	+	+	+	+	70	5	3/68	18
3. 68A-547	59	M	II	3	+	+	0	0	75	0	3/68	?
4. 69A-19	76	F	IV	3	+	+	0	0	120	0	1/68	16
5. 69A-13	26	M	IV	3	0	+	0	+	0	0	9/67	22
6. 69A-577	50	M	II	2	0	+	0	0	38	0	6/68	22
7. 68A-453	50	F	III	3	+	+	+	+	60	10	3/67	20
8. 70A-419	50	M	III	3	+	+	0	0	38	0	2/69	20
9. 70A-509	70	F	IV	3	+	+	0	0	148	0	12/68	16
10. 72A-399	53	M	III	2	+	+	0	0	100	0	5/67	18
11. 71A-209	36	M	III	3	+	+	0	+	15	0	5/68	22
12. 70A-489	43	M	IV	3	+	+	0	+	30	0	10/67	22
13. 73A-87	55	M	III	3	+	+	0	0	100	0	5/68	18

Abbreviations: See Table I.

*Replacement of trileaflet aortic prosthesis eight months before death with a disc prosthesis.

thetic stenosis from this mechanism; uncorrected mitral regurgitation appeared responsible for death in one; postoperative bleeding in one; and severe intravascular hemolysis of uncertain etiology with renal failure in one.

Five of the seven patients who survived more than two days after operation were begun on heparin therapy on the first or second day postoperatively and were either on heparin or warfarin sodium at death. Three of the four patients who died from prosthetic thrombosis in the early (8, 15, and 17 days) postoperative period were on heparin at death, and each had received dipyridamole for several days before operation; the fourth patient, who died two days after operation from a thrombosed prosthetic valve, had not received anticoagulant therapy.

Late deaths

The intervals between operation and death in these 13 patients ranged from 2.1 to 58 months (average 22). The one patient dying 2.1 months after valve replacement had aortic regurgitation from a perivalvular leak. Of the 12 patients with alve replacement

A-V size inside diameter (mm.)	MV operation	Implantation period (days)	Major cause of death	Status of prosthetic aortic valve						Heart weight (Gm.)	LV scarring (SE) (TM)
				Tears	AR	Thrombus	AS	COO	Emboli		
22	0	1	Bleeding	0	0	0	0	0	0	480	SE
24	0	2	AMI	0	0	+	0	+	0	600	SE
22	A	5	MR†	0	0	0	0	0	0	900	0
16	0	8	AMI	0	0	+	+	+	+	470	SE
16	0	15	AMI	0	0	+	+	+	0	580	0
18	R (disc)	16	Hemolysis, massive	0	0	0	0	0	0	700	SE
18‡	0	17	AMI	0	0	+	0	+	+	520	SE

= commissurotomy; CHF = congestive heart failure; COO = coronary ostial occlusion; F = female; LA = left atrium; LV = left ventricle; M = male; peration; PSG = peak systolic gradient; R = replacement; SA = systemic artery; SE = subendocardial; TM = transmural.

valve replacement

MV Operation	Implantation period (months)	Major cause of death	Status of prosthetic aortic valve						Infection	Peribasilar AR	Heart Weight (Gm.)	LV scarring (SE) (TM)
			Tears	AR	Thrombus	AS	COO	Emboli				
A	2.1	AR	0	0	0	0	0	0	0	+	530	0
C	6	AR	+	+	0	0	0	0	0	0	490	0
O	7.5	AR	+	+	0	0	0	0	0	0	600	SE
O	12	Sepsis	+	+	+	0	0	+	+	+	480	TM
A	15	AR	+	+	0	0	0	0	0	0	850	SE
O	18	AMI	0	0	+	+	+	0	0	0	600	SE
R (disc)	18	AR	+	+	0	0	0	0	0	0	450	SE
O	19	AR	+	+	+	0	0	0	0	0	700	SE
O	23	AMI	0	0	0	0	0	0	0	0	470	TM
O	32*	Aortic dissection	+	+	+	0	0	0	0	0	380	SE
A	35	AMI	0	0	+	+	+	+	0	0	690	TM
C	36	AR	+	+	+	0	0	+	0	0	900	SE
O	58	AMI	0	0	+	+	+	+	0	0	700	SE

implantation periods of six months or longer, the aortic prosthesis in eight was torn (Figs. 3 and 4), severely incompetent, and responsible for death (seven patients) or reoperation (one patient); no degeneration of prosthetic material was evident in the other four patients despite long (18 to 58 months [average 29]) implantation periods, but three had large thrombi (Fig. 5) within the prosthetic sinuses causing obstruction to at least one coronary arterial ostium. Histologic examination of the thrombotic material from several patients disclosed it to consist predominantly of fibrin and platelets with only a few erythrocytes. Thus, it was a so-called "white thrombus." The one patient without prosthetic degeneration or thrombosis died of an acute myocardial infarction from severe coronary atherosclerosis 23 months after valve replacement. All patients were discharged from the hospital on warfarin sodium.

Renal hemosiderosis, the anatomic indicator of intravascular hemolysis (in this case the result of trauma to erythrocytes traversing prosthetic aortic valves[10]) was sought for in the late death cases. The kidneys in 11 of the 13 patients dying

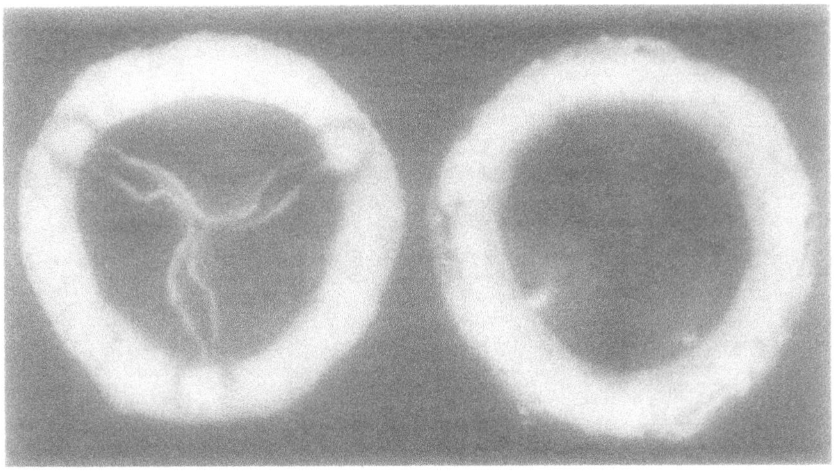

Fig. 1. View of an intact trileaflet prosthesis from the aortic (*left*) and the ventricular aspect (*right*).

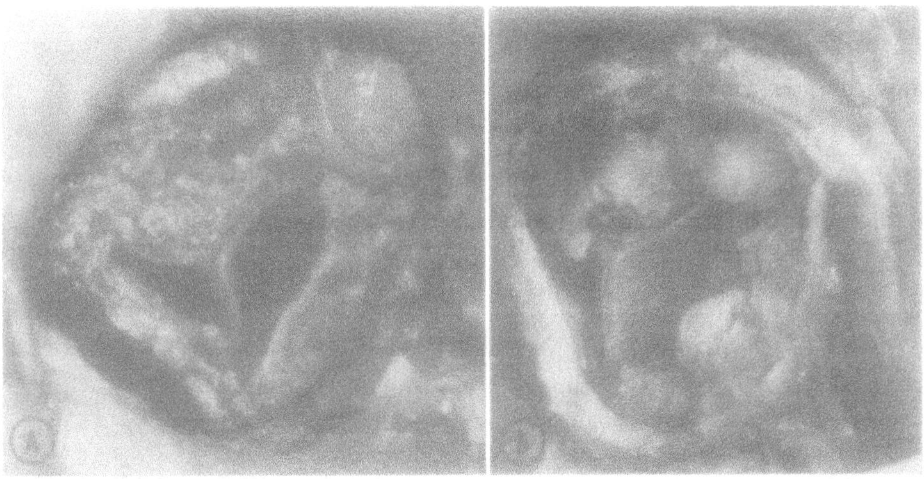

Fig. 2. Patient No. 4, Table I. Prosthesis containing thrombus in each of the three sinuses from a patient dying eight days after valve replacement. The thrombus partially blocked the ostium of the left coronary artery. *Left:* View from aortic aspect about 2 cm. above the prosthesis. *Right:* This view is on a plane corresponding to the cephalad extension of the prosthesis.

late were available for study. All sections were stained by Prussian blue reaction. Four patients had no iron deposits in the kidneys. Of the seven who did, four had had other prosthetic aortic or mitral valves implanted prior to the Hufnagel prosthesis for periods ranging from 16 days to eight years. Two other patients had severe perivalvular leaks, and another had a torn, degenerated, incompetent prosthesis. Thus, of seven patients in whom only trileaflet aortic prostheses were used, four had no renal iron deposits, while each of the remaining three had prosthetic abnormalities which could account for the hemolysis. The pre- and late postoperative blood hematocrit values of all seven patients were similar, indicating that increased hematopoiesis was able to compensate for the intravascular red cell destruction.

Discussion

The trileaflet aortic valve used in the patients described herein consists of three self-suspended flexible leaflets made of polypropylene covered with silicone rubber. The leaflets are supported from the base and do not attach directly to the aortic wall. The base is made of Hepacone (a material which at least in vitro inhibits clotting of blood) except for a small area of Dacron fabric along the suture line (used to stimulate the ingrowth of tissue). Nine to 12 sutures usually are

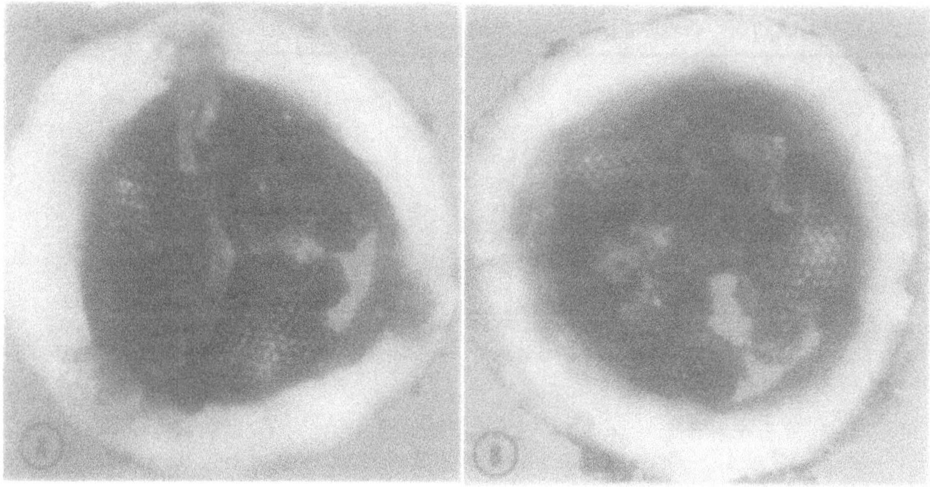

Fig. 3. Patient No. 5, Table II. A severely degenerated prosthesis with extensive tearing of the cusps, from above (*left*), from below (*right*).

used for fixation. This prosthesis has a central flow orifice similar to the normal valve; the cusps are freely pliable, open with low pressure, and initially were believed to have long flex lives. Its central flow characteristic would theoretically make this prosthesis particularly advantageous in patients with small aortas, which might impede rigid-framed poppets or discs. Because it is a central flow valve with smooth-surfaced cusps, hemolysis does not occur. This prosthesis underwent certain changes during its period of clinical application: the late model had more shallow sinuses and shorter vertical struts than did the original model.

Despite these theoretical advantages, use of this trileaflet aortic prosthesis in its present form has been discontinued because of the frequency of cuspal fracture or fibrin-platelet deposition or both. Degeneration (tearing) of the prosthetic cusps occurred in eight of 12 patients surviving six months or longer after valve replacement. Cuspal degeneration occurred as early as six months after implantation (in one patient) and not until nearly six years later (in another patient). Degeneration appears to begin by tearing of a cusp from its most cephalad attachment to a vertical strut. It is apparently at this point that stress is greatest during valve closure. Thrombus formed within one or more of the sinuses of the prosthesis in seven of the 20 patients. All three patients dying late, and three of four dying early from prosthetic thrombosis were on anticoagulants. Although it is impossible to know whether or not these patients were adequately anticoagulated at all times, it appears that the factors of turbulence and difficulties in the control of the equal distribution of stresses in these prostheses are responsible for this frequency of accumulation of thrombi. Similar clotting problems obviously also have been encountered with

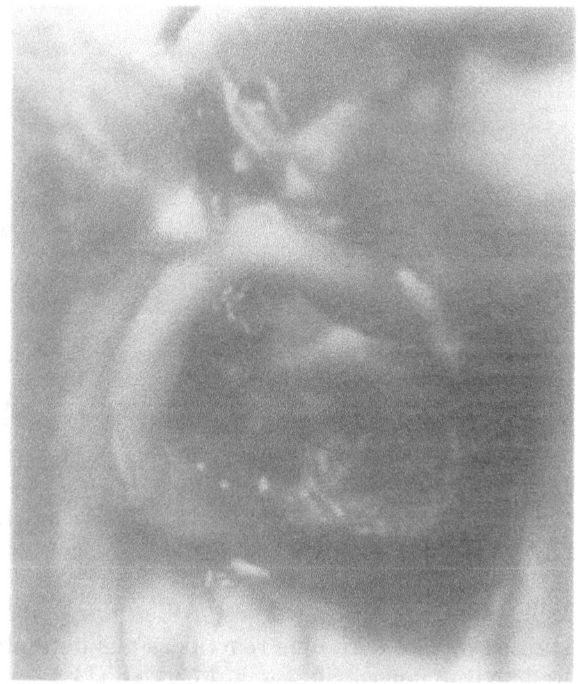

Fig. 4. Same valve as seen in Fig. 3, but from below before the valve was excised at necropsy. The massive degree of incompetence is apparent.

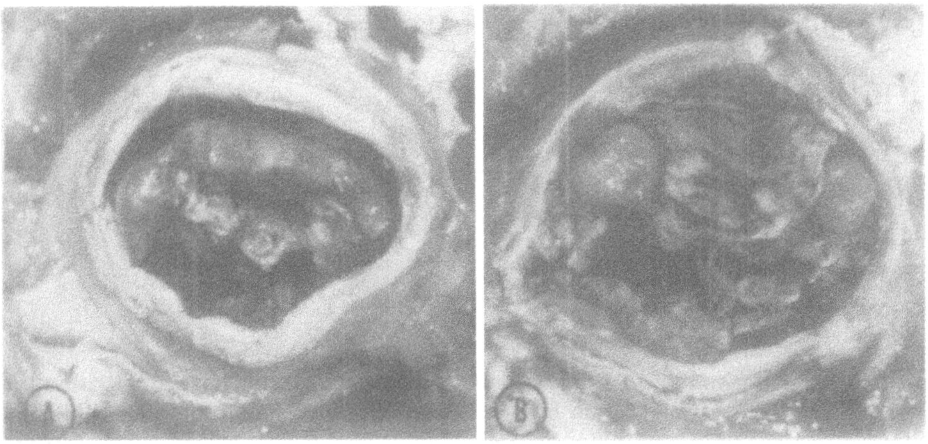

Fig. 5. Patient No. 13, Table II. Prosthetic thrombosis. *Left:* as seen from about 1 cm. above the sinotubular junction of ascending aorta. *Right:* as seen on a plane corresponding to the most cephalad extension of the prosthesis. Thrombus is present in each of the three sinuses and obstructs the ostium of the right coronary artery.

use of other types of prostheses including the caged ball and disc. Because of the central flow feature of this prosthesis, research on the use of new forms of flexible leaflet prosthetic cardiac valves is continuing in an effort to overcome the problems of cuspal fracture and thrombosis.

Summary

Necropsy observations are described in 20 patients dying between October 1967 and March 1973 after replacement of the aortic valve with a Hufnagel trileaflet prosthesis. Seven patients died within two months of operation and 13, between 2.1 and 58 months (average 22). Four of seven patients dying early had extensive prosthetic thrombus causing obstruction of one coronary arterial ostium in each. Of the 12 patients surviving six months or longer after valve replacement, death in eight resulted from degeneration (tearing) of the prosthetic cusps causing severe aortic regurgitation in each, and from thrombosis of the prostheses in three, probably causing prosthetic stenosis and definitely causing narrowing of at least one coronary ostium. Thus, prosthetic degeneration or thrombosis caused death in 11 of the 12 patients surviving six months or longer. In conclusion, this trileaflet aortic prosthesis, although similar in design to the normal aortic valve, is composed of materials not durable enough to withstand the stresses created by blood flow in this position.

REFERENCES

1. Roberts, W. C., Bulkley, B. H., and Morrow, A. G.: Pathologic anatomy of cardiac valve replacement: a study of 224 necropsy patients, Progr. Cardiovasc. Dis. **15**:539, 1973.
2. Yarbrough, J. W., Roberts, W. C., and Reis, R. L.: Structural alterations in tissue cardiac valves implanted in humans and calves, J. Thorac. Cardiovasc. Surg. **65**:364, 1973.
3. Hufnagel, C. A., and Conrad, P. W.: A new approach to aortic valve replacement, Ann. Surg. **167**:791, 1968.
4. Hufnagel, C. A., and Conrad, P. W.: Comparative study of some prosthetic valves for aortic and mitral replacement, Surgery **57**:205, 1965.
5. Falcone, M. V., Roberts, W. C., Morrow, A. G., and Perloff, J. K.: Congenital aortic stenosis resulting from unicommissural valve. Clinical and anatomic features in 21 adult patients, Circulation **44**:272, 1971.
6. Roberts, W. C.: The congenitally bicuspid aortic valve. A study of 85 autopsy patients, Am. J. Cardiol. **26**:72, 1970.
7. Hurwitz, L. E., and Roberts, W. C.: Quadricuspid semilunar valve, Am. J. Cardiol. **31**:623, 1973.
8. Roberts, W. C.: Anatomically isolated aortic valvular disease. The case against it being of rheumatic etiology, Am. J. Med. **49**:151, 1970.
9. Roberts, W. C., Perloff, J. K., and Constantino, T.: Severe valvular aortic stenosis in patients over 65 years of age: a clinico-pathologic study, Am. J. Cardiol. **27**:497, 1971.
10. Roberts, W. C., and Morrow, A. G.: Renal hemosiderosis in patients with prosthetic aortic valves, Circulation **33**:390, 1966.

Cardiac Pathology After Valve Replacement by Disc Prosthesis

A Study of 61 Necropsy Patients

WILLIAM C. ROBERTS, MD, FACC
MICHAEL C. FISHBEIN, MD*
ABNER GOLDEN, MD

Washington, D.C.
Bethesda, Maryland

Clinical and necropsy observations are described in 61 patients who had one or more cardiac valves replaced with a discoid prosthesis of the Hufnagel type. The most common (31 percent) cause of death among the 45 patients who died early (less than 65 days after operation) appeared to be prosthetic disproportion; that is, the prosthesis was too big for the aorta or ventricular cavity into which it was inserted so that inadequate space was present between the margins of the disc and the endocardium of ventricle or intima of aorta. Prosthetic thrombosis occurred in only 3 of the 45 patients who died early, but poppet movement appeared considerably altered in each. In contrast, thrombi were observed on a prosthesis in 14 of the 16 patients who died late (4 to 47 months [average 21] postoperatively), but in none did the thrombi appear of sufficient size to alter poppet function. Excessive bleeding occurred in 11 (24 percent) of the 45 early deaths and was primarily related to the insertion of a patch in the root of the aorta. Uncorrected valvular disease either by itself or by its ability to alter function of the prosthesis appeared responsible for death in 6 (13 percent) of the 45 patients who died early and in 2 (6 percent) of the 16 who died late. Insertion of a mitral poppet disc in a patient with uncorrected aortic regurgitation, even of mild degree, may be hazardous because the aortic regurgitant jet stream may interfere with proper function of the mitral disc. Likewise, insertion of a poppet disc only in the aortic valve position in a patient with combined aortic and mitral regurgitation may considerably increase the degree of mitral incompetence because the aortic prosthesis is intrinsically obstructive.

Disc wear or variance was observed in all but one prosthesis in place for more than 1 year. Although hemolytic anemia of significant degree was not observed in any of the 16 patients who died late, the occurrence of renal hemosiderosis in 13 of the 16 patients indicates that the poppet disc prosthesis is considerably traumatic to erythrocytes. Thus, this type of prosthesis is not an ideal substitute cardiac valve. It clots, despite anticoagulant therapy, it is intrinsically stenotic, portions of it, that is, the disc, degenerate, and it causes hemolysis to erythrocytes.

From the Department of Pathology, Georgetown University Medical Center, Washington, D.C. and the Section of Pathology, National Heart and Lung Institute, National Institutes of Health, Bethesda, Md.

* Present address: Department of Pathology, *Harbor General Hospital, 100 West Carson St.*, Torrance, Calif. 90509.

Address for reprints: William C. Roberts, MD, Bldg. 10A, Rm. 3E30, National Institutes of Health, Bethesda, Md. 20014.

Although numerous clinical and hemodynamic studies of various prosthetic cardiac valves have been reported, comparatively few studies have focused on findings at necropsy in patients with one or more prosthetic valves. Of the latter studies reported, most have been in patients with caged-ball prostheses (mainly of the Starr-Edwards type)[1–8] or tissue valves.[9–14] This report focuses attention on findings at necropsy in 61 patients with replacement of one or more cardiac

TABLE I

Valves Replaced with Discoid Prosthesis of the Hufnagel Type

Valve	Early Deaths (<2 mo)	Late Deaths (>2 mo)	Total
Mitral	21	8	29
Aortic	20	4	24
Aortic + mitral	2	2*	4
Tricuspid	1	2	3
Tricuspid + mitral	1	0	1
Total patients	45	16	61
Total valves	48	18	66

* Hufnagel trileaflet rather than discoid prosthesis used to replace aortic valve in one patient.

valves by a discoid prosthesis of the Hufnael type*[15] and is the first report, to our knowledge, to describe necropsy observations in a large group of patients with prosthetic valves of the disc type.

Patients Studied

Valves Replaced

The 61 patients were classified in two groups: (1) 45 patients who died within 65 days of operation (early deaths), and (2) 16 patients who died 4 to 47 months (average 21 months) after operation (late deaths). The valves replaced are summarized in Table I. Of the 61 patients, 36 (59 percent) were men and 25 (41 percent) were women; their ages ranged from 23 to 77 years (average 49) (Table II). A total of 66 valves were replaced: a disc prosthesis replaced 65 valves and a Hufnagel trileaflet prosthesis[16,17] 1 valve. The

TABLE II

Ages and Sex of Patients with Discoid (Hufnagel Type) Prostheses

	Early Deaths				Late Deaths			
Valve Prosthesis	Male (no.)	Female (no.)	Total (no.)	Age Range & Average (yr)	Male (no.)	Female (no.)	Total (no.)	Age Range & Average (yr)
Mitral	10	11	21	40–68 (50)	2	6	8	38–67 (51)
Aortic	16	4	20	23–77 (50)	4	0	4	51–75 (58)
Aortic + mitral	2	0	2	36–54 (40)	1	1	2	24–50 (37)
Tricuspid	0	1	1	43 (43)	1	1	2	31–49 (40)
Tricuspid + mitral	0	1	1	44 (44)	0	0	0	0 (0)
Totals	28	17	45	23–77 (50)	8	8	16	24–75 (48)

TABLE III

Types of Functional Valve Lesions in Patients with Discoid Prosthesis of the Hufnagel Type (61 patients; 66 valves replaced)

	Early Deaths			Late Deaths		
Valve Prosthesis	S	R	Total	S	R	Total
Mitral Valve						
Mitral	14	7	21	6	2	8
Mitral + aortic	1	1	2	1	1	2
Mitral + tricuspid	1	0	1	0	0	0
Total	16	8	24	7	3	10
Aortic Valve						
Aortic	9	11	20	3	1	4
Aortic + mitral	1	1	2	1	1	2
Total	10	12	22	4	2	6
Tricuspid Valve						
Tricuspid	1	0	1	1	1	2
Tricuspid + mitral	1	0	1	0	0	0
Total	2	0	2	1	1	2
Overall totals	28 (58%)	20 (42%)	48 (100%)	12 (67%)	6 (33%)	18 (100%)

R = pure regurgitation; S = stenosis.

preoperative valvular lesions are summarized in Tables III and IV. Of the 66 valves replaced, 40 (61 percent) had some degree of stenosis, and 26 (39 percent) were purely incompetent. Most stenotic valves also were incompetent, and in a few of them the predominant hemodynamic lesion was regurgitation rather than stenosis. Valves classified as purely incompetent had no pressure gradient across them. Preoperative cardiac catheterization data in the 53 patients with isolated mitral or aortic valve replacement are summarized in Table IV. The preoperative functional classification (New York Heart Association criteria) of the 61 patients was: II = 9 (15 percent); III = 36 (59 percent); and IV = 16 (26 percent).

Etiology

The cause of the valvular disease was variable. Of 29 patients with isolated mitral valve replacement, 20 (69 percent) had stenosis of rheumatic origin.[18] The other nine patients had purely incompetent valves caused by papillary muscle dysfunction or rupture due to myocardial infarction in five,[19] infective endocarditis in two,[20] "spontaneous" rupture of chordae tendineae in one[21] and the "floppy valve syndrome" in one.[22]

* This prosthesis has a polypropylene base completely covered by a Dacron® velour. The cuff contains a central core of "Hepacone," a substance that at least in vitro decreases clotting. The disc itself, disc stops and frame are also made of polypropylene. The polypropylene disc initially was covered by a layer of silicone rubber. The internal diameter of the prosthesis ranges from 13 to 22.5 mm. Several changes, particularly involving the cage legs, have occurred since introduction of this prosthesis in 1962.

TABLE IV

Preoperative Pressures (mm Hg) in 53 Patients with Single Valve Replacement by a Discoid Prosthesis of the Hufnagel Type

	Mitral Valve (mean diastolic gradient [LA*–LV])						Aortic Valve (peak systolic gradient [LV–SA])				
	0–6	7–12	13–20	21–36	no. Cath.	Total	0–20	21–50	51–100	no. Cath.	Total
Early death	7	5	4	3	2	21	5	1	5	9	20
Late death	0	1	2	1	4	8	0	1	2	1	4

* Pulmonary arterial wedge pressure rather than left atrial pressure in some patients.
Cath. = catheterization; LA = left atrium; LV = left ventricle; SA = systemic artery.

TABLE V

Heart Weight in Grams (Range and Average) in 61 Patients with a Discoid (Hufnagel Type) Valve

Valve Replaced	Early Deaths: Men (no. = 28)	Early Deaths: Women (no. = 17)	Early Deaths: Total (no. = 45)	Late Deaths: Men (no. = 8)	Late Deaths: Women (no. = 8)	Late Deaths: Total (no. = 16)
Mitral	350–750 (590)	370–640 (459)	350–750 (528)	400–660 (530)	420–600 (493)	400–660 (502)
Aortic	460–975 (662)	270–800 (557)	460–975 (641)	380–910 (590)	...	380–910 (590)
Aortic + mitral	570–700 (635)	...	570–700 (635)	830 (830)	450 (450)	450–830 (640)
Tricuspid	...	370 (370)	370 (370)	550 (550)	300 (300)	300–550 (425)
Tricuspid + mitral	...	480 (480)	480 (480)	...	...	...
Totals	350–975 (633)	370–800 (496)	350–975 (614)	380–910 (600)	300–600 (464)	300–910 (532)

Figures in parentheses indicate averages.

Of the 24 patients who had isolated aortic valve replacement, 12 had three-cusped stenotic aortic valves. Four of the 12 also had diffusely thickened mitral valves so their disease is considered to be of rheumatic origin[23]; the origin in the other 8 patients is uncertain, but probably degenerative[24,25] in most. Each of the other four stenotic aortic valves was congenitally biscuspid.[26] Of the eight purely incompetent aortic valves, seven were three-cusped and one was two-cusped: the cause of the regurgitation was infective endocarditis in four, rheumatic disease in two, the Marfan syndrome in one and trauma in one.[22]

The valvular disease was of rheumatic origin in each of the three patients who had isolated tricuspid valve replacement and in all five who had more than one valve replaced. In none of the 61 patients were Aschoff bodies found at necropsy in histologic sections of heart.

Myocardial Findings

The heart weights are summarized in Table V. The patients who died late had on the average a smaller heart than did those who died early.

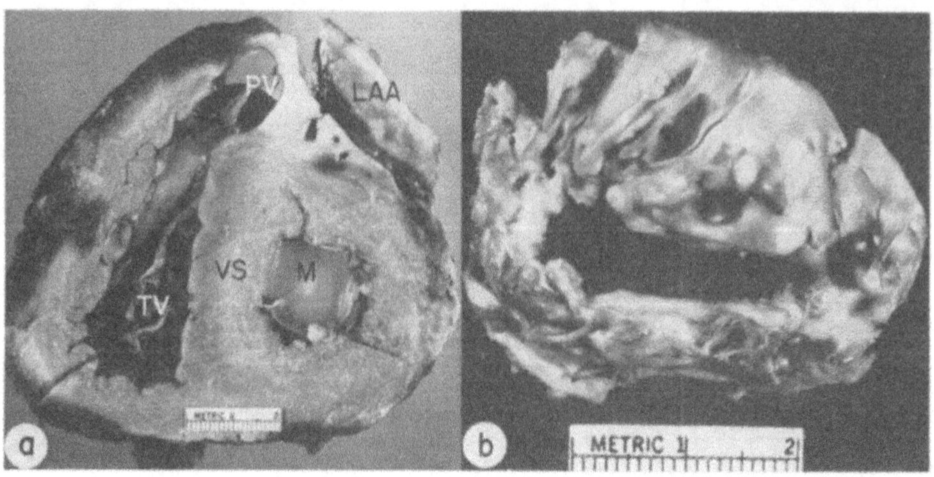

FIGURE 1. *Prosthetic valve dysfunction.* Transverse section of the cardiac ventricles (**a**) and excised stenotic mitral valve (**b**) in a 57 year old woman who died at operation after replacement of the mitral valve with a no. 19 Hufnagel discoid prosthesis (M). The margins of the disc contact the left ventricular endocardium at several sites, and movement of the disc is impeded. In addition to mitral stenosis and severe pulmonary hypertension (90/45 mm Hg), the aortic valve was mildly stenotic (peak systolic pressure gradient 34 mm Hg). LAA = left atrial appendage; PV = pulmonary valve; TV = tricuspid valve; VS = ventricular septum.

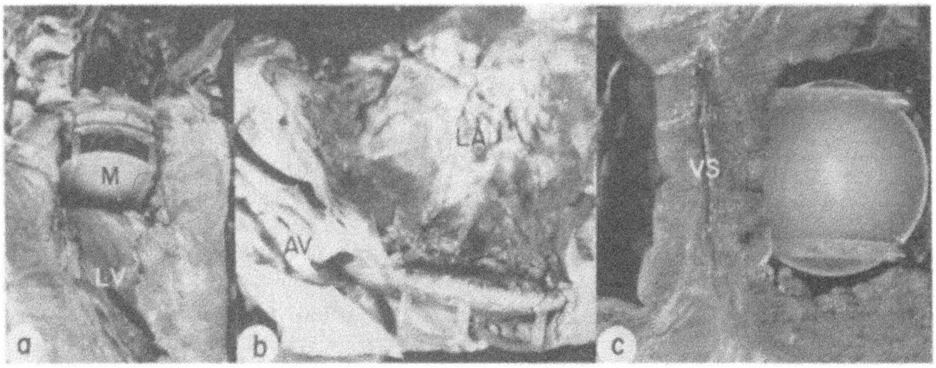

FIGURE 2. *Prosthetic valve dysfunction.* Views of a size 22 mitral valve prosthesis (M) in a 48 year old man who died in the operating room after replacement of the severely stenotic mitral valve (mean diastolic gradient 31 mm Hg between the left atrium and left ventricle). A large thrombus was excised from the left atrium at operation. At necropsy, portions of the margins of the disc and portions of the struts of the mitral valve prosthesis contacted left ventricular endocardium. It appeared that there was inadequate space for flow of blood between the disc margins and left ventricular endocardium. **a,** view of prosthesis (M) from the left ventricle (LV) showing contact of disc margins with endocardium. The prosthesis is very large. (Preoperatively, there was no mitral regurgitation or evidence of aortic valve dysfunction.) **b,** this view shows the left atrium (LA), mitral valve prosthesis and aortic valve (AV). **c,** close-up transverse view of the prosthesis. VS = ventricular septum.

Coronary atherosclerosis of various degrees was observed in most of the 61 patients. The lumen of at least one of the three major coronary arteries (right, left anterior descending and left circumflex) was narrowed by more than 75 percent in 15 patients (25 percent), 9 of whom died early and 6 of whom died late.

Myocardial fibrosis of various degrees also was common. Nearly all patients on histologic examination of sections of the left ventricular free wall or ventricular septum had small foci of interstitial or perivascular fibrosis. Furthermore, on gross examination, focal scars were observed, at least in the apexes, of the left ventricular papillary muscles of most patients. Grossly visible scars limited to the left ventricular free wall or ventricular septum (excluding papillary muscles) were less common, being observed in only 12 patients (20 percent), and were transmural (involving more than half the thickness of the myocardial wall) in 10 (16 percent) of them.

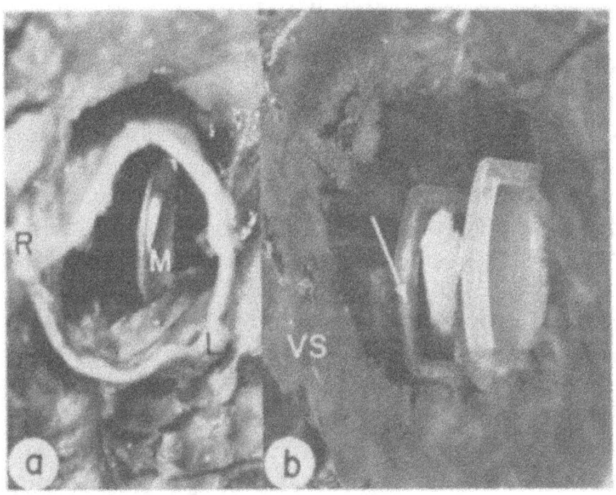

FIGURE 3. *Prosthetic valve dysfunction.* View of mitral valve prosthesis (M) from the aorta (a) and left ventricle (b) in a 46 year old woman who died 3 days after replacement of a severely stenotic mitral valve (pulmonary arterial wedge-left ventricular mean diastolic gradient 18 mm Hg). During the entire postoperative period she had evidence of the low cardiac output syndrome and immediately after valve replacement, complete left bundle branch block was evidenced on the electrocardiogram. This conduction disturbance had not been present preoperatively. **a,** this view shows the mitral disc (M) from the aortic root. The aortic valve cusps have been excised. L = left and R = right coronary artery. **b,** this view shows that one of the prosthetic struts (**arrow**) has burrowed into the ventricular septum (VS). The protrusion of this strut into the septum probably caused the left bundle branch block. Blood exits from the left ventricle only by passing between the strut (contacting the septum) and the disc.

Myocardial necrosis of various degrees also was common. Focal necrosis was observed in the stumps of the left ventricular papillary muscles in all of the 24 patients who died early after mitral valve replacement, including the 6 who died in the operating room. In all of these 24 patients portions of the left ventricular papillary muscles had been excised at operation. Small foci of "contraction bands"[27] also were observed on histologic examination of the left ventricular free wall and ventricular septum in most of the 45 patients who died early. Although on histologic examination a number of patients had small foci of myocardial necrosis limited to the left ventricular subendocardium (involving less than half the thickness of the wall), only six patients, all of whom died early, had grossly visible foci of myocardial necrosis; these were transmural in four and subendocardial in two. Three of the six patients with grossly visible foci of myocardial necrosis also had grossly visible foci of myocardial fibrosis. All six patients with grossly visible foci of myocardial necrosis had greater than 75 percent narrowing of the lumen of at least one of the three major extramural coronary arteries. In contrast, of the nine with grossly visible foci of myocardial fibrosis (without necrosis) only four had coronary arterial luminal narrowing to this degree.

Early Postoperative Deaths

Of the 45 patients, 13 (29 percent) died more than 24 hours after operation, 33 (73 percent) within 1 week and 36 (80 percent) within 2 weeks. The remaining nine patients (20 percent) died 15 to 65 days after operation. Certain anatomic observations in some of these patients are illustrated in Figures 1 to 8.

Low Output Syndrome

Of the 45 patients, 7 died in the operating room. The postoperative course in the other 38 patients was

TABLE VI

Principal Cause of Early Death in 45 Patients After Valve Replacement with Discoid Prosthesis of the Hufnagel Type

Cause	M	A	M+A	T	M+T	Total
Prosthetic dysfunction						17 (38%)
Disproportion*	9	3	1	0	1	
Thrombosis	0	3	0	0	0	
Bleeding	3	7	1	0	0	11 (24%)
No anatomic explanation	3	4	0	0	0	7 (16%)
Uncorrected valvular disease	2	3	0	1	0	6 (13%)
Coronary heart disease	4	0	0	0	0	4 (9%)
Total	21	20	2	1	1	45 (100%)

* Prosthesis too large for left ventricle or aorta into which it was inserted so that flow across prosthesis was partially obstructed.

A = aortic; M = mitral; T = tricuspid.

characterized by evidence of the low cardiac output syndrome.* Although the low cardiac output syndrome was an adequate explanation for death in these patients, a challenge at necropsy was to find the cause or causes of the low cardiac output syndrome in each of the 38 patients surviving the operation. The causes obviously varied (Table VI). In some patients, a clear anatomic cause was found. In others, an anatomic reason for the low cardiac output syndrome or the intraoperative death was less certain or no anatomic explanation for death was discernible.

Postoperative Hemorrhage

Excessive postoperative hemorrhage appeared responsible in 11 (24 percent) of the 45 early deaths (Table VI). The source of the bleeding in 5 of the 11 patients appeared to be diamond-shaped patches that had been utilized to widen the aortic roots to prevent prosthetic valve obstruction.[28] Among the 28 patients whose aortic valve was replaced, 13 had these patches inserted to widen the aortic root. These patches had been utilized in 10 of the 20 patients who died early after aortic valve replacement, and 5 of them died from bleeding at this site (Fig. 4). Of the other six patients who died from hemorrhage, one had had a previous thoracotomy and consequently numerous pleural and pericardial adhesions were present.

Coronary Artery Disease

Although the lumen of at least one of the three major coronary arteries was narrowed by more than 75 percent in 9 (20 percent) of the 45 patients who died early, coronary heart disease was considered the principal cause of death in 4 patients.[29] Each of the four had undergone mitral valve replacement because of severemitral regurgitation, in three from papillary muscle dysfunction resulting from acute myocardial infarction (1 week to 4 months earlier) and in one from infective endocarditis causing rupture of several mitral chordae tendineae. The latter patient had a large embolus to the left circumflex coronary artery causing a huge acute myocardial infarction several days before valve replacement. Three of the four patients died in the operating room because of inadequate ventricular contractions and the fourth died 18 hours after operation.

Associated Uncorrected Valve Disease

The principal cause of death in the remaining 30 patients who died early is less clear. Associated uncorrected valve disease may have been an important factor in as many as 10 patients and was probably a principal cause of death in 6 of them. All 10 patients had both anatomic and clinical evidence of dysfunction of more than one cardiac valve (mitral and aortic in 9 and mitral, aortic and tricuspid in 1), but all had undergone only single valve replacement. Four of the 10 patients had also undergone commissurotomy on at least one of the malfunctioning valves. In these 10 patients the commissurotomy did not appear to relieve adequately the valvular stenosis, or the uncorrected valvular lesion appeared to interfere with proper functioning of the prosthesis, or the use of a prosthesis to replace one malfunctioning valve appeared to worsen the uncorrected valvular lesion, or the use of a prosthesis to replace one malfunctioning valve caused a valve in which a commissurotomy had been performed to be excessively incompetent. Some examples of these four possibilities follow and are illustrated in Figures 5 to 8.

Aortic valve replacement and mitral valve commissurotomy (Fig. 5): In two patients who had aortic valve replacement for pure aortic regurgitation, mitral commissurotomy was performed because of mitral stenosis. Although the preoperative aortic valve lesion in each patient was pure regurgitation, it is likely that use of a discoid prosthesis in the aortic valve position created some systolic pressure gradient between the left ventricle and aorta postoperatively. The mitral valves in these two patients contained considerable calcific deposits and consequently it is likely that each mitral valve was somewhat incompetent after the commissurotomy. The creation of left ventricular outflow obstruction, namely some degree of prosthetic aortic stenosis, combined with commissurotomy on calcific mitral stenosis almost certainly increases the degree of mitral regurgitation. Death in each of the two patients, which came 7 hours and 2 days, respectively, after operation was attributed at necropsy to uncorrected mitral valve disease.

Aortic valve replacement and preoperative mitral regurgitation: In two patients with this combination the aortic valves were replaced because of pure aortic regurgitation and preoperatively the mi-

* All patients at one time had direct systolic pressures of more than 90 mm Hg. Each also had evidence of underperfusion of at least one organ system: brain (disorientation or seizures); bowel (pain or bleeding); kidney (oliguria); lung (alveolar infiltrates, alveolar hemorrhages); liver (hyperbilirubinemia); and skin (peripheral cyanosis or coldness). The hypotension and organ perfusion inadequacy responded poorly or not at all to therapy, including administration of vasopressors.

tral valves were purely incompetent. The degree of mitral regurgitation preoperatively in each was judged to be 1 to 2+/4+. As in the two patients previously described, the insertion of a discoid prosthesis in the aortic valve position probably created some degree of aortic stenosis. The conversion of a purely incompetent aortic valve into a purely obstructive one—of any degree—clearly increases the amount of regurgitation through a purely incompetent mitral valve. In one of these patients there was extremely little space between the margins of the aortic prosthetic disc and the intima of aorta. Thus, almost certainly this patient had considerable prosthetic stenosis. The principal cause of his death is attributed to prosthetic aortic stenosis, although postoperative mitral regurgitation may well have been important. Death in the second patient is attributed to uncorrected mitral regurgitation, probably worsened by

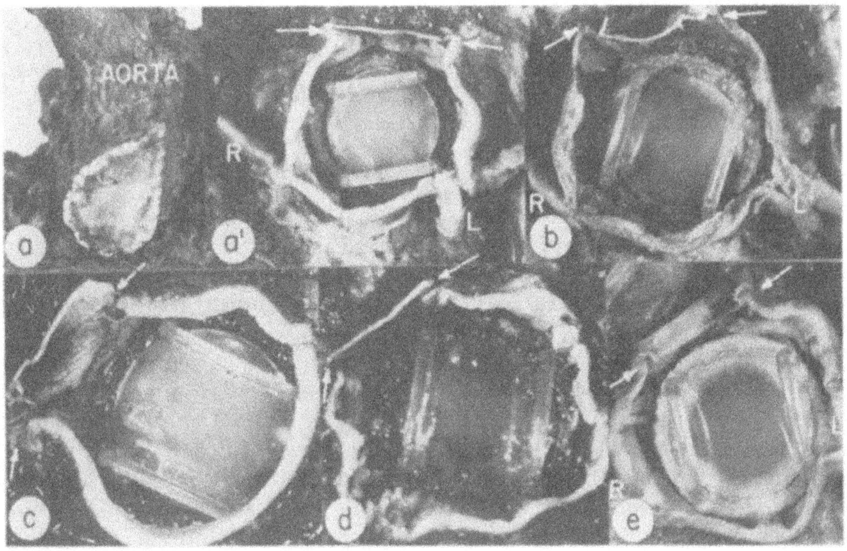

FIGURE 4. *Aortic root patches to widen aorta.* These photographs show aortic root patches and aortic discoid prostheses (all sized 15) in five patients; each prosthesis was inserted in 1971. The patches, designated by the **arrows**, are seen on transverse cuts of the aorta (**a** and **a'**) of a 62 year old man who died 5 days after his stenotic aortic valve was replaced with a disc. The patch has a teardrop shape (**a**). The patient died from extensive bleeding from the area of the aortic root. L = left and R = right coronary artery. **b**, patch and prosthesis in a 66 year old woman who died 20 days after replacement of her stenotic aortic valve. The cause of death was persistent bleeding from the area of the aortic root. She was returned to the operating room on two different occasions to control the hemorrhage. **c**, patch and prosthesis of a 63 year old man who died 2 days after replacement of a purely incompetent aortic valve. Despite the purely regurgitant aortic lesion, the aortic root had to be widened by the patch to provide adequate room for the disc prosthesis. **d**, patch of a 63 year old man who could not be separated from cardiopulmonary bypass after replacement of his stenotic aortic valve. **e**, patch of a 43 year old man who died from massive bleeding in the aortic root area 7 hours after replacement of a purely incompetent aortic valve.

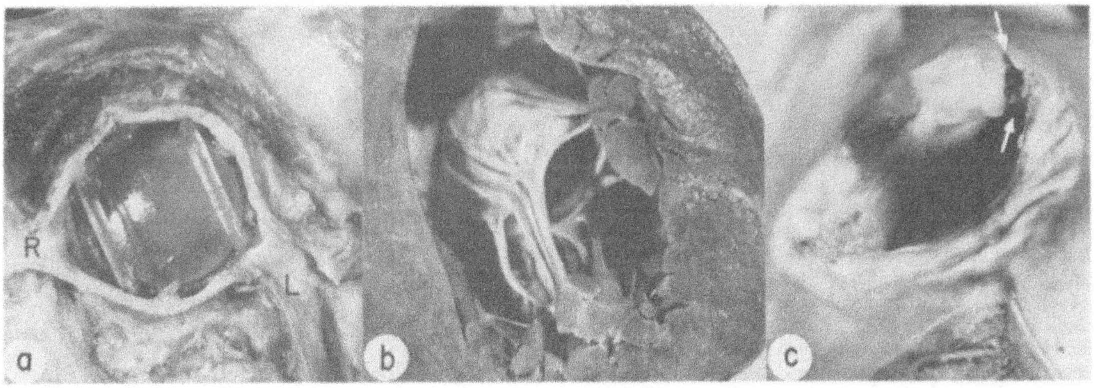

FIGURE 5. *Uncorrected valvular disease.* Aortic valve prosthesis and mitral valve of a 29 year old man who died 7 hours after aortic valve replacement and mitral commissurotomy. Preoperatively, the aortic valve was purely incompetent (3+/4+ aortic regurgitation) and the mitral valve was stenotic (mean diastolic pressure gradient 12 mm Hg). The entire 7 hour postoperative period was characterized by features of the low cardiac output syndrome. **a**, aortic valve prosthesis from above. The margins of struts contact the intima of aorta at three sites and the fourth is located at the orifice of the left (L) coronary artery. The amount of space between the margins of the disc and the intima of the aortic root appears small. R = right coronary artery. **b**, scarred incompetent mitral valve viewed from the left ventricle. **c**, mitral valve viewed from the left atrium. The posteromedial commissure (**arrows**) was incised at operation. The valve orifice appears incompetent. Death in this patient was probably related to the mitral incompetency induced by commissurotomy. Preoperatively, the mitral valve was entirely stenotic. Postoperatively, it appears mainly incompetent. The aortic valve preoperatively was entirely incompetent, but postoperatively it appears stenotic. Obstruction at the aortic valve position may cause mild preoperative mitral regurgitation (from commissurotomy) to become moderate or severe postoperatively.

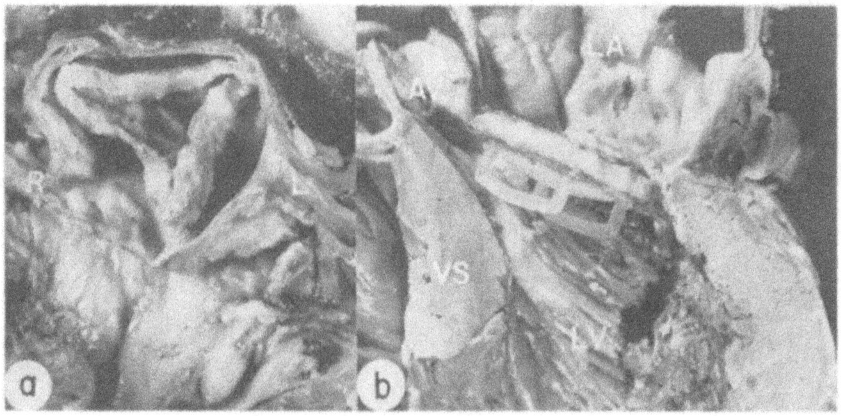

FIGURE 6. *Uncorrected valvular disease.* Views of the heart of a 51 year old woman who died in the operating room after mitral valve replacement and aortic valvuloplasty. Preoperatively, she had mitral stenosis (mean diastolic pressure gradient 12 mm Hg), aortic regurgitation and mild aortic stenosis (peak systolic left ventricular-femoral arterial pressure gradient 23 mm Hg). **a,** aortic valve (AV) from above. It appears that the stenosis has been relieved but the price may have been increased regurgitation. Aortic regurgitation in a patient with a mitral disc can cause the disc to cock and result in intermittent regurgitation between the left atrium (LA) and left ventricle (LV) in systole. L and R = left and right coronary arteries. **b,** coronal section of heart showing the relation of the mitral prosthesis to adjacent structures. VS = ventricular septum.

some degree of obstruction at the level of the prosthetic aortic valve. These two patients lived 1 and 3 days, respectively, after operation.

Mitral valve replacement and aortic valve commissurotomy (Fig 6): In one patient the mitral valve was replaced because of severe mitral stenosis, and aortic valve commissurotomy was performed because of slight (15 mm Hg peak systolic pressure gradient between left ventricle and a systemic artery) aortic stenosis. Examination of the aortic valve at necropsy strongly suggested that it was quite incompetent. It is postulated that the regurgitant stream from the incompetent aortic valve interfered with proper movement of the mitral disc, probably causing it to cock, thus creating prosthetic mitral dysfunction. This patient died in the operating room and death was attributed at necropsy to uncorrected aortic valve disease

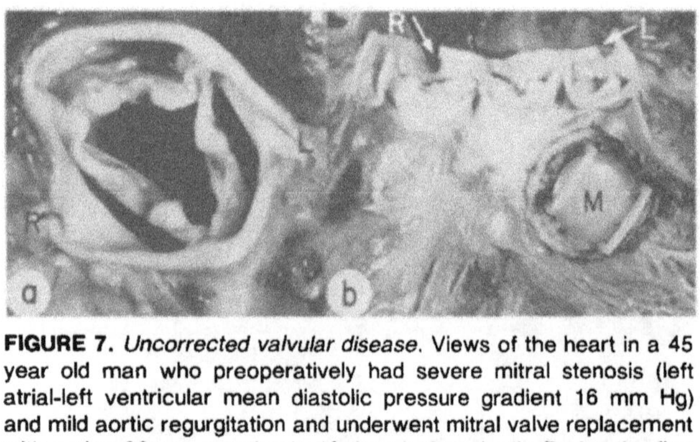

FIGURE 7. *Uncorrected valvular disease.* Views of the heart in a 45 year old man who preoperatively had severe mitral stenosis (left atrial-left ventricular mean diastolic pressure gradient 16 mm Hg) and mild aortic regurgitation and underwent mitral valve replacement with a size 22 mm prosthesis 10 days before death. During the first 24 hours postoperatively, the prosthetic valvular sounds were intermittent (occurring only about 50 percent of the time) and could be altered by change in body position. Because of this intermittent prosthetic valvular dysfunction, the disc mitral valve prosthesis (M) was replaced with a similar but smaller (20 mm) prosthesis. Prosthetic heart sounds thereafter appeared normal. The remaining 8 days of life, however, were characterized by evidence of severely inadequate cardiac output. *At necropsy,* the aortic valve cusps were diffusely fibrotic and the orifice was obviously incompetent (**a** and **b**). There is no anatomic indication that the mitral valve prosthesis (M) functioned abnormally, but intermittent cocking may be missed at necropsy. L and R = left and right coronary arteries or ostia. The necropsy findings suggest that uncorrected aortic regurgitation contributed to the patient's death and also may have been responsible for the intermittent dysfunction of the first mitral valve prosthesis.

Mitral valve replacement and preoperative aortic regurgitation (Fig 7): In each of the four patients with this combination the mitral valve was replaced because of severe mitral stenosis (left atrial to left ventricular mean diastolic pressure gradient ranging from 15 to 31 mm Hg); the aortic valve preoperatively in each was mildly (1 to 2+/4+) incompetent, and in two, mildly stenotic (peak systolic pressure gradients of 16 and 30 mm Hg). In one of these four patients mitral dysfunction was documented postoperatively. It is believed that the aortic regurgitant stream caused his mitral disc to cock, creating considerable mitral prosthetic dysfunction. The mitral prosthetic sounds were quite variable postoperatively in this patient, who was returned to the operating room for replacement of the mitral valve prosthesis with a smaller one. In the other three patients clear clinical evidence that the mitral prosthesis was functioning improperly is lacking. In each of these three patients, however, the prosthesis appeared obstructive (see later); two died in the operating room and the third, 2 days postoperatively.

Tricuspid valve replacement and mitral and aortic valve commissurotomy (Fig 8): In one patient a stenotic and incompetent tricuspid valve was replaced with a discoid prosthesis, and commissurotomy was performed on the mitral and aortic valves because of calcific mitral and aortic stenosis. This patient lived 1 day after operation and at necropsy the stenosis of neither valve appeared relieved by the commissurotomy. Death is attributed, therefore, to uncorrected valvular disease.

Prosthetic Dysfunction

Disproportion: In the remaining 24 patients who died early, prosthetic dysfunction from either disproportion (14 patients) or thrombosis (3 patients) appears the most likely cause of death in 17 (38 percent). Disproportion is defined as too little space between the margins of the prosthetic disc and the wall of either the left ventricle or aorta into which the prosthesis was inserted. If this space between the disc margins and the wall is too small, prosthetic obstruction may result. Of the 14 patients with prosthetic disproportion, 9 had had isolated mitral valve replacement, 1 combined mitral and tricuspid valve replacement, 1 combined mitral and aortic valve replacement, and 3 isolated aortic valve replacement. The mitral prosthesis in 10 and the aortic prosthesis in 4 was judged at necropsy to be obstructive or disproportionate. Prosthetic obstruction is obviously most likely to occur when the cardiac cavity (left ventricle) or great artery (aorta) into which a prosthesis is inserted is not dilated. Such was the case in all 14 patients considered to have prosthetic obstruction. Nine of the 10 patients in whom the mitral prosthesis appeared obstructive had had severe mitral stenosis preoperatively and the 10th patient had had pure mitral regurgitation of recent origin (rupture of chordae tendineae on a previously normal valve). In addition, the latter patient was a small, elderly woman (age 70). Eight of the 10 patients with prosthetic mitral stenosis were women. In all but one the mitral valve prosthesis was judged to interfere with left ventricular inflow (Fig. 1 and 2). Interference to left ventricular outflow occurred in one patient (Fig. 3) and was associated with development of complete left bundle branch block postoperatively, and the ventricular septum was severely indented by the stents or legs of the prosthesis.

Despite severe aortic regurgitation in each (associated with slight stenosis in one) and the insertion of a droplet-shaped patch in the aortic root in one, the ascending aorta was not dilated in any of the four patients judged at necropsy to have prosthetic aortic obstruction (disproportion): two had aortic regurgitation of recent onset (infective endocarditis), and in the other two the mitral valve was stenotic or incompetent, or both. (In combined mitral and aortic valve disease irrespective of the type of aortic lesion, the ascending aorta usually is not dilated.[22]) In one of these four patients prosthetic aortic stenosis was judged to be present at operation when the patient was unable to be separated from cardiopulmonary bypass. A smaller disc was then inserted but the patient showed evidence of extremely depressed cardiac output during the entire 11 hour postoperative period.

Of the 14 patients considered to have prosthetic obstruction, 5 died in the operating room or within 12 hours of operation, 7 between day 2 and 4 postoperatively, 1 on day 6 and 1 on day 8.

Prosthetic thrombosis: All three patients whose prosthetic dysfunction resulted from prosthetic thrombosis had isolated aortic valve replacement. The thrombi in each were large enough to prevent proper movement of the disc, and all three had clinical evidence of systemic emboli postoperatively and systemic infarcts at necropsy. These three patients died 22, 30 and 45 days, respectively, after operation, and all had received anticoagulant agents during that period. It is possible that some type of prosthetic dysfunction preceded the development of prosthetic thrombosis in these three patients.

Deaths Without Adequate Explanation

In the remaining seven patients who died early no reasonable anatomic explanation for death was discernible at necropsy. The mitral valves had been replaced in three (for stenosis in two, pure regurgitation in one) and the aortic valves in four (for stenosis in two, pure regurgitation in two). In each of the

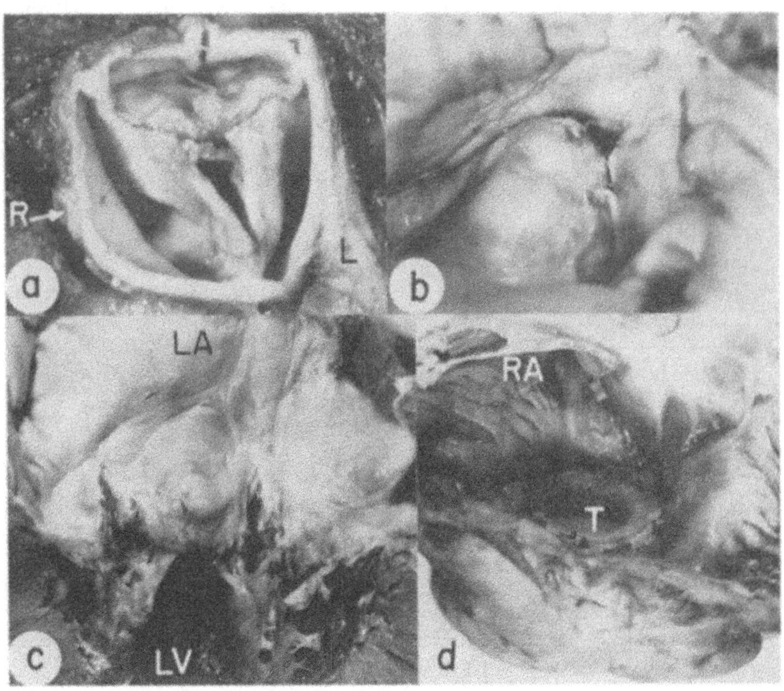

FIGURE 8. *Uncorrected valvular disease.* Aortic valve viewed from above (**a**), mitral valve viewed from the left atrium (**b**) and after being opened (**c**) and replaced tricuspid (T) valve (**d**) in a 43 year old woman who preoperatively had mitral stenosis, aortic stenosis and tricuspid regurgitation. At operation, the tricuspid valve was replaced with a discoid prosthesis and mitral and aortic valvulotomy was performed. Throughout the entire 24 hour postoperative period the patient had evidence of the low cardiac output syndrome. *At necropsy,* the aortic valve cusps were rigid and the orifice appeared quite stenotic (**a**). It seems likely that the commissurotomy on this valve did not accomplish its purpose. L and R = left and right coronary arteries; LA = left atrium; LV = left ventricle; RA = right atrium.

seven patients there was plenty of room to freely accommodate the prosthesis in either the aorta or left ventricle. None of the seven patients had multivalvular disease; the only valve that functioned abnormally preoperatively was the valve replaced. The lumen of at least one of the three major coronary arteries was more than 75 percent narrowed in three of the seven patients and each of them had transmural left ventricular scars. Another patient with nearly clean coronary arteries also had a healed transmural left ventricular infarct at necropsy. It is obviously entirely possible that the healed myocardial infarcts of these four patients, superimposed on the operative trauma of valve replacement, is an adequate explanation for death, but their hearts also were relieved of significant hemodynamic burdens by valve replacement. In none of the other three patients were the coronary arteries significantly narrowed or the left ventricular walls scarred. The average age (56 years) and the average heart weight (663 g) of these seven patients were higher than those of the group as a whole. Of the seven patients, two died in the operating room, two on day 2 postoperatively, one on day 7, one on day 22 and one on day 59.

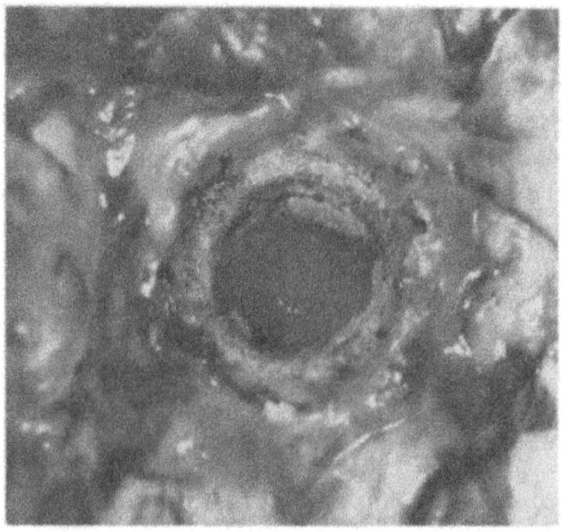

FIGURE 9. *Prosthetic thrombus.* View of prosthesis and thrombus in a 67 year old woman who had had a mitral commissurotomy at age 52 and underwent replacement of the stenotic (pulmonary arterial wedge to left ventricular mean diastolic gradient 9 mm Hg) mitral valve with a size 19 Hufnagel discoid prosthesis 3 months before death. Her condition was not improved by operation and postoperatively, congestive cardiac failure continued to progress until it was fatal. *At necropsy,* a small amount of thrombus was present on the inner margins of the prosthesis, shown here. Disc movement, however, was not hindered by the thrombus. The left ventricular cavity was of normal size, and there was relatively little space between the margins of the disc and the endocardium of left ventricle.

Late Postoperative Deaths

The valves replaced, prosthetic implantation periods and frequency of prosthetic thrombi, clinical equivalents of emboli, peribasilar prosthetic leaks and disc variance or degeneration in the 16 patients are summarized in Table VII, and several of the findings are illustrated in Figures 9 to 17. The implantation periods ranged from 4 to 47 months (average 21). In 10 patients the implantation period was more than 12 months.

Prosthetic thrombi: Of the 17 prosthetic disc valves, 14 (in 14 patients) contained thrombi (Fig. 9 and 11). The thrombi in all 14 patients were attached to the bases of the struts, all four in each of the patients in 13 patients the thrombi were small and probably did not interfere with movement of the discs, but in the 14th, a large thrombus also was located on the atrial aspect of a tricuspid prosthesis and it appeared to interfere with proper disc movement.

Prosthetic valve leaks: Peribasilar prosthetic aorto-left ventricular or left ventricular-left atrial accessory communications (ring leaks) occurred in four patients. These ring leaks involved mitral valve prostheses in three patients and an aortic valve prosthesis in one. None of the ring leaks were produced by in-

TABLE VII

Observations in 16 Patients Who Died Late After Replacement of One or More Cardiac Valves with a Discoid Prosthesis of the Hufnagel Type

			Status of Prosthesis						
Valve Prosthesis	Patients (no.)	Months of Implantation (range and average)	no. with Thrombi	no. with Thrombi on Warfarin	Thrombi Causing Dysfunction	Clinical Emboli	Ring Leak	Disc Wear	Renal Hemosiderosis
Mitral	8	4–47 (15)	8	8	0	4	2	4	7
Aortic	4	9–47 (34)	2	2	0	1	1	3	4
Aortic + mitral	2*	18–33 (26)	2†	2	0	0	1†	2‡	2
Tricuspid	2	18–36 (27)	2	2	1	1	0	1	0
Total 18§	16	4–47 (21)	14	14	1	6	4	10‖	13

* In one of the two patients the aortic valve had been replaced with a Hufnagel trileaflet rather than with a disc prosthesis.

† Mitral prosthesis only.

‡ Of both the mitral and aortic prosthesis in one patient, and in the mitral valve disc in the second. The aortic valve in the latter patient had been replaced with a trileaflet prosthesis.

§ A total of 18 valves actually were replaced, but a trileaflet rather than a discoid prosthesis was utilized in one patient.

‖ In 11 of 15 discoid prostheses, in 10 of 16 patients.

fection. In two of the three patients with mitral leaks, the leak was closed at reoperation but the patient died shortly thereafter. The leaks in the other two patients were minute and neither patient had clinical evidence of prosthetic regurgitation. A left ventricular-to-right ventricular communication was inadvertently created at operation in one patient who underwent aortic valve replacement.

Prosthetic valve degeneration (variance or wear): This was observed in 11 of the 17 discoid prostheses (Fig. 11 to 15)—in 6 of 10 mitral valve prostheses, 4 of 5 aortic valve prostheses and 1 of 2

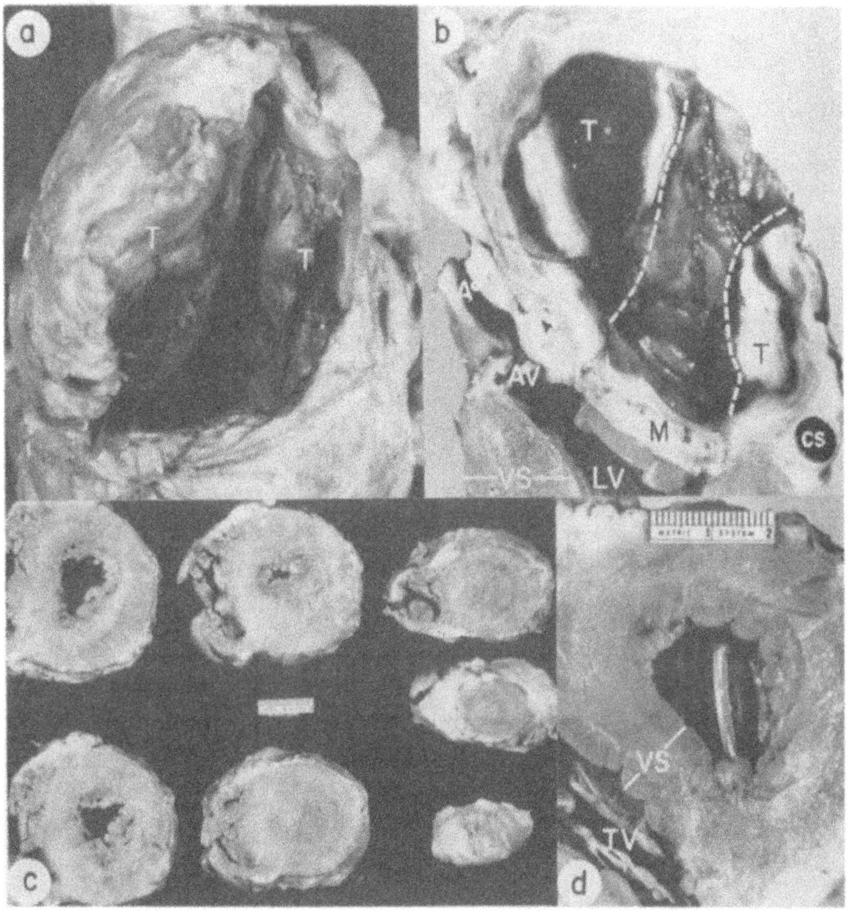

FIGURE 10. *Prosthetic dysfunction causing thrombosis.* Views of the heart in a 46 year old woman who had been well until age 33 when she experienced transient left hemiplegia and was found to have mitral stenosis. Another transient stroke occurred when she was 42 years of age. Because of progressive congestive cardiac failure, mitral valve replacement was performed in February 1973, six months before her death. No left atrial thrombus was observed at operation. Five months after operation right hemiplegia suddenly developed. Physical examination disclosed crisp opening and closing prosthetic sounds. A month later she suddenly had evidence of a larger stroke and died. *Necropsy* disclosed a large thrombus in the body of left atrium and a very small left ventricular cavity. Although the mitral prosthetic disc moved well, the amount of space (for blood to flow) between the margins of the disc and the endocardium of left ventricle was minimal. **a,** left atrium from above showing a large thrombus (T) within its body. **b,** longitudinal section. The channel within the left atrium is outlined by white dashes. No thrombus is present on the mitral prosthesis (M). Ao = aorta; AV = aortic valve; CS = coronary sinus; LV = left ventricle; VS = ventricular septum. **c,** transverse sections of the cardiac ventricles showing the small size of the left ventricular cavity. **d,** close-up view near the left ventricular base showing the small amount of space available for the mitral prosthesis. TV = tricuspid valve orifice.

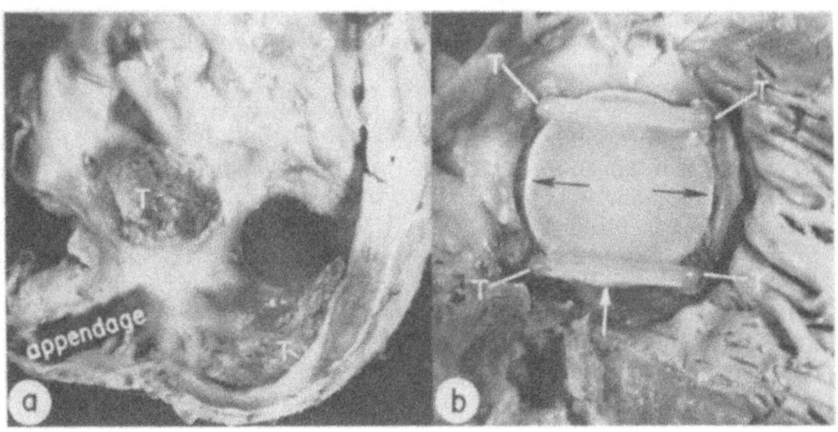

FIGURE 11. *Multiple systemic emboli after mitral valve replacement.* Views of the heart in a 47 year old woman whose stenotic mitral valve was replaced with a size 19 discoid prosthesis and who also underwent a tricuspid anuloplasty for tricuspid regurgitation in July 1969 (19 months before death). At operation, no thrombus was found in the left atrial cavity. One month postoperatively, she had evidence of splenic infarct and 11 months postoperatively right hemiparesis suddenly developed. A month before death she had evidence of another stroke. The prosthetic sounds in the entire postoperative period were always distinct. *At necropsy,* both the brain and spleen were focally infarcted. Thrombus (T) was present in the body of the left atrium (**a**) but not in its appendage. Thrombus also was present on each of the vertical struts of the mitral prosthesis (**b**). The left ventricular cavity was small and the space between the margins of the disc and the endocardium of the left ventricle was small. The margins of the mitral disc were focally grooved (**arrows**). The occurrence of thrombus in the body of the left atrium strongly suggests that the mitral prosthesis was stenotic.

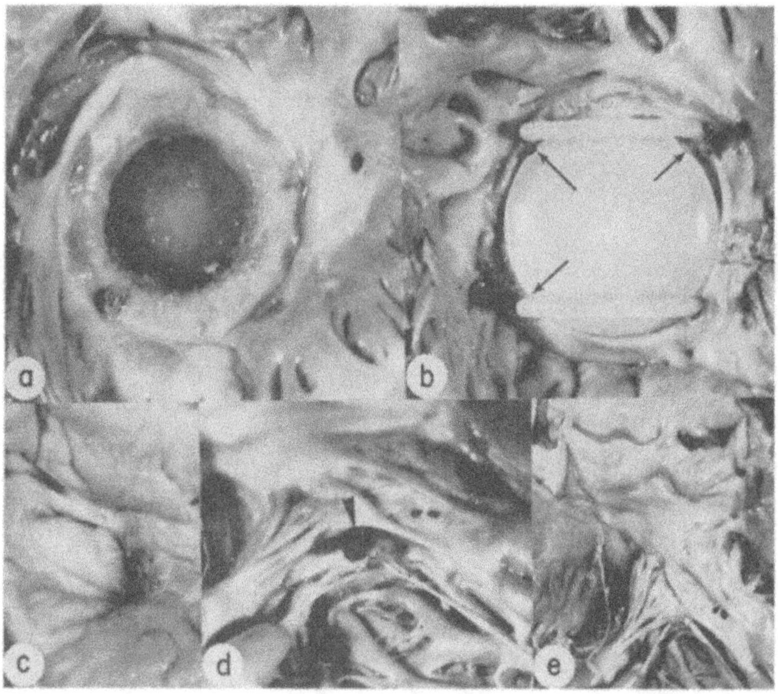

FIGURE 12. *Uncorrected mitral valve disease.* Views of the heart in a 49 year old woman who had signs and symptoms of congestive cardiac failure at age 31 years and underwent mitral commissurotomy. She was thereafter free of symptoms of cardiac dysfunction until age 44 when evidence of congestive cardiac failure reappeared. Studies a year later disclosed mitral stenosis (pulmonary arterial wedge-left ventricular mean diastolic pressure gradient 13 mm Hg) and severe tricuspid valve regurgitation. Mitral commissurotomy and tricuspid anuloplasty were performed (age 45), but her condition did not improve. A year later a third cardiac operation was performed—the tricuspid valve was replaced with a discoid prosthesis. Congestive cardiac failure persisted postoperatively and she died 36 months later. *At necropsy,* the disc of the tricuspid valve prosthesis moved well and there was no evidence of prosthetic dysfunction. A small amount of thrombus was present on the inner rim of the primary orifice. **a,** tricuspid valve prosthesis—in place for 36 months—viewed from the right atrial aspect. **b,** same prosthesis as viewed from right ventricle. Grooves (**arrows**) are present at the margins of the disc. These indentations resulted from contact of the disc margins with the vertical struts and suggest that circular movement of the disc was severely limited. **c,** mitral valve from the left atrium. **d,** mitral valve from the left ventricular aspect. A black probe (**arrow**) is in the mitral orifice. The orifice appears to be severely stenotic. In retrospect, it appears that this valve should have been replaced at the second or the third cardiac operation. **e,** opened left ventricle showing the thickened anterior leaflet of mitral valve and the mildly thickened aortic valve cusps.

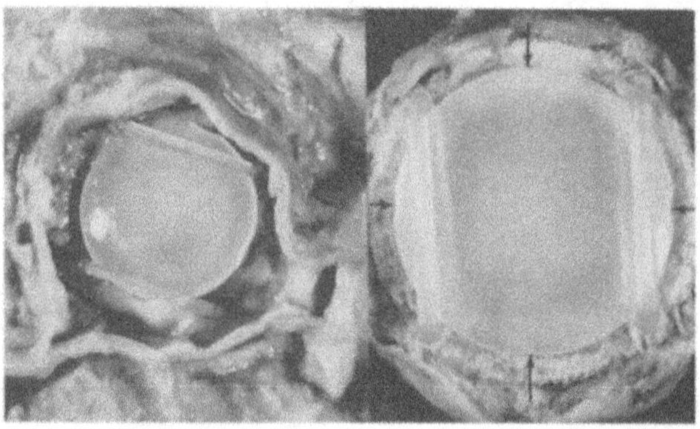

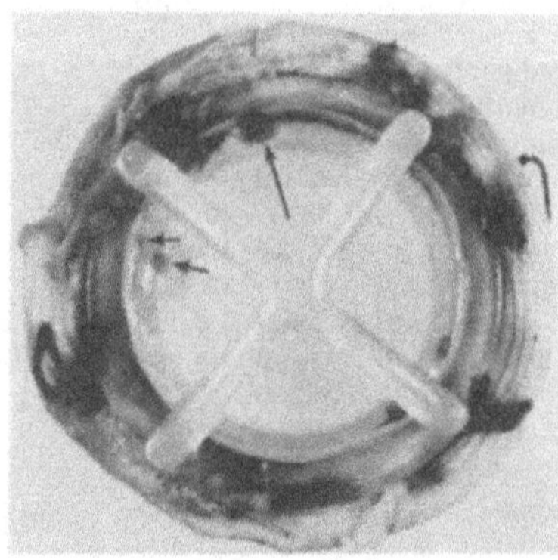

FIGURE 13 (left). *Disc wear (variance).* Shown here are disc prostheses from two patients who had aortic valve replacement 47 and 24 months, respectively, before death. Marginal grooves are present in each disc. There was never clinical evidence of prosthetic dysfunction in either patient. The margins of each disc are indented at four sites (**arrows**), corresponding to the points of contact between the discs and the four vertical struts. Each disc has been rotated to better illustrate the four marginal notches.

FIGURE 14 (right). *Disc wear.* The prosthesis shown here was inserted in January 1970 and the patient died in September 1972. There was no evidence during the 32 month implantation period that the prosthesis functioned abnormally. At necropsy, there is evidence of wear at the margins of the disc: Several small grooves are present and several cysts (**arrows**) containing postmortem blood clot are present.

triscuspid valve prostheses. The degeneration was limited to the disc only; the bases and struts showed no evidence of variance. Of the six prosthetic valves (mitral in five, aortic in one) in place for less than 1 year (range 4 to 9 months [average 7]), disc wear occurred in only one patient and she had had mitral valve replacement 9 months earlier. In the one patient with a prosthetic aortic valve in place for less than 1 year (also 9 months) no disc wear was evident. Of the 11 prosthetic valves (mitral in 5, aortic in 4, tricuspid in 2) in place for more than 1 year (range 18 to 47 months [average 30]), disc wear occurred in 10. The only prosthesis devoid of disc wear had an implantation period of 18 months and was located in the tricuspid valve position. The only other prosthesis utilized for tricuspid valve replacement did show disc wear, but this prosthesis was in place for 36 months.

The degree of disc wear observed in the 11 involved prostheses was variable; in 7 devices (4 mitral, 2 aortic, 1 tricuspid) the wear consisted of four indentations at the margins of the discs. These indenta-

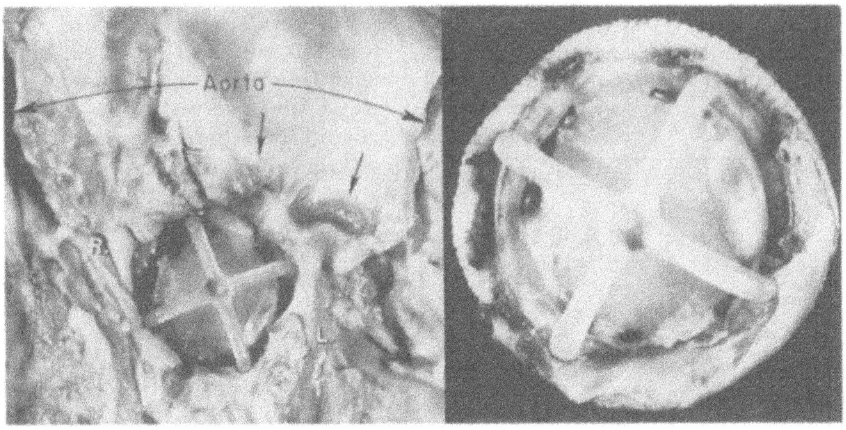

FIGURE 15. *Disc degeneration.* Views of the aortic valve prosthesis in a 24 year old man who underwent replacement of both the mitral and aortic valves in November 1964 (33 months before death) because of severe congestive cardiac failure from combined mitral and aortic regurgitation. Size 22.5 mitral and size 15 aortic valve prostheses were used. Postoperatively, the patient returned to near normal physical activities and appeared well until 2 months before death (31 months after operation) when evidence of congestive cardiac failure reappeared. Examination 3 days beore death disclosed an audible clicking sound within 10 cm of the precordium without use of a stethoscope. A loud (grade 3/6) systolic ejection murmur associated with a thrill, loudest along the left sternal border, was heard. In addition, a grade 2/6 intermittent diastolic blowing murmur was audible over the same area and a grade 2/6 pansystolic blowing murmur was heard at the apex and in the left axilla. During the next 3 days the congestive failure rapidly progressed and a second cardiac operation was performed on an emergency basis. The mitral valve disc showed evidence of severe degeneration and moved poorly. It was replaced with another disc prosthesis. The aortic valve prosthesis was inspected but not replaced. A tricuspid valve anuloplasty also was performed, but the patient could not be weaned from cardiopulmonary bypass. *At necropsy,* the disc of the aortic prosthesis showed considerable evidence of wear. This prosthesis is shown in place on the left and after removal on the right. The margins of the disc are focally eroded and contain several swellings. The largest of the swellings is yellow indicating the presence of lipid material. Several of the swellings are black due to the presence of blood within these cysts. A cyst also is present at the crossing point of the horizontal struts. The aortic root (**left**) contains focal elevated intimal lesions (**arrows**), probably the result of turbulent flow. The kidneys contained large quantities of iron, indicating that hemolysis was occurring intravascularly. L and R = left and right coronary arteries.

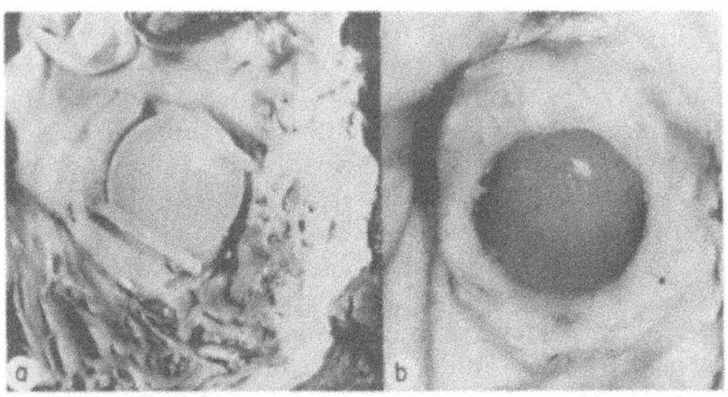

FIGURE 16. *Endocardial fibrosis after mitral valve replacement.* Mitral valve prosthesis in a 61 year old woman who underwent mitral valve replacement in September 1972 because of mitral stenosis. Her condition was improved by the operation but she died 8 months later of uncertain reasons. At necropsy, the endocardium of the left ventricle in the area of the prosthesis was severely thickened. In addition, similar fibrous tissue completely covered the cloth portions of the prosthesis on both the ventricular (**a**) and atrial (**b**) aspects. The disc moved normally.

tions were located equidistant from one another (90°, 180°, 270° and 360°) and corresponded to the locations of the vertical struts. In two of the seven prostheses the disc marginal indentations were minute. It may be assumed that the indentations resulted from contact of the margins of the disc with the vertical struts. The occurrence of four indentations in each disc suggests that the discs moved little or not at all in a circular fashion. The remaining four prostheses not only had marginal indentations, but also multiple, small cystic swelling at the margins of the discs. These cystic swellings contained yellow deposits (lipid). In three of these four prosthetic discs, the numerous cystic swellings appeared large enough to interfere with proper functioning of the prosthesis. It is uncertain whether the indentations by themselves were capable of interfering with proper disc movement in the other seven prosthetic discs.

Renal hemosiderosis: Deposits of iron were present in the cytoplasm of renal tubules in 13 of the 16 patients who died late. The amount of iron deposited in the kidneys was graded on a scale of 0 to 4+. The largest deposits, producing a "blue kidney" after immersion of the cut kidney in Prussian blue solution, occurred in the patients with an aortic valve prosthesis (all six were 3+ or 4+). Large renal ironic deposits occurred in only one of the eight patients with isolated mitral valve replacement, and this patient had a large paramitral ring leak. No renal iron was observed in either of the two patients with isolated tricuspid valve replacement.

Anatomic cardiac changes: *Focal thickening of left ventricular endocardium* was observed in each of the 10 patients who died late after mitral valve replacement (Fig. 16). White fibrous tissue containing numerous elastic fibrils covered the stumps of the amputated left ventricular papillary muscles in all 10 patients. Similar thickening was present in the more basal portions of the left ventricle and focally on the ventricular septum.

The intima of the aortic root was thickened in each of the five patients who died late after aortic valve replacement. This thickening was extensive

TABLE VIII

Principal Cause of Late Death in 16 Patients After Cardiac Valve Replacement with Discoid Prosthesis

Cause	M	A	M+A	T	Total
Prosthesis-related					10 (63%)
Disc degeneration	0	0	1	0	
Peribasibar leak	1	0	0	0	
Atrial thrombus	3	0	0	1	
Infection	1	2	0	0	
Other	0	0	1	0	
Coronary heart disease	1	1	0	0	2 (12%)
Uncertain cause	2	0	0	0	2 (13%)
Uncorrected valvular disease	0	0	0	1	1 (6%)
Miscellaneous	0	1	0	0	1 (6%)
Total	8	4	2	2	16 (100%)

A = aortic; M = mitral; T = tricuspid.

even though focal in each of the four patients with prosthetic implantation periods of 24 months or longer. The ostia of the coronary arteries appeared compromised by this intimal fibrous proliferation in one of the five patients.

Foci of myocardial necrosis were absent in all 16 patients who died late, but foci of left ventricular myocardial fibrosis were observed grossly in four patients. The scarring was transmural in each, "massive" in two. Although gross left ventricular myocardial scarring (excluding that involving only papillary muscles) was present in only four patients (25 percent), severe (greater than 75 percent) luminal narrowing involving one or more of the three major extramural coronary arteries was observed in 6 of the 16 patients, and 3 of them had transmural left ventricular scarring. One patient with transmural left ventricular scarring did not have severe (greater than 75 percent) coronary arterial luminal narrowing.

Causes of Late Deaths

Prosthetic valve-related deaths: The principal cause of death in each of the 16 patients who died late is listed in Table VIII. Death was related to the presence of the prosthesis in 10 of the 16 patients.

Disc wear or degeneration was clearly responsible in one patient. In this patient severe congestive heart failure suddenly developed 33 months postoperatively; reexamination disclosed evidence of mitral and aortic prosthetic valve dysfunction. Reoperation showed severe degeneration of both mitral and aortic prosthetic discs (Fig. 15) and the mitral valve prosthesis was excised and replaced with another.The patient, however, could not be separated from cardiopulmonary bypass.

Parabasilar prosthetic detachment causing large left ventricular-left atrial regurgitation appeared responsible for severe congestive cardiac failure in one patient, who died shortly after operative closure of the accessory communication.

Thrombi in the body of an atrium developed in four patients and three of them had systemic emboli with infarcts (Fig. 10 to 12). Three of these four patients had had mitral valve replacement and one, tricuspid valve replacement. Each mitral valve prosthesis was free of thrombi except on the bases of the struts. The tricuspid valve prosthesis contained obstructing thrombus on the atrial aspect. The finding of thrombus in the body of the atrium, as opposed to that confined to the atrial appendage, in the absence of thrombi before valve replacement, strongly suggests an element of prosthetic obstruction in each patient.[22,30] In none of these four patients, who lived from 5 to 19 months (average 13) postoperatively, did operation result in symptomatic improvement.

Infection was a major factor in causing death in three patients. All three had intermittent septicemia and two during life were considered to have "prosthetic endocarditis." Two had evidence of systemic emboli postoperatively. One, in whom diphtheroid species were cultured from the blood, had an infected vegetation on the ventricular aspect of an aortic prosthesis and extension of the infection beneath the site of attachment but no disruption of the prosthesis. Another patient, who also had diphtheroid species cultured from the blood, had a small thrombus, devoid of organisms, on the primary orifice but no disruption or infection in the prosthetic anulus. The third patient had various gram-negative organisms cultured periodically from the blood during the entire 24 month postoperative period. Death occurred during reoperation to excise a portion of the infected sternum. Despite the periodic septicemia, no vegetations were present on the prosthesis at necropsy and the tissue beneath the site of attachment of the aortic prosthesis was free of infection.

The last patient whose death was related to the prosthesis had undergone double valve replacement 18 months earlier with insertion of a Hufnagel trileaflet aortic valve and a discoid mitral valve. The trileaflet aortic valve cusps tore, causing incompetency, and a ring leak developed in the paramitral region. Reoperation to replace the degenerated trileaflet aortic valve, close the mitral peribasilar leak and replace the incompetent tricuspid valve with a disc prosthesis was unsuccessful.

Coronary artery disease: Two patients, each with a healed large transmural myocardial infarct, clearly died from consequences of severe coronary atherosclerosis. One of them initially had mitral valve replacement because of papillary muscle dysfunction secondary to coronary disease.

Uncertain cause: There was no apparent anatomic cause of death in two patients. Both had undergone mitral valve replacement. One, a 61 year old woman, died suddenly 8 months postoperatively and had severe narrowing of one coronary artery but no myocardial fibrosis or necrosis. The second, a 47 year old woman, lived 47 months after operation. Congestive heart failure appeared several weeks before death and at necropsy the mitral disc contained large indentations but no cysts or lipid infiltrations. Catheterization several days before death showed a small (4 mm Hg) mean diastolic gradient between the left atrium and left ventricle.

Uncorrected associated cardiac valve disease: This appeared responsible for the death of one patient, who had had tricuspid valve replacement and combined mitral and aortic commissurotomy for stenosis 36 months earlier (Fig. 12). Necropsy disclosed that both mitral and aortic valves were quite stenotic.

One patient had a fatal dissecting aortic aneurysm 30 months after successful aortic valve replacement.

Comments

During the past 15 years a number of different prosthetic devices have been introduced to serve as substitutes for malfunctioning cardiac valves. Although nearly 40 differently named prosthetic cardiac valves have been manufactured, most presently used prosthetic valves have one of four basic designs: (1) caged-ball, (2) caged-disc or lens, (3) flap or hinged lens, or (4) tissue valve.[31–33] The most commonly used valvular prosthesis has been the caged-ball. Multiple changes in the design of this prosthesis have occurred during the past 15 years, and numerous reports are now available describing the results and consequences of use of this prosthesis in patients.[34–38] The caged-disc prosthesis has not been as popular as the caged-ball prosthesis and, unlike the latter, its use has been limited by most surgeons to the mitral and tricuspid positions.[39,40] An advantage of the disc mitral valve prosthesis over the caged-ball mitral valve prosthesis has been its applicability to hearts with a "small" left ventricular cavity.[41] In contrast to many hemodynamic studies of the caged-ball prosthesis,[35,37,42–47] however, there have been relatively few hemodynamic studies on the disc prosthesis,[48–55] and to our knowledge no detailed anatomic studies of hearts containing this prosthesis have been reported. The flap or hinged lens prosthesis has been gaining in popularity in the past 5 years.[56–62] In contrast to the caged-ball and disc prostheses, the hinged lens prosthesis resides primarily within the valvular anulus and consequently occupies little space within a ventricular cavity or ascending aorta. Furthermore, flow through this prosthesis is semicentral rather than entirely peripheral. Tissue valves, of either homologous or heterologous origin, although popular in some centers,[63–70] have been less widely used than rigid-frame prostheses. The major advantage of the tissue valve is central flow, as in the normal valve. At present, there is no consensus as to which cardiac valvular prosthesis is best. The fact that so many different ones are being utilized indicates that the search for the best one continues.

In this study we sought information on the disc prosthesis by studying hearts at necropsy of patients who died after replacement of one or more cardiac valves with the disc prosthesis introduced by Hufnagel in 1962.[15] Although the Hufnagel disc prosthesis has certain unique features, much of the information derived from study of this particular discoid prosthesis is also applicable to other prostheses of the disc type.

TABLE IX

Causes of Prosthetic Cardiac Valve Stenosis

1. Intrinsic stenosis of the prosthesis (design problem)
2. Inadequate space in left or right ventricle or in ascending aorta to freely accommodate prosthesis (prosthetic disproportion or tertiary orifice stenosis)
3. Thrombus formation on prosthesis
   A. Prosthetic ring (primary orifice)
   B. Prosthetic struts or legs causing sticking of poppet
4. Prosthetic variance
   A. Swelling, due to lipid infiltration, of poppet causing it to stick either permanently or transiently in the cage
   B. Grooving (notching) of the margins of the poppet also causing sticking or cocking (disc)

Causes of Prosthetic Valve Stenosis

Disc design and inadequate space in ventricle or aorta: Although at one time considered relatively nonobstructive because of its low profile design, the disc type poppet prosthesis, as shown by our study, may be obstructive. Possible causes of prosthetic stenosis are listed in Table IX. It is now well appreciated that the caged-ball prosthesis may obstruct left ventricular outflow or inflow after mitral valve replacement if the left ventricular cavity is small,[2,3,8,30,71–73] and that this device in the aortic position may obstruct if the aorta is small (that is, too little space between the surface of the poppet and the intima of the aorta.[2,3,8,28,74,75]) In this study, 13 (38 percent) of 34 patients with a mitral valve disc prosthesis were judged at necropsy to have insufficient space between the margins of the disc and the ventricular endocardium. In several patients, the disc margins at necropsy contacted left ventricular endocardium and disc mobility appeared limited. Of the 13 patients, 10 died early and 3 late, and all had a "small" or normal-sized left ventricular cavity. Only one was considered at necropsy to have left ventricular outflow obstruction; the others had only inflow obstruction. The worse the obstruction, generally, the shorter the interval between operation and death; patients with the severest anatomic obstruction generally died within 24 hours of operation.

Evidence for prosthetic mitral stenosis in the three patients who died late was the occurrence of large thrombi in the *body* of the left atrium in each. Thrombi frequently occur in the appendage of the atrium in patients with congestive heart failure from any cause, but their presence in the body of the left atrium is infrequent and in our experience occurs only in patients with obstruction to left atrial outflow, that is, mitral stenosis.[18] One of the two patients who died late after tricuspid valve replacement

TABLE X

Hemodynamic Data on Poppet-Disc Prostheses in the Mitral Position

Type	Date of Reference	Patients (no.)	Interval (mo) Postoperatively Range (avg)	Mean LA-LV Mean Diastolic Gradient (mm Hg)			Mean (ml/min per m²) CI		
				Rest		Exercise	Rest		Exercise
				Preop	Postop	Postop	Preop	Postop	Postop
Kay-Shiley	1969[48]	17	3–25 (15)	16	11	18	1.9	2.6	3.9
	1973[54]	14	6–23 (9)	15	8	...	2.2	2.8	
	1973[55]	8	6–27 (12)	...	12	20	2.0	2.6	3.4
Beall	1969[50]	14	... (5)	13	7	20*	2.0	2.3	3.6*
	1971[53]	23	... (9)	18†	8	13	2.4	3.9	4.7
	1972[49]	24	1–34 (...)	...	12	24	2.1	2.5	3.6
Kay-Suzuki	1970[52]	100		...	5	8	...	...	...

* Data from 3 patients only.
† Includes average of 12 patients with mitral stenosis.
CI = cardiac index; LA = left atrium; LV = left ventricle; Postop = postoperatively; Preop = preoperatively.

had a right atrial thrombus obstructing the tricuspid orifice. The occurrence of thrombus in the body of right atrium probably is also indicative of obstruction to right atrial outflow, that is, prosthetic tricuspid valve stenosis.[76] Cardiac catheterization in the latter patient disclosed marked elevation of right atrial pressures.

Prosthetic aortic stenosis was judged to be present at necropsy in 3 (11 percent) of the 28 patients with an aortic valve prosthesis, in 3 of the 22 who died early and in none of the 6 who died late. To prevent the occurrence of prosthetic aortic stenosis a diamond-shaped patch had been inserted in the aortic root in 13 (46 percent) of the 28 patients with a replaced aortic valve.[28,75]

Whenever a judgment is made at necropsy that a prosthetic cardiac valve is obstructive because the ventricular cavity or aortic root is too small to freely accommodate the prosthesis, consideration must be given the possibility that the ventricle or aorta is much smaller at necropsy than during life because the pressure is now zero or because the specimen has been fixed in formalin®*, or both. When dealing with prostheses of the disc type, however, concern is only with the area 1 cm downstream from the site of attachment of the prosthesis. Obviously, there is no contracture of the prosthesis itself between life and death, and the rigidity of the prosthetic ring prevents much contracture of either the aorta or ventricular cavity within 1 cm of the prosthetic anulus. Thus, although contracture of the left or right ventricle or of the aorta does occur between life and death, the amount of space in the immediate area of the prosthesis probably changes relatively little.

Hemodynamic studies of valve obstruction: The only conclusive proof that a prosthetic cardiac valve is obstructive is the demonstration of a pressure gradient across it. Hemodynamic studies in patients with certain disc valves have demonstrated sizable pressure gradients across them. Table X summarizes late hemodynamic observations after replacement of the mitral valve with a Kay-Shiley,[48,54,55] Beall[49,50,53] or Kay-Suzuki[52] prosthesis of the disc type. All three prostheses in this position produced significant mean pressure gradients at rest between the left atrium (or pulmonary arterial wedge position) and left ventricle. Among the 110 patients studied, the mean gradient was 9 mm Hg at rest and 17 mm Hg after exercise. There are no available late hemodynamic studies on the Hufnagel discoid prosthesis in either the mitral or aortic position.

Disc prostheses of the nontilting type have been used infrequently in the aortic valve position, and there is consequently relatively little hemodynamic information on them in this position. Björk et al.[51] performed isolated aortic valve replacement using Kay-Shiley disc prostheses in 60 patients, 4 of whom had an oval-shaped patch inserted to widen the aortic root. Thirteen of the 60 died during the follow-up period of 13 to 33 months (mean 20). Hemodynamic studies in 34 of the 60 patients an average of 12 months postoperatively disclosed peak systolic pressure gradients at rest across the prostheses ranging from 9 to 61 mm Hg (average 27); with exercise these gradients increased to 10 to 100 mm Hg (average 38). The smaller-sized valves produced larger gradients than did the larger-sized valves. Kay et al.[52] utilized Kay-Suzuki discoid prostheses for aortic valve replacement in 74 patients, 11 of whom underwent cardiac catheterization more than a year after valve replacement; in none was the peak systolic pressure gradient between the left ventricle and systemic artery more than 10 mm Hg and in 6 it was zero. Furthermore, the largest gradient produced by exercise was 10 mm Hg. The gradients recorded by Kay et al. across Kay-Suzuki discoid prostheses are considerably smaller than those recorded by Björk et al. across

* Formalin changes the consistency of the tissues—makes them firmer—but does not cause them to contract. The contraction occurs when death appears, not when Formalin is applied.

Kay-Shiley discoid prostheses.[51] Interestingly, the pressure gradients across Starr-Edwards aortic prostheses in patients also studied by Kay et al. were considerably smaller across the caged-ball prostheses than those reported by other authors[35,37,42–47] using similar prostheses.

Late cardiac catheterization findings: Cardiac catheterization was performed late postoperatively in 2 of our 16 patients who died late. In one, whose tricuspid valve had been replaced, the right atrial pressures were enormously elevated, strongly suggesting prosthetic tricuspid valve obstruction; right ventricular pressure was not recorded. In the second patient, cardiac catheterization 47 months after mitral valve replacement disclosed a 4 mm Hg mean diastolic pressure gradient between the pulmonary arterial wedge position and left ventricle. Recently, three living patients with Hufnagel discoid prostheses underwent catheterization late postoperatively: in one, aortic valve replacement was performed in 1964 and study 10 years later showed only a 10 mm Hg peak systolic gradient across the prosthesis when the cardiac index was 2.4 liter/min per m^2. The second also had aortic valve replacement, and cardiac catheterization 45 months later disclosed a 77 mm Hg systolic pressure gradient between the left ventricle and aorta when the cardiac index was 2.5 liters/min per m^2. The third had mitral valve replacement in 1968 and the current mean diastolic gradient between the left atrium and left ventricle in 1974 was 11 mm Hg when the cardiac index was 2.8 liter/min per m^2.

Thrombus formation on prosthesis: Causes of prosthetic cardiac valve stenosis other than prosthetic disproportion and faulty design include prosthetic thrombosis and prosthetic variance (Table IX). Thrombus formation despite anticoagulant therapy is a real or potential complication of all rigid-frame prosthetic valves.[8,13,32,35,39,77] Although the frequency of clinical evidence of emboli may be diminishing with the more recently developed models,[78] most prosthetic cardiac valves at necropsy contain thrombus[8] (14 [88 percent] of our 16 patients who died late). Usually the amount of thrombus on the struts or primary orifice is not sufficient to interfere with proper movement of the poppet[8,13] (in none of the 16 patients described herein), and clinical evidence of systemic emboli are infrequent when the prosthetic thrombi are small. When large, however, the thrombi may obstruct flow through the prosthesis and make the poppet immobile.[79–83] With prostheses of the disc type, the poppet may be tilted in the cage by thrombus on one side, or thrombus may fill the entire space between the disc and ring, causing complete immobility of the poppet.[8,79] Although changes may occur in the opening and closing prosthetic clicking sounds,[81,83] severe obstruction from thrombus may occur in the presence of normal auscultatory sounds[80] and even normal findings on angiography.[80]

Poppet variance causing obstruction: Poppet variance is a well recognized cause of obstruction in prosthetic cardiac valves of the caged-ball type[1,84–96]; the obstruction is due to swelling of the poppet with impaction in the cage. Degeneration of a poppet of the disc type is less well appreciated but is also common.[79,97–105] In contrast to variance of a caged-ball, variance of a poppet of the disc type, to our knowledge, has not been demonstrated hemodynamically to cause prosthetic obstruction (Fig. 13). One patient described herein, however (Fig. 15), was considered at reoperation to have mitral obstruction from severe degeneration of the mitral disc.

TABLE XI

Causes of Prosthetic Cardiac Valve Regurgitation

1. Slight regurgitation intrinsic to design of many prostheses
2. Peribasilar accessory communication
   A. Inadequate number of sutures
   B. Inadequate placement of sutures due to calcific deposits in or adjacent to anulus
   C. Pulling loose of suture(s)
      1. After replacement of anatomically normal or floppy valve
      2. Infection at site of attachment of prosthesis
3. Thrombus formation on prosthetic struts preventing proper seating of poppet or causing it to stick in an open position
4. Prosthetic variance
   A. Atrophy of poppet
      1. Incomplete seating
      2. Dislodgement
   B. Fracture of poppet
      1. Incomplete seating
      2. Dislodgment
   C. Fracture of strut
      1. Dislodgment of poppet
   D. Disruption of ring cloth
5. Mechanical interference to proper seating of poppet by
   A. Unexcised calcific material or chordae tendineae or suture between poppet and ring
   B. Strut of a mitral prosthesis preventing proper seating of the poppet of an aortic prosthesis.
   C. An aortic regurgitant jet stream causing cocking with incomplete closure of a mitral poppet

Prosthetic Valve Regurgitation

Valve design: Although a trace of regurgitation is inherent in most presently available rigid-frame prosthetic cardiac valves, significant regurgitation through or around a prosthetic valve may be less common than stenosis. This situation almost certainly is the case with caged-ball prostheses, but it is possible that regurgitation through a prosthesis of the disc type is more common than generally believed. How often tilting or cocking of a disc or lens occurs is uncertain. Fixed tilting due to thrombus formation, disc wear or jamming of the disc in an open position for no apparent reason quickly leads to clinical evidence of prosthetic malfunction[97–113] (Table XI). Intermittent or transient tilting, however, is probably far more common than fixed tilting, and intermittent cocking may occur without disc thrombosis or disc variance. It is conceivable that acute tilting of a disc could produce sudden death and that the tilting could be missed at necropsy. Because of the possibility of unpredictable tilting, the margin of safety of a poppet valve of the disc type may be less than that of a ball type.

Disc variance: This is probably a major cause of disc cocking. In contrast to ball valves in which the poppet is rotating or spinning during its period of movement so that a different portion of its surface contacts the apex or ring of the cage during each beat, random movement or circular rotation does not occur with the caged-disc poppet prosthesis. Evidence for the lack of disc rotation is the occurrence of four grooves in the margins of the discs. Each groove is directly opposite a vertical strut. This grooving has been described with most disc prostheses including the Kay-Shiley, Cross-Jones, Hufnagel, Kay-Suzuki and Hammersmith types.[97,98,100-106,109] The grooving is most severe in the discs consisting of or covered by silicone rubber,[97,98,101,106,109] but it also has been observed in discs composed of Teflon®[100,102] and polypropylene.[101,105] Whether grooving will occur in the newer discs composed of pyrolite carbon-coated graphite remains to be determined.[78]

Indentations in the margins of the discs were observed in 11 of the 17 prosthetic disc valves described herein with implantation periods of more than 2 months. The grooving involved only the silicone rubber portion of the discs; no wear was evident in the polypropylene portion. With the exception of 1 disc prosthesis in which only two indentations were observed, the other 10 had four marginal indentations, each directly opposite a vertical strut. The earliest evidence of disc wear—small marginal grooves—occurred in a mitral disc in place for 9 months, but no wear was found in an aortic prosthetic disc in place for a similar period of time. Wear was not limited to the discs implanted in the left side of the heart. A disc of a tricuspid valve prosthesis in place for 36 months showed four large marginal grooves. The prostheses in place for the longest periods generally had the greatest amount of disc wear, and the aortic discs in general had more wear than the mitral discs, which had more than the tricuspid discs. The presence of these marginal grooves may cause the disc "to catch" or stick to one or two struts and therefore fail to close properly. Manipulation at necropsy of these grooved discs indicated that sticking or cocking could occur unless the closing pressure was applied directly in the center of the disc.

Not only has disc grooving been observed, but also cracking of the disc margins of both mitral and aortic valve prostheses with infiltration by lipids has occurred. When cracks occur into the disc margins, marginal cysts commonly result. These cysts almost surely increase the tendency for disc cocking.

Dislodgment of silicone rubber aortic poppets is now a recognized complication of caged-ball prostheses.[86,89] Dislodgment of mitral discs also has occurred with and without fracture of a strut.[104,105]

Mitral disc cocking due to aortic regurgitation jet: A not well recognized cause of mitral disc cocking is associated aortic regurgitation.[107-109] When the mitral valve is replaced because of mitral stenosis, the posterior wall of the left ventricle, for reasons unknown, has a shorter longitudinal length than does the anterior left ventricular free wall; that is, the distance between the basal attachment of the posterior mitral leaflet and the left ventricular apex is shorter than the distance between the base of the aortic valve (right anterior cusp) and the left ventricular apex.[114] As a consequence, when the mitral valve is replaced in the setting of a shortened posterior left ventricular wall, the disc (or cage) points directly toward the ventricular septum so that the disc is more or less parallel to the longitudinal axis of the septum and also to that of the ascending aorta. (In contrast, when the preoperative lesion is pure mitral regurgitation, the disc points toward the left ventricular apex rather than toward the ventricular septum.) Thus, during ventricular diastole disc cocking may be produced by contact of the aortic regurgitant jet stream with the atrial side of the disc, thus preventing its complete closure. For normal function it is mandatory that the disc move parallel to the valve seat throughout its entire excursion. In the presence of aortic regurgitation, the mitral disc during ventricular diastole becomes cocked when one edge moves prematurely toward the valve seat while the opposite edge remains in the open position. During the next ventricular systole, the lens or disc may remain tilted, resulting in prosthetic regurgitation. Edgett et al.[107] described prosthetic regurgitation early postoperatively in four patients after mitral valve replacement with a discoid prosthesis and three of their four patients had uncorrected aortic regurgitation. Interestingly, two of the four patients had a Hufnagel discoid prosthesis. These authors clearly demonstrated cocking of the mitral disc by cinefluorography, and the most likely explanation appears to be the associated aortic regurgitation jet's interfering with proper functioning of the disc.

Uncorrected Associated Valve Disease

Not only may uncorrected associated valve disease (aortic regurgitation) interfere with proper functioning of a disc prosthesis (mitral), but also a malfunctioning prosthesis (aortic) may worsen an uncorrected associated valvular lesion (mitral regurgitation). The latter situation occurs primarily in patients who preoperatively have combined pure aortic regurgitation and pure mitral regurgitation. The aortic valve is replaced with a disc but the mitral regurgitation is not considered severe enough to warrant valve replacement. It is well known that after aortic valve replacement with a caged-ball prosthesis a systolic pressure gradient is virtually always produced between the left ventricle and the aorta.[35] An aortic valve disc is usually more obstructive than a caged-ball prosthesis.[51,60,115] The conversion of a purely incompetent aortic valve by disc prosthetic replacement into obstructive aortic valve may increase the degree of mitral regurgitation from mild to moderate or from moderate to severe. Such probably was the case in several patients described herein.

Commissurotomy vs. Valve Replacement

Although a number of patients in our study preoperatively had functional lesions of both the mitral and aortic valves, double valve replacement was carried out in only a few. Several other patients, however, had replacement of one valve and commissurotomy or anuloplasty of the other valve. One patient with combined tricuspid, mitral and aortic stenosis had tricuspid valve replacement and commissurotomy on both the calcified mitral and aortic valves. Whether commissurotomy on any grossly calcified mitral or aortic valve is a proper procedure is debated. In patients with combined valvular disease severe enough to warrant valve replacement, particularly when both left-sided cardiac valves are involved, it may be most reasonable to err on the side of double valve replacement rather than replacement of one valve and commissurotomy or anuloplasty on the other. The functional result of a commissurotomy or anuloplasty is not as predictable as that of valve replacement particularly when the commissurotomy involves a grossly calcified valve.

In general, longevity of patients with replaced mitral and aortic valves is determined by the status of the aortic valve prosthesis. Patients with isolated mitral disease and a mitral valve prosthesis have a better prognosis, in general, than do patients with isolated aortic valve disease and an aortic valve prosthesis. Thus, although there may be an occasional patient with combined mitral and aortic disease in whom mitral valve replacement and aortic valve commissurotomy or anuloplasty may be justified, there appears little indication, as a rule, for the reverse procedure—replacement of the aortic valve and commissurotomy or anuloplasty of the mitral valve. In the latter situation, mitral valve replacement probably more often improves than worsens the prognosis.

Turbulent Flow and Intravascular Hemolysis

In contrast to central flow substitute cardiac valves (tissue valves[9–14] and Hufnagel trileaflet prostheses[16,17]), the caged-ball and caged-disc prosthetic cardiac valves produce turbulent flow and therefore may cause damage to blood cells traversing them. The anatomic indicator for this turbulent flow is proliferation of fibrous tissue in the immediate vicinity of the implanted prosthesis.[1,116] In the case of the mitral valve prosthesis, the adjacent left ventricular endocardium is thickened[116] (Fig. 16); similarly, after aortic valve replacement the intima of the aortic root thickens,[1] and occasionally this thickening extends into the proximal portions of the right and left coronary arteries[1,117–119] (Fig. 17). The thickening of left ventricular endocardium or of aortic root intima was observed in all our patients who died late after disc

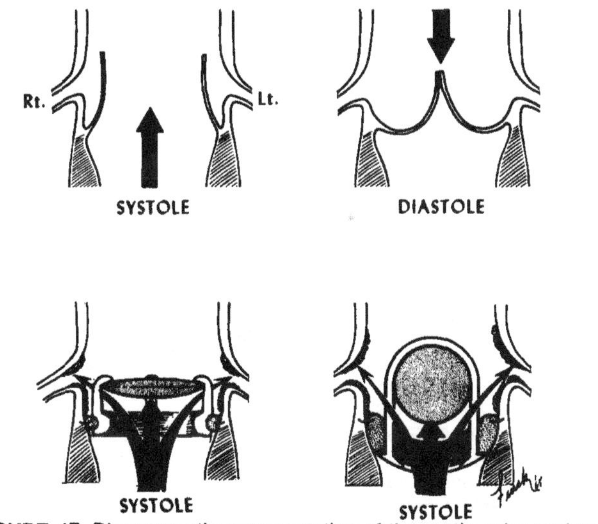

FIGURE 17. Diagrammatic representation of the aortic valve region in the normal heart (**upper panels**) and after valve replacement with a disc or ball poppet prosthesis (**lower panels**). The flow of blood during systole across the normal aortic valve is laminar, and the coronary arteries fill mainly by retrograde flow during diastole. After valve replacement, the flow of blood across the aortic valve area is no longer laminar. The force of left ventricular ejection is directed centrally, as in the normal heart, but the poppet prevents central flow, producing severe turbulence in the area. Thus, during ventricular systole blood between the surface of the poppet and the intima of the aortic root is flowing in a turbulent fashion. The anatomic indicator of turbulent flow under high pressure is intimal proliferation, which was observed in the proximal aorta of each subject who died in the late postoperative period after aortic valve replacement. Since the coronary ostia are no longer "guarded," so to speak, by the aortic cusps during ventricular systole and, since they are in the area of turbulent flow, they also are subject to intimal proliferation.

mitral or aortic valve replacement. Generally, patients with the longest survival times had the greatest degrees of thickening.

When flow through a prosthetic cardiac valve is turbulent, intravascular hemolysis is the consequence.[120–127] The anatomic indicator of intravascular hemolysis is renal hemosiderosis.[128,129] The latter, also called "blue kidney,"[129] was observed in 13 of the 16 patients who died late with disc valves. The most severe intravascular hemolysis occurred after aortic valve replacement and the least, if any, after tricuspid valve replacement. Renal hemosiderosis was observed in all patients who died late after aortic, in seven of eight after mitral but in none of two after tricuspid valve replacement. The amount of iron deposited in the kidneys, however, was far greater after aortic than after mitral valve replacement. In general, the amount of fibrous tissue proliferation in the submitral area after mitral valve replacement or in the aortic root after aortic valve replacement correlated well with the amount of iron deposited in the cytoplasm of the proximal tubules of the kidneys: The greater the fibrous tissue proliferation, indicating turbulence, the greater the amount of renal hemosiderosis, also a consequence of turbulence. The mechanism by which iron is deposited in the kidney is described elsewhere.[128]

References

1. **Roberts WC, Morrow AG:** Late postoperative pathological findings after cardiac valve replacement. Circulation 35 and 36:Suppl I:I-48–I-62, 1967
2. **Roberts WC, Morrow AG:** Causes of early postoperative death following cardiac valve replacement. Clinico-pathologic correlations in 64 patients studied at necropsy. J Thorac Cardiovasc Surg 54:422–437, 1967
3. **Roberts WC, Morrow AG:** Anatomic studies of hearts containing caged-ball prosthetic valves. Johns Hopkins Med J 121: 271–295, 1967
4. **Niles NR, Sandilands JR:** Pathology of heart valve replacement surgery: autopsies of 62 patients with Starr-Edwards prostheses. Dis Chest 56:373–382, 1969
5. **Colapinto ND, Silver MD:** Prosthetic heart valve replacement. Causes of early postoperative death. J Thorac Cardiovasc Surg 61:938–944, 1971
6. **Joassin A, Edwards JE:** Late causes of death after mitral valve replacement. Analysis of 36 cases. J Thorac Cardiovasc Surg 65:255–263, 1973
7. **Joassin A, Edwards JE:** Causes of death within 30 days of mitral valvular replacement. Analysis of 93 cases. Cardiovasc Clin 5:169–184, 1973
8. **Roberts WC, Bulkley BH, Morrow AG:** Pathologic anatomy of cardiac valve replacement: a study of 224 necropsy patients. Prog Cardiovasc Dis 15:539–587, 1973
9. **Davies H, Missen GAK, Blandford G, et al:** Homograft replacement of the aortic valve. A clinical and pathologic study. Am J Cardiol 22:195–217, 1968
10. **Kouchoudos NT, Kerr AR, Sheppard LC, et al:** Heterograft replacement of the mitral valve: clinical, hemodynamic, and pathologic features. Circulation 41 and 42:Suppl II:II-20–II-27, 1970
11. **Ionescu MI, Smith DR, Sutherland TW, et al:** Heart valve replacement with aortic heterografts. Follow-up study. Ann Thorac Surg 13:1–14, 1972
12. **Dubiel WT, Johansson L, Willen R:** Postoperative changes in autologous fascia lata heart valve grafts. A pathological study. Ann Thorac Surg 15:140–155, 1973
13. **Yarbrough JW, Roberts WC, Reis RL:** Structural alterations in tissue cardiac valves implanted in patients and in calves. J Thorac Cardiovasc Surg 65:364–375, 1973
14. **Horowitz MS, Goodman DJ, Fogarty TJ, et al:** Mitral valve replacement with the glutaraldehyde-preserved porcine heterograft. Clinical, hemodynamic, and pathological correlations. J Thorac Cardiovasc Surg 67:885–895, 1974
15. **Hufnagel CA, Conrad PW:** Comparative study of some prosthetic valves for aortic and mitral replacement. Surgery 57: 205–210, 1965
16. **Hufnagel CA, Conrad PW:** A new approach to aortic valve replacement. Ann Surg 167:791–795, 1968
17. **Fishbein MC, Roberts WC, Golden A, et al:** Cardiac pathology after aortic valve replacement using Hufnagel tri-leaflet prostheses: a study of 20 necropsy patients. Am Heart J, in press
18. **Roberts WC, Perloff JK:** Mitral valvular disease. A clinicopathologic survey of the conditions causing the mitral valve to function abnormally. Ann Intern Med 77:939–975, 1972
19. **Roberts WC, Cohen LS:** Left ventricular papillary muscles. Description of the normal and a survey of conditions causing them to be abnormal. Circulation 46:138–154, 1972
20. **Buchbinder NA, Roberts WC:** Left-sided valvular active infective endocarditis. A study of forty-five necropsy patients. Am J Med 53:20–35, 1972
21. **Roberts WC, Braunwald E, Morrow AG:** Acute severe mitral regurgitation secondary to ruptured chordae tendineae. Clinical, hemodynamic, and pathologic considerations. Circulation 33:58–70, 1966
22. **Roberts WC, Dangel JC, Bulkley BH:** Nonrheumatic valvular cardiac disease: a clinicopathologic survey of 27 different conditions causing valvular dysfunction. Cardiovasc Clin 5:333–446, 1973
23. **Roberts WC:** Anatomically isolated aortic valvular disease. The case against its being of rheumatic etiology. Am J Med 49: 151–159, 1970
24. **Roberts WC, Perloff JK, Costantino T:** Severe valvular aortic stenosis in patients over 65 years of age. A clinicopathologic study. Am J Cardiol 27:497–506, 1971
25. **Roberts WC:** The structure of the aortic valve in clinically isolated aortic stenosis. An autopsy study of 162 patients over 15 years of age. Circulation 42:91–97, 1970
26. **Roberts WC:** The congenitally bicuspid aortic valve. A study of 85 autopsy cases. Am J Cardiol 26:72–83, 1970
27. **Reichenbach DD, Benditt EP:** Myofibrillar degeneration. A response of the myocardial cell to injury. Arch Pathol 85:189–199, 1968
28. **Stenseth JH, Danielson GK, McGoon DC:** Pericardial patch enlargement of the aortic outflow tract. J Thorac Cardiovasc Surg 62:442–448, 1971
29. **Roberts WC, Buja LM:** The frequency and significance of coronary arterial thrombi and other observations in fatal acute myocardial infarction. A study of 107 necropsy patients. Am J Med 52:425–443, 1972
30. **Roberts WC, Morrow AG:** Mechanisms of acute left atrial thrombosis after mitral valve replacement. Pathologic findings indicating obstruction to left atrial emptying. Am J Cardiol 18: 497–503, 1966
31. **Kirklin JW, Pacifico A:** Surgery for acquired valvular heart disease. N Engl J Med 288:133–140, 194–199, 1973
32. **Behrendt DM, Austen WG:** Current status of prosthetics for heart valve replacement. Prog Cardiovasc Dis 15:369–401, 1973
33. **Pluth JR, McGoon DC:** Current status of heart valve replacement. Mod Concepts Cardiovasc Dis 43:65–70, 1974
34. **Spencer FC, Reed GE, Clauss RH, et al:** Cloth-covered aortic and mitral valve prostheses. Experiences with 113 patients. J horac Cardiovasc Surg 59:92–108, 1970
35. **Winter TQ, Reis RL, Glancy DL, et al:** Current status of the Starr-Edwards cloth-covered prosthetic cardiac valves. Circulation 45 and 46:Suppl I:I-14–I-24, 1972
36. **Rees JR, Holswade GR, Lillehei CW:** Patient status five or more years after mitral valve replacement. Ann Thorac Surg 14:30–37, 1972
37. **Levine FH, Copeland JG, Morrow AG:** Prosthetic replacement of the mitral valve. Continuing assessments of the 100 patients operated upon during 1961–1965. Circulation 47:518–526, 1973
38. **Bonchek LI, Anderson RP, Starr A:** Mitral valve replacement with cloth-covered composite-seat prostheses. The case for early operation. J Thorac Cardiovasc Surg 67:93–109, 1974
39. **Messmer BJ, Okies JE, Hallman GL, et al:** Early and late thromboembolic complications after mitral valve replacement. A comparative study of various prostheses. J Cardiovasc Surg 13:281–289, 1972
40. **Beall AC Jr, Morris GC Jr, Howell JF Jr, et al:** Clinical experience with an improved mitral valve prosthesis. Ann Thorac Surg 15:601–606, 1973
41. **Kay EB, Suzuki A, Demaney M, et al:** Comparison of ball and disc valves for mitral valve replacement. Am J Cardiol 18: 504–514, 1966
42. **McHenry MM, Smeloff EA, Davey TB, et al:** Hemodynamic results with full-flow orifice prosthetic valves. Circulation 35 and 36:Suppl I:I-24–I-33, 1967
43. **Mason DT, Ross J Jr, Gault JH, et al:** Combined prosthetic replacement of the mitral and aortic valves. Preoperative and postoperative hemodynamic studies at rest and the left ventricular response to muscular exercise. Circulation 35 and 36: Suppl I:I-15–I-23, 1967
44. **Glancy DL, O'Brien KP, Reis RL, et al:** Hemodynamic studies in patients with 2M and 3M Starr-Edwards prostheses: evidence of obstruction to left atrial emptying. Circulation 39 and 40:Suppl I:I-113–I-118, 1969
45. **Rodriquez L:** Haemodynamic and angiographic findings in patients with isolated aortic valvular disease before and after insertion of a Starr-Edwards aortic ball-valve prosthesis. Scand J Thorac Cardiovasc Surg Suppl 5, 1970
46. **Reis RL, Glancy DL, O'Brien K, et al:** Clinical and hemodynamic assessments of fabric-covered Starr-Edwards prosthet-

ic valves. J Thorac Cardiovasc Surg 59:84–91, 104–108, 1970
47. **O'Rourke RA, Peterson KL, Braunwald NS:** Postoperative hemodynamic evaluation of a new fabric-covered ball-valve prosthesis. Circulation 47 and 48:Suppl III:III-74–III-79, 1973
48. **Vogel JHK, Paton BC, Overy HR, et al:** Abnormal hemodynamic function after disc mitral valve replacement. Circulation 39 and 40:Suppl I:I-141–I-147, 1969
49. **Reid JA, Stevens TW, Sigwart U, et al:** Hemodynamic evaluation of the Beall mitral valve prosthesis. Circulation 45 and 46: Suppl I:I-1–I-7, 1972
50. **Linhart JW, Barold SS, Hildner FJ, et al:** Clinical and hemodynamic findings following replacement of the mitral valve with a Beall valve prosthesis (Dacron velour-covered Teflon-disc valve). Circulation 39 and 40:Suppl I:I-127–I-134, 1969
51. **Björk VO, Olin C, Åstrom H:** Results of aortic valve replacement with the Kay-Shiley disc valve. Scand J Thorac Cardiovasc Surg 3:93–106, 1969
52. **Kay EB, Suzuki A, Tambi A, et al:** Comparative analysis of the Starr-Edwards ball valve, the Kay-Suzuki disc valve and transplant valves in the surgical correction of. aortic valve disease. Am J Cardiol 25:535–545, 1970
53. **Ramsey HW, Williams JC Jr, Vernon CR, et al:** Hemodynamic findings following replacement of the mitral valve with the Beall valve prosthesis. J Thorac Cardiovasc Surg 62:624–630, 1971
54. **Shepherd RL, Glancy DL, Reis RL, et al:** Hemodynamic function of the Kay-Shiley prosthetic cardiac valve. Observations after mitral or tricuspid valve replacement. Chest 63:323–326, 1973
55. **Hawe A, Frye RL, Ellis FH Jr:** Late hemodynamic studies after mitral valve surgery. J Thorac Cardiovasc Surg 65:351–358, 1973
56. **Björk VO:** A new central-flow tilting disc valve prosthesis. One year's clinical experience with 103 patients. J Thorac Cardiovasc Surg 60:355–374, 1970
57. **Björk VO, Holmgren A, Olin C, et al:** Clinical and hemodynamic results of aortic valve replacement with the Björk-Shiley tilting disc valve prosthesis. Scand J Thorac Cardiovasc Surg 5: 177–191, 1971
58. **Messmer BJ, Okies JE, Hallman GL, et al:** Mitral valve replacement with the Björk-Shiley tilting-disc prosthesis. J Thorac Cardiovasc Surg 62:938–946, 1971
59. **Wada J, Komatsu S, Kamata K:** Cardiac valve replacement with Wada-Cutter prosthesis. Ann Thorac Surg 14:38–48, 1972
60. **Björk VO, Rodriquez L:** Comparative results of aortic valve replacement with different prosthetic heart valves. J Cardiovasc Surg 13:268–271, 1972
61. **Lepley D, Reuben CF, Flemma RJ, et al:** Experience with the Björk-Shiley prosthetic valve. Circulation 47 and 48:Suppl III:III-51–III-55, 1973
62. **Böök K:** Mitral valve replacement with the Björk-Shiley tilting disc valve. A clinical and haemodynamic study in patients with isolated mitral valve lesions. Scand J Thorac Cardiovasc Surg: Suppl 12:1–28, 1974
63. **Ross DN, Gonzalez-Lavin L, Dalichau H:** A two-year experience with supported autologous fascia lata for heart valve replacement. Ann Thorac Surg 13:97–103, 1972
64. **Gonzalez-Lavin L, Al-Janabi N, Ross DN:** Long-term results after aortic valve replacement with preserved aortic homografts. Ann Thorac Surg 13:594–606, 1972
65. **Angell WW, Shumway NE, Kosek JC:** A five-year study of viable aortic valve homografts. J Thorac Cardiovasc Surg 64: 329–339, 1972
66. **Ross D:** Biologic valves. Their performance and prospects. Circulation 45:1259–1272, 1972
67. **Marcinkevicius A, Sirvydis V, Manelis A, et al:** Degeneration of autogenous fascia lata cardiac valves. J Cardiovasc Surg 14:372–378, 1973
68. **Wallace RB, Londe SP, Titus JL:** Aortic valve replacement with preserved aortic valve homografts. J Thorac Cardiovasc Surg 67:44–52, 1974
69. **Ionescu MI, Pakrashi BC, Mary DAS, et al:** Replacement of heart valves with frame-mounted tissue grafts. Thorax 29: 56–67, 1974
70. **Trimble AS, Gunstensen J, Silver MD, et al:** Aortic valve replacement with fascia lata. An encouraging late study. J Thorac Cardiovasc Surg 68:219–225, 1974
71. **Robicsek F, Sanger PW, Daugherty HK, et al:** Fatal arrhythmias caused by the pressure of the ball-valve prosthesis upon the left ventricular myocardium. Dis Chest 52:813–816, 1967
72. **Kalke B, Korns ME, Goott B, et al:** Engagement of ventricular myocardium by open-cage atrioventricular valvular prosthesis. J Thorac Cardiovasc Surg 58:92–94, 1969
73. **Ibarra-Pérez C, Rodriquez-Trujillo F, Perez-Redondo H:** Engagement of ventricular myocardium by struts of mitral prosthesis. Fatal complication of use of open-cage cardiac valves. J Thorac Cardiovasc Surg 61:403–404, 1971
74. **Quattlebaum FW, Kalke B, Edwards JE, et al:** Obstruction of the aorta by prosthetic aortic valve. J Thorac Cardiovasc Surg 55:231–237, 1968
75. **Najafi H, Ostermiller WE Jr, Javid H, et al:** Narrow aortic root complicating aortic valve replacement. Arch Surg 99:690–694, 1969
76. **Vander Veer JB Jr, Rhyneer GS, Hodam RP, et al:** Obstruction of tricuspid ball-valve prostheses. Circulation 43 and 44: Suppl I:I-62–I-67, 1971
77. **Cooley DA, Okies JE, Wukasch DC, et al:** Ten-year experience with cardiac valve replacement: results with a new mitral prosthesis. Ann Surg 177:818–826, 1973
78. **Beall AC Jr, Morris GC Jr, Noon GP, et al:** An improved mitral valve prosthesis. Ann Thorac Surg 15: 25–34, 1973
79. **Paton BC:** Reoperation for fibrinous stenosis of disc mitral valve prosthesis. J Thorac Cardiovasc Surg 57:726–731, 1969
80. **Mullen DC, Shull WH, Daugherty HK, et al:** Emergency thrombectomy of the prosthetic mitral valve. Vasc Surg 4:137–141, 1970
81. **Demany MA, Zimmerman HA:** Thrombosis of a mitral disc-valve prosthesis: diagnostic importance of the absent opening click. Am Heart J 80:816–819, 1970
82. **Rogers AK, Morgan JR, Forker AD, et al:** Supravalvular stenosis after disc mitral valve replacement. J Thorac Cardiovasc Surg 62:810–812, 1971
83. **Balkoura-Christopoulos MH, Resnekov L, Kittle CF:** Malfunction of a disc mitral valve prosthesis: detection by phonocardiography. Chest 63:624–626, 1973
84. **Starr A, Pierie WR, Raible DA, et al:** Cardiac valve replacement. Experience with the durability of silicone rubber. Circulation 33 and 34:Suppl I:I-115–I-123, 1966
85. **Laforet EG:** Death due to swelling of ball component of aortic ball-valve prosthesis. N Engl J Med 276:1025–1027, 1967
86. **Roberts WC, Morrow AG:** Fatal degeneration of the silicone rubber ball of the Starr-Edwards prosthetic aortic valve. Am J Cardiol 22:614–620, 1968
87. **Sanderson RG, Hall AD, Thomas AN:** The clinical diagnosis of ball variance in a mitral valve prosthesis. Ann Thorac Surg 6: 473–475, 1968
88. **Collins JJ Jr, Berg EJ, Harken DE:** Silicone ball variance. A clinical and pulse duplicator study. Ann Thorac Surg 6:546–551, 1968
89. **Bonnabeau R, Lillehei W:** Mechanical "ball failure" in Starr-Edwards prosthetic valves. A report of three cases. J Thorac Cardiovasc Surg 56:258–264, 1968
90. **Leatherman LL, Leachman RD, McConn RG, et al:** Malfunction of mitral ball-valve prosthesis due to a swollen poppet. J Thorac Cardiovasc Surg 57:160–163, 1969
91. **Hylen JC, Kloster FE, Starr A, et al:** Aortic ball variance: diagnosis and treatment. Ann Intern Med 72:1–8, 1970
92. **Connolly DC, Harrison CE, Ellis FH Jr:** Ball variance in a Starr-Edwards prosthetic mitral valve causing acute pulmonary edema (diagnosis by auscultation before onset of symptoms). Mayo Clin Proc 45:20–24, 1970
93. **Roberts WC, Levinson GE, Morrow AG:** Lethal ball variance in the Starr-Edwards prosthetic mitral valve. Arch Intern Med 126:517–521, 1970
94. **Metzger CC, Magovern GJ, Leonard JJ:** Ball variance in a sutureless mitral valve prosthesis. A report of two cases and a clue to early diagnosis. J Thorac Cardiovasc Surg 61:699–

704, 1971
95. **Schluger J, Mannix EP Jr, Wolf RE:** Auscultatory and phonocardiographic sign of ball variance in a mitral prosthetic valve. Am Heart J 81:809–816, 1971
96. **Hylen JC, Hodam RP, Kloster FE:** Changes in the durability of silicone rubber in ball-valve prostheses. Ann Thorac Surg 13: 324–329, 1972
97. **Carey JS, Hughes RK:** A complication of mitral-valve replacement with caged-lens prosthesis. Ann Thorac Surg 6:77–86, 1968
98. **Vasko JS, Leighton RF:** Acute massive mitral regurgitation resulting from disc-valve malfunction. Ann Thorac Surg 6:564–569, 1968
99. **Samaan HA:** Acute massive mitral regurgitation resulting from disc valve replacement of mitral valve. J Cardiovasc Surg 10: 477–479, 1969
100. **Robinson JJ, Hildner FJ, Greenberg JJ:** Disc variance of Beall mitral valve. Ann Thorac Surg 11:11–17, 1971
101. **Detmer DE, McIntosh CL, Boretos JW, et al:** Polypropylene poppets for low-profile prosthetic heart valves. Ann Thorac Surg 13:122–127, 1972
102. **Berroya RB, Escano FB Jr:** Mitral disc-valve variance. Thorax 27:87–89, 1972
103. **Hildner FJ, Robinson MJ:** Complications of Beall valve prosthesis. Am J Cardiol 30:922, 1972
104. **Nathan MJ:** Strut fracture. A late complication of Beall mitral valve replacement. Ann Thorac Surg 16:610–613, 1973
105. **Shaw TRD, Turner RWD:** Sudden mechanical malfunction of Hammersmith mitral valve prostheses due to wear of polypropylene. J Thorac Cardiovasc Surg 67:579–583, 1974
106. **Low HBC, Lefemine AA:** Acute mitral insufficiency due to jamming of a disc-valve prosthesis. Ann Thorac Surg 4:71–73, 1967
107. **Edgett JW, Nelson WP, Hall RJ, et al:** A complication of valve replacement by a caged-lens prosthesis. Circulation 36:422–426, 1967
108. **Hammermeister KE, Dillard DH, Kennedy JW:** Severe, intermittent, mitral regurgitation in a Cross-Jones valve. Report of a case with angiocardiographic and hemodynamic observations. J Thorac Cardiovasc Surg 58:575–580, 1969
109. **Hopeman AR, Treasure RL, Hall RJ:** Mehanical dysfunction in caged-lens prostheses. J Thorac Cardiovasc Surg 60:51–53, 1970
110. **Oliva PB, Johnson ML, Pomerantz M, et al:** Dysfunction of the Beall mitral prosthesis and its detection by cinefluoroscopy and echocardiography. Am J Cardiol 31:393–396, 1973
111. **Horsley HT, Rappoport WJ, Vigoda PS, et al:** Fatal malfunction of Edwards low-profile mitral valves. Circulation 41 and 42:Suppl II:II-39–II-42, 1970
112. **Gunstensen J:** Acute dysfunction of Starr-Edwards mitral prostheses. Thorax 26:163–166, 1971
113. **Stross JK, Willis PW, Kahn DR:** Diagnostic features of malfunction of disc mitral valve prostheses. JAMA 217:305–308, 1971
114. **Kirch E:** Alterations in size and shape of individual regions of heart in valvular disease. Verh Dtsch Ges Inn Med Kong 41: 324–342, 1929
115. **Olin C:** Evaluation of the Kay-Shiley disc valve prosthesis in the aortic position. Clinical and haemodynamic results, and experimental comparison with other prosthetic aortic valves. Scand J Thorac Cardiovasc Surg: Suppl 7:1–37, 1970
116. **Roberts WC, Morrow AG:** Secondary left ventricular endocardial fibroelastosis following mitral valve replacement. Cause of cardiac failure in the late postoperative period. Circulation 37 and 38:Suppl II:II-101–II-109, 1968
117. **Silver MD, Wigle ED, Trimble AS, et al:** Iatrogenic coronary ostial stenosis. Arch Pathol 88:73–77, 1969
118. **Lesage CH Jr, Vogel JHK, Blount SG:** Iatrogenic coronary occlusive disease in patients with prosthetic heart valves. Am J Cardiol 26:123–129, 1970
119. **Black LL, McComb RJ, Silver MD:** Vascular injury following heart valve replacement. Ann Thorac Surg 16:19–29, 1973
120. **Indeglia RA, Shea MA, Varco RL, et al:** Erythrocyte destruction by prosthetic heart valves. Circulation 37 and 38:Suppl II: II-86–II-93, 1968
121. **Rodgers BM, Sabiston DC Jr:** Hemolytic anemia following prosthetic valve replacement. Circulation 39 & 40:Suppl I:I-155–I-161, 1969
122. **Walsch JR, Starr A, Ritzmann LW:** Intravascular hemolysis in patients with prosthetic valves and valvular heart disease. Circulation 39 and 40:Suppl I:I-135–I-140, 1969
123. **Wallace HW, Kenepp DL, Blakemore WS:** Quantitation of red blood cell destruction associated with valvular disease and prosthetic valves. J Thorac Cardiovasc Surg 60:842–852, 1970
124. **Williams JC Jr, Vernon CR, Dalcoff GR, et al:** Hemolysis following mitral valve replacement with the Beall valve prosthesis. J Thorac Cardiovasc Surg 61:393–396, 1971
125. **Eyster E, Rothchild J, Mychajiw O:** Chronic intravascular hemolysis after aortic valve replacement. Long-term study comparing different types of ball-valve prostheses. Circulation 44: 657–665, 1971
126. **Santinga JT, Kirsh MM, Batsakis JT:** Hemolysis in different series of the Starr-Edwards aortic valve prostheses. Chest 63: 905–908, 1973
127. **Lefemine AA, Miller M, Pinder GC:** Chronic hemolysis produced by cloth-covered valves. The effect of design and valve position. J Thorac Cardiovasc Surg 67:857–862, 1974
128. **Roberts WC, Morrow AG:** Renal hemosiderosis in patients with prosthetic aortic valves. Circulation 33:390–398, 1966
129. **Roberts WC:** Renal hemosiderosis (blue kidney) in patients with valvular heart disease. Am J Pathol 48:409–419, 1966

Late Postoperative Anatomic Observations after Insertion of Hufnagel Caged-ball Prostheses in Descending Thoracic Aorta*

Michael C. Fishbein, M.D. and William C. Roberts, M.D.

Clinical and necropsy observations are described in two patients who died 11 and 13 years, respectively, after implantation of Hufnagel prostheses (the first ever used successfully in humans to treat cardiac valve disease) in descending thoracic aorta. Despite the long implantation periods, there was no evidence of prosthetic degeneration or thrombosis or intravascular hemolysis. Although approximately 4000 Hufnagel descending aortic prostheses were distributed by the manufacturer for human use, data in only 55 patients in whom these prostheses were inserted were found in previous publications, and 26 of them had died. Of the 13 late deaths previously reported, no evidence of prosthetic degeneration or thrombosis was described in the three patients surviving > 3 years (8, 10, 12.5 years, respectively). Since neither our patients nor any of the other three reported long-term survivors had prosthetic-related complications and since the dangers of excising the descending aortic prosthesis are considerable, it appears most reasonable, as a rule, not to remove the descending aortic prosthesis at any time in these patients if aortic valve replacement is subsequently performed.

In 1953 Hufnagel and Harvey[1] described successful implantation of a caged-ball prosthesis into descending thoracic aorta in a patient with severe aortic valvular regurgitation. Similar implantations followed,[2-6] but few reports provided information on long term survivors. The present report attempts to fill this void somewhat by describing certain findings during life and at necropsy in two patients who lived 11 and 13 years, respectively, after implantation of Hufnagel prostheses into descending thoracic aorta. Also, experience during the past 14 years[7-25] with prostheses used to replace malfunctioning cardiac valves, can now be utilized in re-examining or evaluating the first of the caged-ball prostheses.

Description of Prosthesis

In the implantation referred to, the prosthesis consisted of a plastic (plexiglass) tube containing a hollow poppet,[2] the wall of which was composed of nylon, which in turn was covered by a 2 mm thick layer of silicone rubber. The prosthesis was attached to aorta by a nylon multiple-point semiflexible fixation ring. Occasionally, the aorta was wrapped with Orlon after attaching the fixation ring. A pressure of only 5 mm Hg was enough to move the poppet in a completely open or closed position.[2] To insert the prosthesis, a transverse segment of descending thoracic aorta (about 2 cm in width) was excised and the prosthesis (measuring just under 6 cm in length) was inserted into both cut ends of the aorta (Fig 1).

*From the Section of Pathology, National Heart and Lung Institute, National Institutes of Health, Bethesda, Maryland.
Manuscript received October 15; revision accepted November 8.
Reprint requests: Dr. Roberts, Bldg. 10A, Room 3D30, National Institutes of Health, Bethesda 20014

Patients Studied

Certain observations in the two patients are summarized in Table 1. Preoperatively, both had severe aortic regurgitation, and each was in functional class 4 (New York Heart Association classification) from congestive cardiac failure. Postoperatively, both were asymptomatic for several years, and the heart sizes by chest roentgenograms became smaller. Symptoms and signs of congestive cardiac failure recurred in each about one year before death, which shortly followed reoperation (aortic valve replacement). The excised aortic valves in each were three-cusped, diffusely thickened by fibrous tissue, and free of calcific deposits. The Hufnagel prostheses in the descending aorta were not removed at reoperation, but at necropsy both were free of thrombi and no portion of either prosthesis showed evidence of wear or variance. The tissue capsules covering the prostheses consisted of fibrous tissue and lipid. The latter was located adjacent to the prostheses. Several anatomic observations in the two patients are illustrated in Figures 2 to 6.

Comments

Although approximately 4000 Hufnagel prostheses were manufactured and distributed to medical centers in Europe, Africa, Australia and

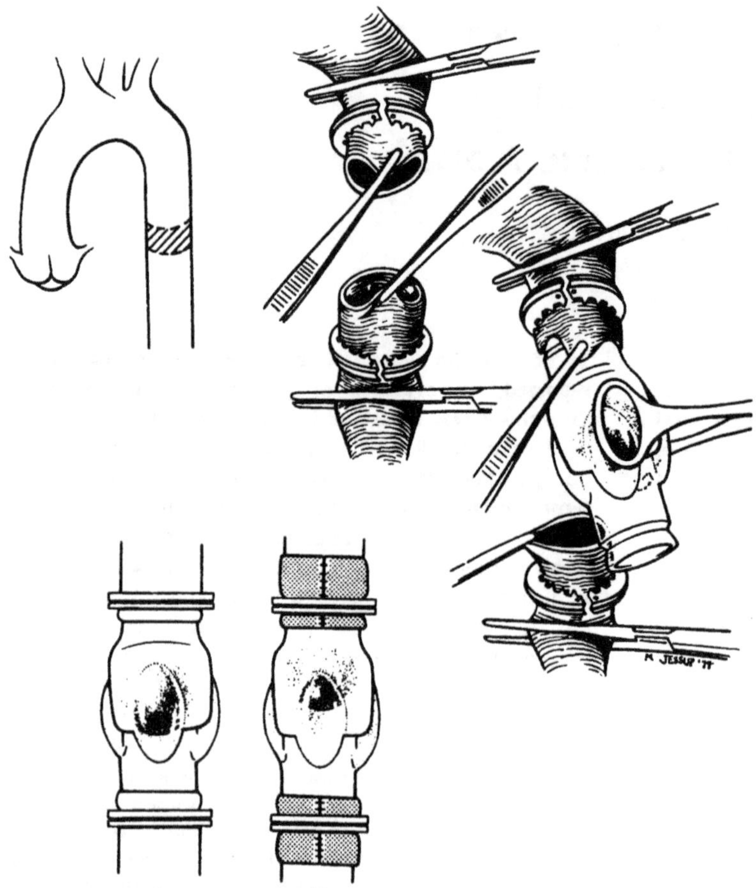

A B

FIGURE 1. Diagram illustrating technique by which the Hufnagel descending aortic prosthesis was usually inserted (see text).

North and South America,[26] clinical, hemodynamic or anatomic observations have been reported previously, to our knowledge, in only 55 patients in whom these prostheses were implanted (Table 2). Of the 55 patients, 13 died within two months of operation (early deaths), and 13 at later periods up to 12.5 years. Of the 13 early deaths, four were due to technical problems (apparently the result of prolonged cross-clamping of the aorta), four to infection (prosthesis infected in only one), and five to uncertain causes. Of the 13 late deaths, four appear to have resulted from prosthetic dysfunction due to prosthetic thrombosis,[2,27] and nine from causes unrelated to the prosthesis. Except for the four with evidences of prosthetic thrombi, the prostheses appear to have functioned properly during the entire postoperative period in the other nine patients. The eventual course in the remaining 21 survivors is unknown, except for the patient reported by Halkier et al.[6] Their patient survived aortic valve replacement and removal of the Hufnagel prosthesis 12.5 years after implantation.

Although, as noted above, dysfunction occurred within this prosthesis, thrombus formation did not occur in any of the reported patients dying within two months of operation or in any survivors with implantation periods longer than three years. Neither of our two patients, surviving 11 and 13 years, respectively, and none of the three previously reported long survivors (eight years,[6] ten years,[5] and

Table 1—*Data in the 2 Patients with Hufnagel Descending Aortic Prostheses*

Patient	Age at death (Yrs)	Sex	History of ARF	Age at onset of symptoms (Yrs)	Age at operation (Yrs)	Implantation period (Yrs)	Pressures (mm Hg) shortly before death: PA (s/d)	PAW (Mean)	LV (s/d)	Aorta (s/d)	CI (L/min/M²)	Body weight (Kg)	Heart weight (Gm)
1*	41	M	+	23	30	11	60/30	19	88/18	90/17	1.8	52	920
2**	40	M	+	26	27	13	24/6	12	190/31	190/60	3.6	64	575

*Case illustrated in Figures 2 and 3.

**Case illustrated in Figures 4 and 5.

Abbreviations: CI = cardiac index; L/min/M² = liters per minute per meter squared; LV = left ventricle; PA = pulmonary artery; PAW = pulmonary arterial wedge; s/d = systole/diastole.

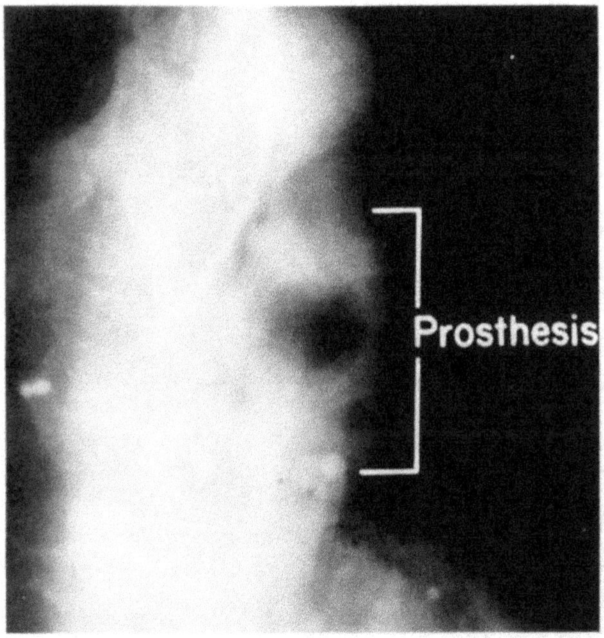

FIGURE 2. Aortogram from patient just before aortic valve replacement and death. The poppet of the prosthesis appears as a non-opacified circle *(bracket).* The poppet excursions appeared to be normal.

12.5 years,[6] respectively) had prosthetic thrombi.

Periprosthetic leakage is a well known complication of implantation of prosthetic cardiac valves.[8,23] Of the 24 patients dying after insertion of Hufnagel prostheses into descending aorta, only one had clinical evidence of leakage, and this resulted in massive hemorrhage and death six weeks after implantation. Infection at the implantation site, however, appears to have been responsible for the suture line disrup-

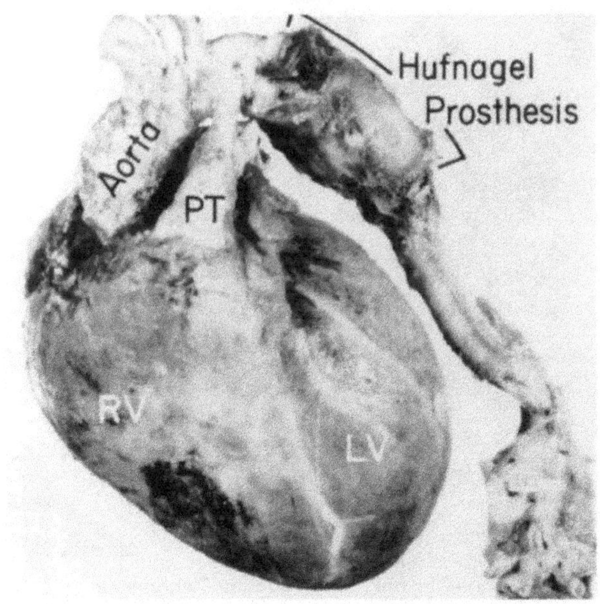

FIGURE 3. Heart and aorta in same patient as in Figure 2. The width of the prosthesis is greater than the width of adjacent aorta. LV=left ventricle; PT=pulmonary trunk; RV=right ventricle.

Table 2—*Previously Reported Studies on Hufnagel Prosthesis in Descending Aorta*

Year (Ref)	No. of patients	Ages at operation (Yrs)	Implantation periods	Early deaths (<2 mo)	Late deaths (>2 mo)
1954[2,28]	23	17-57	op to 11 mos	6	4
1954[3]	1	35	3 mos	0	0
1958[4]	24	10-63	op to 18 mos	5	5
1961[27]	1	37	3 yrs	0	1
1966[5]	1	21	10 yrs	0	1
1970[6]	5	18-45	op to 12.5 yrs	2	2
Totals	55	10-63	op to 12.5 yrs	13	13

Abbreviations: mos = months; op = death during operation; Ref = reference number.

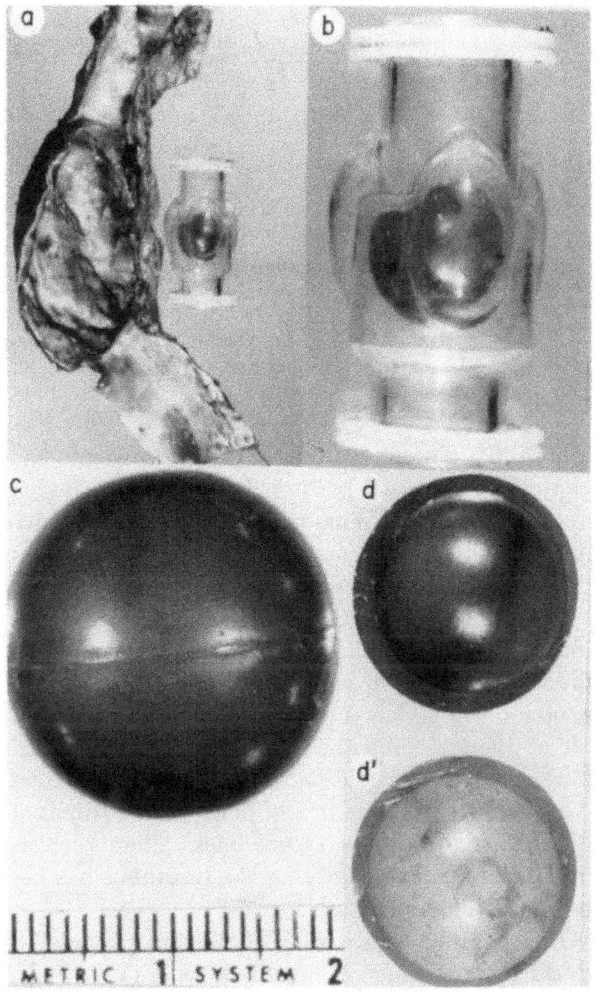

FIGURE 4. Hufnagel descending aortic prosthesis in a second patient. a. Opened aorta showing lining surface of the fibrous capsule which surrounded the prosthesis. Atheromatous plaques are present on the inner lining of the fibrous capsule but not in the adjacent aorta. b. Close-up of Hufnagel prosthesis. c. External surface of poppet, which is brown in color. (The poppet was similar in color when inserted 13 years earlier.) There is no evidence of degeneration of the silicone covering over the polyethylene poppet. d and d[1] One-half of the silicone rubber covering now has been removed (d[1]) demonstrating the polyethylene poppet, which shows no evidence of degeneration.

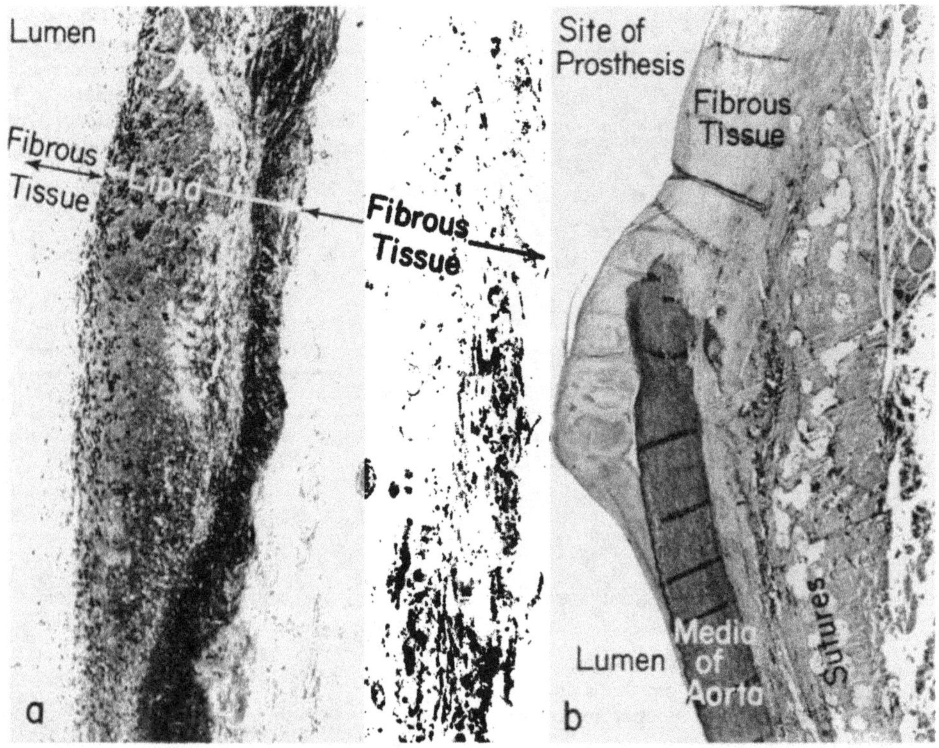

FIGURE 5. Photomicrographs of wall of fibrous capsule covering descending aortic prosthesis (a) and of junction of aorta and fibrous capsule at proximal suture line (b) in second patient (same as in Fig. 4). The inner portion of the tissue capsule surrounding the prosthesis (a) is infiltrated by lipid. The plastic tube containing the poppet had been located to the left. Oil red 0 stain on formalin-fixed frozen section, × 31. b. The junction of aorta and capsule covering the prosthesis. Remnants of Orlon cloth are embedded in dense fibrous tissue where the aorta ends and capsule begins. Elastic–van Gieson stain, × 9.

tion in that patient. Neither of our two patients had clinical evidence of periprosthetic leakage, but at necropsy each had minute separations at the proximal suture lines. Fibrous tissue covered the separations, however, preventing extravasation of blood. Yellow atheromatous plaques were observed on the inner surfaces of the fibrous capsules surrounding the prostheses; their cause is uncertain, but organization of thrombus (the remains of extravasated blood elements) on the luminal surface may well have been responsible. No atherosclerotic plaques were present in the intima of aorta just proximal or distal to the prosthetic suture lines. Atherosclerosis in the fibrous tissue covering the prosthesis has not been described previously.

Degeneration (variance) of silicone poppets[16,19] or discs[25] is common in prosthetic valves used presently to replace malfunctioning mitral and aortic valves. Degeneration of the poppet or the plexiglass housing has not been observed in any of the Hufnagel descending aortic prostheses despite implantation periods of up to 13 years. Furthermore, intravascular hemolysis, an almost invariable consequence of mitral or aortic valve replacement,[8,23,25] has not been observed, to our knowledge, in any patients with only a Hufnagel descending thoracic

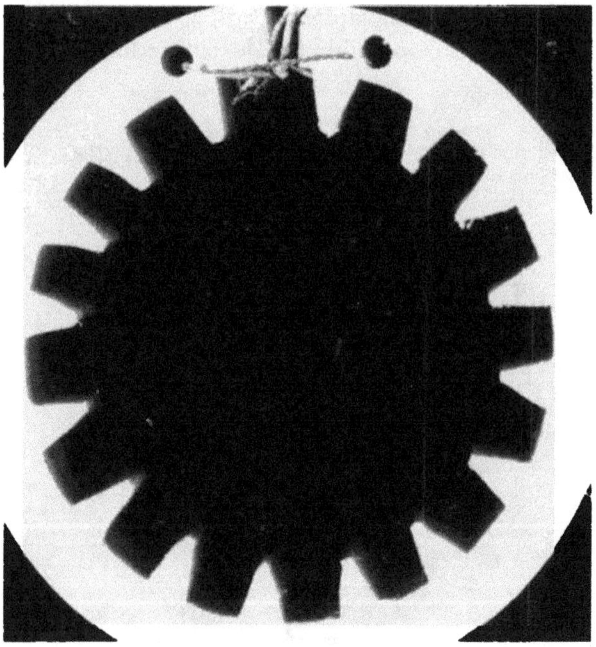

FIGURE 6. Fixation ring, demonstrating "multiple-point fixation" principle, for fixation of prosthesis to aorta. This multiple point fixation device was used rather than a non-point fixation device to prevent possible necrosis or rupture of the wall of the aorta by the constricting holder.

aortic prosthesis. Despite the 11- and 13-year transplantation periods, respectively, in our patients, no clinical (decreased red blood cell survival, elevated reticulocyte count, hemoglobinemia or hemoglobinuria) or anatomic (renal hemosiderosis)[8] evidence of intravascular hemolysis was present.

A caged-ball prosthesis in the descending thoracic aorta obviously only partially diminishes aortic valvular regurgitant flow. Regurgitation from the innominate, left carotid and left subclavian arteries persists, and the pulse pressures in these arteries continue to be wide. The volume of regurgitant flow eliminated by this prosthesis is uncertain. Hufnagel and associates[2] estimated that the prosthesis decreased regurgitant flow by 75 percent. Hemodynamic studies in nine patients postoperatively showed a greater improvement in circulation time (to upper and lower extremities as measured by dye injection curves), cardiac index, and stroke volume than might have been expected by elimination of regurgitant flow from the lower extremities alone. Rose and associates[28] postulated that, because the amount of regurgitation decreased, ventricular contractions became more efficient and stroke volume and cardiac index increased.

Because aortic valvular regurgitation is incompletely relieved by a Hufnagel prosthesis in descending aorta, replacement of the aortic valve usually will be required eventually in the long surviving patients. Halkier and associates[6] and du Plessis and associates[5] each removed a Hufnagel descending aortic prosthesis several weeks after aortic valve replacement for recurrence of congestive heart failure from aortic valvular regurgitation. The Hufnagel prostheses in both patients were removed purely because of uncertainty regarding their eventual fate if left in place. Removal was technically difficult in both patients because of dense fibrous adhesions between aorta and lung and erosion of bony structures adjacent to the prostheses. One patient died shortly after the operation to remove the descending aortic prosthesis;[5] the other required an additional thoracotomy because of postoperative bleeding.[6] Because of the difficulty and danger associated with removal of a Hufnagel descending aortic prosthesis, and because none of the late survivors with this prosthesis, including the patients of Halkier et al[6] and du Plessis et al,[5] had evidence of prosthetic dysfunction, wear, or thrombosis, *excision of a Hufnagel descending aortic prosthesis at any time after aortic valve replacement probably is infrequently justified.*

Although virtually all prostheses now used to correct malfunctioning aortic valves are implanted into the aortic root, certain patients might benefit from at least temporary implantation of a prosthesis into the descending thoracic aorta. Aortic valve replacement may be fruitless in some patients with active infective endocarditis of the aortic valve with ring abscesses or in subjects with endocarditis at sites of attachment of prosthetic aortic valves.[7,29] Such patients might benefit by use of a caged-ball prosthesis implanted into the descending aorta, after excision of the infected natural or prosthetic aortic valve. (Danielson and associates[30] recently implanted a valve prosthesis in the ascending aorta [above the coronary ostia] combined with saphenous vein bypass in a patient with an infected aortic root.)

References

1 Hufnagel CA, Harvey WP: The surgical correction of aortic regurgitation. Preliminary report. Bull Georgetown Univ Med Center 6:60-61, 1953

2 Hufnagel CA, Harvey WP, Rabil PJ, et al: Surgical correction of aortic insufficiency. Surgery 35:673-683, 1954

3 McKusick VA, Hahn DP, Brayshaw JR, et al: Some hemodynamic effects of the Hufnagel operation for aortic regurgitation. Studies in models and a patient. Bull Johns Hopkins Hosp 95:322-377, 1954

4 Conklin WS, Grismer JT, Aalpoel JA: Hufnagel valve surgery for aortic insufficiency. J Thorac Surg 36:238-246, 1958

5 du Plessis LA, Chesler E, Rogers M, et al: Aortic valve replacement in the presence of a Hufnagel valve prosthesis. J Thorac Cardiovasc Surg 51:493-497, 1966

6 Halkier E, Hansen PF, Anderson I: Aortic incompetence: The eventual outcome in a small series treated with Hufnagel's descending aorta ball-valve. Scand J Thorac Cardiovasc Surg 4:52-55, 1970

7 Cohn LH, Roberts WC, Rockoff SD, et al: Bacterial endocarditis following aortic valve replacement. Clinical and pathologic correlations. Circulation 33:209-217, 1966

8 Roberts WC, Morrow AG: Renal hemosiderosis in patients with prosthetic aortic valves. Circulation 36:390-398, 1966

9 Roberts WC, Lambird PA, Gott VL, et al: Fatal aortic regurgitation following replacement of the mitral and aortic valves. A mechanical complication of double valve replacement. J Thorac Cardiovasc Surg 52:189-192, 1966

10 Roberts WC, Morrow AG: Bacterial endocarditis involving prosthetic mitral valves. Clinical and pathologic observations. Arch Pathol 82:164-169, 1966

11 Roberts WC, Morrow AG: Mechanisms of acute left atrial thrombosis after mitral valve replacement. Pathologic findings indicating obstruction to left atrial emptying. Am J Cardiol 18:497-503, 1966

12 Roberts WC, Morrow AG: Late postoperative pathologic findings after cardiac valve replacement. Suppl to Circulation 35 and 36. Suppl 1:48-62, 1967

13 Roberts WC, Morrow AG: Causes of early postoperative death following cardiac valve replacement. Clinicopathologic correlations in 64 patients studied at necropsy. J Thorac Cardiovasc Surg 54:422-437, 1967

14 Roberts WC, Morrow AG: Anatomic studies of hearts containing caged-ball prosthetic valves. Johns Hopkins Med J 121:271-295, 1967

15 Roberts WC, Morrow AG: Secondary left ventricular

endocardial fibroelastosis following mitral valve replacement. Cause of cardiac failure in the late postoperative period. Suppl to Circulation 37 and 38. Suppl 2:101-109, 1968

16 Roberts WC, Morrow AG: Fatal degeneration of the silicone rubber ball of the Starr-Edwards prosthetic aortic valve. Am J Cardiol 22:614-620, 1968

17 Roberts WC, Morrow AG: Compression of anomalous left circumflex coronary arteries by prosthetic valve fixation rings. J Thorac Cardiovasc Surg 57:834-838, 1969

18 Roberts WC, Morrow AG: Late postoperative pathologic findings following cardiac valve replacement with Starr-Edwards prostheses. *In* Proceedings of Second National Conference on Prosthetic Heart Valves. Springfield, Illinois, Charles C Thomas, 1969, p 365-393

19 Roberts WC, Levinson GE, Morrow AG: Lethal ball variance in the Starr-Edwards prosthetic mitral valve. Arch Intern Med 126:517-521, 1970

20 Winter TQ, Reis RL, Glancy DL, et al: Current status of Starr-Edwards cloth-covered prosthetic cardiac valves. Suppl to Circulation 45 and 46. Suppl 1:14-24, 1972

21 Shepherd RL, Glancy DL, Stinson EB, et al: Hemodynamic confirmation of obstruction to left ventricular inflow by a caged-ball prosthetic mitral valve. J Thorac Cardiovasc Surg 65:252-254, 1973

22 Yarbrough JW, Roberts WC, Reis RL: Structural alterations in tissue cardiac valves implanted in patients and in calves. J Thorac Cardiovasc Surg 65:364-375, 1973

23 Roberts WC, Bulkley BH, Morrow AG: Pathologic anatomy of cardiac valve replacement: A study of 224 necropsy patients. Progr Cardiovasc Dis 15:539-587, 1973

24 Fishbein MC, Roberts WC, Golden A, et al: Cardiac pathology after aortic valve replacement using a Hufnagel tri-leaflet prostheses: A study of 20 necropsy patients. Am Heart J (in press)

25 Roberts WC, Fishbein MC, Golden A: Cardiac pathology after valve replacement using disc prostheses. A study of 61 necropsy patients. Am J Cardiol (in press)

26 Personal communication with Mr. Charles Hewson, Brunswick Manufacturing Company, North Quincy, Mass

27 Edwards JE: An Atlas of Acquired Diseases of the Heart and Great Vessels (Vol 3). Philadelphia, Saunders, 1961, p 1065

28 Rose JC, Hufnagel CA, Freis ED, et al: The hemodynamic alterations produced by a plastic valvular prosthesis for severe aortic insufficiency in man. J Clin Invest 33:891-900, 1954

29 Buchbinder NA, Roberts WC: Left-sided valvular active infective endocarditis. A study of 45 necropsy patients. Am J Med 53:20-35, 1972

30 Danielson GK, Titus JL, DuShane JW: Successful treatment of aortic valve endocarditis and aortic root abscesses by insertion of prosthetic valve in ascending aorta and placement of bypass grafts to coronary arteries. J Thorac Cardiovasc Surg 67:443-449, 1974

Cocking of a poppet-disc prosthesis in the aortic position

A cause of intermittent aortic regurgitation

Intermittent aortic regurgitation due to cocking is described for the first time after replacement of the aortic valve with a poppet-disc prosthesis. A combination of disc grooving and strut thrombus produced the cocking with resultant aortic regurgitation.

William J. Hammer, M.D.,* Michael J. Hearne, M.D., and William C. Roberts, M.D.,**
Washington, D. C.

Among patients with prosthetic cardiac valves, a common cause of both early and late death is prosthetic dysfunction.[1] Auscultation and phonocardiographic abnormalities in these patients often are clues to such dysfunction.[2-4] Peribasilar communications or improper seating of the poppet as a result of thrombus or variance are the usual causes of regurgitant type murmurs. This report was prompted by observing intermittent aortic regurgitation after aortic valve replacement with a poppet disc prosthesis. The mechanism of the regurgitation has not been recorded previously after aortic valve replacement.

Case report

A 51-year-old man had been well during the first 6 ½ years after aortic valve replacement with a 16.5 mm. Hufnagel disc prosthesis.[5] Evidence of left ventricular failure then appeared and gradually progressed. Precordial auscultation 7 years after valve replacement disclosed distinct opening and closing prosthetic sounds: a Grade 4/6, harsh, basal systolic murmur and, along the left sternal border, a high-frequency decresendo murmur, which varied from Grade 1/6 to 3/6 in intensity in successive cardiac cycles (Fig. 1). Before cardiac catheterization could be performed, the patient suddenly died.

Necropsy (74A-347) disclosed multiple notches on the margins of the aortic prosthetic disc (Figs. 2 and 3) and thrombus bordering the primary orifice and surrounding two of the four prosthetic struts. No peribasilar communications were present.

From the Department of Medicine (Cardiology) and Pathology, Georgetown University Medical Center, Washington, D. C.

Received for publication May 28, 1975.

*Present address: Division of Cardiology, Department of Medicine, Temple University Health Science Center, Philadelphia, Pa.

**Present address: Section of Pathology, National Heart and Lung Institute, National Institutes of Health, Bethesda, Md.

Comments

Variance of the silicone rubber poppet of a caged-ball prosthetic cardiac valve is well known and usually is characterized by discoloration, grooving, swelling, or shrinkage.[1] Decreased mobility may be the consequence of the poppet's swelling or shrinkage. Either may lead to regurgitation. Grooving of the disc margins is a common late finding after replacement of either mitral or aortic valves with a caged-disc prosthesis. It may cause both fixed and intermittent regurgitation with the prosthesis in the mitral position.[6] Cocking of a disc in the aortic position, however, has not been described. Disc variance, as occurred in our patient, is probably the major cause of such cocking because it allows the disc to stick to one or two of the struts and thereby prevents proper seating.[6] Our patient, who had no peribasilar communication at necropsy, had an obvious aortic regurgitant murmur *of varying intensity* that developed late after valve replacement. Not only were the margins of the disc grooved on our patient, but thrombus surrounded two of the four struts. The combination of poppet grooving and strut thrombus appears responsible for causing the disc to seat differently during each cardiac cycle. Thus there were varying amounts of aortic regurgitant flow (Fig. 3). Because both thrombus and disc variance are common late findings after valve replacement, cocking

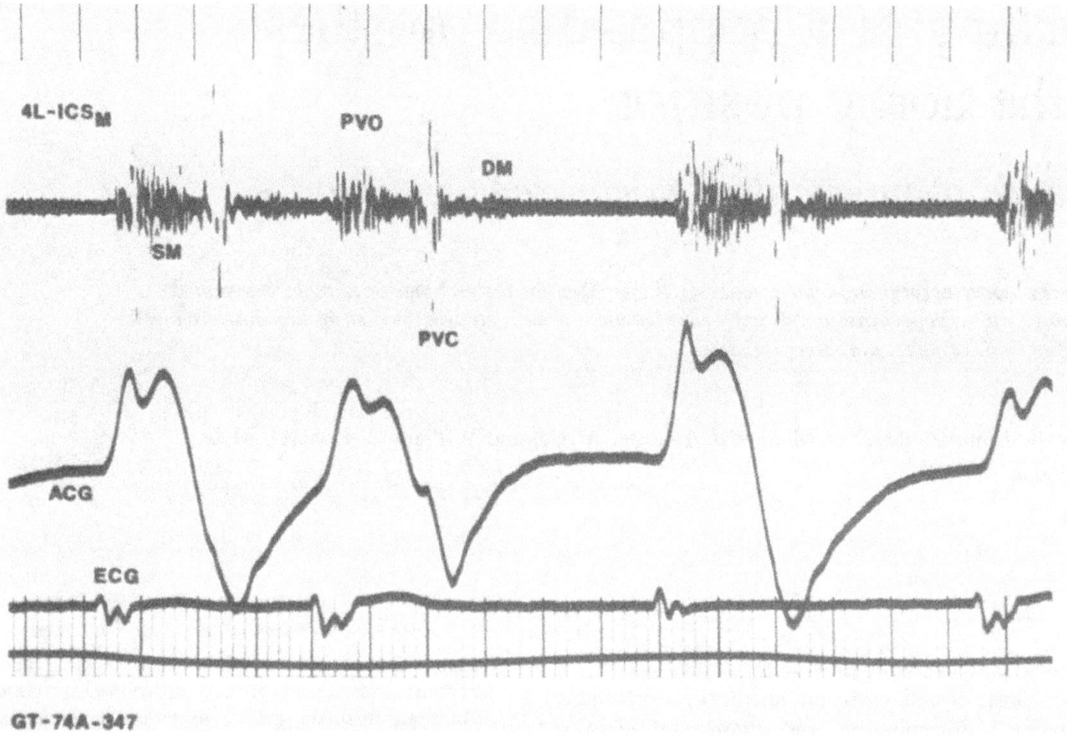

Fig. 1. Phonocardiogram in the patient described showing a prominent systolic murmur *(SM)* and a diastolic murmur *(DM)* of varying intensity. The prosthetic valve opening *(PVO)* and closing *(PVC)* sounds are distinct. This recording was made over the fourth left intercostal space *(ICS)*, at medium *(M)* frequency, and simultaneously an apex cardiogram *(ACG)* and electrocardiogram *(ECG)* (Lead II) were recorded. The latter shows atrial fibrillation and left bundle branch block.

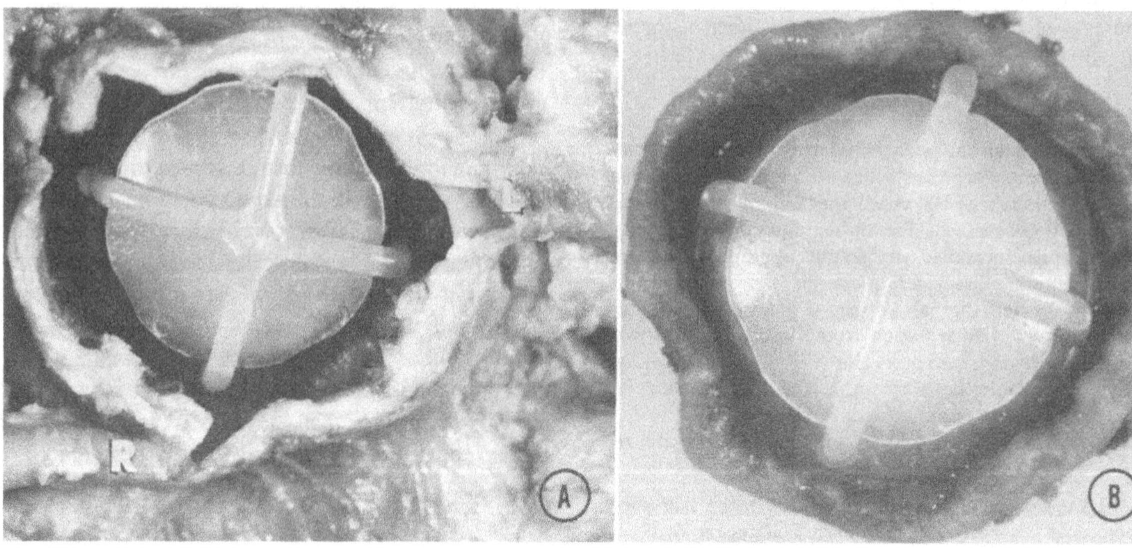

Fig. 2. Views of the aortic disc prosthesis from above. *A,* While situated within the ascending aorta. *R,* Right coronary artery. *L,* Left coronary artery. *B,* After removal of the prosthesis from the aorta. The indentations of the margins of the disc are easily seen.

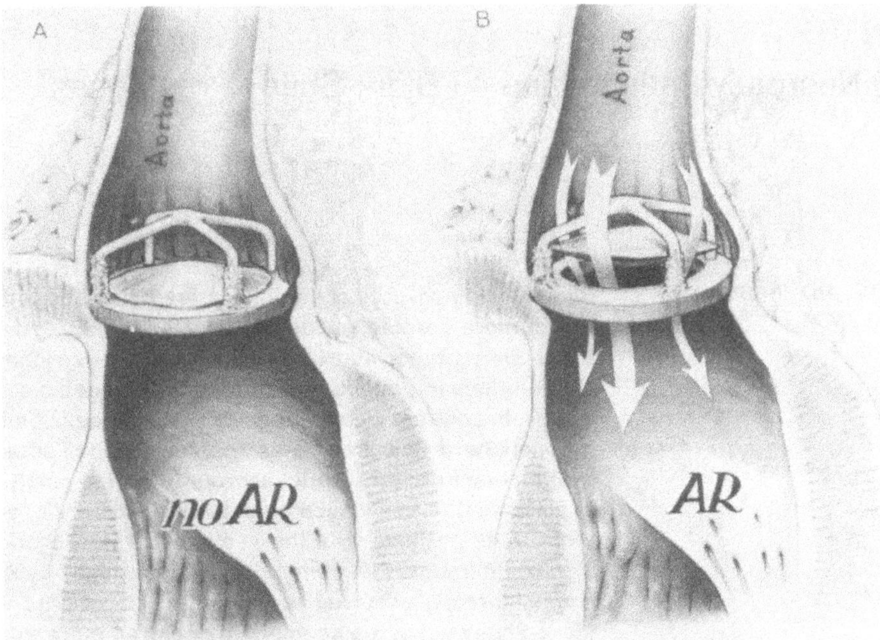

Fig. 3. Drawing showing thrombus on two of the four struts and indentations on the margins of the disc. *A,* The appearance of the prosthesis when the disc is seated properly and there is no aortic regurgitation *(AR)*. *B,* The appearance of the prosthesis when disc-cocking has occurred, allowing aortic regurgitation.

of a poppet disc might be expected to be more common. A poppet-disc prosthesis, however, has been used infrequently in the aortic position.[6]

REFERENCES

1 Roberts, W. C., Bulkley, B. H., and Morrow, A. G.: Pathologic Anatomy of Cardiac Valve Replacement: A Study of 224 Necropsy Patients, Progr. Cardiovasc. Dis. **15:** 539, 1973.

2 Allen, P., and Robertson, R.: The Significance of Intermittent Regurgitation in Aortic Valve Prosthesis, J. Thorac. Cardiovasc. Surg. **54:** 549, 1967.

3 Hylen, J. C., Kloster, F. E., Starr, A., and Griswald, H. E.: Aortic Ball Variance: Diagnosis and Treatment, Ann. Intern. Med. **72:** 1, 1970.

4 Hildner, F. J.: Detection of Prosthetic Valve Dysfunction by Bedside and Laboratory Evaluation, Cardiovasc. Clin. **5:** 289, 1973.

5 Hufnagel, C. A., and Conrad, P. W.: A Comparative Study of Some Prosthetic Valves for Aortic and Mitral Replacement, Surgery **57:** 205, 1965.

6 Roberts, W. C., Fishbein, M. C., and Golden, A.: Cardiac Pathology After Valve Replacement Using Disc Prosthesis: A Study of 61 Necropsy Patients, Am. J. Cardiol. **35:** 740, 1975.

Cardiac Pathology After Valve Replacement With a Tilting Disc Prosthesis (Björk-Shiley Type)

A Study of 46 Necropsy Patients and 49 Björk-Shiley Prostheses

WILLIAM C ROBERTS, MD, FACC
WILLIAM J HAMMER, MD*

Bethesda, Maryland

Clinical and necropsy observations are described in 46 patients who had one or more cardiac valves replaced with a tilting disc prosthesis of the Bjork-Shiley type, and these observations are compared with earlier observations in patients with caged ball, caged disc and trileaflet prostheses. In contrast with its frequent occurrence in patients studied earlier with peripheral flow prostheses, either caged ball or caged disc, prosthetic dysfunction from prosthetic disproportion (too small a ventricular cavity or aortic root to freely accommodate the prosthesis) was observed in only 2 of the 46 patients with the semicentral flow Bjork-Shiley prosthesis. Significant trauma to erythrocytes, as determined by the presence of renal hemosiderosis, occurred in only 1 of 11 patients who died late after Bjork-Shiley valve replacement; it occurred more frequently and with far greater severity in patients who died late after valve replacement with a caged ball or caged disc prosthesis. Prosthetic thrombi may be less frequent after valve replacement with a tilting disc than after replacement with a caged ball or caged disc. They occurred in 7 of 13 patients who died late after Bjork-Shiley valve replacement, but 3 of the 7 patients had infective prosthetic endocarditis, and of the remaining 4, only one had been receiving warfarin sodium. In contrast, prosthetic thrombi were observed in 81 and 88 percent, respectively, of 112 patients who died late after valve replacement with a caged ball or caged disc prosthesis, and most of the 112 patients had received anticoagulant therapy. Although the implantation periods were relatively short (3 to 30 months, average 11), prosthetic wear or variance of the tilting disc prosthesis did not occur in any of the 13 patients who died late.

Although the tilting disc (Bjork-Shiley) prosthesis is prone to clot (and therefore patients with it require long-term anticoagulation), the device is not intrinsically stenotic or significantly incompetent, it is only minimally traumatic to erythrocytes and, at this time, there is no evidence of prosthetic degeneration or variance.

From the Section of Pathology, National Heart and Lung Institute, National Institutes of Health, Bethesda, Md Manuscript accepted November 12, 1975

* Work done while a Fellow in Cardiology, Georgetown University Medical Center, Washington, D C Present address Division of Cardiology, Department of Medicine, Temple University Medical Center, Philadelphia, Pa

Address for reprints William C Roberts, MD, Bldg 10A, Rm 3E30 National Institutes of Health, Bethesda, Md 20014

During the past 15 years many different prosthetic cardiac valves have been introduced, and many clinical and hemodynamic studies on them have appeared. Morphologic studies focusing on findings at necropsy in patients with one or more prosthetic cardiac valves of the caged ball and caged disc type also have appeared.[1–21] Little anatomic information is available, however, on the tilting or pivoting-disc prosthesis[22] This report describes observations at necropsy in 46 patients who had one or more cardiac valves replaced with a tilting disc (Bjork-Shiley type) prosthesis, and compares these observations with those made earlier at necropsy in 298 patients with other types of prosthetic cardiac valves

TABLE I

Total Valves Replaced in the 46 Patients With at Least One Bjork-Shiley Prosthesis

Valve Replaced	Early Deaths (<2 mo)	Late Deaths (>2 mo)	Total Patients	Total Valves	Total Bjork-Shiley Prostheses
Aortic (A)	20	10	30	30	30
Mitral (M)	4	2	6	6	6
A + M	5	0	5	10	6
M + tricuspid (T)	2	0	2	4	2
A + M + T	2	1	3	9	5
Totals	33	13	46	59	49

TABLE II

Valves Replaced by Bjork-Shiley Prostheses

	Early Deaths (<2 mo)	Late Deaths (>2 mo)	Valve Status Preoperatively: Stenotic	Valve Status Preoperatively: Purely Incompetent	Totals
Aortic	26	11	30	7	37
Mitral	6	2	5	3	8
Tricuspid	4	0	1	3	4
Totals	36	13	36	13	49

TABLE III

Types of Prosthetic Valves Inserted in the 46 Patients With at Least One Bjork-Shiley Prosthesis

	Aortic	Mitral	Tricuspid	Totals
Bjork-Shiley	37	8	4	49
Starr-Edwards	1	7	0	8
Hufnagel disc	0	1	0	1
Porcine aortic	0	0	1	1
Totals	38	16	5	59

TABLE IV

Etiology of the Valve Disease in the 46 Patients With at Least One Bjork-Shiley Prosthesis

Etiology	Single Valve Replaced	Multiple Valves Replaced	Totals No	Totals %
Rheumatic	10	8	18	39
Congenital	14*	0	14	30
Infective endocarditis	3†	2*	5	11
Degenerative	4	0	4	9
Unknown	4	0	4	9
Coronary	1	0	1	2
Totals	36	10	46	100

* Aortic valve congenitally bicuspid in all
† Aortic valve congenitally bicuspid in two of the three

TABLE V

Cause (1 per patient) of Death in the 33 Patients Who Died Early (<2 Months) After Replacement of at Least One Cardiac Valve With a Bjork-Shiley Prosthesis

Cause	A	M	A+M	M+T	A+M+T	Totals No	Totals %
No anatomic explanation	7	1	2	1	2	13	40
Bleeding	4	0	1	1	0	6	18
Coronary heart disease	3	1	1	0	0	5	15
Uncorrected associated valve disease	4	0	0	0	0	4	12
Infection	3	0	0	0	0	3	9
Prosthetic dysfunction	0	2	0	0	0	2	6
Totals	21	4	4	2	2	33	100

A = aortic, M = mitral, T = tricuspid

Patients Studied

The 46 patients ranged in age from 25 to 76 years (average 53), 27 were men and 19 were women Preoperatively, 90 percent of the 46 patients were in functional class III or IV (New York Heart Association classification) and 10 percent were in functional class II The 46 patients included 33 who died early (less than 2 months) and 13 who died late (3 to 30 months, average 11) after operation (Table I) The 46 patients had 59 valve prostheses, 49 of the Bjork-Shiley type (Tables II and III) One valve was replaced in 36 patients and more than one valve in 10 None of the 10 patients with more than one valve replacement died of malfunction of any of the prostheses

The replaced valves: Of the 59 valves replaced, 43 (73 percent) had been stenotic and 16 (27 percent) purely incompetent (no element of stenosis). Bjork-Shiley prostheses were utilized to replace 36 of the 43 stenotic valves and 13 of the 16 purely incompetent valves

The causes of the valvular heart disease in the 46 patients are summarized in Table IV The aortic valve was congenitally bicuspid[23–25] in 18 of the 46 patients and in each the aortic valve was replaced, in 15 it was stenotic and in 3 purely incompetent In each of the 15 patients with aortic stenosis the mitral valve was normal. The pure aortic regurgitation in each of the three patients was caused by infective endocarditis[26] Two of them also had mitral valve replacement for pure regurgitation from rupture of chordae tendineae [27] The aortic valve was tricuspid in each of the remaining 28 patients In 15 of them the aortic valve was stenotic, in 5 purely incompetent, and in 8 both anatomically and functionally normal The aortic valve was replaced in each of the 20 with a dysfunctioning aortic valve

Mitral valve replacement (with or without tricuspid valve replacement) was carried out in each of the eight patients with a normal aortic valve and in six of those who also had aortic valve replacement Of the 14 mitral valves replaced, 9 were stenotic and 5 were purely incompetent Of the 28 patients with a tricuspid aortic valve, the mitral valve was diffusely thickened in 17 and anatomically normal in 11 Of the 17 patients with an anatomically abnormal mitral valve, mitral valve replacement was performed in 12, mitral commissurotomy in 3 and mitral anuloplasty in 1 Mitral valve replacement also was carried out in two patients who had severe mitral regurgitation but anatomically normal mitral leaflets and chordae tendineae The cause in one patient was papillary muscle dysfunction from coronary disease[28] and in the second patient was uncertain

Coronary arteries: Coronary arterial atherosclerosis of varying degree was present in all 46 patients. The lumen of at least one of the three major (right, left anterior descending, left circumflex) coronary arteries was narrowed more than 75 percent by atherosclerotic plaques in 13 (28 percent) of the 46 patients, in 12 (36 percent) of the 33 who died early and in 1 (8 percent) of the 13 who died late. Aortocoronary bypass procedures were performed at the time of valve replacement in six patients, five of whom died early and one of whom died late.

Myocardial pathology: Although histologic evidence of myocardial fibrosis—mainly interstitial—was observed in most patients, grossly visible left ventricular myocardial scarring was present in 15 (33 percent) of the 46 patients. The scarring involved subendocardium (inner half of the myocardial wall) or papillary muscle in nine, and it was transmural (more than the inner half of the wall) in six. Grossly visible myocardial necrosis, other than in papillary muscles and in myocardium adjacent to infected prosthetic valves, was observed in two patients who died early: In one, it was limited

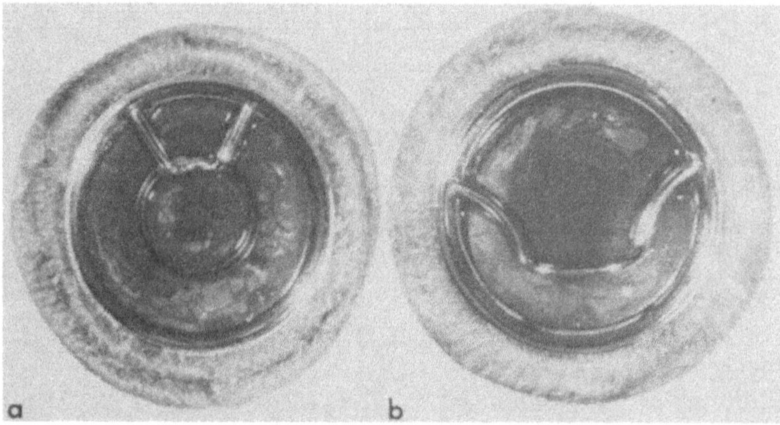

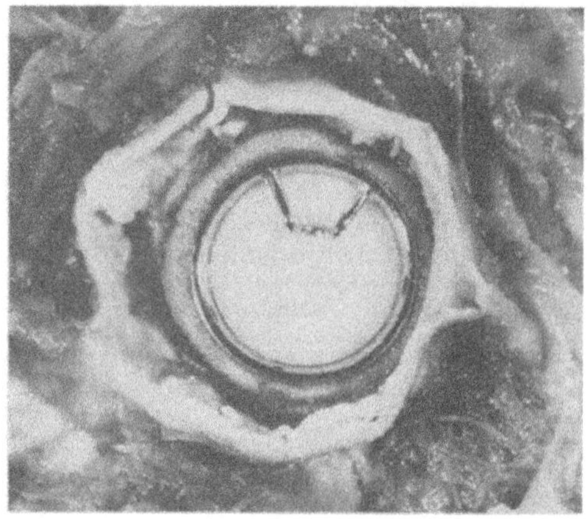

FIGURE 1 (left). Björk-Shiley prosthesis with a pyrolytic carbon disc. This prosthesis was utilized for aortic valve replacement, and the patient died in the operating room. **a,** as viewed from the ascending aorta; **b,** as viewed from the left ventricle.
FIGURE 2 (right). Björk-Shiley prosthesis with a Delrin disc in the aortic position in a 76 year old woman who died in the operating room. The hinge is located posteriorly so that blood flow is primarily anteriorly.

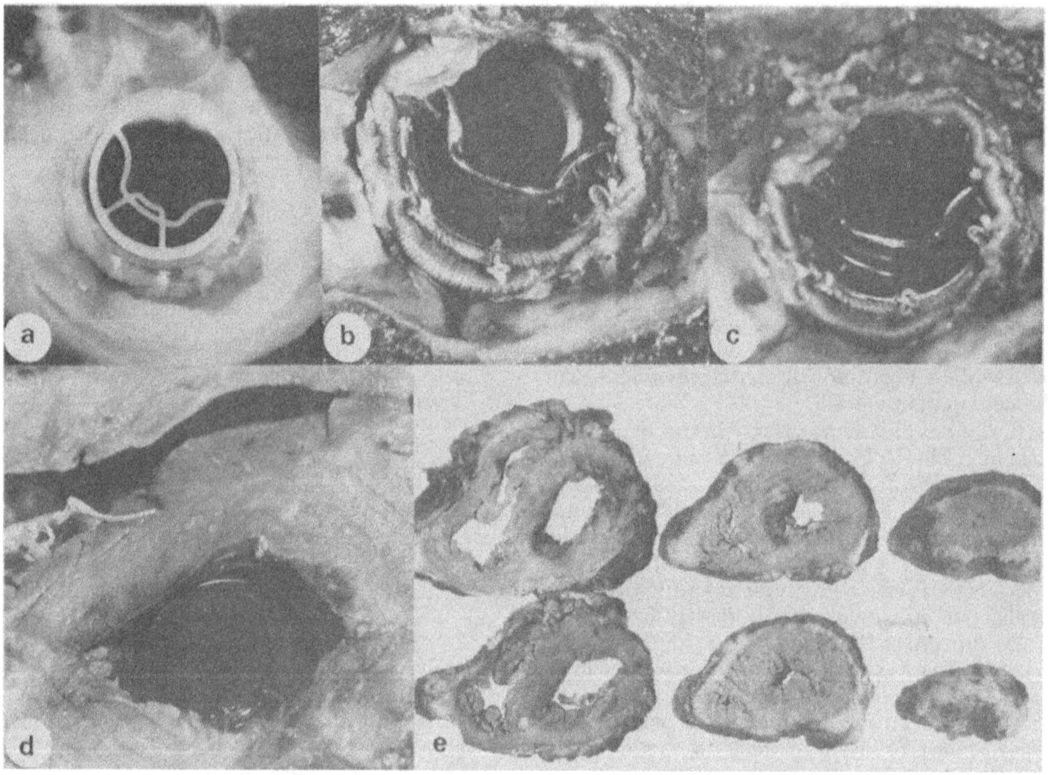

FIGURE 3. Prosthetic dysfunction after mitral valve replacement with the largest-sized Björk-Shiley prosthesis (31 mm) in a 54 year old man with isolated mitral stenosis. Although the prosthesis appeared to have opened well, the disc was prevented from seating by the ventricular septum, which "moved inward" during ventricular systole. The patient could not be separated from cardiopulmonary bypass. **a,** radiograph of heart at necropsy showing the large mitral valve prosthesis. **b,** mitral valve prosthesis from the left atrium *as it should appear* during simulated ventricular systole. **c,** same view showing the mitral disc *as it did appear* during ventricular systole. The disc margins contacted the ventricular septum, preventing seating of the disc. **d,** view from the left ventricle showing the disc margins contacting the ventricular septum. **e,** transverse slices of the ventricles showing a relatively small left ventricular cavity.

to the subendocardium; in the second, it was transmural and circumferential. Severe (more than 75 percent) narrowing of at least one of the three major coronary arteries by atherosclerosis was present in three of the nine patients with subendocardial fibrosis and in five of the six with transmural fibrosis. Of the 13 patients with greater than 75 percent narrowing of at least one of the three major coronary arteries, 9 had grossly visible left ventricular scarring (subendocardial only in 4 and transmural in 5). Six patients had either subendocardial (four patients) or transmural (two patients) fibrosis without severe coronary narrowing.

Results

Patients Who Died Early

Of the 33 patients who died within 2 months of operation, 13 (40 percent) died in the operating room, another within 24 hours and 24 (73 percent) by 7 days. The causes of death in these 33 patients are summarized in Table V, and certain observations are illustrated in Figures 1 to 4.

No anatomic explanation for death was found in 13 patients (40 percent). Five of the 13 could not be separated from cardiopulmonary bypass. One patient died suddenly and unexpectedly at home 30 days postoperatively. Each of the other six patients died after varying periods of inadequate cardiac output. Five of these 13 patients had more than one valve replaced, and each of the other 7 had isolated aortic valve replacement. Only two had coronary luminal narrowing greater than 75 percent, but in each only one of the three major coronary arteries was narrowed to this degree. Only 2 of the 13 had left ventricular scarring, but in each it was limited to subendocardium. None had left ventricular necrosis.

Massive bleeding caused death in six patients (19 percent). Between 1,200 and 6,800 ml of extravasated blood was measured at necropsy in the chest of these six patients.

Severe coronary arterial narrowing from atherosclerosis was considered the major cause of death in five patients, four of whom also had aortocoronary bypass grafts inserted. All five patients had "three vessel disease" (more than 75 percent narrowing of the lumen of all three major coronary arteries). One of the five had extensive left ventricular circumferential hemorrhagic necrosis. Four of these five patients preoperatively had valvular aortic stenosis[30]; the fifth had mitral regurgitation after healing of a myocardial infarct.

Uncorrected associated valve disease appeared responsible for death in four patients, all of whom had aortic valve replacement and either mitral commissurotomy (three patients) or mitral anuloplasty (one pa-

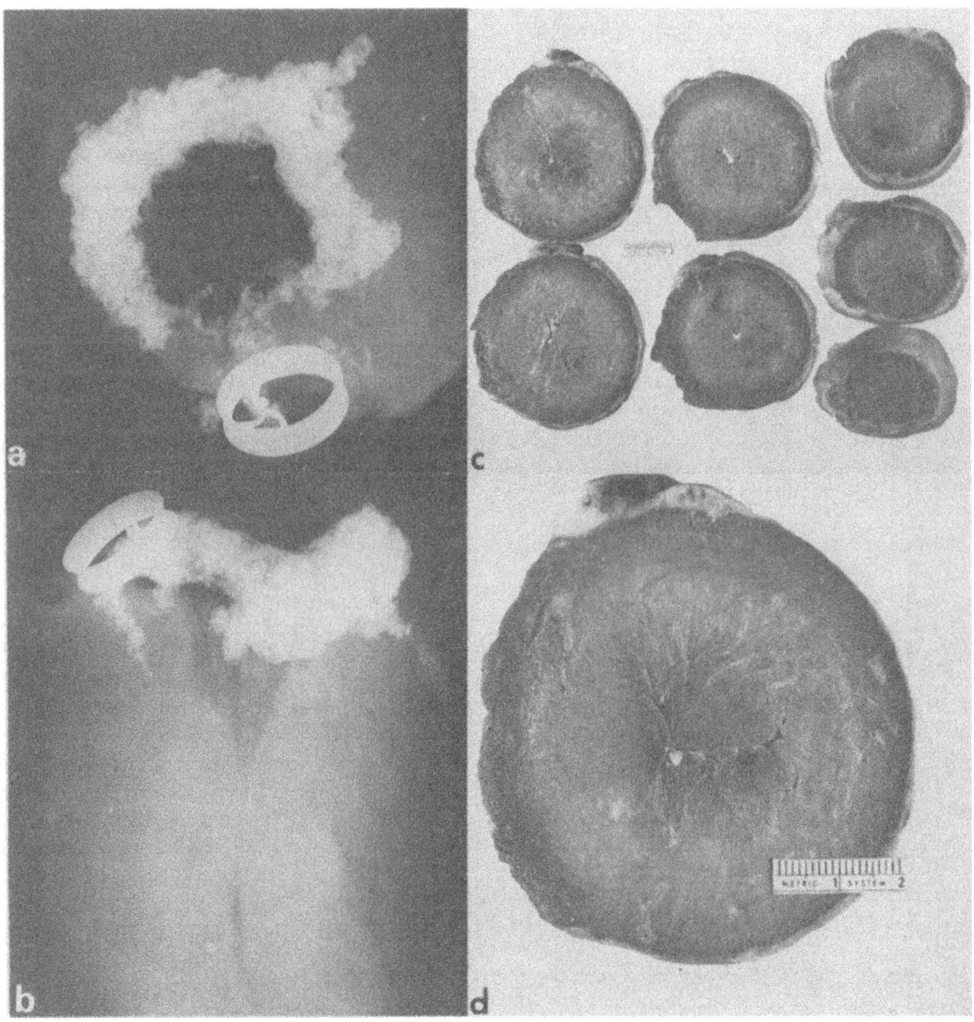

FIGURE 4. Radiographs of heart (**a** and **b**) and transverse sections of the left ventricle (**c** and **d**) in a 70 year old woman. The radiographs demonstrate "massive" amounts of calcific deposits in the mitral anulus in addition to the Björk-Shiley prosthetic aortic valve. Preoperatively, a 7 mm Hg mean diastolic gradient was recorded between the pulmonary arterial wedge position and the left ventricle. The "slices" of the left ventricle show considerable hypertrophy of the ventricular wall but virtual absence of a left ventricular cavity. **d** is a close-up of the left upper slice in **c**. There are no myocardial foci of necrosis and only minute focal scars. This patient's 3 day postoperative course was characterized by features of the low cardiac output syndrome. The heart appears to have stopped during peak ventricular systole, and this heart is probably characteristic of what clinically has been called *"the stone heart"*.[29]

TABLE VI

Observations in Patients Who Died Late (>2 Months) After Bjork-Shiley Valve Replacement

Case no	Age (yr) & Sex	Pressures (mm Hg) Preop LA-LV (mdg)	Preop LV-SA (psg)	Postop LA-LV (mdg)	Postop LV-SA (psg)	Valve Replaced A	Valve Replaced M	Size* of Prosthesis (mm)	Implantation Period (mo)	Heart Weight (g)	Anticoagulant	Prosthetic Valve Thrombus	Prosthetic Valve Endocarditis	Prosthetic Valve Ring Leak	Hematocrit (%) Preop	Hematocrit (%) Postop	Renal Iron (0–4+)	Cause of Death
1	52M	0	80	—	—	+	0	23	3	650	W,D	+†	+	+‖	40	38	0	PVE
2	68F	5	80	—	80	+	0	19	3	430	W	0	0	0	40	41	0	?
3	49M	0	45	—	—	+‡	0	—	4	—	W	0	0	0	—	—	—	CHD
4	46M	0	80	—	—	+	0	19	6	620	D	+	0	0	45	—	0	PVT
5	63F	0	125	—	35	+	0	19	9	320	D	+	0	0	40	36	1	PVT
6	40M	0	0	0	0	+	0	25	11	530	W	+†	+	0	—	32	4	PVE
7	54M	0	↑	—	—	+	0	23	12	620	W	+†	+	+‖	44	—	0	PVE
8	48M	15	50	—	—	+	+§	23	15	850	W	0	0	0	47	43	0	?
9	40M	0	0	—	—	+	0	20	23	750	D	0	0	0	44	43	0	?
10	61M	0	60	0	10	+	0	—	24	—	W	0	0	+	—	—	—	AR
11	50F	7	80	—	5	+	0	21	30	400	D	+	0	0	—	—	0	PVT
12	36M	0	0	0	0	0	+	21	3	440	W	0	+	+‖	41	42	1	PVE
13	36F	↑	0	25	—	0	+	27	3	710	W,D	+	0	0	42	31	0	AR¶

*Size range of Bjork-Shiley prosthesis = 19 to 31 mm †Infected thrombus ‡Aortocoronary bypass grafts also §Mitral valve replacement with a Starr-Edwards prosthesis, also tricuspid valve replacement with a porcine xenograft ‖This leak was secondary to infective endocarditis postoperatively ¶Induced at time of mitral valve replacement 3 months earlier
↑ = increased, — = not measured or information not available, + = positive, 0 = absent
A = aortic valve, AR = aortic regurgitation, CHD = coronary heart disease, D = dipyridamole, LA = left atrial, LV = left ventricular, M = mitral valve, mdg = mean diastolic gradient, postop = postoperative, preop = preoperative, PVE = prosthetic valve endocarditis, PVT = prosthetic valve thrombosis, ? = uncertain, SA = systemic arterial, psg = peak systolic gradient, W = warfarin sodium

tient). In none of the three patients with mitral commissurotomy was the mitral valve judged at necropsy to be adequately opened.

Infection appeared to be responsible for death in three patients All three had septicemia: Two had wound infections (gram-negative organisms) with extensive mediastinal and pulmonary infection; the third had infection (*Staphylococcus aureus*) behind the site of attachment of the prosthesis with partial disruption, severe aortic regurgitation and congestive heart failure.

Prosthetic dysfunction appeared responsible for death in two patients, both of whom died in the operating room A purely stenotic mitral valve was replaced in each but the left ventricular cavity in each was too small to accommodate the prosthesis, which was not able to open or close well because its margins contacted the ventricular septum. One of these two patients, a 50 year old woman, was a pituitary dwarf who weighed only 22.5 kg, and she had the smallest left ventricular cavity of any patient we have studied at necropsy after valve replacement. The second patient, a 50 year old man, had the largest size prosthesis (31 mm), and his left ventricle was too small to accommodate it. Although the disc appeared to open adequately during ventricular diastole, contraction of the ventricle caused the margins of the disc to contact the ventricular septum and this contact prevented closure and allowed severe prosthetic regurgitation (Fig 3)

Patients Who Died Late

Of the 13 patients who died late, single valve replacement was carried out in 12 and triple valve replacement in 1 (Table VI, Fig 5 to 9). *Noninfective prosthetic valve thrombi* were present in four patients, causing total obstruction in three. *Prosthetic valve endocarditis* occurred in four patients, causing in each fatal regurgitation from partial detachment. *A peribasilar leak unassociated with prosthetic infection* caused fatal aortic regurgitation in one patient. *Mechanical interference to mitral disc opening from "massive" aortic regurgitation* occurred in one patient (Case 13, Table VI) Aortic regurgitation was inadvertently produced at mitral valve replacement 103 days before death and cardiac catheterization performed 90 days after mitral valve replacement revealed a mean diastolic gradient of 25 mm Hg across the prosthesis. The patient died in the operating room at the time of aortic valve replacement, and at necropsy there was no evidence of mitral prosthetic dysfunction. It is likely, however, that during life the large aortic regurgitant jet stream interfered with proper opening of the mitral disc

Hemosiderosis: Sections of kidney were available in 9 of the 13 patients (Table VI). Stains for iron (Prussian blue reaction) disclosed renal hemosiderosis[31] in 3 of the 9 patients, but only one patient (Case 6, Table VI) had massive iron deposits

Hemodynamics: Cardiac catheterization was performed late postoperatively in four patients In the three with aortic valve prostheses, the peak systolic pressure gradient between the left ventricle and systemic artery was 10, 35 and 80 mm Hg, respectively. The two patients (both women) with the highest gradients had small-sized (no. 19) Björk-Shiley prostheses; both women were small (40 and 51 kg, respectively), and both had a relatively small-sized ascending aorta. In the one patient with a mitral valve prosthesis, the mean diastolic gradient between the pulmonary arterial wedge position and the left ventricle was 25 mm Hg. This patient had uncorrected severe aortic regurgitation, and it is suspected that the aortic regurgitant jet contacted the disc of the mitral prosthesis during ventricular diastole preventing adequate opening of the mitral prosthesis.

No evidence of degeneration or variance was observed in any of the 13 Björk-Shiley prostheses studied late postoperatively.

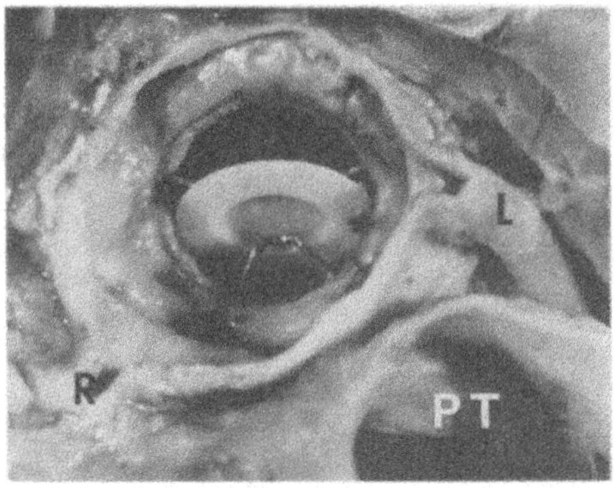

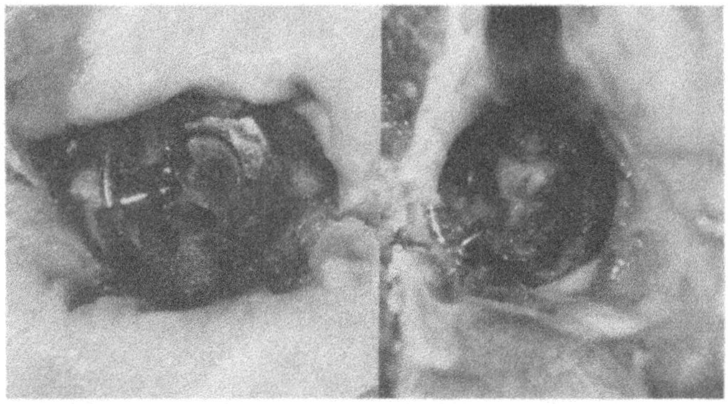

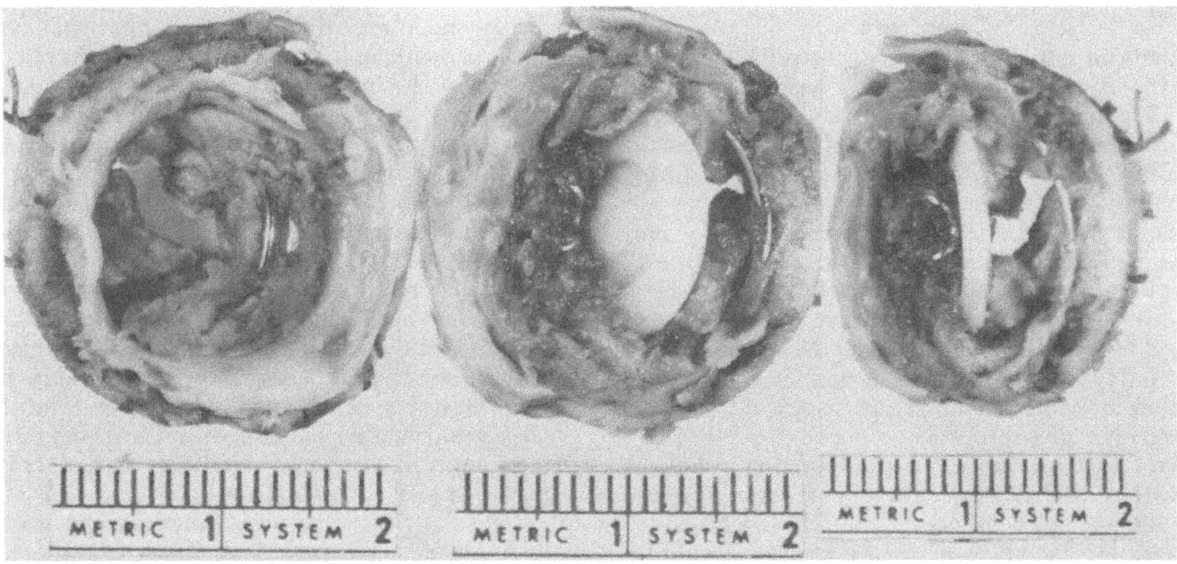

FIGURE 5 (upper left). Well functioning Björk-Shiley aortic valve prosthesis in Patient 8 (Table VI). This prosthesis had been in place for 15 months and functioned well. The disc is of Delrin. L = left and R = right coronary artery; PT = pulmonary trunk.
FIGURE 6 (bottom). Three views of thrombosed (noninfected) Björk-Shiley aortic valve prosthesis in Patient 2 (Table VI). This prosthesis had been in place for 270 days and the patient had not been receiving warfarin sodium. **Left,** view from ventricular side. **Center,** view from aortic side showing immobilization of the Delrin disc. **Right,** view from aortic side showing orifice in its maximal dimension. Severe prosthetic obstruction was present.
FIGURE 7 (upper right). Prosthetic thrombosis in Patient 11 (Table VI). This patient died from severe obstruction to the aortic prosthesis by thrombus. The patient had not been receiving warfarin sodium. **Left,** from above. **Right,** from the left ventricle. Thrombus is located on both sides of the prosthesis, causing it to be immobile.

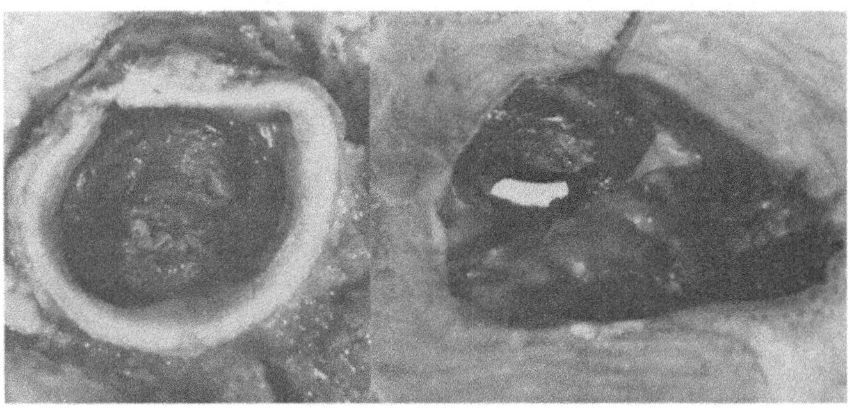

FIGURE 8. Prosthetic thrombosis in Patient 4 (Table VI). This patient died from severe obstruction to the aortic prosthesis by thrombus. The patient had not been receiving warfarin sodium. **Left,** from the aorta. **Right,** from the left ventricle. Thrombus is located on both sides of the prosthesis, causing it to be immobile.

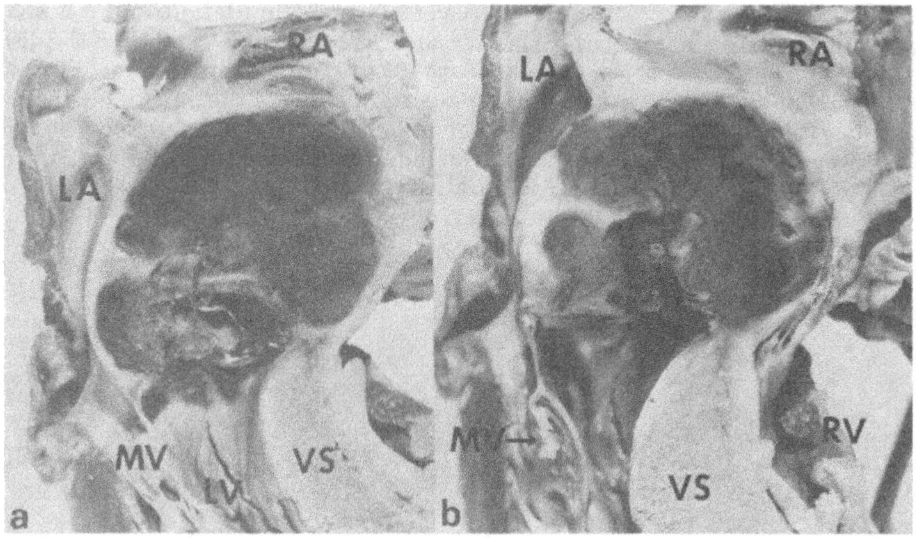

FIGURE 9. Prosthetic endocarditis. Disc of Björk-Shiley aortic valve prosthesis immobilized by infected thrombus in Patient 6 (Table VI). These photographs were taken of the anterior half of the heart as viewed from the back. The prosthesis was in place for 330 days. The patient had evidence of infective endocarditis for about 2 weeks before death. **a,** with prosthesis in place. **b,** after removal of the prosthesis. LA = left atrium; LV = left ventricle; MV = mitral valve; RA = right atrium; RV = right ventricle; VS = ventricular septum.

Comments

Since its introduction as a valve substitute in January 1969, the Björk-Shiley prosthesis has progressively gained in popularity among surgeons and it is now used in many cardiovascular surgical clinics throughout the world.[32–43] Clinical studies from several centers during the subsequent 6 years have indicated that this tilting-disc prosthesis has excellent hemodynamic characteristics,[33,40] is minimally traumatic to erythrocytes,[44] and, at least since the substitution of pyrolytic carbon for Delrin® as the material of the disc, does not degenerate (at least at this point in time). Nevertheless, the Björk-Shiley prosthesis is not a perfect one because thrombus may form on it and anticoagulant therapy is required on a long-term basis.[45]

Valve dysfunction: The preceding morphologic observations in the 46 patients support the clinical observations reported by others that the Björk-Shiley prosthesis is a good prosthetic cardiac valve. Death related to the size of the prosthesis is uncommon: in only 2 of the 33 patients who died early (less than 2 months after operation) was the prosthesis too large for the cavity (left ventricle or aorta) into which it was inserted. Death in none of the other patients could be related to interference with disc movement by the wall of the left ventricle or aorta. Among patients who died late (more than 2 months after operation), there was no evidence of degeneration, wear or variance of the prosthesis up to 30 months after insertion. Hemolysis, as evidenced by renal hemosiderosis,[31] was absent or minimal except in one patient who had prosthetic aortic obstruction and incompetence due to the presence of a huge infected thrombus.

Cause of death: In this study, as in previous studies from this laboratory, an attempt has been made to pinpoint a single principal cause of death of each patient after valve replacement. In some cases possibly more than one explanation is proper, but a judgment has been made as to which factor appeared to be the initial or at least the dominant cause. Although there may be some disagreement regarding a particular patient's principal cause of death, as long as the same person is making the judgment the information is useful in comparing one prosthesis, or one patient with a prosthesis, with another. During the past 14 years one of us (W.C.R.) has examined at necropsy the hearts of approximately 400 patients who died after replacement of one or more cardiac valves with prostheses, and the same investigator has assigned a principal cause of death to each case. The prostheses inserted in these 400 patients included the caged ball prosthesis (mainly Starr-Edwards type) valves,[16] caged disc prosthesis (Hufnagel and Kay-Shiley types),[20] tissue valves (mainly porcine type)[46] and synthetic trileaflet valve (Hufnagel).[47] Observations in the patients with tilting-disc prostheses are compared with those in patients with other types of prostheses in Tables VII and VIII.

Causes of death after cardiac valve replacement may be subdivided into three general types: (1) those related to the prosthesis, (2) those related to the underlying cardiac condition, and (3) those related neither to the prosthesis nor to the heart. Although superficial examination of Table VII might tend to indicate relatively similar percentages of death related to the prosthesis and heart disease among patients with any of the four valve prostheses analyzed, closer examination of the group with "prosthesis-related" death shows a striking difference between the central or semicentral flow prostheses (tilting or pivoting disc [Björk-Shiley] and trileaflet) and the peripheral flow prostheses (caged ball and caged disc). This difference was the frequency of prosthetic dysfunction produced by prosthetic disproportion. A major cause of death early after replacement with a caged ball or caged disc type of prosthesis was inadequate space in the cardiac ventricle or ascending aorta to accommodate the prosthesis readily. If the space for peripheral flow is inadequate the consequence may be inflow or outflow obstruction, or both, produced by the prostheses itself. Prosthetic disproportion was judged to be the cause of early death in 29 of 125 pa-

TABLE VII

Causes of Death (1 per patient) After Cardiac Valve Replacement

Patients	Caged Ball no	Caged Ball %	Caged Disc no	Caged Disc %	Trileaflet no	Trileaflet %	Tilting Disc no	Tilting Disc %
Early deaths (<2 months)								
Prosthesis-related	60	48	17	38	3	42	5	15
Disproportion	29		14		0		1	
Infection	3		0		0		3	
Other	28		3		3		0	
No anatomic cause	30	24	7	16	1	14	13	40
Coronary heart disease	10	8	4	9	1	14	5	15
Uncorrected valve disease	7	6	6	13	1	14	4	12
Bleeding	12	10	11	24	1	14	6	18
Miscellaneous	6	4	0		0		0	
Totals	125	100	45	100	7	100	33	100
Late deaths (>2 months)								
Prosthesis-related	52	57	10	63	8	62	9	69
Degeneration	18		1		6		0	
Stenosis	6		1		0		0	
Regurgitation	2		1		1		1	
Infection	5		3		1		5	
Thrombosis	1		3		0		2	
Other	20		1		0		1	
No anatomic cause	14	15	2	13	0		3	23
Coronary heart disease	10	11	2	12	4	30	1	8
Uncorrected valve disease	4	4	1	6	0		0	
Myocardial disease	3	3	0		0		0	
Miscellaneous	9	10	1	6	1	8	0	
Totals	92	100	16	100	13	100	13	100

TABLE VIII

Observations at Necropsy in 135 Patients Who Died Late (more than 2 months) After Replacement of One or More Cardiac Valves With Various Prostheses

	Caged Ball no	Caged Ball %	Caged Disc no	Caged Disc %	Trileaflet no	Trileaflet %	Tilting Disc no	Tilting Disc %
Patients	96		16		13		13	
Months from operation to death								
Range	2 1–116		4–47		2 1–58		3–30	
Average		28		21		22		11
Prosthetic thrombi (noninfected)								
Patients with thrombi	71	81	14	88	7	54	4	31
Patients taking warfarin with thrombi	49		14		7		1	
Thrombi causing dysfunction	21		1		3		3	
Clinical emboli	16	17	6	37	4	31	0	
Prosthetic variance	22/42	52*	10/11	91†	6/10	60†	0/6†	
Renal hemosiderosis	36/51	71	13/16	81	3/7	43‡	3/9	33§
Prosthetic endocarditis	5	5	2	12	1	8	4/13	31
Prosthetic ring leaks (noninfective)	11	11	4	25	2	15	1/13	8
Coronary atherosclerosis (>75% narrowing of 1 or more of the 3 major coronary arteries)	17	18	6	38	2	15	1/13	8
Myocardial fibrosis								
Transmural (TM)	27	28	4	25	3	23	2	20
Subendocardial (SE)	15	16	0		8	61	3	30
Either TM or SE	42	44	4	25	11	84	5	50

*Implantation period >2 years and variance of silicone rubber poppet only To date there are no reports describing variance of the Stellite 21 poppet Wear of the cloth of the struts, however, is common in the prostheses with hollow metal poppets

†Implantation period >1 year

‡Only in patients with malfunctioning (incompetent) protheses

§Quantity in 2 of the 3 patients was minute, whereas the quantity of renal iron in the patients with caged ball or caged disc prostheses was generally heavy tients (23 percent) after valve replacement with a caged ball prosthesis[13] and in 14 of 45 patients (31 percent) after valve replacement with a caged disc prosthesis.[20] In contrast, prosthetic disproportion was judged to be the cause of early death in only 2 of 33 patients (6 percent) who died early after valve replacement with a Bjork-Shiley prosthesis (Table VII). This low rate of early death from prosthetic disproportion among patients with a tilting disc prosthesis probably explains the greater percent with "no anatomic explanation" in this group compared with patients with peripheral flow prostheses. The percent with underlying severe coronary atherosclerosis, myocardial fibrosis and associated uncorrected valvular heart disease was similar among the four groups. The greater frequency of excessive bleeding after caged disc valve replacement may be attributed to the frequent use of a widening patch in the aortic root.[48]

Thromboembolism: Although thromboembolism may occur after cardiac valve replacement with a tilting disc prosthesis, it occurs no more frequently, and possibly less frequently, than with either the caged ball or caged disc prosthesis. Prosthetic thrombi were observed at necropsy in 7 of the 13 patients with Bjork-Shiley prostheses who died late (Table VIII), but 3 of the 7 had prosthetic endocarditis. Thus, it is possible that only 4 of the 13 had noninfected prosthetic thrombi. In three of the four patients with noninfected thrombi, the clots obstructed the prostheses but none of these three patients had been receiving warfarin sodium. Of the five patients receiving warfarin and without prosthetic endocarditis, only one had thrombus on the prosthesis at necropsy, and the thrombus was small and did not interfere with disc movement. In contrast, prosthetic valve thrombi were observed at necropsy in 71 (74 percent) of 96 patients who died late after valve replacement with a caged ball prosthesis[16]; 49 of the 71 had been receiving warfarin sodium.

Advantages of the tilting disc prosthetic valve: This valve has three distinct advantages over the caged ball or caged disc prosthesis, and two of these are summarized in Table VIII. (1) Thus far, the tilting or pivoting disc[49] prosthesis has shown no evidence of wear or variance (since the Delrin® disc has been replaced with a pyrolytic carbon one). Both the caged ball and caged disc prostheses have shown evidence of prosthetic degeneration that at times has been fatal. (2) The tilting disc prosthesis is relatively nonobstructive in most patients. The caged ball and caged disc prostheses, in contrast, nearly always produce some pressure gradient, at times a large one. (3) The tilting disc prosthesis causes only a minimal degree of hemolysis to erythrocytes. With the exception of our patient with an immobile infected prosthesis, renal hemosiderosis, the anatomic indicator of intravascular hemolysis,[31] was either absent or minimal in the remaining 10 patients whose kidney was examined. In contrast, renal hemosiderosis was found in 36 (71 percent) of 51 patients with caged ball prostheses and in 27 of them it was heavy (3+ or 4+ on a scale of 4[16]); likewise, renal hemosiderosis was observed in 13 of 16 patients who died late after valve replacement with a caged disc prosthesis.[20] The frequency of prosthetic valve endocarditis was surprisingly large (4 of 13 patients) in the patients who died late after valve replacement with Bjork-Shiley prostheses. The reason for the greater frequency in this group than in patients with the other three prostheses (Table VIII) is uncertain. The frequencies of prosthetic ring leaks, severe (greater than 75 percent luminal narrowing) coronary atherosclerosis and myocardial fibrosis are not dependent on the type of prosthetic valve utilized; nevertheless, these factors are shown in Table VIII for comparison.

A caution might be mentioned regarding mitral valve replacement with a tilting disc prosthesis in association with uncorrected, although mild, aortic regurgitation. It has been pointed out previously that aortic regurgitation may cause cocking of a mitral disc of a caged disc prosthesis.[16,50,51] It would appear from study of our Patient 13 (Table VI) that aortic regurgitation also may prevent proper opening of a mitral tilting disc prosthesis and lead to mitral prosthetic dysfunction.

References

1. **Roberts WC, Morrow AG:** Mechanisms of acute left atrial thrombosis after mitral valve replacement. Pathologic findings indicating obstruction to left atrial emptying. Am J Cardiol 18: 497–503, 1966
2. **Roberts WC, Morrow AG:** Late postoperative pathological findings after cardiac valve replacement. Circulation 35, 36: Suppl I: I-48–I-62, 1967
3. **Roberts WC, Morrow AG:** Causes of early postoperative death following cardiac valve replacement. Clinico-pathologic correlations in 64 patients studied at necropsy. J Thorac Cardiovasc Surg 54: 422–437, 1967
4. **Roberts WC, Morrow AG:** Anatomic studies of hearts containing caged-ball prosthetic valves. Johns Hopkins Med J 121: 271–295, 1967
5. **Quattlebaum FW, Kalke B, Edwards JE, et al:** Obstruction of the aorta by prosthetic aortic valve. J Thorac Cardiovasc Surg 55: 231–237, 1968
6. **Roberts WC, Morrow AG:** Secondary left ventricular endocardial fibroelastosis following mitral valve replacement. Cause of cardiac failure in the late postoperative period. Circulation 37, 38: Suppl II: II-101–II-109, 1968
7. **Roberts WC, Morrow AG:** Fatal degeneration of the silicone rubber ball of the Starr-Edwards prosthetic aortic valve. Am J Cardiol 22: 614–620, 1968
8. **Kalke B, Korns ME, Goott B, et al.** Engagement of ventricular myocardium by open-cage atrioventricular valvular prosthesis. J Thorac Cardiovasc Surg 58: 92–94, 1969
9. **Niles NR, Sandilands JR:** Pathology of heart valve replacement surgery: autopsies of 62 patients with Starr-Edwards prostheses. Dis Chest 56: 373–382, 1969
10. **Roberts WC, Levinson GE, Morrow AG.** Lethal ball variance in the Starr-Edwards prosthetic mitral valve. Arch Intern Med 126: 517–521, 1970
11. **Ibarra-Perez C, Rodriguez-Trujillo F, Perez-Redondo H:** Engagement of ventricular myocardium by struts of mitral prosthesis. Fatal complication of use of open-cage cardiac valves. J Thorac Cardiovasc Surg 61: 403–404, 1971
12. **Colapinto ND, Silver MD:** Prosthetic heart valve replacement. Causes of early postoperative death. J Thorac Cardiovasc Surg

61 938–944, 1971
13 **Roberts WC, Morrow AG:** Causes of death and other anatomic observations after cardiac valve replacement Adv Cardiol 7 226–247, 1972
14 **Winter TQ, Reis RL, Glancy DL, et al:** Current status of the Starr-Edwards cloth-covered prosthetic cardiac valves Circulation 45, 46 Suppl I I-14–I-24, 1972
15 **Joassin A, Edwards JE:** Late causes of death after mitral valve replacement Analysis of 36 cases J Thorac Cardiovasc Surg 65 255–263, 1973
16 **Roberts WC, Bulkley BH, Morrow AG:** Pathologic anatomy of cardiac valve replacement a study of 224 necropsy patients Prog Cardiovasc Dis 15 539–587, 1973
17 **Joassin A, Edwards JE:** Causes of death within 30 days of mitral valvular replacement Analysis of 93 cases Cardiovasc Clin 5 169–184, 1973
18 **Bulkley BH, Morrow AG, Roberts WC.** Calcification of prosthetic valve anuli a late complication of cardiac valve replacement Am Heart J 87 129–133, 1974
19 **Seningen RP, Bulkley BH, Roberts WC.** Prosthetic aortic stenosis A method to prevent its occurrence by measurement of aortic size from preoperative aortogram Circulation 49 921–924, 1974
20 **Roberts WC, Fishbein MC, Golden A:** Cardiac pathology after valve replacement by disc prosthesis A study of 61 necropsy patients Am J Cardiol 35 740–760, 1975
21 **Fishbein MC, Roberts WC.** Late postoperative anatomic observations after insertion of Hufnagel caged-ball prostheses in descending thoracic aorta Chest 68 6–11, 1975
22 **Henze A, Carlsson S, Bjork VO:** Mortality and pathology following aortic valve replacement with the Bjork-Shiley tilting disc valve Scand J Thorac Cardiovasc Surg 7 7–16, 1973
23 **Roberts WC:** The congenitally bicuspid aortic valve A study of 85 autopsy cases Am J Cardiol 26 72–83, 1970
24 **Roberts WC:** The structure of the aortic valve in clinically isolated aortic stenosis An autopsy study of 162 patients over 15 years of age Circulation 42 91–97, 1970
25 **Roberts WC:** Anatomically isolated aortic valvular disease The case against its being of rheumatic etiology Am J Med 49 151–159, 1970
26 **Buchbinder NA, Roberts WC:** Left-sided valvular active infective endocarditis A study of forty-five necropsy patients Am J Med 53 20–35, 1972
27 **Roberts WC, Braunwald E, Morrow AG:** Acute severe mitral regurgitation secondary to ruptured chordae tendineae Clinical, hemodynamic, and pathologic considerations Circulation 33 58–70, 1966
28 **Roberts WC, Cohen LS:** Left ventricular papillary muscles Description of the normal and a survey of conditions causing them to be abnormal Circulation 46 138–154, 1972
29 **Cooley DA, Reul CJ, Wukasch DC:** Ischemic contracture of the heart "stone heart" Am J Cardiol 29 575–577, 1972
30 **Roberts WC, Perloff JK, Constantino T** Severe valvular aortic stenosis in patients over 65 years of age A clinicopathologic study Am J Cardiol 27 497–506, 1971
31 **Roberts WC, Morrow AG:** Renal hemosiderosis in patients with prosthetic aortic valves Circulation 33 390–398, 1966
32 **Bjork VO:** A new central-flow tilting disc valve prosthesis One year's clinical experience with 103 patients J Thorac Cardiovasc Surg 60 355–374, 1970
33 **Bjork VO, Holmgren A, Olin C, et al·** Clinical and hemodynamic results of aortic valve replacement with the Bjork-Shiley tilting disc valve prosthesis Scand J Thorac Cardiovasc Surg 5 177–191, 1971
34 **Messmer BJ, Okies JE, Hallman GL, et al:** Mitral valve replacement with the Bjork-Shiley tilting-disc prosthesis J Thorac Cardiovasc Surg 62 938–946, 1971
35 **Bjork VO, Olin C, Rodriguez L·** Comparative results of aortic valve replacement with different prosthetic heart valves J Cardiovasc Surg 13 268–271, 1972
36 **Messmer BJ, Okies JE, Hallman GL, et al:** Early and late thrombo-embolic complications after mitral valve replacement A comparative study of various prostheses J Cardiovasc Surg 13 281–289, 1972
37 **Messmer BJ, Okies JE, Hallman GL, et al:** Aortic valve replacement two years' experience with the Bjork-Shiley tilting-disc prosthesis Surgery 72 772–779, 1972
38 **Fernandez J, Maranhao V, Gooch AS, et al:** The Bjork-Shiley prosthesis A significant advance in aortic valve replacement Ann Thorac Surg 14 527–538, 1972
39 **Lepley D, Reuben CF, Flemma RJ, et al·** Experience with the Bjork-Shiley prosthetic valve Circulation 47, 48 Suppl III III-51–III-55, 1973
40 **Bjork VO, Book K, Cernigliaro C, et al:** The Bjork-Shiley tilting disc valve in isolated mitral lesions Scand J Thorac Cardiovasc Surg 7 131–148, 1973
41 **Nitter-Hauge S, Hall K-V, Froysaker T, et al:** Aortic valve replacement one-year results with Lillehei-Kaster and Bjork-Shiley disc prosthesis Am Heart J 88 23–28, 1974
42 **Bjork VO, Henze A, Holmgren A.** Five years' experience with the Bjork-Shiley tilting-disc valve in isolated aortic valvular disease J Thorac Cardiovasc Surg 68 393–404, 1974
43 **Bjork VO, Henze A, Holmgren A:** Long-term results with the Bjork-Shiley tilting disc valve in aortic valvular disease Isr J Med Sci 11 161–172, 1975
44 **Slater SD, Sallam IA, Bain WH, et al:** Haemolysis with Bjork-Shiley and Starr-Edwards prosthetic heart valves a comparative study Thorax 29 624–631, 1974
45 **Ben-Zvi J, Hildner FJ, Chandraratna PA, et al:** Thrombosis on Bjork-Shiley aortic valve prosthesis Clinical, arteriographic, echocardiographic and therapeutic observations in seven cases Am J Cardiol 34 538–544, 1974
46 **Yarbrough JW, Roberts WC, Reis RL:** Structural alterations in tissue cardiac valves implanted in patients and in calves J Thorac Cardiovasc Surg 65 364–375, 1973
47 **Fishbein MC, Roberts WC, Golden A, et al:** Cardiac pathology after aortic valve replacement using Hufnagel trileaflet prostheses a study of 20 necropsy patients Am Heart J 89 443–448, 1975
48 **Stenseth JH, Danielson GK, McGoon DC.** Pericardial patch enlargement of the aortic outflow tract J Thorac Cardiovasc Surg 62 442–448, 1971
49 **Lillehei CW, Kaster RL, Coleman M, et al:** Heart-valve replacement with Lillehei-Kaster pivoting disc prosthesis NY State J Med 8 1426–1438, 1974
50 **Edgett JW, Nelson WP, Hall RJ, et al:** A complication of valve replacement by a caged-lens prosthesis Circulation 36 422–426, 1967
51 **Hammermeister KE, Dillard DH, Kennedy JW.** Severe, intermittent, mitral regurgitation in a Cross-Jones valve Report of a case with angiocardiographic and hemodynamic observations J Thorac Cardiovasc Surg 58 575–580, 1969

Prosthetic Valve Endocarditis

Clinicopathologic Analysis of 22 Necropsy Patients With Comparison of Observations in 74 Necropsy Patients With Active Infective Endocarditis Involving Natural Left-Sided Cardiac Valves

ERNEST N. ARNETT, MD
WILLIAM C. ROBERTS, MD, FACC

Bethesda, Maryland

Clinical and morphologic features are described in 22 necropsy patients with endocarditis involving rigid-framed prosthetic valves: aortic in 15 patients and mitral in 7. The interval from valve replacement to onset of symptoms of prosthetic valve endocarditis was less than 2 months in 8 patients and longer than 2 months in 14 patients. The most frequent infecting organism was the Staphylococcus (13 patients). In each of the 22 patients the infection was located behind the site of attachment of the prosthesis to the valve ring, and the infection spread to adjacent structures in 13 patients, 11 of whom had aortic prostheses. Prosthetic detachment causing severe regurgitation occurred in 12 of the 15 patients with an infected aortic valve prosthesis, and in 2 of the 7 with an infected mitral valve prosthesis. Prosthetic obstruction by vegetative material occurred in 5 of 7 patients with prosthetic mitral infection and in only 1 of 15 with prosthetic aortic infection. High degrees of conduction defects developed in seven patients with aortic prosthetic valve endocarditis: complete heart block in five, and complete left bundle branch block in two.

Comparison of observations in the 22 patients with prosthetic valve endocarditis with those in 74 patients with active infective endocarditis involving natural left-sided cardiac valves revealed significant ($P < 0.05$) differences in the percent with ring abscess, hemodynamic consequences of the endocarditis (valve stenosis), frequency of Staphylococcus as the causative organism and percent with complete heart block or left bundle branch block. No significant differences were observed between the two groups when comparing age, sex, type of underlying valve disease or frequency of organ infarcts or splenomegaly.

From the Pathology Branch, National Heart and Lung Institute, National Institutes of Health, Bethesda, Md. Manuscript received January 16, 1976; revised manuscript received March 29, 1976, accepted March 31, 1976.

Address for reprints: William C. Roberts, MD, Bldg. 10A, Room 3E-30, National Institutes of Health, Bethesda, Md. 20014.

Among 450 consecutive patients with one or more rigid-framed prosthetic cardiac valves studied by us at necropsy,[1–7] 22 (5 percent) had infection involving a prosthetic valve. These 22 patients represent 17 percent of the 127 patients with active valvular infective endocarditis studied in this laboratory.[8–10] Although many reports are available on patients with fatal active infective endocarditis involving natural cardiac valves, surprisingly little information is available on the morphologic features of endocarditis involving prosthetic cardiac valves. This report consequently focuses on the clinicopathologic features in 22 patients with prosthetic valve endocarditis and compares them with the features we observed in 74 nonsurgical necropsy patients with active infective endocarditis involving natural left-sided cardiac valves.

Patients Studied

Clinical observations: Clinical and morphologic observations in the 22 patients with prosthetic valve

TABLE I

Prosthetic Valve Endocarditis: Type of Prosthesis Infected

	Aortic Valve	Mitral Valve	Totals
Caged ball	9*	6*	15*
Tilting disc	5†	0	5†
Poppet disc	1‡	1§	2
Totals	15	7	22

* Starr-Edwards; † Björk-Shiley; ‡ Hufnagel; § Kay-Shiley.

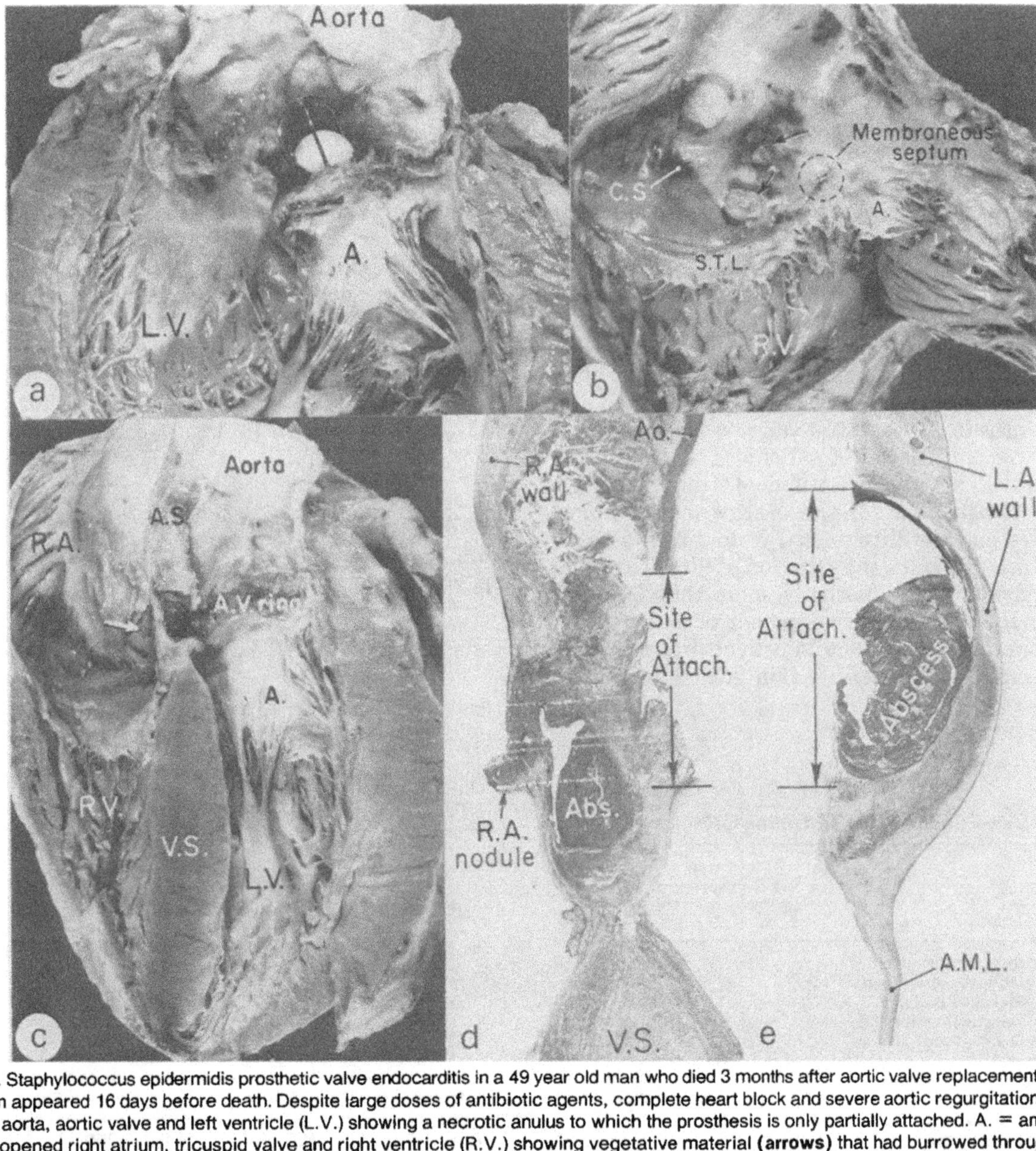

FIGURE 1. Staphylococcus epidermidis prosthetic valve endocarditis in a 49 year old man who died 3 months after aortic valve replacement. Symptoms of infection appeared 16 days before death. Despite large doses of antibiotic agents, complete heart block and severe aortic regurgitation developed. **a,** opened aorta, aortic valve and left ventricle (L.V.) showing a necrotic anulus to which the prosthesis is only partially attached. A. = anterior mitral leaflet. **b,** opened right atrium, tricuspid valve and right ventricle (R.V.) showing vegetative material **(arrows)** that had burrowed through the atrial septum from the necrotic aortic valve ring. C.S. = ostium of coronary sinus; S.T.L. = septal tricuspid leaflet; A. = anterior tricuspid leaflet. **c,** longitudinal section of the heart with the anterior portion removed. The necrotic aortic valve (A.V.) ring is again seen and the penetration of the infective process through the atrial septum (A.S.) is apparent. An **arrow** indicates the vegetation in the right atrium (R.A.). V.S. = ventricular septum. **d** and **e,** histologic sections through the ring abscess. The site of attachment (Attach.) of the prosthesis, which has been removed, is indicated. The infected nodule, an extension of the ring abscess (Abs.), is showing in the right atrium. Ao. = aortic wall; L.A. = left atrium; A.M.L. = anterior mitral leaflet.

TABLE II

Prosthetic Endocarditis: Clinical Observations in 22 Cases

Prosthesis Infected	Patients: no.	Patients: Age Range and Average (yr)	Patients: Sex: M	Patients: Sex: F	Preop Lesion: Stenosis	Preop Lesion: Pure Regurgitation	Interval From Valve Replacement to Infection: <2 mo	Interval From Valve Replacement to Infection: >2 mo	Duration of Signs and Symptoms of Infection: <60 Days	Duration of Signs and Symptoms of Infection: >60 Days	Patients Receiving Antibiotics >7 Days (no.)	Conduction Disturbance: LBBB	Conduction Disturbance: CHB	Prosthetic Dysfunction: Regurgitation	Prosthetic Dysfunction: Stenosis
Aortic	15	37–69 (54)	13	2	12	3	5	10	10	5	9	2	5	11	1
Mitral	7	37–65 (52)	3	4	7	0	3	4	6	1	2	0	0	0	0
Totals	22	37–69 (53)	16	6	19	3	8	14	16	6	13	2	5	11	1

CHB = complete heart block; LBBB = left bundle branch block; Preop = preoperative.

endocarditis are summarized in Tables I to V, and some of the morphologic features are illustrated in Figures 1 to 11. Certain observations in several of these patients have appeared elsewhere.[1–3,11–13] Patients with active infective endocarditis at the time of valve replacement were excluded. The 22 patients had 27 prosthetic cardiac valves; 17 patients had one prosthetic valve and 5 had two prosthetic valves. Of the 27 prosthetic valves, 22 were infected (Table I): the aortic prosthesis in 15 patients and the mitral in 7. Clinical evidence of infective endocarditis was present less than 2 months after operation in 8 patients (early deaths) (Table II), and from 3 months to 10 years after valve replacement in 14 patients. In 6 of the latter 14 patients clinical evidence of infection did not appear until more than 1 year after valve replacement. The duration of signs and symptoms of infective endocarditis ranged from 14 days to 13 months. In 16 patients, the duration of illness was less than 60 days and, in 6 patients, more than 60 days. Factors predisposing to development of endocarditis were apparent in only 5 of the 14 patients who died late: tooth extraction (2 patients), skin graft infection (1 patient), prolonged use of an intravenous catheter (1 patient) and prolonged use of a transthoracic pacing wire (1 patient). It is presumed that the infection in the eight patients who died early either was incurred at operation or was secondary to a wound infection.

The infecting organisms (cultured from the blood during life in 20 patients) are listed in Table III. Staphylococcus was the responsible organism in 13 patients, and a different organism in each of the other 9. Fungi caused the endocarditis in two patients who had negative blood cultures during life. Evidence of prosthetic dysfunction was present clinically in 12 of the 15 patients with an infected aortic valve prosthesis

TABLE III

Prosthetic Valve Endocarditis: Infecting Organism

Organism	Onset From Valve Replacement: <2 mo	Onset From Valve Replacement: >2 mo	Totals
I. Gram-positive bacterium	6	11	17
Staphylococcus epidermidis	3	7	10
Staphylococcus aureus	2	1	3
Streptococcus pneumoniae	0	1	1
Group-D streptococcus	0	1	1
Diphtheroids	1	0	1
Listeria monocytogenes	0	1	1
II. Gram-negative bacterium	1	2	3
Proteus mirabilis	1	0	1
Klebsiella species	0	1	1
Serratia marcescens	0	1	1
III. Fungus	1	1	2
Candida species	0	1	1
Aspergillus fumigatus	1	0	1
Totals	8	14	22

TABLE IV

Prosthetic Valve Endocarditis: Necropsy Observations in 22 Cases

Prosthesis Infected	Patients (no.)	Ring Abscess	Ring Organisms	Prosthetic Valve Detachment (Regurgitation)	Prosthetic Valve Stenosis
Aortic	15	15	8	12	1
Mitral	7	7	5	2	5
Totals	22	22	13	14	6

TABLE V

Prosthetic Valve Endocarditis: Organ Weights and Infarcts in 22 Cases

Prosthesis Infected	Patients (no.)	Organ Weight (g) (range and average): Spleen	Organ Weight (g) (range and average): Liver	Gross Infarcts (no. of patients): Spleen	Gross Infarcts (no. of patients): Kidney	Gross Infarcts (no. of patients): Brain
Aortic	15	120–1000 (470)	1450–2950 (2140)	7	3	3
Mitral	7	170–920 (370)	1350–2000 (1755)	5	4	4
Totals	22	120–1000 (460)	1350–2950 (2050)	12	7	7

(regurgitation in 11 and stenosis plus regurgitation in 1), but in none of the 7 patients with an infected mitral valve prosthesis. High grade conduction disturbances occurred in 7 patients, all in the group of 15 with an infected aortic prosthesis: left bundle branch block in 2 and complete heart block in 5. Thirteen of the 22 patients received appropriate antibiotic therapy for more than 7 days. Three patients underwent valve replacement for prosthetic endocarditis. The principal causes of death in the 22 patients were congestive heart failure (19 patients), central nervous system embolus (2 patients) and generalized infection (1 patient).

Morphologic observations: Among the 22 patients, 17 had one valve prosthesis and 5 had two valve prostheses. In each of the five latter patients, only the "downstream" prosthesis was infected: the aortic prosthesis in the three patients with mitral and aortic prostheses, and the mitral prosthesis in the two patients with tricuspid and mitral prostheses. Twelve of the 15 infected aortic valve prostheses and 2 of the 7 infected mitral valve prostheses were partially or completely detached. In contrast, 5 of the 7 infected mitral prostheses and only 1 of the 15 infected aortic prostheses were obstructed by vegetative material.

Ring abscesses (Table IV) were present in each of the 22 infected prostheses; in one the abscess was visible only by histologic examination. The ring abscess involved the entire valve anulus in 14 patients and only portions of the anulus in the other 8. In 13 of the 22 patients the infective process spread to adjacent

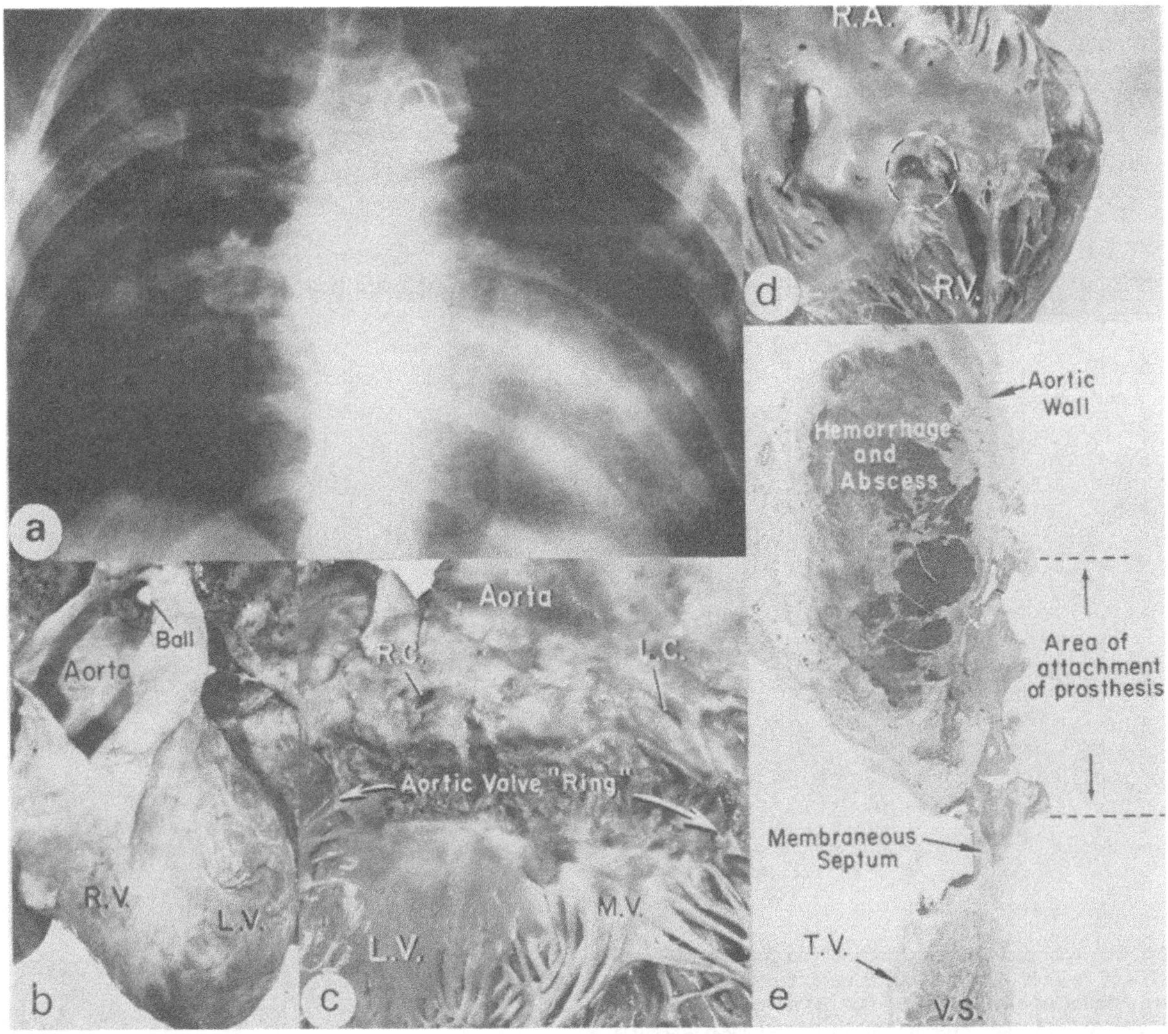

FIGURE 2. Staphylococcus epidermidis prosthetic aortic valve endocarditis in a 48 year old man. He had been well for 11 months after insertion of the Starr-Edwards prosthesis when, 1 month before death and 6 weeks after dental extraction, shaking chills appeared and blood cultures were positive for Staphylococcus epidermidis. Despite intensive antibiotic therapy, signs of aortic regurgitation appeared, and minutes before death he complained of "feeling funny." **a,** chest roentgenogram immediately after death revealed that the prosthesis had dislodged and migrated to the aortic arch. **b,** anterior view of the heart and opened ascending aorta. The detached prosthesis ball is visible, lodged in the transverse aorta. L.V. = left ventricle; R.V. = right ventricle. **c,** opened aorta, aortic valve "ring" and left ventricle showing a totally necrotic aortic anulus. L.C. = ostium of left coronary artery; M.V. = anterior mitral leaflet; R.C. = ostium of right coronary artery. **d,** opened right atrium (R.A.), tricuspid valve and right ventricle showing a ring abscess **(dashed circle)** that had extended from the prosthetic aortic valve anulus. **e,** photomicrograph through the aortic valve "ring" showing a large ring abscess and the necrotic aortic anulus material that extended through the membranous ventricular septum into the right atrium. T.V. = tricuspid valve leaflet; V.S. = ventricular septum. (Hematoxylin-eosin X2, reduced by 24 percent.)

structures. In 11 of the 15 patients with an infected aortic aortic valve prosthesis the ring abscess burrowed into adjacent structures: through the ascending aorta into the periaortic space (7 patients); through the atrial septum into the right atrium (9 patients) or into the left atrium (2 patients); through the ventricular septum into the right ventricle (8 patients); and into the anterobasal left ventricular wall (2 patients). In two patients with an infected mitral valve prosthesis the ring abscess burrowed through the atrial wall into the pericardial space. Histologic examination of the infected rings disclosed colonies of organisms in 13 of the 22 patients.

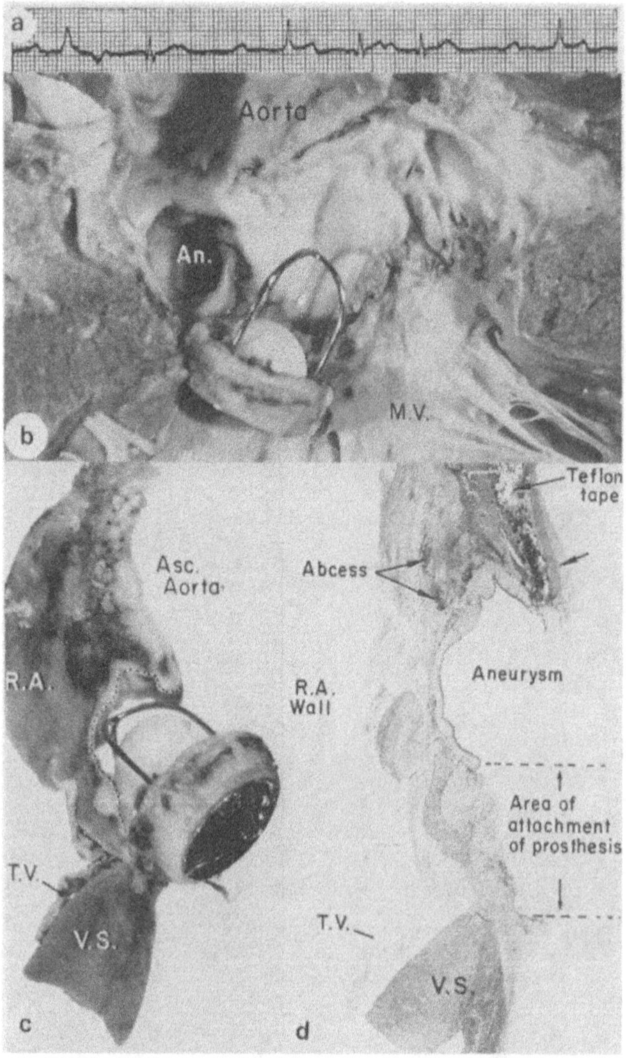

FIGURE 3. Staphylococcus epidermidis prosthetic aortic valve endocarditis in a 55 year old man. The Starr-Edwards prosthesis was used to replace an infected trileaflet Teflon® (Muller) valve 45 days before death. **a,** electrocardiogram revealing complete heart block and signs of massive aortic regurgitation that appeared despite antibiotic therapy. **b,** opened aorta, aortic valve and left ventricle. The aortic valve ring is necrotic, and the prosthesis is almost totally detached. The cage of the prosthesis has burrowed into the wall of the aorta causing a saccular aneurysm (An.). M.V. = mitral valve. **c,** longitudinal section showing the caged ball prosthesis burrowing into the ascending (Asc.) aorta, producing the aneurysm. R.A. = right atrium; T.V. = septal tricuspid valve leaflet; V.S. = ventricular septum. **d,** photomicrograph through the same area after removal of the prosthesis. (Hematoxylin-eosin ×2, reduced by 25 percent.)

Both arterial emboli and gross organ infarcts were common with both prosthetic aortic and prosthetic mitral valve endocarditis (Table V). Grossly visible infarcts were present in the spleen in 12, the kidney in 7 and the brain in 7 of the 22 patients. Two patients had a bowel infarct, one a pancreatic infarct and one a transmural myocardial infarct. In addition, mycotic aneurysms were present in the ascending aorta of three patients: in two patients, aneurysms resulted from jet lesions from the infected prosthesis and, in the third, the cage of the partially detached prosthesis burrowed into the wall of a weakened aorta (after an aortotomy performed weeks earlier) causing a sacular aneurysm.

The spleen ranged in weight from 120 to 1,000 g (average 460) and in 14 of the 22 patients it weighed more than 300 g. The liver ranged in weight from 1,350 to 2,950 g (average 2,050).

Comments

Clinical Features

Incidence: Study of our 22 necropsy patients and analysis of more than 150 necropsy cases of prosthetic valve endocarditis reported by others[14–47] allows certain general conclusions regarding this condition. It is a devastating complication of cardiac valve replacement,

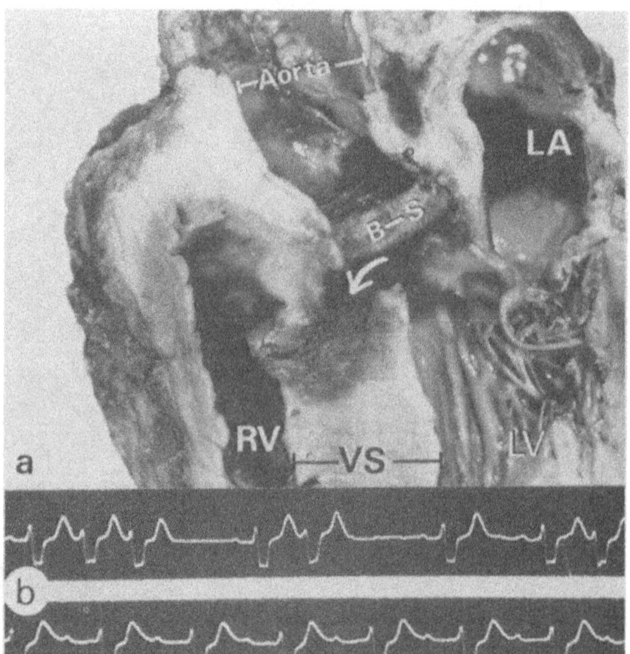

FIGURE 4. Staphylococcus epidermidis prosthetic aortic valve endocarditis in a 51 year old man. The stenotic bicuspid aortic valve had been replaced with a Björk-Shiley prosthesis 83 days before death. Fever was present in the early postoperative period, and shortly before death complete heart block and signs of congestive heart failure appeared. **a,** longitudinal section of the heart with the anterior portion removed. The Björk-Shiley (B-S) prosthesis is partially detached and the ring abscess **(arrow)** has burrowed through the ventricular septum (VS) into the right ventricle (RV). LA = left atrium; LV = left ventricle. **b,** rhythm strip obtained shortly before death revealing complete heart block.

but fortunately it is infrequent. The exact incidence rate is uncertain but it is clearly less than 1 percent annually among patients with prosthetic cardiac valves.[37,39,45,48] Although prospective studies[49,50] have been inconclusive, retrospective studies[16,17,51,52] have shown a reduction in the frequency of early (less than 2 months after valve replacement) endocarditis coincident with the use of prophylactic antibiotic therapy. Late prosthetic valve infection now appears to be more common than early infection,[37,45] presumably because there are now so many persons with prosthetic cardiac valves. Although the mortality rate is high for both groups,

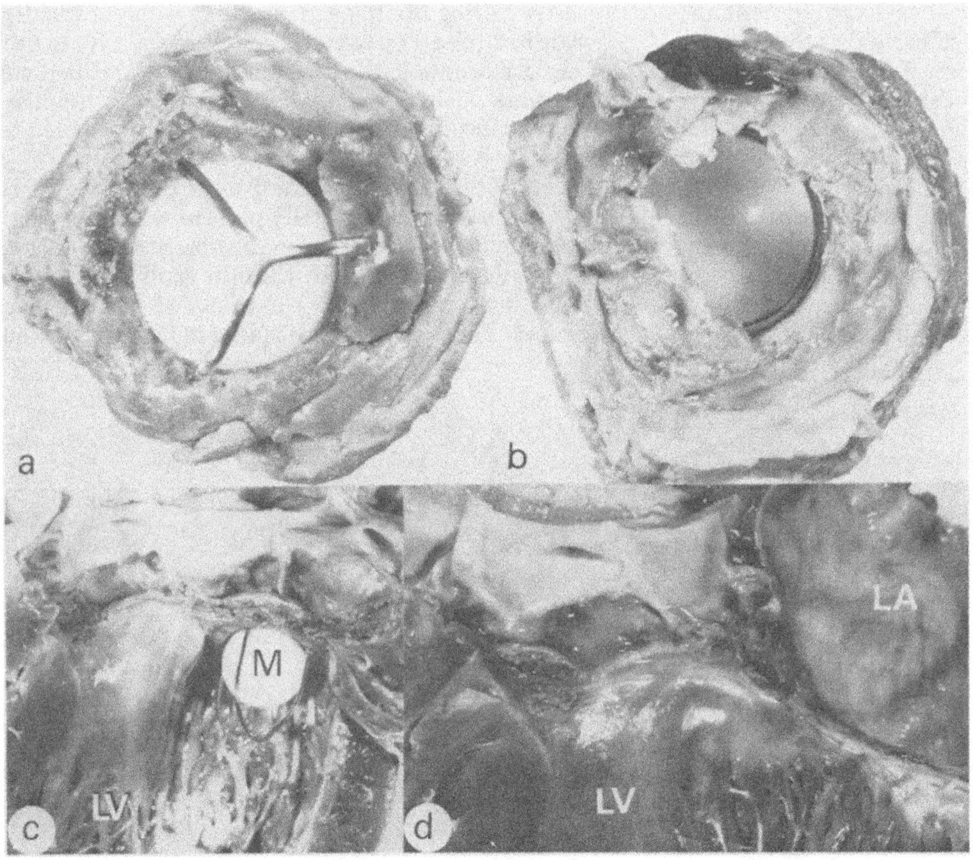

FIGURE 5. Serratia marcescens prosthetic aortic valve endocarditis in a 57 year old man whose infection occurred 4 months after replacement of both aortic and mitral valves. The apparent source of the infection was an intravenous catheter. Left bundle branch block and signs of aortic regurgitation appeared and, despite massive doses of antibiotic agents, he died 3 months after the onset of symptoms of infection. **a,** view of the aortic prosthesis from above. Infected thrombus is present on its anulus. **b,** view of the prosthesis as it appeared from the left ventricle. Some of the infected thrombus became detached during excision of this prosthesis at necropsy. The primary orifice is partially obstructed by the infected material. **c,** opened aortic root, aortic valve and left ventricle (LV) after removal of the aortic prosthesis. Most of the aortic ring is necrotic. In addition, the portion of mitral (M) prosthesis in direct apposition to the aortic anulus also is infected. **d,** view after excision of the mitral prosthesis showing extension of the aortic anular infection into the junctional area between the aortic and mitral anuli. LA = left atrium.

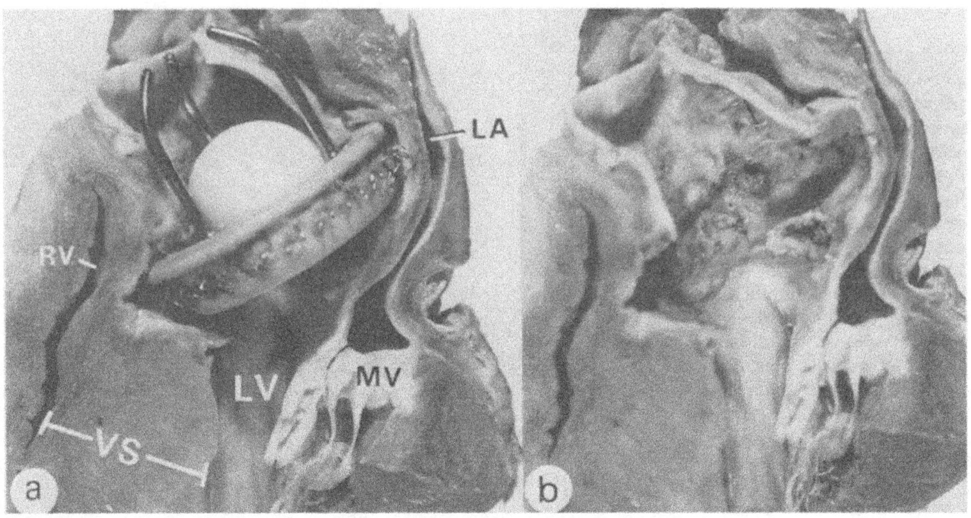

FIGURE 6. Staphylococcus epidermidis endocarditis originally involving a Björk-Shiley aortic valve prosthesis that was excised and replaced with a Magovern prosthesis 28 days before death in a 69 year old man. Fever and signs of aortic regurgitation appeared 7 months after aortic valve replacement with the Björk-Shiley prosthesis. After replacement with the Magovern prosthesis, a murmur of aortic regurgitation reappeared. At necropsy, the sewing ring of the Magovern prosthesis had burrowed deeply into the necrotic anulus, causing the ball of the prosthesis to strike the nonnecrotic portion of the aortic wall, probably producing prosthetic aortic stenosis. **a,** longitudinal section of the heart through the aortic anulus with the Magovern prosthesis in place; **b,** section after removal of the prosthesis. The frame of the prosthesis has burrowed deeply into the necrotic anulus. LA = left atrium; LV = left ventricle; MV = mitral valve; RV = right ventricular cavity; VS = ventricular septum.

early prosthetic valve infection apparently is more often fatal than late infection.[37,39,45,48]

Etiology: Most early infections either are incurred at operation or result from a wound infection.[25,29,37,39,48] Those at operation appear to result from contamination of the cardiopulmonary bypass equipment.[53,54] Staphylococcus is the organism cultured most frequently from cardiopulmonary bypass equipment and it is the most frequent cause of early prosthetic valve endocarditis.[14,16–18,25,30,37,39,44,45] When gram-negative bacteria or fungi cause endocarditis early, they are usually also recovered from the operating room equipment or from a wound infection.[28,39] Late infections usually result from transient bacteremias.[37,39,45,48] Although both staphylococci and streptococci are frequent causes of clinically diagnosed late prosthetic valve endocarditis,[37,39,45] the former have caused most cases of necropsy-proved late endocarditis and the latter relatively few. In none of our 22 necropsy patients was the infection caused by Streptococcus. Staphylococcus was the most common cause of endocarditis in our patients whether the infection occurred early or late.

Blood cultures: Among patients with prosthetic valve endocarditis, blood cultures are almost always positive, except when the infections are caused by certain fungi.[27,28,31,32,37,39,44,45,48] Blood cultures were positive during life in each of our 20 patients with endocarditis caused by bacteria and were negative in each of our 2 patients with fungal endocarditis. Blood cultures were positive in only 3 of 39 patients with endocarditis caused by Aspergillus species in a series reviewed by Kammer and Utz.[55]

Prosthetic valve dysfunction: Signs of prosthetic valve dysfunction are usually present when the aortic prosthesis is infected and usually absent when the mitral prosthesis is infected. Clinical signs of aortic regurgitation were present in 11 of our 15 patients with an infected aortic valve prosthesis. In three of the four

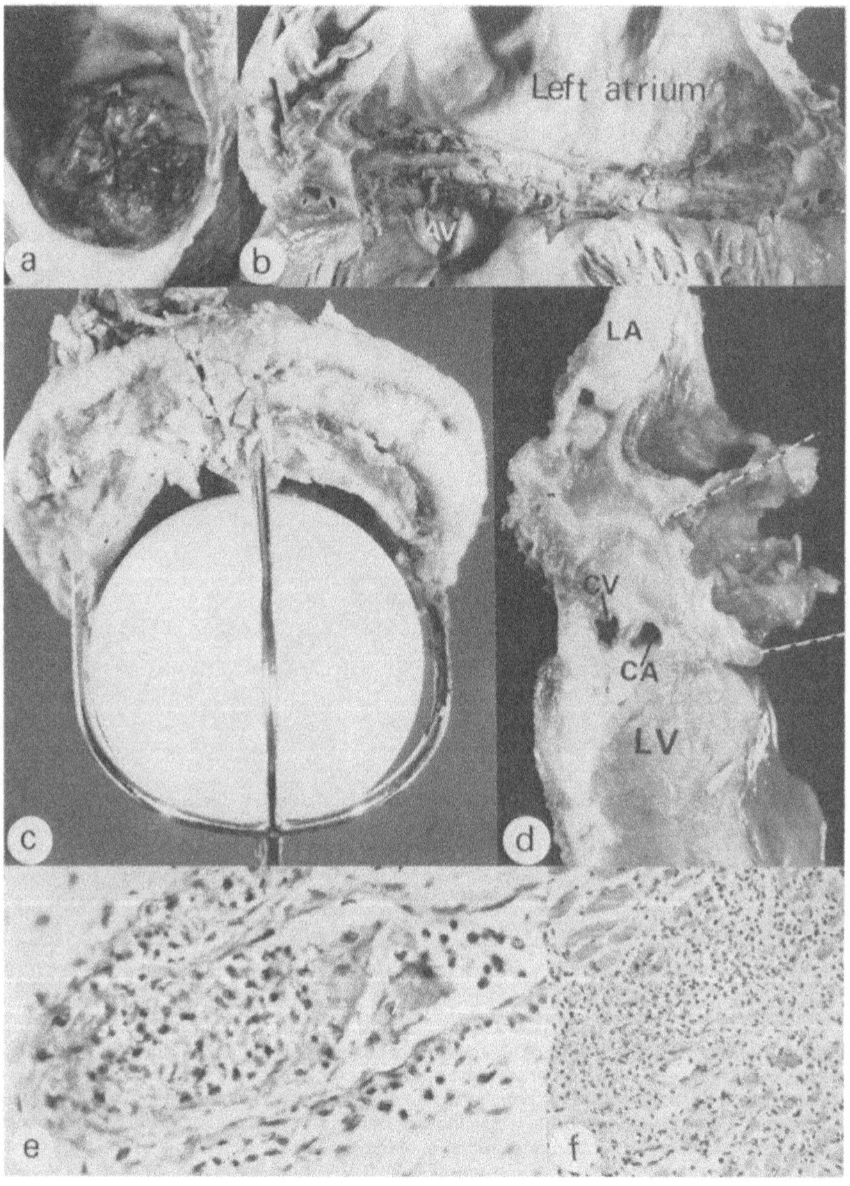

FIGURE 7. Staphylococcus aureus prosthetic mitral valve endocarditis in a 47 year old man who had the onset of symptoms of infective endocarditis 4 months after valve replacement. He had done well during the first 3 months after operation, but symptoms of infection developed after grafting of a cutaneous ulcer. Signs of prosthetic dysfunction were never detected clinically. **a,** prosthetic mitral valve orifice obstructed by vegetative material, as viewed from the left atrium. **b,** opened left atrium, mitral anulus and left ventricle after removal of the mitral prosthesis. The entire anulus is necrotic. AV = aortic valve. **c,** mitral valve prosthesis showing infected thrombus at its base. **d,** longitudinal section through the left atrium (LA), mitral anulus and left ventricle (LV). The former site of attachment of the prosthesis is designated by the **dashed lines.** The infective process burrowed through the wall of the heart and caused pericarditis. CA = coronary artery; CV = coronary vein in the right atrioventricular sulcus. **e** and **f,** hematoxylin-eosin-stained histologic sections of the left ventricle remote from the infected mitral anulus. **e,** infected embolus in an intramural coronary artery. **f,** microscopic-sized myocardial abscess. (×400 [**e**] and ×160 [**f**], reduced by 24 percent.)

patients without clinical signs of aortic regurgitation, the prosthesis was not detached at necropsy. Among patients with acute aortic regurgitation, however, classic signs of aortic regurgitation may be absent.[56–59] Signs of aortic regurgitation were not detected in three of nine necropsy patients with prosthetic aortic valve endocarditis described by Madison et al.,[44] but all three had prosthetic detachment at necropsy.

In contrast, patients with infection involving the mitral valve prosthesis usually have no clinical signs of prosthetic mitral valve dysfunction. Clinical signs of such dysfunction were not detected in any of our seven patients with prosthetic mitral valve endocarditis although the prosthesis was significantly obstructed by vegetative material in five of the seven and partially detached from the anulus in two.[12] McAllister et al.[43] reported on two patients with virtual total obstruction of the mitral prosthesis.

Morphologic Features

Valve ring abscess: The most consistent morphologic feature of prosthetic valve infection in our 22 patients was infection behind the site of attachment of the valve prosthesis, resulting in valve ring abscess. Ring abscess was present in each of our 22 patients, and in 14 the infection involved the entire circumference of the valve anulus. In several patients, however, only a portion of the circumference of the valve anulus was involved and, in one patient, histologic examination of the anulus disclosed infection that had not been apparent on gross examination. Extension of the ring infection to adjacent cardiac structures was common, especially when the aortic prosthesis was infected. This extension resulted in the frequent occurrence of both intracardiac fistulas and complete heart block or left bundle branch block. Among nine necropsy patients with prosthetic aortic valve endocarditis described by Madison et al.,[44] each had infection at the site of attachment of the prosthesis, and atrioventricular conduction defects developed in 7 (44 percent) of their entire group of 16 patients with prosthetic aortic valve endocarditis. Obviously, it is the occurrence of the infection behind the site of attachment of the prosthesis that makes reoperation so hazardous. Were the infection limited to the interior por-

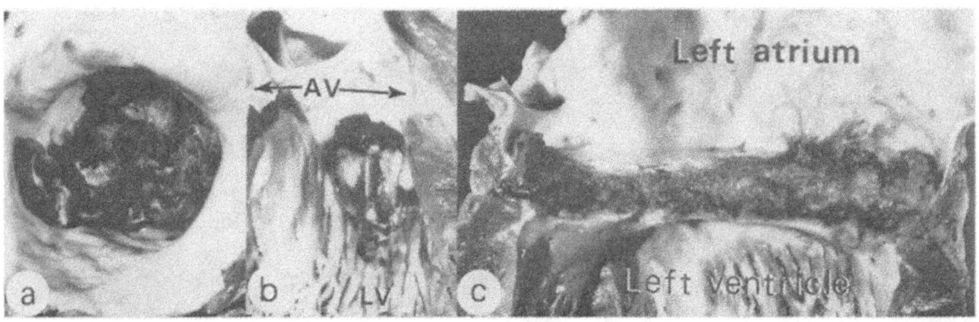

FIGURE 8. Staphylococcus epidermidis prosthetic mitral valve endocarditis in a 46 year old man who died 16 months after mitral valve replacement with a Starr-Edwards prosthesis. Eight months postoperatively, when he was asymptomatic, cardiac catheterization disclosed normal left atrial pressure and cardiac output. Signs of infection appeared 15 months after valve replacement. Despite antibiotic therapy, fatal congestive heart failure developed. **a,** mitral valve prosthesis as viewed from the left atrium. A large infected thrombus virtually occludes the mitral valve orifice. **b,** opened aorta, aortic valve (AV) and left ventricle (LV) showing infected thrombus on the cage of the mitral prosthesis. **c,** opened left atrium and ventricle showing a completely necrotic mitral valve anulus. The prosthesis has been removed.

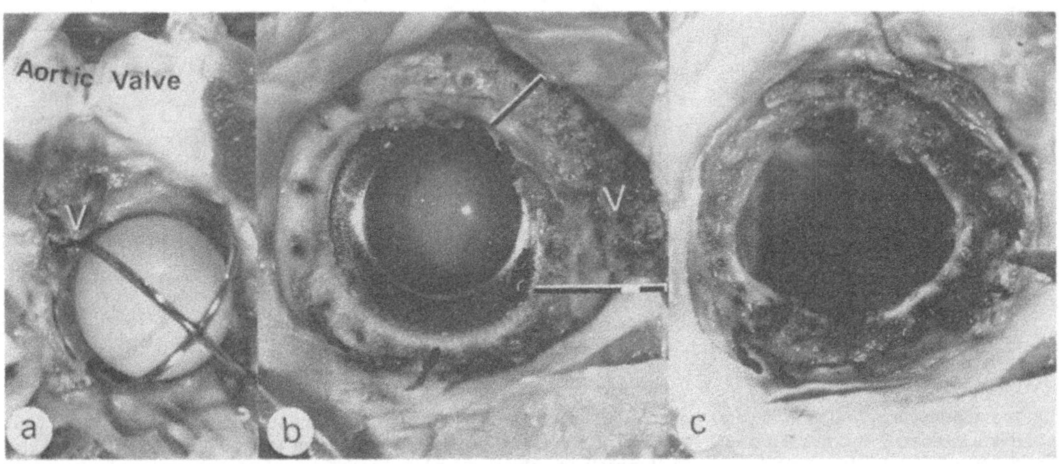

FIGURE 9. Staphylococcus epidermidis prosthetic mitral valve endocarditis in a 59 year old woman. The infection appeared 10 years after replacement of both mitral and tricuspid valves. At necropsy, only the mitral prosthesis was infected. **a,** infected mitral valve prosthesis viewed from the left ventricle. Vegetative material (V) is present on the prosthetic anulus just below the aortic valve. **b,** prosthesis as viewed from the left atrium showing vegetations (V) at the junction of the prosthetic and natural valve anuli. **c,** same view after removal of the prosthesis showing even greater extensiveness of the infection at the site of attachment of the prosthesis.

tion of the prosthesis, excision of the prosthesis should eliminate the infection. Unfortunately, as demonstrated in our patients and in those described by others,[20,35,38,43,44,47] the tissues behind the site of attachment of the prosthesis usually are involved by the infective process.

Treatment

Replacement of infected prosthesis: The occurrence of a grossly necrotic anulus at the time of reoperation for prosthetic valve endocarditis does not necessarily mean that valve replacement will be fruitless. Although it may be grossly necrotic, the anulus may be free of colonies of organisms and cultures of the necrotic anulus may be negative. In 9 of our 22 patients with prosthetic valve endocarditis and ring abscess, no stainable organisms were found in histologic sections from the prosthetic anulus.

One hazard of inserting a prosthesis in a necrotic anulus at the time of valve replacement for prosthetic valve endocarditis is burrowing of the sewing ring of the new prosthesis into the necrotic anulus with resulting impingement on movement of the poppet of the prosthesis by adjacent tissue. This sequence occurred in one of our patients and resulted in prosthetic aortic stenosis from inability of the ball to ascend in the cage (Fig. 6).

Tissue valve endocarditis: Although prosthetic valve endocarditis in patients with rigid-framed prostheses (the kind present in our 22 patients) usually indicates infection behind the site of attachment of the prosthesis, that is, the sewing ring, ring abscess may be less frequent with endocarditis involving tissue valves. Indeed, in animals and in man, the infective process may be limited to the cusps of the tissue valve, as when infective endocarditis involves natural valves.[60,61] Thus, the chance of cure, either by antibiotic therapy or valve replacement, or both, when infective endocarditis is superimposed on a homograft or heterograft (porcine valve, for example) is much better than when endocarditis involves a rigid-framed prosthesis.[61] This, then, is an advantage, although a small one, of the tissue valve (porcine) over the rigid-framed prosthesis.

Diagnosis: Establishment of the diagnosis of prosthetic valve endocarditis, particularly in the early postoperative period at times may be difficult, as pointed out by several investigators.[48,62,63] Diagnosis in the late postoperative period, in contrast, is usually

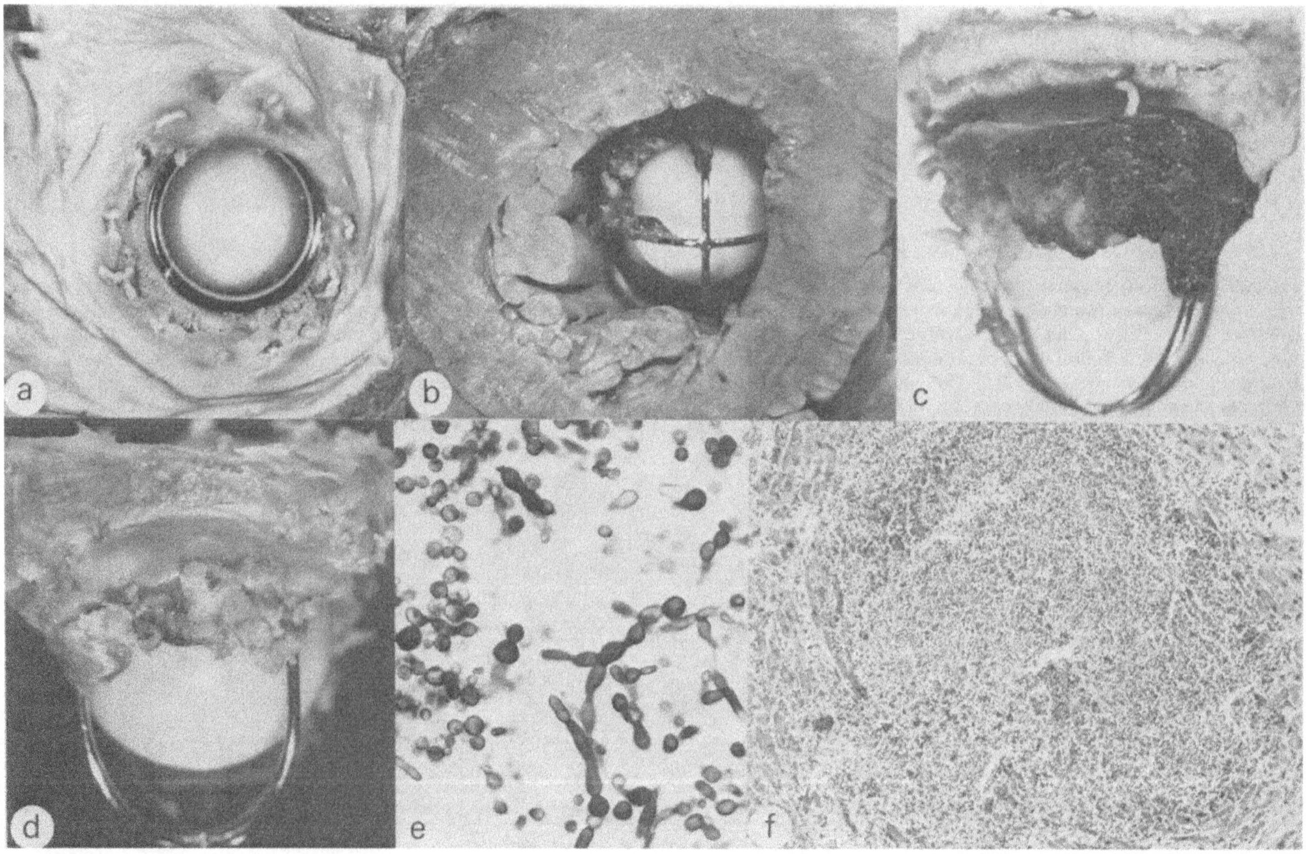

FIGURE 10. Candida species prosthetic mitral valve endocarditis in a 37 year old woman who underwent valve replacement 125 months before death because of mitral stenosis (mean mitral gradient 7 mm Hg) and regurgitation. Her tricuspid valve was replaced with a porcine xenograft because of severe tricuspid regurgitation 66 days before death. Postoperatively, she required prolonged use of a transthoracic pacing wire, which was the apparent source of the infection. She died from central nervous system embolism. Necropsy disclosed infection of the mitral valve prosthesis. **a,** mitral valve prosthesis viewed from the left atrium; **b,** prosthesis viewed from the left ventricle. Large vegetations are present on the base and struts of the prosthesis. **c** and **d,** removed mitral valve prosthesis viewed from two different sides showing large vegetations. **e,** photomicrograph of Candida species in the mitral vegetations. (Methenemine silver stain ×860, reduced by 23 percent.) **f,** photomicrograph of microabscess in the left ventricular myocardium. (Hematoxylin-eosin ×80, reduced by 23 percent.)

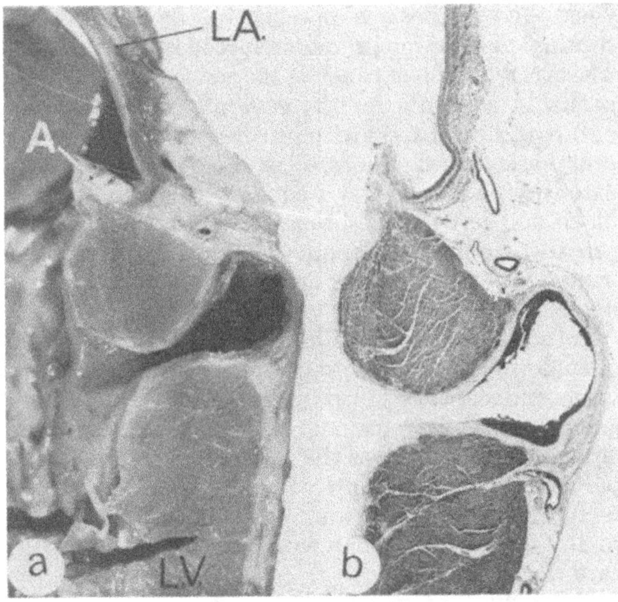

FIGURE 11. Left ventricular aneurysm simulating prosthetic valve endocarditis in a 46 year old woman. She had almost daily fever after mitral valve replacement 4 months before death and one of many blood cultures grew Staphylococcus epidermidis and diphtheroids. The clinical diagnosis was prosthetic valve endocarditis and she was treated with prolonged intravenous antibiotic therapy. She died from central nervous system embolism. At necropsy, an aneurysm was present in the basal portion of the left ventricular free wall. The prosthesis and its anulus were free of signs of infection. **a,** longitudinal cut of the left atrial (LA.) wall, mitral anulus (A) and left ventricular (L.V.) wall through the aneurysm. **b,** histologic section of the aneurysm (Movat stain). Thrombus is present in the aneurysm.

made quite readily.[48,62,63] It is worth emphasizing, however, that the combination of fever and a positive blood culture in a patient with a prosthetic cardiac valve does not always indicate the presence of prosthetic valve infection. We recently studied a patient at necropsy who was diagnosed during life as having prosthetic mitral valve endocarditis on the basis of fever, cerebral episodes consistent with emboli, and one blood culture that grew Staphylococcus epidermidis and diphtheroids. She received antibiotic treatment during most of her 4 month postoperative period and at necropsy no endocarditis was found. A left ventricular aneurysm was present immediately caudal to the mitral anulus and a sterile thrombus was present in the aneurysm (Fig. 11). The latter was the likely source of the cerebral emboli.

Antibiotic agents: There seems to be a general view that prosthetic valve endocarditis can at times be cured by antibiotic drugs. For such cure to be established, however, it is necessary that prosthetic valve endocarditis be confirmed during life, and this unequivocal confirmation can be obtained only by examination of the prosthetic valve and its anulus (site of attachment) at reoperation. In other words, to establish cure of prosthetic valve endocarditis it is necessary to be absolutely positive of the diagnosis. Although this confirmation is usually not obtained, it has now been obtained in enough patients to support the view that prosthetic valve endocarditis can indeed be cured in some patients.[16,17,21,23,24,29,30,37,39,44,45,48,64,65]

TABLE VI

Comparison between Active Infective Endocarditis (IE) Involving Prosthetic Cardiac Valves and Natural Cardiac Valves

	Mitral Valve				Aortic Valve			
	Prosthetic		Natural		Prosthetic		Natural	
	no.	%	no.	%	no.	%	no.	%
Necropsy patients (no.)	7		22		15		52*	
Age (yr) (range and average)	37–65 (52)		15–74 (43)		37–69 (54)		17–83 (45)	
Sex ratio (male:female)	3:4		12:10		13:2		41:11	
Underlying valve disease	7	100	7	32	15	100	26	50
Rheumatic	—	—	6	27	—	—	4	8
Congenital	—	—	0	0	—	—	12	23
Other	—	—	1†	5	—	—	10‡	19
None	—	—	15	68	—	—	26	50
Previous episode IE	1	14	0	0	1	7	3	6
Infecting organism								
Staphylococcus§	4	57	7	32	9	60	13	25
Alpha streptococcus	0	0	0	0	0	0	9	17
Pneumococcus	0	0	2	9	1	7	6	12
Valve regurgitation (from IE)	2	29	14	64	12	80	36	69
Valve stenosis (from IE)§	5	71	1	5	1	7	1	2
Valve-ring abscess§	7	100	1	5	15	100	21	40
Complete heart block§	0	0	1	5	5	33	4	8
Left bundle branch block§	0	0	0	0	2	13	0	0
Organ infarcts	5	71	17	77	9	60	31/47	66
Spleen >300 g	2/6	33	3	20	12	80	19/38	50

* Eighteen of the 52 also had infection of the mitral valve, but in at least 13 of them the mitral valve infection appeared to be secondary to the aortic valve infection.
† Floppy mitral valve.
‡ Degenerative (5 patients); previous infective endocarditis that healed (3 patients) and uncertain origin (2 patients).
§ $P < 0.05$.

Comparison With Endocarditis Involving Natural Valves

Comparison of observations in our 22 patients with prosthetic valve endocarditis with our observations in 74 nonsurgically treated necropsy patients with active infective endocarditis involving natural left-sided cardiac valves disclosed certain clear differences between the two groups (Table VI): (1) Ring abscess was always present in patients with prosthetic valve endocarditis regardless of the site of the prosthesis, but was present in only 30 percent of the comparison group and then, with rare exception, only when the aortic valve was infected. (2) The hemodynamic consequences were different. Prosthetic valve endocarditis caused valve obstruction nearly as often as valve regurgitation, whereas valve stenosis from active infective endocarditis involving natural cardiac valves was extremely rare.[10,66] (3) Spread of ring abscess was more extensive in patients with prosthetic valve endocarditis than in patients with natural valve endocarditis, and consequently the frequency of high grade conduction defects was much greater in the former patients. (4) The infecting organism in fatal prosthetic valve endocarditis was most commonly the Staphylococcus. Alpha streptococcus, which remains a common cause of fatal active infective endocarditis in patients with natural cardiac valves, is a rare cause of fatal prosthetic valve endocarditis.

Valve ring abscess: Among patients with infective endocarditis involving native cardiac valves, ring abscess when present almost always (95 percent of cases) involves the aortic valve.[67] Among our necropsy patients with active infective endocarditis involving a natural aortic valve, 40 percent had a valve ring abscess, whereas only 5 percent of patients with endocarditis involving a natural mitral valve had a ring abscess. In contrast, each of our 22 patients with prosthetic valve endocarditis had a ring abscess. Thus, valve ring abscess is the usual morphologic feature of prosthetic valve endocarditis, regardless of the valve infected.

Ring abscesses in patients with infection involving prosthetic valves are generally more extensive than those in patients with active infective endocarditis involving natural cardiac valves. This appears to be a consequence of the rigid nature of the prosthetic frame. Once the prosthesis is loosened by the infection, the rocking-rigid frame promotes spread of the infection. The greater turbulence across the aortic valve prosthesis probably accounts for the generally more extensive nature of ring abscess with prosthetic aortic than with prosthetic mitral endocarditis. A consequence of this extension is the greater frequency of complete heart block and left bundle branch block in patients with prosthetic aortic valve endocarditis (32 percent) than in patients with natural aortic valve endocarditis (8 percent).

Infecting organism: *Staphylococcus* (either aureus or epidermidis) is the most common cause of prosthetic valve endocarditis (59 percent). Many different organisms cause the remainder of the infections. Although alpha streptococcus was the responsible organism in 17 percent of our 74 patients with natural aortic valve infection, this bacterium was not the causative organism in any of our 22 patients with prosthetic valve endocarditis.

Valve dysfunction: The hemodynamic consequences of prosthetic valve endocarditis vary with the site of the infected prosthesis. Valve regurgitation developed in 12 of the 15 patients (80 percent) with prosthetic aortic valve endocarditis and in 2 of the 7 patients (28 percent) with prosthetic mitral valve infection. In contrast, valve obstruction developed from the infection in 5 of the 7 patients (71 percent) with prosthetic mitral valve endocarditis, and in 1 of the 15 patients (7 percent) with prosthetic aortic valve endocarditis. Among patients with natural left-sided valve infection, 65 percent (64 percent of those with mitral valve disease and 69 percent of those with aortic valve disease) had valve regurgitation from active infective endocarditis, and relatively few (3 percent) had valve obstruction from the endocarditis.[10] Thus, aortic prosthetic valve endocarditis almost alv 1ys causes valve regurgitation and mitral prosthetic valve endocarditis most often causes valve obstruction.

Splenomegaly (greater than 300 g) is common both in patients with prosthetic valve endocarditis (64 percent) and in patients with native left-sided valve endocarditis (37 percent). The frequency of infarcts in other body organs is similar in both groups (64 and 70 percent, respectively).

References

1. **Roberts WC, Morrow AG:** Anatomic studies of hearts containing caged-ball prosthetic valves. John Hopkins Med J 121:271–295, 1967
2. **Roberts WC, Morrow AG:** Causes of death and other anatomic observations after cardiac valve replacement. Adv Cardiol 7: 226–247, 1972
3. **Roberts WC, Bulkley BH, Morrow AG:** Pathologic anatomy of cardiac valve replacement: a study of 224 necropsy patients. Prog Cardiovasc Dis 15:539–587, 1973
4. **Fishbein MC, Roberts WC, Golden A, et al:** Cardiac pathology after aortic valve replacement using Hufnagel trileaflet prostheses: a study of 20 necropsy patients. Am Heart J 89:443–448, 1975
5. **Roberts WC, Fishbein MC, Golden A:** Cardiac pathology after valve replacement by disc prosthesis. A study of 61 necropsy patients. Am J Cardiol 35:740–760, 1975
6. **Fishbein MC, Roberts WC:** Late postoperative anatomic observations after insertion of Hufnagel caged-ball prosthesis in descending thoracic aorta. Chest 68:6–11, 1975
7. **Roberts WC, Hammer WJ:** Cardiac pathology after valve replacement with a tilting disc prosthesis (Björk-Shiley type): a study of 46 necropsy patients and 49 Björk-Shiley prostheses. Am J Cardiol 37:1024–1033, 1976
8. **Roberts WC, Buchbinder NA:** Right-sided valvular infective endocarditis. A clinicopathologic study of twelve necropsy patients. Am J Med 53:7–19, 1972
9. **Buchbinder NA, Roberts WC:** Left-sided valvular active infective endocarditis. A study of forty-five necropsy patients. Am J Med 53:20–35, 1972
10. **Arnett EN, Roberts WC:** Pathology of active infective endocarditis. A clinicopathologic study of 137 necropsy patients. Current

Problems in Cardiology, in press.
11. **Cohn LH, Roberts WC, Rockoff SD, et al:** Bacterial endocarditis following aortic valve replacement. Clinical and pathological correlations. Circulation 33:209–217, 1966
12. **Roberts WC, Morrow AG:** Bacterial endocarditis involving prosthetic mitral valves. Clinical and pathologic observations. Arch Pathol 82:164–169, 1966
13. **Arnett EN, Roberts WC:** Prosthetic valve endocarditis. A study of 18 patients at necropsy (abstr). Am J Cardiol 35:120, 1975
14. **Björk VO:** Aortic valve replacement. Thorax 19:369–378, 1964
15. **Newman WH, Cordell AR:** Aspergillus endocarditis after open-heart surgery. Report of a case and review of literature. J Thorac Cardiovasc Surg 48:652–660, 1964
16. **Amoury RA, Bowman FO Jr, Malm JR:** Endocarditis associated with intracardiac prostheses. Diagnosis, management and prophylaxis. J Thorac Cardiovasc Surg 51:36–48, 1966
17. **Stein PD, Harken DE, Dexter L:** The nature and prevention of prosthetic valve endocarditis. Am Heart J 71:393–407, 1966
18. **Fraser RS, Rossall RE, Dvorkin J:** Bacterial endocarditis occurring after open heart surgery. Can Med Assoc J 96:1551–1558, 1967
19. **Leffert RC, Hackett RL:** Aspergillus aortitis following replacement of aortic valve. J Thorac Cardiovasc Surg 53:866–874, 1967
20. **McConnell EM, Roberts C:** Pathological findings in three cases of fungal endocarditis complicating open-heart surgery. J Clin Pathol 20:555–560, 1967
21. **Geraci JE, Forth RJ, Ellis FH:** Postoperative prosthetic valve endocarditis due to *Corynebacterium xerosis*. Mayo Clin Proc 42: 736–743, 1967
22. **Cheng TO, Kinhal V, Tice DA:** Fatal thrombosis of the Starr-Edwards mitral valve prosthesis associated with bacterial endocarditis. Diagnostic significance of a disappearing prosthetic click. Chest 57:151–155, 1970
23. **Hairston P, Lee WH Jr:** Management of infective prosthetic heart valves. Ann Thorac Surg 9:229–237, 1970
24. **Killen DA, Collins HA, Koenig MG, et al:** Prosthetic cardiac valves and bacterial endocarditis. Ann Thorac Surg 9:238–246, 1970
25. **Shafer RB, Hall WH:** Bacterial endocarditis following open heart surgery. Am J Cardiol 25:602–607, 1970
26. **Sutton GC, Wright JEC:** Major detachment of aortic prosthetic valves. Br Heart J 32:337–343, 1970
27. **Chaudhuri MR:** Fungal endocarditis after valve replacements. J Thorac Cardiovasc Surg 60:207–214, 1970
28. **Gage AA, Dean DC, Schimert G, et al:** Aspergillus infection after cardiac surgery. Arch Surg 101:384–387, 1970
29. **Block PC, DeSanctis RW, Weinberg AN, et al:** Prosthetic valve endocarditis. J Thorac Cardiovasc Surg 60:540–548, 1970
30. **Okies JE, Viroslav J, Williams TW Jr:** Endocarditis after cardiac valvular replacement. Chest 59:198–202, 1971
31. **Ostermiller WE Jr, Dye WS, Weinberg M:** Fungal endocarditis following cardiovascular surgery. J Thorac Cardiovasc Surg 61: 670–675, 1971
32. **Lawrence T, Shockman AT, Macvaugh H 3rd:** Aspergillus infection of prosthetic aortic valves. Chest 60:406–414, 1971
33. **Robinson MJ, Greenberg JJ, Korn M, et al:** Infective endocarditis at autopsy: 1965–1969. Am J Med 52:492–498, 1972
34. **Levin S, Balagtas R, Susmano A, et al:** Meningococcus endocarditis at the site of Starr-Edwards mitral prosthesis. Arch Intern Med 129:963–966, 1972
35. **Joassin A, Edward JE:** Late causes of death after mitral valve replacement. J Thorac Cardiovasc Surg 65:255–263, 1973
36. **Vlachakis ND, Gazes PC, Hairston P:** Nocardial endocarditis following mitral valve replacement. Chest 63:276–278, 1973
37. **Slaughter L, Morris JE, Starr A:** Prosthetic valvular endocarditis. A 12-year review. Circulation 47:1319–1326, 1973
38. Case records of the Massachusetts General Hospital. Weekly clinicopathological exercises. Case 24, 1973. N Engl J Med 288:1290–1296, 1973
39. **Dismukes WE, Karchmer AW, Buckley MJ, et al:** Prosthetic valve endocarditis. Analysis of 38 cases. Circulation 48:365–377, 1973
40. **Jackson G, Saunders K:** Prosthetic valve diphtheroid endocarditis treated with sodium fusidate and erythromycin. Br Heart J 35: 931–936, 1973
41. **Harris JA, Cobbs CG:** Serratia endocarditis in patients with a Starr-Edwards valve: report of a case of bacteriologic cure with antimicrobial therapy. South Med J 66:1117–1120, 1973
42. **Hall WJ 3rd:** Penicillium endocarditis following open heart surgery and prosthetic valve insertion. Am Heart J 87:501–506, 1974
43. **McAllister RG, Samet J, Mazzoleni A, et al:** Endocarditis on prosthetic mitral valves. Fatal obstruction to left ventricular inflow. Chest 66:682–686, 1974
44. **Madison J, Wang K, Gobel FL, et al:** Prosthetic aortic valvular endocarditis. Circulation 51:940–949, 1975
45. **Wilson WR, Jaumin PM, Danielson GK, et al:** Prosthetic valve endocarditis. Ann Intern Med 82:751–756, 1975
46. **Rubenstein E, Noriega ER, Simberkoff MS, et al:** Fungal endocarditis: analysis of 24 cases and review of the literature. Medicine 54:331–344, 1975
47. **Robboy SJ, Kaiser J:** Pathogenesis of fungal infection on heart valve prostheses. Human Pathol 6:711–715, 1975
48. **Kloster FE:** Diagnosis and management of complications of prosthetic heart valves. Am J Cardiol 35:872–885, 1975
49. **Conte JE, Cohen SN, Roe BB, et al:** Antibiotic prophylaxis and cardiac surgery. A prospective double-blind comparison of single-dose versus multiple-dose regimens. Ann Intern Med 76: 943–949, 1972
50. **Goodman JS, Schaffner W, Collins HA, et al:** Infection after cardiovascular surgery: clinical study including examination of antimicrobial prophylaxis. N Engl J Med 287:117–123, 1968
51. **Nelson RM, Jenson CB, Peterson CA, et al:** Effective use of prophylactic antibiotics in open-heart surgery. Arch Surg 90:731–735, 1965
52. **Herr R, Starr A, McCord CW, et al:** Special problems following valve replacement. Embolus, leak, infection, red cell damage. Ann Thorac Surg 1:403–415, 1965
53. **Ankeney JL, Parker RF:** Staphylococcal endocarditis following open heart surgery related to positive intraoperative blood cultures. In, Prosthetic Heart Valves (Brewer LA III, ed). Springfield, Ill, Charles C Thomas, 1969, p 719–730
54. **Blakemore WS, McGarrity GJ, Thurer RJ, et al:** Infection by airborne bacteria with cardiopulmonary bypass. Surgery 70: 830–838, 1971
55. **Kammer RB, Utz JP:** Aspergillus species endocarditis. The new face of a not so rare disease. Am J Med 56:506–521, 1974
56. **Wigle ED, Labrosse CJ:** Sudden, severe aortic insufficiency. Circulation 32:708–720, 1965
57. **Wise JR, Bentall HH, Cleland WP, et al:** Urgent aortic-valve replacement for acute aortic regurgitation due to infective endocarditis. Lancet 2:115–121, 1971
58. **Wise JR Jr, Oakley CM, Goodwin JF:** Acute aortic regurgitation in patients with infective endocarditis. The distinctive clinical features and the role of premature mitral valve closure. J Maine Med Assoc 63:273–278, 1972
59. **Mann T, McLaurin L, Grossman W, et al:** Assessing the hemodynamic severity of acute aortic regurgitation due to infective endocarditis. N Engl J Med 293:108–113, 1975
60. **Yarbrough JW, Roberts WC, Reis RL:** Structural alterations in tissue cardiac valves implanted in patients and in calves. J Thorac Cardiovasc Surg 65:364–375, 1973
61. **Clarkson PM, Barratt-Boyes BG:** Bacterial endocarditis following homograft replacement of the aortic valve. Circulation 42:987–991, 1970
62. **Sande MA, Johnson WD Jr, Hook EW, et al:** Sustained bacteremia in patients with prosthetic cardiac valves. N Engl J Med 286: 1067–1070, 1972
63. **Weinstein L:** Infected prosthetic valves: a diagnostic and therapeutic dilemma. N Engl J Med 286:1108–1109, 1972
64. **Watanakunakorn C, Hamburger M:** Staphylococcus epidermidis endocarditis complicating a Starr-Edwards prosthesis. A therapeutic dilemma. Arch Intern Med 126:1014–1018, 1970
65. **Walker SR, Shumway NE, Merigan TC:** Management of infected cardiac valve prostheses. JAMA 208:531–533, 1969
66. **Roberts WC, Ewy GA, Glancy DL, et al:** Valvular stenosis produced by active infective endocarditis. Circulation 36:449–451, 1967
67. **Arnett EN, Roberts WC:** Valve ring abscess in active infective endocarditis. Frequency, location, and clues to clinical diagnosis from the study of 95 necropsy patients. Circulation 54:140–145, 1976

Choosing a Substitute Cardiac Valve: Type, Size, Surgeon

WILLIAM C. ROBERTS, MD, FACC

Bethesda, Maryland

Certain ideal characteristics of substitute cardiac valves are analyzed for each of the four basic types of available substitute cardiac valves. Of the four, the caged disc prosthesis is the least desirable: It obstructs, it clots and it degenerates. Each of the other three types of substitute cardiac valves has more favorable characteristics. Ideally, the caged ball prosthesis might be limited to patients with predominantly regurgitant lesions because of the problem of prosthetic disproportion. The tilting disc has favorable hemodynamic and wear characteristics, but long-term anticoagulant therapy is essential, as with the caged ball and caged disc types of prosthesis. The porcine xenograft appears to be desirable, but patients with sufficient implantation time (more than 5 years) for proper evaluation are just beginning to be studied and, therefore, final judgment must be reserved. Assuming that valve replacement is to be carried out in a large medical center by a surgical team experienced in this procedure, the results of this operation today are dependent more on the type and size of substitute valve inserted than on the surgeon who inserts the valve. It is therefore important for the cardiologist to become more informed about the various types of prosthetic cardiac valves and to become a member of the team deciding which type and size of cardiac valve are most suitable for his (or her) patient.

In the annals of cardiology the decade of the 1960's will probably be remembered most as the decade during which cardiac valve replacement became a successful reality. This tremendous accomplishment has brought new life to several hundred thousand persons since the first successful (survival more than 3 months) cardiac valve replacement in September 1960. Despite this success, the ideal cardiac valve is still not available or, if available, not adequately tested. This review will examine the various advantages and disadvantages of available substitute cardiac valves and, in addition, will examine the determinants of the results of cardiac valve replacement.

Available Prosthetic Valves

Of the nearly 50 different substitute cardiac valves introduced during the past 2 decades, many have been discarded and, of those remaining, usually several modifications have been made. At present, four basic types of substitute cardiac valves are in use: (1) caged ball, (2) caged disc, (3) tilting disc, and (4) tissue valve. The caged ball was the first prosthesis used successfully for the treatment of cardiac valve disease; it was placed in the descending thoracic aorta by Hufnagel in 1953 for treatment of severe aortic regurgitation.[1,2] Although utilized unsuccessfully for aortic valve replacement (subcoronary insertion) in 1960 by Harken et al.,[3,4] the caged ball was first used successfully for mitral valve replacement in the same year by Starr and Edwards.[5] Although first utilized in the descending thoracic aorta as treatment for aortic regurgitation in 1956,[6–8] the aortic valve homograft was introduced for aortic valve replacement

From the Pathology Branch, National Heart, Lung, and Blood Institute, National Institutes of Health, Bethesda, Md. 20014. Manuscript received March 17, 1976; accepted March 31, 1976.

Address for reprints: William C. Roberts, MD, National Institutes of Health, Bldg 10A, Rm. 3E 30, Bethesda, Md. 20014.

in 1962[9–12] (later[13] for mitral valve replacement), and the heterograft aortic valve was first used for aortic valve replacement in 1967.[14–16] The caged disc appeared in 1965[17,18] and the tilting disc in 1967.[19–22] Flow through the caged ball and caged disc is peripheral, through the tilting disc semicentral, and through the tissue valve central.

Characteristics of Prosthetic Valves

There are at least six ideal characteristics of a good prosthetic cardiac valve (Table I): (1) It has good hemodynamic characteristics, that is, it is *nonobstructive* or nearly so, and completely *competent* or nearly so; (2) it is *nonthrombogenic;* (3) it *does not degenerate,* wear out or vary; (4) it *does not significantly alter blood components;* (5) *it can be inserted without undue difficulty* (that is, exquisite technical skill is not required

TABLE I

Substitute Cardiac Valves: General Characteristics

Type	Year Intro-duced	Ob-struc-tive	In-com-petent	Throm-botic	Hemo-lytic	De-gener-ates
Caged ball	1960	+	0	+	+	+
Caged disc	1965	+	0	+	+	+
Tilting disc	1967	+	0	+	0	0
Tissue valve						
Homograft	1962	0	+	0	0	+
Xenograft	1965	+	0	0	0	?

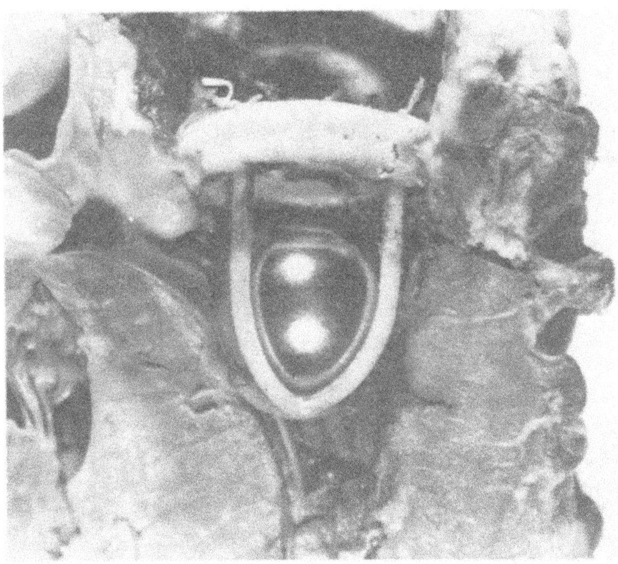

FIGURE 1. Prosthetic mitral stenosis after replacement with a ball valve prosthesis. Shown is longitudinal section of the heart of a woman with severe isolated mitral stenosis. The valve was replaced in July 1974 with a size 3M Starr-Edwards prosthesis. The prosthesis is too large for the normal-sized left ventricular cavity, and both struts and poppet contact the endocardium of the left ventricle causing obstruction to left ventricular inflow. The patient could not be separated from cardiopulmonary bypass.

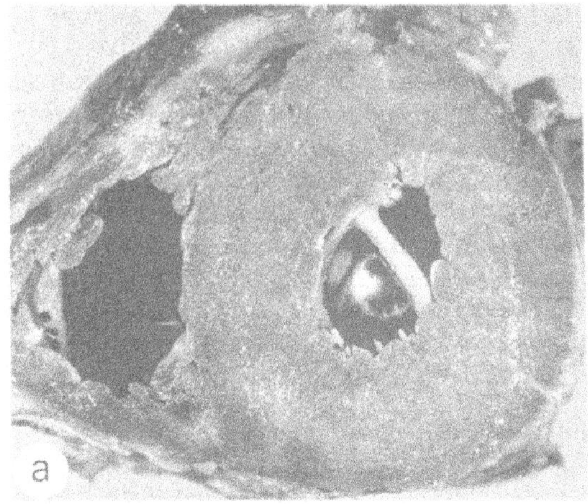

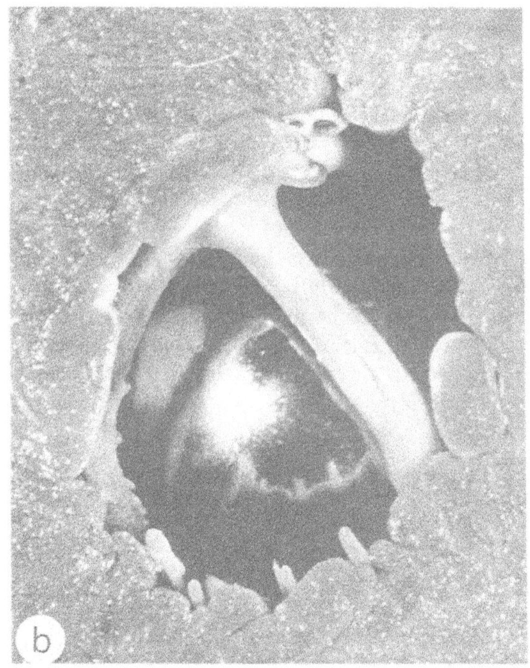

FIGURE 2. Prosthetic mitral stenosis after replacement of a stenotic mitral valve (7 mm Hg mean diastolic gradient between left ventricle and pulmonary capillary wedge position) with a size 4M model 6320 Starr-Edwards prosthesis. This 58 year old man also had his stenotic aortic valve (103 mm Hg peak systolic pressure gradient between left ventricle and brachial artery) replaced with a size 9A model 2320 Starr-Edwards prosthesis. The immediate postoperative period was complicated by the low cardiac output syndrome. Late postoperatively, however, the patient became asymptomatic. At cardiac catheterization 6 1/2 months postoperatively, the mean diastolic gradient across the mitral prosthesis was 11 mm Hg and no systolic gradient was present across the aortic prosthesis. The mitral valve area preoperatively was 2.0 and, postoperatively, 1.6 cm^2. The patient died suddenly 5 days after the postoperative catheterization. *At necropsy,* as shown in the above photographs, the mitral prosthesis is too large for the normal-sized left ventricular cavity (shown here as it appears during ventricular systole). Thus, not only did the mitral prosthesis appear obstructive at necropsy but the pressure gradient was considerably greater postoperatively than preoperatively. Although this patient had been asymptomatic postoperatively, he had considerable prosthetic mitral stenosis. **a,** transverse section of the cardiac ventricles. Each of the cloth-covered struts contacts endocardium of the left ventricle and the metal poppet occupies too much space in the left ventricular cavity, as seen in the closer view (**b**).

for its insertion); and (6) it *does not disturb the patient.*

Analysis of each of the four types of substitute cardiac valves for the first four of these ideal characteristics should separate the good ones from the bad ones. The degree of difficulty or ease in inserting each of the four basic types of currently employed substitute valves is similar because all have rigid or semirigid frames and cloth-covered sewing rings. Furthermore, with the possible exception of the recent metal track Starr-Edwards prosthesis, none of the substitute valves now used make noise audible to the patient.

Caged Ball Valve

The caged ball prosthesis (Harken, Starr-Edwards, Magovern, Smeloff-Cutter, Braunwald-Cutter, De Bakey) clearly belongs in the "good" category. More information on it is available than on any of the other prostheses because it has been the one used most widely and for the longest time; however, it is not necessarily the best prothesis. It has had a number of modifications (a word not always synonymous with "improvements") during the past 16 years, and generally has adequate but not the best hemodynamic characteristics.[23–35] Although the introduction of cloth covering on the struts and base has diminished the incidence of clinical events compatible with emboli, this prosthesis continues to have a tendency to form thrombus, and anticoagulant agents are required.[35] It hemolyzes erythrocytes, more frequently and more severely after aortic than after mitral valve replacement and also more frequently and more severely with the cloth-covered than with non-cloth-covered models.[36–43] Hemolysis, however, is rarely a major clinical problem with any prosthesis because the bone marrow is capable of replacing the destroyed erythrocytes without development of anemia or thrombocytopenia.

Degeneration of the silicone rubber poppet was common in the caged ball prostheses inserted before 1967,[44–62] but no degeneration or variance has been reported in the metallic (stellite 21) hollow poppet introduced at that time. The silicone rubber poppet models continue to be employed in some major centers and it is likely that poppet degeneration eventually will occur in them. Such was the case with the Braunwald-Cutter aortic valve prosthesis, which has been withdrawn from the market.[63] Wear of cloth covering on both struts and orifice occurred in some of the completely cloth-covered caged ball prostheses, but strut cloth wear has not been observed since introduction of the metal track in the latest Starr-Edwards models.

Obstructive complications: A problem with the caged ball prosthesis is that it may occupy too much space within either the ventricle or aortic root, and, because flow is entirely peripheral, there may not be adequate space between the surface of the poppet and the endocardium of the ventricle or the intima of the ascending aorta to accommodate blood flow adequately[64–78] (Fig. 1 to 3). This situation occurs most frequently when mitral valve replacement is performed in a patient, usually a woman, with pure mitral stenosis and a normal aortic valve. In this circumstance the left ventricle may not be of adequate size to accommodate the mitral prosthesis, and one or more struts of the

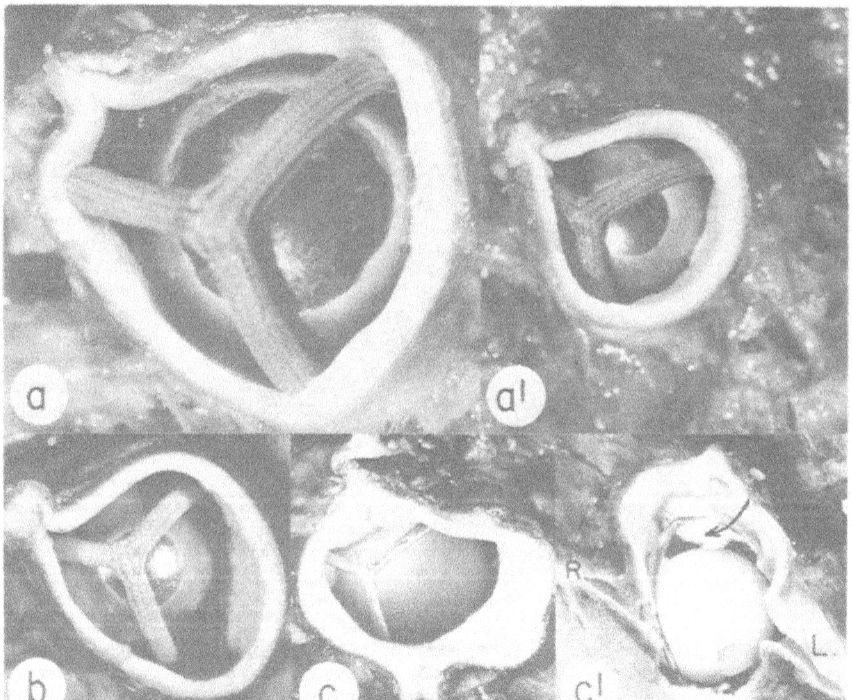

FIGURE 3. Prosthetic aortic stenosis secondary to disproportion between the size of the caged ball prosthesis and the size of the ascending aorta. The aortic prostheses, even though small (8A, Starr-Edwards), are too large for the aortas into which they had been placed. The struts of the cages contact the aortic walls, which protrude between the struts to contact the poppets and restrict their movement. **a, a**[1], from a 45 year old woman who had had mitral stenosis (11 mm Hg mean diastolic gradient between the left atrium and left ventricle) and pure aortic regurgitation (2+/4+). She died several hours after operation. **b,** from a 55 year old woman who also had severe mitral stenosis (17 mm Hg mean diastolic gradient between the left atrium and left ventricle) and pure aortic regurgitation (4+/4+). She died in the operating room. **c, c**[1], from a 25 year old man also with severe mitral stenosis (18 mm Hg mean diastolic gradient between the left atrium and left ventricle) and pure aortic regurgitation (2+/4+). The patient also died on the day of operation several hours after entering the recovery room.

prosthesis may burrow into the myocardial wall preventing adequate descent of the poppet, with resulting obstruction to left atrial emptying.[64] This occurrence is obviously most likely when a large prosthesis is utilized, but it may occur when even the smallest caged ball prosthesis is used to replace a purely stenotic mitral valve. Fatal obstruction to left ventricular outflow occurs most commonly in the patient with combined mitral and aortic valve disease. In most such patients, whether the aortic valve lesion is stenosis or pure regurgitation, the aortic root is usually not dilated and consequently the space available in the aortic root to accommodate the caged ball may be limited. A particularly dangerous circumstance is combined mitral and aortic stenosis. In this circumstance, the left ventricular wall is hypertrophied but its cavity is not dilated. Insertion of a mitral caged ball into a hypertrophied nondilated left ventricle may obstruct left ventricular inflow or outflow. Because ventricular inflow obstruction is probably even more common after tricuspid than after mitral valve replacement with a caged ball prosthesis, utilization of this prosthesis in the tricuspid position may be unwise.[74–78]

Real and potential prosthetic disproportion (prosthesis too large or ventricular cavity or aorta too small) occur most frequently with the caged ball prosthesis although none of the various types of substitute cardiac valves are completely immune from it (Fig. 4 to 7). Therefore, it may be most wise to limit the use of this type of prosthesis to patients with purely incompetent or at least predominantly incompetent valve lesions, that is, to patients in whom volume overload has produced a large left ventricular cavity or ascending aorta. Use of the caged ball prosthesis in patients with purely stenotic or predominantly stenotic valve lesions appears unnecessary because of the availability of other excellent substitute cardiac valves.

Caged Disc Valve

The caged disc prosthesis (Kay-Shiley, Cross-Jones, Hufnagel, Kay-Suzuki, Beall, Harken, Cooley-Bloodwell-Cutter, Cooley-Cutter) is in my view the least desirable prosthetic cardiac valve now in use. Because of its "low profile" configuration, this prosthesis was introduced as an alternative to the caged ball prosthesis and was initially believed to be particularly useful in the patient with the "small left ventricle," (pure mitral stenosis). This device, however, has proved to be highly thrombogenic[79–85] and the most obstructive of all the prosthetic valves now in use.[86–99] In a recent study, although the pulmonary arterial pressures had decreased and the cardiac indexes had increased, the mean diastolic pressure gradient across the mitral prosthesis (Beall type) was not significantly different from preoperative values.[99] In addition, the nonmetallic discs have shown evidence of degeneration,[87,97,100–113] and strut fracture of uncertain cause with dislodgment of the disc occluder has been reported.[96,107] Hemolysis with this prosthesis is universal.[97,114] This device was

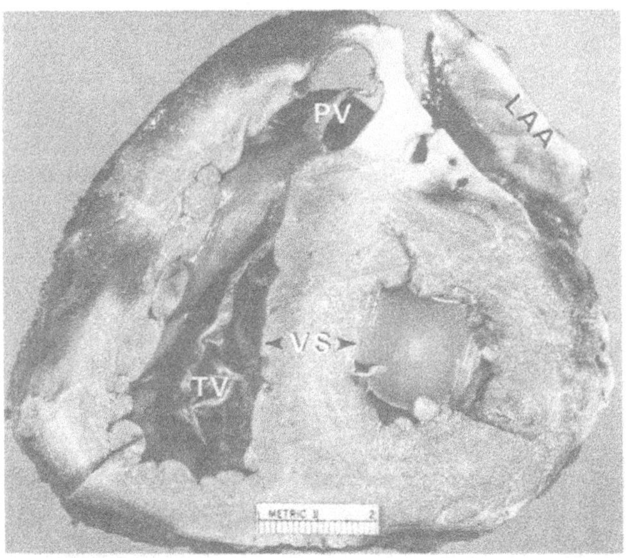

FIGURE 4. Prosthetic stenosis after replacement of the mitral valve with a caged disc prosthesis. Shown is a transverse section of the cardiac ventricles in a 57 year old woman who died in the operating room after replacement of a severely stenotic mitral valve with a no. 19 Hufnagel discoid prosthesis. The margins of the disc contact the left ventricular endocardium at several sites and movement of the disc is impeded. In addition to mitral stenosis and severe pulmonary hypertension (95/45 mm Hg), the aortic valve was mildly stenotic (peak systolic pressure gradient 34 mm Hg). LAA = left atrial appendage; PV = pulmonary valve; TV = tricuspid valve; VS = ventricular septum.

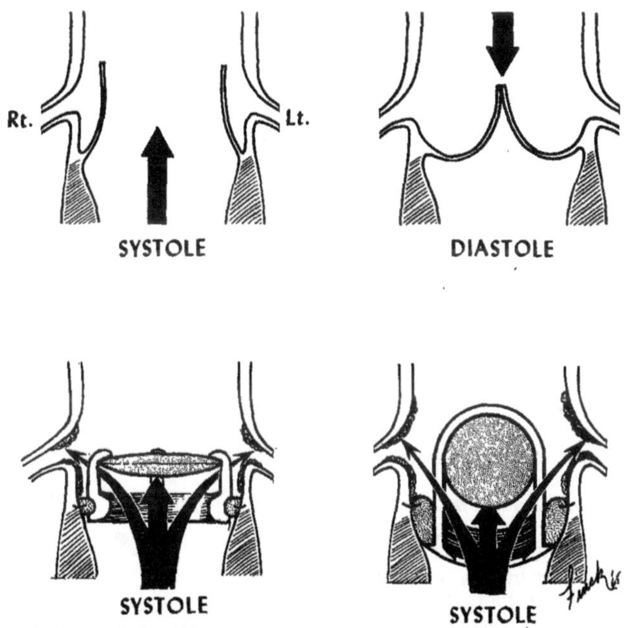

FIGURE 5. Diagram delineating flow across the normal aortic valve (**upper**) and across a caged disc and caged ball prosthesis (**lower**). Normally, flow across the aortic valve is central and nearly laminar. Flow across the prostheses is entirely peripheral and therefore turbulent. Intimal proliferation in the proximal ascending aorta is an expected consequence of this peripheral flow.[45,46] On rare occasion, this intimal proliferation may extend into one or both coronary arteries. It is likely that this intimal proliferation will progressively increase with time. Flow across a tissue valve is certainly more laminar than across either the caged disc or caged ball. Lt. = left; Rt. = right.

utilized briefly in the aortic position[89,90,97] but its use in this location was abandoned because of its obstructive, thrombogenic and wear characteristics.

More recently, a new type of caged disc, the Cooley-Cutter biconical disc, has been introduced for use in both atrioventricular and semilunar valve positions.[115–117] This newer prosthesis, which has a semidiamond-shaped occluder rather than a flat one (like all other caged discs) also has entirely peripheral flow characteristics and is therefore unlikely to have ideal hemodynamic features. Furthermore, intimal proliferation in the aortic root (where the coronary ostia are located) remains a potential problem with the peripheral flow type of prosthesis and is probably most severe with use of the caged disc[97] (Fig. 5). Also very worrisome is disc cocking, a potential problem with all caged discs[80,82,83,102,110–113,118,119] including the newly introduced one, and its frequency of occurrence is entirely unknown (Fig. 8). Possibly, nonfatal transient cocking is common, and fatal cocking of the caged disc may occur and be totally unrecognized at necropsy.

Tilting Disc Valve

The tilting disc prosthesis (Wada-Cutter, Lillehei-Kastor, Björk-Shiley) of the latter two types (the first type has been discontinued[120]) has proved to be a good prosthesis for replacement of tricuspid, mitral and aortic valves. Its semicentral flow usually allows minimal gradients,[121–127] its effect on red blood cell survival is minimal[128,129] and there has been no evidence of disc wear (variance) since the introduction of the carbon pyrolyte disc. This prosthesis, however, has a tendency to clot, and anticoagulant agents are required.[129–135] Because movement of the disc is in close proximity to the sewing ring, the chances of interference to it by contact with adjacent mural endocardium or aortic intima is small, but, as with all prostheses, a potential problem if a large model is utilized in a small ventricle or aorta[129] (Fig. 6 and 7).

Tissue Valves

Tissue valves, in the form of aortic homografts, were first utilized for aortic valve replacement in 1962.[9–12]

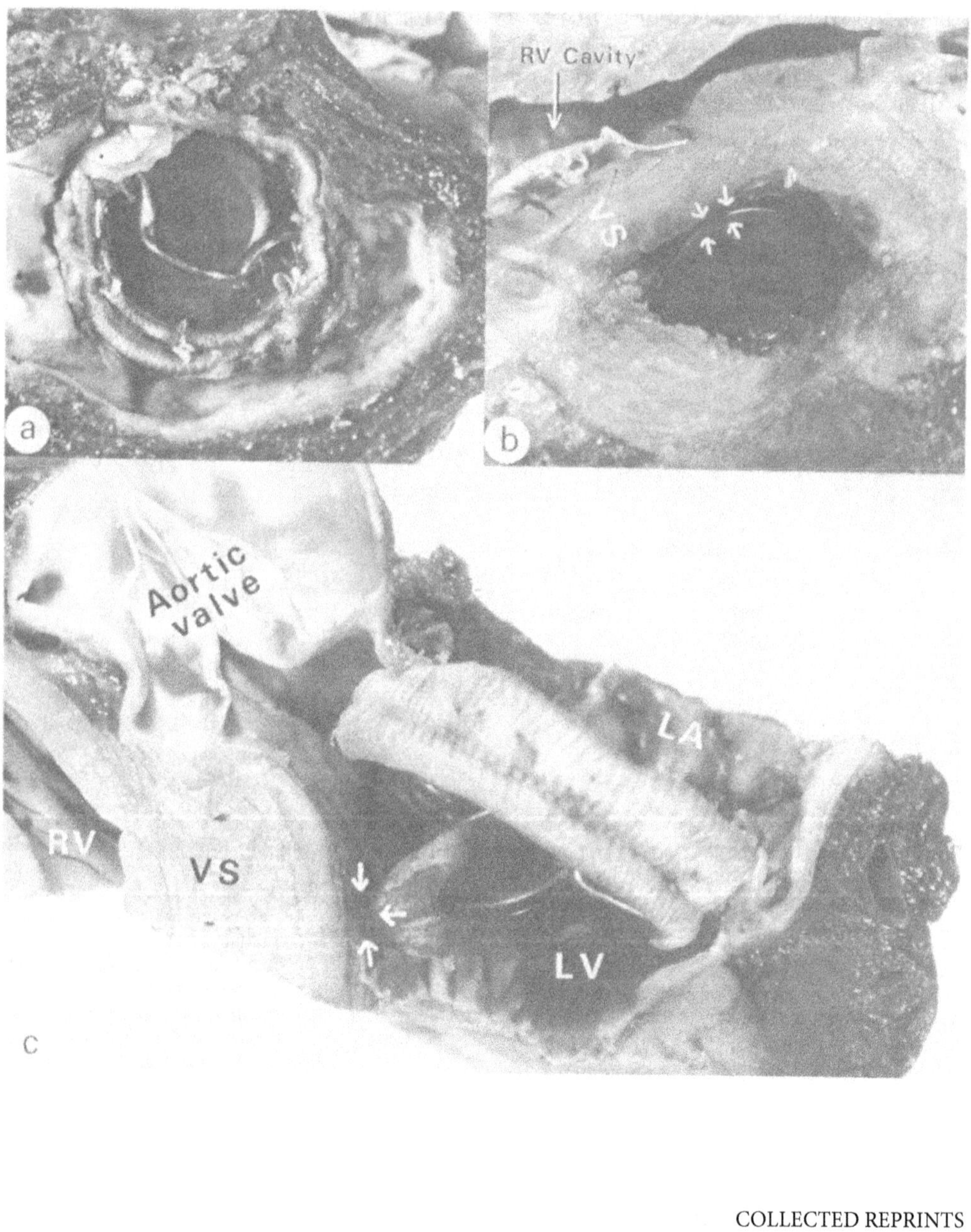

FIGURE 6. Prosthetic malfunction after replacement of a severely stenotic mitral valve with the largest-sized (31 mm) Björk-Shiley prosthesis in a 54 year old man. Although the prosthesis appears to have opened well, the occluder (disc) was prevented from seating by the ventricular septum, which "moved inward" during ventricular systole. The patient could not be separated from cardiopulmonary bypass. **a,** prosthesis as it *should appear* when viewed from left atrium during simulated ventricular systole. It fills most of the "floor" of this chamber. **b,** view of mitral prosthesis from below as it *did appear* during ventricular systole. The margin (**arrows**) of the disc contracted the ventricular septum (VS), preventing seating of the disc. RV = right ventricular. **c,** longitudinal cut of the heart again showing the disc as it appeared during ventricular systole. The margins (**arrows**) of the disc contact the ventricular septum. LA = left atrium; LV = left ventricle.

The initial results were gratifying: The valve lesions were usually ameliorated, and anticoagulant therapy was not required. The problem proved to be accelerated wear and tear with development of incompetency.[136–140] Other tissue valves followed—namely, fascia lata, dura mater, parietal pericardium—but all proved to be poor valve substitutes because they became stiff and relatively immobile.[141–145] The fresh antibiotic-sterilized homograft remains in use, but now the most commonly employed tissue valve is the porcine xenograft attached to a semiflexible stent[146] and preserved by a glutaraldehyde process.[146–153] (The graft failed when preserved in formalin.[141,154])

Porcine xenograft: Enthusiasm for this substitute valve is increasing. Although relatively few late postoperative hemodynamic studies have been reported, a pressure gradient across the porcine bioprosthesis has been recorded in all three valve positions despite its central flow. Among 56 patients studied late postoperatively after mitral valve replacement, the mean diastolic gradient averaged 6 mm Hg,[148,151,152] but of 37 patients studied at the National Heart, Lung, and Blood Institute, no gradient was recorded across the mitral porcine valve in 16 patients. Of 11 patients studied late postoperatively after tricuspid valve replacement with a porcine xenograft, the mean diastolic gradient averaged 4 mm Hg.[152] Hemodynamic data after aortic valve replacement with the porcine xenograft are virtually nonexistent: Among five patients studied late postoperatively at the National Heart, Lung, and Blood Institute, the peak systolic pressure gradients ranged from 10 to 35 mm Hg (average 18).[146] Other data are not available, to my knowledge.

Clinical episodes compatible with emboli are rare after valve replacement with the porcine xenograft and, therefore, its use rarely requires anticoagulant therapy. The porcine xenograft does not damage blood elements. The major concern is its wear characteristics. The en-

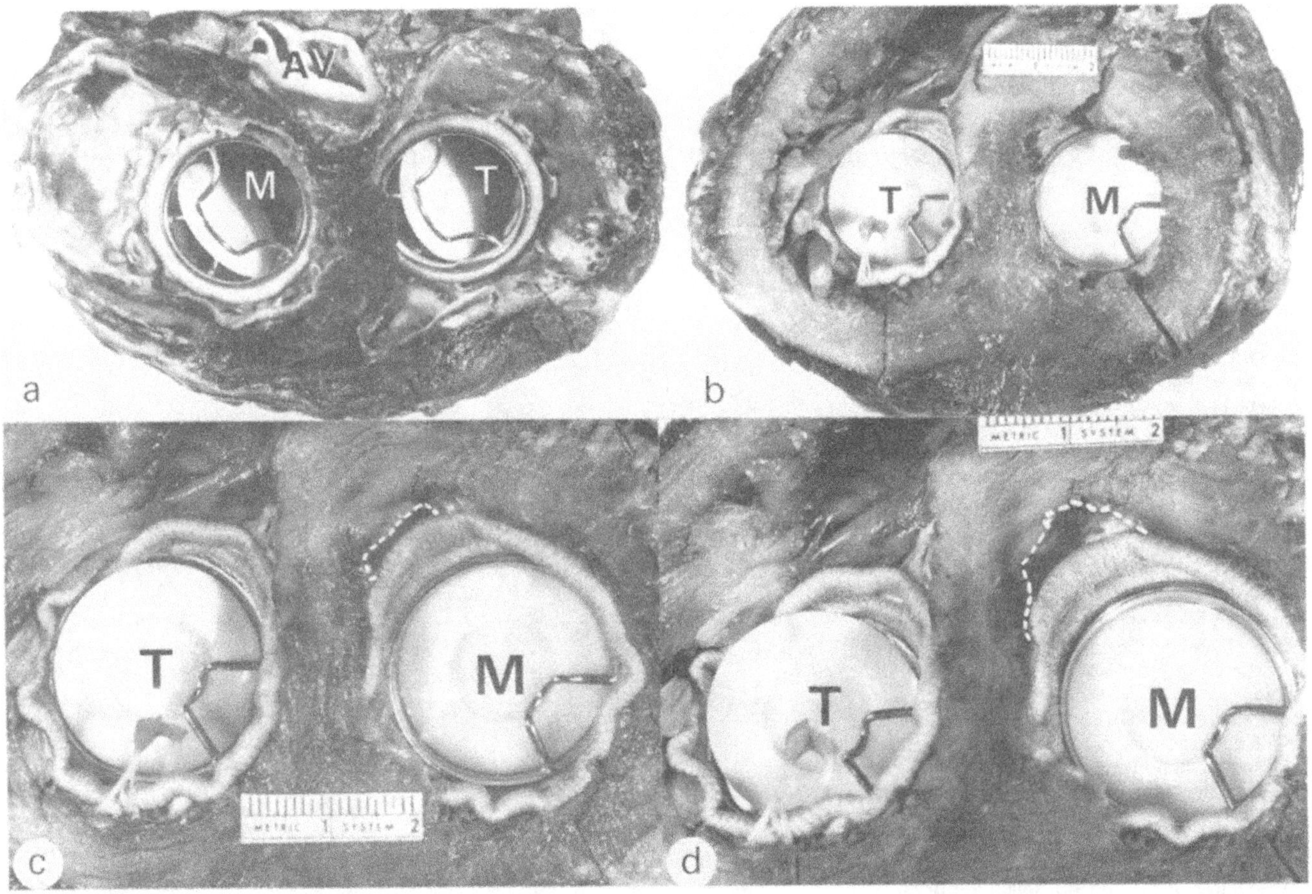

FIGURE 7. Prosthetic-ventricular chamber disproportion after replacement of both mitral and tricuspid valves with tilting-disc (Björk-Shiley) prostheses in a 64 year old woman with severe mitral stenosis, severe pulmonary hypertension and functional tricuspid regurgitation. At operation in April 1975, both mitral and tricuspid anuli readily accepted a 31 mm Björk sizer and, consequently, size 31 mm Björk-Shiley prostheses were inserted in both positions. The patient died in the operating room. At necropsy, the major problem appeared to be obstruction to left ventricular emptying (**b, c, d**) and, of lesser importance, failure of the tricuspid valve occluder to seat completely (**b, c, d**). **a,** heart during simulated ventricular diastole from the atrial aspect after most of the atrial walls have been excised. Both prostheses occupy most of the "floor" of each atrium. AV = aortic valve; M = mitral valve prosthesis; T = tricuspid valve prosthesis. **b,** view of both prostheses from below. The left ventricular outflow tract is nearly completely obliterated in this view by the mitral prosthesis. The tricuspid valve disc is prevented from seating completely. **c** and **d,** close-up views of both prostheses from the ventricular aspects showing interference to closure of the tricuspid occluder and severe obstruction to left ventricular outflow by the mitral prosthesis. The retained fragment of right ventricular papillary muscle and chordae tendineae potentially could have interfered with movement of the tricuspid valve occluder. The aortic valve was normal and the left ventricular cavity was of normal size.

couraging feature at this time is that there have been extremely few "valve failures"[146–153] and, indeed, no other substitute valve has had so few problems in its first 5 years. Nevertheless, relatively few patients (estimated to be about 500) have had this substitute valve in place for longer than 5 years, and signs of cusp degeneration, should they occur, are likely to occur after this period.

It is likely that the cusps of the porcine valve will be subject to changes that affect all natural left-sided cardiac valves, namely, lipid deposition and calcification.[155–157] These changes occur on the native valves, on the aortic aspects of the aortic valve cusps and on the ventricular aspects of the mitral valve cusps. Such changes will probably occur more rapidly in this substitute valve than in the natural valve, but, at least by 5 years, calcific deposits in the substitute valve cusps have been infrequent and minimal.[158] Small thrombi have been observed on the sinus aspects of the porcine cusps and possibly it is the organization of these minute thrombi that has led to the calcific deposits, at this point almost entirely microscopic in size.[141]

Factors Determining Outcome of Valve Replacement

At least six major factors appear to determine the result of valve replacement in a particular patient: (1) the type of the substitute valve inserted; (2) the size of the substitute valve inserted; (3) the experience and technical skill of the surgeon; (4) the adequacy of the "pump team," anesthesiologists and surgeons, physicians and nurses providing postoperative care; (5) the presence of associated (diagnosed or undiagnosed) or uncorrected cardiac disease or previous pericardiotomy; and (6) the preoperative status of the patient. The relative effect of each of these factors on the outcome of valve replacement will be examined next.

Assuming that the cardiac operation will take place in a large medical center where several cardiac operations are performed weekly by a surgeon or group of surgeons experienced in cardiac valve replacement, the most important factor determining the long-term outcome of valve replacement is the type of substitute valve inserted. At a conference on prosthetic valves for cardiac surgery held in Chicago[159] on September 9 and 10, 1960, it was observed that there were no living survivors of total cardiac valve replacement. After Starr's successful replacement of the mitral valve with a caged ball prosthesis on September 21, 1960, survival after valve replacement using the caged ball prosthesis rapidly became commonplace. The caged ball was the first prosthesis used for cardiac valve replacement by many surgeons whose previous valve operations had consisted entirely of mitral commissurotomy and yet, nearly from

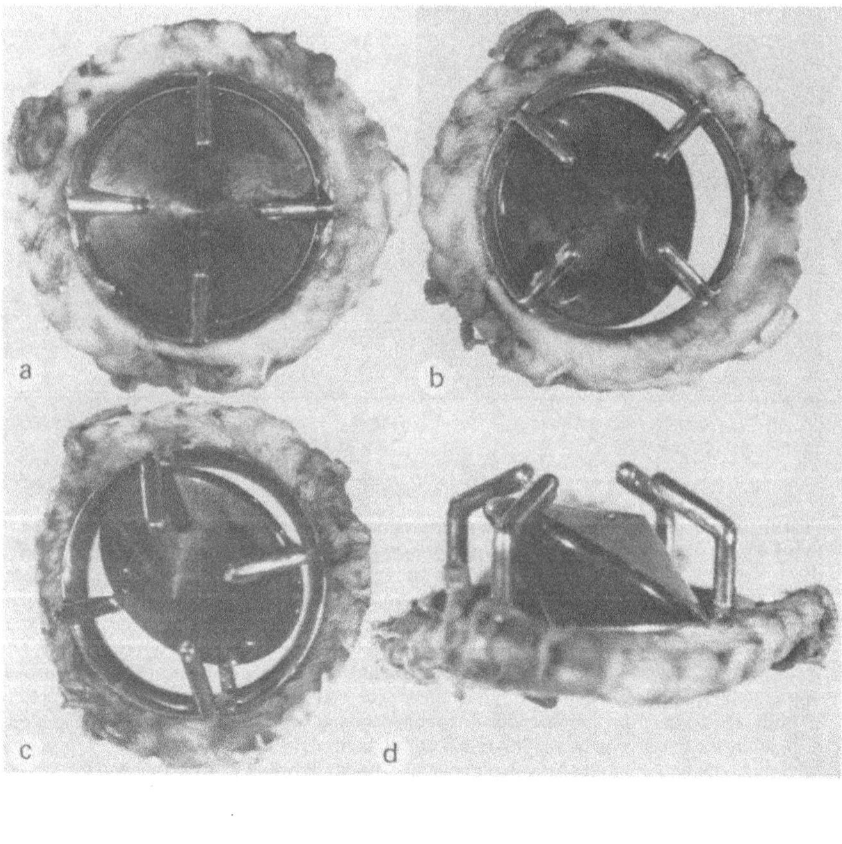

FIGURE 8. Various views of the Cooley-Cutter biconical caged disc prosthesis that had been inserted in the aortic valve position 4 months earlier in a 30 year old man because of severe pure aortic regurgitation. Late postoperatively the patient had severe aortic regurgitation (blood pressure 170/20 mm Hg) and fatal pulmonary edema. At necropsy, half of the circumference of the prosthesis had detached from the anulus, and there was no evidence of active infective endocarditis. The cause of the detachment, therefore, is uncertain, but at operation, continuous sutures had been utilized except for four interrupted sutures (one in each of the four quadrants). These four views of this prosthesis show potential types of cocking that are possible with any type of caged disc prostheses. A photograph of the closed prosthesis as it should appear in ventricular diastole is shown in **a.** For the occluder to ascend in the aortic position properly, pressure must be exerted on all portions of the occluder more or less equally. If pressure is exerted unequally for any reason, cocking may occur (**b, c, d**). One of the good features of the caged ball prosthesis is that the poppet ascends, in the aortic position, irrespective of the angle at which the blood is ejected from the left ventricle. Not so with the caged disc. If the prosthesis is inserted at a non-right angle to the aortic "anulus," the force of ejection may not be applied equally to all portions of the disc occluder. The result may be asymmetric opening of the prosthesis, and systolic cocking may be a precursor to diastolic cocking. In other words, the range of error for insertion of a caged disc in the aortic position is probably not as great as that inherent to the other three types of substitute cardiac valves discussed.

the beginning, rapid success was achieved using this device.

Choice of Valve Prosthesis

Choice of type of prosthesis: Because the decision regarding the type of substitute valve to be chosen for a particular patient is crucial, consideration might be given to the following questions: (1) Who *does* choose the type of prosthesis to be inserted? and (2) Who *should* choose the type of prosthesis to be inserted? From the beginning, that is, 1960, the surgeon has determined the type of prosthesis to be inserted in a particular patient. What are factors that determine a surgeon's preference for a prosthesis? The major one is previous experience, including personal experience and that of colleagues. The choice of prosthesis by a particularly prominent surgeon or by the trainer of a new cardiovascular surgeon may be especially influencing. Some surgeons who started with the caged ball, for example, and had satisfactory results are reluctant to change. One is simply more comfortable with the device one has used before. Change of prosthesis or model when it proves not to be ideal is admirable, and best exemplified by Cooley's experience with 34 different types or models of prosthetic cardiac valves.[116]

The choice of prosthesis by some surgeons has been influenced by personal involvement in the development of a particular prosthesis. Admitting that a prosthesis of someone else's design is better than one of one's own design is, at best, difficult. There may be inherent conflict when the same surgeon participates in the design of, and in the insertion of, a particular prosthesis. There have been many examples of this potential conflict during the past 16 years.

Again, assuming that valve replacement is to be performed in a large medical center with an experienced cardiovascular surgical team, long-term survival is more dependent on the type of prosthesis inserted than on the surgeon who inserts the prosthesis. Thus, if I personally were to undergo valve replacement, I would first choose the type of prosthesis and, second, the surgeon whose results with this particular prosthesis were excellent. In my view, the referring cardiologist is not fulfilling his responsibility by simply referring his patient to a surgeon irrespective of the type of prosthesis the surgeon most frequently utilizes. To use a caged disc, at least one of those with a flat occluder, is unwise in my view and, to date, few hemodynamic or other data are available to allow proper evaluation of the biconical type of caged disc. Although some surgeons periodically employ all four types of available substitute cardiac valves, most generally use only one or two types. If the patient has mitral stenosis or combined mitral and aortic valve disease (and in this circumstance the aortic "root" is usually small) or if the patient is small, referral to a surgeon who only, or nearly always, uses the caged ball prosthesis would not appear ideal. The fewest problems with valve replacement now appear to be with the porcine xenograft, but this too may change. Patients requiring valve replacement who have real or potential bleeding tendencies should have a porcine xenograft because anticoagulant therapy is required with use of any of the other three substitute valves.

Cardiologists in large medical centers usually refer their patients requiring valve replacement to the surgeons in the same medical center even though they may not necessarily be pleased with or involved in the choice of the substitute valve to be used. Ideally this choice would be made by both the cardiologist and the surgeon in light of all the data known about a particular patient. Greater participation by cardiologists in valve selection would require their acquisition of greater knowledge of such valves than they now generally have. Obviously, who chooses the type of substitute valve for a particular patient is not important so long as the choice is the right one, but surgeons do not necessarily have a monopoly on that right choice. The point is that the era of the "one-valve surgeon" may be over: "... Selection of the most favorable valve substitute for implantation should be individualized to each patient's specific anatomical, hemodynamic, and hematological needs".[160] It no longer appears proper for a surgeon to use only one type of substitute valve for all patients.

Determination of the size of prosthesis to insert: This determination, to my knowledge, has always been made in the operating room with the patient on cardiopulmonary bypass and after the insertion of various sizers placed through the valve orifice after excision of the native valve. But does this method best determine the size of a prosthesis to be inserted? My view is no. With the patient on cardiopulmonary bypass and with various retractors pulling on the heart, the surgeon may be able to insert large sizing devices and, therefore be led to insert a large prosthesis when, in actuality, with the patient off cardiopulmonary bypass and all retractors withdrawn, the valve orifice is much smaller (Fig. 6 and 7). Therefore, the size of the valve to be inserted might best be determined, not exclusively on the basis of sizing devices at operation, but at least in part on the basis of the hemodynamic valve lesion or lesions before operation with consideration of the lean weight of the patient. A small woman with pure mitral stenosis and a normally functioning aortic valve should have a relatively small prosthesis. Recently (1975), I saw the hearts at necropsy of two patients with severe isolated mitral stenosis who each had the largest tilting disc prosthesis (Björk-Shiley 31 mm). At operation in each, the sizing devices had apparently indicated that the valve orifice was capable of accommodating this large prosthesis. Yet fatal malfunction of the prosthesis because of its large size and each patient's "small" left ventricle occurred by mechanisms delineated in Figures 6 and 7. If the largest prosthesis is used in a small woman with pure mitral stenosis, what size of device should be used in a large man with pure mitral regurgitation? Thus, the decision regarding the size of prosthesis to insert might roughly be determined at the preoperative conference or consultation and based on the hemodynamic valve lesion and body weight and not entirely on the dimensions measured in the operating room.

Surgical Skill and Experience

Although I have thus far placed greatest emphasis on the type and size of the prosthetic valve inserted, the technical skill and experience of the surgeon are obviously extremely important and experience is probably more important than technical skill. (One of the finest examples of technical skill in the field of cardiac valve surgery is the placing of a porcine xenograft on a semiflexible cloth-covered stent. This procedure is performed by women before the tissue valve is shipped to surgeons.) There is no question that results of valve replacement are better among experienced than among nonexperienced surgeons, although the technical skills of the latter might be greater. The "occasional open heart surgeon," as emphasized by Eiseman and Spencer,[161] no matter how great his technical skill, is not the ideal cardiac surgeon. Certain technical factors, however, might be taken into consideration by the referring physician. Should prosthetic valves be inserted with continuous or interrupted sutures? It appears most reasonable that interrupted sutures would be less likely to be associated with "massive" prosthetic regurgitation (prosthetic disruption), and yet continuous or nearly continuous sutures are commonly employed by some surgeons.[162] If the world's "best" surgeon uses the world's worst prosthesis or inserts it by noninterrupted suture, the result may not be ideal.

Other Determinants of Results

The three other determinants of the results of cardiac valve replacement are self-evident. Obviously, the entire surgical team must be a good one. The patients with associated heart disease—for example, coronary heart disease or previous thoracotomy—do not do as well as patients without these complications.[61,62] The less sick the patient before operation the greater are his (or her) chances of survival after operation, but the sicker the patient before operation, usually the more dramatic is the change after operation.

Acknowledgment

I thank Dr. Johanna M. van der Bel-Kahn, Associate Professor of Pathology, University of Cincinnati, Cincinnati, Ohio, for allowing me to study with her two patients with a biconical disc prosthesis in the aortic valve position.

Addendum

Recently, some hemodynamic data have been reported concerning patients with a porcine (Hancock) xenograft valve in the aortic position. Cohn et al.[163] studied seven patients postoperatively and found they had a peak systolic pressure gradient at rest of 5 to 32 mm Hg (average 16 mm Hg). Morris[164] studied 23 patients postoperatively whose peak systolic pressure gradient at rest ranged from 6 to 58 mm Hg (mean 23 mm Hg). The higher pressure gradients tended to occur in the patients who had the smaller bioprostheses.

References

1. **Hufnagel CA, Harvey WP:** The surgical correction of aortic regurgitation. Preliminary report. Bull Georgetown Univ Med Center 6:60–61, 1953
2. **Hufnagel CA, Harvey WP, Rabil PJ, et al:** Surgical correction of aortic insufficiency. Surgery 35:673–683, 1954
3. **Harken DE, Soroff HS, Taylor WJ, et al:** Partial and complete prostheses in aortic insufficiency. J. Thorac Cardiovasc Surg 40:744–762, 1960
4. **Harken DE, Taylor WJ, Lefemine AA, et al:** Aortic valve replacement with a caged ball valve. Am J Cardiol 9:292–299, 1962
5. **Starr A, Edwards ML:** Mitral replacement: clinical experience with a ball-valve prosthesis. Ann Surg 154:726–740, 1961
6. **Murray G:** Homologous aortic-valve-segment transplants as surgical treatment for aortic and mitral insufficiency. Angiology 7:446–471, 1956
7. **Kerwin AJ, Lenkei SC, Wilson DR:** Aortic-valve homograft in the treatment of aortic insufficiency. Report of nine cases, with one followed for six years. N Engl J Med 266:852–857, 1962
8. **Beall AC, Morris GC, Cooley DA, et al:** Homotransplantation of aortic valve. J Thorac Cardiovasc Surg 42:497–506, 1961
9. **Ross DN:** Homograft replacement of the aortic valve. Lancet 2:487, 1962
10. **Duran CG, Gunning AJ:** A method for placing a total homologous aortic valve in the subcoronary position. Lancet 2:488–489, 1962
11. **Barratt-Boyes BG:** Homograft aortic valve replacement in aortic incompetence and stenosis. Thorax 19:131–150, 1964
12. **Barratt-Boyes BG, Lowe JB, Cole DS, et al:** Homograft valve replacement for aortic valve disease. Thorax 20:495–504, 1965
13. **Angell WW, Wuerflein RD, Shumway NE:** Mitral valve replacement with the fresh aortic valve homograft: experimental results and clinical application. Surgery 62:807–813, 1967
14. **Binet JP, Duran CG, Carpentier A, et al:** Heterologous aortic valve transplantation. Lancet 2:1275, 1965
15. **Ionescu MI, Wooler GH, Smith DR, et al:** Mitral valve replacement with aortic heterografts in humans. Thorax 22:305–313, 1967
16. **Carpentier A, Blondeau Ph, Laurens B, et al:** Mitral valve replacement with frame-mounted aortic heterografts. J Thorac Cardiovasc Surg 56:388–394, 1968
17. **Hufnagel CA, Conrad PW:** Comparative study of some prosthetic valves for aortic and mitral replacement. Surgery 57:205–210, 1965
18. **Kay EB, Suzuki A, Demaney M, et al:** Comparison of ball and disc valves for mitral valve replacement. Am J Cardiol 18:504–514, 1966
19. **Wada J:** Knotless suture method and Wada hingeless valve. Jpn J Thorac Surg 15:88–94, 1967
20. **Wada J, Komatsu S, Kamata K:** Cardiac valve replacement with Wada-Cutter prosthesis. Ann Thorac Surg 14:38–46, 1972
21. **Kaster RL, Lillehei CW:** A new cageless free-floating pivoting disc prosthetic heart valve: design, development and evaluation. In, Digest of the 7th International Conference on Medical and Biological Engineering. Stockholm, 1967, p 387
22. **Björk VO:** A new tilting disc valve prosthesis. Scand J Thorac Cardiovasc Surg 3:1–10, 1969
23. **Mason DT, Ross J Jr, Gault JH, et al:** Combined prosthetic replacement of the mitral and aortic valves. Preoperative and postoperative hemodynamic studies at rest and the left ventricular response to muscular exercise. Circulation 35, 36:Suppl I:I-15–I-23, 1967

24. **McHenry MM, Smeloff EA, Davey TB, et al:** Hemodynamic results with full-flow orifice prosthetic valves. Circulation 35, 36:Suppl I:I-24–I-33, 1967
25. **Glancy DL, O'Brien KP, Reis RL, et al:** Hemodynamic studies in patients with 2M and 3M Starr-Edwards prostheses: evidence of obstruction to left atrial emptying. Circulation 39, 40:Suppl I:I-113–I-118, 1969
26. **Reis RL, Glancy DL, O'Brien K, et al:** Clinical and hemodynamic assessments of fabric-covered Starr-Edwards prosthetic valves. J Thorac Cardiovasc Surg 59:84–91, 104–108, 1970
27. **Rodriguez L:** Haemodynamic and angiographic findings in patients with isolated aortic valvular disease before and after insertion of a Starr-Edwards aortic ball-valve prosthesis. Scand J Thorac Cardiovasc Surg [Suppl] 5:1–39, 1970
28. **Winter TQ, Reis RL, Glancy DL, et al:** Current status of the Starr-Edwards cloth-covered prosthetic cardiac valves. Circulation 45, 46:Suppl I:I-14–I-24, 1972
29. **Björk VO, Olin C, Rodriguez L:** Comparative results of aortic valve replacement with different prosthetic heart valves. J Cardiovasc Surg 13:268–271, 1972
30. **Levine FH, Copeland JG, Morrow AG:** Prosthetic replacement of the mitral valve. Continuing assessments of the 100 patients operated upon during 1961–1965. Circulation 47:518–526, 1973
31. **O'Rourke RA, Peterson KL, Braunwald NS:** Postoperative hemodynamic evaluation of a new fabric-covered ball-valve prosthesis. Circulation 47, 48:Suppl III:III-74–III-79, 1973
32. **Bonchek LI, Anderson RP, Starr A:** Mitral valve replacement with cloth-covered composite-seat prostheses. The case for early operation. J Thorac Cardiovasc Surg 67:93–109, 1974
33. **Bonchek LI, Starr A:** Ball valve prostheses: current appraisal of late results. Am J Cardiol 35:843–854, 1975
34. **Brawley RK, Donahoo JS, Gott VL:** Current status of the Beall, Björk-Shiley, Braunwald-Cutter, Lillehei-Kaster and Smeloff-Cutter cardiac valve prostheses. Am J Cardiol 35:855–865, 1975
35. **Smithwick W III, Kouchoukos NT, Karp RB, et al:** Late stenosis of Starr-Edwards cloth-covered prostheses. Ann Thorac Surg 20:249–255, 1975
36. **DeCesare W, Rath C, Hufnagel C:** Hemolytic anemia of mechanical origin with aortic-valve prosthesis. N Engl J Med 272: 1045–1050, 1965
37. **Walsch JR, Starr A, Ritzmann LW:** Intravascular hemolysis in patients with prosthetic valves and valvular heart disease. Circulation 39, 40:Suppl I:I-135–I-140, 1969
38. **Wallace HW, Kenepp DL, Blakemore WS:** Quantitation of red blood cell destruction associated with valvular disease and prosthetic valves. J Thorac Cardiovasc Surg 60:842–852, 1970
39. **Roberts WC, Morrow AG:** Renal hemosiderosis in patients with prosthetic aortic valves. Circulation 36:390–398, 1966
40. **Roberts WC, Morrow AG:** Causes of death and other anatomic observations after cardiac valve replacement. Adv Cardiol 7: 226–247, 1972
41. **Weily HS, Genton E:** Altered platelet function in patients with prosthetic mitral valves. Effects of sulfinpyrazone therapy. Circulation 42:967–972, 1970
42. **Steele PP, Weily HS, Davies H, et al:** Platelet survival time following aortic valve replacement. Circulation 51:358–362, 1975
43. **Ahmad R, Manohitharajah SM, Deverall PB, et al:** Chronic hemolysis following mitral valve replacement. A comparative study of the Björk-Shiley, composite-seat Starr-Edwards, and frame-mounted aortic homograft valves. J Thorac Cardiovasc Surg 71:212–217, 1976
44. **Starr A, Pierie WR, Raible DA, et al:** Cardiac valve replacement. Experience with the durability of silicone rubber. Circulation 33, 34:Suppl I:I-115–I-123, 1966
45. **Roberts WC, Morrow AG:** Late postoperative pathological findings after cardiac valve replacement. Circulation 35, 36:Suppl I:I-48–I-62, 1967
46. **Roberts WC, Morrow AG:** Anatomic studies of hearts containing caged-ball prosthetic valves. Johns Hopkins Med J 121:271–295, 1967
47. **Laforet EG:** Death due to swelling of ball component of aortic ball-valve prosthesis. N Engl J Med 276:1025–1027, 1967
48. **Roberts WC, Morrow AG:** Fatal degeneration of the silicone rubber ball of the Starr-Edwards prosthetic aortic valve. Am J Cardiol 22:614–620, 1968
49. **Sanderson RG, Hall AD, Thomas AN:** The clinical diagnosis of ball variance in a mitral valve prosthesis. Ann Thorac Surg 6: 473–475, 1968
50. **Collins JJ Jr, Berg EJ, Harken DE:** Silicone ball variance. A clinical and pulse duplicator study. Ann Thorac Surg 6:546–551, 1968
51. **Bonnabeau R, Lillehei W:** Mechanical "ball failure" in Starr-Edwards prosthetic valves. A report of three cases. J Thorac Cardiovasc Surg 56:258–264, 1968
52. **Leatherman LL, Leachman RD, McConn RG, et al:** Malfunction of mitral ball-valve prostheses due to a swollen poppet. J Thorac Cardiovasc Surg 57:160–163, 1969
53. **Roberts WC, Morrow AG:** Late postoperative pathologic findings following cardiac valve replacement with Starr-Edwards prostheses. In, Proceedings of Second National Conference on Prosthetic Heart Valves. Springfield, Ill, Charles C Thomas, 1969, p 365–393
54. **Hylen JC, Kloster FE, Starr A, et al:** Aortic ball variance: diagnosis and treatment. Ann Intern Med 72:1–8, 1970
55. **Roberts WC, Levinson GE, Morrow AG:** Lethal ball variance in the Starr-Edwards prosthetic mitral valve. Arch Intern Med 126:517–521, 1970
56. **Connolly DC, Harrison CE, Ellis FH Jr:** Ball variance in a Starr-Edwards prosthetic mitral valve causing acute pulmonary edema (diagnosis by auscultation before onset of symptoms). Mayo Clin Proc 45:20–24, 1970
57. **Metzger CC, Magovern GJ, Leonard JJ:** Ball variance in a sutureless mitral valve prosthesis. A report of two cases and a clue to early diagnosis. J Thorac Cardiovasc Surg 61:699–704, 1971
58. **Schluger J, Mannix EP Jr, Wolf RE:** Auscultatory and phonocardiographic sign of ball variance in a mitral prosthetic valve. Am Heart J 81:809–816, 1971
59. **Hylen JC, Hodam RP, Kloster FE:** Changes in the durability of silicone rubber in ball-valve prostheses. Ann Thorac Surg 13: 324–329, 1972
60. **Roberts WC, Bulkley BH, Morrow AG:** Pathologic anatomy of cardiac valve replacement: a study of 224 necropsy patients. Prog Cardiovasc Dis 15:539–587, 1973
61. **Barnhorst DA, Oxman HA, Connolly DC, et al:** Isolated replacement of the mitral valve with the Starr-Edwards prosthesis. An eleven-year review. J Thorac Cardiovasc Surg 71:230–237, 1976
62. **Barnhorst DA, Oxman HA, Connolly DC, et al:** Long-term follow-up of isolated replacement of the aortic or mitral valve with the Starr-Edwards prosthesis. Am J Cardiol 35:228–233, 1975
63. **Pluth JR, Broadbent JC, Barnhorst DA, et al:** Aortic and mitral valve replacement with cloth-covered Braunwald-Cutter prosthesis. A three-year follow up. Ann Thorac Surg 20:239–248, 1975
64. **Roberts WC, Morrow AG:** Mechanisms of acute left atrial thrombosis after mitral valve replacement. Pathologic findings indicating obstruction to left atrial emptying. Am J Cardiol 18: 497–503, 1966
65. **Roberts WC, Lambird PA, Gott VL, et al:** Fatal aortic regurgitation following replacement of the mitral and aortic valves. A mechanical complication of double valve replacement. J Thorac Cardiovasc Surg 52:189–192, 1966
66. **Roberts WC, Morrow AG:** Causes of early postoperative death following cardiac valve replacement. Clinico-pathologic correlations in 64 patients studied at necropsy. J Thorac Cardiovasc Surg 54:422–437, 1967
67. **Robicsek F, Sanger PW, Daugherty HK, et al:** Fatal arrhythmias caused by the pressure of the ball-valve prosthesis upon the left ventricular myocardium. Dis Chest 52:813–816, 1967
68. **Quattlebaum FW, Kalke B, Edwards JE, et al:** Obstruction of the aorta by prosthetic aortic valve. J Thorac Cardiovasc Surg 55: 231–237, 1968
69. **Kalke B, Korns ME, Goott B, et al:** Engagement of ventricular myocardium by open-cage atrioventricular valvular prosthesis. J Thorac Cardiovasc Surg 58:92–94, 1969
70. **Najafi H, Ostermiller WE Jr, Javid H, et al:** Narrow aortic root

complicating aortic valve replacement. Arch Surg 99:690–694, 1969
71. **Ibarra-Pérez C, Rodriguez-Trujillo F, Perez-Redondo H:** Engagement of ventricular myocardium by struts of mitral prosthesis. Fatal complications of use of open-cage cardiac valves. J Thorac Cardiovasc Surg 61:403–404, 1971
72. **Shepherd RL, Glancy DL, Stinson EB, et al:** Hemodynamic confirmation of obstruction to left ventricular inflow by a caged-ball prosthetic mitral valve. J Thorac cardiovasc Surg 65:252–254, 1973
73. **Seningen RP, Bulkley BH, Roberts WC:** Prosthetic aortic stenosis. A method to prevent its occurrence by measurement of aortic size from preoperative aortogram. Circulation 49:921–924, 1974
74. **Vander Veer JB Jr, Rhyneer GS, Hodam RP, et al:** Obstruction of tricuspid ball-valve prostheses. Circulation 43, 44:Suppl I:I-62–I-67, 1971
75. **Bache RJ, From AHL, Castaneda AR, et al:** Late thrombotic obstruction of Starr-Edwards tricuspid valve prosthesis. Chest 61:613–616, 1972
76. **Assad-Morrell JL, Tajik AJ, Anderson MW, et al:** Malfunctioning tricuspid valve prosthesis. Clinical, phonocardiographic, echocardiographic and surgical findings. Mayo Clinic Proc 49:443–447, 1974
77. **Baxter RH, Bain WH, Rankin RJ, et al:** Tricuspid valve replacement: a five-year appraisal. Thorax 30:158–161, 1975
78. **Malcolm AD, Ahuja SP, Chamberlain MJ:** Malfunction of tricuspid valve prosthesis shown by isotope angiocardiography. J Thorac Cardiovasc Surg 71:134–136, 1976
79. **Paton BC:** Reoperation for fibrinous stenosis of disc mitral valve prosthesis. J Thorac Cardiovasc Surg 57:726–731, 1969
80. **Horsley HT, Rappoport WJ, Vigoda PS, et al:** Fatal malfunction of Edwards low-profile mitral valves. Circulation 41, 42:Suppl I:II-39–II-42, 1970
81. **Mullen DC, Shull WH, Daugherty HK, et al:** Emergency thrombectomy of the prosthetic mitral valve. Vasc Surg 4:137–141, 1970
82. **Demany MA, Zimmerman HA:** Thrombosis of a mitral disc-valve prosthesis: diagnostic importance of the absent opening click. Am Heart J 80:816–819, 1970
83. **Gunstensen J:** Acute dysfunction of Starr-Edwards mitral prostheses. Thorax 26:163–166, 1971
84. **Stross JK, Willis PW, Kahn DR:** Diagnostic features of malfunction of disc mitral valve prostheses. JAMA 217:305–308, 1971
85. **Balkoura-Christopoulos MH, Resnekov L, Kittle CF:** Malfunction of a disc mitral valve prosthesis: detection by phonocardiography. Chest 63:624–626, 1973
86. **Linhart JW, Barold SS, Hildner FJ, et al:** Clinical and hemodynamic findings following replacement of the mitral valve with a Beall valve prosthesis (Dacron velour-covered Teflon-disc valve). Circulation 39, 40:Suppl I:I-127–I-134, 1969
87. **Vogel JHK, Paton BC, Overy HR, et al:** Abnormal hemodynamic function after disc mitral valve replacement. Circulation 39, 40:Suppl I:I-141–I-147, 1969
88. **Björk VO, Olin C, Aström H:** Results of aortic valve replacement with the Kay-Shiley disc valve. Scand J Thorac Cardiovasc Surg 3:93–106, 1969
89. **Kay EB, Suzuki A, Tambi A, et al:** Comparative analysis of the Starr-Edwards ball valve, the Kay-Suzuki disc valve and transplant valves in the surgical correction of aortic valve disease. Am J Cardiol 25:535–545, 1970
90. **Olin C:** Evaluation of the Kay-Shiley disc valve prosthesis in the aortic position. Clinical and haemodynamic results, and experimental comparison with other prosthetic aortic valves. Scand J Thorac Cardiovasc Surg [Suppl] 7:1–37, 1970
91. **Ramsey HW, Williams JC Jr, Vernon CR, et al:** Hemodynamic findings following replacement of the mitral valve with the Beall valve prosthesis. J Thorac Cardiovasc Surg 62:624–630, 1971
92. **Rogers AK, Morgan JR, Forker AD, et al:** Supravalvular stenosis after disc mitral valve replacement. J Thorac Cardiovasc Surg 62:810–812, 1971
93. **Reid JA, Stevens TW, Sigwart U, et al:** Hemodynamic evaluation of the Beall mitral valve prosthesis. Circulation 45, 46:Suppl I: I-1–I-7, 1972
94. **Shepherd RL, Glancy DL, Reis RL, et al:** Hemodynamic function of the Kay-Shiley prosthetic cardiac valve. Observations after mitral or tricuspid valve replacement. Chest 63:323–326, 1973
95. **Hawe A, Frye RL, Ellis FH Jr:** Late hemodynamic studies after mitral valve surgery. J Thorac Cardiovasc Surg 65:351–358, 1973
96. **Beall AC Jr, Morris GC Jr, Howell JF Jr, et al:** Clinical experience with an improved mitral valve prosthesis. Ann Thorac Surg 15: 601–606, 1973
97. **Roberts WC, Fishbein MC, Golden A:** Cardiac pathology after valve replacement by disc prosthesis. A study of 61 necropsy patients. Am J Cardiol 35:740–760, 1975
98. **Wellons HA Jr, Strauch RS, Nolan SP, et al:** Isolated mitral valve replacement with the Kay-Shiley disc valve. Actuarial analysis of the long-term results. J Thorac Cardiovasc Surg 70:862–868, 1975
99. **Fernandez J, Morse D, Spagna P, et al:** Results of mitral valve replacement with the Beall prosthesis in 209 patients. J Thorac Cardiovasc Surg 71:218–225, 1976
100. **Behrendt DM, Austen WG:** Current status of prosthetics for heart valve replacement. Prog Cardiovasc Dis 15:369–401, 1973
101. **Carey JS, Hughes RK:** A complication of mitral-valve replacement with caged-lens prosthesis. Ann Thorac Surg 6:77–81, 1968
102. **Vasko JS, Leighton RF:** Acute massive mitral regurgitation resulting from disc-valve malfunction. Ann Thorac Surg 6:564–569, 1968
103. **Robinson JJ, Hildner FJ, Greenberg JJ:** Disc variance of Beall mitral valve. Ann Thorac Surg 11:11–17, 1971
104. **Detmer DE, McIntosh CL, Boretos JW, et al:** Polypropylene poppets for low-profile prosthetic heart valves. Ann Thorac Surg 13:122–127, 1972
105. **Berroya RB, Escana FB Jr:** Mitral disc-valve variance. Thorax 27:87–89, 1972
106. **Hildner FJ, Robinson MJ:** Complications of Beall valve prosthesis. Am J Cardiol 30:922, 1972
107. **Nathan MJ:** Strut fracture. A late complication of Beall mitral valve replacement. Ann Thorac Surg 16:610–613, 1973
108. **Shaw TRD, Turner RWD:** Sudden mechanical malfunction of Hammersmith mitral valve prostheses due to wear of polypropylene. J Thorac Cardiovasc Surg 67:579–583, 1974
109. **Hughes DA, Leatherman LL, Norman JC, et al:** Late embolization of prosthetic mitral valve occluder with survival following reoperation. Ann Thorac Surg 19:212–215, 1975
110. **Low HBC, Lefemine AA:** Acute mitral insufficiency due to jamming of a disc-valve prosthesis. Ann Thorac Surg 4:71–73, 1967
111. **Hopeman AR, Treasure RL, Hall RJ:** Mechanical dysfunction in caged-lens prostheses. J Thorac Cardiovasc Surg 60:51–59, 1970
112. **Oliva PB, Johnson ML, Pomerantz M, et al:** Dysfunction of the Beall mitral prosthesis and its detection by cinefluoroscopy and echocardiography. Am J Cardiol 31:393–396, 1973
113. **Hammer WJ, Hearne MJ, Roberts WC:** Cocking of a poppet disc prosthesis in the aortic position. A cause of intermittent aortic regurgitation. J Thorac Cardiovasc Surg 71:259–261, 1976
114. **Williams JC Jr, Vernon CR, Daicoff GR, et al:** Hemolysis following mitral valve replacement with the Beall valve prosthesis. J Thorac Cardiovasc Surg 61:393–396, 1971
115. **Cooley DA, Okies JE, Wukasch DC, et al:** Ten-year experience with cardiac valve replacement: results with a new mitral prosthesis. Ann Surg 177:818–826, 1973
116. **Wukasch DC, Sandiford FM, Reul GJ Jr, et al:** Complications of cloth-covered prosthetic valves: results with a new mitral prosthesis. J Thorac Cardiovasc Surg 69:107–116, 1975
117. **Cooley DA, Sandiford FM, Wukasch DC, et al:** Mitral valve replacement with a new prosthesis. Experience with 366 patients. J Cardiovasc Surg (Torino): special no:378–383, 1975
118. **Edgett JW, Nelson WP, Hall RJ, et al:** A complication of valve replacement by a caged-lens prosthesis. Circulation 36:422–426, 1967
119. **Hammermeister KE, Dillard DH, Kennedy JW:** Severe, intermittent, mitral regurgitation in a Cross-Jones valve. Report of a case with angiocardiographic and hemodynamic observations. J Thorac Cardiovasc Surg 58:575–580, 1969

120. **Roe BB, Fishman NH, Hutchinson JC, et al:** Occluder disruption of Wada-Cutter valve prosthesis. Ann Thorac Surg 20:256–264, 1975
121. **Björk VO, Holmgren A, Olin C, et al:** Clinical and hemodynamic results of aortic valve replacement with the Björk-Shiley tilting disc valve prosthesis. Scand J Thorac Cardiovasc Surg 5: 177–191, 1971
122. **Lepley D, Reuben CF, Flemma RJ, et al:** Experience with the Björk-Shiley prosthetic valve. Circulation 47, 48:Suppl III:III-51–III-55, 1973
123. **Böök K:** Mitral valve replacement with the Björk-Shiley tilting disc valve. A clinical and haemodynamic study in patients with isolated mitral valve lesions. Scand J Thorac Cardiovasc Surg [Suppl] 12:1–28, 1974
124. **Lillehei CW, Kaster RL, Coleman M, et al:** Heart-valve replacement with Lillehei-Kaster pivoting disk prosthesis. NY State J Med 8:1426–1438, 1974
125. **Björk VO, Henze A, Holmgren A:** Five years' experience with the Björk-Shiley tilting-disc valve in isolated aortic valvular disease. J Thorac Cardiovasc Surg 68:393–404, 1974
126. **Björk VO, Henze A, Holmgren A:** Long-term results with the Björk-Shiley tilting disc valve in aortic valvular disease. Isr J Med Sci 11:161–172, 1975
127. **Starek PJK, Wilcox BR, Murray GF:** Hemodynamic evaluation of the Lillehei-Kaster pivoting disc valve in patients. J Thorac Cardiovasc Surg 71:123–128, 1976
128. **Slater SD, Sallam IA, Bain WH, et al:** Haemolysis with Björk-Shiley and Starr-Edwards prosthetic heart valves: a comparative study. Thorax 29:624–631, 1974
129. **Roberts WC, Hammer WJ:** Cardiac pathology after valve replacement with a tilting disc prosthesis (Björk-Shiley type): a study of 46 necropsy patients and 49 Björk-Shiley prostheses. Am J Cardiol 37:1024–1033, 1976
130. **Messmer BJ, Okies JE, Hallman GL, et al:** Mitral valve replacement with the Björk-Shiley tilting-disc prosthesis. J Thorac Cardiovasc Surg 62:938–946, 1971
131. **Messmer BJ, Okies JE, Hallman GL, et al:** Early and late thromboembolic complications after mitral valve replacement. A comparative study of various prostheses. J Cardiovasc Surg 13:281–289, 1972
132. **Messmer BJ, Okies JE, Hallman GL, et al:** Aortic valve replacement: two years' experience with the Björk-Shiley tilting-disc prosthesis. Surgery 72:772–779, 1972
133. **Henze A, Carlsson S, Björk VO:** Mortality and pathology following aortic valve replacement with the Björk-Shiley tilting disc valve. Scand J Thorac Cardiovasc Surg 7:7–16, 1973
134. **Ben-Zvi J, Hildner FJ, Chandraratna PA, et al:** Thrombosis on Björk-Shiley aortic valve prosthesis. Clinical, arteriographic, echocardiographic and therapeutic observations in seven cases. Am J Cardiol 34:538–544, 1974
135. **Byrd CL, Yahr WZ, Greenberg JJ:** Long-term results of "simple" thrombectomy for thrombosed Björk-Shiley aortic valve prostheses. Ann Thorac Surg 20:265–273, 1975
136. **Ross D:** Biologic valves. Their performance and prospects. Circulation 45:1259–1272, 1972
137. **Angell WW, Shumway NE, Kosek JC:** A five-year study of viable aortic valve homografts. J Thorac Cardiovasc Surg 64:329–339, 1972
138. **Wallace RB, Londe SP, Titus JL:** Aortic valve replacement with preserved aortic valve homografts. J Thorac Cardiovasc Surg 67:44–52, 1974
139. **Wallace RB:** Tissue valves. Am J Cardiol 35:866–871, 1975
140. **Moore CH, Martelli V, Al-Janabi N, et al:** Analysis of homograft valve failure in 311 patients followed up to 10 years. Ann Thorac Surg 20:274–281, 1975
141. **Yarbrough JW, Roberts WC, Reis RL:** Structural alterations in tissue cardiac valves implanted in patients and in calves. J Thorac Cardiovasc Surg 65:364–375, 1973
142. **Ionescu MI, Pakrashi BC, Mary DAS, et al:** Replacement of heart valves with frame-mounted tissue grafts. Thorax 29:56–67, 1974
143. **Nuno-Conceicão A, Puig LB, Verginelli G, et al:** Homologous dura mater cardiac valves. Structural aspects of eight implanted valves. J Thorac Cardiovasc Surg 70:499–508, 1975
144. **Mary DAS, Pakrashi BC, Catchpole RW, et al:** Tissue valves in the mitral position. Five years' experience. Br Heart J 37: 1123–1132, 1975
145. **Olsen EGJ, Al-Janabi N, Salamáo CS, et al:** Fascia lata valves: a clinicopathological study. Thorax 30:528–534, 1975
146. **Reis RL, Hancock WD, Yarbrough JW, et al:** The flexible stent. A new concept in the fabrication of tissue heart valve prostheses. J Thorac Cardiovasc Surg 62:683–695, 1971
147. **Stinson EB, Griepp RB, Shumway NE:** Clinical experience with a porcine aortic valve xenograft for mitral valve replacement. Ann Thorac Surg 18:391–401, 1974
148. **Horowitz MS, Goodman DJ, Fogarty TJ, et al:** Mitral valve replacement with the glutaraldehyde-preserved porcine heterograft. Clinical, hemodynamic, and pathological correlations. J Thorac Cardiovasc Surg 67:885–895, 1974
149. **Carpentier A, Deloche A, Relland J, et al:** Six-year follow-up of glutaraldehyde-preserved heterografts. With particular reference to the treatment of congenital valve malformations. J Thorac Cardiovasc Surg 68:771–782, 1974
150. **Brown JW, Myerowitz PD, Cann MS, et al:** Clinical and hemodynamic comparisons of Kay-Shiley, Starr-Edwards no. 6520, and Reis-Hancock porcine xenograft mitral valves. Surgery 76:983–991, 1974
151. **Johnson AD, Daily PO, Peterson KL, et al:** Functional evaluation of the porcine heterograft in the mitral position. Circulation 50, 51:Suppl I:I-40–I-48, 1975
152. **McIntosh CL, Michaelis LL, Morrow AG, et al:** Atrioventricular valve replacement with the Hancock porcine xenograft: a five year clinical experience. Surgery 78:768–775, 1975
153. **Pipkin RD, Buch WS, Fogarty TJ:** Evaluation of aortic valve replacement with a porcine xenograft without long-term anticoagulation. J Thorac Cardiovasc Surg 71:179–186, 1976
154. **Zudhi N, Hawley W, Voehl V, et al:** Porcine aortic valves as replacement for human heart valves. Ann Thorac Surg 17:479–491, 1974
155. **Roberts WC, Perloff JK, Constantino T:** Severe valvular aortic stenosis in patients over 65 years of age. A clinicopathologic study. Am J Cardiol 27:497–506, 1971
156. **Roberts WC, Perloff JK:** Mitral valvular disease. A clinicopathologic survey of the conditions causing the mitral valve to function abnormally. Ann Intern Med 77:939–975, 1972
157. **Roberts WC, Dangel JC, Bulkley BH:** Nonrheumatic valvular cardiac disease: a clinicopathologic survey of 27 different conditions causing valvular dysfunction. Cardiovasc Clin 5:333–446, 1973
158. **Hancock WD:** Personal communication, November 1975
159. **Merendino KA, Morrow AG, Lillehei CW, et al:** Prosthetic Valves for Cardiac Surgery. Springfield, Ill, Charles C Thomas, 1961, p 86
160. **Braunwald NS:** The fabric-covered prosthetic heart valve. Present status and future development. Ann Thorac Surg 20:360–363, 1975
161. **Eiseman B, Spencer FC:** The occasional open-heart surgeon. Circulation 31:161–162, 1965
162. **Fernandez J:** Insertion of Björk-Shiley aortic prosthesis by continuous suture technique. Ann Thorac Surg 17:587–590, 1974
163. **Cohn LH, Sanders JH Jr, Collins JJ Jr:** Aortic valve replacement with the Hancock porcine xenograft. Presented at the Society of Thoracic Surgeons, Washington, DC, January, 1976
164. **Morris DC:** Hemodynamic evaluation of porcine xenograft valve. Presented at the Annual Scientific Sessions of the American College of Cardiology, New Orleans, February, 1976

Clinical pathologic conference

A conversation on prosthetic valve endocarditis

Ernest N. Arnett, M.D.*
David G. Kastl, M.D.
A. Julian Garvin, M.D., Ph.D.
William C. Roberts, M.D.
Bethesda, Md.

DR. ROBERTS: The starting point for this discussion on prosthetic valve endocarditis will be a description of a patient with this fatal complication of cardiac valve replacement.

DR. KASTL: This 47-year-old man (J.G. #1123701) was in good health until 11 months before death when symptoms of fatigue and exertional dyspnea appeared four weeks after a dental procedure. Hospitalization four months after onset of symptoms (seven months before death) revealed anemia, a colonic filling defect, periodic fever, and *Streptococcus bovis* in several blood cultures. Penicillin, 20 million units intravenously per day, was administered for six weeks; the fever rapidly disappeared, but murmurs of mitral and aortic regurgitation and signs of congestive heart failure appeared. Digoxin and diuretic therapy resulted in transient improvement of the congestive heart failure, and the colonic mass, which proved to be a benign polyp, was resected. He returned home, but heart failure quickly returned and he was hospitalized, now in functional Class IV (New York Heart Association classification), 55 days before death. Digoxin, furosemide, and aldactone produced a 20 pound weight loss. Subsequently, at cardiac catheterization, the pressures in mm. Hg were: pulmonary artery wedge mean 35, a wave 35, v wave 55; pulmonary artery 60/35 (mean 50); right ventricle 60/15; and right atrial mean 15, a wave 22, and v wave 17. Multiple blood cultures during that hospitalization were negative. He was transferred to the National Heart, Lung and Blood Institute (NHLI) 37 days before death.

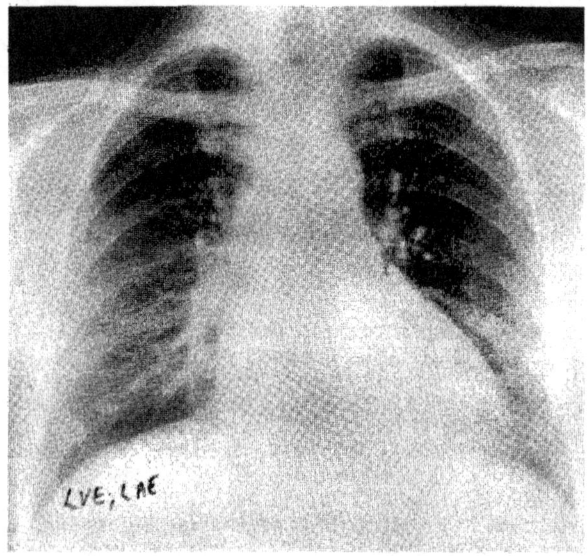

Fig. 1. Posteroanterior chest roentgenogram 4 days before valve replacement.

The blood pressure was 140/70 mm. Hg, cardiac rate, 90 beats per minute, and respiratory rate, 20 breaths per minute. The jugular venous pressure was elevated, and the carotid upstroke was rapid but weak. Basilar râles were present in both lungs. The second heart sound split paradoxically and both third and fourth heart sounds were present. A Grade 3/6 decrescendo diastolic murmur was present along the left sternal border, and a Grade 2/6 holosystolic murmur and a Grade 2/6 middiastolic rumbling murmur were present at the apex. The anteroinferior edge of the liver was palpable 4 cm. below the right costal margin. Chest roentgenograms (Fig. 1) showed marked cardiac enlargement and electrocardio-

From the Pathology Branch and Clinic of Surgery, National Heart, Lung and Blood Institute, and the Laboratory of Pathology, National Cancer Institute, National Institutes of Health, Bethesda, Md.

Received for publication June 9, 1976.

Reprint requests: W. C. Roberts, M.D., Bldg. 10A Rm 3E-30, National Institutes of Health, Bethesda, Maryland 20014.

*Present address: Department of Medicine, The Johns Hopkins Hospital, Baltimore, Maryland.

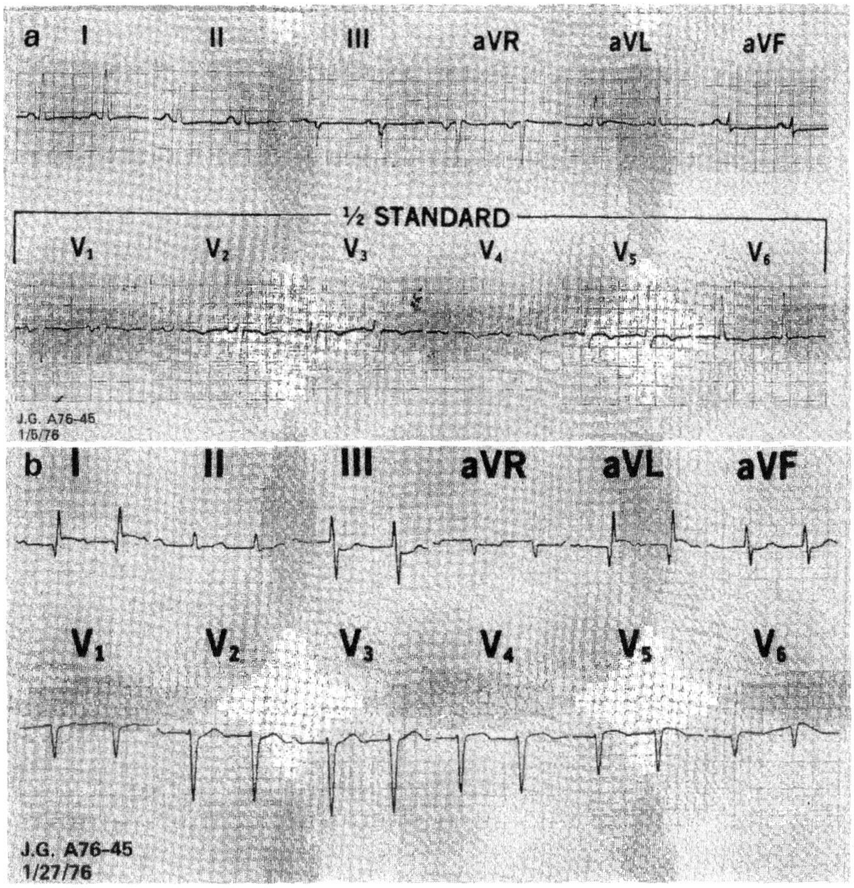

Fig. 2. Electrocardiograms. *a,* Four days before valve replacements showing changes of left ventricular hypertrophy and left atrial enlargement. *b,* Eighteen days postoperatively (10 days before death). Q waves are present in Leads I, aVR, aVL and V_6, the R waves in the precordial leads are of markedly diminished amplitude, and the ST segments are elevated in Leads I, aVL and V_4 through V_6. In addition, the P-R interval is prolonged.

gram (Fig. 2*a*) showed left ventricular hypertrophy. The hematocrit was 37 per cent, and the white blood count 11,900 per cubic millimeter. Simultaneous aortic and left ventricular pressures were 120/50 and 120/30 mm. Hg, respectively. Cineangiography revealed severe aortic and mitral valve regurgitation, but good left ventricular function.

The aortic valve was replaced with a No. 10A model 2320, Starr-Edwards prosthesis and the mitral valve, with a 33 mm. Hancock xenograft 28 days before death. Both the excised aortic valve and the excised mitral valve (Fig. 3) contained one or more perforations in the cusps. Histologic examination of the excised valves revealed no evidence of active infection.

During the first 24 hours postoperatively, excessive bleeding necessitated repeat thoracotomy. Although no specific bleeding sites were found, a large quantity (2,000 ml.) of blood was evacuated from the mediastinum. Oxacillin, 4 Gm. intravenously per day, and streptomycin, 1 Gm. intramuscularly per day, were started at the time of the initial operation and continued for 10 and 7 days, respectively. All chest tubes were removed on the fourth postoperative day. Two days later fever (38.5° C.) was noted but he otherwise appeared to be doing well. Nine days postoperatively ventricular fibrillation occurred, but electroshock was successful in restoring sinus rhythm. Electrocardiograms following this episode showed diffuse nonspecific ST segment and T wave abnormalities. Over the ensuing 4 days, he continued to have frequent ventricular premature beats. On the 17th postoperative day his temperature rose to 39.5° C., the white blood cell

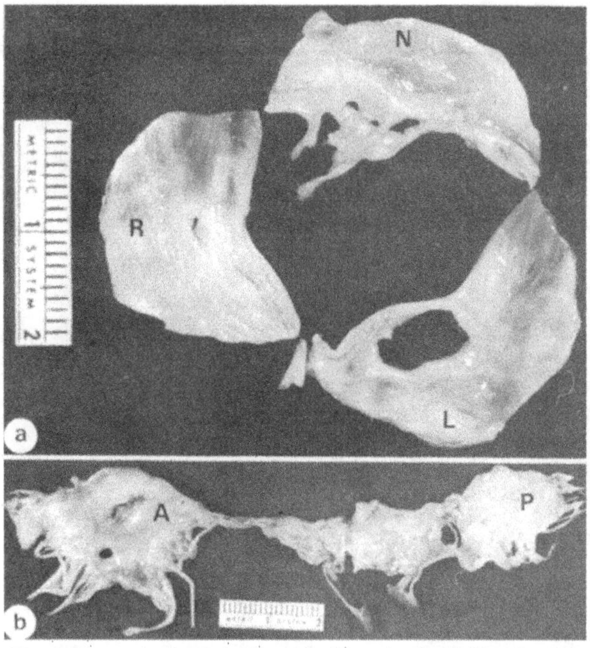

Fig. 3. Operatively excised aortic *(a)* and mitral *(b)* valves. A single perforation is present in the left *(L)* and right *(R)* coronary cusp, and multiple ones are present in the noncoronary *(N)* cusp. A perforation is present in the anterior *(A)* mitral leaflet, and several chordae tendineae from the posterior *(P)* mitral leaflet are absent.

count was 14,500 per cubic millimeter, and blood cultures were positive for *Staphylococcus epidermidis.* Oxacillin, 12 Gm. intravenously per day, was reinstituted. The following day the blood pressure dropped to 95/70 mm. Hg and the electrocardiogram (Fig. 2*b*) showed changes of an acute anterolateral myocardial infarction. On the nineteenth postoperative day, splinter hemorrhages were noted, the white blood cell count was 17,000 per cubic millimeter, and blood cultures again were positive for *S. epidermidis,* resistant to penicillin but sensitive to both oxacillin and cephalosporin. On the twenty-first postoperative day he lost consciousness, his temperature rose to 39° C., and his systolic blood pressure fell to 90 mm. Hg. During insertion of a catheter into a jugular vein, a collection of pus was entered, and Gram stain and culture of the aspirated material disclosed *S. epidermidis.* Exploration of the mediastinum revealed no focal collections of pus. Oxacillin was stopped and cephalosporin, 12 Gm. intravenously per day, was started. Over the next four days consciousness returned, the blood pressure rose to 110/60 mm. Hg, but the white blood count was 27,000 per cubic millimeter, and fever and positive blood cultures continued. On the twenty-seventh postoperative day, his blood pressure suddenly dropped and he died the next day.

Dr. Garvin: Necropsy (A76-45) disclosed no residual pus in the chest. The heart weighed 660 Gm., and the anterolateral left ventricular wall from midportion to apex was necrotic. Large vegetations closed the primary orifice of the aortic valve prosthesis, and a fibrin thrombus was present at the apex of its cage (Fig. 4). Although the aortic prosthesis remained attached, the site of attachment of the prosthesis was necrotic. Necrosis of the valve anulus, however, was apparent only after removal of the prosthesis (Fig. 5). The ring infection extended through the atrial spetum into the right atrium and into the adjacent portion of the prosthetic mitral anulus. Histologic sections from the site of attachment of the aortic prosthesis revealed numerous colonies of Gram-positive cocci. Examination of subserial sections of the extramural coronary arteries revealed total obstruction of the lumen of the left anterior descending coronary artery by a septic embolus (Fig. 6). Sections of myocardium showed numerous foci of suppurating and nonsuppurating inflammation. The lungs were edematous and contained foci of acute inflammation. The walls of the small muscular pulmonary arteries were thick. Both the liver (2,600 grams) and spleen (670 grams) were enlarged, and multiple infarcts were present in the spleen. Focal collections of mononuclear cells were present in the renal interstitium, but otherwise the kidneys were normal.

Dr. Roberts: The above-described patient provides an opportunity to apply information previously derived from a study of 22 necropsy patients with fatal prosthetic valve endocarditis to the present patient.[1] To begin this discourse, Dr. Arnett, how do you define "Prosthetic Valve Endocarditis?"

Dr. Arnett: "Prosthetic valve endocarditis" is an infection involving a prosthetic cardiac valve in a patient in whom no active infective endocarditis was present at the time of prosthetic valve insertion. In other words, the infection was acquired after valve replacement. Although the present patient's valvular disease resulted from infective endocarditis, the infection was healed at the time of valve replacement.

Dr. Roberts: Dr. Kastl, in your presentation of this patient, you mentioned that the cause of

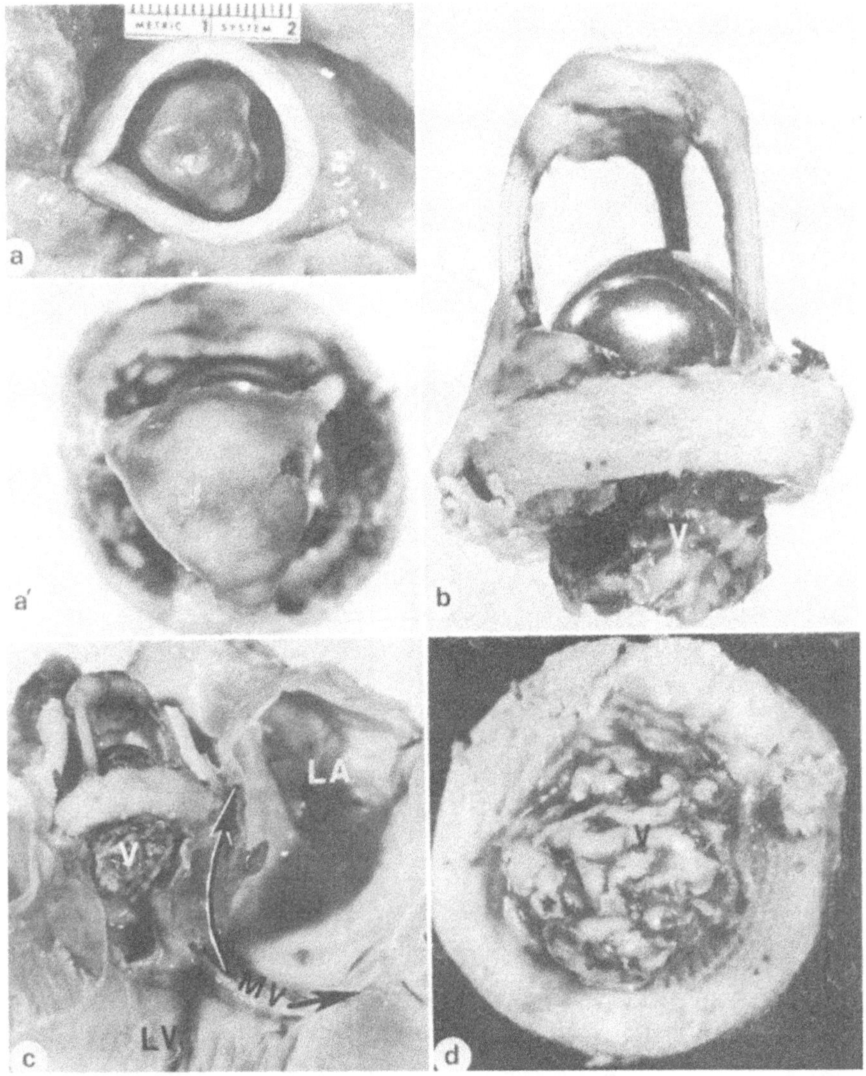

Fig. 4. Infected aortic valve prosthesis. *a,* Prosthesis, viewed from above, in place, and *a'* after removal. Thrombus covers the apex of the cage. *b,* Excised prosthesis viewed laterally. *c,* Longitudinal section showing aortic prosthesis in place. The mitral valve prosthesis has been excised. The aortic "anulus" is necrotic and so is the adjacent portion of mitral anulus. A large vegetation *(V)* is present in the primary orifice of the prosthesis; its obstructive nature is better seen in *d,* a view of the prosthesis from the left ventricular *(LV)* aspect. *LA* = left atrium.

this patient's infective endocarditis, which had involved presumably both anatomically and functionally normal valves, was *Streptococcus bovis.* The cause of the prosthetic valve endocarditis in him, however, was *Staphylococcus epidermidis.* Dr. Arnett, could you summarize the organisms found in our previous 22 patients with prosthetic valve endocarditis?

Dr. Arnett: Among our 22 previous necropsy patients with prosthetic valve endocarditis, *Staphylococcus (epidermidis* in 10 and *aureus* in three) caused the infection in 13 (59 per cent.) In the other nine patients, nine different organisms caused the infection. Of these later nine organisms, three were Gram-negative bacteria, and two were fungi.

Dr. Roberts: We have found it useful to subdivide patients with prosthetic valve endocarditis into those with early infection, i.e., appearing within two months of valve replacement, and those with infection appearing later, i.e., those with signs of cardiac infection appearing longer than two months after operation. Dr. Arnett, have there been any differences in the types of infecting organisms in patients with early prosthetic valve endocarditis as contrasted to those in

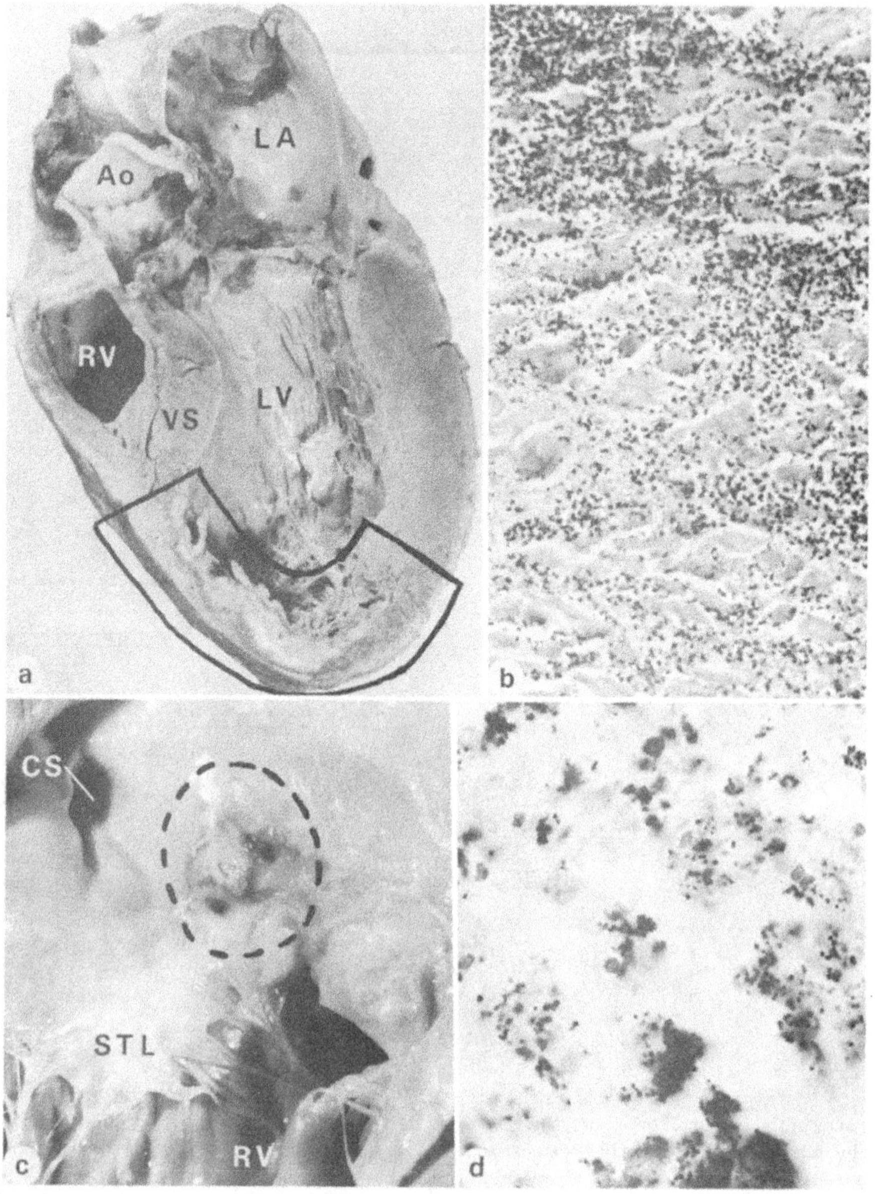

Fig. 5. Ring abscess and acute myocardial infarct. *a,* Longitudinal section of heart showing the ring abscess involving the entire aortic "anulus" and the portion of mitral anulus adjacent to the aortic valve. A large transmural infarct is present in the anterior wall of left ventricle (in brackets). *Ao* = aorta; *LA* = left atrium; *LV* = left ventricle; *RV* = right ventricle; *VS* = ventricular septum. *b,* Histologic section of the anterior left ventricular wall. The myocardial cells are necrotic and numerous polymorphonuclear leukocytes are present. (Hematoxylin and eosin stain; × 330). *c,* Opened right atrium, tricuspid valve, and right ventricle *(RV).* The aortic ring abscess has extended through the adjacent atrial septum and is visible in right atrium *(dashed circle). CS* = ostium of coronary sinus; *STL* = septal tricuspid leaflet. *d,* Histologic section showing colonies of Gram-positive cocci in the necrotic aortic valve anulus (Brown and Brenn stain; × 880).

whom the infection appeared months or years after valve replacement?

Dr. Arnett: Among patients with early prosthetic valve endocarditis, *Staphylococcus epidermidis* has been the most frequent causative organism.[2-4] Among patients with late prosthetic valve endocarditis both staphylococci and streptococci have been frequent causes; however, the former have caused most cases of necropsy-proven late prosthetic valve endocarditis, and the latter, relatively few.

Dr. Roberts: Among patients with early prosthetic valve endocarditis it is presumed that the infection either was incurred at operation or resulted from a wound infection. The former may result from contamination of cardiopulmonary bypass equipment.[5, 6] Dr. Arnett, what have been the predisposing factors in patients with late prosthetic valve endocarditis?

DR. ARNETT: Late prosthetic valve endocarditis presumably results from transient bacteremia, and the source of the bacteremia is often obscure.[3, 7] Among our previous 22 necropsy patients with prosthetic valve endocarditis, 14 had the onset of symptoms of prosthetic endocarditis longer than two months after operation. Predisposing factors were apparent in only five of them: dental procedures in two, and in one patient each, skin graft infection, prolonged use of an intravenous catheter, and prolonged use of a transthoracic pacing wire.

DR. ROBERTS: Dr. Arnett, you mentioned a similarity between early and late prosthetic endocarditis in regard to the types of infecting organisms. Are there distinct clinical differences between patients with prosthetic valve endocarditis appearing early after operation as contrasted to those with infection appearing late?

DR. ARNETT: Prosthetic valve endocarditis occurring in the early postoperative period is often more difficult to diagnose.[7] Signs of prosthetic infection may be masked by other more common postoperative complications, and transient bacteremia may be attributed to another cause. That was the situation in the present patient: persistent staphylococcal bacteremia was attributed to the known mediastinal infection and the diagnosis of prosthetic valve endocarditis was never established during life. When fever and bacteremia appear suddenly in an otherwise well patient months or years after cardiac valve replacement, however, a diagnosis of prosthetic valve endocarditis is usually made quite readily.

DR. ROBERTS: It is worth emphasizing, however, that the combination of fever and positive blood culture in a patient with a prosthetic cardiac valve, especially in the early postoperative period, does not always indicate the presence of prosthetic valve endocarditis.[8] We recently studied at necropsy a patient who was diagnosed during life as having mitral prosthetic valve endocarditis on the basis of fever, cerebral episodes consistent with emboli, and a blood culture which grew *Staphylococcus epidermidis*. She received antibiotics during most of her four-month postoperative period and, at necropsy, no prosthetic valve endocarditis was found. A left ventricular aneurysm, however, was present immediately

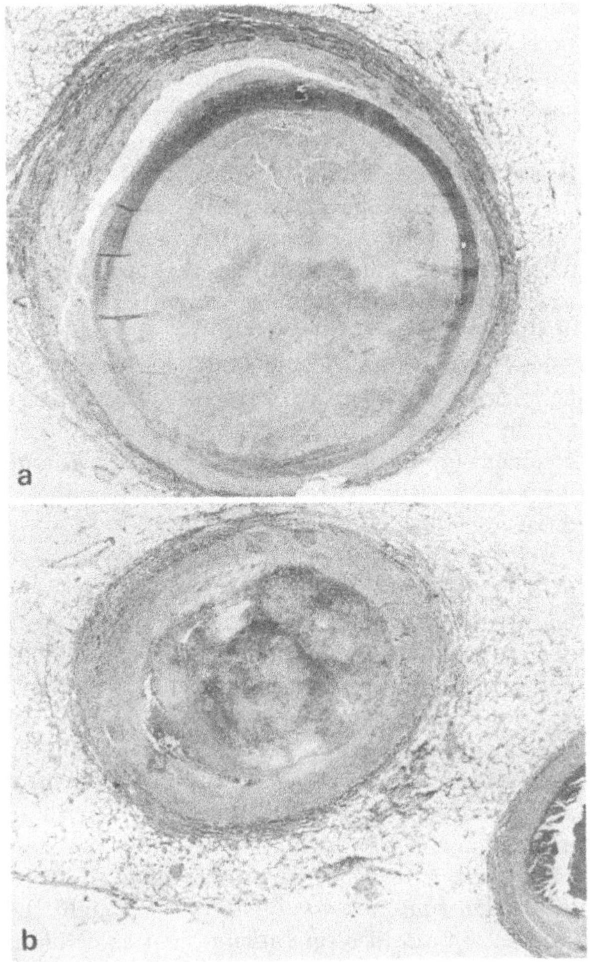

Fig. 6. Left anterior descending coronary artery. *a,* Proximal 1 cm. and *b,* a distal branch. The lumen is totally obstructed by a septic embolus. (*a,* Elastic van Gieson stain; *b,* hematoxylin and eosin stain; both × 12.)

caudal to the mitral anulus and a thrombus, which presumably had been infected at one time, was present in the aneurysm. The latter appeared to have been the source of cerebral emboli.

Although the present patient's aortic valve prosthesis was almost totally obstructed by vegetative material, a diagnosis of endocarditis was never established, presumably because signs of prosthetic dysfunction were absent. Dr. Arnett, do patients with prosthetic valve endocarditis usually have signs of prosthetic dysfunction?

DR. ARNETT: This patient was somewhat unusual. Infection of an aortic valve prosthesis usually results in detachment of the prosthesis, not obstruction, and signs of aortic regurgitation are usually present. Eleven of our previous 15 necropsy patients with aortic prosthetic infection had signs of aortic regurgitation, and in each of them the prosthesis was at least partially detached. Only one previous patient had aortic prosthetic obstruction from infection, and he had clinical signs of aortic valve obstruction. In contrast to aortic prosthetic infection, mitral infection usually causes obstruction of the prosthesis, but signs of mitral obstruction usually are not detected. None of our seven patients with mitral prosthetic endocarditis had clinical signs of prosthetic dysfunction, but at necropsy five of them had large vegetations obstructing the orifice of the prosthesis.

DR. ROBERTS: This patient had infection behind the site of attachment of the prosthesis, i.e., in the valve ring. Dr. Arnett, would you comment on the frequency of ring abscess among necropsy patients with prosthetic valve endocarditis?

DR. ARNETT: Infection behind the sewing ring, or ring abscess, is a consistent morphologic feature of prosthetic valve endocarditis. Ring abscess was present in each of our 22 previous patients, all of whom had rigid-framed prosthesis. In two thirds of them the entire circumference of the valve anulus was necrotic. Extension of the ring infection into adjacent cardiac structures also is common, especially in the patients with an infected aortic prosthesis. In nine of our previous 15 patients with aortic prosthetic valve endocarditis, the ring abscess burrowed through the cardiac septum into ring atrium, just as it did in the present patient.

DR. ROBERTS: Thus ring abscess is to be expected in patients with infection involving rigid-frame prostheses. Indeed, the infection in these patients nearly always involves the site of attachment of the prosthesis, and this is why patients with prosthetic valve endocarditis are so difficult to treat. If the infection was limited to the prosthesis, an infected prosthesis could be excised and replaced with another prosthesis. In the present patient, as in most of the others, the entire valve anulus was necrotic, and although he had received appropriate antibiotic therapy, intravenously for four weeks, numerous colonies of viable-appearing Gram positive cocci were present in the valve ring at necropsy. This patient developed prolongation of the PR interval, presumably from extension of the aortic ring abscess into the cephalad portion of the ventricular septum. Dr. Arnett, how common are atrioventricular conduction defects in patients with aortic prosthetic endocarditis?

DR. ARNETT: Among our previous 15 patients with aortic valve prosthetic endocarditis, five developed complete heart block and two others developed left bundle branch block. In each of these patients the ring abscess had extended into the basal portion of the ventricular septum.

DR. ROBERTS: The present patient had multiple infarcts in the spleen as well as a transmural acute myocardial infarct. Are systemic emboli common in patients with prosthetic valve endocarditis?

DR. ARNETT: Fourteen of our 22 previous necropsy patients (64 per cent) had gross infarcts in other organs. The organs most frequently involved were: spleen (12 patients), kidney (7 patients), and brain (7 patients). Only one of the previous 22 patients, however, had a transmural acute myocardial infarct from a coronary arterial embolus.

DR. ROBERTS: We have not touched on the frequency of prosthetic valve endocarditis. We have examined at necropsy approximately 450 patients in whom one or more cardiac valves had been replaced by prostheses. Twenty-three of them (5 per cent), including the patient described herein, had infection involving a prosthetic valve. Thus, although prosthetic valve endocarditis is a devastating complication of cardiac valve replacement, fortunately, it is infrequent. Although its exact frequency is uncertain, it may be less than 1 per cent per year among patients with prosthetic cardiac valves. In the early days of cardiac valve replacement, prosthetic infection in the early postoperative period was more common than in the late postoperative period. Now, however, it is likely that infection occurring late is more common than that occurring early, simply because there are large numbers of patients with prosthetic valves.

Dr. Arnett and I have studied 74 patients with active infective endocarditis involving natural left-sided cardiac valves. Dr. Arnett, would you summarize the major differences between our patients with prosthetic endocarditis and those with natural valve infective endocarditis.

DR. ARNETT: Comparison of observations in the 22 patients with prosthetic valve endocarditis to those in the 74 patients with active left-sided valvular endocarditis revealed two major differences. *Ring abscess* was present in each of the patients with prosthetic valve endocarditis, regardless of the site of the prosthesis. Among the patients with natural valve endocarditis, ring abscess was common only in patients with aortic valve infection.[9] Because heart block in patients with infective endocarditis is usually due to extension of ring abscess into the ventricular septum, it is more frequent in patients with prosthetic endocarditis than in patients with natural valve endocarditis.

The second major difference between patients with prosthetic endocarditis, and those with natural valve endocarditis is the frequency of *valvular obstruction* from infective endocarditis. The hemodynamic consequence of natural valve endocarditis is almost always regurgitation; valvular obstruction is rare.[10, 11] The hemodynamic consequence of prosthetic valve infection often is obstruction, especially when a mitral prosthesis is infected.

REFERENCES

1. Arnett, E. N., and Roberts, W. C.: Prosthetic valve endocarditis. A clinico pathologic analysis of 22 necropsy patients with comparison of observations to 74 necropsy patients with active infective endocarditis involving natural left-sided cardiac valves, Am. J. Cardiol. **38**:281, 1976.
2. Slaughter, L., Morris, J. E., and Starr, A.: Prosthetic valvular endocarditis. A 12-year review, Circulation **47**:1319, 1973.
3. Dismukes, W. E., Karchmer, A. W., Buckley, M. J., Austen, W. G., and Swartz, M. N.: Prosthetic valve endocarditis. Analysis of 38 cases, Circulation **48**:365, 1973.
4. Wilson, W. R., Jaumin, P. M., Danielson, G. K., Giuliani, E. R., Washington, J. A., and Geraci, J. E.: Prosthetic valve endocarditis, Ann. Intern. Med. **82**:751, 1975.
5. Ankeney, J. L., and Parker, R. F.: Staphylococcal endocarditis following open heart surgery related to positive intraoperative blood cultures, *in* Prosthetic heart valves, edited by Brewer, L. A., III, Springfield, Ill., 1969, Charles C Thomas, Publisher, pp. 719-730.
6. Blakemore, W. S., McGarrity, G. J., Thurer, R. J., Wallace, H. W., MacVaugh, H., III, and Coriell, L. L.: Infection by air-borne bacteria with cardiopulmonary bypass, Surgery **70**:830, 1971.
7. Kloster, F. E.: Diagnosis and management of complications of prosthetic heart valves, Am. J. Cardiol. **35**:872, 1975.
8. Sande, M. A., Johnson, W. D., Jr., Hook, E. W., and Kaxe, D.: Sustained bacteremia in patients with prosthetic cardiac valves, N. Engl. J. Med. **286**:1067, 1972.
9. Arnett, E. N., and Roberts, W. C.: Valve ring abscess in active infective endocarditis. Frequency, location, and clues to clinical diagnosis from study of 95 necropsy patients, Circulation **54**:140, 1976.
10. Roberts, W. C., Ewy, G. A., Glancy, D. L., and Marcus, F. I.: Valvular stenosis produced by active infective endocarditis, Circulation **36**:449, 1967.
11. Arnett, E. N., and Roberts, W. C.: Active infective endocarditis. A clinico pathologic analysis of 137 necropsy patients. Current Concepts in Cardiology (In press, October, 1976 issue).

Structural Changes in Porcine Xenografts Used as Substitute Cardiac Valves

Gross and Histologic Observations in 51 Glutaraldehyde-Preserved Hancock Valves in 41 Patients

THOMAS L. SPRAY, MD*
WILLIAM C. ROBERTS, MD, FACC

Bethesda, Maryland

Gross and histologic changes are described in 51 Hancock glutaraldehyde-preserved porcine heterograft bioprostheses from 41 patients: 33 valves from 25 patients had been in place for less than 2 months ("early") and 18 valves from 17 patients were examined at later periods up to 75 months ("late") after implantation. The major gross changes were thrombosis (five bioprostheses) and degeneration (three bioprotheses) of the cusps. Major histologic changes observed in 44 bioprostheses (26 early and 18 late) examined histologically were: (1) fibrin deposits on inflow and outflow surfaces of the cusps; (2) inflammatory cell infiltrates; (3) histiocyte deposition; (4) giant cell formation, and (5) focal disruption of the fibrocollagenous structure of the cusps. These observations indicate that porcine bioprostheses are not biologically inert in the human circulation. However, valve failure is rare at the implantation periods studied.

The glutaraldehyde-preserved stented porcine xenograft is now widely used as a substitute cardiac valve,[1–10] yet relatively little information is available on structural changes in this bioprosthesis.[3–10] This report describes gross and histologic observations in 51 Hancock glutaraldehyde-preserved porcine cardiac valve bioprostheses (Hancock Laboratories, Anaheim, California) from 41 patients whose bioprostheses had been in place for up to 75 months.

Materials and Methods

Of the 51 valves, 47 were examined at necropsy in 38 patients; 33 valves from 25 patients (10 men and 15 women) had been in place for less than 2 months ("early") (range 0 to 50 days, mean 12) and 18 valves from 17 patients (8 men and 9 women) were examined more than 2 months ("late") after implantation (range 2.1 to 75 months, mean 15). Seven of the 18 late valves had been in place for longer than 12 months. Each bioprosthesis was fixed in either 10 percent buffered formalin or 3 percent glutaraldehyde. In 44 of the 51 valves a section was taken for histologic examination from each of the three cusps. The sections were processed in alcohols and xylene, embedded in paraffin, cut and stained. One section from each cusp was stained by the hematoxylin-eosin, Verhoeff-van Gieson, calcium, phosphotungstic-acid hematoxylin and Movat's pentachrome methods. Each section was examined with both light and polarization microscopy.

Of the 33 early valves, 19 were in the mitral position and they ranged in size from 25 to 35 mm (average 29 mm), 10 were in the tricuspid position (range 29 to 35 mm, average 33 mm), 3 were in the aortic position (27, 27 and 29 mm, respectively) and 1 was in the pulmonary position (21 mm) as part of a composite conduit.

Of the 18 late valves, 12 were in the mitral position (size range 25 to 35 mm, average 29 mm), 5 in the tricuspid position (31 to 35 mm, average 33 mm) and 1 was in the aortic position (25 mm). Four valves (three mitral and one tricuspid) were removed at operation because of prosthetic regurgitation caused in three

From the Pathology Branch, National Heart, Lung, and Blood Institute, National Institutes of Health, Bethesda, Maryland. Manuscript received January 26, 1977; revised manuscript received March 11, 1977, accepted March 16, 1977.

* Present address: Department of Surgery, Duke University Medical Center, Durham, North Carolina 27710.

Address for reprints: William C. Roberts, MD, Bldg. 10A, Rm. 3E30, National Heart, Lung, and Blood Institute, National Institutes of Health, Bethesda, Maryland 20014.

TABLE I

Prosthetic Dysfunction or Prosthesis-Related Complications

Type of Dysfunction	no.	Affected Bioprostheses: Valve Site	Affected Bioprostheses: Duration of Implantation
Leaflet degeneration (regurgitation)	3	Mitral	56 months
		Mitral	75 months
		Tricuspid	3 months
Thrombosis (stenosis)	5	Mitral and tricuspid	32 days
		Mitral	8 days
		Aortic	5 months
		Tricuspid	2 months
Strut in outflow tract	3	Mitral	1 day
		Mitral	4 days
		Mitral	6 days
Prosthetic disproportion	3	Tricuspid and mitral	4 days
		Aortic	1 day
Coronary ostial obstruction	1	Aortic	1 day

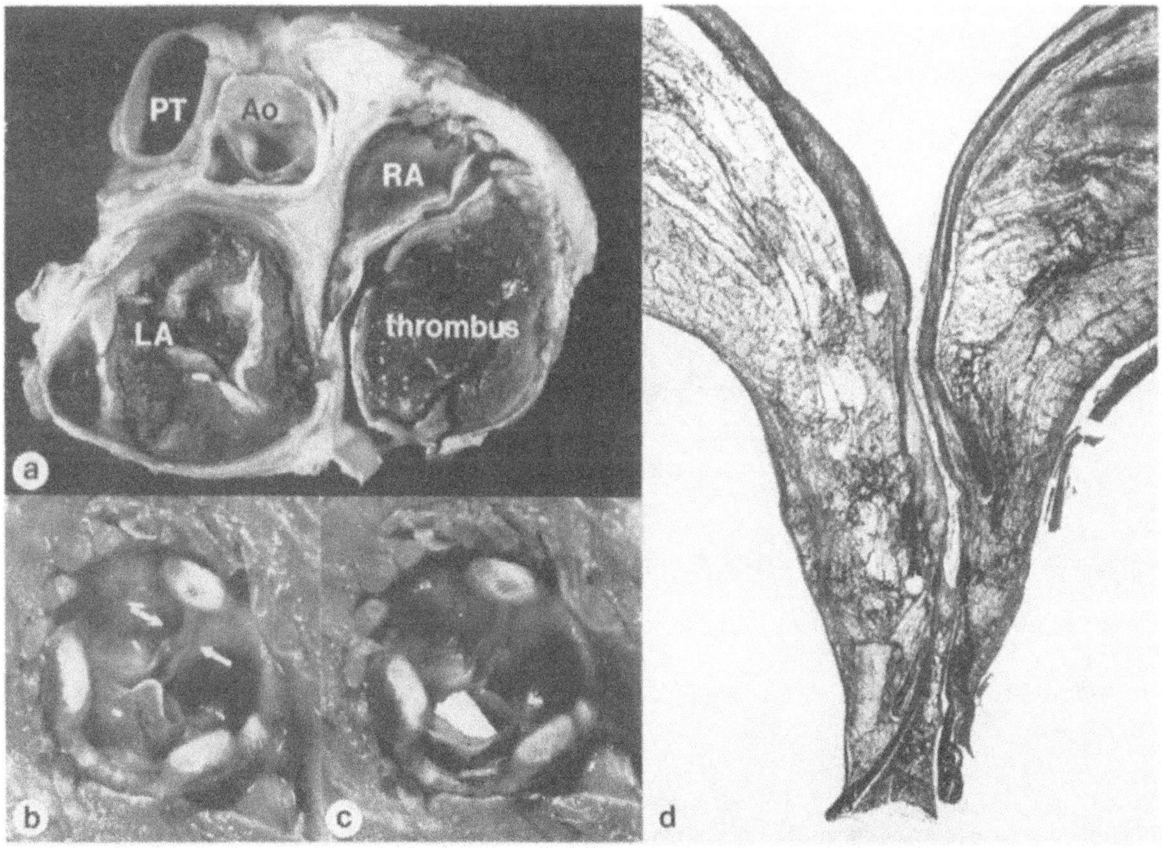

FIGURE 1. Stenosis of porcine bioprostheses implanted 32 days earlier in a 61 year old woman who had had rheumatic mitral stenosis and tricuspid regurgitation. The patient sustained an air embolus intraoperatively and remained comatose with severe low cardiac output after operation. **a,** at necropsy, both the right (RA) and left (LA) atria were filled with organizing thrombi. Ao = aortic root; PT = pulmonary trunk. **b,** view of the 31 mm porcine bioprosthesis in the tricuspid position from the ventricular aspect as seen in systole. Thrombus is present in two of the three cusp sinuses and there is fusion of the commissure between these leaflets **(arrows)**. **c,** bioprosthesis in simulated ventricular diastole. The fusion of two leaflets permits opening of only the one mobile leaflet with resulting valve stenosis. **d,** section through fused leaflets at level of arrows in **b** showing adherence of the leaflets by fibrin thrombus. (Phosphotungstic acid-hematoxylin stain ×16, reduced by 24 percent [**d**].)

by prosthetic degeneration and in the fourth by a parabasilar leak. The two mitral valves with the longest implantation time (56 and 75 months, respectively) were removed because of severe regurgitation secondary to leaflet degeneration; at reoperation, these two valves were replaced with fresh Hancock xenografts. One of these two patients died 14 days later of respiratory complications.

Results

Gross Observations

Of the 33 bioprostheses with implantation periods of less than 2 months, 30 were entirely normal on visual inspection at necropsy, and the remaining 3 showed some gross alterations (discussed later). Of the 18 bioprostheses implanted for more than 2 months, 13 were normal on visual inspection at necropsy, and the remaining 5 showed some gross alteration either at necropsy or reoperation. The major gross changes observed in these eight bioprostheses included thrombosis (both early and late) and degeneration (late only) of the cusps (Table I).

Cusp thrombus: This was present in five bioprostheses (two mitral, two triscuspid and one aortic). Bioprostheses were implanted in both the mitral and

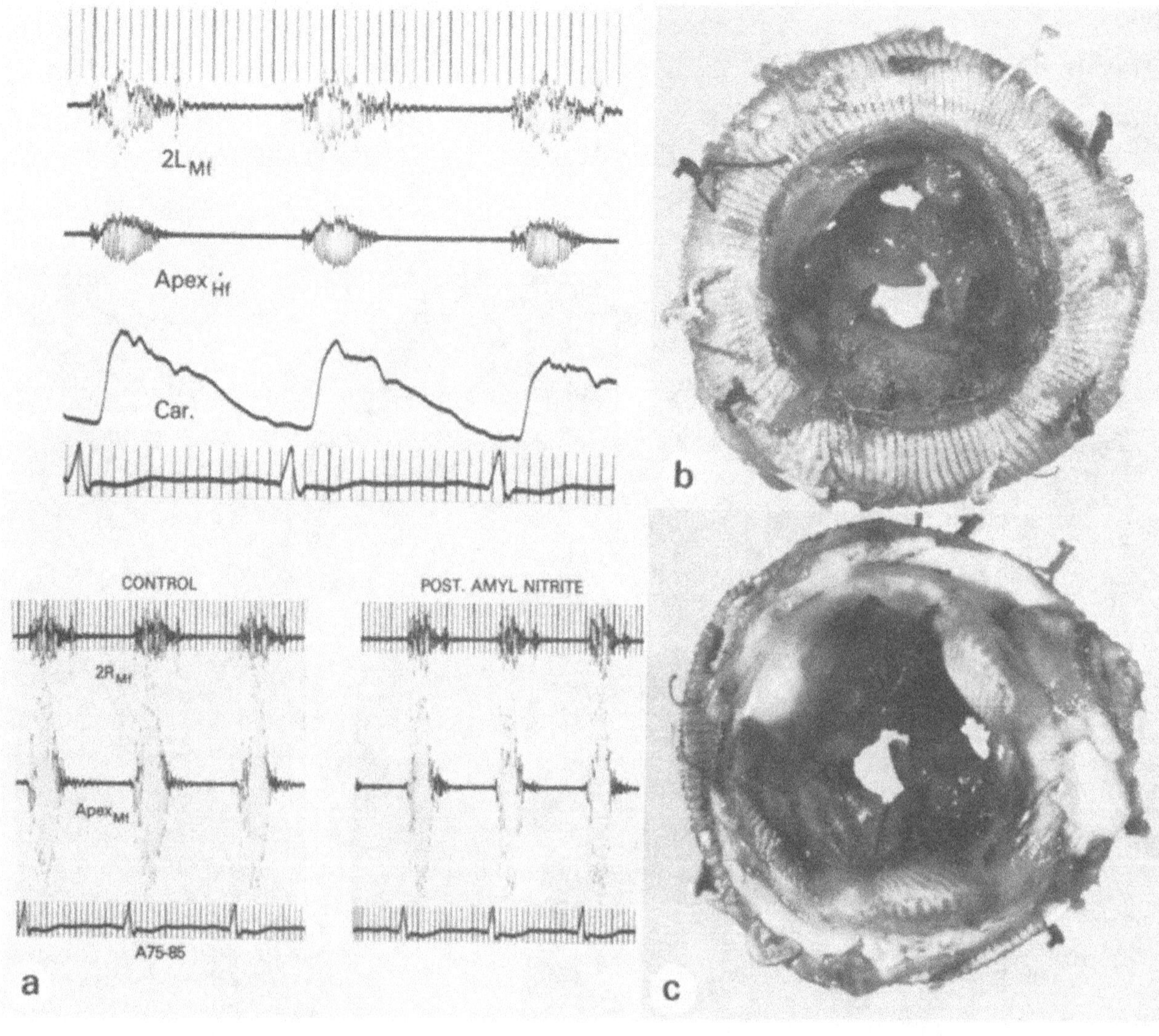

FIGURE 2. Tissue degeneration in a 56 month old porcine bioprosthesis in the mitral position. The patient had undergone mitral valve replacement and aortic and tricuspid valve commissurotomy for mitral, aortic and tricuspid stenosis. She did well for 56 months (without anticoagulant therapy) when she had the sudden onset of left-sided chest pain and dyspnea, and a murmur of mitral regurgitation was heard for the first time postoperatively. At no time was evidence for infective endocarditis present. Phonocardiograms **(a)** now showed a systolic precordial murmur consistent with mitral regurgitation (no increase with amyl nitrite). Cardiac catheterization revealed 4+/4+ mitral regurgitation, and at reoperation the 29 mm porcine mitral bioprosthesis **(b,c)** showed extensive disruption of the leaflets and adherent thrombotic material. At reoperation, the porcine mitral valve was replaced with a new porcine bioprosthesis. The tricuspid valve, which was stenotic, also was replaced with a porcine bioprosthesis, and the aortic valve, which was both stenotic and regurgitant, was replaced with a size 7A, model 2320 Starr-Edwards prosthesis. The patient did well for the first 2 weeks postoperatively but experienced sudden chest pain on the 14th postoperative day and died.

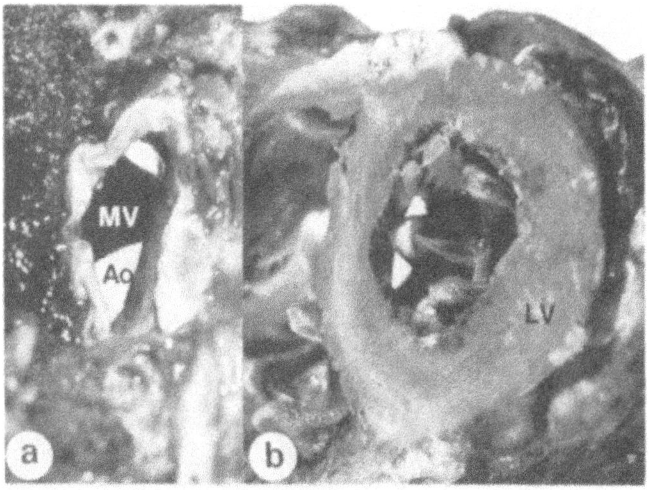

FIGURE 3. Strut of porcine bioprosthesis in the mitral position partially obstructing left ventricular (LV) outflow in a 54 year old woman who had undergone tricuspid and mitral valve (MV) replacement with mechanical prostheses for valve stenosis 3 days before death. She had a low cardiac output requiring pressor agents postoperatively. The prosthetic valve sounds were poorly heard and reexploration performed on the third postoperative day revealed that the mechanical tricuspid prosthesis had thrombosed. Both mechanical prostheses in the tricuspid and mitral positions were replaced with porcine bioprostheses, but the patient could not be separated from cardiopulmonary bypass. At necropsy, one strut of the mitral prosthesis partially obstructed left ventricular outflow **(a)**. **b**, ventricular aspect, showing placement of the porcine valve strut in the outflow tract.

tricuspid valve positions in one patient, who died 32 days postoperatively after a prolonged period of inadequate cardiac output (Fig. 1). At necropsy, thrombus filled the sinuses of two of the three cusps of the tricuspid valve prosthesis, and one of the three commissures had fused; only one of the three cusps remained pliable and consequently the prosthetic orifice appeared stenotic. The bioprosthesis in the mitral position in the same patient also contained thrombus in two of the three cusps, but none of the commissures had fused. Both atria at necropsy were filled with organizing thrombus. In a second patient with a bioprosthesis in the mitral position, a large thrombus, which filled the body and appendage of the left atrium, was attached to the atrial aspects of each of the three cusps; in addition, thrombus also filled the sinus portions of each of the

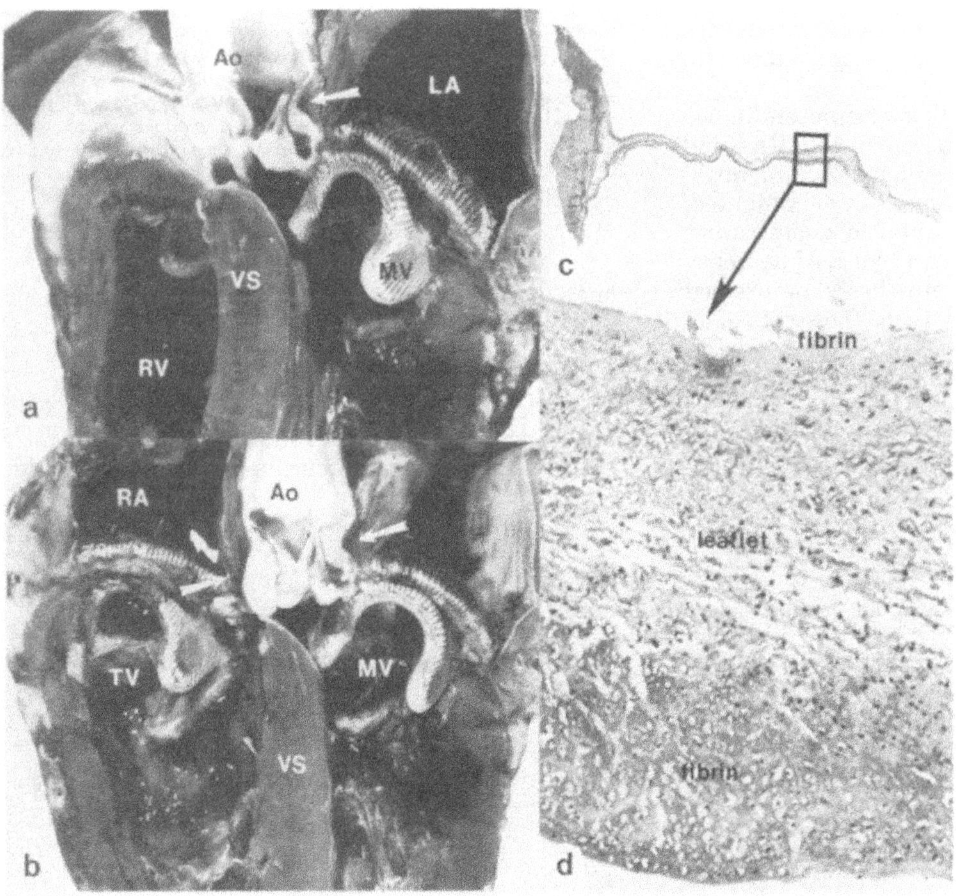

FIGURE 4. Prosthetic disproportion in a 50 year old woman who had had mitral (MV) and tricuspid (TV) valve replacements with porcine bioprostheses 4 days before death for mitral and tricuspid valve stenosis. She was in a low cardiac output state despite vasopressors during the entire postoperative period. At necropsy, one strut of the mitral bioprosthesis partially obstructed left ventricular outflow. In addition, the sewing ring of the 31 mm bioprosthesis in the mitral position appeared to indent the aorta (Ao) just above the valve **(arrow)** **(a)**. **b**, the 31 mm bioprosthesis in the tricuspid valve position also compressed **(arrow)** the aortic root, possibly causing some aortic regurgitation. At necropsy, thrombus was present in the left atrium (LA). RA = right atrium; RV = right ventricle; VS = ventricular septum. **c**, section of one leaflet of the bioprosthesis in the mitral position showing fibrin deposits. **d**, higher power view of area enclosed by the box in **c**, showing fibrin on both surfaces. (Hematoxylin-eosin stains ×6.5 [**c**] and ×220 [**d**], reduced by 30 percent.)

three cusps, thereby producing severe prosthetic obstruction. This patient lived 8 days postoperatively and the cause of the thrombosis was not determined. One bioprosthesis in the tricuspid valve position for 2 months had gross thrombi in the cusps with only mild limitation of movement of the leaflets. In one bioprosthesis in the aortic valve position for 5 months, thrombus was present in two of the three sinuses.

Clinical or morphologic evidence for thromboembolism was present in four patients with late bioprostheses, but all four patients had mechanical prostheses in addition to porcine bioprostheses, and three had thrombus present on the mechanical prostheses. In one patient who had a 31 mm tricuspid valve bioprosthesis implanted 21 months earlier, evidence of pulmonary embolism occurred 3 months postoperatively. The origin of the embolus is unclear, but at necropsy fibrin thrombus was present in the sinuses of the bioprosthesis although she had had long-term warfarin sodium therapy.

Cusp degeneration: Degeneration of the cusp tissue with resulting regurgitation was present in three valves, two mitral (with an implantation period of 56 and 75 months, respectively) (Fig. 2) and one tricuspid valve with a 3 month implantation period. All three bioprostheses showed tears of the cusps with adherent thrombus. In the 56 and 75 month old mitral bioprostheses, gross nodular calcific deposits were present.

In three mitral valves, one of the three struts of the flexible stent was in the left ventricular outflow tract (Fig. 3). All three patients were hypotensive throughout the postoperative period and died 1, 4 and 6 days, respectively, after operation.

Prosthetic disproportion: This was present in two patients (three valves). In one, a woman with tricuspid regurgitation and severe mitral stenosis, 31 mm mitral and 33 mm tricuspid valve prostheses were implanted. Postoperatively, she had evidence of inadequate cardiac output and, finally, complete heart block. At necropsy (Fig. 4), the sewing rings of the prostheses compressed the aortic root. In the second patient, the struts of an aortic bioprosthesis obstructed both coronary ostia; this patient died soon after operation from circumferential myocardial necrosis (Fig. 5).

Fatal endocarditis was present on a mechanical prosthesis in two patients (aortic in one and mitral in one), but the porcine bioprostheses (mitral and tricuspid, respectively) were uninvolved (Fig. 6).

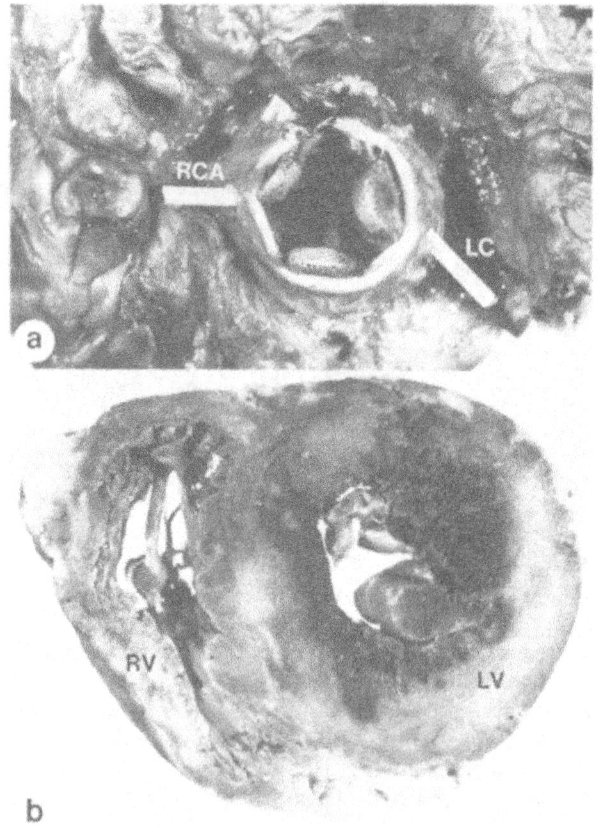

FIGURE 5. Coronary ostial occlusion by a 27 mm porcine bioprosthesis in the aortic position in a 63 year old woman who had had aortic stenosis. The patient died with pulmonary edema 36 hours after operation. **a,** view of aortic prosthesis from above. A Teflon® patch was used to attempt to widen the aorta. White sticks designate the origins of the right (RCA) and left main (LC) coronary arteries. The origins of both major coronary arteries are occluded by the struts of the prosthesis. **b,** section of ventricles showing extensive circumferential hemorrhagic necrosis. LV = left and RV = right ventricle.

Histologic Observations

Of the 51 porcine bioprostheses, 44 were examined histologically (Table II). In addition, two unimplanted glutaraldehyde-fixed porcine valves were sectioned to

TABLE II

Histologic Findings in 44 Porcine Xenograft Cardiac Valve Bioprostheses

	Fibrin in Cusps*		Fibrin on Inflow Surface†		WBC‡		Histiocytes		Giant Cells		Leaflet Disruption§	
	no.	%	no.	%	no.	%	no.	%	no.	%	no.	%
Early (no. = 26)	18	69	12	46	16	62	14	54	7	27	4	15
Late (no. = 18)	14	78	9	50	13	72	14	78	12	67	8	45

* Ventricular surface of tricuspid and mitral valves; aortic surface of aortic valves.
† Atrial surface of tricuspid and mitral valves, ventricular surface of aortic valves.
‡ Plasma cells, polymorphonuclear leukocytes, lymphocytes.
§ Focal invasion of leaflets by host cells or disruption.

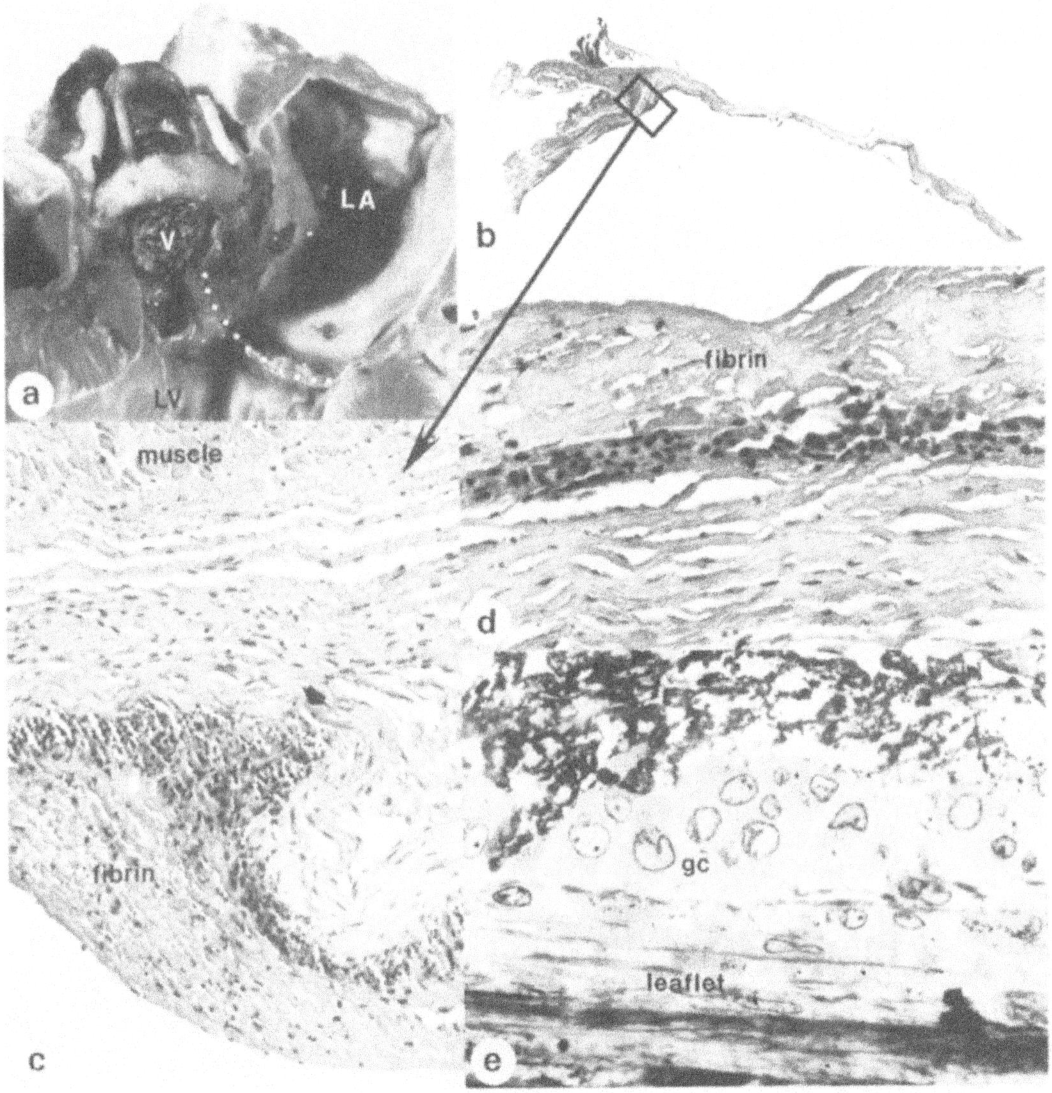

FIGURE 6. Staphylococcus epidermidis endocarditis on a mechanical prosthesis implanted 28 days before death in a 47 year old man with aortic and mitral regurgitation and replacement of the mitral valve with a porcine bioprosthesis. The patient received warfarin daily postoperatively. **a,** view of mechanical aortic valve prosthesis showing obstruction of the primary orifice by vegetations (V). The anulus of the mitral valve prosthesis **(dotted line)** is designated. LA = left atrium; LV = left ventricle. **b,** section of one leaflet of the removed bioprosthesis in the mitral position showing intact leaflet structure. **c,** area enclosed by box in **b** near hinge of leaflet showing fibrin and inflammatory cell deposition with focal invasion of the valve tissue **(arrow)**. **d,** high power view of the atrial surface of the leaflet showing fibrin and inflammatory cell deposition. **e,** thin section of surface of the leaflet showing giant cells (gc) and histiocytes under a fibrin layer. Stains for bacteria and fungi did not reveal infection of the tissue valve. (Hematoxylin-eosin stains ×7.5 [**b**], ×220 [**c**], ×350 [**d**] and toluidine blue stain ×860 [**e**], all reduced by 21 percent.)

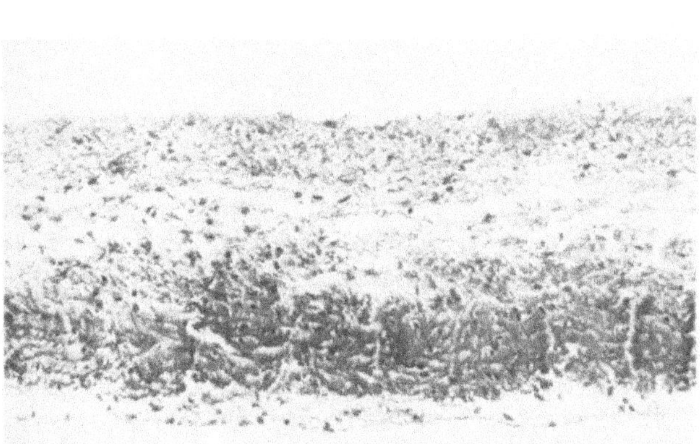

FIGURE 7. Normal unprocessed and unimplanted porcine valve. Bundles of fibrocollagenous tissue within a matrix of ground substance are present. Cells with elongated nuclei are scattered throughout the leaflet. Thin delicate endothelium is present on one surface. (Hematoxylin-eosin stain ×220, reduced by 28 percent.)

serve as controls.* Of the three cusps in the normal porcine aortic valve, the right one is attached to a "muscle shelf" that consequently limits the pliability of this cusp.[11] Each of the three cusps is composed of multiple layers of cells with elongated nuclei, collagen bundles arranged radially and short elastic fibers (Fig. 7).

"Early" valves: Of the 33 valves with implantation periods of less than 2 months, 26 were examined histologically. *Fibrin deposits* were present on the outflow surfaces of the cusps in 18 (69 percent) (Fig. 4), and on the inflow surfaces of 12 (46 percent) bioprostheses. Occasionally, the fibrin deposits were large enough to limit cusp mobility (Fig. 1). Collections of platelets and erythrocytes were associated with the fibrin deposits in a few patients. Three patients whose bioprostheses had been implanted for 13, 14 and 19 days, respectively, received warfarin daily postoperatively. Two of the three valves from these patients showed moderate fibrin deposits on the cusps of the bioprostheses. Leukocytes, lymphocytes and, occasionally, plasma cells were

* Courtesy of Warren D. Hancock, Hancock Laboratories, Anaheim, California.

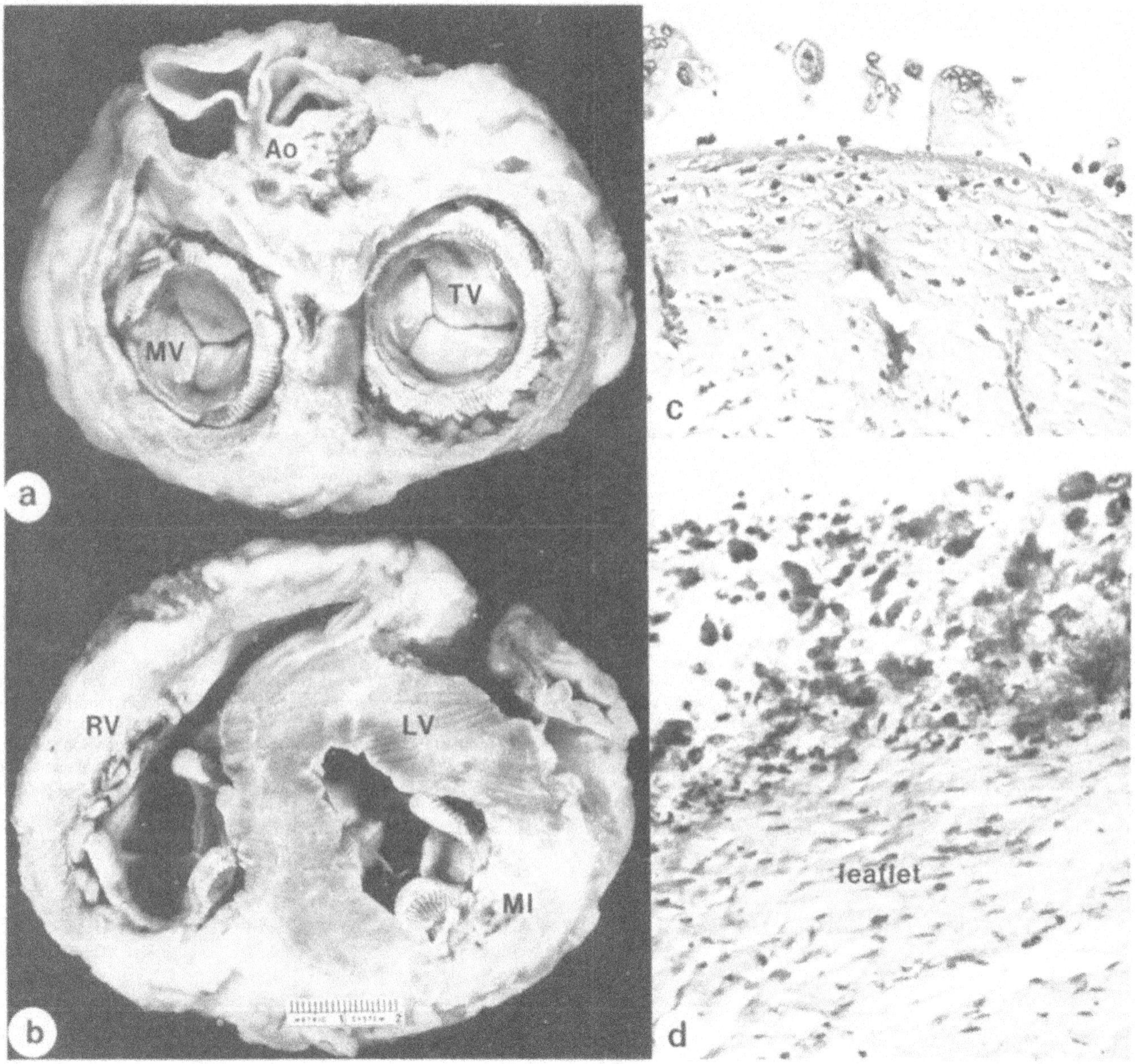

FIGURE 8. Same patient as in Figure 3. The porcine bioprostheses in the mitral and tricuspid valve positions had been implanted 14 days earlier. Postoperatively, the function of both bioprostheses was normal. **a,** view from above showing the tricuspid (TV), mitral (MV) and aortic (Starr-Edwards) (Ao) prostheses. **b,** view from below showing posterobasal transmural myocardial infarct (MI) of the left ventricle (LV). RV = right ventricle. **c,** section of one leaflet of the 14 day old bioprosthesis in the mitral position. Marked giant cell reaction and a few lymphocytes and plasma cells line the surface of the leaflet. **d,** section of one leaflet of the bioprosthesis in the tricuspid valve position. Histiocytes, inflammatory cells and fibrin cover the leaflet's surface, and its interior is invaded by the inflammatory cells. (Hematoxylin-eosin stains [**c** and **d**], ×330, reduced by 17 percent.)

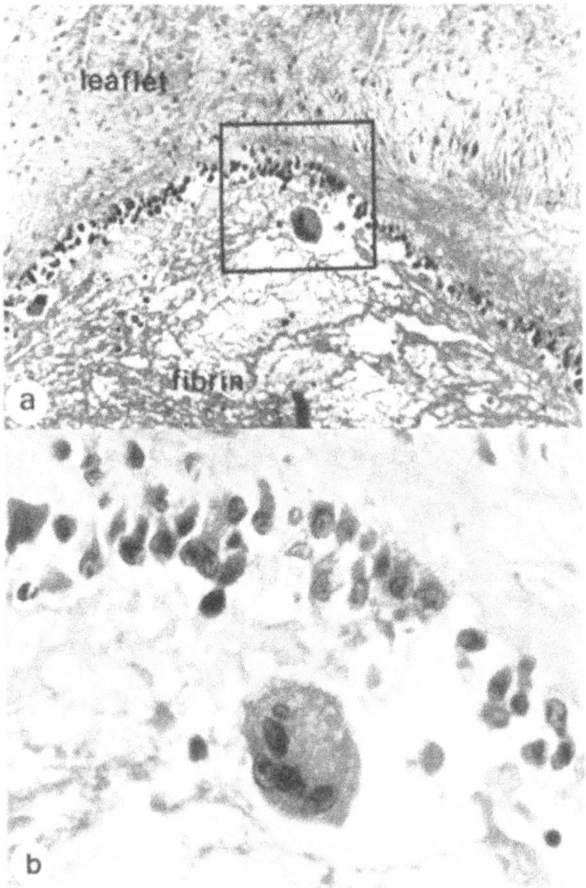

FIGURE 9 (left). Histiocyte, giant cell and inflammatory cell reaction in the cusp of a bioprosthesis in the mitral position. It had been implanted 7 months earlier. **a,** closeup of area enclosed by the box in **a** is shown in **b.** A large giant cell is present in the fibrin matrix. (Hematoxylin-eosin stains ×220 [**a**] and ×860 [**b**], reduced by 28 percent.)

FIGURE 10 (below). Porcine bioprosthesis in the mitral position implanted 14 months earlier. **a,** longitudinal view of heart showing moderate host tissue overgrowth on the struts of the bioprosthesis **(arrow),** and the relation of the bioprosthesis to the mechanical prosthesis in the aortic valve (AV) position. LA = left atrium; VS = ventricular septum. **b,** section of one leaflet of the bioprosthesis showing a thin, delicate leaflet. **c** and **d,** higher-power view of area enclosed by box in **b. c,** atrial side; a thin fibrin layer with histiocytic cells lines the surface of the leaflet. Little nuclear staining of the glutaraldehyde-fixed porcine leaflet cells is present. **d,** ventricular side; a thick fibrin coat with enclosed giant cells, plasma cells and histiocytes is present with mild surface invasion of the leaflet. (Hematoxylin-eosin stains ×8 [**b**], ×330 [**c**], ×350 [**d**], reduced by 24 percent.)

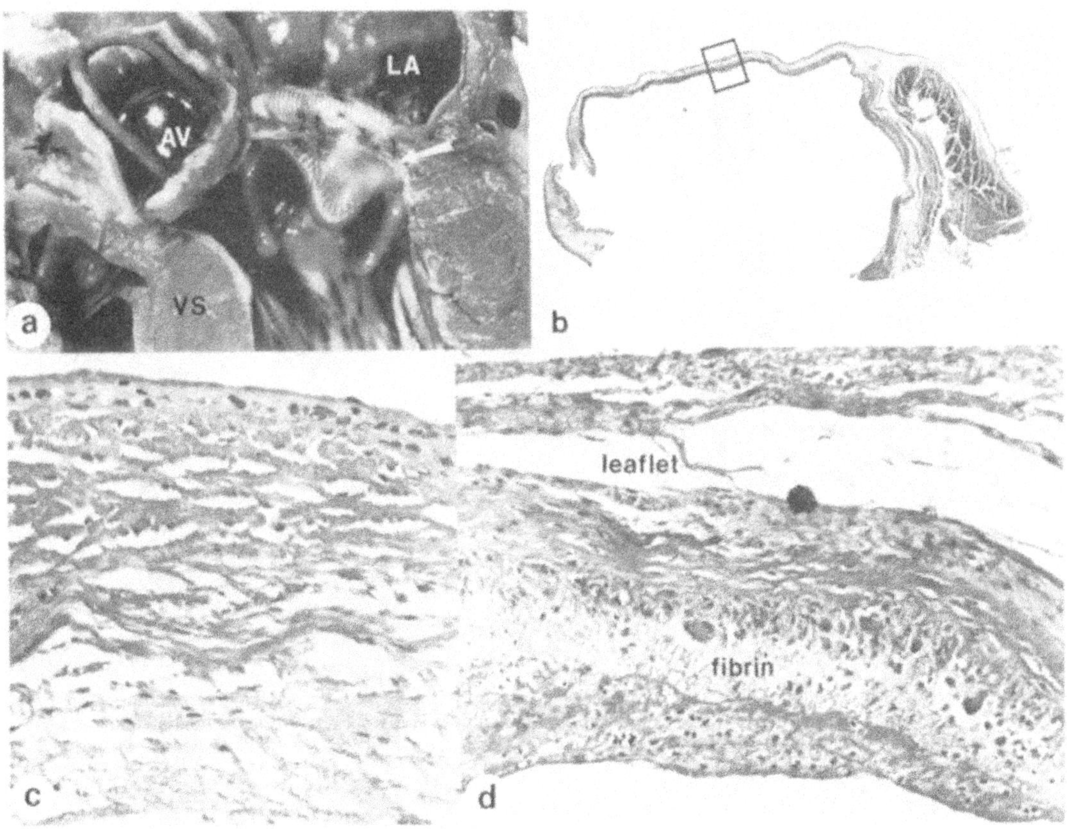

present in the fibrin matrix or along the leaflet surface in 16 (62 percent) of the 26 bioprostheses. Often leukocytes infiltrated the porcine aortic wall behind the cusps.

Macrophages with histologic characteristics of histiocytes lined portions of the cusps in 14 (54 percent) of the 26 bioprostheses, and in 7 of the 14 valves histiocytes had collected together forming giant cells. The histiocytes occasionally were present in the outermost portions of the fibrocollagenous structure of the cusps. On polarization microscopy, talc and other foreign bodies were absent. Of the seven bioprostheses that showed a giant cell reaction, giant cells were present in small numbers in three patients with bioprostheses in place for less than 30 days, whereas in the three patients with bioprostheses in place from 30 to 60 days, they were present in abundance. In one patient, two bioprostheses (one mitral, one tricuspid), each in place for 14 days, showed marked inflammatory cell reaction, histiocyte accumulation and giant cell formation (Fig. 8). In this patient a 56 month old bioprosthesis was removed from the mitral position because disruption of the cusps had resulted in regurgitation. The mitral and tricuspid valves were then replaced with fresh bioprostheses. In 4 (15 percent) of 26 bioprostheses, the substance of the cusps contained inflammatory cells or histiocytes. However, none of these four bioprostheses showed either clinical or necropsy evidence of dysfunction.

The fibrocollagenous structure of the remaining 22 bioprostheses was intact and appeared unchanged from the structure of the 2 control valves. Despite good ingrowth of tissue over the struts and the sewing rings of the prostheses, host cell ingrowth was absent on the leaflet surfaces of all bioprostheses in place for less than 2 months. Host cell ingrowth extended only a few millimeters beyond the sewing ring over the porcine tissue.

"Late" valves: All 18 valves that had been in place for more than 2 months were available for histologic study (Table II). *Fibrin deposits* were present on the

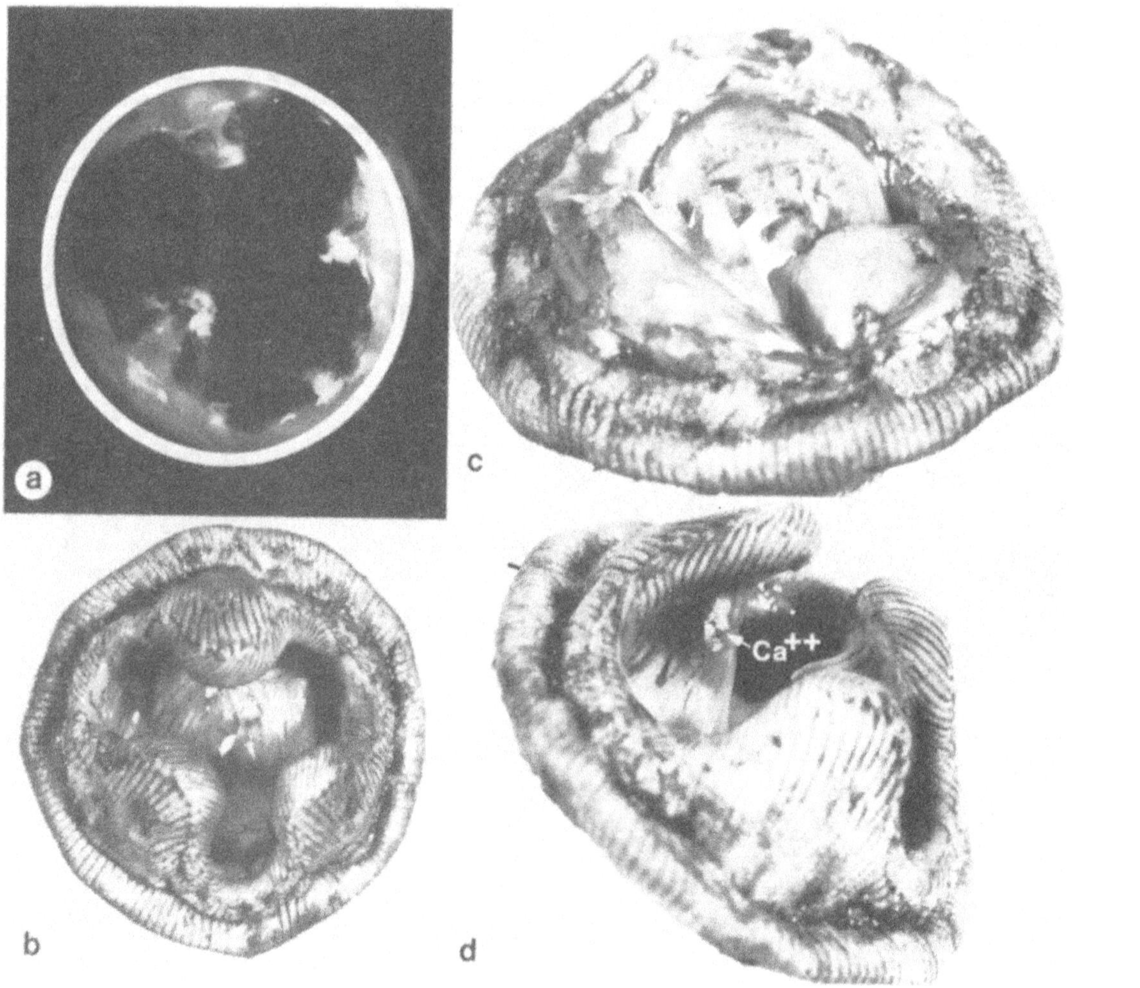

FIGURE 11. Tissue degeneration and calcification in a 75 month old porcine bioprosthesis that had been in the mitral position. **a,** roentgenogram of the removed bioprosthesis showing focal calcific deposits in the leaflets. **b,** view of the bioprosthesis from the ventricular aspect showing bowing-in of all three struts. **c,** view of the bioprosthesis from the atrial aspect showing tears and fraying of two of the three leaflets and prolapse of the leaflets toward the atrial side of the valve. The resulting regurgitation required reoperation and replacement of the bioprosthesis with a fresh bioprosthesis. **d,** side view showing nodular calcific deposits (Ca^{++}) at the commissural attachment of two leaflets.

outflow surface of the cusps in 14 (78 percent) of the 18 bioprostheses and on the inflow surface in 9 (50 percent). *Leukocytes* were present in 13 bioprostheses (72 percent) and *histiocytes* lined the cusp surfaces in 14 (78 percent). *Giant cell* formation was frequent (Fig. 9); 12 (67 percent) showed giant cells, and focal invasion of the cusps by host cells and giant cells was present in 8 (45 percent) (Fig. 10). In three valves, a 3 month old tricuspid and two much later (56 and 75 months, respectively) mitral valves, complete disruption of cusp tissue occurred (Fig. 2). The two mitral valves also had calcific deposits in the cusps (Fig. 11). Except for a few giant cells, cell elements were absent and collagen was degenerated in these two bioprostheses.

Marked host cell endothelialization of the cusps was observed in one bioprosthesis in place in the tricuspid position for 21 months (Fig. 12); however, the endothelial cells were present over a thin layer of fibrin and

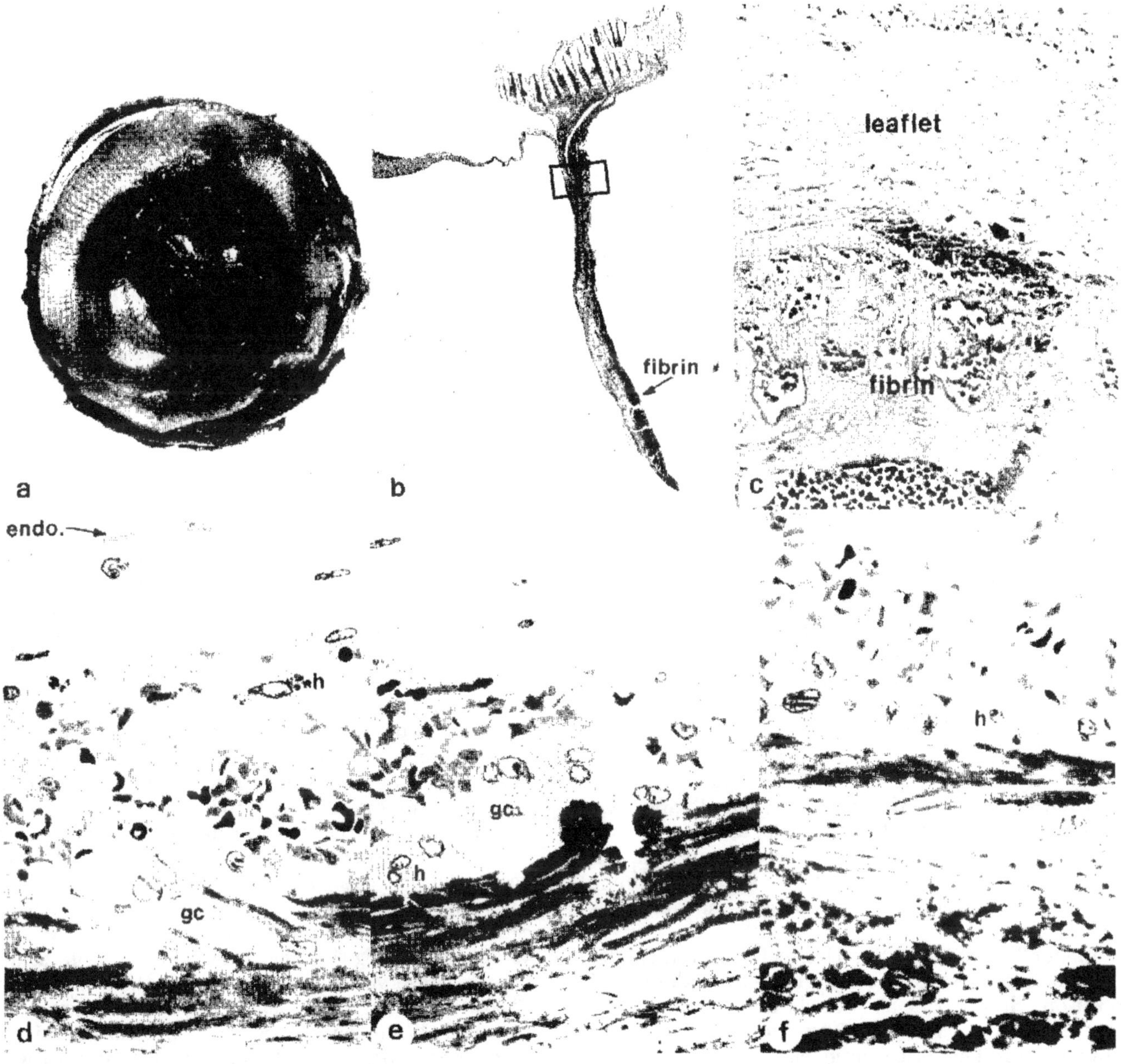

FIGURE 12. A 31 mm bioprosthesis that was in the tricuspid valve position for 21 months in a 57 year old woman who also had Starr-Edwards aortic and mitral prostheses. She received warfarin daily during her entire postoperative period. At cardiac catheterization shortly before she died, a 4 mm Hg end-diastolic pressure gradient was noted between the right atrium and right ventricle. **a,** view of excised bioprosthesis from the atrial surface showing overgrowth of host tissue over the sewing ring and over the leaflets of the bioprosthesis. All three leaflets were slightly stiffer than normal. **b,** section of one leaflet showing thickening due to host ingrowth and fibrin deposition. **c,** high-power view of area enclosed by the box in **b,** showing fibrin deposits on the leaflet and inflammatory cells **(arrow). d, e** and **f,** high-power views of 1 μ thick sections of the atrial (inflow) surface of the leaflet showing endothelialization (endo.) of the fibrin and red cell thrombus that covers the leaflet. Histiocytes (h) and giant cells (gc) line the leaflet, and the surface of the fibrocollagenous structure is disrupted. (Hematoxylin-eosin stains ×7 [**b**], ×220 [**c**]; toluidine blue stain: ×860 [**d, e** and **f**], all reduced by 25 percent.)

therefore appeared to represent endothelialization of thrombus rather than of the porcine tissue. No other late bioprostheses showed endothelialization of the cusps (Fig. 13). Polarization microscopy revealed no foreign bodies in any cusp of any bioprosthesis.

Five of the 18 porcine bioprostheses were in patients who postoperatively were receiving either warfarin sodium (three patients) or aspirin plus dipyridamole (two patients) because they also had mechanical prostheses. In all five bioprostheses in these five patients various degrees of fibrin deposits were evident on the cusps (Fig. 12).

Comments

Previous observations on porcine bioprostheses: Good clinical and usually adequate hemodynamic results have been reported by several groups of investigators in patients who have had porcine heterograft bioprostheses implanted for up to 5 years.[1-9] These studies have shown low rates of clinical episodes suggestive of thromboembolism although long-term anticoagulant agents have rarely been used.[1,4,6,12] Reports of failure of these bioprostheses have been rare.[1,6,9] However, most studies of porcine heterograft prostheses have concerned formalin-fixed tissue or tissue treated with various glutaraldehyde preservation techniques.[3,10,13-19] Few descriptions of structural changes have been reported in valves processed by the Hancock stabilized-glutaraldehyde process, and few bioprostheses prepared by this fixative have been studied late.[10,13]

Examination of formalin-treated porcine bioprostheses showed a high frequency of structural failure. Zuhdi et al.[3] noted structural failure in 20 of 31 stented formalin-fixed porcine bioprostheses within 4 years after implantation. Histologic studies showed inflammatory-cell infiltrates in the cusps, fibrin deposits and histiocyte and giant cell accumulation. However, no degenerative changes were seen in eight glutaraldehyde-preserved bioprostheses in place from 8 days to 16 months.[3]

Carpentier et al.,[6] utilizing a different glutaraldehyde fixation technique and rigid stents, noted valve dysfunction in seven patients with implantation periods of 1 to 5 years. No immunologic reaction was seen, but collagen degeneration with cusp perforation and lining of cusps with histiocytes, macrophages and giant cells was observed.

In 4 of 32 patients with a Hancock glutaraldehyde-fixed bioprosthesis on a semirigid stent in the mitral position, Horowitz et al.[5] noted "normal" histologic features in four valves removed 4 to 29 months after implantation. They also mentioned "moderate numbers of macrophages and a few giant cells" at the base of the muscle shelf of the right coronary cusp in a valve in place for 18 months. Yarbrough et al.[10] noted essentially normal valve structure in six Hancock glutaraldehyde-preserved bioprostheses in place for 14 to 180 days. Mild fibrin deposits and layers of "mesothelial-like cells" were noted in a bioprosthesis in the tricuspid position for 39 days.[10]

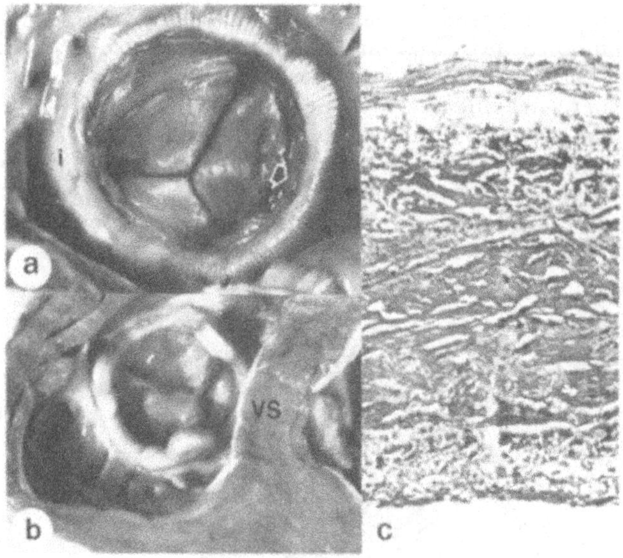

FIGURE 13. Porcine bioprosthesis implanted in the tricuspid valve position 15 months earlier. **a,** view from right atrium. Host connective tissue (i) covers the sewing ring but stops abruptly at the porcine tissue **(arrow). b,** view from right ventricle showing ingrowth of whitish host tissue over struts but not onto the valve leaflets. VS = ventricular septum. **c,** section of one leaflet of the bioprosthesis showing lack of host endothelialization of the leaflet surfaces. (Hematoxylin-eosin stain ×220 **[c]**, reduced by 29 percent.)

Present observations on structural changes: Our study of 51 Hancock bioprostheses (44 examined histologically) showed a high frequency of structural changes, but most of these changes did not affect valve function. Fibrin deposits on the cusp outflow surfaces and inflammatory cells were present in nearly 70 percent of all bioprostheses studied. Almost half of the prostheses showed fibrin deposits on the inflow surfaces. The similar frequency of these changes in both early (implanted for less than 2 months) and late (implanted for more than 2 months) bioprostheses and the lack of organization of the fibrin deposits suggests that fibrin and inflammatory cells begin to be deposited soon after implantation. Perhaps fibrin deposition occurs as a response to structural stresses. However, histiocyte accumulation was slightly less frequent (54 percent) in early than in late (76 percent) bioprostheses, and giant cell formation was more than twice as common in late valves, suggesting that these reactions to the glutaraldehyde-preserved tissue occur later than the fibrin deposits. Although gross leaflet disruption was present in only 3 (17 percent) of 18 late bioprostheses, microscopic-sized focal cusp disruption by host cells was present in 45 percent of the late bioprostheses.

Although the observed histologic changes in the glutaraldehyde-fixed bioprostheses are qualitatively similar to those described in formalin-fixed heterografts, the magnitude of the cell reaction is less. Thus, the Hancock bioprostheses are not biologically inert in man. These findings suggest that the Hancock stabilized-glutaraldehyde preservation technique creates more stable cross-linking of collagen and less tissue antigenicity than formalin fixation.[3] Collagen degeneration, with valve failure, was noted in the two valves that were in place for the longest periods, thus raising the possibility that cusp fatigue ultimately may occur in many of these bioprostheses. Although clinical studies of the Hancock bioprostheses for up to 5 years are encouraging,[1,9] longer periods of follow-up of patients with such valves will be necessary to ascertain the ultimate fate of the glutaraldehyde-treated valves.

Thromboembolism: implications for anticoagulant therapy: Despite the frequency of gross and microscopic-sized fibrin thrombi, no clear evidence of valve-related thromboemboli was found. Reendothelialization of the valve cusps did not occur, and long-term anticoagulation therapy did not prevent fibrin thrombi. These results suggest that such therapy, at least with warfarin, is not necessary when Hancock bioprostheses are used. Thrombosis with stenosis occurred in 3 of our 41 patients (four bioprostheses). Two of the three had very low cardiac output immediately after operation, and this factor may have contributed to the thrombus formation; the third patient had a 42 mm Hg peak systolic pressure gradient between the left ventricle and a systemic artery, and this gradient may have altered flow in the vicinity of the bioprosthesis and therefore allowed thrombus formation. Horowitz et al.[12] have listed five indications for a 6 week course of anticoagulation after bioprosthetic valve replacement: (1) atrial fibrillation; (2) thrombus in the left atrium at operation; (3) history of thromboembolism; (4) absence of a smooth suture line; and (5) low cardiac output. Our data appear to reinforce at least the last of these indications.

Prosthetic dysfunction: In our study prosthetic dysfunction usually was secondary to technical factors. The struts of a mitral bioprosthesis partially obstructed left ventricular outflow in three patients; all died soon after operation. In only three patients was valve failure the result of degeneration of leaflet tissue.

Of the early bioprostheses studied, the greatest inflammatory reaction seen was in 14 day old tricuspid and mitral bioprostheses from a patient who had removal of an incompetent disrupted mitral bioprosthesis that had been in place for 56 months. This finding suggests that perhaps host sensitization to bioprosthetic antigen was present after destruction of the first bioprosthesis. In the rare patient with bioprosthetic dysfunction, therefore, replacement with a mechanical prosthesis rather than another bioprosthesis may be advisable.

References

1. **McIntosh CL, Michaelis LL, Morrow AG, et al:** Atrioventricular valve replacement with the Hancock porcine xenograft: a five-year clinical experience. Surgery 78:768–775, 1975
2. **Stinson EB, Griepp RB, Shumway NE:** Clinical experience with a porcine aortic valve xenograft for mitral valve replacement. Ann Thorac Surg 18:391–401, 1974
3. **Zuhdi N, Hawley W, Voehl V, et al:** Porcine aortic valves as replacement for human heart valves. Ann Thorac Surg 17:479–491, 1974
4. **Pipkin RD, Buch WS, Fogarty TJ:** Evaluation of aortic valve replacement with a porcine xenograft without long-term anticoagulation. J Thorac Cardiovasc Surg 71:179–186, 1976
5. **Horowitz MS, Goodman DJ, Fogarty TJ, et al:** Mitral valve replacement with the glutaraldehyde-preserved porcine heterograft: Clinical, hemodynamic, and pathological correlations. J Thorac Cardiovasc Surg 67:885–895, 1974
6. **Carpentier A, Deloche A, Relland J, et al:** Six-year follow-up of glutaraldehyde-preserved heterografts with particular reference to the treatment of congenital valve malformations. J Thorac Cardiovasc Surg 68:771–782, 1974
7. **Brown JW, Myerowitz PD, Cann MS, et al:** Clinical and hemodynamic comparisons of Kay-Shiley, Starr-Edwards No. 6520, and Reis-Hancock porcine xenograft mitral valves. Surgery 76: 983–991, 1974
8. **Bowman FO Jr, Hancock WD, Malm JR:** A valve-containing dacron prosthesis. Its use in restoring pulmonary artery-right ventricular continuity. Arch Surg 107:724–728, 1973
9. **Hannah H, Reis RL:** Current status of porcine heterograft prostheses: A 5-year appraisal. Circulation 54:Suppl III:III-27–III-31, 1976
10. **Yarbrough JW, Roberts WC, Reis RL:** Structural alterations in tissue cardiac valves implanted in patients and in calves. J Thorac Cardiovasc Surg 65:364–375, 1973
11. **Mohri H, Reichenbach DD, Merendino KA:** Biology of homologous and heterologous aortic valves. In, Biological Tissue in Heart Valve Replacement (Ionescu MI, Ross DN, Wooler GH, ed). London, Butterworth, 1972, p 137–194
12. **Horowitz MS, Goodman DJ, Hancock EW, et al:** Noninvasive diagnosis of complications of the mitral bioprosthesis. J Thorac Cardiovasc Surg 71:450–457, 1976
13. **Reis RL, Hancock WD, Yarbrough JW, et al:** The flexible stent. A new concept in the fabrication of tissue heart valve prostheses. J Thorac Cardiovasc Surg 62:683–695, 1971
14. **Rose AG:** Pathology of the formalin-treated heterograft porcine aortic valve in the mitral position. Thorax 27:401–409, 1972
15. **Buch WS, Angell WW, Shumway NE:** Deterioration of formalin-treated aortic valve heterografts. J Thorac Cardiovasc Surg 60: 673–682, 1970
16. **O'Brien MF, Neilson GH, Galea EG, et al:** Heterograft valves. An analysis of clinical results of valve replacement. Circulation 41, 42:Suppl II:II-16–II-19, 1970
17. **Kouchoukos NT, Kerr AR, Sheppard LC, et al:** Heterograft replacement of the mitral valve: clinical, hemodynamic and pathological features. Circulation 41, 42:Suppl II:II-2–II-28, 1970
18. **Ionescu MI, Smith DR, Sutherland TW, et al:** Heart valve replacement with aortic heterografts: followup study. Ann Thorac Surg 13:1–14, 1972
19. **Kaiser GA, Hancock WD, Lukban SB, et al:** Clinical use of a new design stented xenograft heart valve prosthesis. Surg Forum 20: 137–138, 1969

Prosthetic Heart Valves: Which Ones and Why

WILLIAM C. ROBERTS *National Heart, Lung and Blood Institute*

The type and to some extent the size of prosthesis are by far the most important factors determining the patient's prognosis. Extensive necropsy experience shows that in terms of hemodynamics, thrombogenesis, and deterioration – the three major criteria – none of the four main types of prosthetic valves in use today is ideal. Emphasis is placed on the role of the referring cardiologist in the choice of surgeon and prosthesis.

About half a million people have had surgical replacement of a heart valve, the great majority successfully, since the procedure came into general use in the 1960s. Currently, a good estimate is that prostheses of various types are being inserted in close to 40,000 individuals a year.

Over the past 15 years at the National Institutes of Health, I have studied at necropsy approximately 500 persons who died after valve replacement at intervals ranging from minutes to years. These studies, like others from other vantage points, have led to certain conclusions – notably, the crucial importance of the type of prosthesis employed. It appears that, other things being approximately equal (i.e., the skill and experience of the surgeon and his team), the type and, to some extent, the size of prosthesis inserted are by all odds the most important factors determining the patient's prognosis. As a corollary, the choice of prosthesis should not be automatically left to the surgeon, as is currently the rule, but should also involve the cardiologist who recommended the patient for surgery.

The ideal valve prosthesis should possess at least six qualities: 1) it should have good hemodynamic characteristics, meaning that it should obstruct blood flow minimally when open and be fully competent when shut; 2) it should not be thrombogenic; 3) it should not degenerate, wear out, or vary during the expected lifetime of the patient; 4) it should not significantly alter blood components, e.g., by inducing hemolysis; 5) it should be insertable without undue difficulty, that is, without requiring exquisite, and therefore rare, technical skills; and 6) it should not disturb the patient by making audible noise.

Of these six criteria, however, the first three are most important. While some types of prostheses produce more hemolysis than others, this is seldom of clinical significance, in that the bone marrow can generally replace the losses without the development of anemia or thrombocytopenia. With regard to difficulty of insertion, this is much the same for all existing types, since most now used have rigid or semirigid frames with cloth-covered sewing rings. Finally, with the possible exception of one recently introduced model, no current prosthesis produces noise audible to the patient.

Considered in terms of the three important criteria – hemodynamics, thrombogenesis, and degeneration – none of the existing types of prostheses can be considered ideal. However, the criteria do provide a measuring rod for comparing one type with another. The four types we shall consider – the ones in wide use today – are the caged ball, the nontilting caged disc, the tilting disc, and the xenograft (porcine).

The caged-ball prosthesis, currently available in half a dozen makes, has been longest in use and, mainly for this reason, is the one on which the most voluminous data are available. This device, however, has undergone numerous modifications during the 17 years it has been employed. Nonetheless, enough information currently exists to permit some firm conclusions on its characteristics.

Its hemodynamic properties are adequate, though not as good as those of another, more recent type. The most useful measurement of cardiac hemodynamics is the pressure gradient between one side of the open valve and the other, obtained by catheterization. In the normal heart, these gradients are zero, i.e., once the valve is open it interposes no barrier to the flow of blood. With the caged ball installed in, e.g., the mitral position, the pressure difference

Dr. Roberts is Chief, Pathology Branch, National Heart, Lung and Blood Institute, National Institutes of Health, Bethesda, and Clinical Professor of Pathology and Medicine (Cardiology), Georgetown University, Washington, D.C.

averages about 6 mm Hg (compared with 4 mm Hg for another type of valve, which we shall discuss below.)

The pressure difference reflects the fact that with the caged ball, blood flow through the valve is peripheral, around the circumference of the ball, and is therefore turbulent; this contrasts with flow through the normal (anatomic) valve, which is central and nearly smooth ("laminar"). When a caged-ball prosthesis is installed in the aortic position, this turbulent flow is likely to induce proliferation of the aortic intima in the vicinity of the prosthesis. Occasionally, this overgrowth may narrow one or both coronary ostia.

Initially, the caged-ball prosthesis had a rather pronounced tendency to induce clotting. This has been somewhat ameliorated by the introduction of cloth covering on the struts and ring-shaped seat of the prosthesis, but all patients must be maintained on anticoagulants indefinitely. The cloth covering appears to increase hemolysis somewhat, though (as noted earlier) seldom to the point of posing clinical problems. Wear of the cloth has sometimes occurred. One recent model seeks to obviate this problem by placing a metal "track" on the interior of the struts. However, the track can produce an audible noise when struck by the ball, which some patients find disturbing.

The initial models of the caged-ball prosthesis employed a silicone rubber poppet. It soon became apparent that this was liable to degeneration – cracking and/or swelling, sometimes to the point where it could no longer move freely within the cage. This problem was eliminated with the introduction of a hollow, metallic ball made of the alloy Stellite-21. Nonetheless, the silicone balls continue to be used in some centers, even though they can be expected to degenerate eventually.

Perhaps the major problem with the caged-ball prosthesis is the amount of space it occupies. If the left ventricle is small, a mitral prosthesis may project far enough into the ventricle to obstruct the aortic outflow; if part of the cage burrows into the ventricular wall, movement of the ball may also be partially blocked, leading to obstructed ventricular filling. This problem can be even more severe in patients with stenosis of both mitral and aortic valves, where there may not be enough space at either position to accommodate a caged-ball prosthesis.

The problem of too large a prosthesis for the available space obviously emphasizes the importance of proper size selection on the surgeon's part. However, in some patients the problem can occur even with the smallest size of caged ball available.

In summary, in my view the caged-ball prosthesis should be reserved for patients with predominant or pure valvular incompetence, those in whom volume overload has produced a large ventricular cavity or ascending aorta. Where the lesions are purely or predominantly stenotic, this type of prosthesis should be avoided in favor of other and better substitutes that are available. These prostheses are not ideal in the right ventricle because of the tendency of the struts to burrow into the free wall of the ventricle or into the ventricular septum.

The space problem with the caged-ball prosthesis was one of the factors that led to development of the caged-disc type, in which the ball was replaced with a "flat" (actually, lens-shaped) disc. The resulting "low profile," it was thought, would obviate the space problem. Unfortunately, the device's other characteristics have more than offset the advantage resulting from its smaller size. It is more thrombogenic than the caged-ball type, and more obstructive. The latter is a consequence of its design, which allows less space between disc and base than exists between ball and base in earlier prostheses; this is reflected in a higher pressure gradient – in the mitral position, an average of 8 mm Hg as against 6 for the caged ball.

In the caged-ball prosthesis, the ball, assuming no obstructions exist, will move normally regardless of the angle at which the blood strikes it. With the caged disc, however, unless the bloodstream strikes more or less at right angles to the disc, it may "cock," opening much more on one side than the other, with consequent further obstruction to blood flow. There is reason to suspect that this may in some cases result in jamming the disc permanently in the cocked, half-open position, which can prove fatal.

More recently, a new type of caged disc has been introduced in which the "flat" disc has been replaced by a biconical disc whose cross section is a flattish diamond. However, there is no evidence that this modification is any less obstructive than the older version, or indeed that it represents any sort of improvement. Thus in default of evidence that the caged disc – of either type – possesses important advantages over other prostheses, its use, in my view, should be avoided.

The tilting-disc prosthesis, as its name implies, operates on a somewhat different principle from those previously discussed. Instead of a ball or disc moving back and forth within a cage, it employs a lens-shaped disc that twists or tilts at an angle of about 60° to 80° when the valve opens, returning to the flat position during closure. Thus, blood flow through it is not peripheral – as in the caged-ball or caged-disc prosthesis – but semicentral. This fact is reflected in low pressure gradients, e.g., an average of 4 mm Hg when the valve is installed in the mitral position. Its hemolytic char-

Prosthetic Heart Valves: A Box Score

Type	*Year Introduced*	*Obstructive*	*Incompetent*	*Thrombotic*	*Hemolytic*	*Degenerates*
Caged ball	1960	+ +	0	+ +	+	+
Caged disc	1965	+ +	0	+ +	+	+
Tilting disc	1967	+	0	+ +	0	0
Bioprostheses						
Homograft	1962	0	+	0	0	+
Xenograft	1965	+ +	0	0	0	?

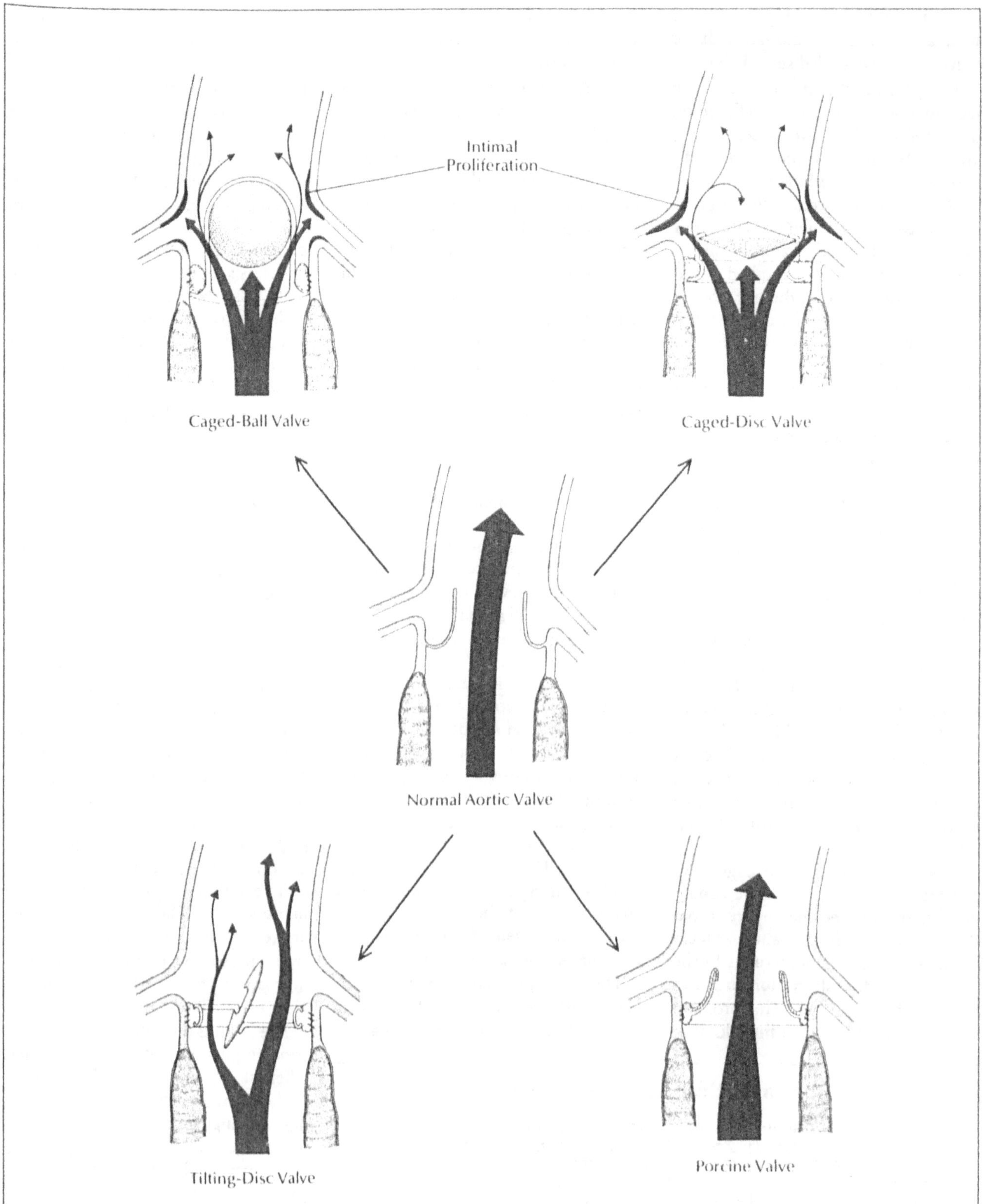

Different types of prostheses are evaluated against schematized normal valve, in which central flow produces no pressure gradient when valve is open. With caged ball, flow is peripheral and turbulent, producing pressure gradient and sometimes intimal overgrowth around coronary ostia; these problems are encountered also with caged disc. Flow through tilting disc is semi-central, with minimal gradient. Porcine valve has central flow, but significant pressure gradient owing to its smaller size.

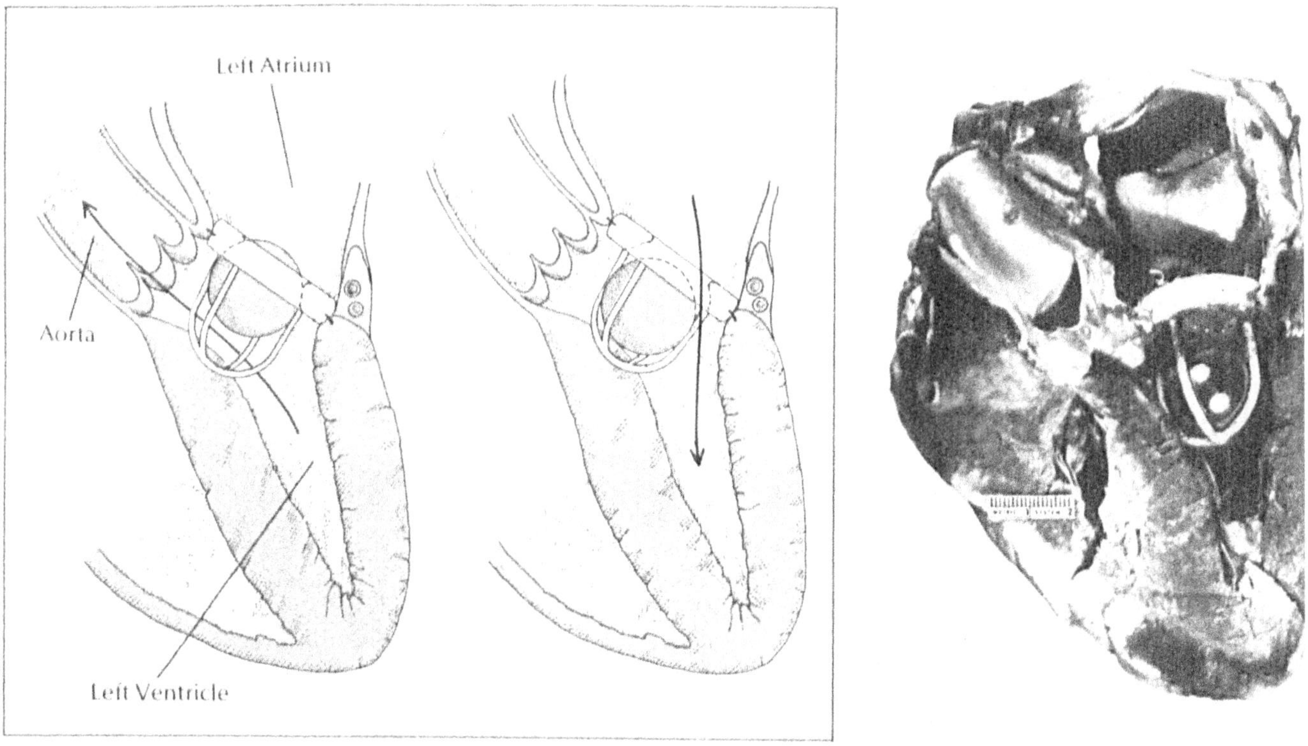

Shortened rear wall of the ventricle, secondary to mitral stenosis without significant aortic valvular disease, may cause a prosthetic mitral valve to lie transversely within the ventricle. This occasionally obstructs outflow (left) or, more commonly, inflow (center). An oversized prosthesis can produce similar obstruction even when it is correctly positioned (right).

acteristics are good, as is its resistance to wear. Its only defect is that, like the caged-ball and nontilting disc prostheses, it stimulates thrombogenesis, so that the patient must be maintained on anticoagulants. (It is worth noting that thrombogenesis is dangerous not just for the obvious reason – the likelihood of an embolism if the clot breaks loose from the prosthesis – but also because clots remaining in situ can seriously obstruct the proper functioning of the device.)

Because of the design of this prosthesis, no part of the disc moves very far from its seat, meaning that the chances of interference with movement through contact with the ventricular wall or aortic intima are minimal. Such interference can occur, though, if a large-sized prosthesis is installed in a small ventricle or aorta. In my judgment, the tilting disc can, with certain reservations, be considered the prosthesis of choice in most cases, whether installed in the aortic, mitral, or tricuspid position.

Tissue-valve prostheses, in the form of aortic valve replacement using cadaver material, have been used since 1962. However, though the initial results were gratifying, these and other kinds of human tissue prostheses (fascia lata, dura mater, or parietal pericardium) eventually proved disappointing owing to accelerated wear, with development of incompetency, or to stiffening, with resulting immobility. Currently, the favored type of tissue valve is a porcine xenograft. The pig valves are carefully trimmed of most muscle and fixed in glutaraldehyde (earlier valves treated with formaldehyde proved disastrous; the leaflets simply tore apart).

Since blood flow through the porcine valve is entirely central, comparable to that through a natural valve, one would expect that the pressure drop across it would be minimal. In fact, it approximates the drop across the caged-ball prosthesis, an average of 6 mm Hg in the mitral position. The reason seems to be that when mounted on its attachment ring, the porcine valve is somewhat smaller than the human valve. The result is a degree of stenosis. The porcine xenograft, however, is essentially nonhemolytic and certainly less thrombogenic than are the completely rigid-formed prostheses, and therefore anticoagulant maintenance is not necessary. This fact alone would make the porcine graft the prosthesis of choice, were it not for some unresolved questions about its wear characteristics.

Thus far, few porcine xenografts in place for more than five years have been studied morphologically. Functionally, this prosthesis seems to operate very well during at least the first five years. However, postmortem examination of porcine valves has revealed some disquieting changes. At gross examination, the valves usually appear normal. Under light microscopy, however, they do not look as good, with evidence of minor degeneration and areas of calcification, though seldom to the point of functional impairment. Under electron microscopy or scanning electron microscopy, they look worse, with degeneration of collagen and tiny tears, which seem likely to be the precursors of more serious degeneration later on. While we cannot be certain until more data covering longer periods are available, the weight of present evidence is that the porcine valves will tend to develop serious degeneration in possibly from seven to 10 years. The odds are against their functioning well for as long as 20 years.

The degeneration problem makes it impossible to recommend the porcine valve unreservedly. As things now stand, one must weigh the risk of ultimate degeneration against the risks of maintaining the patient on anticoagulants if another type of prosthesis is used. Ordinarily, patients on anticoagulants can be expected to develop major bleeding complications at the rate of about 1% per year, and of course this risk is markedly enhanced in individuals with a preexisting clotting disorder. Broadly speaking, where this or some other contraindication to anticoagulants exists, the surgeon – and the cardiologist – should consider using the porcine valve, with the expectation that it may have to be replaced in seven to 10 years. Absent such contraindications, it might perhaps be best to use some other type of prosthesis (notably the tilting disc) until more, and more encouraging, long-term data on the porcine valve become available.

Before concluding this account, there are a couple of other points that need to be discussed. The first is the size of the prosthesis. Normally, this is decided on the spot by the surgeon, often by inserting a trocar dilator into the "hole" where the prosthesis will be implanted. Most surgeons prefer to insert the largest prosthesis possible, feeling – not unreasonably – that the larger the prosthesis, the better the resulting blood flow. However, this is true *only* if there is space within the ventricle (or the aorta) for the poppet of the prosthesis to move freely.

As already noted, if the ventricle is not enlarged (as in mitral stenosis), space will be at a premium, and this will be true also in a small patient. In such cases, it should be assumed a priori that the patient must receive a relatively small prosthesis, regardless of the nominal size of the attachment site. In the case of a large individual with pure mitral or aortic regurgitation, on the other hand, prosthetic size is far less critical.

The second point concerns the method of attachment of the prosthe-

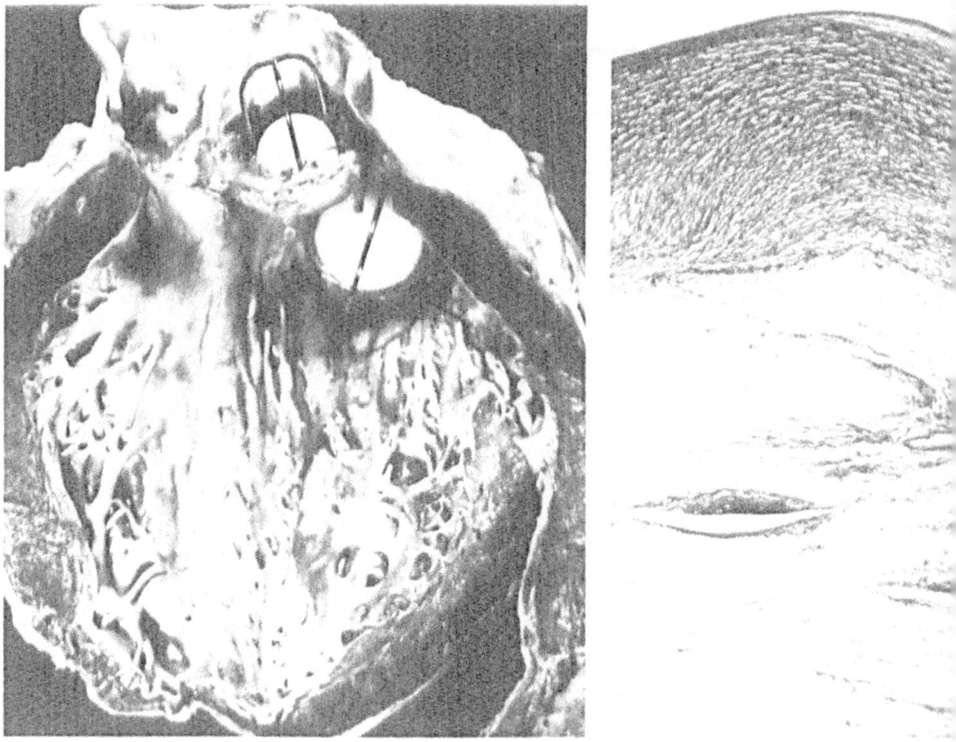

Turbulent flow through mitral prosthesis can produce fibroelastosis of ventricular endocardium, apparent here in both gross view and enlarged section. Patient died 11 months postoperatively of congestive failure, probably related to endocardial thickening.

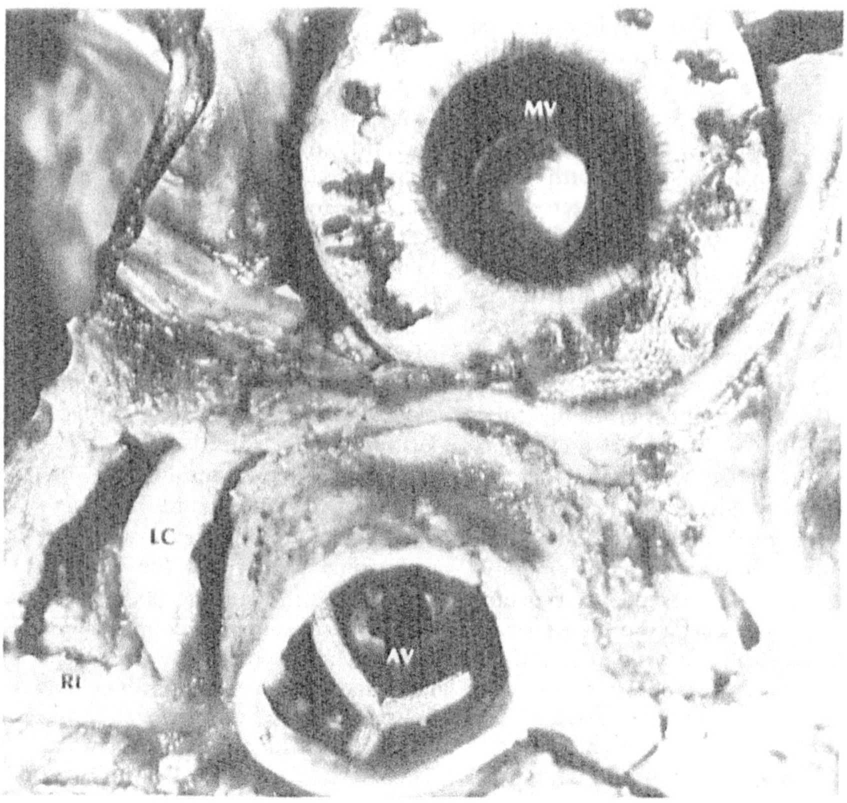

When left circumflex coronary artery (LC) rises anomalously, from right coronary (Rt), double-valve replacement can compress it, with fatal results. This patient died 10 days postoperatively; necropsy showed acute infarction of left ventricular wall.

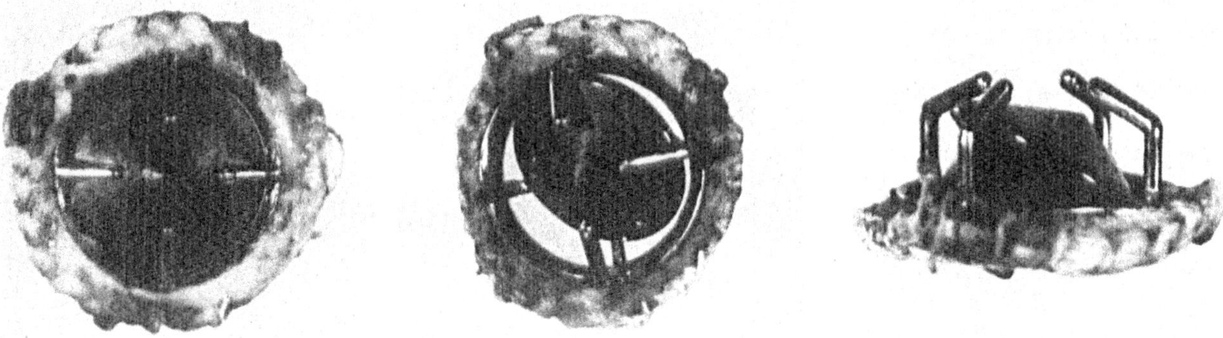

Asymmetric flow through the caged-disc prosthesis can produce "cocking" (center, right), with the disc twisted from the normal closed position (left). If the valve becomes stuck in cocked position, the resulting incompetence is likely to prove fatal.

sis. Some surgeons employ only four interrupted sutures, placed at angles of 90° around the ring, with the intervening areas closed by continuous sutures. The rationale for this is that continuous sutures can be inserted more quickly, thereby decreasing the patient's time on the heart-lung machine. My own opinion is that this rationale is faulty, in that it neglects the much-enhanced risk if a suture fails – a leak through something like 25% of the parabasilar area, as against, say, 5% if 20 or so interrupted sutures are used. This risk, it seems to me, more than offsets a gain of a few minutes off the pump.

To sum up the question of choice of prosthesis, it is my view that when the operation is done in a large medical center where several valve replacements are performed weekly, differences in technical skill among surgeons will play a minor role in patient survival. This statement is unlikely to win me friends among surgical colleagues, but I think it is accurate. The most obvious evidence of this is found in the early years of valve replacement. Until development of the caged-ball prosthesis, few patients survived more than several days. Following the introduction of the caged-ball prosthesis, most patients survived even though, at the beginning, the operation was necessarily being performed by many surgeons who had never done a valve replacement, their experience of valve surgery being limited to mitral commissurotomy. A more recent case concerns a young surgeon I know who had assisted at many valve replacements but had never actually done one himself. He nonetheless went on to perform about 90 operations without a death. His success was due in considerable measure, I think, to the fact that he held strong opinions on the importance of selecting a prosthesis of the proper size, particularly favoring the smaller-sized ones over the larger-sized ones.

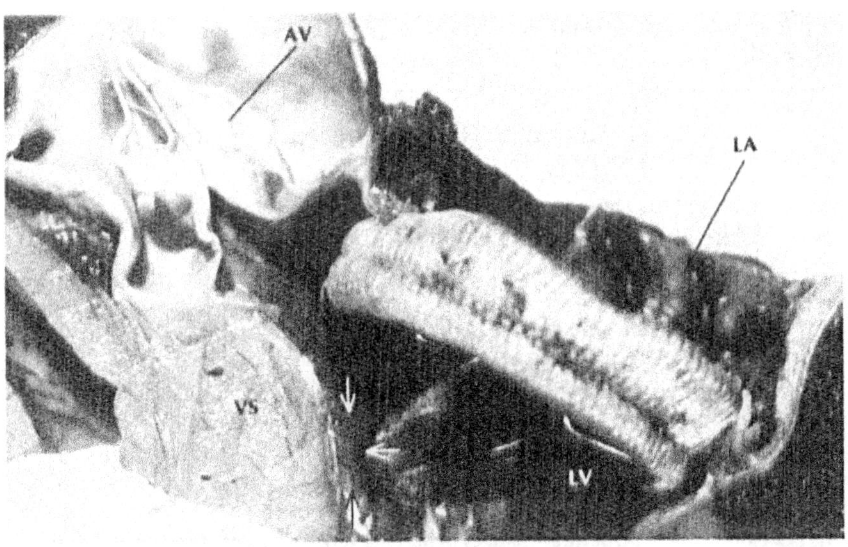

Oversize tilting-disc mitral prosthesis failed to seat properly because edge of disc impinged on ventricular septum (arrows) as it moved inward during systole. Patient died during the operation; he could not be separated from cardiopulmonary bypass.

If, as I believe, it is the type and size of prosthesis chosen that primarily influences the patient's survival, then who should choose it? At present, the choice is up to the surgeon. He is likely to give preference to the type of prosthesis he has already worked with. He is also likely to be influenced by the experience of particularly prominent members of his specialty or by that of the surgeon who trained him. Finally, if he has himself played a role in the development of a particular type of prosthesis, he is likely to prefer that one. A surgeon who has developed a given prosthesis, and at the same time has the sole responsibility for deciding whether or not to use it, is involved in a sort of conflict of interest.

The obvious conclusion is that the decision on which prosthesis to employ should not be solely that of the surgeon but should involve input from the cardiologist who has referred the patient. Once the patient has been referred, it is the surgeon who decides not only whether to operate – which is perfectly reasonable – but also *how* to operate, in the sense of which prosthesis to use – which is not so reasonable. In my view, the referring physician owes it to his patient to exercise his own judgment in this area.

Attempts by a nonsurgeon to express opinions on a matter traditionally considered within the surgeon's sole competence can obviously raise delicate questions of professional relationships. Many of these can be avoided *ab initio*, however, by giving prior thought to which surgeon the patient is being referred to, not simply in terms of technical competence (a criterion that one takes for granted) but in terms of which prosthesis or prostheses he habitually employs, and on *how appropriate these may be for the patient in question.*

For example, a patient with mitral stenosis or combined mitral and aortic valve disease (when the root of the aorta is usually small) should probably not be referred to a surgeon who always or nearly always uses the caged ball. Equally, patients should probably not be referred to surgeons using only the caged (non-tilting) disc, at least until much more information is available on the long-term results of this prosthesis. Finally, a patient with real or potential bleeding problems should not be referred to a surgeon who never uses the porcine valve, which, as I have indicated above, should be considered the prosthesis of choice in such cases.

And finally, for a cardiologist to exercise his responsibility fully toward his patient, he must take the trouble to become more sophisticated on the advantages and disadvantages of the different types of prosthetic valves. The decision regarding type and also size of prosthesis chosen for his patient no longer should rest entirely with the surgeon. □

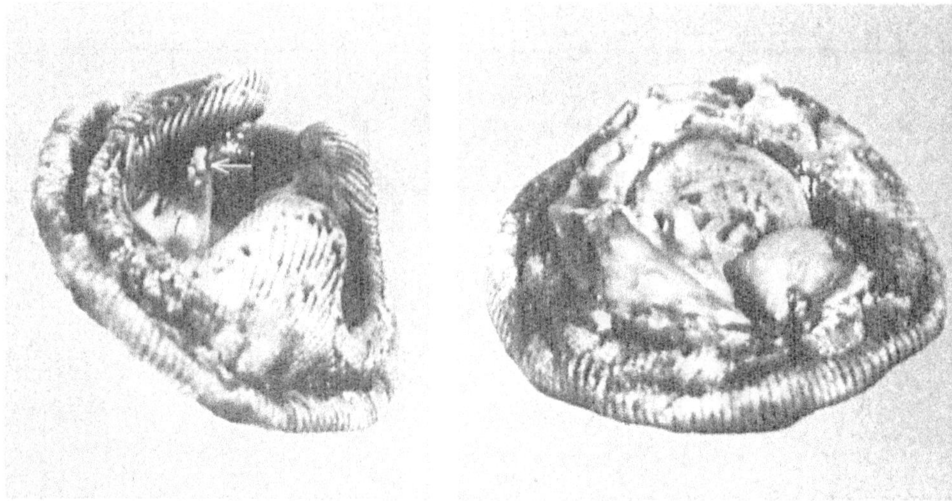

Porcine prosthesis (above), replaced successfully 75 months after implantation, showed calcium deposits (left, arrow) and tears and fraying of two leaflets (right). Another such prosthesis, part of a double-valve replacement (below, left) showed inflammatory changes under microscope 14 months later (below, right). Had these progressed, they could eventually have caused trouble; however, patient died of other causes.

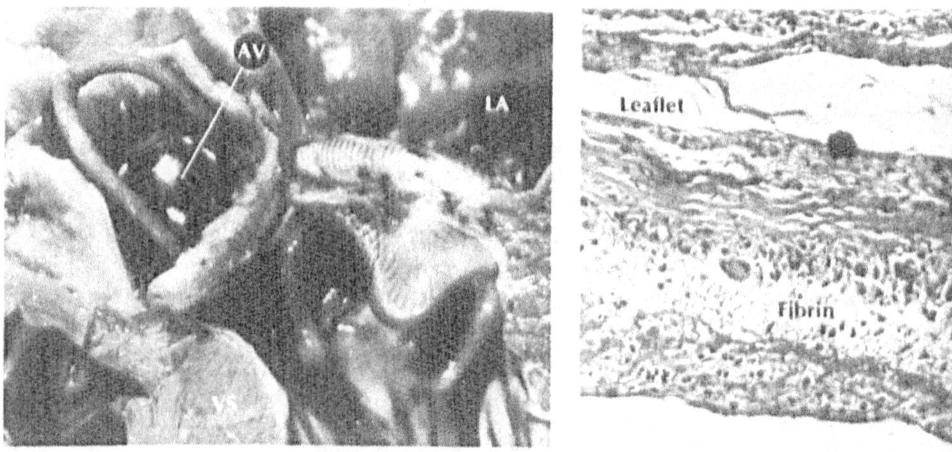

Selected Reading

Roberts WC, Bulkey BH, Morrow AG: Pathologic anatomy of cardiac valve replacement: a study of 224 necropsy patients. Prog Cardiovasc Dis 15:539, 1973

Fishbein MC, Roberts WC, Golden A, Hufnagel CA: Cardiac pathology after aortic valve replacement using a Hufnagel tri-leaflet prosthesis: a study of 20 necropsy patients. Am Heart 89:443, 1975

Roberts WC, Fishbein MC, Golden A: Cardiac pathology after valve replacement by disc prosthesis. A study of 61 necropsy patients. Am J Cardiol 35:740, 1975

Roberts WC, Hammer WJ: Cardiac pathology after valve replacement with a tilting disc prosthesis (Bjork-Shiely type). A study of 46 necropsy patients and 49 Bjork-Shiley prostheses. Am J Cardiol 37:1024, 1976

Roberts WC: Choosing a substitute cardiac valve: type size, surgeon. Am J Cardiol 38:633, 1976

Spray TL, Roberts WC: Structural changes in porcine xenografts used as substitute cardiac valves. Gross and histologic observations in 51 gluteraldehyde-preserved Hancock valves in 41 patients. Am J Cardiol 40:319, 1977

A complete list of references for this article is available on request to Box TC, HOSPITAL PRACTICE.

Structural Changes in Hancock Porcine Xenograft Cardiac Valve Bioprostheses

THOMAS L. SPRAY and WILLIAM C. ROBERTS

Pathology Branch, National Heart, Lung, and Blood Institute, National Institutes of Health, Bethesda, Md.

Introduction

The glutaraldehyde-preserved, stented porcine xenograft is now widely used as a substitute cardiac valve [1–10]. Despite its wide use, however, relatively little information on structural changes in this bioprosthesis is available [3–6, 10]. This report describes gross and histologic findings in 51 Hancock (Hancock Laboratories, Anaheim, Calif.) glutaraldehyde-preserved, porcine, cardiac valve bioprostheses from 41 patients in whom the bioprostheses had been in place for periods up to 75 months [11].

Patients Studied and Methods

The 51 bioprostheses from 41 patients (table I) were divided into two groups: (1) 33 valves with implantation periods of < 2 months (early valves), and (2) 18 valves with implantation periods of > 2 months (late valves). The means and ranges of implantation periods, the mean sizes of the prostheses used, and the positions in which the valves were implanted are shown in tables II (early valves) and III (late valves). 4 (all late) of the 51 valves were removed at operation (3 mitral, 1 tricuspid); all 4 valves were removed because of severe regurgitation, 3 (2 mitral, 1 tricuspid) for tissue degeneration and 1 (mitral) because of a paravalvular leak. The 2 mitral valves in this series with the longest implantation times (56 and 75 months) were removed because of tissue degeneration of the leaflets with resulting regurgitation, and in each the removed valve was replaced with a new Hancock bioprosthesis. 1 of these patients died 14 days later of respiratory complications. 1 tricuspid valve was removed because of leaflet degeneration after 3 months, and was replaced with a mechanical valve. The mitral valve removed because of paravalvular leak was replaced with a fresh porcine xenograft.

Table I. Structural changes in porcine xenograft cardiac valve bioprostheses (Hancock stabilized glutaraldehyde process)

Number of patients	41
Valves	
Mitral	31
Tricuspid	15
Aortic	4
Pulmonary	1
Total	51

Table II. Structural changes in porcine xenograft cardiac valve bioprostheses: early valves (< 2 months), range: 0–50 days, mean 12 days

Valve	Number	Size range, mm	Mean size, mm
Mitral	19	25–35	29
Tricuspid	10	29–35	33
Aortic	3	27–29	27
Pulmonary	1	21	–
Total	33		

Table III. Structural changes in porcine xenograft cardiac valve bioprostheses: late valves (> 2 months), range: 2.1–75 months, mean 14 months (7> 1 year)

Valve	Number	Size range, mm	Mean size, mm
Mitral	12	25–35	29
Tricuspid	5	31–35	33
Aortic	1	25	–
Pulmonary	0	–	–
Total	18		

Table IV. Structural changes in porcine xenograft cardiac valve bioprostheses: gross observations

Observation	Early	Late
Normal	30	13
Thrombosis (stenosis)	3	2
Leaflet degeneration (regurgitation)	0	3
Strut in outflow tract	3	0
Prosthetic disproportion	3	0
Coronary ostial obstruction by struts	1	0

Gross Observations (table IV)

Of the 33 bioprostheses with implantation periods of less than 2 months, 30 were entirely normal by visual inspection at necropsy, and the remaining 3 showed some gross structural changes. Of the 18 bioprostheses with implantation periods of greater than 2 months, 13 were normal by visual inspection at necropsy, and the remaining 5 showed some gross alteration either at necropsy or reoperation. The major gross changes observed in these 8 bioprostheses included cuspal thrombosis (both early and late) and cuspal degeneration (late only). In addition, 7 instances of prosthetic-related complications or evidence for prosthetic dysfunction were noted (table IV).

Cuspal *thrombus* was present grossly in 5 bioprostheses (2 mitral, 2 tricuspid and 1 aortic) from 4 patients. In 1 of these patients, bioprostheses were implanted in both the mitral and tricuspid valve positions and the patient died 32 days postoperatively after a prolonged period of low cardiac output. At necropsy, thrombus filled the sinuses of 2 of the 3 cusps of the tricuspid valve prosthesis, and 1 of the 3 commissures had fused; only 1 of the 3 cusps remained pliable and consequently the prosthetic orifice appeared stenotic. The bioprosthesis in the mitral position in the same patient also contained thrombus in 2 of the 3 cusps, but none of the commissures had fused. Both atria at necropsy were filled with organizing thrombus. In a second patient with a bioprosthesis in the mitral position, a large thrombus, which filled the body and appendage of the left atrium, was attached to the atrial aspects of each of the 3 cusps. Thrombus also filled the sinus portions of each of the 3 cusps, thereby producing severe prosthetic obstruction. This patient lived 8 days postoperatively and the cause of the thrombosis was not determined. In a third patient a bioprosthesis in the tricuspid valve position for 2 months showed gross thrombi in the cusps, but only mild limitation of movement of the leaflets. Thrombus was present in 2 of the 3 sinuses of a bioprosthesis in the aortic position for 5 months in a fourth patient.

Degeneration of the cuspal tissue with resulting regurgitation was present in 3 valves from 3 patients – 2 mitral (implantation periods 56 months and 75 months) and 1 tricuspid (3 months). All 3 bioprostheses showed tears of the cusps with adherent thrombus. In the 56- and 75-month-old mitral bioprostheses, gross nodular calcific deposits were present.

Clinical or morphologic evidence for thromboembolism was present in 4 patients with 'late' bioprostheses, but each patient had mechanical prostheses in addition to porcine bioprostheses, and in 3 patients thrombus was present on the mechanical prostheses. In 1 patient who had a 31-mm tricuspid valve bioprosthesis implanted 21 months earlier, evidence of pulmonary embolism occurred 3 months postoperatively. The origin of the embolus in her is unclear, but at necropsy fibrin thrombus was present in the sinus of the bioprosthesis despite long-term warfarin sodium therapy.

In 3 mitral valves, 1 of the 3 struts of the flexible stent was situated directly in the left ventricular outflow tract. All 3 patients were hypotensive throughout the postoperative period and died 1, 4 and 6 days, respectively, after operation.

In 2 patients (3 valves), prosthetic disproportion was present. In 1, 31-mm mitral and 33-mm tricuspid valve prostheses were implanted in a woman with tricuspid regurgitation and severe mitral stenosis. Postoperatively, she had evidence of inadequate cardiac output and finally complete heart block. At necropsy, the sewing rings of the prostheses compressed the aortic root. In the second patient, the struts of an aortic bioprosthesis obstructed both coronary ostia and she died soon after operation from circumferential myocardial necrosis.

In 2 patients, fatal infective endocarditis was present on a mechanical prosthesis (aortic in 1 and mitral in 1) and the porcine bioprostheses (mitral and tricuspid) were uninvolved.

Histologic Observations

Of the 51 porcine bioprostheses, 44 were examined histologically (table V). In addition, 2 unimplanted glutaraldehyde-fixed porcine valves were sectioned to serve as controls (courtesy of Warren D. Hancock, Hancock Lab-

Table V. Structural changes in porcine xenograft cardiac valve bioprostheses

	Histology (44 valves)											
	fibrin in cusps [1]		fibrin on inflow surface [2]		WBC [3]		histiocytes		giant cells		leaflet disruption [4]	
	No.	%	No.	%	No.	%	No.	%	No.	%	No.	%
Early	18/26	69	12/26	46	16/26	62	14/26	54	7/26	27	4/26	15
Late	14/18	78	9/18	50	13/18	72	14/18	78	12/18	67	8/18	45

[1] Ventricular surface of tricuspid and mitral valves; aortic surface of aortic valves.

[2] Atrial surface of tricuspid and mitral valves, ventricular surface of aortic valves.

[3] Plasma cells, polymorphonuclear leukocytes, lymphocytes.

[4] Focal invasion of leaflets by host cells or disruption.

oratories). Of the 3 cusps in the normal porcine aortic valve, the right one is attached to a 'muscle shelf' which consequently limits the pliability of this cusp [12]. Each of the 3 cusps is composed of multiple layers of cells with elongated nuclei, collagen bundles arranged radially, and short elastic fibers.

Early Valves

Of the 33 valves with implantation periods less than 2 months, 26 were examined histologically. *Fibrin deposits* were present on the outflow surfaces of the cusps in 18 (69 %), and on the inflow surfaces of 12 (46 %) bioprostheses. Occasionally, the fibrin deposits were large enough to limit cuspal mobility. Collections of platelets and erythrocytes were associated with the fibrin deposits in a few patients. 3 patients with 'early' (13, 14, 19 days) bioprostheses received warfarin daily postoperatively. 2 of the 3 valves from these patients showed moderate fibrin deposits on the cusps of the bioprostheses. Leukocytes, lymphocytes and occasionally plasma cells were present in the fibrin matrix or along the leaflet surface in 16 (62 %) of the 26 bioprostheses. Often leukocytes infiltrated the porcine aortic wall behind the cusps.

Macrophages, with histologic characteristics of *histiocytes* lined portions of the cusps in 14 (54 %) of the 26 bioprostheses and in 7 of the 14 histiocytes had collected together forming *giant cells*. The histiocytes occasionally were present in the outermost portions of the fibrocollagenous structure of the cusps. By polarization microscopy, talc and other foreign bodies were absent. Of the 7 bioprostheses which showed a giant cell reaction, giant cells were present in small numbers in 3 patients with bioprostheses in place for less than 30 days, whereas in the 3 patients with bioprostheses in place from 30 to 60 days, they were present in abundance. In 1 patient, 2 bioprostheses (1 mitral, 1 tricuspid), each in place for 14 days, showed marked inflammatory cell reaction, histiocyte accumulation and giant cell formation. This patient had a 56-month-old bioprosthesis removed from the mitral position due to disruption of the cusps causing regurgitation. The mitral and tricuspid valves were then replaced with fresh bioprostheses. In 4 (15%) of 26 bioprostheses, the substance of the cusps contained inflammatory cells or histiocytes. None of these 4 bioprostheses, however, showed either clinical or necropsy evidence of dysfunction. The fibrocollagenous structure of the remaining 22 bioprostheses was intact and appeared unchanged from the structure of the 2 control valves. Despite good ingrowth of tissue over the struts and the sewing rings of the prostheses, host cell ingrowth was absent on the leaflet surfaces of all bioprostheses in place for less than 2 months. Host cell ingrowth extended only a few millimeters beyond the sewing ring over the porcine tissue.

Late Valves

All 18 valves which had been in place for more than 2 months were available for histologic study (table V). *Fibrin deposits* were present on the outflow surface of the cusps in 14 (78%) of the 18 bioprostheses and on the inflow surface in 9 (50%). *Leukocytes* were present in 13 bioprostheses (72%) and *histiocytes* lined their cuspal surfaces in 78%. *Giant cell* formation was frequent: 12 (67%) of 18 showed giant cells, and in 8 (45%), focal invasion of the cusps by host cells and giant cells was present. In 3 valves (3-month-old tricuspid, 56- and 75-month-old mitrals) complete disruption of cuspal tissue occurred. In the 56- and 75-month-old valves, calcific deposits also were present in the cusps. Except for a few giant cells, cellular elements were absent and collagen was degenerated in each of the 2 patients with mitral bioprostheses in place for 56 and 75 months, respectively.

One bioprosthesis in place in the tricuspid position for 21 months showed marked host cellular endothelialization of the cusps; the endothelial cells, however, were present over a thin layer of fibrin and, therefore, appeared to represent endothelialization of thrombus rather than of the porcine tissue. No other late bioprostheses showed endothelialization of the cusps. Polarization microscopy showed no foreign bodies in any cusp of any bioprosthesis.

5 of the 18 porcine bioprostheses were in patients who postoperatively were either on warfarin sodium (3 patients) or aspirin plus dipyridamole (2 patients) because of also having mechanical prostheses. All 5 bioprostheses in these 5 patients showed fibrin deposits of varying degree on their cusps.

Comments

Good clinical and usually adequate hemodynamic results have been reported by several groups of investigators in patients in whom porcine heterograft bioprostheses have been implanted for up to 5 years [1–9]. These studies have shown low rates of clinical episodes suggestive of thromboembolism despite rare use of long-term anticoagulants [1, 4, 6, 13]. Furthermore, reports of failure of the bioprostheses have been rare [1, 6, 9]. Most studies of porcine heterograft prostheses, however, have concerned formalin-fixed tissue or tissue treated with various different glutaraldehyde preservation techniques [3, 10, 14–20]. Few descriptions of structural changes have been reported in valves processed by the Hancock stabilized-glutaraldehyde process, and few bioprostheses prepared by this fixative have been studied late [10, 11, 14].

Examination of formalin-treated porcine bioprostheses showed a high frequency of structural failure. Zuhdi *et al.* [3] noted structural failure in 20 of 31 stented formalin-fixed porcine bioprostheses within 4 years after implantation. Histologic studies showed inflammatory cell infiltrates in the cusps, fibrin deposits, and histiocyte and giant cell accumulation. No degenerative changes were seen, however, in 8 glutaraldehyde-preserved bioprostheses in place from 8 days to 16 months [3].

Carpentier *et al.* [6], utilizing a different glutaraldehyde fixation technique and rigid stents, noted valve dysfunction in 7 patients with implantation periods from 1 to 5 years. No immunologic reaction was seen, but collagen degeneration with cuspal perforation, and lining of cusps with histiocytes, macrophages and giant cells was observed.

In 4 of 32 patients with Hancock glutaraldehyde-fixed bioprostheses on a semirigid stent in the mitral position, Horowitz *et al.* [5] noted 'normal' histology in 4 valves removed 4–29 months after implantation. They also mentioned 'moderate numbers of macrophages and a few giant cells' at the base of the muscle shelf of the right coronary cusp in a valve in place for 18 months. Yarbrough *et al.* [10] noted essentially normal valve structure in 6 Hancock glutaraldehyde-preserved bioprostheses in place from 14 to 180 days. Mild fibrin deposits and layers of 'mesothelial-like cells' were noted in a bioprosthesis in the tricuspid position for 39 days [10].

The present study of 51 Hancock bioprostheses (44 examined histologically) shows a high frequency of structural changes, but most of the changes did not affect valvular function [11]. Fibrin deposits on the cuspal outflow surfaces and inflammatory cells were present in nearly 70% of both early and late bioprostheses. Almost half of the prostheses showed fibrin deposits on the inflow surfaces. The similar frequency of these changes in both early (< 2 months) and late (> 2 months) bioprostheses and the lack of organization of the fibrin deposits suggests that fibrin and inflammatory cells begin to be deposited soon after implantation. Perhaps fibrin deposition occurs as a response to structural stresses. Histiocyte accumulation, however, was slightly less frequent (54%) in early than in late (76%) bioprostheses, and giant cell formation was more than twice as common in late valves, suggesting that these reactions to the glutaraldehyde-preserved tissue occur later than the fibrin deposits. Although gross leaflet disruption was present in only 3 (17%) of 18 late bioprostheses, microscopic-sized focal cuspal disruption by host cells was present in 45% of the late valves.

Although the observed histologic changes in the glutaraldehyde-fixed bioprostheses are qualitatively similar to those described in formalin-fixed heterografts, the magnitude of the cellular reaction is less. Thus, the Hancock bioprostheses are not biologically inert in the human. These findings suggest that the Hancock stabilized-glutaraldehyde preservation technique creates more stable cross-linking of collagen and less tissue antigenicity than formalin fixation [3]. Collagen degeneration, with valve failure, was noted in the 2 valves which were in place for the longest periods, raising the possibility that cuspal fatigue ultimately may occur in many of these bioprostheses at long implantation periods. Although clinical studies of the Hancock bioprostheses for up to 5 years are encouraging [1, 9], longer periods of follow-up of patients with such valves will be necessary to ascertain the ultimate fate of the glutaraldehyde-treated valves.

Despite the frequency of gross and microscopic-sized fibrin thrombi, no clear evidence of valve-related thromboemboli was found. Reendothelialization of the valve cusps did not occur, and fibrin thrombi were not prevented by chronic anticoagulation. These results suggest that chronic anticoagulation therapy, at least with warfarin, is not necessary when Hancock bioprostheses are used. Thrombosis with stenosis occurred in 3 of our 41 patients (4 bioprostheses). 2 of them had very low cardiac outputs immediately after operation and this factor may have contributed to the thrombus formation; the thrid patient had a 42 mm Hg peak systolic pressure gradient between left ventricle and a systemic artery and this gradient may have altered flow in the vicinity of the bioprosthesis and therefore allowed thrombus formation. HOROWITZ *et al.* [13] have listed 5 indications for a 6-week course of anticoagulation after bioprosthetic valve replacement: (1) atriàl fibrillation; (2) thrombus in the left atrium at operation; (3) history of thromboembolism; (4) absence of a smooth suture line, and (5) low cardiac output. The present study appears to reinforce at least the last of these 'indications'.

Prosthetic dysfunction in this study usually was secondary to technical factors. The struts of a mitral bioprosthesis partially obstructed left ventricular outflow in 3 patients; all died soon after operation. In only 3 patients was valve failure the result of degeneration of leaflet tissue.

Of the early bioprostheses studied, the greatest inflammatory reaction seen was in 14-day-old tricuspid and mitral bioprostheses from a patient who had removal of an incompetent, disrupted mitral bioprosthesis which had been in place for 56 months. This finding suggests that perhaps host sensitization to bioprosthetic antigen was present after destruction of the first bioprosthesis. In the rare patient with bioprosthetic dysfunction, therefore, replacement with a mechanical prosthesis rather than another bioprosthesis may be advisable.

Summary

Gross and histologic observations are described in 51 Hancock glutaraldehyde-preserved porcine heterograft bioprostheses from 41 patients: 33 valves from 25 patients had been in place for <2 months *(early)* and 18 valves from 17 patients were examined at later periods up to 75 months *(late)* after implantation. The major gross changes were cuspal thrombosis (5 bioprostheses) and cuspal degeneration (3 bioprostheses). Major histologic changes observed in 44 bioprostheses (26 early and 18 late) examined histologically were: (1) fibrin deposits on inflow and outflow surfaces of the cusps; (2) inflammatory cell infiltrates; (3) histiocyte deposition; (4) giant cell formation, and (5) focal disruption of the fibrocollagenous structure of the cusps. These observations indicate that porcine bioprostheses are not biologically inert in the human circulation. Valve failure, however, is rare at the implantation periods studied.

References

1 McINTOSH, C. L.; MICHAELIS, L. L.; MORROW, A. G.; ITSCOITZ, S. R.; REDWOOD, D. R., and EPSTEIN, S. E.: Atrioventricular valve replacement with the Hancock porcine xenograft. A five-year clinical experience. Surgery *78:* 768–775 (1975).

2 Stinson, E. B.; Griepp, R. B., and Shumway, N. E.: Clinical experience with a porcine aortic valve xenograft for mitral valve replacement. Ann. thorac. Surg. *18:* 391–401 (1974).

3 Zuhdi, N.; Hawley, W.; Voehl, V.; Hancock, W.; Carey, J., and Greer, A.: Porcine aortic valves as replacement for human heart valves. Ann. thorac. Surg. *17:* 479–491 (1974).

4 Pipkin, R. D.; Buch, W. S., and Fogarty, T. J.: Evaluation of aortic valve replacement with a porcine xenograft without long-term anticoagulation. J. thorac. cardiovasc. Surg. *71:* 179–186 (1976).

5 Horowitz, M. S.; Goodman, D. J.; Fogarty, T. J., and Harrison, D. C.: Mitral valve replacement with the glutaraldehyde-preserved porcine heterograft. Clinical, hemodynamic, and pathological correlations. J. thorac. cardiovasc. Surg. *67:* 885–895 (1974).

6 Carpentier, A.; Deloche, A.; Relland, J.; Fabiani, J. N.; Forman, J.; Camilleri, J. P.; Soyer, R., and Dubost, C. H.: Six-year follow-up of glutaraldehyde-preserved heterografts with particular reference to the treatment of congenital valve malformations. J. thorac. cardiovasc. Surg. *68:* 771–782 (1974).

7 Brown, J. W.; Myerowitz, P. D.; Cann, M. S.; Colvin, S. B.; McIntosh, C. L., and Morrow, A. G.: Clinical and hemodynamic comparisons of Kay-Shiley, Starr-Edwards No. 6520, and Reis-Hancock porcine xenograft mitral valves. Surgery *76:* 983–991 (1974).

8 Bowman, F. O., jr.; Hancock, W. D., and Malm, J. R.: A valve-containing dacron prosthesis. Its use in restoring pulmonary artery-right ventricular continuity. Archs Surg. *107:* 724–728 (1973).

9 Hannah, H. and Reis, R. L.: Current status of porcine heterograft prostheses. A 5-year appraisal. Circulation *54:* suppl. III, pp. 27–31 (1976).

10 Yarbrough, J. W.; Roberts, W. C., and Reis, R. L.: Structural alterations in tissue cardiac valves implanted in patients and in calves. J. thorac. cardiovasc. Surg. *65:* 364–375 (1973).

11 Spray, T. L. and Roberts, W. C.: Structural changes in porcine xenografts used as substitute cardiac valves. Gross and histologic observations in 51 glutaraldehyde-preserved Hancock valves in 41 patients. Am. J. Cardiol. (in press).

12 Mohri, H.; Reichenbach, D. D., and Merendino, K. A.: Biology of homologous and heterologous aortic valves; in Ionescu, Ross and Wooler Biological tissue in heart valve replacement, pp. 137–194 (Butterworth, London 1972).

13 Horowitz, M. S.; Goodman, D. J.; Hancock, E. W., and Popp, R. L.: Noninvasive diagnosis of complications of the mitral bioprosthesis. J. thorac. Cardiovasc. Surg. *71:* 450–457 (1976).

14 Reis, R. L.; Hancock, W. D.; Yarbrough, J. W.; Glancy, D. L., and Morrow, A. G.: The flexible stent. A new concept in the fabrication of tissue heart valve prostheses. J. thorac. cardiovasc. Surg. *62:* 683–695 (1971).

15 Rose, A. G.: Pathology of the formalin-treated heterograft porcine aortic valve in the mitral position. Thorax *27:* 401–409 (1972).

16 Buch, W. S.; Angell, W. W., and Shumway, N. E.: Deterioration of formalin-treated aortic valve heterografts. J. thorac. cardiovasc. Surg. *60:* 673–682 (1970).

17 O'Brien, M. F.; Neilson, G. H.; Galea, E. G.; Molphy, R.; Power, W.; Lomas, C., and Stephens, B. J.: Heterograft valves. An analysis of clinical results of valve replacement. Circulation *41/42:* suppl. II, pp. 16–19 (1970).

18 Kouchoukos, N. T.; Kerr, A. R.; Sheppard, L. C.; Ceballos, R., and Kirklin, J. W.: Heterograft replacement of the mitral valve. Clinical, hemodynamic and pathological features. Circulation *41/42:* suppl. II, pp. 2–28 (1970).

19 Ionescu, M. I.; Smith, D. R.; Sutherland, T. W., and Wooler, G. H.: Heart valve replacement with aortic heterografts. Follow-up study. Ann. thorac. Surg. *12:* 1–14 (1972).

20 Kaiser, G. A.; Hancock, W. D.; Lukban, S. B., and Litwak, R. S.: Clinical use of a new design stented xenograft heart valve prosthesis. Surg. Forum *20:* 137–138 (1969).

Substitute Cardiac Valves

Advantages and Disadvantages of Four Commonly Used Ones

William C. Roberts

Pathology Branch, National Heart and Lung Institute, National Institutes of Health, Bethesda, Md.

In the annals of cardiology the decade of the 1960s will probably be remembered most as the decade during which cardiac valve replacement became a successful reality. This tremendous accomplishment has brought new life to several hundred thousand individuals since the first successful (survival > 3 months) cardiac valve replacement in September 1960. Despite this success, the ideal cardiac valve is still not available, or at least, if available, not adequately tested. This piece will examine the various advantages and disadvantages of the presently available substitute cardiac valves, and, in addition, will examine the determinants of the results of cardiac valve replacement.

Of the nearly 50 different substitute cardiac valves introduced during the past two decades, many have been discarded, and of those remaining, usually several modifications have been made. At present, four basic types of substitute cardiac valves are in use: (1) caged ball; (2) caged disc; (3) tilting disc, and (4) tissue valve. The caged ball was the first prosthesis used successfully for treatment of valvular heart disease; it was placed in the descending thoracic aorta by Hufnagel in 1953 for treatment of severe aortic regurgitation [1, 2]. Although utilized unsuccessfully for aortic valve replacement (subcoronary insertion) in 1960 by Harken *et al.* [3, 4] the caged-ball was first used successfully for cardiac valve replacement (in the mitral position) in the same year by Starr and Edwards [5]. Although first utilized in the descending thoracic aorta as treatment for aortic regurgitation in 1956 [6–8] the aortic valve homograft was introduced for aortic valve replacement in 1962 [9–12] (later [131], for mitral valve replacement), and the heterograft aortic valve for aortic valve replacement in 1967 [15, 16]. The caged disc appeared in 1965 [17, 18] and the tilting disc, in 1967 [19–22]. Flow through

Table I. Substitute cardiac valves: general characteristics

Type	Year introduced	Hemodynamics obstructive	incompetent	thrombotic	hemolytic	degenerates
Caged ball	1960	++	0	++	+	+
Caged disc	1965	++	0	++	+	+
Tilting disc	1967	+	0	++	0	0
Tissue valve						
Homograft	1962	0	++	0	0	++
Xenograft	1965	+	0	0	0	?

the caged ball and caged disc is peripheral, through the tilting disc, semicentral, and through the tissue valve, central.

There are at least six ideal characteristics of a good prosthetic cardiac valve (table I): (1) it has good hemodynamic characteristics, i.e., it is *nonobstructive* or nearly so, and completely *competent* or nearly so; (2) it is *nonthrombogenic;* (3) it *does not degenerate,* wear out or vary; (4) it *does not significantly alter blood components;* (5) it *can be inserted without undue difficulty,* i.e., exquisite technical skill is not required for its insertion, and (6) it *does not disturb the patient.*

Analysis of each of the four types of substitute cardiac valves for the first four of these ideal characteristics should separate the good ones from the bad ones. The degree of difficulty or ease in inserting each of the four basic types of presently employed substitute valves is similar because all have rigid or semirigid frames and cloth-covered sewing rings. Furthermore, with the possible exception of the recent metal-track Starr-Edwards prosthesis, none of the presently used substitute valves make noise audible to the patient.

The *caged ball prosthesis* (Harken, Starr-Edwards, Magovern, Smeloff-Cutter, Braunwald-Cutter, De Bakey) clearly belongs in the 'good' category. More information on it is available than on any of the other prostheses because it has been more widely used and used for the longest time. Because the most information is available on this prosthesis and because it has been the one most widely employed, however, does not mean that it necessarily is the best prosthesis. This prosthesis, which has had a number of modifications (the word 'modification' unfortunately is not synonymous with the word 'improvement') during the past 16 years, in general, has adequate but not the best hemodynamic characteristics [23–35]. Although the introduction of cloth-covering on the struts and base has diminished the incidence of clinical events compatible with emboli, this prosthesis, nevertheless, continues to have a tendency to form thrombus, and anticoagulants are required [35]. It hemolyzes erythrocytes, more frequently and more severely after aortic than after mitral valve replacement, and, also, more frequently and more severely after replacement which the cloth-covered models than with the noncloth-covered models [36–43]. Hemolysis, however, is rarely a major clinical problem with this prosthesis or with any of them because the bone marrow is capable of replacing the destroyed erythrocytes without development of anemia or thrombocytopenia.

Degeneration of the silicone rubber poppet was common in the caged-ball prostheses inserted before 1967 [44–62], but no degeneration or variance has been reported in the metallic (stellite 21) hollow poppet introduced at that time. The silicone-rubber poppet models continue to be employed in some major centers and it is likely that poppet degeneration eventually will occur in them. Such was the case with the Braunwald-Cutter aortic valve prosthesis which has been withdrawn from the market [63]. Wear of cloth-covering on both struts and orifice occurred in some of the completely cloth-covered caged-ball prostheses, but strut-cloth wear has not been observed since introduction of the metal track in the latest Starr-Edwards models.

A problem with the caged-ball prosthesis is that it may occupy too much space within either the cardiac ventricle or the aortic root, and, because flow is entirely peripheral, there may not be adequate space between the surface of the poppet and the endocardium of the ventricle or the intima of ascending aorta to adequately accommodate blood flow [64–78]. This situation occurs most frequently when mitral replacement is performed in a patient, usually a woman, with pure mitral stenosis and a normal aortic valve. In this circumstance the left ventricle may not be of adequate size to accommodate the mitral prosthesis, and one or more struts of the prosthesis burrows into the myocardial wall preventing adequate descent of the poppet, with resulting obstruction to left atrial emptying [64]. This occurrence, obviously, is most likely when larger-sized prosthetics are utilized, but it may occur when even the smallest-sized caged ball prostheses are employed to replace purely stenotic mitral valves. The most common circumstance in which fatal obstruction to left ventricular outflow occurs is in the patient with combined mitral and aortic valve disease. In most of these patients, irrespective of the type of aortic valve lesion, i.e., whether stenosis or pure regurgitation, the aortic root usually is not dilated and consequently the space available in the aortic root to accommodate the caged ball may be limited. A particularly dangerous cricumstance is combined mitral and aortic stenosis. In this circumstance, the left ventricular wall is hypertrophied but its cavity is not dilated. Insertion of a mitral caged ball into a hypertrophied, nondilated left ventricle may obstruct left ventricular inflow or outflow. Ventricular inflow obstruction is probably even more common after replacement of the tricuspid valve than the mitral valve with a caged-ball prosthesis, and, therefore, utilization of this prosthesis in this position may be unwise [74–78].

Although none of the various types of substitute cardiac valves are completely immune from it, prosthetic disproportion (prosthesis too large or ventricular cavity or aorta too small), both real and potential, is most frequent with the caged-ball prosthesis. Therefore, it may be most wise to limit the use of this type prosthesis to patients with purely incompetent or at least predominately incompetent valve lesions, i.e., to those patients in whom volume overload has produced large-sized left ventricular cavities or ascending aortas. Use of the caged-ball prosthesis in patients with purely stenotic or predominately stenotic valve lesions appears unnecessary because of the availability of other excellent substitute cardiac valves.

The *caged-disc prosthesis* (Kay-Shiley, Cross-Jones, Hufnagel, Kay-Suzuki, Beall, Harken, Cooley-Bloodwell-Cutter, Cooley-Cutter), in my view, is the least desirable prosthetic cardiac valve presently in use. This prosthesis, because of its 'low profile' configuration, was introduced as an alternative to the caged-ball prosthesis and believed intitially to be particularly useful in the patient with the 'small left ventricle', i.e., pure mitral stenosis. This initial hope, however, was ill-fated. This device has proved to be highly thrombogenic [79–85] and the most obstructive of all the prosthetic valves presently in use [86–99]. In a recent study, although the pulmonary arterial pressures had decreased and the cardiac indices increased, the mean diastolic pressure gradients across the mitral prosthesis (Beall type) was not significantly different postoperatively compared to the preoperative values [99]. In addition, the nonmetallic discs have shown evidence of degeneration [87, 97, 100–113], and strut fracture, of uncertain cause, with dislodgment of the disc occluder, has been reported [96, 107]. Hemolysis with this prosthesis is universal [97, 114]. This device was utilized briefly in the aortic position [89, 90, 97] but its use in this location was abandoned because of its obstructive, thrombogenic and wear characteristics. More recently, a new type of caged disc, the Cooley-Cutter biconical disc, has been introduced for use in both atrioventricular and similunar valve positions [115–117]. This newer prosthesis, which has a semi-diamond-shaped occluder rather than a flat one (like all other caged discs), nevertheless continues to have entirely peripheral flow characteristics, and therefore, the hemodynamic features are unlikely to be ideal. Furthermore, intimal proliferation in the aortic root (where the coronary ostia are located) remains a potential problem with the peripheral flow type prostheses, probably most extensive with use of the caged disc [97]. Also very worrisome is disc cocking, a potential problem with all caged discs [80, 82, 83, 102, 110–113, 118, 119] including the newly introduced one, and its frequency of occurrence is entirely unknown. Possibly, nonfatal transient cocking is common and fatal cocking of the caged disc may occur during life and be totally unrecognized at necropsy.

The *tilting-disc prosthesis* (Wada-Cutter, Lillehei-Kastor, Björk-Shiley) of the latter two types (the first type has been discontinued) [120] has proved to be a good prosthesis for replacement of tricuspid, mitral and aortic valves. Its semicentral flow usually allows minimal gradients [121–127], its effect on red blood cell survival is minimal [128, 129], and there has been no evidence of disc wear (variance) since the introduction of the carbon pyrolyte disc. This prosthesis, however, has a tendency to clot and anticoagulants are required [129–135]. Because movement of the disc is in close proximity to the sewing ring, the chances of interference to it by contact with adjacent mural endocardium or aortic intima is small, but, nevertheless, as with all prostheses, a potential problem if large-sized models are utilized in small-sized ventricles or aortas [129].

Tissue valves, in the form of aortic homografts, were first utilized for aortic valve replacement in 1962 [9–12]. The initial results were gratifying: the valve lesions were usually ameliorated and anticoagulants were not required. The problem, however, proved to be accelerated wear and tear with development of incompetency [136–140]. Other tissue valves followed, namely fascia lata, dura mater, parietal pericardium, but all proved to be poor valve substitutes because of their becoming stiff and relatively immobile [141–145]. At present, the fresh antibiotic-sterilized homograft remains in use, but now the most commonly employed tissue valve is the *porcine xenograft* attached to a semi-flexible stint [146] and preserved by a glutaraldehyde process [146–153]. (It failed when preserved in formalin [141, 154].) This substitute valve is receiving increasingly greater enthusiasm. Although relatively few hemodynamic studies late postoperatively have been reported, pressure gradients across the porcine bioprosthesis have been recorded in all three valve positions despite its central flow. Of 56 patients studied late postoperatively after mitral replacement, the mean diastolic gradient averaged 6 mm Hg [148, 151, 152], but of 37 patients studied at the National Heart and

Lung Institute no gradient was recorded across the mitral porcine valve in 16 patients. Of 11 patients studied late postoperatively after tricuspid valve replacement with a porcine xenograft, the mean diastolic gradient averaged 4 mm Hg [152]. Hemodynamic data after aortic valve replacement with the porcine xenograft is minimal: of 5 patients studied late postoperatively at the National Heart and Lung Institute, the peak systolic pressure gradients ranged from 10 to 35 mm Hg (average 18) [146].

With few exceptions [152, 153], the porcine xenograft does not clot and, therefore, anticoagulants are not required. This substitute valve does not damage blood elements. The major concern with this substitute valve, of course, is its wear characteristics. The encouraging feature at this time is that there have been relatively few 'valve failures' [146–153] and, indeed, none of the other substitute valves cited have had so few problems in their first 5 years. Although results achieved with the porcine xenograft continue to be encouraging, relatively few patients, estimated to be less than 500, have had this substitute valve in place for longer than 5 years and it will probably be after this period before signs of cuspal degeneration will appear, if indeed they do.

It is likely that the cusps of the porcine valve will be subject to changes which affect all natural left-sided cardiac valves, namely lipid deposition and calcification [155–157]. The changes occur on the native valves on the aortic aspects of the aortic valve cusps and on the ventricular aspects of the mitral valve cusps. It is likely that these changes will be accelerated in this substitute valve compared to the natural valve [158]. Small thrombi have been observed on the sinus aspects of the porcine cusps and possibly it is the organization of these minute thrombi which has led to the calcific deposits [141].

After discussing the various types of prosthetic cardiac valves, a consideration of the factors which determine the outcome of valve replacement in a particular patient appears appropriate. At least six major factors appear to determine the result: (1) the type substitute valve inserted; (2) the size of the prosthesis inserted; (3) the experience and technical skill of the surgeon; (4) adequacy of the 'pump team', anesthesiologists, and surgeons, physicians and nurses providing postoperative care; (5) the presence of associated (diagnosed or undiagnosed) or uncorrected cardiac disease or previous pericardiotomy, and (6) the preoperative status of the patient. The remainder of this piece will examine the relative effect of each of these factors on the outcome of valve replacement.

Assuming that the cardiac operation is to be performed in a large medical center where several cardiac operations are performed weekly by a surgeon or group of surgeons experienced in cardiac valve replacement, the most important factor at present determining the long-term outcome of valve replacement is *the type of substitute valve inserted.* On September 9 and 10, 1960, a conference on prosthetic valves for cardiac surgery was held in Chicago [159]. At that time it was observed that there were no living survivors of total cardiac valve replacement. After STARR's successful replacement of the mitral valve with a caged-ball prosthesis on September 21, 1960, survival after valve replacement using the caged-ball prosthesis rapidly became commonplace. The caged-ball was the first prosthesis used for cardiac valve replacement by numerous surgeons whose previous valve operations had consisted, in many cases, entirely of mitral commissurotomy, and yet, nearly from the beginning, rapid success was achieved using this device.

Because the decision regarding the type of substitute valve to be chosen for a particular patient is crucial, consideration might be given to the following questions: (1) Who *does* choose the type of prosthesis to be inserted? and (2) Who *should* choose the type of prosthesis to be inserted? From the beginning, i. e. 1960, the surgeon has determined the type of prosthesis to be inserted in a particular patient. What are factors which determine a surgeon's preference of a prosthesis? The major one, of course, is previous experience, including personal and that of colleagues. The choice of prosthesis by a particularly prominent surgeon or the choice used by the trainer of a new cardiovascular surgeon may be especially influencing. Some surgeons who started with the caged-ball, for example, and had satisfactory results, are reluctant to change. One is simply more comfortable with the device he or she has used before. Change of prosthesis or model when the one being used proves not be ideal, however, is obviously admirable, and best exemplified by COOLEY's experience with 34 different types or models of prosthetic cardiac valves [115].

Choice of prosthesis used, by some surgeons, has been influenced by personal involvement in the development of a particular prosthesis. Admitting that a prosthesis of someone else's design is better than one of one's own designs is, at best, difficult. There may be inherent conflict when the same surgeon participants in the design of, and in the insertion of, a particular prosthesis. There have been abundant examples of this potential conflict during the past 16 years.

Again, assuming that valve replacement is to be performed in a large medical center with an experienced cardiovascular surgical team, long-term survival is more dependent on the type of prosthesis inserted than on the surgeon who inserts the prosthesis. Thus, if I personally were to undergo valve replacement, I would first choose the type of prosthesis, and secondly, the surgeon whose results with this particular prosthesis were excellent. In my view, the referring cardiologist is not fully fulfilling his responsibility by simply referring his patient to a surgeon irrespective of the type of prosthesis the surgeon most frequently utilizes. To use a caged disc, at least those with a flat occluder, in my view, is unwise, and to date little hemodynamic or other data is available to allow proper evaluation of the biconical type of caged disc. Although some surgeons periodically employ all four types of presently available substitute cardiac valves, most generally use only one or two of them. If the patient has mitral stenosis or combined mitral and aortic valve disease (and in this circumstance the aortic 'root' is usually small), or if the patient is small, referral to a surgeon who uses only, or nearly always, the caged-ball prosthesis would not appear ideal. The fewest problems with valve replacement *at the moment* appear to be with the porcine xenograft, but, as mentioned earlier, that too may change. Patients with bleeding tendencies, real or potential, requiring valve replacement, should have a porcine xenograft, because patients with the other types of substitute valves usually receive anticoagulants.

The cardiologists in large medical centers usually refer their patients requiring valve replacement to the surgeons in the same medical center even though they may not be necessarily pleased or involved in the choice of valve prosthesis used in their patients. The choice of substitute cardiac valve ideally should be a mutually agreeable one for a particular patient. Of course, for cardiologists to become more involved in the decision making process for type of substitute valve for a particular patient would require him to acquire considerably more knowledge regarding substitute valves than is presently available by this group of specialists. Obviously, it makes no difference who chooses the type of substitute valve for a particular patient just as long as the choice is the right one. The point here is that the era of the 'one-valve surgeon' is over, '...Selection of the most favorable valve substitute for implantation should be individualized to each patient's specific anatomical, hemodynamic, and hematological needs' [160]. It no longer appears proper for a surgeon to use only one type of substitute valve for all individuals.

Now to *the size of the prosthesis to insert.* This determination, to my knowledge, has always been made in the operating room with the patient on cardiopulmonary bypass, by the insertion of various sizers placed through the valve orifice after excision of the native valve. But does this method best determine the size of a prosthesis to be inserted? My view is no. With the patient on cardiopulmonary bypass and with various retractors pulling on the heart, the surgeon may be able to insert large-sized sizing devices and, therefore, be led to insert a large-sized prosthesis, when, in actuality, with the patient off cardiopulmonary bypass and all retractors withdrawn, the valve orifice is much smaller. Therefore, the size valve to be inserted might best be determined not exclusively on the basis of sizing devices at operation, but at least in part on the basis of the hemodynamic valve lesion(s) before operation with consideration of the lean weight of the patient. A small woman with pure mitral stenosis and a normally functioning aortic valve should have a relatively small-sized prosthesis inserted. Recently (1975), I saw the hearts at necropsy of 2 patients with severe, isolated mitral stenosis and both had had the largest sized tilting disc prostheses (Björk-Shiley, 31 mm) inserted. At operation in each, however, the sizing devices apparently had indicated that the valve orifices were capable of accommodating devices of such large size. Fatal malfunction of the prosthesis due to its large size and the patient's 'small' left ventricle, however, occurred in each patient. If the largest sized prosthesis is used in a small woman with pure mitral stenosis, what sized devices should be used in a large man with pure mitral regurgitation? Thus, the decision regarding the size of prosthesis to insert might roughly be determined at the preoperative conference or consultation and be based on the hemodynamic valve lesion and body weight and not entirely on the dimensions measured in the operating room.

Although the greatest emphasis here regarding determinants of results of valve replacement has been placed on the type and size of the prosthetic valve inserted, *the technical skill and experience of the surgeon* is obviously extremely important. Of these two, experience probably is more important than technical skill. (One of the finest examples of technical skill in the field of cardiac valve surgery is the placing of a porcine xenograft on a semi-flexible cloth-coverd stint. This procedure is performed by women before the tissue valve is shipped to surgeons.) There is no question that results of valve replacement are better by experienced surgeons than by nonexperienced ones, although the technical skills of the latter might even be greater. The 'occasional open-heart surgeon', as emphasized by EISEMAN and SPENCER [161], no matter how great his technical skill, is not the ideal cardiac surgeon. Certain technical factors, however, might be taken into consideration by the referring physician. Should prosthetic valves be inserted with continuous or interrupted sutures? It appears most reasonable that interrupted sutures would be less likely to be associated with 'massive' prosthetic regurgitation (prosthetic disruption), and yet continuous or nearly continuous sutures are commonly employed by some surgeons [162]. If the world's 'best' surgeon uses the world's worst prosthesis or inserts it by noninterrupted suture, the result may not be ideal.

The three other determinants of the results of cardiac valve replacement are self-evident. Obviously, the entire surgical team must be a good one. The patients with associated heart disease, for example coronary heart disease or previous throacotomy, do not do as well as those without these complications [61, 62]. The less sick the patient before operation, the greater are his (or her) chances of survival after operation, but the sicker the patient before operation, obviously, the more dramatic the change after operation.

In *summary,* certain ideal characteristics of substitute cardiac valves have been analyzed for each of the four basic types of presently available substitute cardiac valves. Of these four, the caged-disc prosthesis, in my judgment, is the least desirable: it obstructs, it clots, it degenerates, and each of the other three types of substitute cardiac valves have more favorable characteristics. Ideally, the caged-ball prosthesis might be limited to those patients with volume lesions, i.e., pure or at least predominant regurgitation, because of the problem of prosthetic disproportion. The tilting disc has favorable hemodynamic and wear characteristics, but long-term anticoagulants are essential, as with the caged-ball and caged-disc types of prosthesis. The porcine xenograft, at this time, appears quite favorable, but sufficient (> 5 years) implantation periods for proper evaluation are just beginning to appear and, therefore, final judgment must be reserved. Assuming that valve replacement is to be carried out in a large medical center by a surgical team experienced in this procedure, the results of this operation today are most dependent upon the type of, and size of, substitute valve inserted rather than on the surgeon who inserts the valve. Therefore, it is important for the cardiologist to become more informed on the various types of prosthetic carciac valves and to become a member of the team deciding which type and size of cardiac valve is most proper for his (or her) patient.

References

1 Hufnagel, C. A. and Harvey, W. P.: The surgical correction of aortic regurgitation. Preliminary report. Bull. Georgetown Univ. med. Cent. *6:* 60–61 (1953).

2 Hufnagel, C. A.; Harvey, W. P.; Rabil, P. J., *et al.:* Surgical correction of aortic insufficiency. Surgery *35:* 673–683 (1954).

3 Harken, D. E.; Soroff, H. S.; Taylor, W. J., *et al.:* Partial and complete prostheses in aortic insufficiency. J. thorac. cardiovasc. Surg. *40:* 744–762 (1960).

4 Harken, D. E.; Taylor, W. J.; Lefemine, A. A., *et al.:* Aortic valve replacement with a caged ball valve. Am. J. Cardiol. *9*: 292–299 (1962).

5 Starr, A. and Edwards, M. L.: Mitral replacement: clinical experience with a ball-valve prosthesis. Ann. Surg. *154:* 726–740 (1961).

6 Murray, G.: Homologous aortic-valve-segment transplants as surgical treatment for aortic and mitral insufficiency. Angiology *7:* 446–471 (1956).

7 Kerwin, A. J.; Lenkei, S. C., and Wilson, D. R.: Aortic-valve homograft in the treatment of aortic insufficiency. Report of nine cases, with one followed for six years. New Engl. J. Med. *266:* 852–857 (1962).

8 Beall, A. C.; Morris, G. C.; Tooley, D. A., *et al.:* Homotransplantation of aortic valve. J. thorac. cardiovasc. Surg. *42:* 497–506 (1961).

9 Ross, D. N.: Homograft replacement of the aortic valve. Lancet *ii:* 487 (1962).

10 Duran, C. G. and Gunning, A. J.: A method for placing a total homologous aortic valve in the subcoronary position. Lancet *ii:* 488–489 (1962).

11 Barratt-Boyes, B. G.: Homograft aortic valve replacement in aortic incompetence and stenosis. Thorax *19:* 131–150 (1964).

12 Barratt-Boyes, B. G.; Lowe, J. B.; Cole, D. S., *et al.:* Homograft valve replacement for aortic valve disease. Thorax *20:* 495–504 (1965).

13 Angell, W. W.; Wuerflein, R. D., and Shumway, N. E.: Mitral valve replacement with the fresh aortic valve homograft: experimental results and clinical application. Surgery *62:* 807–813 (1967).

14 Binet, J. P.; Duran, C. G.; Carpentier, A., *et al.:* Heterologous aortic valve transplantation. Lancet *ii:* 1275 (1965).

15 Ionescu, M. I.; Wooler, G. H.; Smith, D. R., *et al.:* Mitral valve replacement with aortic heterografts in humans. Thorax *22:* 305–313 (1967).

16 Carpentier, A.; Blondeau, P.; Laurens, B., *et al.:* Mitral valve replacement with frame-mounted aortic heterografts. J. thorac. cardiovasc. Surg. *56:* 388–394 (1968).

17 Hufnagel, C. A. and Conrad, P. W.: Comparative study of some prosthetic valves for aortic and mitral replacement. Surgery *57:* 205–210 (1965).

18 Kay, E. B.; Suzuki, A.; Demaney, M., *et al.:* Comparison of ball and disc valves for mitral valve replacement. Am. J. Cardiol. *18:* 504–514 (1966).

19 Wada, J.: Knotless suture method and Waga hingeless valve. Jap. J. thorac. Surg. *15:* 88–94 (1967).

20 Wada, J.; Komatsu, S., and Kamata, K.: Cardiac valve replacement with Wada-Cutter prosthesis. Ann. thorac. Surg. *14:* 38–46 (1972).

21 Kaster, R. L. and Lillehei, C. W.: A new cageless free-floating pivoting disc prosthetic heart valve: design, development and evaluation. Digest 7th Int. Conf. on Medical and Biological Engineering, Stockholm 1967, p. 387.

22 Björk, V. O.: A new tilting disc valve prosthesis. Scand. J. thorac. cardiovasc. Surg. *3:* 1–10 (1969).

23 Mason, D. T.; Ross, J., jr.; Gault, J. H., *et al.:* Combined prosthetic replacement of the mitral and aortic valves. Preoperative and postoperative hemodynamic studies at rest and the left ventricular response to muscular exercise. Circulation *35/36:* suppl. I, pp. 15–23 (1967).

24 McHenry, M. M.; Smeloff, E. A.; Davey, T. B., *et al.:* Hemodynamic results with full-flow orifice prosthetic valves. Circulation *35/36:* suppl. I, pp. 24–33 (1967).

25 GLANCY, D. L.; O'BRIEN, K. P.; REIS, R. L., *et al.:* Hemodynamic studies in patients with 2M and 3M Starr-Edwards prostheses: Evidence of obstruction to left atrial emptying. Circulation *39/40:* suppl. I, pp. 113–118 (1969).

26 REIS, R. L.; GLANCY, D. L.; O'BRIEN, K., *et al.:* Clinical and hemodynamic assessments of fabric-covered Starr-Edwards prosthetic valves. J. thorac. cardiovasc. Surg. *59:* 84–91, 104–108 (1970).

27 RODRIGUEZ, L.: Haemodynamic and angiographic findings in patients with isolated aortic valvular disease before and after insertion of a Starr-Edwards aortic ball-valve prosthesis. Scanc. J. thorac. cardiovasc. Surg., suppl. 5 (1970).

28 WINTERT, R. O.; REIS, R., L.; GLANCY, D. L., *et al.:* Current status of the Starr-Edwards cloth-covered prosthetic cardiac valves. Circulation *45/46:* suppl. I, pp. 14–24 (1972).

29 BJÖRK, V. O.; OLIN, C., and RODRIGUEZ, L.: Comparative results of aortic valve replacement with different prosthetic heart valves. J. cardiovasc. Surg. *13:* 268–271 (1972).

30 LEVINE, F. H.; COPELAND, J. G., and MORROW, A. G.: Prosthetic replacement of the mitral valve. Continuing assessment of the 100 patients operated upon during 1961–1965. Circulation *47:* 518–526 (1973).

31 O'ROURKE, R. A.; PETERSON, K. L., and BRAUNWALD, N. S.: Postoperative hemodynamic evaluation of a new fabric-covered ball-valve prosthesis. Circulation *47/48:* suppl. III, pp. 74–79 (1973).

32 BONCHEK, L. I.; ANDERSON, R. P., and STARR, A.: Mitral valve replacement with cloth-covered composite-seat prostheses. The case for early operation. J. thorac. cardiovasc. Surg. *67:* 93–109 (1974).

33 BONCHEK, L. I. and STARR, A.: Ball valve prostheses: current appraisal of late results. Am. J. Cardiol. *35:* 843–854 (1975).

34 BRAWLEY, R. K.; DONAHOO, J. S., and GOTT, V. L.: Current status of the Beall, Björk-Shiley, Braunwald-Cutter, Lillehei-Kaster and Smeloff-Cutter cardiac valve prostheses. Am. J. Cardiol. *35:* 855–865 (1975).

35 SMITHWICK, W., III; KOUCHOUKOS, N. T.; KARP, R. B., *et al.:* Late stenosis of Starr-Edwards cloth-covered prostheses. Ann. thorac. Surg. *20:* 249–255 (1975).

36 DECESARE, W.; RATH, C., and HUFNAGEL, C.: Hemolytic anemia of mechanical origin with aortic-valve prosthesis. New Engl. J. Med. *272:* 1045–1050 (1965).

37 WALSCH, J. R.; STARR, A., and RITZMANN, L. W.: Intravascular hemolysis in patients with prosthetic valves and valvular heart disease. Circulation *39/40:* suppl. I, pp. 135–140 (1969).

38 WALLACE, H. W.; KENEPP, D. L., and BLAKEMORE, W. S.: Quantitation of red blood cell destruction associated with valvular disease and prosthetic valves. J. thorac. cardiovasc. Surg. *60:* 842–852 (1970).

39 ROBERTS, W. C. and MORROW, A. G.: Renal hemosiderosis in patients with prosthetic aortic valves. Circulation *36:* 390–398 (1966).

40 ROBERTS, W. C. and MORROW, A. G.: Causes of death and other anatomic observations after cardiac valve replacement. Adv. Cardiol., vol. 7, pp. 226–247 (Karger, Basel 1972).

41 WEILY, H. S. and GENTON, E.: Altered platelet function in patients with prosthetic mitral valves. Effects of sulfinpyrazone therapy. Circulation *42:* 967–972 (1970).

42 Steele, P. P.; Weily, H. S.; Davies, H., *et al.:* Platelet survival time following aortic valve replacement. Circulation *51:* 358–362 (1975).

43 Ahmad, R.; Manohitharajah, S. M.; Deverall, P. B., *et al.:* Chronic hemolysis following mitral valve replacement. A comparative study of the Björk-Shiley, composite-seat Starr-Edwards, and frame-mounted aortic homograft valves. J. thorac. cardiovasc. Surg. *71:* 212–217 (1976).

44 Starr, A.; Pierie, W. R.; Raible, D. A., *et al.:* Cardiac valve replacement. Experience with the durability of silicone rubber. Circulation *33/34:* suppl. I, pp. 115–123 (1966).

45 Roberts, W. C. and Morrow, A. G.: Late postoperative pathological findings after cardiac valve replacement. Circulation *35/36:* suppl. I, pp. 48–62 (1967).

46 Roberts, W. C. and Morrow, A. G.: Anatomic studies of hearts containing caged-ball prosthetic valves. Johns Hopkins med. J. *121:* 271–295 (1967).

47 Laforet, E. G.: Death due to swelling of ball component of aortic ball-valve prosthesis. New Engl. J. Med. *276:* 1025–1027 (1967).

48 Roberts, W. C. and Morrow, A. G.: Fatal degeneration of the silicone rubber ball of the Starr-Edwards prosthetic aortic valve. Am. J. Cardiol. *22:* 614–620 (1968).

49 Sanderson. R. G.; Hall, A. D., and Thomas, A. N.: The clinical diagnosis of ball variance in a mitral valve prosthesis. Ann. thorac. Surg. *6:* 473–475 (1968).

50 Collins, J. J., jr.; Berg, E. J., and Harken, D. E.: Silicone ball variance. A clinical and pulse duplicator study. Ann. thorac. Surg. *6:* 546–551 (1968).

51 Bonnabeau, R. and Lillehei, W.: Mechanical 'ball failure' in Starr-Edwards prosthetic valves. A report of three cases. J. thorac. cardiovasc. Surg. *56:* 258–264 (1968).

52 Leatherman, L. L.; Leachman, R. D.; McConn, R. G., *et al.:* Malfunction of mitral ball-valve prostheses due to a swollen poppet. J. thorac. cardiovasc. Surg. *57:* 160–163 (1969).

53 Roberts, W. C. and Morrow, A. G.: Late postoperative pathologic findings following cardiac valve replacement with Starr-Edwards prostheses; in Proc. 2nd Nat. Conf. Prosthetic Heart Valves, pp. 365–393 (Thomas, Springfield 1969).

54 Hylen, J. C.; Kloster, F. E.; Starr, A., *et al.:* Aortic ball variance: diagnosis and treatment. Ann. intern. Med. *72:* 1–8 (1970).

55 Roberts, W. C.; Levinson, G. E., and Morrow, A. G.: Lethal ball variance in the Starr-Edwards prosthetic mitral valve. Archs intern. Med. *126:* 517–521 (1970).

56 Connolly, D. C.; Harrison, C. E., and Ellis, F. H., jr.: Ball variance in a Starr-Edwards prosthetic mitral valve causing acute pulmonary edema (diagnosis by auscultation before onset of symptoms). Mayo Clin. Proc. *45:* 20–24 (1970).

57 Metzger, C. C.; Magovern, G. J., and Leonard, J. J.: Ball variance in a sutureless mitral valve prosthesis. A report of two cases and a clue to early diagnosis. J. thorac. cardiovasc. Surg. *61:* 699–704 (1971).

58 Schluger, J.; Mannix, E. P., jr., and Wolf, R. E.: Auscultatory and phonocardiographic sign of ball variance in a mitral prosthetic valve. Am. Heart J. *81:* 809–816 (1971).

59 Hylen, J. C.; Hodam, R. P., and Kloster, F. E.: Changes in the durability of silicone rubber in ball-valve prostheses. Ann. thorac. Surg. *13:* 324–329 (1972).

60 Roberts, W. C.; Bulkley, B. H., and Morrow, A. G.: Pathologic anatomy of cardiac valve replacement: a study of 224 necropsy patients. Prog. cardiovasc. Dis. *15:* 539–587 (1973).

61 Barnhorst, D. A.; Oxman, H. A.; Connolly, D. C., *et al.:* Isolated replacement of the mitral valve with the Starr-Edwards prosthesis. An eleven-year review. J. thorac. cardiovasc. Surg. *71:* 230–237 (1976).

62 Barnhorst, D. A.; Oxman, H. A.; Connolly, D. C., *et al.:* Long-term follow-up of isolated replacement of the aortic or mitral valve with the Starr-Edwards prosthesis. Am. J. Cardiol. *35:* 228–233 (1975).

63 Pluth, J. R.; Broadbent, J. C.; Barnhorst, D. A., *et al.:* Aortic and mitral valve replacement with cloth-covered Braunwald-Cutter prosthesis. A three-year follow-up Ann. thorac. Surg. *20:* 239–248 (1975).

64 Roberts, W. C. and Morrow, A. G.: Mechanisms of acute left atrial thrombosis after mitral valve replacement. Pathologic findings indicating obstruction to left atrial emptying. Am. J. Cardiol. *18:* 497–503 (1966).

65 Roberts, W. C.; Lambird, P. A.; Gott, V. L., *et al.:* Fatal aortic regurgitation following replacement of the mitral and aortic valves. A mechanical complication of double valve replacement. J. thorac. cardiovasc. Surg. *52:* 189–192 (1966).

66 Roberts, W. C. and Morrow, A. G.: Causes of early postoperative death following cardiac valve replacement. Clinico-pathologic correlations in 64 patients studied at necropsy. J. thorac. cardiovasc. Surg. *54:* 422–437 (1967).

67 Robicsek, F.; Sanger, P. W.; Daugherty, H. K., *et al.:* Fatal arrhythmias caused by the pressure of the ball-valve prosthesis upon the left ventricular myocardium. Dis. Chest. *52:* 813–816 (1967).

68 Quattlebaum, F. W.; Kalke, B.; Edwards, J. E., *et al.:* Obstruction of the aorta by prosthetic aortic valve. J. thorac. cardiovasc. Surg. *55:* 231–237 (1968).

69 Kalke, B.; Korns, M. E.; Goott, B., *et al.:* Engagement of ventricular myocardium by open-cage atrioventricular valvular prosthesis. J. thorac. cardiovasc. Surg. *58:* 92–94 (1969).

70 Najafi, H.; Ostermiller, W. E., jr.; Javid, H., *et al.:* Narrow aortic root complicating aortic valve replacement. Archs Surg. *99:* 690–694 (1969).

71 Ibarra-Pérez, C.; Rodriguez-Trujillo, F., and Perez-Redondo, H.: Engagement of ventricular myocardium by struts of mitral prosthesis. Fatal complications of use of open-cage cardiac valves. J. thorac. cardiovasc. Surg. *61:* 403–404 (1971).

72 Shepherd, R. L.; Glancy, D. L.; Stinson, E. B., *et al.:* Hemodynamic confirmation of obstruction to left ventricular inflow by a caged-ball prosthetic mitral valve. J. thorac. cardiovasc. Surg. *65:* 252–254 (1973).

73 Seningen, R. P.; Bulkley, B. H., and Roberts, W. C.: Prosthetic aortic stenosis. A method to prevent its occurrence by measurement of aortic size from preoperative aortogram. Circulation *49:* 921–924 (1974).

74 Vander Veer, J. B., jr.; Rhyneer, G. S.; Hodam, R. P., *et al.:* Obstruction of tricuspid ball-valve prostheses. Circulation *43/44:* suppl. I, pp. 62–67 (1971).

75 Bache, R. J.; From, A. H. L.; Castaneda, A. R., *et al.:* Late thrombotic obstruction of Starr-Edwards tricuspid valve prosthesis. Chest *61:* 613–616 (1972).

76 Assad-Morrell, J. L.; Tajik, A. I.; Anderson, M. W., *et al.:* Malfunctioning

tricuspid valve prosthesis. Clinical phonocardiographic echocardiographic and surgical findings. Mayo Clin. Proc. *49:* 443–447 (1974).

77 BAXTER, R. H.; BAIN, W. H.; RANKIN, R. J., *et al.:* Tricuspid valve replacement: a five-year appraisal. Thorax *30:* 158–161 (1975).

78 MALCOLM, A. D.; AHUJA, S. P., and CHAMBERLAIN, M. J.: Malfunction of tricuspid valve prosthesis shown by isotope angiocardiography. J. thorac. cardiovasc. Surg. *71:* 134–136 (1976).

79 PATON, B. C.: Reoperation for fibrinous stenosis of disc mitral valve prosthesis. J. thorac. cardiovasc. Surg. *57:* 726–731 (1969).

80 HORSLEY, H. T.; RAPPOPORT, W. J.; VIGODA, P. S., *et al.:* Fatal malfunction of Edwards low-profile mitral valves. Circulation *41/42:* suppl. II, pp. 39–42 (1970).

81 MULLEN, D. C.; SHULL, W. H.; DAUGHERTY, H. K., *et al.:* Emergency thrombectomy of the prosthetic mitral valve. Vasc. Surg. *4:* 137–141 (1970).

82 DEMANY, M. A. and ZIMMERMAN, H. A.: Thrombosis of a mitral disc-valve prosthesis: diagnostic importance of the absent opening click. Am. Heart J. *80:* 816–819 (1970).

83 GUNSTENSEN, J.: Acute dysfunction of Starr-Edwards mitral prostheses. Thorax *26:* 163–166 (1971).

84 STROSS, J. K.; WILLIS,, and KAHN, D. R.: Diagnostic features of malfunction of disc mitral valve prostheses. J. Am. med. Ass. *217:* 305–308 (1971).

85 BALKOURA-CHRISTOPOULOS, M. H.; RESNEKOV, L., and KITTLE, C. F.: Malfunction of a disc mitral valve prosthesis. Detection by phonocardiography. Chest *63:* 624–626 (1973).

86 LINHART, J. W.; BAROLD, S. S.; HILDNER, F. J., *et al.:* Clinical and hemodynamic findings following replacement of the mitral valve with a Beall valve prosthesis (Dacron velour-covered Teflon-disc valve). Circulation *39/40:* suppl. I, pp. 127–134 (1969).

87 VOGEL, J. H. K.; PATON, B. C.; OVERY, H. R., *et al.:* Abnormal hemodynamic function after disc mitral valve replacement. Circulation *39/40:* suppl. I, pp. 141–147 (1969).

88 BJÖRK, V. O.; OLIN, C., and ASTRÖM, H.: Results of aortic valve replacement with the Kay-Shiley disc valve. Scand. J. thorac. cardiovasc. Surg. *93–106 (1969).*

89 KAY, E. B.; SUZUKI, A.; TAMBI, A., *et al.:* Comparative analysis of the Starr-Edwards ball valve, the Kay-Suzuki disc valve and transplant valves in the surgical correction of aortic valve disease. Am. J. Cardiol. *25:* 535–545 (1970).

90 OLIN, C.: Evaluation of the Kay-Shiley disc valve prosthesis in the aortic position. Clinical and haemodynamic results, and experimental comparison with other prosthetic aortic valves. Scand. J. thorac. cardiovasc. Surg., suppl. 7, pp. 1–37 (1970).

91 RAMSEY, H. W.; WILLIAMS, J. C., jr.; VERNON, C. R., *et al.:* Hemodynamic findings following replacement of the mitral valve with the Beall valve prosthesis. J. thorac. cardiovasc. Surg. *62:* 624–630 (1971).

92 ROGERS, A. K.; MORGAN, J. R.; FORKER, A. D., *et al.:* Supravalvular stenosis after disc mitral valve replacement. J. thorac. cardiovasc. Surg. *62:* 810–812 (1971).

93 REID, J. A.; STEVENS, T. W.; SIGWART, U., *et al.:* Hemodynamic evaluation of the Beall mitral valve prosthesis. Circulation *45/46:* suppl. I, pp. 1–7 (1972).

94 Shepherd, R. L.; Glancy, D. L.; Reis, R. L., *et al.:* Hemodynamic function of the Kay-Shiley prosthetic cardiac valve. Observations after mitral or tricuspid valve replacement. Chest *63:* 323–326 (1973).

95 Hawe, A.; Frye, R. L.;, and Ellis, F. H., jr.: Late hemodynamic studies after mitral valve surgery. J. thorac. cardiovasc. Surg. *65:* 351–358 (1973).

96 Beall, A. C., jr.; Morris, G. C., jr.; Howell, J. F., jr., *et al.:* Clinical experience with an improved mitral valve prosthesis. Ann. thorac. Surg. *15:* 601–606 (1973).

97 Roberts, W. C.; Fishbein, M. C., and Golden, A.: Cardiac pathology after valve replacement by disc prosthesis. A study of 61 necropsy patients. Am. J. Cardiol. *35:* 740–760 (1975).

98 Wellons, H. A., jr.; Strauch, R. S.; Nolan, S. P., *et al.:* Isolated mitral valve replacement with the Kay-Shiley disc valve. Actuarial analysis of the long-term results. J. thorac. cardiovasc. Surg. *70:* 862–868 (1975).

99 Fernandez, J.; Morse, D.; Spagna, P., *et al.:* Results of mitral valve replacement with the Beall prosthesis in 209 patients. J. thorac. cardiovasc. Surg. *71:* 218–225 (1976).

100 Behrendt, D. M. and Austen, W. G.: Current status of prosthetics for heart valve replacement. Prog. cardiovasc. Dis. *15:* 369–401 (1973).

101 Carey, J. S. and Hughes, R. K.: A complication of mitral-valve replacement with caged-lens prosthesis. Ann. thorac. Surg. *6:* 77–81 (1968).

102 Vasko, J. S. and Leighton, R. F.: Acute massive mitral regurgitation resulting from disc-valve malfunction. Ann. thorac. Surg. *6:* 564–569 (1968).

103 Robinson, J. J.; Hildner, F. J., and Greenberg, J. J.: Disc variance of Beall mitral valve. Ann. thorac. Surg. *11:* 11–17 (1971).

104 Detmer, D. E.; McIntosh, C. L.; Boretos, J. W., *et al.:* Polypropylene poppets for low-profile prosthetic heart valves. Ann. thorac. Surg. *13:* 122–127 (1972).

105 Berroya, R. B. and Escana, F. B., jr.: Mitral disc-valve variance. Thorax *27:* 87–89 (1972).

106 Hildner, F. J. and Robinson, M. J.: Complications of Beall valve prosthesis. Letters to the Editor. Am. J. Cardiol. *30:* 922 (1972).

107 Nathan, M. J.: Strut fracture. A late complication of Beall mitral valve replacement. Ann. thorac. Surg. *16:* 610–613 (1973).

108 Shaw, T. R. D. and Turner, R. W. D.: Sudden mechanical malfunction of Hammersmith mitral valve prostheses due to wear of polyprophylene. J. thorac. cardiovasc. Surg. *67:* 579–583 (1974).

109 Hughes, D. A.; Leatherman, L. L.; Norman, J. C., *et al.:* Late embolization of prosthetic mitral valve occluder with survival following reoperation. Ann. thorac. Surg. *19:* 212–215 (1975).

110 Low, H. B. C. and Lefemine, A. A.: Acute mitral insufficiency due to jamming of a disc-valve prosthesis. Ann. thorac. Surg. *4:* 71–73 (1967).

111 Hopeman, A. R.; Treasure, R. L., and Hall, R. J.: Mechanical dysfunction in caged-lens prostheses. J. thorac. cardiovasc. Surg. *60:* 51–59 (1970).

112 Oliva, P. B.; Johnson, M. L.; Pomerantz, M., *et al.:* Dysfunction of the Beall mitral prosthesis and its detection by cinefluoroscopy and echocardiography. Am. J. Cardiol. *31:* 393–396 (1973).

113 Hammer, W. J.; Hearne, M. J., and Roberts, W. C.: Cocking of a poppet disc

prosthesis in the aortic position. A cause of intermittent aortic regurgitation. J. thorac. Cardiovasc. Surg. *71:* 259–261 (1976).

114 WILLIAMS, J. C., jr.; VERNON, C. R.; DAICOFF, G. R., *et al.:* Hemolysis following mitral valve replacement with the Beall valve prosthesis. J. thorac. cardiovasc. Surg. *61:* 393–396 (1971).

115 COOLEY, D. A.; OKIES, J. E.; WUKASCH, D. C., *et al.:* Ten-year experience with cardiac valve replacement. Results with a new mitral prosthesis. Ann. Surg. *177:* 818–826 (1973).

116 WUKASCH, D. C.; SANDIFORD, F. M.; REUL, G. J., jr., *et al.:* Complications of cloth-covered prosthetic valves: results with a new mitral prosthesis. J. thorac. cardiovasc. Surg. *69:* 107–116 (1975).

117 COOLEY, D. A.; SANDIFORD, F. M.; WUKASCH, D. C., *et al.:* Mitral valve replacement with a new prosthesis. Experience with 366 patients. J. cardiovasc. Surg., Spec. No., pp. 378–383 (1975).

118 EDGETT, J. W.; NELSON, W. P.; HALL, R. J., *et al.:* A complication of valve replacement by a caged-lens prosthesis. Circulation *36:* 422–426 (1967).

119 HAMMERMEISTER, K. E.; DILLARD, D. H., and KENNEDY, J. W.: Severe, intermittent, mitral regurgitation in a Cross-Jones valve. Report of a case with angiocardiographic and hemodynamic observations. J. thorac. cardiovasc. Surg. *58:* 575–580 (1969).

120 ROE, B. B.; FISHMAN, N. H.; HUTCHINSON, J. C., *et al.:* Occluder disruption of Wada-Cutter valve prosthesis. Ann. thorac. Surg. *20:* 256–264 (1975).

121 BJÖRK, V. O.; HOLMGREN, A.; OLIN, C., *et al.:* Clinical and hemodynamic results of aortic valve replacement with the Björk-Shiley tilting disc valve prosthesis. Scand. J. thorac. cardiovasc. Surg. *5:* 177–191 (1971).

122 LEPLEY, D.; REUBEN, C. F.; FLEMMA, R. J., *et al.:* Experience with the Björk-Shiley prosthetic valve. Circulation *47/48:* suppl. III, pp. 51–55 (1973).

123 BÖÖK, K.: Mitral valve replacement with the Björk-Shiley tilting disc valve. A clinical and haemodynamic study in patients with isolated mitral valve lesions. Scand. J. thorac. cardiovasc. Surg., suppl. 12, pp. 1–28 (1974).

124 LILLEHEI, C. W.; KASTER, R. L.; COLEMAN, M., *et al.:* Heart-valve replacement with Lillehei-Kaster pivoting disk prosthesis. N.Y. St. J. Med. *8:* 1426–1438 (1974).

125 BJÖRK, V. O.; HENZE, A., and HOLMGREN, A.: Five years' experience with the Björk-Shiley tilting-disc valve in isolated aortic valvular disease. J. thorac. cardiovasc. Surg. *68:* 393–404 (1974).

126 BJÖRK, V. O.; HENZE, A., and HOLMGREN, A.: Long-term results with the Björk-Shiley tilting disc valve in aortic valvular disease. Israel J. med. Scis *11:* 161–172 (1975).

127 STAREK, P. J. K.; WILCOX, B. R., and MURRAY, G. F.: Hemodynamic evaluation of the Lillehei-Kaster pivoting disc valve in patients. J. thorac. cardiovasc. Surg. *71:* 123–128 (1976).

128 SLATER, S. D.; SALLAM, I. A.; BAIN, W. H., *et al.:* Haemolysis with Björk-Shiley and Starr-Edwards prosthetic heart valves. A comparative study. Thorax *29:* 624–631 (1974).

129 ROBERTS, W. C. and HAMMER, W. J.: Cardiac pathology after valve replacement with a tilting disc prosthesis (Björk-Shiley type). A study of 46 necropsy patients and 49 Björk-Shiley prostheses. Am. J. Cardiol. *7:* 1024–1032 (1976).

130 MESSMER, B. J.; OKIES, J. E.; HALLMAN, G. L., *et al.*: Mitral valve replacement with the Björk-Shiley tilting-disc prosthesis. J. thorac. cardiovasc. Surg. *62:* 938–946 (1971).

131 MESSMER, B. J.; OKIES, J. E.; HALLMAN, G. L., *et al.*: Early and late thromboembolic complications after mitral valve replacement. A comparative study of various prostheses. J. cardiovasc. Surg. *13:* 281–289 (1972).

132 MESSMER, B. J.; OKIES, J. E.; HALLMAN, G. L., *et al.*: Aortic valve replacement: two years' experience with the Björk-Shiley tilting-disc prosthesis. Surgery *72:* 772–779 (1972).

133 HENZE, A.; CARLSSON, S., and BJÖRK, V. O.: Mortability and pathology following aortic valve replacement with the Björk-Shiley tilting disc valve. Scand. J. thorac. cardiovasc. Surg. *7:* 7–16 (1973).

134 BEN-ZVI, J.; HILDNER, F. J.; CHANDRARATNA, P. A., *et al.*: Thrombosis on Björk-Shiley aortic valve prosthesis. Clinical arteriographic, echocardiographic and therapeutic observations in seven cases. Am. J. Cardiol. *34:* 538–544 (1974).

135 BYRD, C. L.; YAHR, W. Z., and GREENBERG, J. J.: Long-term results of 'simple' thrombectomy for thrombosed Björk-Shiley aortic valve prostheses. Ann. thorac. Surg. *20:* 265–273 (1975).

136 ROSS, D.: Biologic valves. Their performance and prospects. Circulation *45:* 1259–1272 (1972).

137 ANGELL, W. W.; SHUMWAY, N. E., and KOSEK, J. C.: A five-year study of viable aortic valve homografts. J. thorac. cardiovasc. Surg. *64:* 329–339 (1972).

138 WALLACE, R. B.; LONDE, S. P., and TITUS, J. L.: Aortic valve replacement with preserved aortic valve homografts. J. thorac. cardiovasc. Surg. *67:* 44–52 (1974).

139 WALLACE, R. B.: Tissue valves. Am. J. Cardiol. *35:* 866–871 (1975).

140 MOORE, C. H.; MARTELLI, V.; AL-JANABI, N., *et al.*: Analysis of homograft valve failure in 311 patients followed up to 10 years. Ann. thorac. Surg. *20:* 274–281 (1975).

141 YARBROUGH, J. W.; ROBERTS, W. C., and REIS, R. L.: Structural alterations in tissue cardiac valves implanted in patients and in calves. J. thorac. cardiovasc. Surg. *65:* 364–375 (1973).

142 IONESCU, M. I.; PAKRASHI, B. C.; MARY, D. A. S., *et al.*: Replacement of heart valves with frame-mounted tissue grafts. Thorax *29:* 56–67 (1974).

143 NUNO-CONCEICÃO, A.; PUIG, L. B.; VERGINELLI, G., *et al.*: Homologous dura mater cardiac valves. Structural aspects of eight implanted valves. J. thorac. cardiovasc. Surg. *70:* 499–508 (1975).

144 MARY, D. A. S.; PAKRASHI, B. C.; CATCHPOLE, R. W., *et al.*: Tissue valves in the mitral position. Five years' experience. Br. Heart J. *37:* 1123–1132 (1975).

145 OLSEN, E. G. J.; AL-JANABI, N.; SALAMÁO, C. S., *et al.*: Fascia lata valves: a clinicopathologcial study. Thorax *30:* 528–534 (1975).

146 REIS, R. L.; HANCOCK, W. D.; YARBROUGH, J. W., *et al.*: The flexible stent. A new concept in the fabrication of tissue heart valve prostheses. J. thorac. cardiovasc. Surg. *62:* 683–695 (1971).

147 STINSON, E. B.; GRIEPP, R. B., and SHUMWAY, N. E.: Clinical experience with a porcine aortic valve xenograft for mitral valve replacement. Ann. thorac. Surg. *18:* 391–401 (1974).

148 Horowitz, M. S.; Goodman, D. J.; Fogarty, T. J., *et al.:* Mitral valve replacement with the glutaraldehyde-preserved porcine heterograft. Clinical, hemodynamic, and pathological correlations. J. thorac. cardiovasc. Surg. *67:* 885–895 (1974).
149 Carpentier, A.; Deloche, A.; Relland, J., *et al.:* Six-year follow-up of glutaraldehyde-preserved heterografts. With particular reference to the treatment of congenital valve malformations. J. thorac. cardiovasc. Surg. *68:* 771–782 (1974).
150 Brown, J.W.; Myerowitz, P.D.; Cann, M. S., *et al.:* Clinical and hemodynamic comparisons of Kay-Shiley, Starr-Edwards. No. 6520, and Reis-Hancock porcine xenograft mitral valves. Surgery *76:* 983–991 (1974).
151 Johnson, A.D.; Daily, P. O.; Peterson, K. L., *et al.:* Functional evaluation of the porcine heterograft in the mitral position. Circulation *50/51:* suppl. I, pp. 40–48 (1975).
152 McIntosh, C. L.; Michaelis, L. L.; Morrow, A.G. *et al:* Atrioventricular valve replacement with the Hancock porcine xenograft: a five year clinical experience. Surgery *78:* 768–775 (1975).
153 Pipkin, R. D.; Buch, W. S., and Fogarty, T. J.: Evaluation of aortic valve replacement with a porcine xenograft without long-termo anticoagulation. J. thorac. cardiovasc. Surg. *71:* 179–186 (1976).
154 Zuhdi, N.; Hawley, W.; Voehl, V., *et al.:* Porcine aortic valves as replacement for human heart valves. Ann. thorac. Surg. *17:* 479–491 (1974).
155 Roberts, W.C.; Perloff, J.K., and Constantino, T.: Severe valvular aortic stenosis in patients over 65 years of age. A clinicopathologic study. Am. J. Cardiol. *27:* 497–506 (1971).
156 Roberts, W.C. and Perloff, J.K.: Mitral valvular disease. A clinicopathologic survey of the conditions causing the mitral valve to function abnormally. Ann. intern. Med. *77:* 939–975 (1972).
157 Roberts, W.C.; Dangel, J.C., and Bulkley, B. H.: Nonrheumatic valvular cardiac disease: a clinicopathologic survey of 27 different conditions causing valvular dysfunction. Cardiovasc. Clin. *5:* 333–446 (1973).
158 Hancock, W. D.: Personal commun. (November 1975).
159 Merendino, K.A.; Morrow, A.G.; Lillehei, C.W. *et al.:* Prosthetic valves for cardiac surgery, p. 86. (Thomas, Springfield 1961).
160 Braunwald, N. S.: The fabric-covered prosthetic heart valve. Present status and future development. Ann. thorac. Surg. *20:* 360–363 (1975).
161 Eiseman, B. and Spencer, F.C.: The occasional open-heart surgeon. Circulation *31:* 161–162 (1965).
162 Fernandez, J.: Insertion of Björk-Shiley aortic prosthesis by continuous suture technique. Ann. thorac. Surg. *17:* 587–590 (1974).

Prosthetic-valve Endocarditis Due to Listeria monocytogenes

ROBERT H. BREYER, M.D., ERNEST N. ARNETT, M.D., THOMAS L. SPRAY, M.D., AND WILLIAM C. ROBERTS, M.D.

From the Clinic of Surgery and the Pathology Branch, National Heart, Lung and Blood Institute, National Institutes of Health, Bethesda, Maryland

Breyer, Robert H., Arnett, Ernest N., Spray, Thomas L., and Roberts, William C.: Prosthetic-valve endocarditis due to *Listeria monocytogenes*. Am J Clin Pathol 69: 186–187, 1978. Clinical and necropsy observations in the case of a patient with prosthetic-valve endocarditis due to *Listeria monocytogenes* are presented. Although rare cases of *L. monocytogenes* infection of natural cardiac valves have been reported, this represents the first known case of infection of a prosthetic cardiac valve by this organism. (Key words: Prosthetic heart valves; Endocarditis; *Listeria monocytogenes*.)

PROSTHETIC-VALVE ENDOCARDITIS has been caused by a variety of unusual organisms, but, to our knowledge, there has been no report of its being caused by *Listeria monocytogenes*. Such was the case, however, in the patient to be described herein.

Report of a Case

A 64-year-old man who died November 13, 1974, had had his heavily calcified, stenotic, tricuspid aortic valve replaced with a Starr-Edwards prosthesis on January 11, 1973 (22 months before death). His early postoperative course had been complicated by temporary paresis of the right arm. Although the patient had had transient cerebral signs and symptoms 3 months after operation, he had been in functional class II status (New York Heart Association classification) until March 1974 (8 months before death) when he had noticed increasing exertional fatigue.

On September 24, 1974, the patient had had fever and sweats, and two days later he had been hospitalized. Oral temperature at that time was 39.2 C. Examination disclosed the expected prosthetic valve opening and closing sounds and a basal systolic ejection murmur. The leukocyte count was 17,000 cu mm. *Listeria monocytogenes* was grown from each of ten blood cultures of samples drawn serially over a two-day period. The organism was identified and speciated according to growth characteristics standardized by the Center for Disease Control. Minimal inhibitory concentrations (MIC) of antibiotics against this organism were (all in μg/ml): penicillin 0.2, ampicillin 0.2, cephalothin 1.6, erythromycin <0.4, tetracycline <0.4, kanamycin 3.0, gentamicin 1.6, intravenous administration of penicillin, 20 million units daily, was begun, and within 24 hours the fever had subsided. Serum bactericidal titers confirmed the adequacy of the antibiotic therapy (>99.9% bactericidal at 1:8 dilution 30 minutes before the scheduled dose of penicillin; 100% bactericidal at 1:32 dilution 10 minutes after the intravenous penicillin injection).

On October 13, 1974, however, the patient suddenly vomited, and had a severe headache. Two hours later, acute pulmonary edema appeared, followed by shock and finally, cardiac arrest. Although resuscitated, the patient never fully regained consciousness, and he died 30 days later. He had received penicillin intravenously during the entire period, and all further blood cultures were negative.

Received November 29, 1976; received revised manuscript January 25, 1977; accepted for publication January 25, 1977.

Address reprint requests to Dr. Roberts: Chief, Pathology Branch, National Heart, Lung and Blood Institute, National Institutes of Health, Bethesda, Maryland 20014.

At necropsy (A74-296), thrombus rimmed the primary orifice of the Starr-Edwards aortic prosthesis (Fig. 1). The site of attachment of the prosthesis was focally necrotic and the prosthesis partially detached (Fig. 1). The necrotic process had burrowed through the wall of the aorta into the space between the aorta and left atrium. Histologic examination of the site of prosthetic attachment disclosed polymorphonuclear leukocytes and fibrin, but no colonies of organisms, and cultures of cardiac blood were negative. Examination of the brain at necropsy revealed subarachnoid hemorrhage over the right cerebellar hemisphere and cavitary lesions in the left frontal and right parietal lobes.

Comments

Although *Listeria monocytogenes* is an infrequent cause of human infection, it is known to cause infection of the meninges and the female pelvic organs. It also may produce infection in newborns and in patients who have lymphoreticular malignancies.[3] This organism is a rare cause of infective endocarditis; only 12 patients with *L. monocytogenes* endocarditis involving native cardiac valves have been reported.[2] Before the infection, five of the 12 patients had had normal cardiac valves, five others were known to have underlying valvular disease, and in two cases the status of the valve before the infection was not mentioned. None had a debilitating disease.

In our patient, the infection was present behind the site of attachment of the prosthesis but colonies of organisms were absent, and postmortem heart blood cultures were negative, presumably because of the intravenous administration of antibiotic therapy for more than 40 days. Organisms may be absent, however, in patients with fatal prosthetic valve endocarditis treated with antibiotics.[1] Although clinical signs of aortic regurgitation were never apparent, partial detachment of the prosthesis occurred. Our patient died, however, not from the effect of prosthetic endocarditis on the heart, but as a result of a central

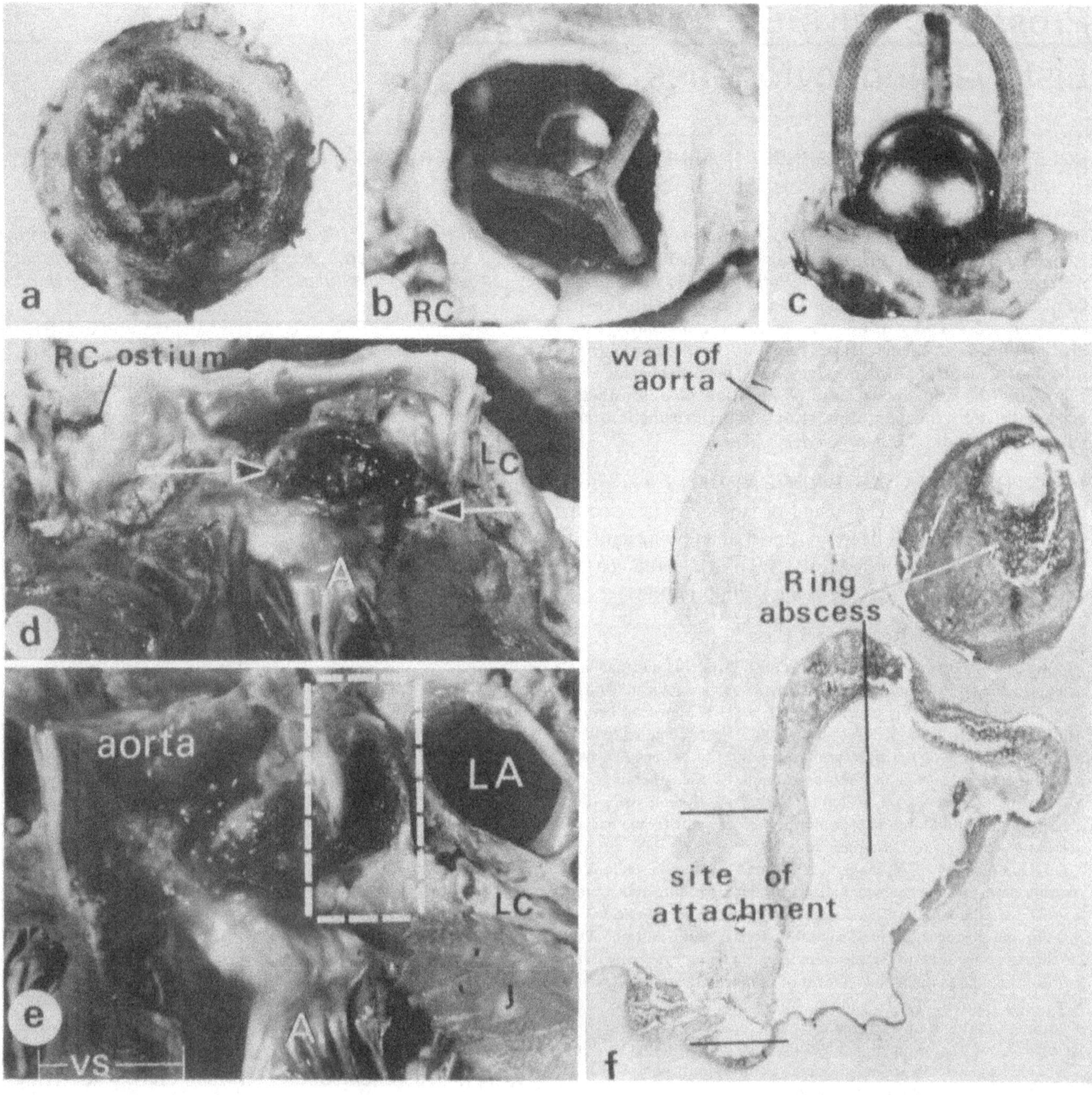

FIG. 1. Infected Starr-Edwards aortic valve prosthesis. *a*, Prosthesis as viewed from left ventricle. Thrombus devoid of organisms and inflammatory cells is present on the margins of the primary orifice. *b*, Prosthesis as viewed from above. RC = right coronary artery. *c*, Prosthesis as viewed laterally. The struts are devoid of thrombus. *d*, Opened aortic valve after removal of the prosthesis. A ring abscess (between the arrows) involves nearly half of the former site of attachment of the prosthesis. A = anterior mitral leaflet; LC = left coronary artery. *e*, Longitudinal cut through the ring abscess, showing extension through the full thickness of the wall of the aorta. Extravasation of blood did not occur because of marked fibrous thickening of the aortic adventitia. LA = left atrium; VS = ventricular septum. *f*, Histologic section through the area enclosed by dashed lines in *e*. Histologic section through the ring abscess, which represents an extension from the site of attachment of the prosthesis. No colonies of organisms were seen in the ring abscess or in the prosthetic anulus. Brown and Brenn stain: ×6.2.

nervous system catastrophe, presumably due to an embolus from the infected prosthetic valve.

References

1. Arnett EN, Roberts WC: Prosthetic valve endocarditis: A clinicopathologic analysis of 22 necropsy patients with comparison of observations to 74 necropsy patients with active infective endocarditis involving natural left-sided cardiac valves. Am J Cardiol 38:281–292, 1976
2. Bassan R: Bacterial endocarditis produced by *Listeria monocytogenes*. Am J Clin Pathol 63:522–527, 1975
3. Buckner LH, Schneierson SS: Clinical and laboratory aspects of *Listeria monocytogenes* infection. Am J Med 45:904–921, 1968

Structural Changes in Glutaraldehyde-Treated Porcine Heterografts Used As Substitute Cardiac Valves

Transmission and Scanning Electron Microscopic Observations in 12 Patients

VICTOR J. FERRANS, MD, PhD, FACC*
THOMAS L. SPRAY, MD*
MARGARET E. BILLINGHAM, MD†
WILLIAM C. ROBERTS, MD, FACC*

Bethesda, Maryland
Stanford, California

Scanning and transmission electron microscopic studies were made of (1) 12 glutaraldehyde-treated porcine valvular heterografts that had been implanted in patients for 2 days to 76 months; (2) 3 unimplanted commercially processed porcine aortic valves; and (3) 1 unprocessed porcine aortic valve. Comparison of unprocessed porcine valves and unimplanted commercially processed valves showed loss of endothelium and acid mucopolysaccharides during preimplantation processing. Short-term (less than 2 months) changes after implantation consisted of insudation of plasma proteins, penetration of erythrocytes into surface crevices, formation of a thin surface layer of fibrin, and deposition of macrophages, giant cells and a few platelets. Longer-term (more than 2 months) changes were proportional to the time interval after implantation and consisted of progressive disruption of collagen, erosion of the valve surfaces, formation of aggregates of platelets and accumulation of lipid. The surfaces of the leaflets did not become covered with endothelium or with a fibrous sheath. Calcific deposits were found in one valve and bacterial organisms in another. Thus, progressive breakdown of collagen appears to be a critical factor in determining the long-term durability of glutaraldehyde-treated porcine valvular heterografts.

Although porcine aortic valve heterografts have been used extensively during the past few years, little is known of the structural changes that these valves undergo after implantation for various periods of time. Gross anatomic and histologic changes have been described in a few porcine valve heterografts,[1–5] and one recent study[6] described a large series of these valves, including several that had been implanted for more than 1 year. These studies have suggested that degeneration of collagen, with loss of integrity of the fibrous framework of the cusps, may become a major cause of structural and functional failure of porcine valve heterografts implanted for long periods of time. An ultrastructural study of this problem seemed necessary because degenerative changes in collagen cannot be appreciated properly at the light microscopic level, and because no detailed reports have been published of the ultrastructure of porcine valvular heterografts after implantation.

This communication reports histologic and electron microscopic observations on porcine valve heterografts that had been treated with a stabilized glutaraldehyde process (Hancock Laboratories, Anaheim, California) and had been implanted in patients for 2 days to 76 months. These observations are compared with those on (1) fully processed but nonimplanted porcine valve heterografts, and (2) a normal porcine aortic valve that was fixed according to the usual procedure for histologic and ultrastructural study but not subjected to the stabilized glutaraldehyde process by which these valves are prepared for clinical use.

From the Pathology Branch, National Heart, Lung, and Blood Institute, National Institutes of Health, Bethesda, Maryland,* and the Department of Pathology, Stanford University School of Medicine, Stanford, California.† Manuscript received September 29, 1977, accepted November 16, 1977.

Address for reprints: Victor J. Ferrans, MD, Building 10, Room 7N208, National Heart, Lung, and Blood Institute, National Institutes of Health, Bethesda, Maryland 20014.

Materials and Methods

The morphologic studies to be described were made on 12 porcine valve heterografts obtained either at necropsy (nine patients) or reoperation for valve replacement (three patients). Pertinent clinical and hemodynamic data on these 12 patients are given in Table I. Similar morphologic studies were made of (1) two nonimplanted porcine aortic valves (Hancock Laboratories), (2) one nonimplanted Carpentier-Edwards valve, and (3) one normal porcine aortic valve. Both Hancock valves (obtained by courtesy of Hancock Laboratories, Anaheim, California) were subjected to the full process of preservation with stabilized glutaraldehyde; one valve was mounted on a flexible stent, as for clinical use; the other valve was unmounted. The Carpentier-Edwards valve was mounted as for clinical use. A grossly and histologically normal aortic

TABLE I

Clinical Data on 12 Patients Who Had Had Cardiac Valve Replacement With Porcine Heterografts

Case no.	Age (yr) & Sex	Preop. Valve Lesion	Operation	Size of PPV	Duration of PPV Implant (days)	Reason for Removal of PPV	Infected PPV	Infection Elsewhere	Cause of Death
1	65 F	MS, MR	MVR-P	33	2	Necropsy	0	0	Hemorrhage into right hemithorax
2	64 F	MS, MR	MVR-P, SVBG	29	3	Necropsy	0	0	Recurrent VT, shock
3	62 F	AS	AVR-P	23	28	Necropsy	0	Skin incision	Renal failure
4	47 M	MR	AVR-SE, MVR-P	33	28	Necropsy	0	On aortic SE prosthesis	PVE, septic shock
5	63 F	MS, MR	MVR-P	29	35	Necropsy	0	0	Recurrent VT
6	63 M	AS, MS	AVR-SE, MVR-P	31	60	Necropsy	0	Sepsis	Sepsis
7	61 M	MS	MVR-P	29	90	Perivalve leak	0	0	. . .
8	34 M	AS, AR, MS	MVR-P	29	210	Necropsy	0	0	CAD
9	57 F	MS, MR, AS, TR	AVR-SE, MVR-SE, TVR-P	31	630	Necropsy	0	0	CHF
10	44 M	MR	MVR-P	35	900	Dysfunction (regurgitation)	+	0	. . .
11	63 M	MR	MVR-P	33	900	Necropsy	0	0	CHF, CAD
12	61 F	MS, MR	MVR-P	31	2,280	Dysfunction (regurgitation)	0	0	. . .

0 = absent; + = present; AR = aortic regurgitation; AS = aortic stenosis; AVR-P = aortic valve replacement with porcine valve; AVR-SE = aortic valve replacement with Starr-Edwards valve; CAD = coronary artery disease; CHF = congestive heart failure; MR = mitral regurgitation; MS = mitral stenosis; MVR-P = mitral valve replacement with porcine valve; MVR-SE = mitral valve replacement with Starr-Edwards valve; PPV = porcine prosthetic valve; Preop. = preoperative; PVE = prosthetic valve endocarditis; SVBG = saphenous vein aortocoronary bypass graft; TR = tricuspid regurgitation; TVR-P = tricuspid valve replacement with porcine valve; VT = ventricular tachycardia.

TABLE II

Postimplantation Changes in 12 Porcine Valve Heterografts

		Changes in Valve Surfaces											Changes in Collagen					
		Fib. L.		RBC		Pl. A.		Macr.										
Case no.	Duration of Implant (days)	IS	OS	IS	OS	IS	OS	IS	OS	Tears in Leaflets	Thrombi	Fin. Fibr. Mat.	Loose Bundle	Disr. Fibr.	Gran. Fibr.	Punct. Dens.	Lip. Dep.	Other Changes
1	2	+	+	0	0	0	0	0	0	0	0	+	+	0	0	0	0	
2	3	+	+	+	+	+	+	0	0	0	0	++	+	0	0	0	0	
3	28	+	+	+	+	0	0	+	+	0	0	++	+	0	0	0	0	
4	28	++	++	++	++	0	0	+	++	0	+	++	++	+	+	0	0	Num. giant cells
5	35	+	++	0	++	0	+	+	++	0	+	++	+	+	+	0	0	Num. giant cells
6	60	+	++	0	0	–	–	+	++	0	+	–	–	–	–	–	–	
7	90	0	+	+	0	0	0	++	+++	0	0	+	+	+	+	0	0	
8	210	+	++	0	+	0	0	+	++	0	+	++	++	++	+	0	+	
9	630	+	++	0	++	+	+	+	++	0	+	++	+++	+++	++	+	0	Endo. thrombus
10	900	++	++	+	+	0	0	+	+	0	+	+++	+++	+++	+++	+++	+++	Bacterial infection
11	900	+	+	+	0	0	0	+	+	0	+	++	++	++	+	0	0	
12	2,280	0	0	+	++	+	+	+	+	++	+	+++	+++	+++	+++	++	++	Surface erosion

0 = change absent; + = minimal change; ++ = moderate change; +++ = severe change; – = data not available (valve from patient 6 was not examined with transmission electron microscopy); Disr. Fibr. = disruption of collagen fibrils; Endo. = endothelialized; Fib. L. = layer of fibrin; Fin. Fibr. Mat. = finely fibrillar material possibly representing insudated plasma proteins; Gran. Fibr. = abnormal granular appearance of collagen fibrils; IS = inflow surface; Impl. = implant; Lip. Dep. = lipid deposits; Loose Bundle = loosening of the arrangement of bundles of collagen fibrils; Macr. = macrophages; Num. = numerous; OS = outflow surface; Pl. A. = platelet aggregates (these were very scarce in Patients 2 and 5); Punct. Dens. = punctate densities; RBC = red blood cells adherent to surface.

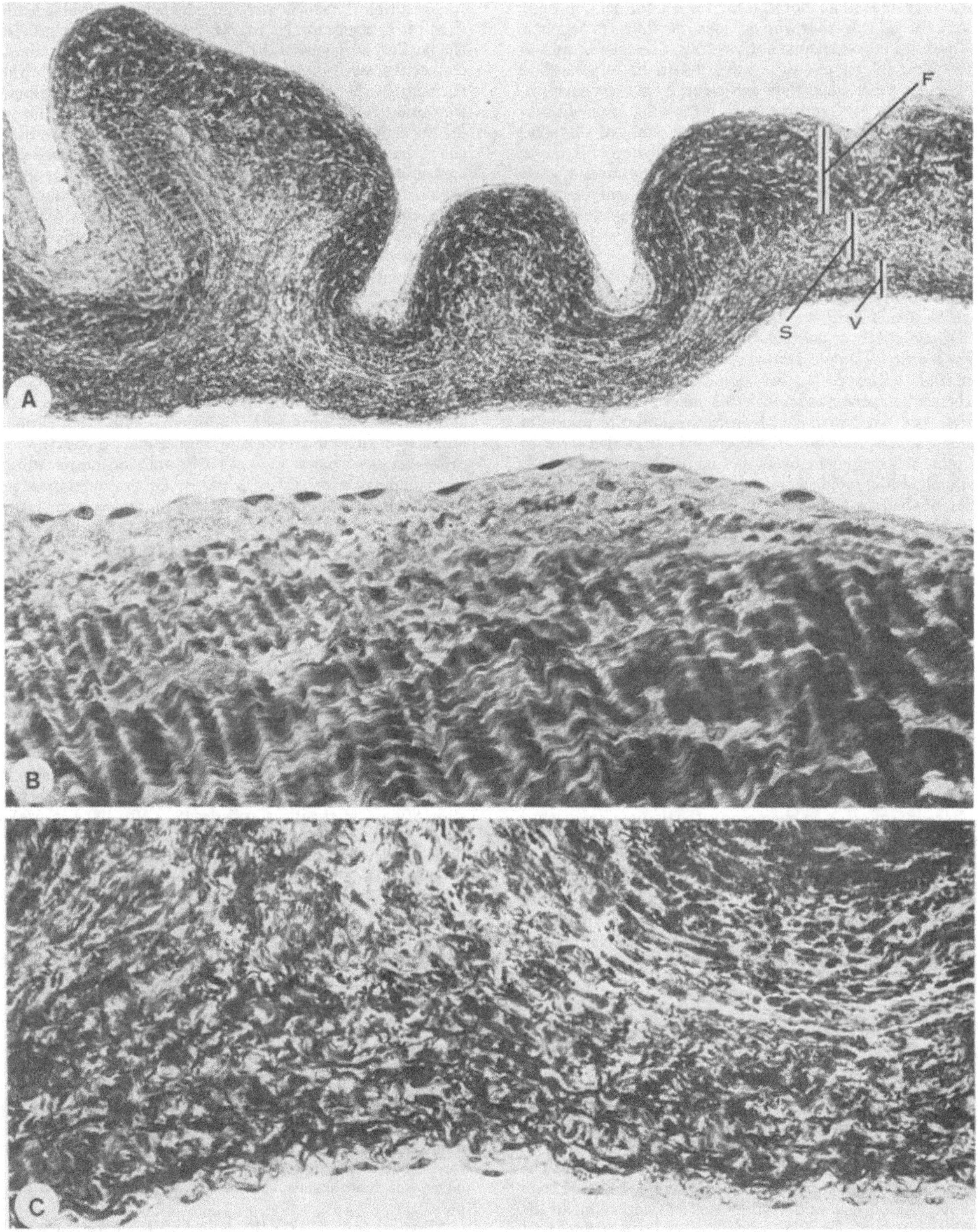

FIGURE 1. Light micrographs of 0.5 μ-thick plastic sections, stained with alkaline toluidine blue, of normal porcine aortic valve leaflet. **A,** Low power view showing layered arrangement of leaflet. F = fibrosa, S = spongiosa and V = ventricularis. The base of the leaflet is toward the left and the free edge toward the right. The inflow surface is at bottom; the outflow surface, which displays several prominent transversely oriented folds (compare with Fig. 4C), is at top. **B,** higher magnification view of outflow surface, showing fibrosa, composed of dense bundles of collagen (compare with Fig. 2), and overlying layer of endothelial cells. **C,** view of the inflow surface, showing surface endothelium and adjacent layer (ventricularis) rich in elastic fibers and collagen (compare with Fig. 3). (**A** ×125, **B** ×600, **C** ×600, all reduced by 3 percent.)

valve was removed at thoracotomy from a normal pig (body weight 101 kg), together with adjacent portions of the aortic root and the left ventricular outflow tract. Special precautions were taken not to touch the valve during its removal and subsequent processing. Care was taken to remove each implanted valve by handling only its sewing ring without touching the leaflets. Immediately after removal, all valves were fixed with cold 3 percent glutaraldehyde in 0.1 molar phosphate buffer, pH 7.2. After fixation, central strips of valve tissue extending from the anulus to the free margin of the leaflet were removed from each valve and processed for light microscopy and for transmission and scanning electron microscopy (Table II).

For light microscopy, the tissues were embedded in paraffin, sectioned and stained according to the following methods: hematoxylin-eosin, von Kossa, phosphotungstic acid hematoxylin, Movat pentachrome and elastica-van Gieson.

For transmission electron microscopy, the strips of tissue were cut into three pieces (base, middle and tip of the leaflet), washed with 5 percent sucrose in 0.1 molar phosphate buffer, pH 7.2, postfixed with cold 1 percent osmium tetroxide in Millonig's phosphate buffer, dehydrated in a graded series of ethanols and propylene oxide and embedded in Maraglas®. Flat embedding molds were used to maintain proper orientation of the tissue blocks. For optimal embedding of these large blocks of tissue, the dehydration and plastic infiltration steps were carried out with continuous agitation, using an REM-20B Automatic Tissue Processor (Sakura Finetechnical Co., Tokyo, Japan). Half-micron thick sections of the Maraglas-embedded tissue blocks were cut, stained with alkaline toluidine blue and examined with a light microscope to select areas for ultrathin sectioning and to make appropriate light electron microscopic correlations. Ultrathin sections were cut with an LKB Ultrotome III, stained with uranyl acetate and lead citrate, and examined with a JEOL 100B electron microscope. Selected ultrathin sections were collected on uncoated, 300 mesh gold grids and stained for the ultrastructural demonstration of elastic tissue with the method of Kajikawa et al.[7]

For scanning electron microscopy, the tissues were washed with cold 5 percent sucrose in 0.1 molar phosphate buffer, pH 7.2, rinsed with distilled water, dehydrated with acetone to the critical point of carbon dioxide, coated with gold-palladium and examined with a Hitachi HHS-2R scanning electron microscope. Two adjacent strips of each valve were prepared for scanning electron microscopy in order to allow examination of the two surfaces of the leaflets.

Results

Morphologic Features of the Normal Porcine Aortic Valve

The leaflets in a normal porcine aortic valve are unequal in size, the noncoronary leaflet being smaller than the other two. The right coronary leaflet differs from the other two by having a small shelf of muscle extending into its base.[8]

Inflow and outflow surfaces and layers of leaflets: The two surfaces of the porcine aortic cusp will be referred to in this paper as inflow and outflow surfaces according to the definitions that follow. The inflow surface is the surface that faces the ventricular cavity when the valve is in its normal anatomic (semilunar) position. When the valve is implanted in the atrioventricular (A-V) position, the inflow surface faces the atrium. The outflow surface faces the aortic root when the valve is in its normal anatomic (semilunar) position; this surface faces the ventricle when the valve is implanted in the A-V position. The basic structure of each aortic valve leaflet (Fig. 1 to 3) consists of (1) an *endothelial cell layer* that covers the outflow surface; (2) the *fibrosa,* a layer of dense fibrous connective tissue subjacent to the endothelium of the outflow surface; (3) the *spongiosa,* a layer of more loosely arranged fibrous and elastic connective tissue adjacent to the fibrosa; (4) the *ventricularis,* a thin layer of fibrous connective tissue that is subjacent to the inflow surface, shows a localized increase in the density of its connective tissue and tapers off gradually toward the free edge of the cusp; and (5) the *endothelial cell layer* that covers the inflow surface. This arrangement is similar to that in human aortic valves.[9]

Endothelial cell layer: This is a monolayer of cells that form a continuous covering and are joined to one another by intercell junctions (Fig. 1 to 3). These junctions are similar to those of endothelial cells elsewhere in the vascular system. The shapes of aortic valve endothelial cells are variable. Some are thin, elongated and attenuated with flattened nuclei, whereas others are thicker and their nuclei bulge into the lumen. These variations are dependent upon the state of relaxation of the leaflet.[10–12] The surfaces of endothelial cells have variable numbers of small microvilli-like cytoplasmic processes. These processes are evident on both transmission and scanning electron microscopy (Fig. 4, A and B). On examination at low magnification with scanning electron microscopy, the inflow surface appears considerably smoother than the outflow surface. The latter surface has numerous ridges that are oriented transversely (that is, parallel to the free edge of the cusp) and resemble those described by Clark and Finke[10,11] in human aortic valves. The basement membranes of valve endothelial cells are composed of finely filamentous material of moderate electron density. The basement membrane that invests endothelial cells in the inflow surface is thin and poorly defined (Fig. 3); in contrast, the basement membrane in the outflow surface is prominent and reduplicated or multilayered (Fig. 2). This feature is helpful in distinguishing between the two valve surfaces.

The spongiosa: This layer contains loosely arranged connective tissue in which fibroblasts, collagen fibrils, small elastic fibers, microfibrils, spicules (200 Å to 400 Å in size) of highly electron-dense material and a network of poorly defined extremely delicate filaments (~ 50 Å in diameter) are present. Histochemical and ultrastructural studies in other tissues[13,14] have shown that dense spicules of this type are composed of acid mucopolysaccharides. The collagen fibrils course in various directions and show periodic banding similar to that of normal collagen elsewhere. Elastic fibers are more numerous and considerably larger (up to 2 μ in diameter) in the area subjacent to the inflow surface (Fig. 3) than in other areas of the valves. As in other tissues, elastic fibers in porcine valves have two structural components: a centrally located amorphous component (elastin) and peripherally located microfibrils. The elastin component is selectively demonstrated by staining with the method of Kajikawa et al.[7] The microfibrils are not stained selectively with this method. Small bundles of microfibrils appear to provide points of reinforcement to the attachment of endothelial cells and their basement membranes to underlying connective tissue fibers.

Fibrosa: In this layer the collagen fibrils are much more abundant and more densely packed, and show a tendency to form parallel bundles. These bundles are arranged in interwoven layers. Spicules of acid mucopolysaccharides are much less abundant in the fibrosa than in the spongiosa. Fibroblasts (Fig. 2) are present in both the fibrosa and the spongiosa. These cells appear similar to fibroblasts in other organs; they

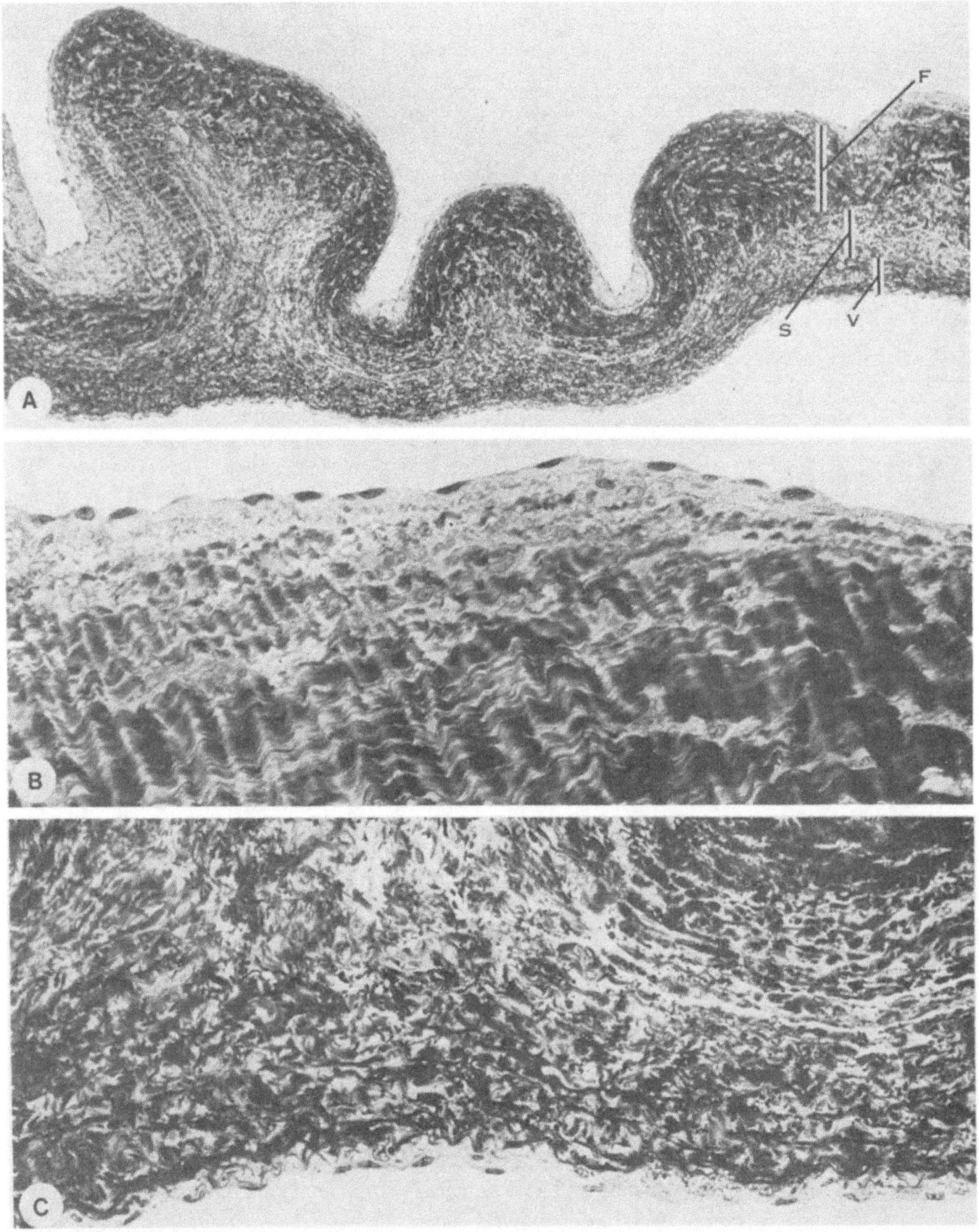

FIGURE 2. Transmission electron micrographs of outflow surface of normal porcine aortic valve leaflet. Sections stained according to method of Kajikawa et al.[7] for elastic tissue. **A,** low magnification view showing endothelial cells connected by junctions **(arrowheads)**, and part of several subjacent valve fibroblasts surrounded by densely packed bundles of collagen in fibrosa. Elastic fibers, stained black, are few and small. **B,** higher magnification view showing thin attenuated cytoplasm of endothelial cell and reduplicated layers of basement membrane material **(arrowheads)**. Elastic fibers have two components: centrally located dark amorphous material (elastin) and peripherally located microfibrils. A delicate network of spicules and filaments of acid mucopolysaccharide material is present throughout the interstitium. (**A** ×72,000, **B** ×27,400, each reduced by 4 percent.)

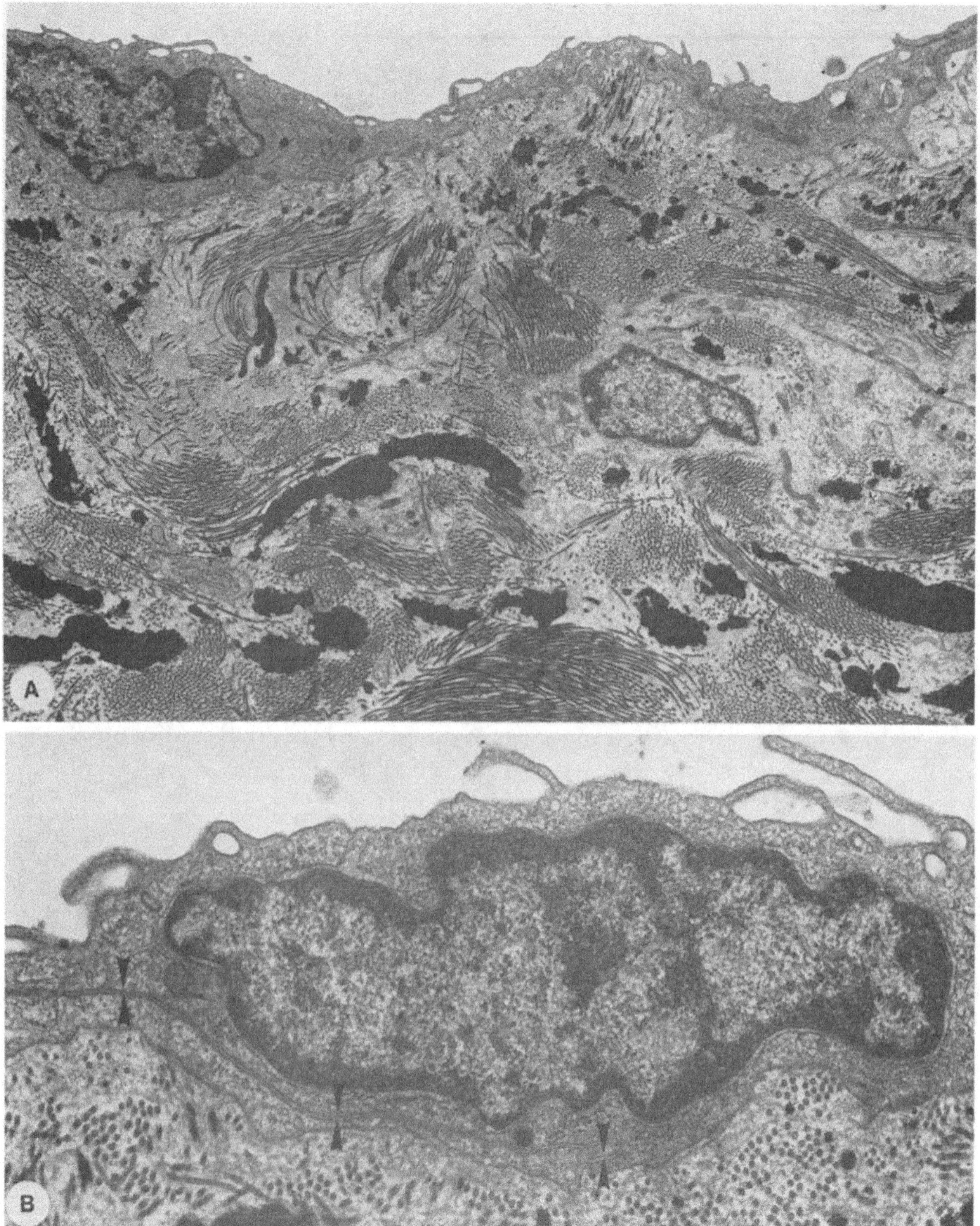

FIGURE 3. Electron micrographs of the inflow surface of a normal porcine aortic valve leaflet. Tissue stained for elastin as in Figure 2. **A,** low magnification view of endothelium and adjacent layer (ventricularis) rich in elastic fibers. Cytoplasmic projections protrude from the endothelial surface (compare with scanning electron micrographs in Fig. 4, A and B). Elastic fibers are larger and more numerous than in the outflow surface (compare with Fig. 2A). **B,** endothelial cell in the inflow surface shows indistinct basement membrane (compare with Fig. 2B). This cell overlaps the adjacent endothelial cell, with which it forms extended area of apposition **(arrowheads)**. (**A** ×7200, **B** ×26,400, each reduced by 1 percent).

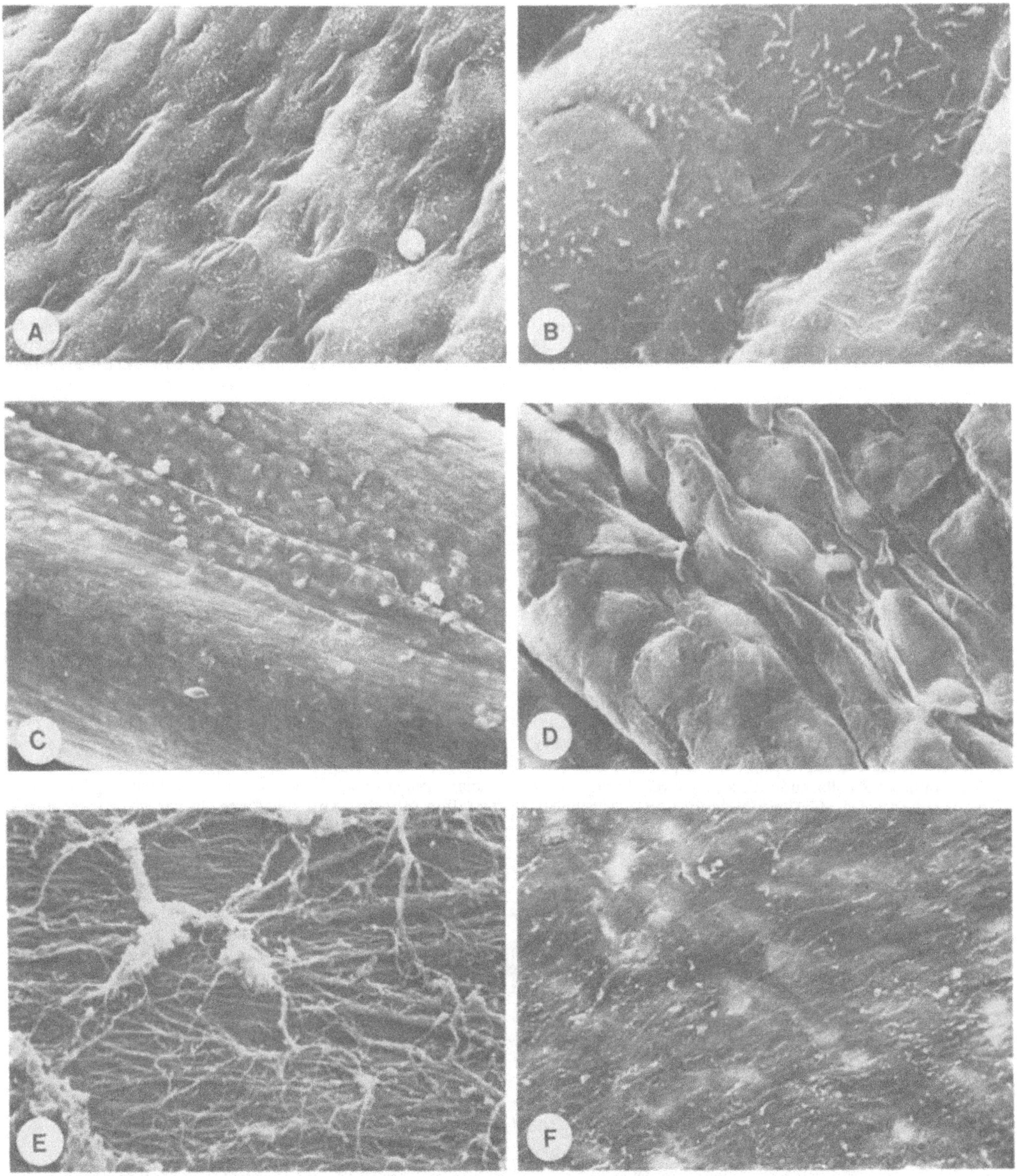

FIGURE 4. Scanning electron micrographs of normal (**A** and **B**) and processed but unimplanted (**C, D, E** and **F**) porcine aortic valves. **A** and **B** show low and high magnification views of endothelium in the outflow surface of the normal leaflet. Note the slight irregularity of surfaces, numerous cytoplasmic processes (filopodia) and areas of cell to cell apposition. **C,** outflow surface of leaflet from a valve that was treated by Hancock process but was not mounted on a stent. Typical transversely oriented ridges are partially denuded of endothelium. **D,** higher magnification view of area similar to that in **C**. Endothelial cells lack filopodia and are partially separated and detached. **E,** inflow surface of unimplanted Carpentier-Edwards valve is completely denuded of endothelium (compare with the light micrograph in Fig. 5 and the transmission electron micrograph in Fig. 6A) and is composed of frayed bundles of collagen. **F,** outflow surface of Hancock valve. Although also denuded of endothelium, this surface is much smoother than the inflow surface shown in **E**. (**A** ×1,000, **B** ×5,000, **C** ×300, **D** ×1,000, **E** ×2,000, **F** × 1,000, all reduced by 1 percent.)

lack basement membranes and contain prominent cisterns of rough-surfaced endoplasmic reticulum and Golgi elements, and variable numbers of actin-like cytoplasmic filaments. In some cells, the cytoplasmic filaments are present in such large numbers that these cells resemble smooth muscle cells. We regard such cells as myofibroblasts.

Structure of Unimplanted Hancock and Carpentier-Edwards Porcine Valves

Endothelial surface changes: Because morphologic studies revealed no significant differences between two unimplanted Hancock porcine valves (one mounted and one unmounted) and one mounted unimplanted Carpentier-Edwards porcine valve, the observations on these three valves will be described together. However, major structural alterations were evident when the morphologic features of these three valves were compared with those of the unprocessed porcine valve. The most important alteration was disruption of the endothelial cell layer (Fig. 4 to 6), with fairly complete loss of endothelial cells from the inflow surface and only partial loss from the outflow surface (Fig. 4, C and D). Preservation of valve endothelium was better in the unmounted than in the mounted Hancock valve. The mounted Hancock valve and the Carpentier-Edwards valve were similar in their surface structure. Because of the loss of endothelium, the two valve surfaces were constituted of subendothelial connective tissue components, including basement membrane-like material, collagen fibrils and a few elastic fibrils (Fig. 5 and 6). Nevertheless, the two surfaces of the valves had a completely different appearance. This difference was clearly evident on study with scanning electron microscopy at medium to high magnifications (Fig. 4), although at very low magnifications (less than ×100) the two surfaces appeared similar.

On scanning electron microscopic examination, the inflow surfaces (Fig. 4E) of the Hancock valves and the Carpentier-Edwards valve appeared much rougher than the outflow surfaces (Fig. 4F) and appeared to be composed of small, cylindrical bundles of collagen fibrils and of larger bundles that represented either elastic fibers or large masses of collagen fibrils. In contrast, the outflow surface (Fig. 4F) of each valve appeared smoother, more homogeneous and composed of material resembling basement membrane; it did not exhibit large numbers of exposed collagen fibrils. This surface layer appeared to correspond to the reduplicated endothelial basement membrane observed in the outflow surfaces of unprocessed valves with transmission electron microscopy (Fig. 2).

Connective tissue changes: The unimplanted valves showed loss of the ground substance of connective tissue, including the dense spicules of acid mucopolysaccharides and the network of less dense fine filaments associated with the spicules (Fig. 6). As a consequence, the collagen fibrils and elastic fibers, both of which remained structurally normal, appeared surrounded by a matrix of greatly increased electron lucency (Fig. 6), with some "loosening" of their arrangement. These changes were particularly pronounced in the spongiosa. As judged by the usual standard of electron microscopic fixation with glutaraldehyde, the quality of the structural preservation of valve fibroblasts was poor in all three valves treated with the stabilized glutaraldehyde process. Fibroblasts in these valves showed loss of integrity of cytoplasmic membranes and disruption of organelles (Fig. 6).

Morphology of Short-Term (less than 2 months) Implanted Hancock Valves

Comparison of unimplanted and short-term implanted Hancock valves revealed that several structural alterations had developed in the surfaces and substances of the valves after implantation.

Alterations involving the valve surfaces consisted of: (1) deposition of fibrin on both surfaces (more on the outflow than on the inflow surface) with formation of small thrombi that were visible only microscopically; (2) entrapment of erythrocytes in a meshwork of fibrin and direct adherence of erythrocytes to the denuded surfaces of the valves (again more on the outflow than on the inflow surface); (3) occasional adherence of platelets to the surfaces, and (4) deposition of macrophages and giant cells on the surfaces, without penetration into the valve substance. The relative frequency of occurrence of these changes is indicated in Table II.

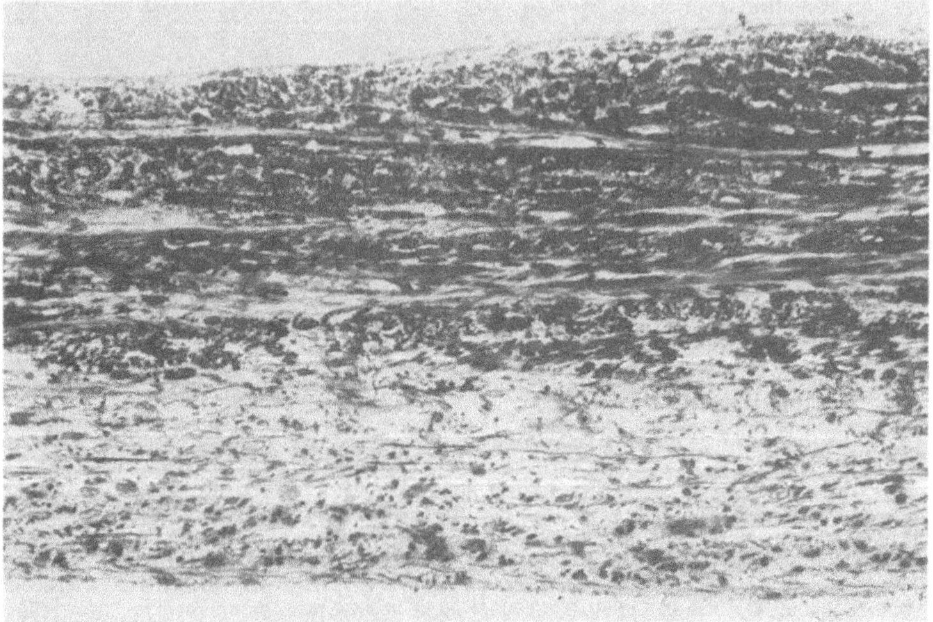

FIGURE 5. Light micrograph of plastic section, stained with alkaline toluidine blue, of unimplanted Carpentier-Edwards valve. The fibrosa appears dense; the spongiosa is more loosely arranged than normal, and the ventricularis is indistinct. Both the outflow **(top)** and inflow **(bottom)** surfaces are denuded of endothelium. The inflow surface appears more frayed than the outflow surface. (×300, reduced by 29 percent.)

Changes involving the connective tissue components of the valves (Fig. 7 and 8) included: (1) insudation of plasma proteins into the substance of the leaflets; (2) penetration of erythrocytes and leukocytes into the spongiosa, presumably through crevices in surfaces that were denuded of endothelium; (3) loosening of the arrangement of the bundles of collagen in the spongiosa and to a lesser extent in the fibrosa, and (4) evidence of mild disruption of collagen.

Valves implanted for 2 to 3 days: In the two valves that had been implanted for only 2 and 3 days, respectively (Fig. 7 and 8), structural changes were minimal and consisted of deposition of a thin (less than 10 μ in thickness) layer of fibrin and occasional erythrocytes and platelets on the exposed collagen surfaces. No macrophages were observed. In spite of these short periods after implantation, some insudation of plasma proteins, manifested by very fine fibrillar material between the collagen fibers, was already evident in superficial layers of the valves. This material surrounded the collagen fibrils, which before implantation were surrounded by a characteristically lucent matrix.

Valves implanted for 1 to 2 months: In the four valves that had been in place for 1 to 2 months, the layers of fibrin

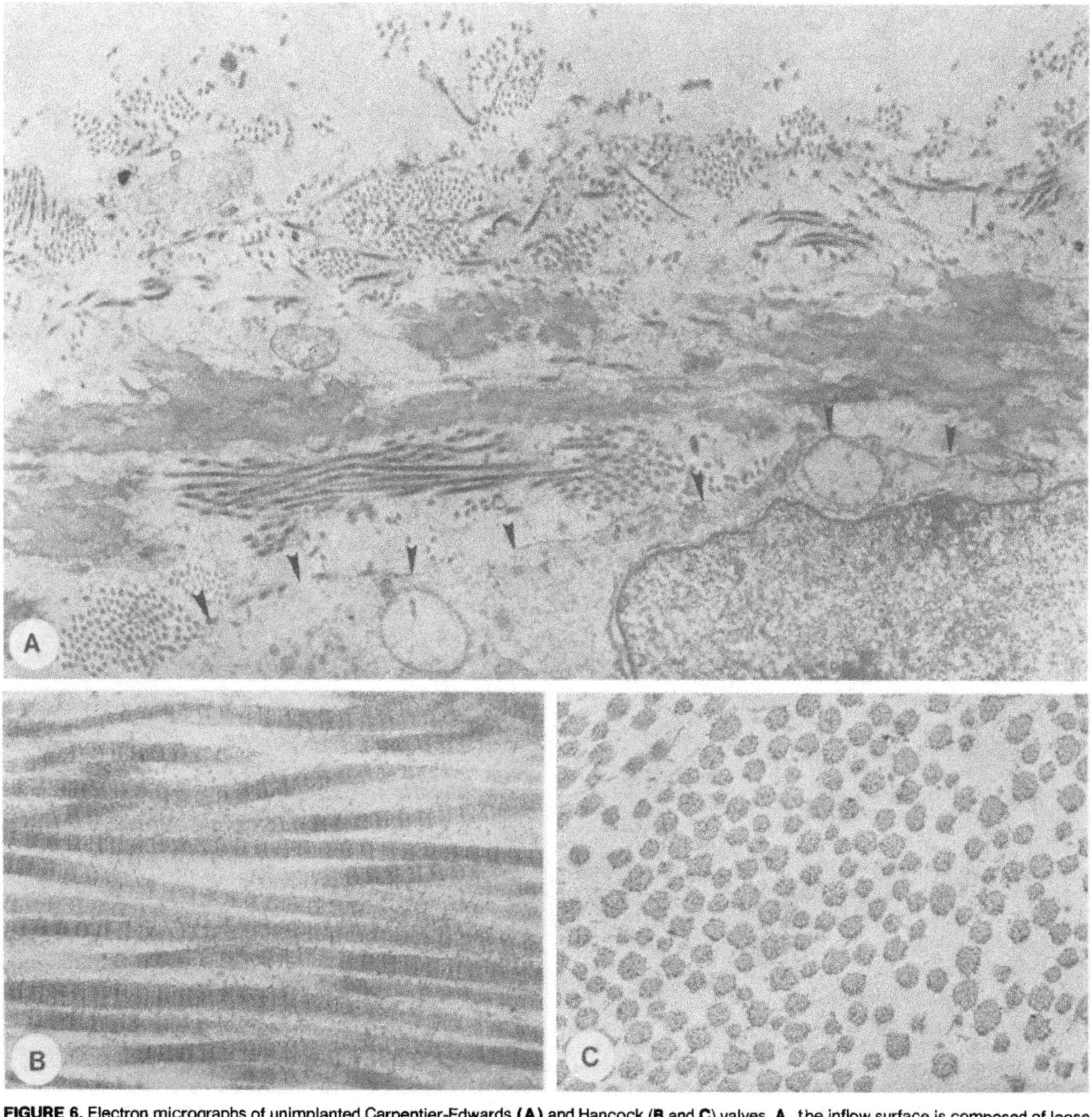

FIGURE 6. Electron micrographs of unimplanted Carpentier-Edwards (**A**) and Hancock (**B** and **C**) valves. **A,** the inflow surface is composed of loose bundles of collagen and of deeper elastic fibers. The morphologic features of the valve fibroblast (outlined by **arrowheads**) is poorly preserved, and there are damaged mitochondria and broken plasma membranes. **B** and **C**, longitudinally (**B**) and transversely (**C**) sectioned collagen fibrils in the fibrosa appear normal, but their surrounding matrix is abnormally lucent. (**A** ×22,000, **B** and **C** × 54,000, all reduced by 1 percent.)

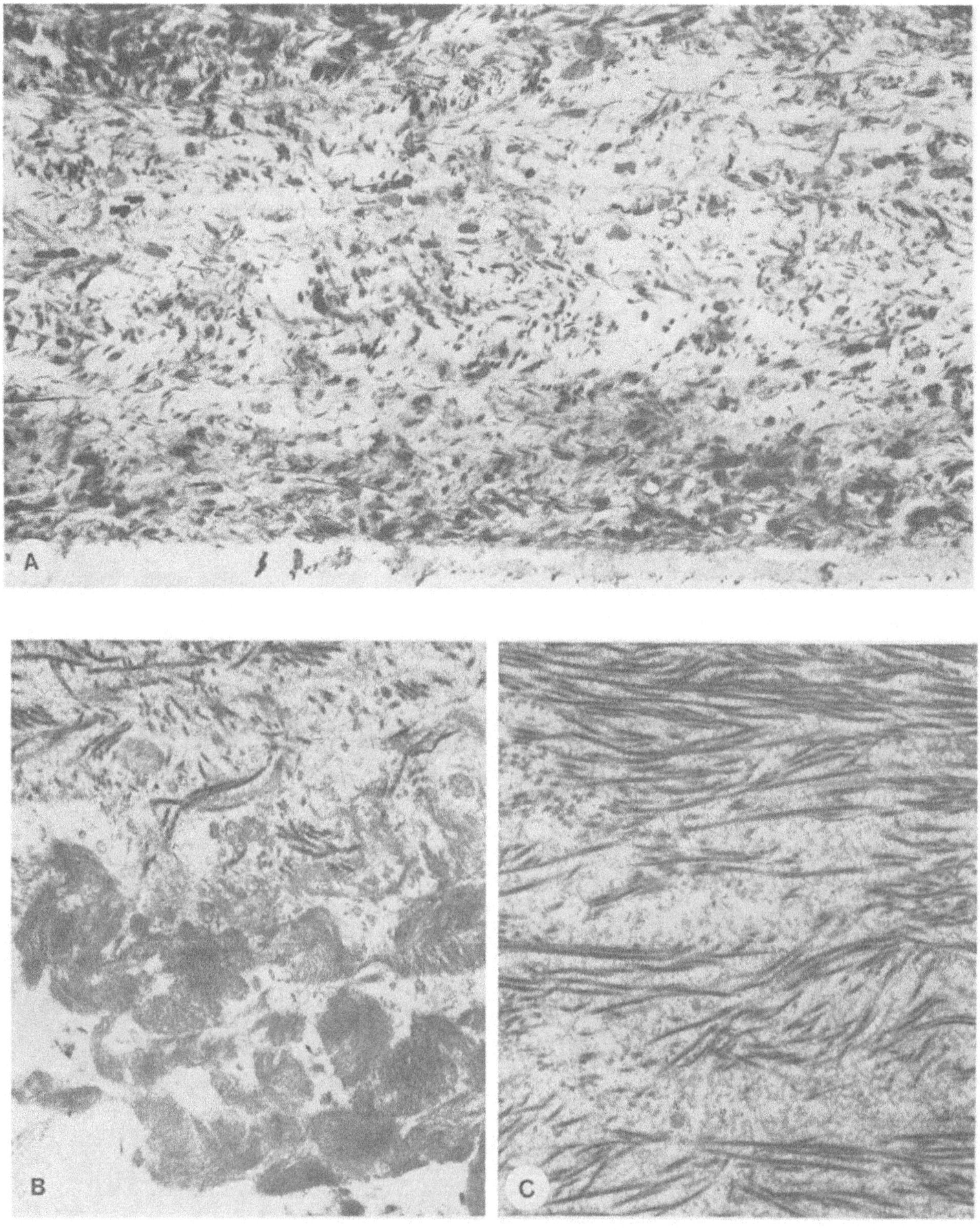

FIGURE 7. Light **(A)** and electron (**B** and **C**) micrographs of porcine valve heterografts implanted for short periods of time (**A** and **B,** from Patient 2, valve implanted for 3 days; **C,** from Patient 3, valve implanted for 28 days). **A,** inflow surface **(bottom)** is covered by thin layer of fibrin. Arrangement of connective tissue in ventricularis and spongiosa is looser than normal, and a number of red blood cells **(arrowheads)** are found at an appreciable distance from the surface. **B,** area similar to that in **A,** showing typical strands of fibrin adjacent to collagen in inflow surface. Fine fibrillar material is present between collagen fibrils. **C,** after 28 days of implantation, collagen in this area of fibrosa appears less compactly arranged than normal and is surrounded by finely fibrillar material presumed to represent plasma proteins. (**A**, toluidine blue stain ×500, **B** ×79,700, **C** ×18,000, all reduced by 8 percent.)

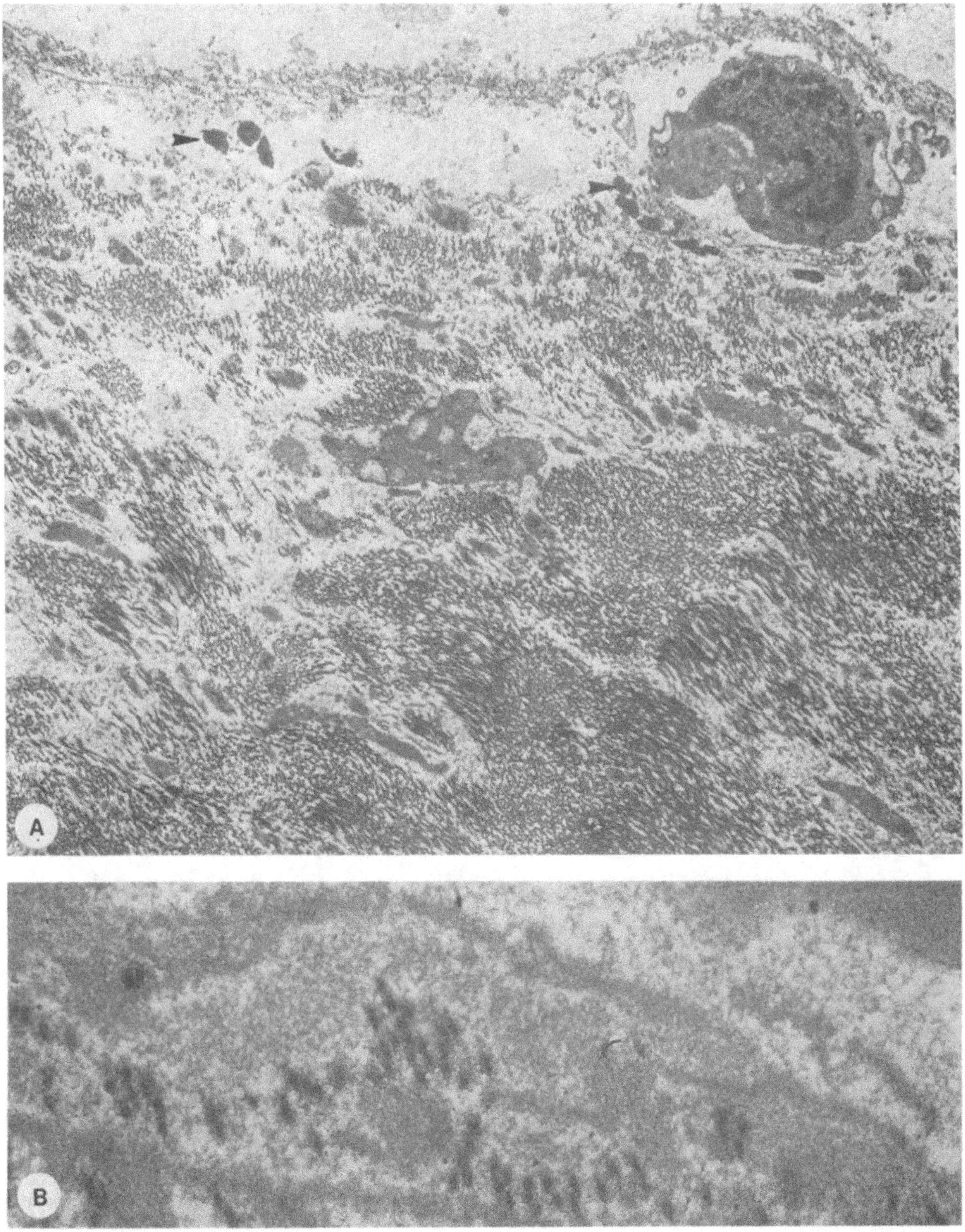

FIGURE 8. Electron micrographs of outflow surface of valve (implanted for 3 days) from Patient 3. **A**, the surface is denuded of endothelium and is composed of collagen and multilayered basement membrane material. Platelets **(arrowheads)** are present just beneath the surface in the area of separation between basement membrane and underlying fibrosa. Finely fibrillar material is seen between collagen bundles. **B**, high magnification view of the surface shown in **A**. Note the layers of basement membrane material (compare with fibrosa of the normal valve in Fig. 2A) and the gray halo surrounding each collagen fibril. (**A** × 5,200, **B** ×59,000, both reduced by 3 percent.)

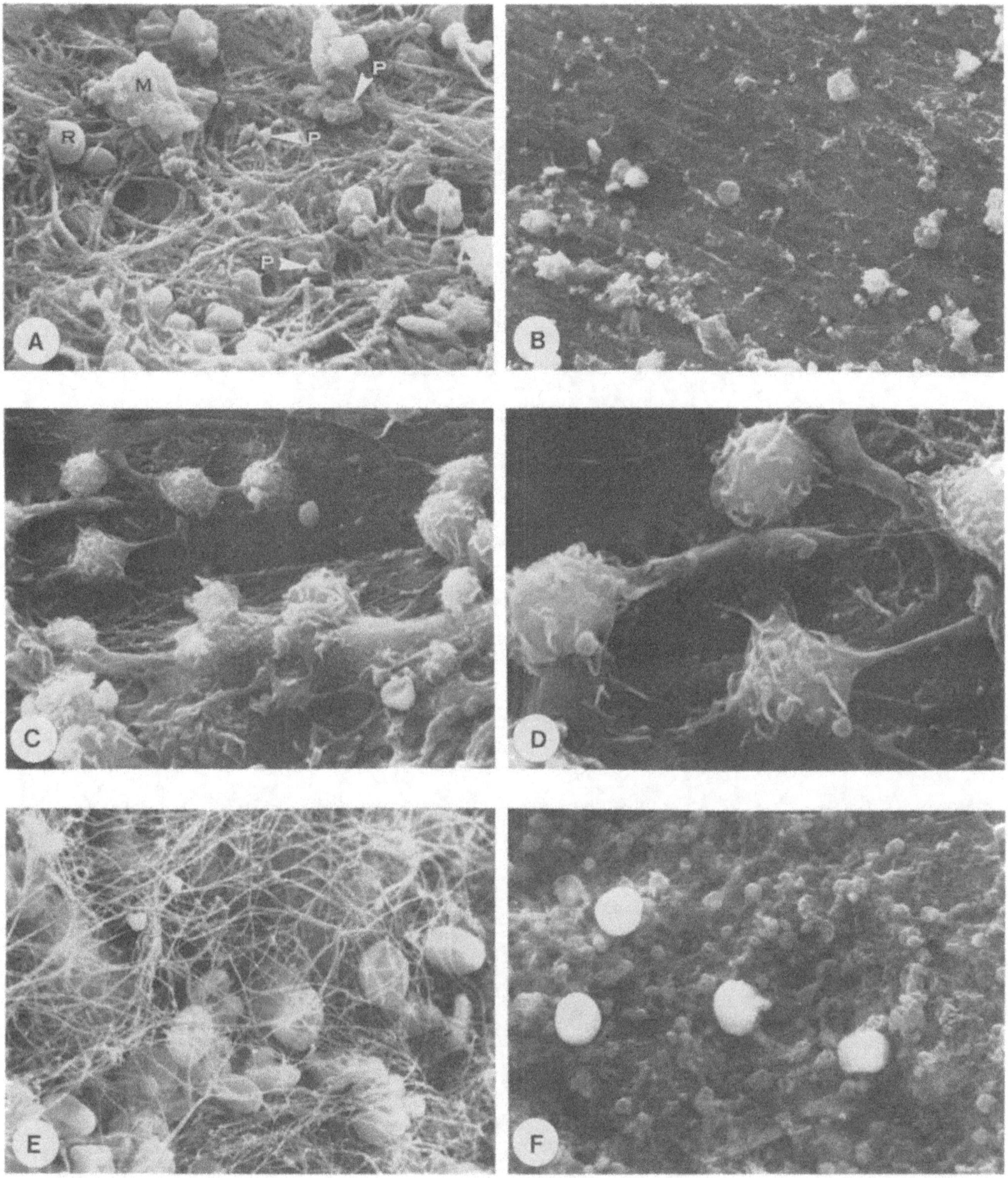

FIGURE 9. Scanning electron micrographs of postimplantation changes in porcine valve heterografts. **A,** red blood cells (R), macrophages (M) and platelets (P) are deposited on top of coarse bundles of collagen (compare with Fig. 4E) forming the inflow surface of a valve (implanted for 28 days) from Patient 4. **B,** scattered red blood cells and macrophages are superimposed upon a relatively smooth outflow surface (compare with Fig. 4F) of a valve (implanted for 35 days) from Patient 5. **C** and **D,** two views of macrophages on the outflow surface of a valve (implanted for 3 months) from Patient 7. These cells (compare with Fig. 11A) have ruffled surfaces and elongated cytoplasmic projections. **E,** red blood cells are trapped in a mesh of fibrin near the torn edge of the leaflet in a valve (replaced, because of regurgitation caused by leaflet tears, 76 months after implantation) from Patient 12. **F,** same valve as in **E,** showing several red blood cells and numerous platelets that cover the surface almost completely. (**A** ×1,000, **B** ×600, **C** ×1,200, **D** ×3,000, **E** ×2,000, **F** ×2,000, all reduced by 1 percent.)

were thicker, especially on the outflow surfaces, and macrophages lined the surfaces of the leaflets, usually forming a monolayer. Macrophages were consistently more numerous on the outflow than on the inflow surfaces. In these four valves, and in those in place for longer periods (Fig. 9), fibrin deposits (that were visible only microscopically) and larger thrombi tended to be much greater on the outflow than on the inflow surfaces. Multinucleated giant cells were present together with the macrophages on the outflow surfaces (Fig. 9 to 11). The macrophages on the valve surfaces had the following morphologic features: (1) prominent surface folds (filopodia); (2) moderate numbers of small mitochondria, cisterns of endoplasmic reticulum and cytoskeletal (100 Å in diameter) filaments, and (3) variable numbers of lysosomes and residual bodies. No phagocytosis of collagen by macrophages was observed. Multinucleated giant cells had organelles similar to those in macrophages (Fig. 10 and 11). These giant cells showed greatly complex surface folds, which interdigitated extensively with those of adjacent cells, and had from two to six irregularly arranged nuclei. Scanning electron microscopic examination (Fig. 9) confirmed the impression gained from light microscopy and transmission electron microscopy that the leaflets did not endothelialize but became covered with a discontinuous layer of fibrin, blood cells and macrophages, all of which were directly superimposed upon the collagen fibrils and basement membranes of the previously denuded valvular surfaces.

Alterations involving collagen fibrils consisted of increased granularity, irregularity of staining, and disruption of the fibrils (Fig. 12, A and B). The latter change was associated with fraying or tufting of the ends of the collagen fibrils and with the appearance of finely fibrillar or granular material, presumed to be derived from disrupted collagen. In valves implanted for short periods of time, these changes were minimal and involved mostly the more superficial areas of the cusps.

Morphology of Hancock Valves Implanted for 3 to 76 Months

Disruption of collagen: The most significant change observed in Hancock valves implanted for long periods of time (3 to 76 months) was disruption of collagen (Fig. 13). The extent to which this change occurred correlated with the length of time the valve had been in place. Breakdown of collagen was of mild to moderate severity in valves examined after 3 and 7 months of implantation; however, this change was severe in all valves that had been implanted for 21 months or longer. On light microscopy, collagen breakdown was manifested by disappearance of the bundles of collagen fibrils and by the formation of a homogeneous hyaline-appearing, pale-staining matrix that was free of fibrillar elements and showed no birefringence. Although macroscopically normal, the valves removed 21 and 30 months after implantation showed severe collagen breakdown.

In addition to the ultrastructural changes observed in the short-term implants, the collagen in the long-term implants showed extensive disruption and marked variability in the intensity of staining. Areas of disrupted collagen were characterized by the presence of either extremely fine, short,

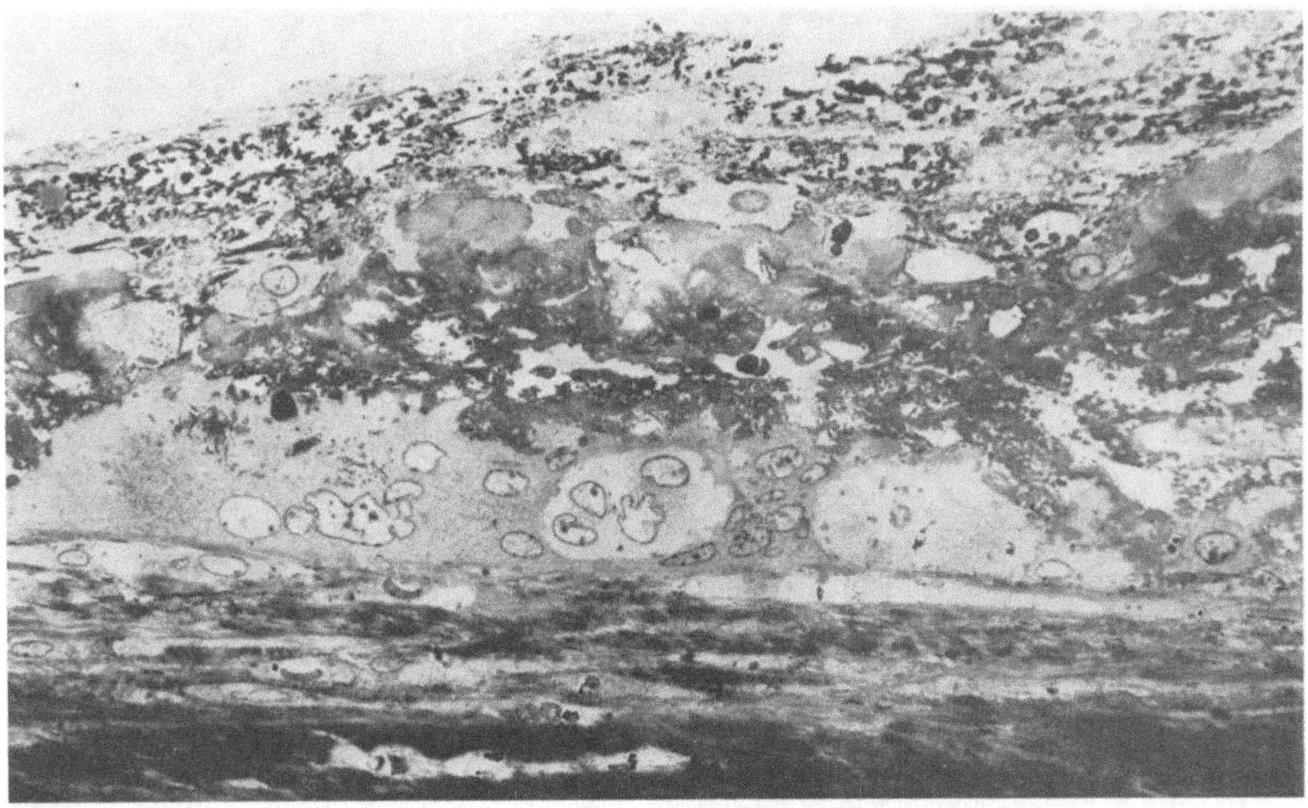

FIGURE 10. Light micrograph of the outflow surface of a valve (implanted for 28 days) from Patient 4, showing several multinucleated giant cells located on top of the fibrosa (dark layer at bottom) and beneath the layered fibrin thrombus. Compare with Fig. 11B. (Alkaline toluidine blue stain ×600.)

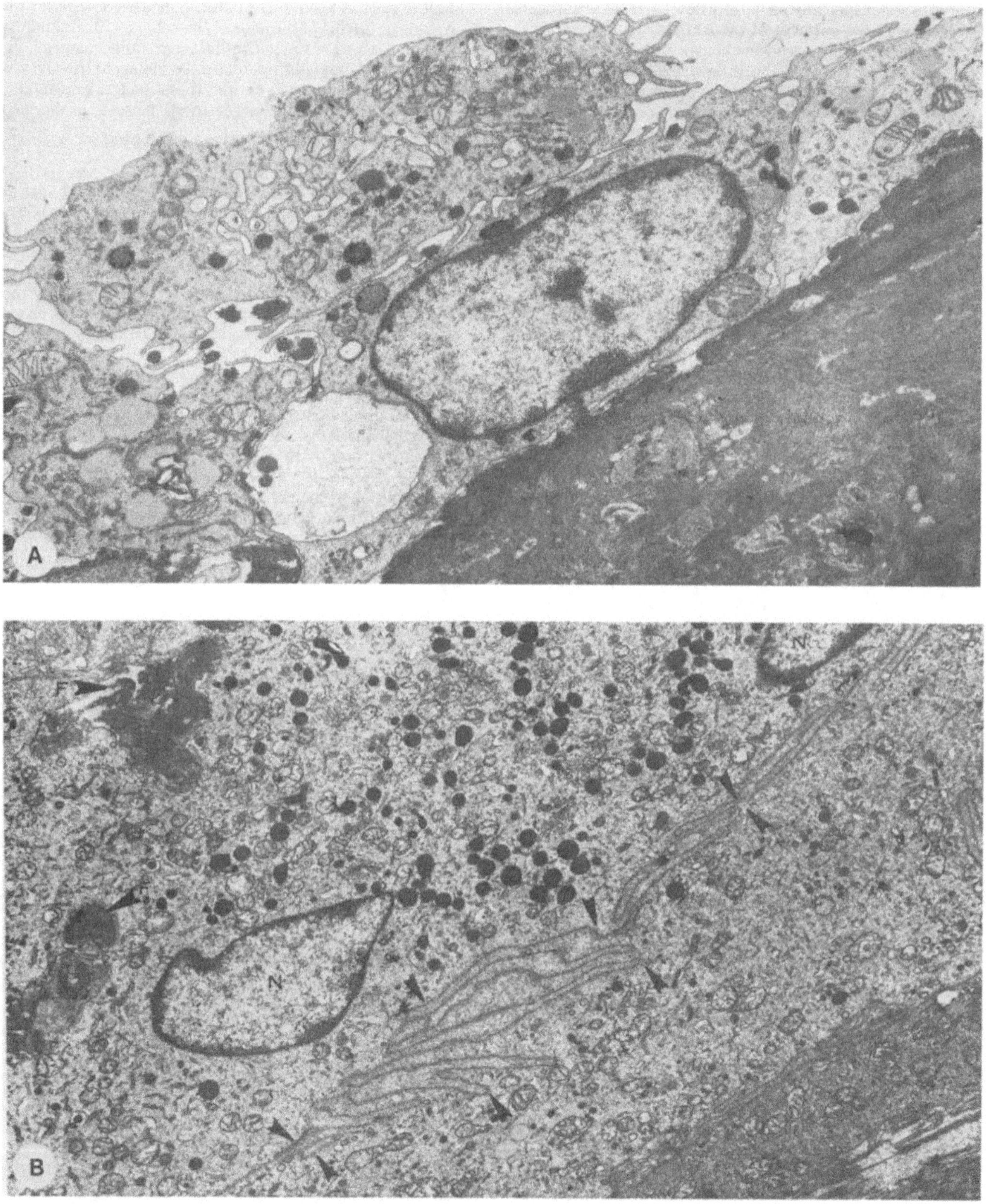

FIGURE 11. Electron micrographs of macrophages **(A)** and multinucleated giant cells **(B)** in thrombus shown in the light micrograph of Figure 10. **A,** view of several macrophages that have numerous surface projections, contain abundant dense bodies and some lipid droplets, and overlie a large mass of fibrin at **lower right. B,** complex interdigitations of plasma membranes **(arrowheads)** connect several adjacent giant cells. The cell in **upper left** and **center** is multinucleated (note parts of 2 nuclei [N]) and contains numerous dense bodies and several membrane-bound strands of fibrin (F). (**A** ×13,500, **B** ×1,900, both reduced by 1 percent.)

threadlike fibrils (Fig. 13, A to D) or irregular clumps of coarsely granular material resembling fibrinoid (Fig. 13F). Peculiar punctate densities were often present in collagen fibrils in the process of undergoing disruption (Fig. 13E). These structures consisted of clusters of electron-dense particles, ~50 Å, in diameter, that were distributed throughout the collagen fibrils without showing a definite relation to the banding patterns of these fibrils. These punctate densities occurred in three of four valves in place for 21 months or longer, and were not present in any of those in place for shorter periods.

Lipid particles: Electron-lucent particles ranging in size from 1,000 Å to 1 μ and resembling lipid droplets were present in three of five valves in place for 7 months or longer (Fig. 13, C and D). The valve in which these particles were most frequent had been in place for 30 months and was the site of infection; the second valve containing lipid particles had been in place for 76 months and had to be removed because of severe disruption; the third valve was removed at necropsy from a 34 year old man who also had type IV hyperlipoproteinemia and died of coronary heart disease; this valve had been in place for only 7 months. Confirmation of the presence of lipid droplets in these valves was obtained with light microscopic study of frozen sections stained with oil red O.

Surface changes: As in short-term implants, the surfaces of the long-term implants were associated with variable amounts of fibrin and variable numbers of erythrocytes, macrophages and giant cells. The latter cells were uncommon in the two valves implanted for the longest periods (30 to 76 months). Endothelial cells were found only in one valve (implanted for 21 months), in which they formed part of the surface of an incompletely organized thrombus (Fig. 14). Except for this, all valves were denuded of endothelium. Valve fibroblasts, which appeared poorly preserved and structurally indistinguishable from those in nonimplanted valves, were still present in all implanted valves. Because of their morphologic features, these cells were regarded as porcine fibroblasts. No evidence of fibroblastic ingrowth of host tissue (fibrous

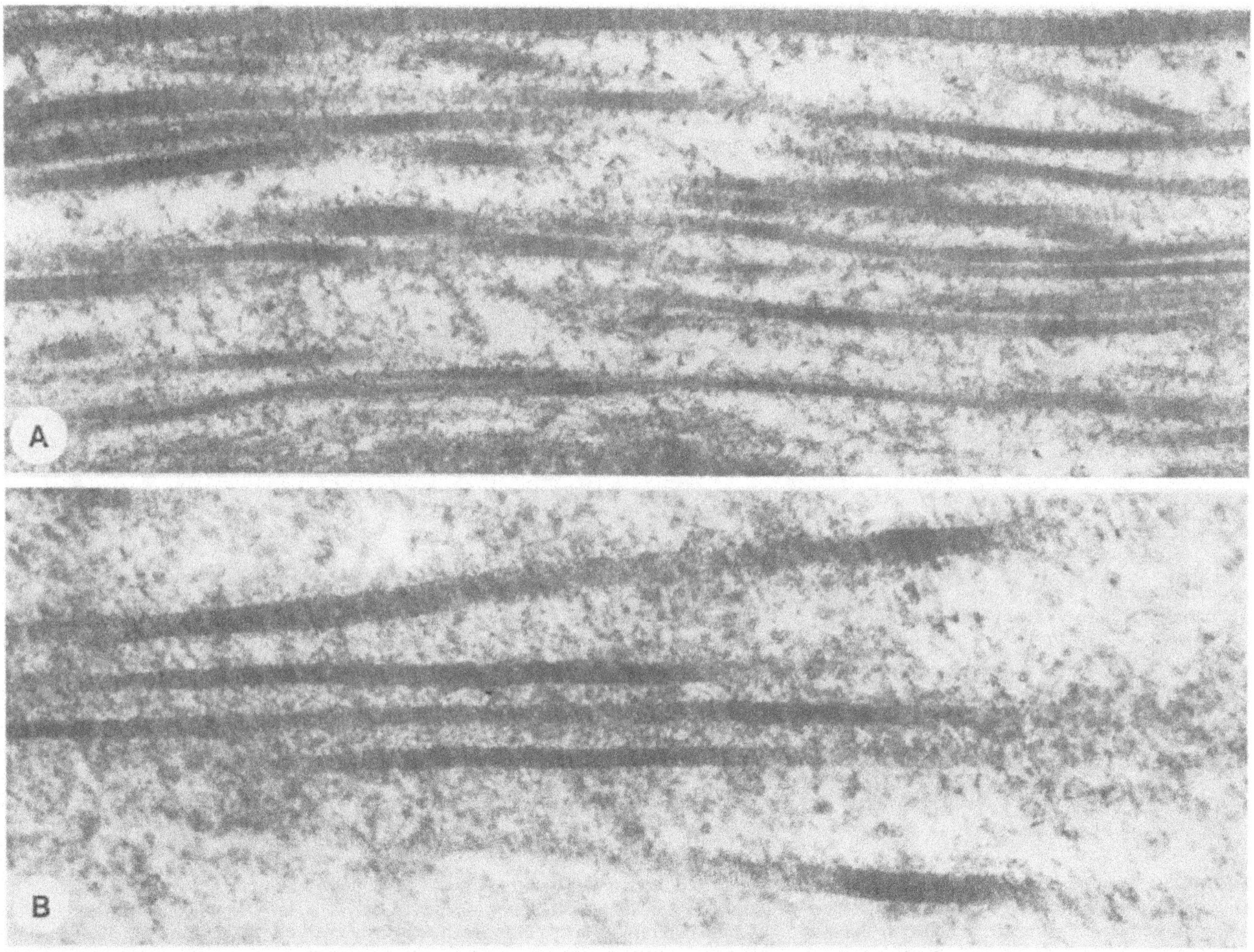

FIGURE 12. Electron micrographs of early changes in collagen in porcine valve heterografts. **A**, collagen fibrils in the fibrosa of a valve (implanted for 28 days) from Patient 4 begin to show disintegration, with focal loss of banding and with formation of finely granular material. Much of the latter material seems to coat nondisrupted collagen fibrils. **B**, higher magnification view of collagen in the fibrosa of a valve (implanted for 35 days) from Patient 5, showing fraying of the free ends of fibrils that seem to terminate in tufts of granular material. (**A** ×49,500, **B** × 84,500, both reduced by 1 percent.)

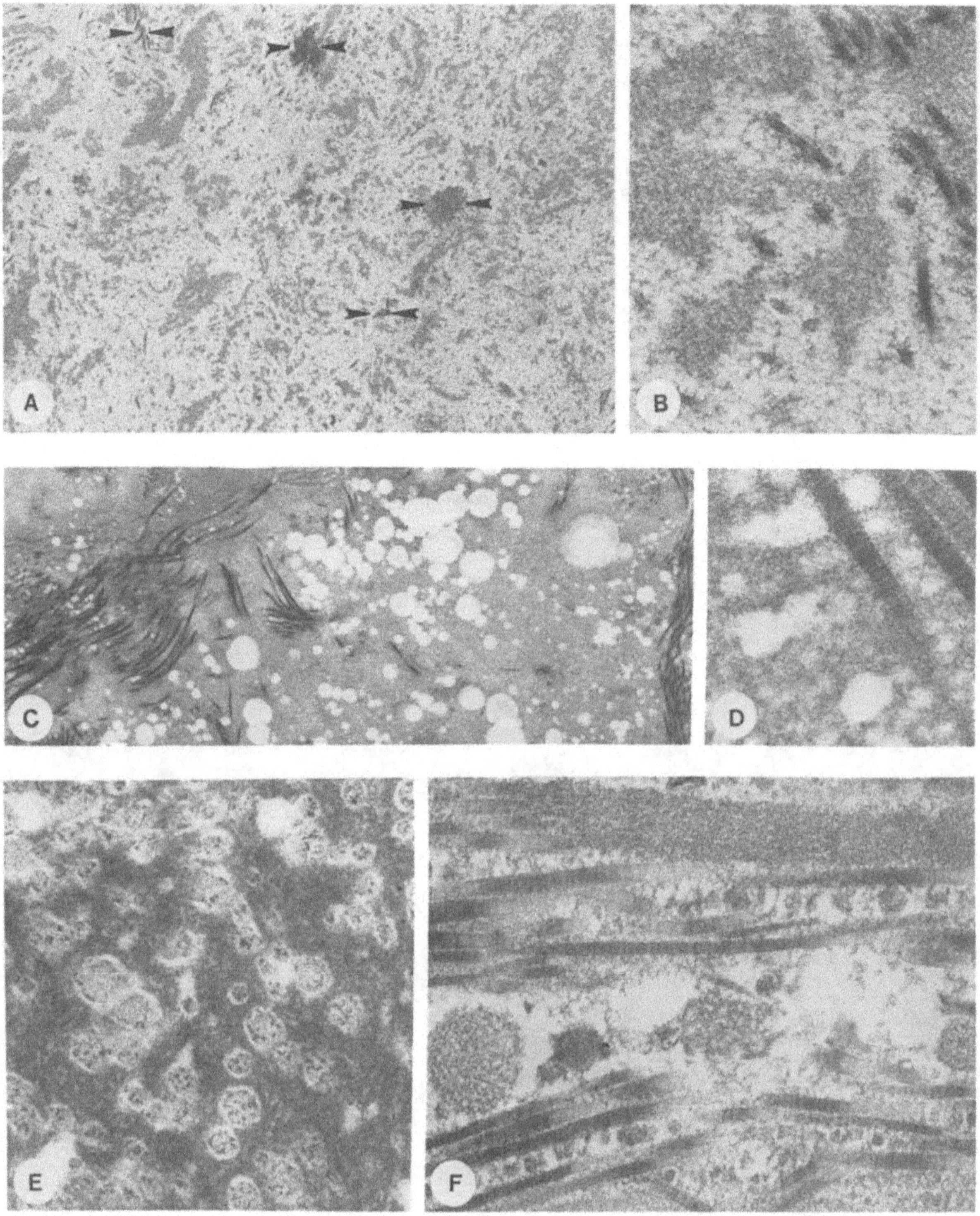

FIGURE 13. Electron micrographs of late changes in collagen in porcine valve heterografts. **A** and **B,** two views of collagen adjacent to area of tear in valve (implanted for 76 months) from Patient 12 (compare with light micrographs in Fig. 15 and 17). **A,** low magnification view of an area of almost complete destruction of collagen. Bundles of collagen that remain in this area are indicated by **arrowheads. B,** high magnification view of area shown in **A**. Collagen fibrils are surrounded by fine fibrils, some of which form patches of irregular shapes. **C** and **D,** two views of another area of the same valve as in **A** and **B,** showing lipid accumulation and severe loss of collagen fibrils, of which only a few darkly stained bundles remain. Granular material, present throughout in large amounts and shown at high magnification in **D,** is thought to represent the end stage of collagen destruction. **E,** punctate densities are present in transversely sectioned collagen fibrils in valve (implanted for 30 months) from Patient 10. Surrounding areas of matrix appear extremely dense, except for small lucent areas that probably represent lipid. **F,** fraying and disruption of collagen in a valve (implanted for 21 months) from Patient 9 are associated with marked variation in intensity of staining of fibrils and with formation of granules of fibrinoid-like material. (**A** ×9,600, **B** ×33,750, **C** ×11,500, **D** ×60,000, **E** ×75,000, **F** ×45,000, all reduced by 8 percent.)

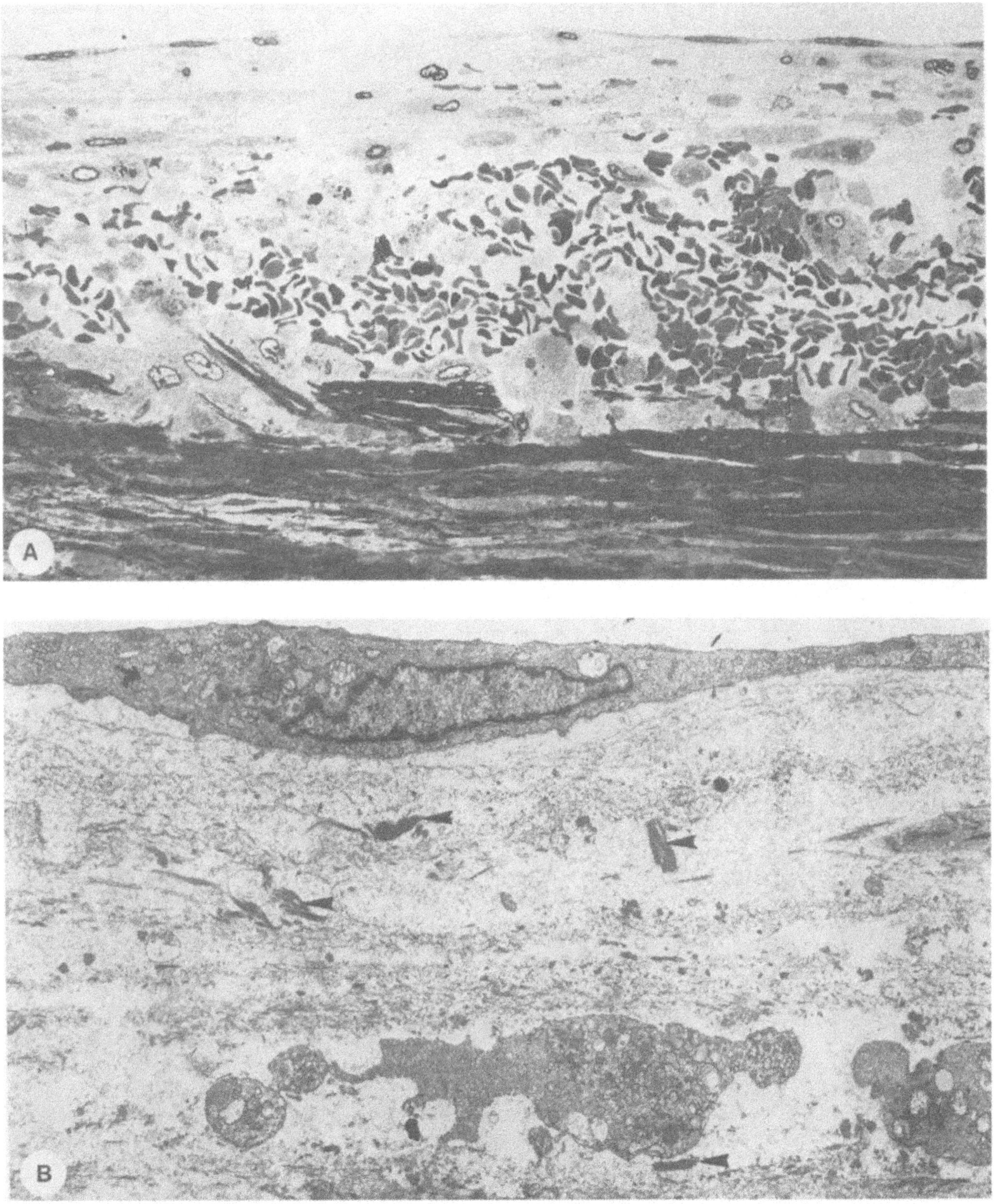

FIGURE 14. Light **(A)** and electron **(B)** micrographs of endothelial cells covering thrombus on outflow surface of a valve (implanted for 21 months) from Patient 9. **A,** mononuclear cells lie within thrombus that is covered with a monolayer of flattened, elongated endothelial cells. Collagen bundles in the area of the fibrosa immediately subjacent to thrombus are fragmented. **B,** endothelial cell, connected **(upper right)** to adjacent cell by a small area of intercell junction, overlies layered thrombus that contains strands of fibrin **(arrowheads)** and several fragments of necrotic cells. (*Toluidine blue stain ×600[**A**], ×11,400[**B**], both reduced by 1 percent.)

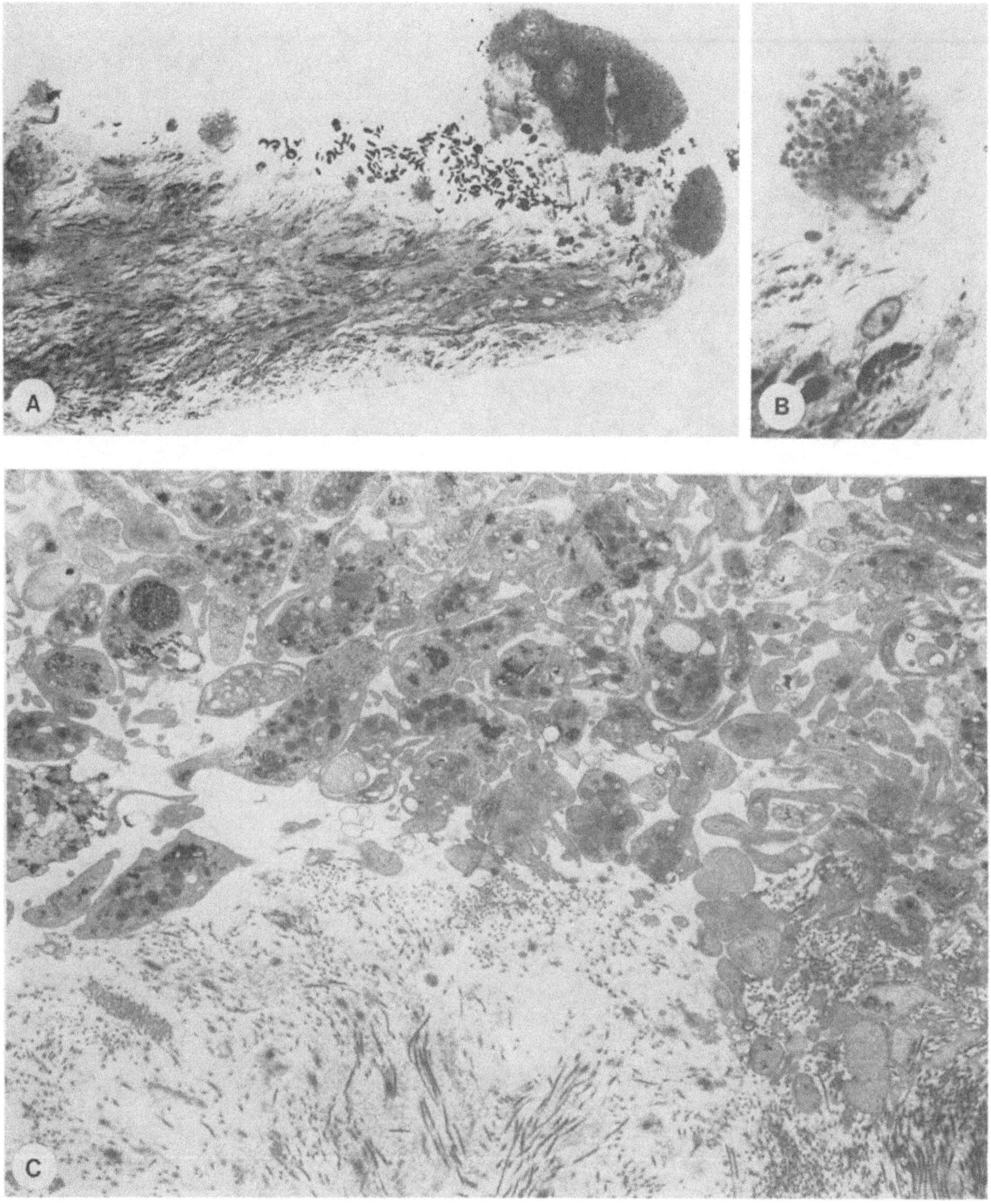

FIGURE 15. Light (**A** and **B**) and electron (**C**) micrographs of aggregates of platelets in a valve from Patient 12. **A,** section through the area adjacent to a tear (the edge of which is seen at **far right**) in the leaflet. Collagen in this area is greatly disrupted, and layers of valve connective tissue are not recognizable. The outflow surface **(top)** is covered with red blood cells and with several aggregates of platelets. **B,** aggregate of platelets (shown at upper left in **A**) is connected to the surface of the valve by a narrow pedicle. **C,** base of a platelet aggregate similar to that shown in **B.** The platelets are in direct contact with severely disrupted collagen in the valve surface; they are well preserved and contain abundant glycogen. (**A** and **B** alkaline toluidine blue stain ×250 and ×750, respectively; **C** ×13,000.)

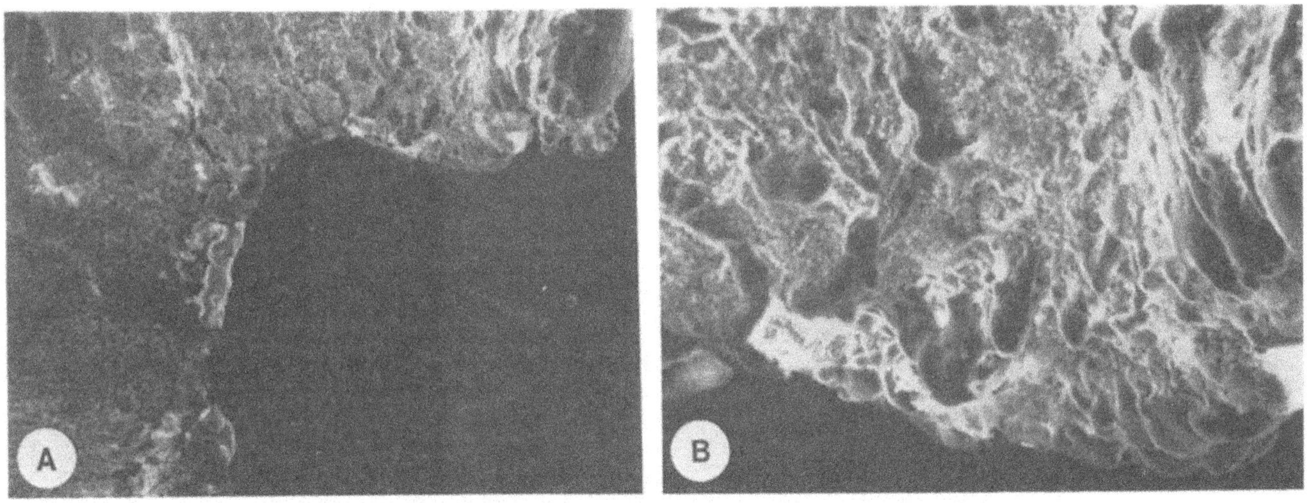

FIGURE 16. Scanning electron micrographs of the V-shaped tear in the free edge of the leaflet of the valve shown in Figure 15. These are severe damage and erosion of the valve surface, with considerable loss of valve tissue. (**A** ×30, **B** ×150, both reduced by 1 percent.)

sheath) was observed in any valve leaflet. Ingrowth of host fibrous tissue into the sewing ring is known to develop in implanted Hancock valves.[6]

Platelet aggregates: Platelet aggregates (as opposed to simple adherence of single platelets to the surfaces) were observed in 2 valves; one of these had been implanted for 21 months, the other for 75 months. These aggregates consisted of spherical masses of clumped platelets that appeared morphologically normal, contained abundant glycogen, showed extensive surface processes and were not associated with fibrin (Fig. 15). The platelets at the base of the aggregates were in direct contact with valve collagen and with finely fibrillar material presumed to be derived from disrupted collagen. Such aggregates were very frequent and large (up to 60 μ in diameter) in the valve that had been implanted for 76 months. This valve also showed several tears in the leaflets (Fig. 16 and 17). Scanning electron microscopic examination (Fig. 16) revealed extensive erosion of the valve surfaces at, and adjacent to, the edges of these tears. Study by transmission electron microscopy (Fig. 13, A and B) confirmed the occurrence of this erosion and showed that the collagen in large areas of the fibrosa had undergone almost complete disruption and transformation into finely fibrillar material. Apparently unaltered elastic fibers were observed in the midst of severely disrupted collagen.

Valve infection: One valve showed anatomic evidence of infection, characterized by the presence of colonies of bacteria deep in the substance of the cusps. This valve, which grossly appeared shaggy and necrotic, was removed from the mitral position at operation from a 44 year old man who had signs of valve dysfunction and a mean diastolic pressure gradient of 34 mm Hg across the prosthesis. Although febrile at the time of admission, the patient did not receive antibiotic therapy. Repeated blood cultures and culture of the cuspal tissue removed at reoperation gave negative results. Similarly negative results were obtained on multiple attempts to demonstrate organisms by means of special light microscopic stains. Nevertheless, ultrastructural study (Fig. 18) of pieces of this valve fixed with glutaraldehyde immediately after removal disclosed a number of colonies of spore-forming rod-like bacilli measuring up to 1.5 μ in length and 0.3 μ in width. Some of these organisms appeared dead and consisted mainly of empty shells. Others showed good preservation of internal structure and could have been viable. The organisms were present in deep areas of the cusps and were associated with evidence of severe necrosis of connective tissue, with large deposits of fibrin and with polymorphonuclear leukocytes.

Discussion

Structure of the normal porcine aortic valve and structural changes produced in it by the Hancock process: The normal porcine aortic valve consists of a sheet of connective tissue whose two surfaces are covered by a continuous layer of endothelial cells. the distribution of various connective tissue elements within this sheet of connective tissue is asymmetric, as it is in the human aortic valve,[9-11] with larger and more numerous elastic fibers in areas subjacent to the inflow surface. Our observations show that the structure of the endothelial basement membranes differs in the inflow and outflow surfaces of the porcine aortic valve. The basement membrane is poorly defined in the inflow surface, but it is prominent and reduplicated or multilayered in the outflow surface, where collagen is denser and elastic fibers are small and sparse. The two surfaces also appear different on scanning electron microscopic examination: The inflow surface is much smoother than the outflow surface, which shows a series of transversely oriented ridges that are clearly visible at low magnification (×100 or less). These ridges appear to provide important structural support to the cusps, particularly when they close.

The loss of endothelium from the surfaces of processed but implanted valves, especially from the inflow surface, presumably is a consequence of postmortem autolysis and of handling of the valves during processing. Thus, the endothelial barrier is largely destroyed in these valves. The two surfaces of processed, unimplanted valves appeared markedly different when examined by scanning electron microscopy at magnifications of ×2,000 or higher. The very smooth appearance of the outflow surface is attributable to the fact that endothelium covering this surface is detached along a plane of cleavage that extends relatively smoothly between reduplicated layers of basement membrane material. Conversely, the rough appearance of the inflow surface appears to be a consequence of the lack of reduplication of the basement membrane, for which reason the plane of cleavage for endothelial detachment

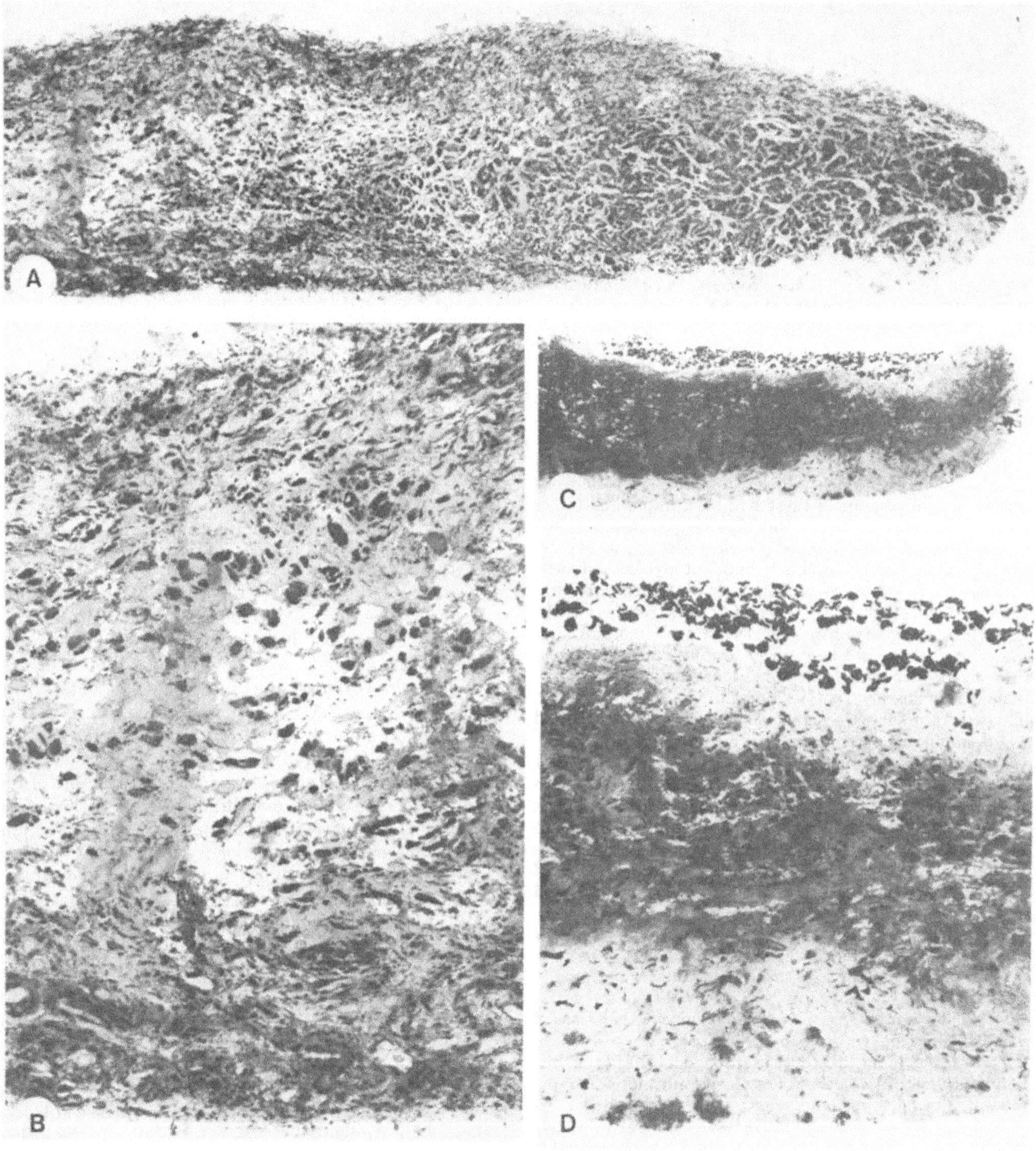

FIGURE 17. Light micrographs of structural changes in areas adjacent to edges of two tears in the valve shown in Figures 15 and 16. **A** and **B,** low and high magnification views of an area showing clear spaces, indicative of loss of tissue, in the middle of the leaflet. The collagen is markedly altered (compare with electron micrographs of this area, shown in Fig. 13, A and B), and much of it appears homogeneously gray. The tear presumably developed as a consequence of disruption of collagen and erosion of leaflet substance. **C** and **D,** views of another tear in the leaflet. Valve tissue in this area is different from that shown in **A** and **B** in that normal-appearing bundles of collagen are virtually absent. Instead, a central dense layer (remnant of fibrosa?) of homogeneous material and two peripheral, less dense layers of severely disrupted collagen are evident. Collagen in this area was ultrastructurally similar to that in **A** and **B.** (**A** ×100, **B** ×400, **C** ×50, **D** ×200, all reduced by 1 percent.)

extends in an irregular manner between the most superficial layers of collagen and elastin of the inflow surface. These findings were confirmed by transmission electron microscopic study of processed, unimplanted valves.

Other than the loss of endothelium, two observations on processed unimplanted valves are noteworthy: the loss of acid mucopolysaccharide spicules and finely filamentous components of connective tissue, and the poor quality of preservation of the membranes and organelles of valve fibroblasts. Loss of acid mucopolysaccharide material may be the first step in the loosening that the connective tissue framework of the valve undergoes after implantation. This loss is not surprising, given the extreme solubility in water of acid mucopolysaccharides and the known difficulty in retaining these components in tissues during the process of fixation with histologic reagents.[15] It is obvious that the concentration of glutaraldehyde used either in the Hancock or in the Carpentier-Edwards process is not sufficiently great to produce tissue fixation of a quality comparable with that needed for ultrastructural study.

Postimplantation changes in porcine aortic valves: Postimplantation changes observed in our study of Hancock valves are qualitatively similar in many respects to those described in structural studies of other types of bioprostheses, including variously processed valve homografts, formalin-treated valve heterografts and fascia lata valves.[12,16–30] Ultrastructural observations thus far published on biologic tissue valves are summarized in Table III. We are aware of only one ultrastructural study of glutaraldehyde-treated porcine aortic valves[28]; this study, which described valves that had been treated with the Carpentier process, alluded briefly to changes resembling those reported herein.

Stages of postimplantation changes: Although postimplantation changes in porcine aortic valves represent a continuum of alterations, they can be classified into three stages. The first is characterized by the deposition of a thin microscopically visible layer of fibrin on the valve surfaces and by penetration of plasma proteins into the valve substance. During the second stage, macrophages are deposited upon the valve surfaces, erythrocytes penetrate into crevices into the more superficial areas of the cusps, and collagen breakdown begins. During the third stage, severe breakdown of collagen occurs and lipid is deposited in the cusps. Foci of calcium were observed in only one valve studied by us. These foci were present at and near the commissures and were also identified on radiography. For technical reasons, these foci were not examined with electron microscopy. Similar foci have been described in a previous study[6] of Hancock valves in place for long periods. Thus, deposition of calcium also appears to be a feature of the third stage of changes after implantation.

Deposition of fibrin on the surface of Hancock valves: This was an early alteration, as shown by its occurrence in valves that had been implanted for only 2 and 3 days. Fibrin deposits appeared to be laid down in direct contact with the most superficial layers of valve collagen and frequently were not associated with blood cells. These deposits formed a thin discontinuous layer that did not endothelialize and showed little tendency to increase in thickness with time. These findings are in accord with clinical observations showing that thromboembolism is not a major problem in the clinical use of glutaraldehyde-treated porcine valve hetero-

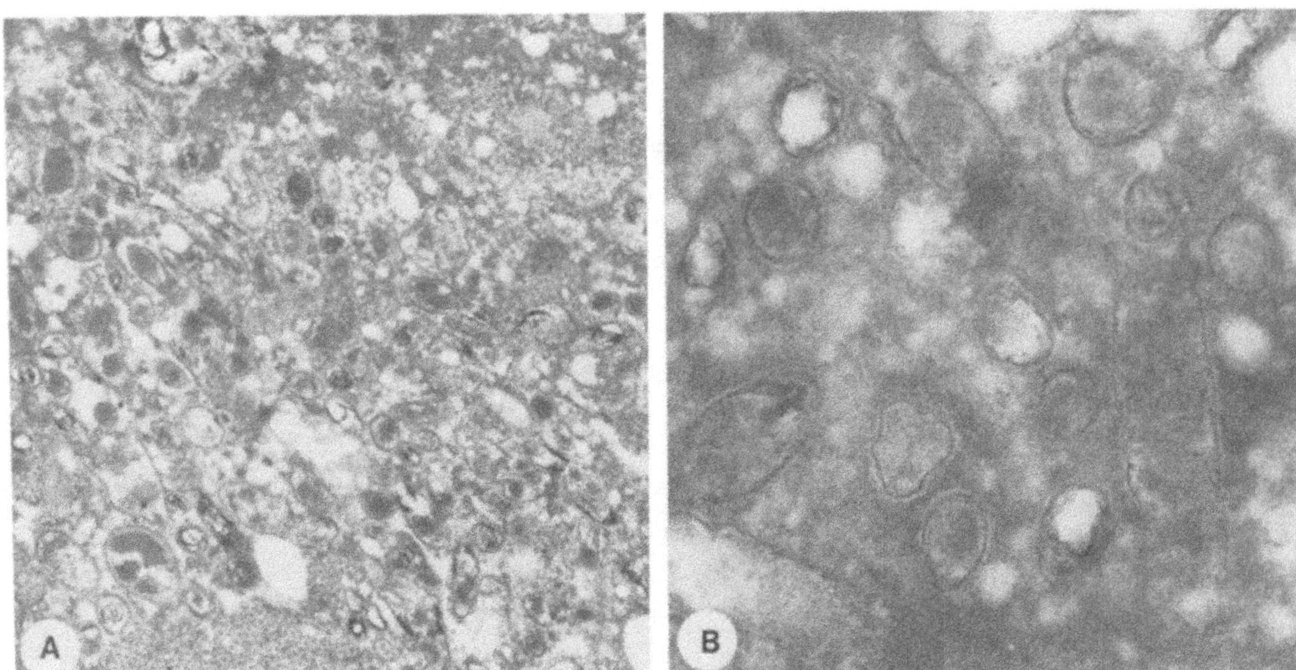

FIGURE 18. Low **(A)** and high **(B)** magnification views of colonies of rod-shaped bacteria that had invaded the valve heterograft of Patient 10 and were located in an area of marked breakdown of connective tissue. (**A** ×20,800, **B** ×64,000, both reduced by 1 percent.)

TABLE III

Ultrastructural Observations on Cardiac Valve Bioprostheses

Author	Type of Valve	Species	Preimplantation Treatment	Implantation Into: Species	Implantation Into: Site	Implant Duration (Days)	Morphologic Changes: Endothelial Cells	Fibrin Dep.	Cell Infiltr.	Breakdown of Coll.	Breakdown of El.	Other
Gavin *et al.*[16]	AV, PV	Dog	(a) None; (b) antibiotics; (c) antibiotics, CM	Not implanted	–	–	–	–	–	–	–	Death of fibroblasts
Girinath et al.[17]	AV, PV	Dog	Antibiotics	None. Kept in CM up to 35 days	–	–	–	–	–	–	–	Death of fibroblasts
Gavin and Monro[18]	AV, PV	Dog	(a) None; (b) antibiotics	Dog	MV	Up to 636	Growth over fibrous sheath	+	RBC, PMN, Macr.	+	+	loss of fibroblasts
Hammon et al.[12]	AV	Dog	Antibiotics	Dog	MV	7–365	Gradual loss	+	Few round cells	–	–	Exposed, disordered Coll. bundles
Reichenbach et al.[19]	AV, PV	Human	(a) BPL, Fr.; (b) Fr.-D	Human	AV	21–900	0	+	RBC, Macr., PLC	+	–	Granular hyaline matrix along Coll.
Gavin et al.[20]	AV, PV	Human	(a) BPL; (b) EO, Hanks' or Fr.-D.	Human	AV, MV	182–455	0	+	Macr, Lym., RBC	0	0	Fibrinoid change
Wheeler *et al.*[21]	AV, PV	Human	(a) Antibiotics; (b) BPL	Human	AV, MV, TV	300–1855	0	+	RBC, Macr. PMN	–	–	–
Gavin et al.[22]	AV, PV	Human	Antibiotics	Human	AV, MV, TV	<1–1176	0	+	RBC, Macr.	0	0	Loss of fibroblasts
Gavin et al.[23]	AV	Human	Hanks'	Human	AV	98–3094	Growth over fibrous sheath	+	Macr., Lym., PLC	0	0	Loss of fibroblasts
Gersbach & Wegmann[24]	Fascia lata	Human	None	Human	AV	410–2820	0	+	Lym., monocytes	+	0	Areas of necrosis and Ca++
Willén et al.[25]	Fascia lata	Human	None	Human	AV, MV	540–1230	Discontinuous	+	Mononuclear cells, Macr.	–	–	Granular material on surface
Willén et al.[26]	Fascia lata	Human	None	Human	AV, MV	540–1230	–	–	–	0	0	Viable fibrocytes
Rose[27]	AV	Pig	Form.	Human	MV	2–960	–	+	Mononuclear cells, PLC	+	0	
Yaroshinsky et al.[28]	AV	Human, pig	(a) None; (b) BPL; (c) form; (d) glut.; (e) rad. & Fr.	Human	MV, TV	365–1740	–	–	Fibroblast-like cells	+	0	Coll. changes greater in BPL- and Form.- than in Glut.-treated valves

TABLE III (cont'd)

Ultrastructural Observations on Cardiac Valve Bioprostheses

Author	Type of Valve	Species	Preimplantation Treatment	Implantation Into: Species	Implantation Into: Site	Implant Duration (Days)	Morphologic Changes: Endothelial Cells	Fibrin Dep.	Cell Infiltr.	Breakdown of Coll.	Breakdown of El.	Other
Aparicio et al.[29]	AV, PV	Human	(a) BPL, Fr.-D; (b) Rad.	Human	AV, MV	3–1620	0	+	RBC, PMN, "Eosinophilic cells"	+	+	Fibrinoid change in Coll.
		Pig	(a) BPL, Fr.-D; (b) Rad.	Human	AV, MV	3–1620	0	+	RBC,PMN Macr.	+	–	Coll. preservation reasonable; phagocytosis of Coll.
Okamura et al.[30]	AV, PV	Pig	Hanks', MP, EG, glut.	Dog	TV	7–183	0	+	Mononuclear cells, Lym., Macr.	+	0	Ca++
Present study	AV	Pig	Glut.	Human	AV, MV, TV	2–2280	0	+	Macr., Lym., RBC, Plat.	+	0	

+ = present; 0 = absent; – = data not available; AV = aortic valve; BPL = β-propiolactone; Ca++ = calcific deposits; CM = culture medium; Coll. = collagen; Dep. = deposits; EG = ethylene glycol; EL = elastin; EO = ethylene oxide; Form. = formaldehyde; Fr. = freezing; Fr.-D. = freeze-drying; glut. = glutaraldehyde; Infiltr. = infiltrate; Lym. = lymphocytes; MP = metaperiodate; MV = mitral valve; Macr. = macrophages; PLC = plasma cells; PMN = polymorphonuclear leukocytes; PV = pulmonary valve; Plat. = platelets; Rad. = γ-irradiation; RBC = red blood cells; TV = tricuspid valve.

grafts.[31-38] These findings can be interpreted as suggesting that glutaraldehyde-treated porcine valve heterografts have very little tendency to induce formation of fibrin deposits, aggregates of platelets, or thrombi. To a certain extent this appears to be true, and it seems reasonable to believe that the glutaraldehyde treatment reduces the thrombogenic properties of the connective tissue components of these valves. Nevertheless, the study of Spray and Roberts[6] showed that fibrin thrombi on the outflow surfaces of Hancock valves are common, in spite of the low incidence of clinically apparent thromboembolic episodes. As summarized in Table III, fibrin deposition on the surfaces of leaflets is a consistent finding in many different types of prosthetic tissue valves. Therefore, such a deposition does not seem to depend upon the type of preimplantation treatment of the valve.

Our ultrastructural observations point to the possibility that small fibrin deposits and platelet aggregates form continuously on the surfaces of Hancock valves and that, because of the mechanical forces to which they are subjected, the large majority of such deposits or aggregates are shed from the surfaces into the bloodstream before they have had an opportunity to grow to a large size. Thus, the brief period of adherence to the valve surfaces may be the reason why many of the fibrin deposits found on the surfaces of porcine valve heterografts show no evidence of organization or endothelialization. The fact that fibrin deposits and cells were more numerous on the outflow surfaces is in agreement with the concept that the forces of flow (shear stress) are greater on the inflow than on the outflow surfaces of the valves. Therefore, fibrin deposits on the outflow surfaces would be less easily removed and would be expected to be larger and to show evidence of organization, as indeed was found in this study.

Platelet aggregates on valve surface: A situation similar to that just described may be involved in the formation and detachment of aggregates of platelets, such as those we observed in two of the valves in place for long periods. It appears unlikely that platelet aggregates such as those shown in Figure 15 would remain attached for a long time to the cusp surfaces, to which they are anchored by only a few strands of collagen. The association of these platelet aggregates with collagen is not surprising because collagen is well known to induce aggregation of platelets. In fact, these valves might be expected to be much more extensively covered with platelets. The fact that they are not covered with platelets suggests that the ability of collagen to induce platelet aggregation is diminished by treatment of the valves with the glutaraldehyde process, and that this ability again becomes significant after collagen breakdown has occurred. Because of the association of collagen with platelet aggregates and fibrin deposits, it appears likely that some collagen forming part of the valve surface becomes detached together with these deposits, and that this loss of collagen contributes to erosion of the valve surface. It should be pointed out that aggregates of platelets are not unique to tissue valves: Similar aggregates have been observed on the surfaces of Silastic poppets in mechanical prostheses of the ball-valve type[39,40] and on the surfaces of native aortic valves that have become stenotic.[41]

Thus, these findings suggest that (1) in patients with porcine valve heterografts fibrin or platelet microemboli may develop more frequently than is clinically suspected; (2) many of these microemboli are too small to produce clinical signs or symptoms, and (3) morphologic methods reveal the presence of platelet aggregates on the surfaces of valves only when their rate of formation is very high.

Diffusion of plasma proteins into valve substance: In the absence of direct demonstration (that is, by immunofluorescence) of the presence of plasma proteins in the valvular substance, it can only be presumed that these proteins diffuse into the matrix spaces between the collagen fibrils. That such a diffusion does occur, and that it begins at a very early stage (by 2 or 3 days after implantation), is suggested by the appearance of a finely filamentous or amorphous, moderately electron-dense material in matrix areas that were electron-lucent before implantation of the valve. This material differed morphologically from the acid mucopolysaccharide spicules and filaments present in unprocessed unimplanted valves but appeared similar to that we have observed in edematous myocardial interstitium in various conditions associated with extravascular leakage of plasma proteins.[42] Such diffusion of plasma proteins, which would be expected to occur because of the loss of the endothelial barrier, would make it possible for the proteolytic enzymes in plasma to attack the connective tissue components of the valves. Accordingly, one would expect the consequences of the activity of such proteolytic enzymes to become manifest only after long intervals after implantation. Thus, the penetration of plasma proteins into the cusps eventually may become an important cause of lysis of collagen. The presence of lipid in the cusps may be related to the penetration of plasma lipoproteins. This phenomenon was observed only after long intervals after implantation, which suggests that it occurs only when the permeability of the surfaces is increased to the point of permitting the passage of very large macromolecules, such as lipoprotein particles, which then become trapped within the cusp substance. The coarse electron-dense granules found in some areas of collagen damage resembled the "fibrinoid" material described by others[43–45] as resulting from the combination of altered collagen with insudated plasma proteins.

Presence of erythrocytes in deep areas of the cusps soon after implantation: This was a somewhat surprising finding, even though this change has been described in homografts.[19] These erythrocytes were morphologically normal and had not been phagocytosed. Therefore, these erythrocytes probably penetrated into the valves through crevices in their surfaces. It is possible that the opening and closing of these crevices during the motion of the cusps in each phase of the cardiac cycle would tend to trap the erythrocytes in these crevices and push them into deeper areas of the valves.

Macrophages and giant cells: The earliest interval after implantation at which macrophages and giant cells were evident on the valve surfaces was 28 days. In other studies of Hancock valves these cells have been observed as early as 14 days.[6] The morphologic features of the organelles were similar in macrophages and giant cells, suggesting a derivation of the latter cells from macrophages. Such a derivation, mediated by cell fusion, has been suggested with respect to giant cells in granulomas,[46–47] cells that in many ways are similar to the giant cells in porcine valve heterografts. Two features of the inflammatory cells in valve heterografts were of unusual interest: (1) The inflammatory cell population was composed almost exclusively of macrophages and giant cells, with few lymphocytes or plasma cells, and (2) the macrophages and giant cells remained on or near the surfaces, with very little tendency to penetrate into deeper areas of the valves. The latter phenomenon may be a manifestation either of a repellent effect of glutaraldehyde-fixed tissue on macrophages or of an inability of macrophages to penetrate into a tissue in which the cross-linking of stromal proteins has been artificially increased by the glutaraldehyde treatment.

Other inflammatory cells: The paucity of other types of inflammatory cells suggests that porcine valve heterografts elicit a foreign body type of reaction rather than a strong immunologic reaction. It has been suggested[30] that the glutaraldehyde treatment reduces the antigenicity of porcine valve heterografts. Plasma cells and lymphocytes form a more prominent component of the cell reaction in homografts.[19,20,23] However, macrophages form a significant part of the cell infiltrate on the leaflet surfaces in other types of tissue valves, including fascia lata valves, homografts and porcine heterografts (Table III) regardless of the preimplantation treatment given to the valves. The presence of numerous plasma cells in porcine heterograft valves treated with formalin[2,27] suggests that formalin fixation is less successful than glutaraldehyde fixation in reducing the antigenicity of the heterologous tissue. The relatively small numbers of macrophages on Hancock valves implanted for long periods of time suggest that after a certain time the valve components that elicit the foreign body type of reaction become dissipated. It is also possible, however, that these cells become more easily detached from the valves as the collagen in the surfaces becomes more extensively disrupted. A direct participation of macrophages in the process of collagen disruption is indicated by the known ability of these cells to produce large amounts of collagenase.[48]

Breakdown of collagen framework of valves: Our most significant finding in relation to valve function is the gradual and progressive breakdown of the collagen framework of the valves with time. Although the breakdown of collagen was of only mild or moderate severity in the valves in place for 3 to 7 months, all valves in place for longer than 21 months showed severe breakdown of collagen. One valve in place for 76 months (the longest interval after implantation in this study) showed tears of the valve cusps, presumably due to failure of the damaged fibrocollagenous framework of the valve to withstand the hemodynamic stress of valve opening and closure. However, in spite of ultrastructural evidence of severe breakdown of collagen, on macroscopic examination most valves appeared unchanged from unimplanted valves. This observation emphasizes two facts: (1) Macroscopic examination of porcine valve heterografts is inadequate to evaluate their state of structural integrity, and (2) these heterografts may continue to function normally, for a yet undetermined period of time, after their collagen is extensively altered.

The ultrastructural findings of collagen breakdown in glutaraldehyde-preserved porcine heterografts are qualitatively similar to the changes seen in other tissue valves (Table III). Fragmentation of collagen, with accumulation of granular material and with loss of staining and periodic banding of collagen, has been observed in homografts treated with various methods of preservation,[19,20] in formalin- and glutaraldehyde-treated porcine heterografts[27,28,30] and in autologous fascia lata valves.[24] However, this process appears to occur more slowly in glutaraldehyde-treated valves than in other types of tissue valves.

Causes of damage to collagen framework: Several possible causes of damage to the collagen in porcine heterograft valves can be suggested: (1) reversal of glutaraldehyde-mediated cross-linking effect, with conversion of collagen from the fibrillar to the soluble form; (2) binding of plasma proteins to collagen, with formation of "fibrinoid"-like material; (3) hydrolysis of collagen by specific collagenases from inflammatory cells and by nonspecific proteolytic enzymes in inflammatory cells and in blood plasma; (4) breakdown of collagen fibrils by mechanical forces of valve motion; (5) erosion of superficial layers of valve collagen by the forces of blood flow (shear stress), and (6) immunologic or foreign-body reaction to the heterologous tissue. Each of these causes may contribute to the overall effect of collagen breakdown. Because the glutaraldehyde-mediated cross-linking of collagen is quite stable in comparison with that produced by other histologic fixatives, the breakdown of collagen by solubilization of the fibrillar form can be expected to be a slow process that might be accelerated by the interaction with other disruptive forces such as hemodynamic stresses and hydrolytic enzymes from plasma and inflammatory cells. In addition, glutaraldehyde fixation increases the brittleness of tissues and, therefore, may contribute to the mechanism of mechanical disruption of collagen.

Absence of endothelialization: The lack of host endothelialization of glutaraldehyde-preserved heterograft valves is in contrast to the development of a so-called "intimal fibrous sheath" in some human aortic valve homografts.[22,23] These sheaths of avascular host tissue extend from the anulus of the valve for varying distances and to varying thicknesses along the surfaces of the valves, causing thickening and stiffening of the cusps. Although these fibrous sheaths may reinforce the structure of the homograft valves by thickening their leaflets, retraction of the avascular fibrous tissue "scar" may lead to deformation of the cusps and resultant regurgitation.[23] Infection contributed to the breakdown of connective tissue in one valve we studied. This infection was detected only with electron microscopic examination, which revealed colonies of organisms with characteristics suggestive of gram-positive bacteria. The cause and duration of this infection could not be determined.

Implications: Although a relatively small number of valves was examined, this study shows that the collagenous framework of glutaraldehyde-treated Hancock porcine valve heterografts undergoes progressive deterioration with time. Glutaraldehyde-treated heterologous tissue valves do not contain viable cells and, therefore, do not have a mechanism for the replacement of the collagen that has broken down. Consequently, deterioration of collagen probably will be the critical factor in determining the durability of these valves.

Acknowledgment

We express our appreciation for the skilled assistance of Mrs. Octavia Dejoie (electron microscopy), Mrs. Esther Wilhoite (photography), Mrs. Dorothy Veigle (secretarial and editorial work) and Mr. Randolph Ross (scanning electron microscopy).

References

1. **Yarbrough JW, Roberts WC, Reis RL:** Structural alterations in tissue cardiac valves implanted in patients and in calves. J Thorac Cardiovasc Surg 65:364–375, 1973
2. **Zuhdi N, Hawley W, Voehl V, et al:** Porcine aortic valves as replacements for human heart valves. Ann Thorac Surg 17:479–491, 1974
3. **Horowitz MS, Goodman DJ, Fogarty TJ, et al:** Mitral valve replacement with glutaraldehyde-preserved porcine heterograft. Clinical, hemodynamic and pathological correlations. J Thorac Cardiovasc Surg 67:885–895, 1974
4. **Pipkin RD, Buch WS, Fogarty TJ:** Evaluation of aortic valve replacement with a porcine xenograft without long-term anticoagulation. J Thorac Cardiovasc Surg 71:179–186, 1976
5. **Fishbein MC, Gissen SA, Collins JJ Jr, et al:** Pathology in patients with glutaraldehyde-fixed porcine cardiac valves. Am J Cardiol 40:331–337, 1977
6. **Spray TL, Roberts WC:** Structural changes in porcine xenografts used as substitute cardiac valves. Gross and histologic observations in 51 glutaraldehyde-preserved Hancock valves in 41 patients. Am J Cardiol 40:319–330, 1977
7. **Kajikawa K, Yamaguchi T, Katsuda S, et al:** An improved electron stain for elastic fibers using tannic acid. J Electron Microsc (Tokyo) 24:287–289, 1975
8. **Binet JP, Planche C, Weiss M:** Heterograft replacement of the aortic valve. In, Biological Tissue in Heart Valve Replacement (Ionescu MI, Ross DN, Wooler GH, ed). London, Butterworths, 1972, p 409
9. **Gross L, Kugel MA:** Topographic anatomy and histology of the valves in the human heart. Am J Pathol 7:445–473, 1931
10. **Clark RE, Finke EH:** Scanning and light microscopy of human aortic leaflets in stressed and relaxed states. J Thorac Cardiovasc Surg 67:792–804, 1974
11. **Clark RE, Finke EH:** The morphology of stressed and relaxed human aortic leaflets. Trans Am Soc Artif Intern Organs 20B:

437–448, 1974
12. **Hammon JW Jr, O'Sullivan MJ, Oury J, et al:** Allograft cardiac valves. A view through the scanning electron microscope. J Thorac Cardiovasc Surg 68:352–360, 1974
13. **Ferrans VJ, Roberts WC:** Structural features of cardiac myxomas. Histology, histochemistry and electron microscopy. Hum Pathol 4:111–146, 1973
14. **Wight TN, Ross R:** Proteoglycans in primate arteries. I. Ultrastructural localization and distribution in the intima. J Cell Biol 67:660–674, 1975
15. **Pearse AGE:** Histochemistry, Theoretical and Applied. Boston, Little, Brown, 1968, p 99
16. **Gavin JB, Monro JL, Wall FM, et al:** Fine structural changes in the fibroblasts of canine heart valves prepared for grafting. Thorax 28:748–755, 1973
17. **Girinath MR, Gavin JB, Strickett MG, et al:** The effects of antibiotics and storage on the viability and ultrastructure of fibroblasts in canine heart valves prepared for grafting. Aust NZ J Surg 44: 170–172, 1974
18. **Gavin JB, Monro JL:** The pathology of pulmonary and aortic valve allografts used as mitral valve replacements in dogs. Pathology 6:119–127, 1974
19. **Reichenbach DD, Mohri H, Merendino KA:** Pathological changes in human aortic valve homografts. Circulation 39: Suppl I:47–56, 1969
20. **Gavin JB, Herdson PB, Barratt-Boyes BG:** The pathology of chemically-sterilized human heart valve allografts. Pathology 4: 175–183, 1972
21. **Wheeler EE, Gavin JB, Herdson PB:** A scanning electron microscopy study of human heart valve allografts. Pathology 4: 185–192, 1972
22. **Gavin JB, Herdson PB, Monro JL, et al:** Pathology of antibiotic-treated human heart valve allografts. Thorax 28:473–481, 1973
23. **Gavin JB, Barratt-Boyes BG, Hitchcock GC, et al:** Histopathology of 'fresh' human aortic valve allografts. Thorax 28:482–487, 1973
24. **Gersbach P, Wegmann W:** Aorta valve replacement using autologous fascia lata transplants. Late morphological changes: an electron microscopic study. Virchows Arch [Pathol Anat] 364: 235–247, 1974
25. **Willén R, Dubiel WT, Johansson L:** Viability and surface properties of autologous fascia lata heart valve grafts. A radioautographic and scanning electron microscopical study. Ann Thorac Surg 18: 597–607, 1974
26. **Willén R, Dubiel WT, Johansson L:** Viability properties in autologous fascia lata heart valve grafts. A transmission electron microscopical study. Ann Thorac Surg 19:494–502, 1975
27. **Rose AG:** pathology of the formalin-treated heterograft porcine aortic valve in the mitral position. Thorax 401–409, 1972
28. **Yaroshinsky YN, Shekhter AB, Artyukhina TV, et al:** Electron microscopy study of the aortic valve allo- and xenotransplants following their prolonged functioning in the human heart. Biull Eksp Biol Med 78:116–119, 1974
29. **Aparicio SR, Donnelly RJ, Dexter F, et al:** Light and electron microscopy studies on homograft and heterograft heart valves. J Pathol 115:147–162, 1975
30. **Okamura K, Yuge I, Kawazoe K, et al:** A comparative study between glutaraldehyde-preserved aortic and pulmonary heterograft valves in the tricuspid position in dogs. J Cardiovasc Surg 17: 178–185, 1976
31. **Carpentier A, Deloche A, Relland J, et al:** Six-year follow-up of glutaraldehyde-preserved heterografts with particular reference to the treatment of congenital valve malformations. J Thorac Cardiovasc Surg 68:771–782, 1974
32. **Horowitz MS, Goodman DJ, Fogarty TJ, et al:** Mitral valve replacement with the glutaraldehyde-preserved porcine heterograft: clinical, hemodynamic, and pathological correlations. J Thorac Cardiovasc Surg 67:885–895, 1974
33. **Stinson EB, Griepp RB, Shumway NE:** Clinical experience with a porcine aortic valve xenograft for mitral valve replacement. Ann Thorac Surg 18:391–401, 1974
34. **McIntosh CL, Michaelis LL, Morrow AG, et al:** Atrioventricular valve replacement with the Hancock porcine xenograft: a five-year clinical experience. Surgery 78:768–775, 1975
35. **Cohn LH, Sanders JH Jr, Collins JJ Jr:** Aortic valve replacement with the Hancock porcine xenograft. Ann Thorac Surg 22:221–226, 1976
36. **Hannah H, Reis RL:** Current status of porcine heterograft prostheses: a 5-year appraisal. Circulation 54: Suppl III:III-27–III-31, 1976
37. **Horowitz MS, Goodman DJ, Hancock EW, et al:** Noninvasive diagnosis of complications of the mitral bioprosthesis. J Thorac Cardiovasc Surg 71:450–456, 1976
38. **Stinson EB, Griepp RB, Oyer PE, et al:** Long-term experience with porcine aortic valve xenografts. J Thorac Cardiovasc Surg 73: 54–62, 1977
39. **Rodman NF, Doty DB, Caughey RC:** Surface ultrastructural studies of mitral valve prosthetic devices. In, Scanning Electron Microscopy 1974, part III: Proceedings of the Workshop on Advances in Biomedical Applications of the SEM, IIT Research Institute, Chicago, 1974, p 729–736
40. **Allwork SP, Norton R:** Surface ultrastructure of silicone rubber aortic valve poppets after long-term implantation. A scanning electron microscope study of four poppets. Thorax 31:742–752, 1976
41. **Stein PD, Sabbah HN, Pitha JV:** Continuing disease process of calcific aortic stenosis: role of microthrombi and turbulent flow. Am J Cardiol 39:159–163, 1977
42. **Ferrans VJ, Levitsky S, Buja LM, et al:** Histological and ultrastructural studies on preserved hearts. Circulation 41: Suppl II: II-104–II-109, 1970
43. **Gitlin D, Craig JM, Janeway JA:** Studies on the nature of fibrinoid in the collagen diseases. Am J Pathol 33:55–77, 1957
44. **Lannigan R, Zaki SA:** Ultrastructure of lesions of rheumatic carditis. J Pathol Bacteriol 93:449–461, 1967
45. **Mohos SC, Wagner BM:** Damage to collagen in corneal immune injury: observation of connective tissue structure. Arch Pathol 88:3–20, 1969
46. **Sutton J, Weiss L:** Transformation of monocytes in tissue culture into macrophages, epithelioid cells, and multinucleated giant cells. An electron microscope study. J Cell Biol 28:303–332, 1966
47. **Black MM, Epstein WL:** Formation of multinucleate giant cells in organized epithelioid cell granulomas. Am J Pathol 74:263–274, 1974
48. **Horwitz AL, Crystal RG:** Collagenase from rabbit pulmonary alveolar macrophages. Biochem Biophys Res Commun 69:296–303, 1976

Ultrastructure of Hancock Porcine Valvular Heterografts

Pre- and Post-Implantation Changes

VICTOR J. FERRANS, M.D., PH.D., THOMAS L. SPRAY, M.D., MARGARET E. BILLINGHAM, M.D., AND WILLIAM C. ROBERTS, M.D.

SUMMARY Scanning and transmission electron microscopic studies were made of: 1) 15 glutaraldehyde-treated porcine valvular heterografts that had been implanted in patients for periods of time ranging from 2 days to 76 months; 2) unimplanted, commercially processed porcine aortic valves; and 3) unprocessed porcine aortic valves. Unimplanted, commercially processed valves showed loss of endothelium and acid mucopolysaccharides. Short-term (< 2 months) post-implantation changes consisted of insudation of plasma proteins, penetration of erythrocytes into surface crevices, formation of a thin surface layer of fibrin, and deposition of macrophages, giant cells and a few platelets. Longer term (> 2 months) changes consisted of progressive disruption of collagen, erosion of valvular surfaces, formation of aggregates of platelets, and accumulation of lipid. The surfaces of the leaflets did not become covered with endothelium or with a fibrous sheath. It is concluded that progressive breakdown of collagen is a critical factor in determining the long-term durability of glutaraldehyde-treated porcine valvular heterografts.

LITTLE IS KNOWN of the structural changes that develop in porcine aortic valvular heterografts after implantation for long periods of time, although gross anatomical and histological studies[1, 2] have suggested that degeneration of collagen may become a major cause of long-term structural and functional failure of these valves. We are reporting our histological and electron microscopic observations on porcine valvular heterografts that had been treated by a stabilized glutaraldehyde process (Hancock Laboratories, Anaheim, California) and had been implanted in patients for different periods of time.

Materials and Methods

The morphologic studies described in detail below were made on 15 porcine valve heterografts obtained either at necropsy (9 patients) or reoperation for valvular replacement (6 patients). These patients (8 women, 7 men) ranged in age from 10 to 65 years. Twelve of the valves had been implanted in the mitral position, two in the aortic position, and one in the tricuspid position. The period of time between implantation and removal of the valves ranged from 2 days to 76 months. Four of the valves had been implanted for less than 1 month, and four others for longer than 2 years.

Morphologic studies were also made of: 1) two non-implanted porcine aortic valves (Hancock Laboratories) one mounted on a flexible stent, the other unmounted; 2) one non-implanted Carpentier-Edwards valve, also mounted on a stent; and 3) one normal porcine aortic valve, which was removed at thoracotomy from an adult animal and was not subjected to the glutaraldehyde processing by which these valves are prepared for implantation. Immediately after removal, all valves were fixed with cold 3% glutaraldehyde in 0.1 M phosphate buffer, pH 7.2. After fixation, central strips extending from the anulus to the free margin of the leaflet were removed from each valve and processed for light microscopy and for transmission and scanning electron microscopy. For transmission electron microscopy, the strips of tissue were washed with buffered sucrose, postfixed with OsO_4, dehydrated and embedded in Maraglas. Sections of this tissue 0.5 μ thick were examined with a light microscope to select areas for ultrathin sectioning. Ultrathin sections were stained either with uranyl acetate and lead citrate, or with the Kajikawa method for demonstration of elastic tissue.[3]

For scanning electron microscopy, the tissues were washed with buffered sucrose, rinsed with distilled water, dehydrated with acetone to the critical point of CO_2, coated with gold-palladium, and examined with a scanning electron microscope.

Results

Morphology of the Normal Porcine Aortic Valve

The two surfaces of the porcine aortic cusp will be referred to in this paper as inflow and outflow surfaces. When the valve is in its normal anatomical (semilunar) position, the inflow surface faces the ventricular cavity, and the outflow surface faces the aortic root. Each aortic valvular leaflet consists of: 1) an *endothelial cell layer* that covers the outflow surface; 2) the *fibrosa,* a layer of dense fibrous connective tissue subjacent to the endothelium of the outflow surface; 3) the *spongiosa,* a layer of more loosely arranged fibrous and elastic connective tissue adjacent to the fibrosa; 4) the *ventricularis,* a thin layer of fibrous connective tissue that is subjacent to the inflow surface and tapers off gradually toward the free edge of the cusp; and 5) the *endothelial cell layer* that covers the inflow surface. This arrangement (figs. 1–4) is similar to that in human aortic valves.[4]

From the Pathology Branch, National Heart, Lung, and Blood Institute, National Institutes of Health, Bethesda, Maryland, and Department of Pathology, Stanford University School of Medicine, Stanford, California.

Address for reprints: Dr. Victor J. Ferrans, Building 10 Room 7N208, National Heart, Lung, and Blood Institute, National Institutes of Health, Bethesda, Maryland 20014.

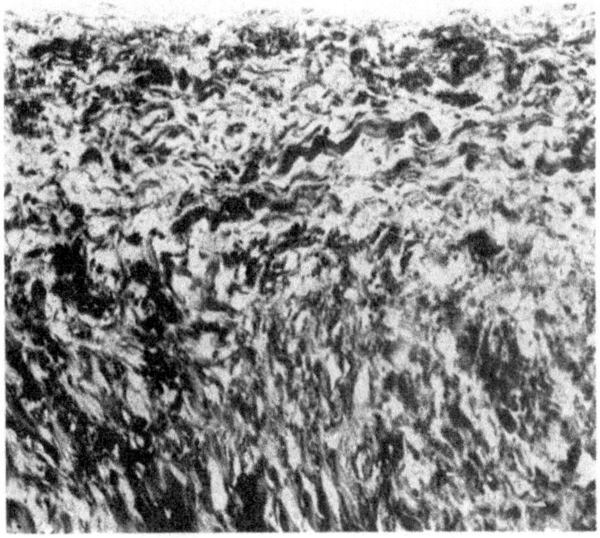

FIGURE 1. *Light micrograph of half-micron-thick section of outflow surface of normal porcine aortic valve, showing densely packed fibrous connective tissue (fibrosa) and endothelial surface layer. Alkaline toluidine blue, × 400.*

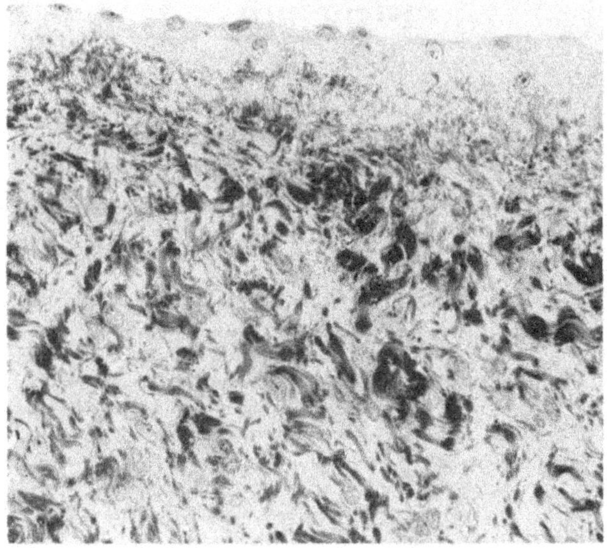

FIGURE 2. *Inflow surface (preparation as in fig. 1) of normal porcine aortic valve, showing loosely arranged connective tissue and surface endothelium. Alkaline toluidine blue, × 400.*

FIGURE 3. *Electron micrograph of outflow surface of normal porcine aortic valve (compare with fig. 1). Note: surface projections from endothelium; junction (J) between adjacent endothelial cells; reduplicated basement membrane (BM); small, sparse elastic fibers (here selectively stained black with Kajikawa method); valvular fibroblast (F) with cisterns of rough-surfaced reticulum; densely packed collagen fibrils (C) and delicate fibrils and spicules of acid mucopolysaccharide material. × 27,000.*

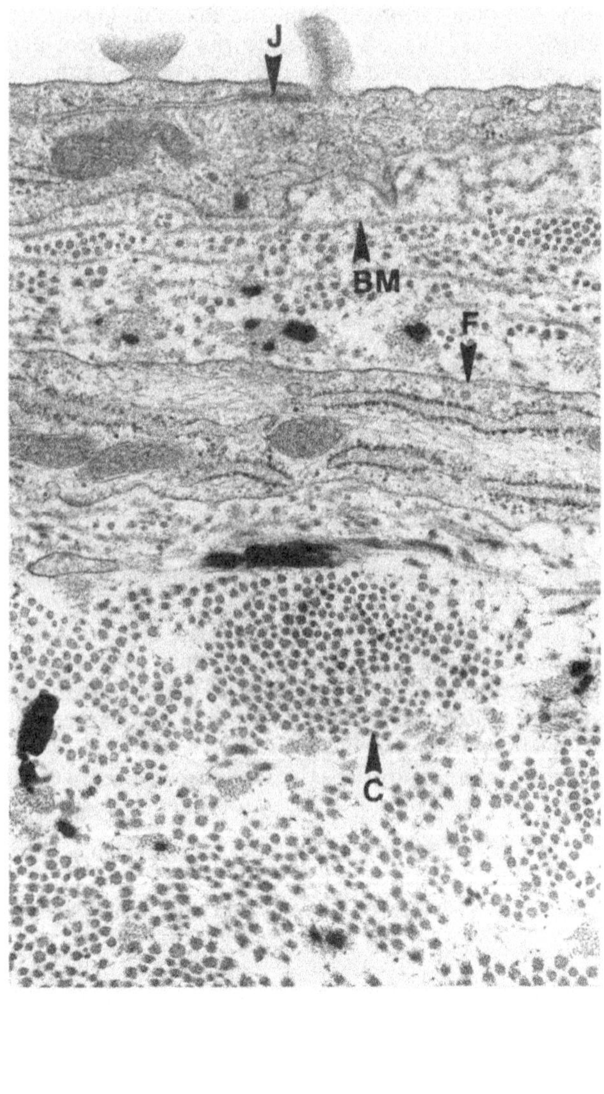

Structure of Unimplanted Hancock and Carpentier-Edwards Porcine Valves

Morphologic studies did not reveal any significant differences between two unimplanted Hancock porcine valves (one mounted and one unmounted) and one mounted, unimplanted Carpentier-Edwards valve. All three valves showed disruption of the endothelial cell layer (fig. 5), with fairly complete loss of endothelial cells from the inflow surface and only partial loss from the outflow surface. On scanning electron microscopic examination, the inflow surfaces of the Hancock valves and the Carpentier-Edwards valve appeared much rougher than the outflow surfaces, appearing composed of small, cylindrical bundles of collagen fibrils and of larger bundles that represented either elastic fibers or large masses of collagen fibrils. In contrast, the outflow surface of each valve appeared smoother, more homogeneous, and composed of material resembling basement membrane; it did not exhibit large numbers of exposed collagen fibrils.

The unimplanted valves also showed loss of the ground substance of connective tissue (fig. 6), in-

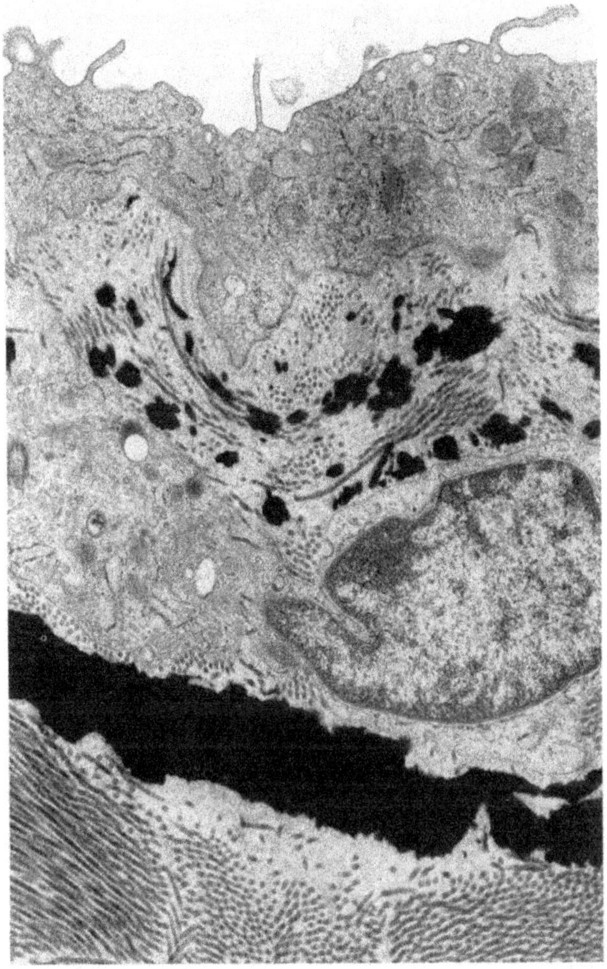

FIGURE 4. *View of inflow surface of normal porcine aortic valve (compare with fig. 3). Note: surface endothelium, valvular fibroblast, large (stained black) elastic fibers (this feature is helpful in identifying the inflow surface of the valve) and subjacent collagen (bottom). Endothelial basement membrane on this surface is not reduplicated. Kajikawa stain. × 15,000.*

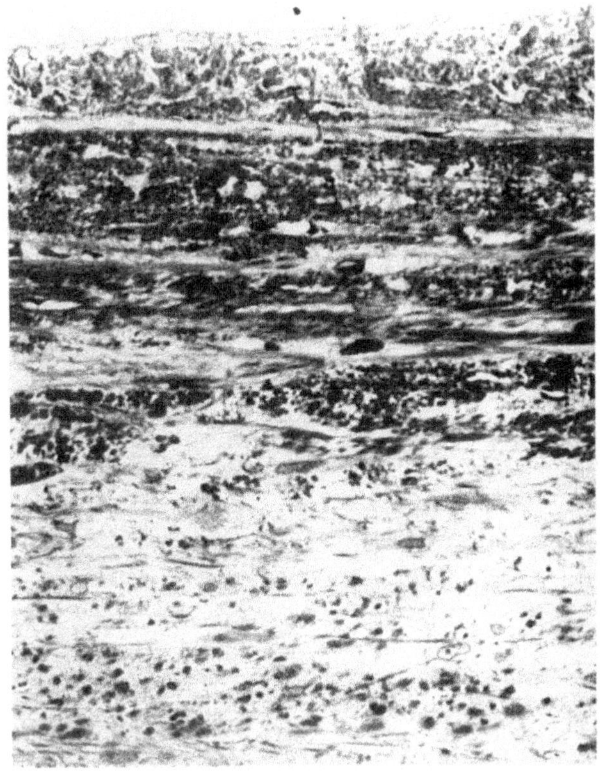

FIGURE 5. *Light micrograph of 0.5 μ thick plastic section, stained with toluidine blue, of unimplanted Carpentier-Edwards valve. Fibrosa (top) appears dense. Spongiosa (bottom) is loosely arranged. Both the outflow (top) and inflow (bottom) surfaces are denuded of endothelium (compare with figs. 1–4). × 250.*

cluding the dense spicules of acid mucopolysaccharides and the network of fine filaments associated with the spicules, so that the collagen fibrils and elastic fibers (both of which remained structurally normal) appeared surrounded by a matrix of greatly increased electron lucency, with some "loosening" of their arrangement. Fibroblasts in these valves showed loss of integrity of cytoplasmic membranes and disruption of organelles.

Morphology of Short-Term (< 2 Months) Implanted Hancock Valves

Structural alterations developed in the surfaces and substances of the valves after implantation (fig. 7). Alterations involving the valvular surfaces consisted of: 1) deposition of fibrin on both surfaces (more on the outflow than on the inflow surface), with formation of small thrombi; 2) entrapment of erythrocytes in a meshwork of fibrin; 3) adherence of erythrocytes, and occasionally of platelets, to the denuded surfaces of the valves; and 4) deposition of macrophages and giant cells on the surfaces, without penetration into the valvular substance.

Changes involving the connective tissue components of the valves included: 1) insudation of plasma proteins into the substance of the leaflets; 2) penetration of erythrocytes and leukocytes into the spongiosa, presumably through crevices in the surfaces; 3) loosening of the arrangement of the bundles of collagen in the spongiosa and to a lesser extent in the fibrosa; and 4) evidence of mild disruption of collagen.

In the two valves that had been implanted for only 2 and 3 days, respectively, structural changes were minimal and consisted of deposition of a thin (< 10 μ in thickness) layer of fibrin (fig. 7) and occasional erythrocytes and platelets on the exposed collagen surfaces. Some insudation of plasma proteins, manifested by the finding of very finely fibrillar material between the collagen fibers, was already evident in superficial layers of the valves (fig. 7).

In the four valves that had been in place for 1 to 2 months, the layers of fibrin were thicker, especially on the outflow surfaces, and macrophages and multi-

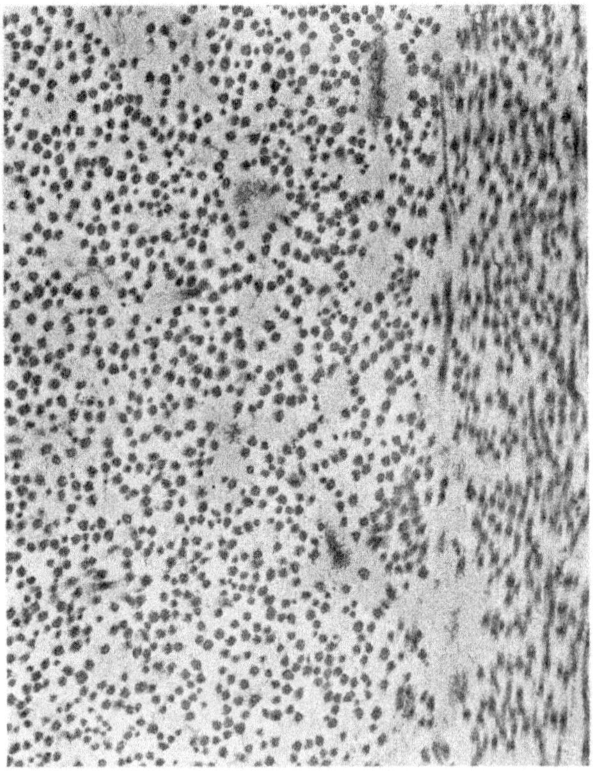

FIGURE 6. *Collagen in fibrosa of unimplanted Hancock valve is associated with electron-lucent matrix.* × *27,000.*

nucleated giant cells lined the surfaces of the leaflets. No phagocytosis of collagen by macrophages was observed. Multinucleated giant cells had organelles similar to those in macrophages. These giant cells showed greatly complex, interdigitating surface folds, and had from two to six irregularly arranged nuclei. Scanning electron microscopic examination confirmed that the leaflets did not endothelialize but became covered with a discontinuous layer of fibrin, blood cells, and macrophages.

Alterations involving collagen fibrils consisted of increased granularity, irregularity of staining, and disruption of the fibrils. The latter change was associated with fraying or tufting of the ends of the collagen fibrils and with the appearance of finely fibrillar or granular material, presumed to be derived from disrupted collagen.

Morphology of Hancock Valves Implanted for 3 to 76 Months

The most significant change observed in Hancock valves implanted for long periods of time (3 to 76 months) was disruption of collagen. The extent to which this change occurred correlated with the length of time the valve had been in place. By light microscopy, collagen breakdown was manifested by disappearance of the bundles of collagen fibrils and by the formation of a homogeneous, hyaline-appearing, pale-staining matrix (fig. 8). By electron microscopy,

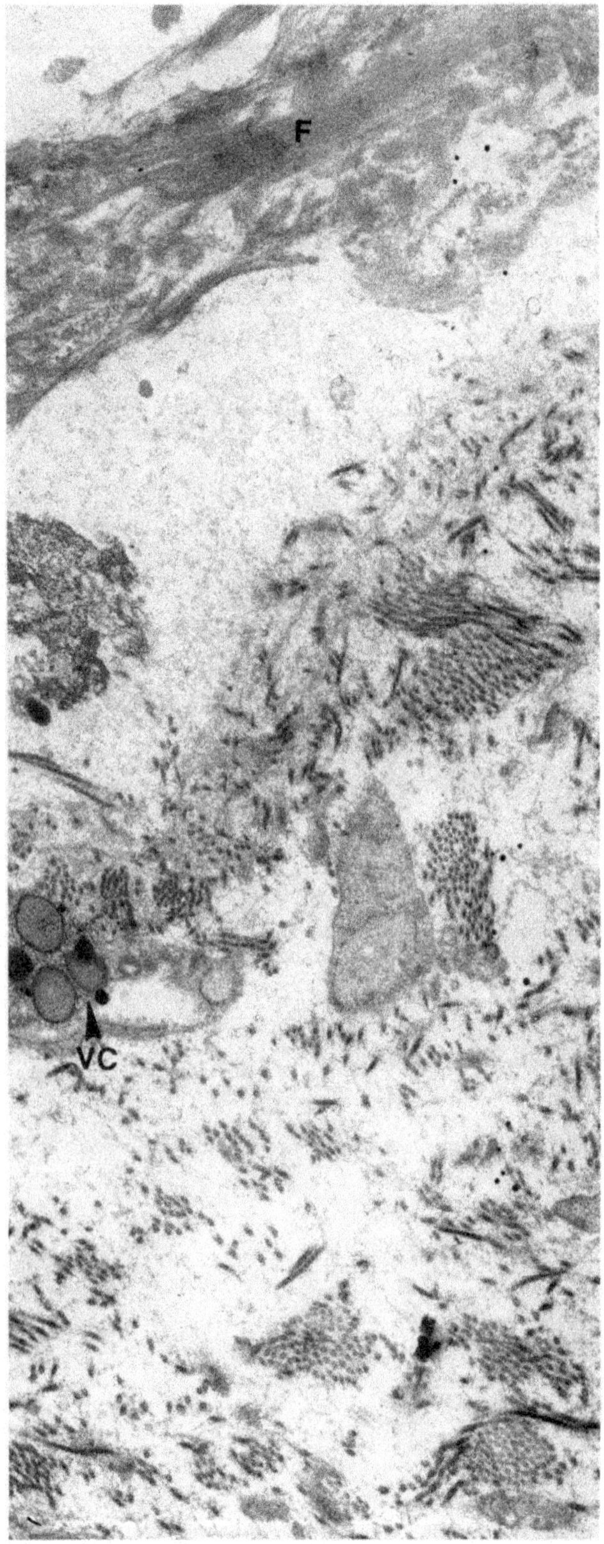

FIGURE 7. *Inflow surface of Hancock valve removed at necropsy 3 days after implantation in the mitral position. Cause of death was recurrent ventricular tachycardia. Note the layer of fibrin (F) at top, the partially disrupted collagen at the surface of the valve, the fine fibrillar material between the collagen fibrils, and fragments of valvular (porcine) cells (VC).* × *18,000.*

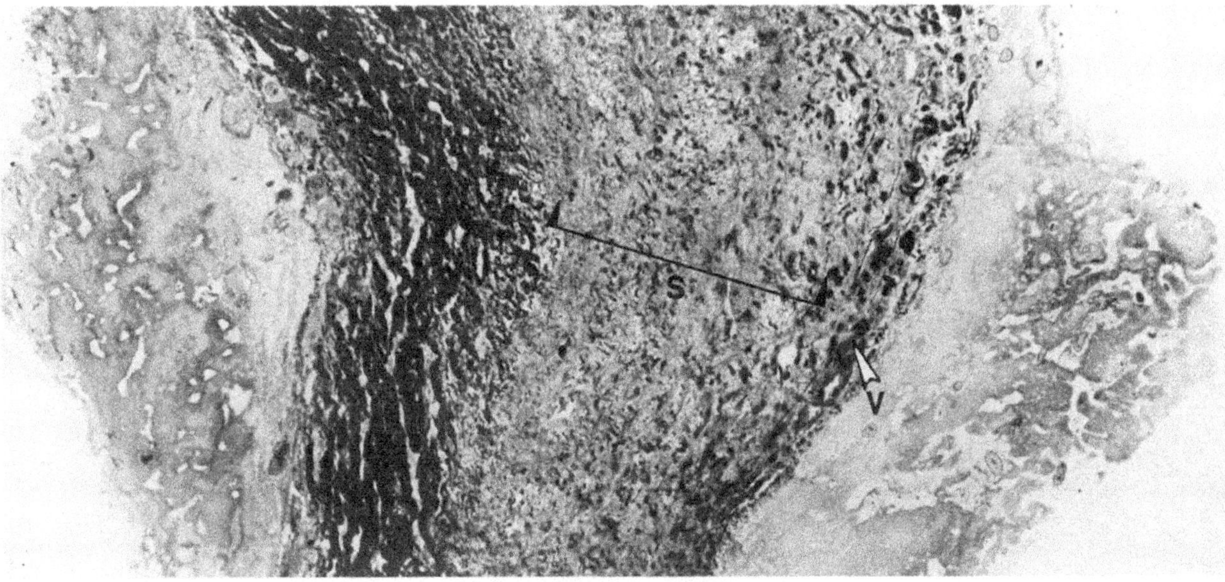

FIGURE 8. *Thick layers of fibrin cover both surfaces (inflow at right, outflow at left) of porcine valve (mitral position) removed because of development of regurgitation 36 months after implantation Ventricularis (V) and spongiosa (S) contain areas in which the darkly stained collagen bundles have been replaced by gray, homogeneous material. Ultrastructurally, such areas resemble those shown in figure 9. × 200.*

areas of disrupted collagen were characterized by the presence of either extremely fine, short, threadlike fibrils or irregular clumps of coarsely granular material resembling fibrinoid (fig. 9). Peculiar punctate densities, ∼ 50 Å in diameter, were often present in collagen fibrils in the process of undergoing disruption. Electron-lucent particles ranging in size from 1000 Å to 1 μ and resembling lipid droplets were present in six of eight valves in place for 7 months or longer. Confirmation of the presence of lipid droplets in these valves was obtained by light microscopic study of frozen sections stained with oil red O.

The surfaces of long-term implants also were associated with variable amounts of fibrin (fig. 8) and variable numbers of erythrocytes, macrophages, and giant cells. Endothelial cells were found only in one valve (implanted for 21 months), in which they formed part of the surface of an incompletely organized thrombus. Valvular (porcine) fibroblasts, which appeared poorly preserved, were still present in all implanted valves. No evidence of fibroblastic ingrowth of host tissue (fibrous sheath) was observed in any valve leaflet.

Platelet aggregates (as opposed to simple adherence of single platelets to the surfaces) were observed in two valves; one of these had been implanted for 21 months, the other for 75 months. These aggregates (fig. 10) consisted of spherical masses of clumped platelets that were not associated with fibrin. The platelets at the base of the aggregates were in direct contact with valvular collagen and with finely fibrillar material presumed to be derived from disrupted collagen. Such aggregates were very frequent and large (up to 60 μ in diameter) in the valve that had been implanted for 76 months. This valve also showed several tears in the leaflets, extensive erosion of the valvular surfaces, and disruption and transformation of collagen in large areas of the fibrosa into finely fibrillar material.

One valve that was removed because of dysfunction 2½ years after implantation showed anatomical evidence of infection, characterized by the presence of colonies of bacteria (spore-forming rod-like bacilli measuring up to 1.5 μ in length and 0.3 μ in width) deep in the substance of the cusps (fig. 11). No growth was obtained on culture of this valve or on blood cultures taken preoperatively.

Discussion

Loss of endothelium from the surfaces of processed but unimplanted valves presumably is a consequence of postmortem autolysis and of handling of the valves during processing. Thus, the endothelial barrier is destroyed in these valves. Loss of acid mucopolysaccharide material from unimplanted valves may be the first step in the loosening that the connective tissue framework of the valve undergoes after implantation. It is obvious that the concentration of glutaraldehyde used either in the Hancock or in the Carpentier-Edwards process is not sufficiently high to produce tissue fixation of a quality comparable to that needed for ultrastructural study.

Post-implantation changes observed in the present study of Hancock valves are qualitatively similar in many respects to those described in structural studies of other types of bioprostheses, including variously processed valvular homografts, formalin-treated valvular heterografts and fascia lata valves.[5-20] We are aware of only one ultrastructural study of glutaraldehyde-treated porcine aortic valves.[18] This study

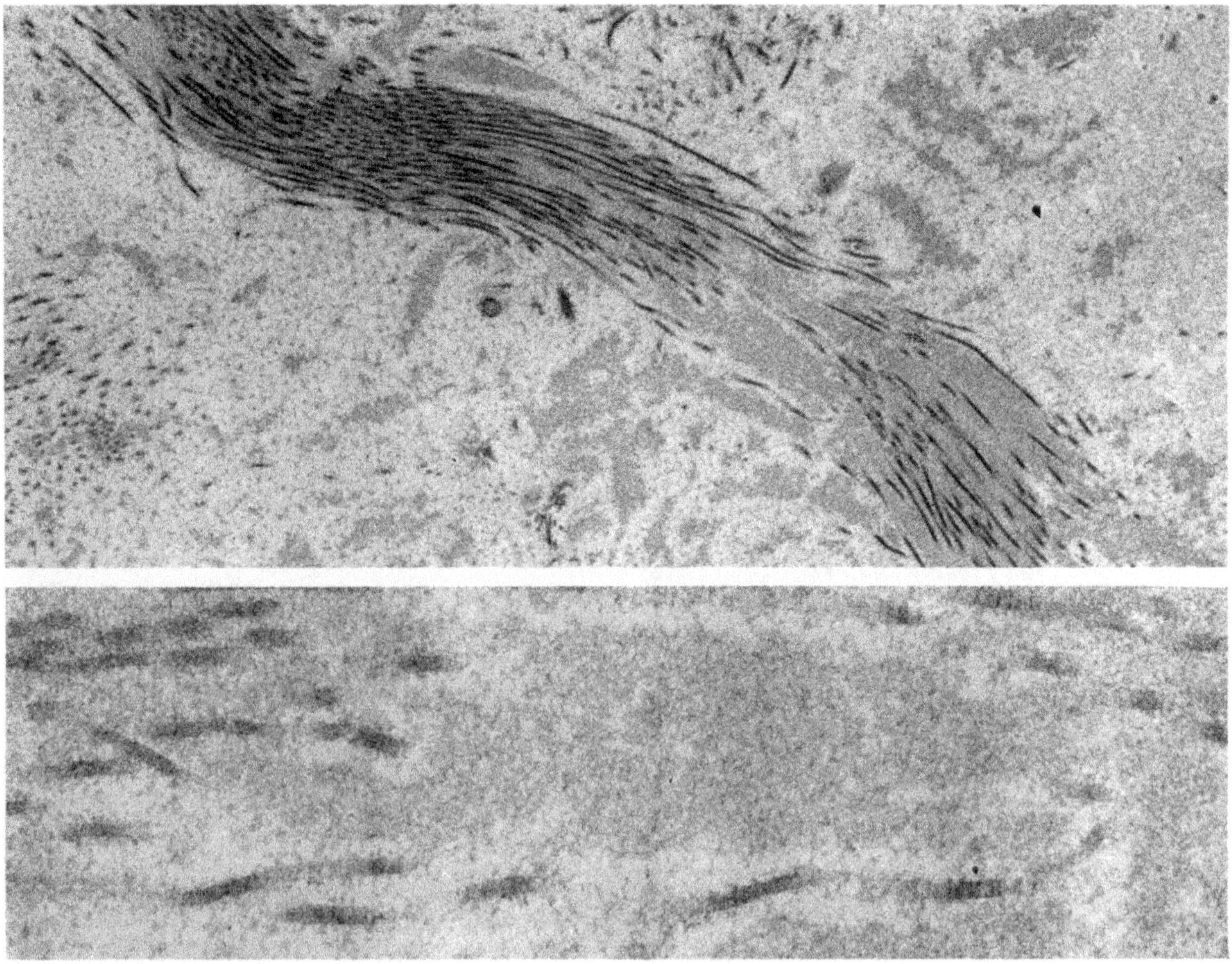

FIGURE 9. *Low (upper) and high (lower) magnification views of fibrosa in porcine valve removed because of dysfunction 76 months after implantation in mitral position. Much of the collagen has been replaced by amorphous or finely filamentous material of low electron density. Disintegrating collagen fibrils that appear to form this material are shown in the lower view. Upper, × 16,500. Lower, × 38,300.*

described valves that had been treated with the Carpentier process, and alluded briefly to changes resembling those reported herein.

Although they represent a continuum of alterations, post-implantational changes in porcine aortic valves can be classified into three stages. The first is characterized by the deposition of a thin, microscopically visible layer of fibrin on the valvular surfaces and by penetration of plasma proteins into the valvular substance. During the second stage, macrophages are deposited upon the valvular surfaces, erythrocytes penetrate into crevices into the more superficial areas of the cusps, and collagen breakdown begins. During the third stage, severe breakdown of collagen occurs, and lipid is deposited in the cusps.

The *deposition of fibrin* on the surface of Hancock valves was an early alteration, as shown by its occurrence in valves that had been implanted for only 2 and 3 days. Fibrin deposits appeared to be laid down in direct contact with the most superficial layers of valvular collagen, forming a thin, discontinuous layer that did not endothelialize and showed relatively little tendency to increase in thickness with time. It seems reasonable to believe that the glutaraldehyde treatment reduces the thrombogenic properties of the connective tissue components of these valves. Nevertheless, the study of Spray and Roberts[1] showed that fibrin thrombi on the outflow surfaces of Hancock valves are common, in spite of the low incidence of clinically apparent thromboembolic episodes. The ultrastructural observations in this report point to the possibility that small fibrin deposits and platelet aggregates form continuously on the surfaces of Hancock valves and that, because of the mechanical forces to which they are subjected, the large majority of such deposits or aggregates are shed from the surfaces into the bloodstream before they have had an opportunity to grow to a large size. It appears unlikely that platelet aggregates would remain attached for a long time to the cuspal surfaces, to which they are anchored only by a few strands of collagen. The association of these platelet aggregates with collagen is not surprising, since collagen is well known to induce aggregation of platelets. The ability of collagen to induce platelet

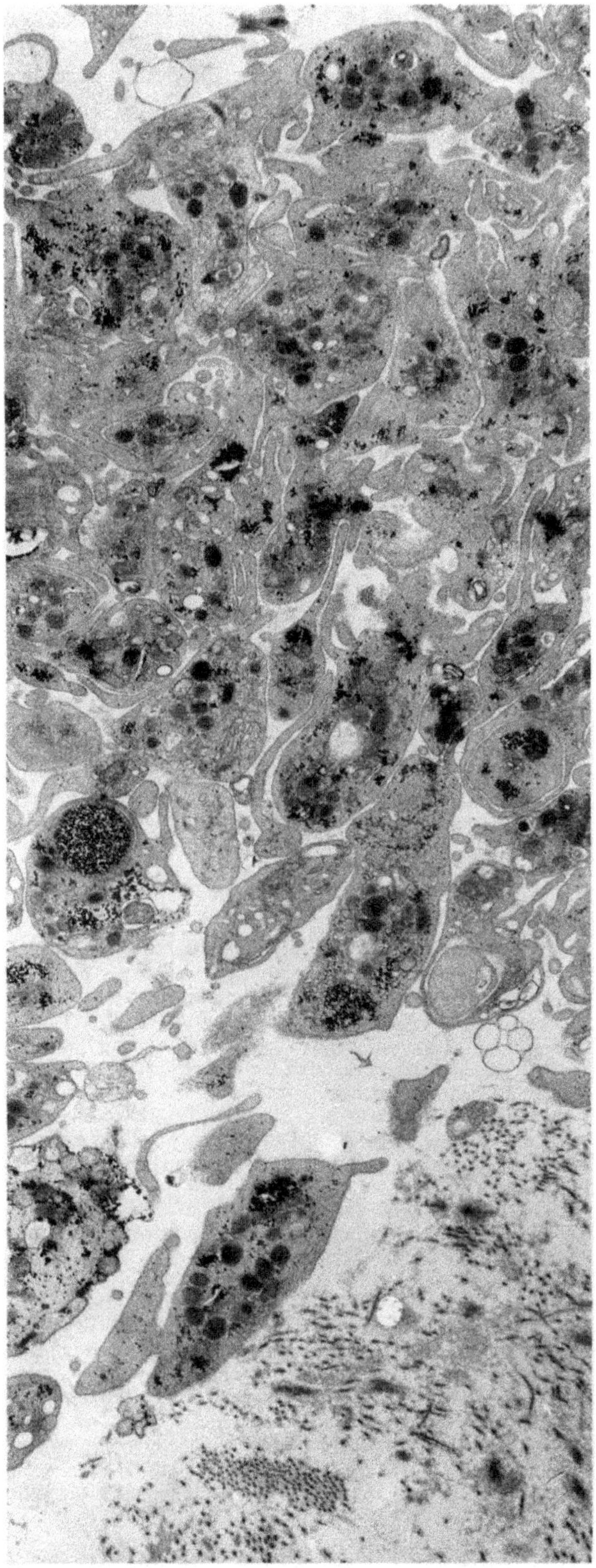

FIGURE 10. *Part of aggregate of platelets attached to disrupted collagen (lower right) in outflow surface of same valve as in figure 9.* × *15,000.*

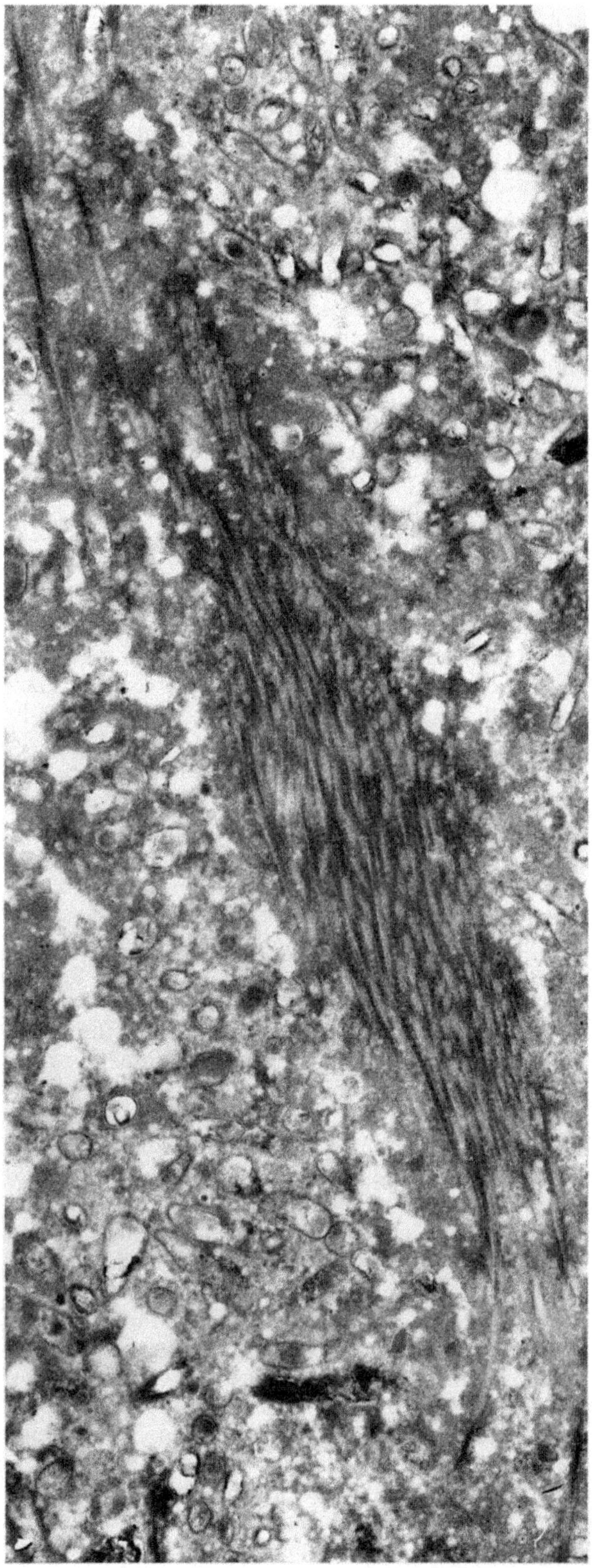

FIGURE 11. *Masses of rod-shaped bacteria are present in severely disrupted connective tissue of valve removed, because of dysfunction, 2½ years after being implanted in mitral position.* × *18,000.*

aggregation appears to be diminished by treatment of the valves with glutaraldehyde, and to again become significant after collagen breakdown has occurred.

That diffusion of plasma proteins into the valvular substance does occur, and that it begins at a very early stage (by 2 or 3 days after implantation), is suggested by the appearance of a finely filamentous or amorphous, moderately electron-dense material in matrix areas that were electron-lucent before implantation of the valve. This material appeared similar to that which we have observed in edematous myocardial interstitium in various conditions associated with extravascular leakage of plasma proteins.[21] Such diffusion of plasma proteins would make it possible for the proteolytic enzymes in plasma to attack the connective tissue components of the valves. Thus, penetration of plasma proteins into the cusps eventually may become an important cause of lysis of collagen. The presence of lipid in the cusps may be related to the penetration of plasma lipoproteins.

Two features of the inflammatory cells in valvular heterografts were of unusual interest. These features were: 1) the inflammatory-cell population was composed almost exclusively of macrophages and giant cells, with few lymphocytes or plasma cells, and 2) the macrophages and giant cells remained on or near the surfaces, with very little tendency to penetrate into deeper areas of the valves. The latter phenomenon may be a manifestation of: 1) a repellent effect of glutaraldehyde-fixed tissue on macrophages, or 2) an inability of macrophages to penetrate into a tissue in which the cross-linking of stromal proteins has been artificially increased by the glutaraldehyde treatment.

In terms of valvular function, the most significant finding of the present study is the gradual and progressive breakdown of the collagenous framework of the valves with time. Although the breakdown of collagen was of only mild or moderate severity in the valves in place for 3 to 7 months, all valves in place for longer than 21 months showed severe breakdown of collagen. One valve in place for 76 months (the longest interval after implantation in this study) showed cuspal tears, presumably due to failure of the damaged fibrocollagenous framework of the valve to withstand the hemodynamic stresses of valvular opening and closure. In spite of ultrastructural evidence of severe breakdown of collagen, however, on macroscopic examination most valves appeared unchanged from unimplanted valves.This observation emphasizes that macroscopic examination of porcine valvular heterografts is inadequate to evaluate their state of structural integrity, and that these heterografts may continue to function normally, for a yet undetermined period of time, after their collagen is extensively altered.

The ultrastructural findings of collagen breakdown in glutaraldehyde-preserved porcine heterografts are qualitatively similar to the changes seen in other tissue valves. Fragmentation of collagen, with accumulation of granular material and with loss of staining and periodic banding of collagen, has been observed in homografts treated by various methods of preservation,[8, 9] in formalin- and glutaraldehyde-treated porcine heterografts,[18, 20] and in autologous fascia lata valves.[14] It would appear, however, that this process occurs more slowly in glutaraldehyde-treated valves than in other types of tissue valves.

Several possible causes of damage to the collagen in porcine heterograft valves can be suggested: 1) reversal of glutaraldehyde-mediated cross-linking effect, with conversion of collagen from the fibrillar to the soluble form; 2) binding of plasma proteins to collagen, with formation of "fibrinoid"-like material; 3) hydrolysis of collagen by specific collagenases from inflammatory cells and by nonspecific proteolytic enzymes in inflammatory cells and in blood plasma; 4) breakdown of collagen fibrils by mechanical forces of valvular motion; 5) erosion of superficial layers of valvular collagen by the forces of blood flow (shear stress); and 6) immunologic or foreign-body reaction to the heterologous tissue. Each of these causes may contribute to the overall effect of collagen breakdown.

In conclusion, this study shows that the collagenous framework of glutaraldehyde-treated Hancock porcine valvular heterografts undergoes progressive deterioration with time. These valves do not contain viable cells and do not have a mechanism for the replacement of the collagen that has broken down. Consequently, deterioration of collagen probably will be the critical factor in determining the durability of these valves.

References

1. Spray TL, Roberts WC: Structural changes in porcine xenografts used as substitute cardiac valves. Gross and histologic observations in 51 glutaraldehyde-preserved Hancock valves in 41 patients. Am J Cardiol **40**: 319, 1977
2. Fishbein MC, Gissen SA, Collins JJ Jr, Barsamian EM, Cohn LH: Pathologic findings after cardiac valve replacement with glutaraldehyde-fixed porcine valves. Am J Cardiol **40**: 331, 1977
3. Kajikawa K, Yamaguchi T, Katsuda S, Miwa A: An improved electron stain for elastic fibers using tannic acid. J Electron Microsc (Tokyo) **24**: 287, 1975
4. Gross L, Kugel MA: Topographic anatomy and histology of the valves in the human heart. Am J Pathol **7**: 445, 1931
5. Hammon JW Jr, O'Sullivan MJ, Oury J, Fosburg RG: Allograft cardiac valves. A view through the scanning electron microscope. J Thorac Cardiovasc Surg **68**: 352, 1974
6. Gavin JB, Monro JL, Wall FM, Chalcroft SCW: Fine structural changes in the fibroblasts of canine heart valves prepared for grafting. Thorax **28**: 748, 1973
7. Girinath MR, Gavin JB, Strickett MG, Barratt-Boyes BG: The effects of antibiotics and storage on the viability and ultrastructure of fibroblasts in canine heart valves prepared for grafting. Aust NZ J Surg **44**: 170, 1974
8. Gavin JB, Monro JL: The pathology of pulmonary and aortic valve allografts used as mitral valve replacements in dogs. Pathology **6**: 119, 1974
9. Reichenbach DD, Mohri H, Merendino KA: Pathological changes in human aortic valve homografts. Circulation **39** (suppl I): I-47, 1969
10. Gavin JB, Herdson PB, Barratt-Boyes BG: The pathology of chemically-sterilized human heart valve allografts. Pathology **4**: 175, 1972
11. Wheeler EE, Gavin JB, Herdson PB: A scanning electron microscopy study of human heart valve allografts. Pathology **4**: 185, 1972

12. Gavin JB, Herdson PB, Monro JL, Barratt-Boyes BG: Pathology of antibiotic-treated human heart valve allografts. Thorax **28**: 473, 1973
13. Gavin JB, Barratt-Boyes BG, Hitchcock GC, Herdson PB: Histopathology of 'fresh' human aortic valve allografts. Thorax **28**: 482, 1973
14. Gersbach P, Wegmann W: Aorta valve replacement using autologous fascia lata transplants. Late morphological changes: an electron microscopic study. Virchows Arch [Pathol Anat] **364**: 235, 1974
15. Willén R, Dubiel WT, Johansson L: Viability and surface properties of autologous fascia lata heart valve grafts. A radioautographic and scanning electron microscopical study. Ann Thorac Surg **18**: 597, 1974
16. Willén R, Dubiel WT, Johansson L: Viability properties in autologous fascia lata heart valve grafts. A transmission electron microscopical study. Ann Thorac Surg **19**: 494, 1975
17. Rose AG: Pathology of the formalin-treated heterograft porcine aortic valve in the mitral position. Thorax **27**: 401, 1972
18. Yaroshinsky YN, Shekhter AB, Artyukhina TV, Glagoleva EV, Fursov BA: [Electron microscopy study of the aortic valve allo- and xenotransplants following their prolonged functioning in the human heart]. Biull Eksp Biol Med **78**: 116, 1974
19. Aparicio SR, Donnelly RJ, Dexter F, Watson DA: Light and electron microscopy studies on homograft and heterograft heart valves. J Pathol **115**: 147, 1975
20. Okamura K, Yuge I, Kawazoe K, Kitamura N, Imamura E, Koyanagi H, Konno S: A comparative study between glutaraldehyde-preserved aortic and pulmonary heterograft valves in the tricuspid position in dogs. J Cardiovasc Surg **17**: 178, 1976
21. Ferrans VJ, Levitsky S, Buja LM, Williams WH, McIntosh CL, Roberts WC: Histological and ultrastructural studies on preserved hearts. Circulation **41** (suppl II): II-104, 1970

Factors Determining Outcome of Cardiac Valve Replacement

William C. Roberts, M.D.

From 1960 through 1976, approximately 466,500 substitute cardiac valves were implanted for treatment of patients with malfunctioning cardiac valves. Some patients benefited enormously from the cardiac valve replacement and others did not. During this same period I examined more than 500 hearts postmortem in patients in whom 1 or more substitute cardiac valves had been inserted [4, 6–9]. From these studies, certain conclusions were drawn about factors considered most important in determining the long-term result of cardiac valve replacement. These factors are examined in this paper.

There are at least six factors that are very important in determining the result of cardiac valve replacement in a given patient: (1) the type of substitute valve inserted; (2) the size of the substitute valve; (3) the experience and technical skill of the surgeons; (4) the adequacy of the "pump team," the anesthesiologists and surgeons, and the physicians and nurses providing postoperative care; (5) the presence of associated (diagnosed or undiagnosed) or uncorrected cardiac disease or previous pericardiotomy; and (6) the preoperative status of the patient. The relative effect of each of these factors on the outcome of valve replacement is examined here.

Assuming that the cardiac operation takes place in a large medical center where several cardiac operations are performed weekly by a surgeon or group of surgeons experienced in cardiac valve replacement, the most important factor determining the long-term outcome of valve replacement is *the type of substitute valve inserted.* Before 1960, no patient had survived longer than 3 months after total excision of a native cardiac valve and replacement with a prosthesis. Then the caged-ball prosthesis was used successfully, on March 10, 1960, by Harken and associates [5] for aortic valve replacement and on September 21, 1960, by Starr and Edwards [10] for mitral valve replacement. Thereafter, valve replacement using the caged-ball prosthesis quickly became commonplace. The caged ball was the first prosthesis used for cardiac valve replacement by many surgeons whose previous valve operations had consisted entirely of mitral commissurotomy. Yet, almost from the beginning, rapid success was achieved with this device.

Because the decision regarding the type of substitute valve to be chosen for each patient is crucial, consideration might be given to two closely related questions. Who *does* choose the type of prosthesis to be inserted? Who *should* choose the type of prosthesis to be inserted? From the beginning, that is, 1960, the surgeon has determined the type of prosthesis. What factors determine a surgeon's preference for a particular prosthesis? The major one, I presume, is previous experience, both personal and that of colleagues. Some surgeons who started with the caged ball, for example, and had satisfactory results are reluctant to change. (One is simply more comfortable with the device one has used before.) Also, the choice of prosthesis by a prominent surgeon may be especially influential. If a prosthesis or model proves not to be ideal, despite high recommendations and previous experience, it should be changed, a difficult but admirable decision for a surgeon.

For some surgeons the choice of prosthesis has been influenced by personal involvement in the development of a particular prosthesis. Admitting that a prosthesis designed by someone else is better than one's own is hard. There may be inherent conflict when the same surgeon participates in the design of and insertion of the same prosthesis, and many instances of this potential conflict have occurred during the past 17 years.

From the Pathology Branch, National Heart, Lung, and Blood Institute, National Institutes of Health, Building 10A, Room 3E-30, Bethesda, MD 20014.

Several thoracic surgical journals each month carry manufacturers' advertisements delineating the virtues of particular substitute cardiac valves. One prominent surgeon has advocated a particular prosthesis by "massive" letter mailing, even though no postoperative hemodynamic or long-term follow-up information is available on patients in whom this particular prosthesis had been inserted. It is to be hoped that the choice of a cardiac valve prosthesis is not influenced by the manufacturer's advertising with or without the assistance of a surgeon who utilizes that particular prosthesis.

Again assuming that valve replacement is to be performed in a large medical center with an experienced cardiovascular surgical team, long-term survival is more dependent on the type of prosthesis inserted than on the surgeon who inserts it. Thus, if I were to undergo valve replacement, I would choose first the type of prosthesis and then the surgeon whose results with that prosthesis were excellent. In my view, the referring cardiologist is not fulfilling his responsibility if he simply refers the patient to a surgeon irrespective of the type of prosthesis the surgeon most frequently utilizes. To use a caged disc, at least 1 with a flat nontilting occluder, is unwise, in my view, and, to date, little hemodynamic or other data are available to allow proper evaluation of the biconical type of caged disc. Although some surgeons periodically employ all 4 types of available substitute cardiac valves (caged ball, caged [nontilting] disc, tilting disc, and aortic valve tissue), most generally use only 1 or 2 types. If the patient has mitral stenosis or combined mitral and aortic valve disease (and in this circumstance the aortic "root" is usually small) or if the patient is small, referral to a surgeon who only, or nearly always, uses the caged-ball prosthesis would not appear ideal. Patients who require valve replacement and who have real or potential bleeding tendencies should have a tissue valve because anticoagulant therapy is necessary with use of all rigid-framed substitute valves.

Cardiologists in large medical centers usually refer patients requiring valve replacement to surgeons in the same medical center even though they may not necessarily be pleased with, or involved in, the choice of the substitute valve. Ideally, this choice would be made by both the cardiologist and the surgeon in light of all the data known about a particular patient. Greater participation by cardiologists in valve selection would require, however, the acquisition of much more knowledge of such valves than they now generally have. Obviously, who chooses the type of substitute valve for a given patient is not important as long as the choice is the right one, but surgeons do not necessarily have a monopoly on that correct choice.

The second most important factor determining long-term survival after cardiac valve replacement is *the size of the prosthesis inserted.* This determination, to my knowledge, has always been made in the operating room with the patient on cardiopulmonary bypass and after placing various sizers through the valve orifice after excision of the native valve. But does this method best determine the proper size of a prosthesis to be inserted? In my opinion, the answer is no. With the patient on cardiopulmonary bypass and with various retractors pulling on the heart, the surgeon may be able to insert large sizing devices and, therefore, choose a large prosthesis when in actuality, the valve orifice is much smaller. It seems to me that the size of the valve to be inserted might best be determined in part on the basis of the hemodynamic valve lesion or lesions before operation with consideration of the lean weight of the patient, and not exclusively on the basis of sizing devices at operation. For example, a small woman with pure mitral stenosis and a normally functioning aortic valve should have a relatively small prosthesis.

In 1975, I saw postmortem the hearts of 2 patients with severe isolated mitral stenosis in each of whom the largest tilting-disc prosthesis (Björk-Shiley, 31 mm) had been inserted. At operation, the sizing devices had apparently indicated that the valve orifices were capable of accommodating these large-sized prostheses; but, fatal malfunction of the prosthesis because of prosthetic disproportion (prosthesis too large for occluder to move properly within the left ventricle) occurred in each patient. If the largest prosthesis is used in a small woman with pure mitral stenosis, what size of device should be used in a large man with pure mitral regurgitation? The decision regarding what size of prosthesis to insert might roughly be determined at the preoperative consultation and be based on the hemodynamic valve lesion and lean body weight and not entirely on the dimensions measured in the operating room.

Although I have placed greatest emphasis on the type and size of the prosthetic valve inserted, *the technical skill and experience of the surgeon* are obviously extremely important, experience probably being more important than technical skill. (One of the finest examples of technical skill in the field of cardiac valve replacement is the placing of a porcine xenograft on a semiflexible cloth-covered stent. This procedure is done by women before the tissue valves are shipped to surgeons.) Without question, results of valve replacement are better among experienced than nonexperienced surgeons, although the technical skills of the latter might be greater. The "occasional open-heart surgeon," as emphasized by Eiseman and Spencer [2], no matter how great his technical skill, is not the ideal cardiac surgeon. Certain technical factors, however, might be taken into consideration by the referring physician. Should prosthetic valves be inserted with continuous suture or interrupted sutures? It appears most reasonable that interrupted sutures would be less likely to be associated with "massive" prosthetic regurgitation (prosthetic disruption), and yet continuous or nearly continuous sutures are commonly employed by some surgeons [3]. If the world's "best" surgeon uses the world's worst prosthesis or inserts it by noninterrupted suture, the result is not ideal.

The three other determinants of the results of cardiac valve replacement are self-evident. Obviously, the entire surgical team must be good. Patients with associated heart disease, for example, coronary heart disease or previous thoracotomy, do not do as well as patients without these associated conditions [1]. The less sick the patient before operation, the greater are the chances of survival after operation; but the sicker the patient before operation, usually the more dramatic is the change after operation.

References

1. Barnhorst DA, Oxman HA, Connolly DC, et al: Long-term follow-up of isolated replacement of the aortic or mitral valve with the Starr-Edwards prosthesis. Am J Cardiol 35:228, 1975
2. Eiseman B, Spencer FC: The occasional open-heart surgeon. Circulation 31:161, 1965
3. Fernandez J: Insertion of Björk-Shiley aortic prosthesis by continuous suture technique. Ann Thorac Surg 17:587, 1974
4. Fishbein MC, Roberts WC, Golden A, et al: Cardiac pathology after aortic valve replacement using Hufnagel trileaflet prostheses: a study of 20 necropsy patients. Am Heart J 89:443, 1975
5. Harken DE, Taylor WJ, Lefemine AA, et al: Aortic valve replacement with a caged ball valve. Am J Cardiol 9:292, 1962
6. Roberts WC, Bulkley BH, Morrow AG: Pathologic anatomy of cardiac valve replacement: a study of 224 necropsy patients. Prog Cardiovasc Dis 15:539, 1973
7. Roberts WC, Fishbein MC, Golden A: Cardiac pathology after valve replacement by disc prosthesis. A study of 61 necropsy patients. Am J Cardiol 35:740, 1975
8. Roberts WC, Hammer WJ: Cardiac pathology after valve replacement with a tilting disc prosthesis (Björk-Shiley type). A study of 46 necropsy patients and 49 Björk-Shiley prostheses. Am J Cardiol 37:1024, 1976
9. Spray TL, Roberts WC: Structural changes in porcine xenografts used as substitute cardiac valves. Gross and histologic observations in 51 glutaraldehyde-preserved Hancock valves in 41 patients. Am J Cardiol 40:319, 1977
10. Starr A, Edwards ML: Mitral replacement: clinical experience with a ball-valve prosthesis. Ann Surg 154:726, 1961

Calcific Pulmonic Stenosis in Adulthood*

Treatment by Valve Replacement (Porcine Xenograft) With Postoperative Hemodynamic Evaluation

Edgar A. Covarrubias, M.D.; Mazhar U. Sheikh, M.D.; Jeffrey M. Isner, M.D.; Mario Gomes, M.D., F.C.C.P.; Charles A. Hufnagel, M.D., F.C.C.P.; and William C. Roberts, M.D., F.C.C.P.

Clinical and morphologic features are described in a 56-year-old man in whom severe, isolated pulmonic valve stenosis was treated by valve replacement with a porcine prosthesis. The calcific deposits were located on the ventricular aspect of the pulmonic valve, opposite the location (arterial aspect) of calcific deposits on stenotic aortic valves, and calcific deposits also were present in the tricuspid valve anulus.

Isolated pulmonic valve stenosis of severe degree in persons over 50 years of age is rare.[1-4] Calcific deposits in stenotic pulmonic valves also are rare,[24] and calcific deposits in the tricuspid valve anulus are even more rare.[5,6] Treatment of isolated pulmonic valve stenosis by valve replacement has not been reported. Although each of the above occurrences is rare, all of them occurred together in our patient. In addition, the patient had postoperative hemodynamic evaluation after pulmonic valve replacement with a porcine xenograft.

Case Report

A 56-year-old man was easily fatigued during his teens and was denied military service because of a "heart murmur." He was asymptomatic until age 46 years when exertional dyspnea occurred, and he was digitalized. At age 52, atrial fibrillation was noted, and cardioversion was done. During the next four years, the exertional dyspnea gradually progressed so that by age 56, he had considerable dyspnea when walking three flat blocks at a normal pace or climbing one flight of stairs.

Examination in November 1977 (age 56) disclosed a prominent "a" wave in the jugular veins, no precordial thrills, a decreased pulmonic component of the second heart sound at the base, a grade 3/6 harsh, systolic precordial murmur loudest over the upper left sternal border, and no organomegaly or subcutaneous edema. Electrocardiogram showed sinus rhythm and right bundle branch block. Chest roentgenogram (Fig 1) disclosed cardiomegaly and heavy calcific deposits in the pulmonic valve. The catheterization data are summarized in Table 1.

At operation on Feb 2, 1978, palpation via the right atrium disclosed calcific deposits in the tricuspid valve anular region. The pulmonary trunk was dilated, and a thrill was palpated.

*From the Georgetown Cardiology Service, District of Columbia Hospital, and the Departments of Surgery, Medicine, and Pathology, Georgetown University Hospital, Washington, DC; and the Pathology Branch, National Heart, Lung, and Blood Institute, National Institutes of Hea'th, Bethesda.
Reprint requests: Dr. Roberts, Chief, Pathology Branch, NHLBI, Bldg 10A, Room 3E30, 9000 Rockville Pike, Bethesda 20014

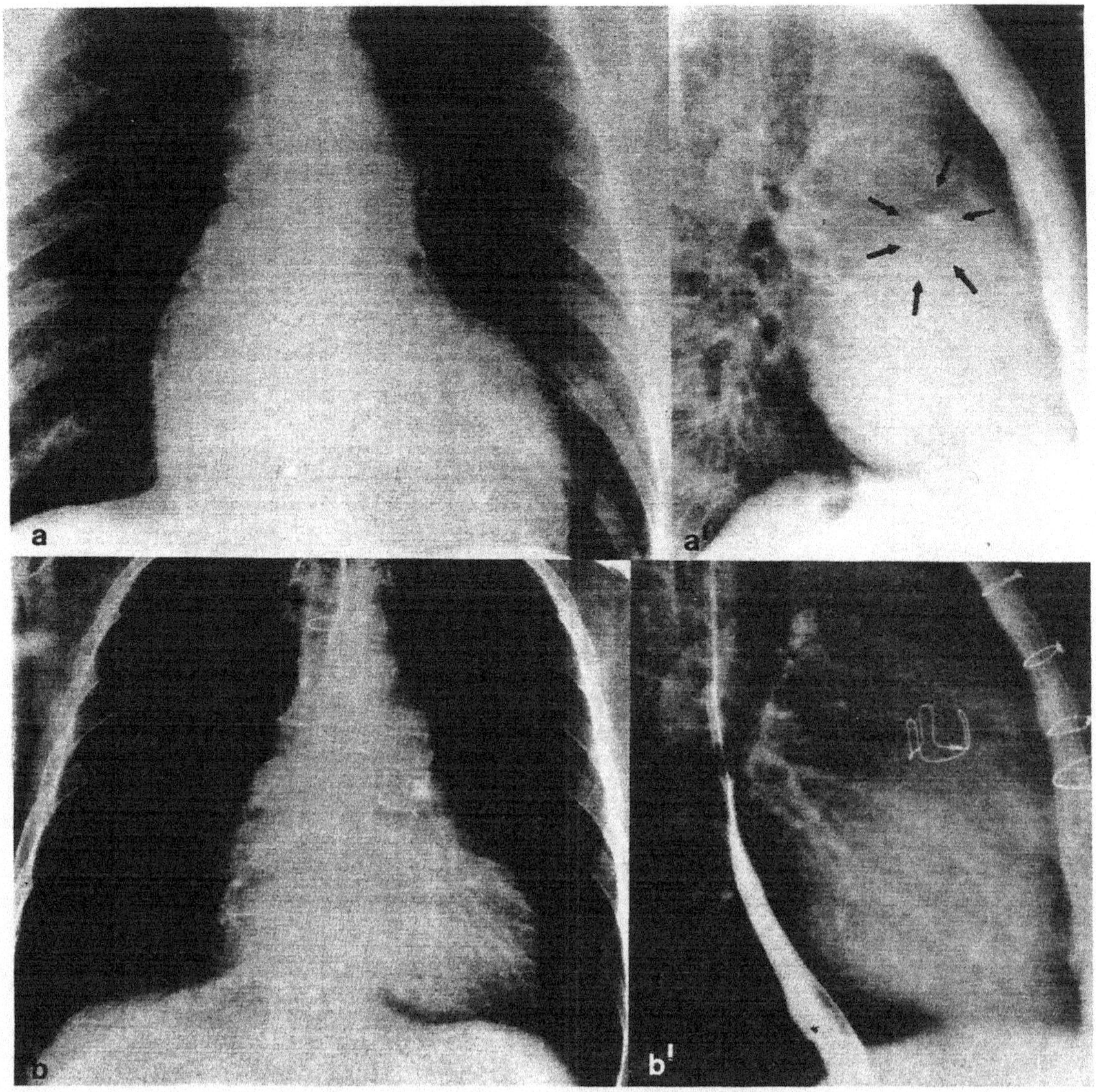

FIGURE 1. Three days before (*a* and *a'*) and 75 days after (*b* and *b'*) valve replacement. In preoperative lateral view, (a'), calcific deposits (*arrows*) are apparent. In postoperative roentgenograms (b and b'), wire of prosthetic cage is readily visible.

Table 1—*Cardiac Catheterization Data*

Date	RA	RV (s/d)	PT (s/d)	PAW mean	LV (s/d)	SA	CI liters/min/sq meter
		Pressures, mm Hg					
12/15/77	a=18 v=14 Mean=12	150/11	. . .	. . .	150/8	150/80	2.7
2/2/78*	. . .	106/16	17/5	. . .	. . .	. . .	. . .
2/2/78**	. . .	59/7	30/18	. .	. . .	. . .	. . .
4/26/78	a=14 v=10 Mean=10	60/12	24/14	10	. . .	140/85	3.0

CI=cardiac index; LV=left ventricle; PAW=pulmonary artery wedge; PT=pulmonary trunk; RA=right atrium; RV=right ventricle; SA=systemic artery; and s/d=systole/diastole.

*During operation, before cardiopulmonary bypass.

**During operation, after discontinuing bypass.

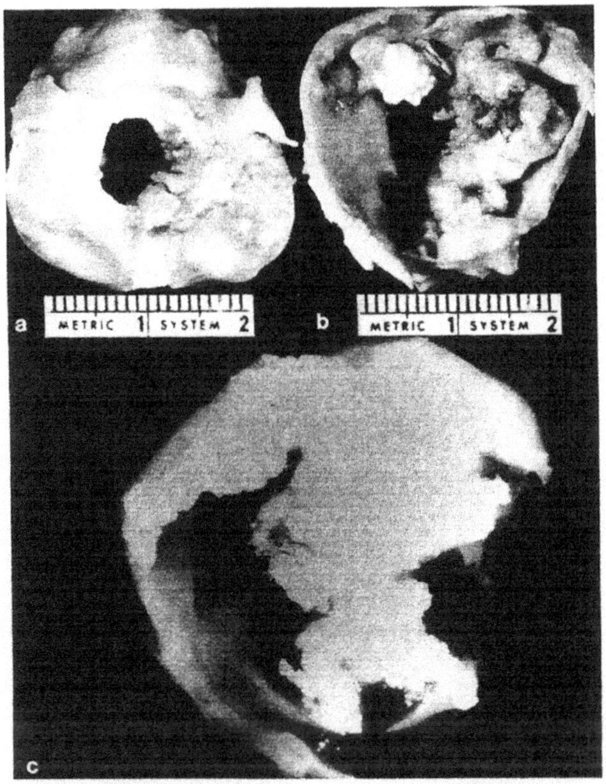

FIGURE 2. Operatively excised pulmonic valve. *a,* View from pulmonary arterial aspect; *b,* view from right ventricular aspect showing heavy calcific deposits on this undersurface; and *c,* roentgenogram again showing heavy calcific deposits.

The pulmonic valve was dome-shaped with a central stenotic orifice and heavy calcific deposits on its ventricular aspect (Fig 2). The infundibulum by palpation appeared narrowed, and therefore, several fragments of crista supraventricularis muscle were excised. The pulmonic valve was replaced with a 25-mm Hancock porcine xenograft via an incision in the pulmonary trunk. The postoperative course was smooth. The QRS complex on the ECG widened from 0.12 to 0.16 sec.

When evaluated nearly three months postoperatively, the patient stated that he had noted no change in his exercise tolerance. The precordial systolic ejection-type murmur was now of grade 2/6 intensity. Chest roentgenogram (Fig 1) showed a decrease in the size of the cardiac silhouette. Repeat catheterization disclosed a 36 mm Hg peak systolic pressure gradient at the level of the porcine valve and no subvalvular gradient.

Discussion

Calcific deposits in stenotic pulmonic valves have been reported previously in at least 27 patients,[2-4] 15 (56 percent) with intact ventricular septa and 12 (44 percent) with associated ventricular septal defect. A prerequisite for calcium deposition in this valve is a severe degree of valvular stenosis, and with rare exception,[3] an age of greater than 30 years, usually greater than 40 years. Both of these requirements were fulfilled by our patient.

Calcific deposits on dome-shaped stenotic *pulmonic* valves appear to occur on the undersurface or ventricular aspect of the cusp, whereas calcific deposits on stenotic *aortic* valves are located entirely or predominantly on the arterial (aortic) aspect of the cusps. The following two reasons appear to account for these differences in location: (1) the low diastolic pressure in the pulmonary trunk as contrasted to the relatively high diastolic pressure in the aorta; and (2) the difference in configuration of the stenotic pulmonic valve compared to that of the stenotic aortic valve. Blood ejected from the right ventricle during systole initially contacts the concave surface of a stenotic dome-shaped pulmonic valve, whereas that ejected from the left ventricle contacts initially the convex surface of a stenotic aortic valve. Deposition of calcium on a convex surface appears to be more difficult than on a concave surface. Despite the location of the calcific deposits on the ventricular aspect of the pulmonic cusp and the high (150 mm Hg) right ventricular systolic pressure preoperatively, intravascular hemolysis was either absent or insignificant in our patient.

Calcific deposits in the mitral valve anulus are common, particularly in persons over 65 years of age, and they may occur at an earlier age at this site in patients with elevated left ventricular systolic pressures (systemic hypertension, aortic stenosis, hypertrophic cardiomyopathy).[5] In contrast, calcific deposits in the tricuspid valve anulus, as occurred in our patient, are rare.[6] The prerequisite for tricuspid valve anular calcification appears to be a right ventricular systolic pressure equal to or higher than the normal left ventricular systolic pressure and an age greater than 40 years. Because our patient's stenotic pulmonic valve was accommissural, it is likely that the valve in him was considerably stenotic from the time of birth and that his right ventricular systolic pressure was similar to his left ventricular systolic pressure for his entire 56 years before operation. A systolic closing pressure on the tricuspid valve five times that of normal for 56 years appears to be an adequate explanation for the tricuspid valve anular calcification.

Our patient is the first, to our knowledge, to undergo pulmonic valve replacement with a porcine xenograft for isolated pulmonic valve stenosis. Although this procedure reduced the right ventricular systolic pressure from 150 to 60 mm Hg, and the right ventricular outflow peak systolic pressure gradient from approximately 125 to 36 mm Hg, the right ventricular diastolic pressure remained unchanged and elevated (12 mm Hg). Because of the heavy calcific deposits in the pulmonic valve, partial valvulotomy would not have been feasible, and valve replacement appears to have been a better option than total valvulectomy despite the 36 mm Hg systolic pressure gradient across the prosthesis three months postoperatively. This degree of right ventricular outflow obstruction, however, should not in itself be responsible for symptoms of cardiac dysfunction. Possibly, there is considerable right ventricular fibrosis as a consequence of the severe elevation of the right ventricular systolic pressure for nearly six decades.

References

1 Tinker J, Howitt G, Markman P, et al: The natural history of isolated pulmonary stenosis. Br Heart J 27:151-160, 1965

2 Dinsmore RE, Sanders CA, Harthorne JW, et al: Calcification of the congenitally stenotic pulmonary valve. N Engl J Med 275:99-100, 1966

3 Roberts WC, Mason DT, Morrow AG, et al: Calcific pulmonic stenosis. Circulation 37:973-978, 1968

4 Rodriguez GR, Bennett KR, Lehan PH: Calcification of the pulmonary valve. Chest 59:160-164, 1971

5 Roberts WC, Perloff JK: Mitral valvular disease: A clinicopathologic survey of the conditions causing the mitral valve to function abnormally. Ann Intern Med 77:939-975, 1972

6 Arnold JR, Ghahramani AR, Hernandez FA, et al: Calcification of annulus of tricuspid valve (observation in two patients with congenital pulmonary stenosis). Chest 60: 229-232, 1971

Infection of Glutaraldehyde-Preserved Porcine Valve Heterografts

VICTOR J. FERRANS, MD, PhD
STEVEN W. BOYCE, BA
MARGARET E. BILLINGHAM, MD
THOMAS L. SPRAY, MD
WILLIAM C. ROBERTS, MD, FACC

Bethesda, Maryland
Stanford, California

Gross, histologic and ultrastructural changes associated with bacterial infection are described in four porcine valve heterografts that had been in place in patients for 6 days to 28 months. In one patient, culture of the aortic tissue tag included in the heterograft container grew Mycobacterium chelonei; however, examination of the heterograft, recovered at necropsy 6 days after implantation, revealed small colonies of bacteria that differed morphologically from mycobacteria. A second heterograft was the site of staphylococcal infection associated with extensive destruction of collagen in the leaflets. Similar destruction was observed in a third heterograft, which was found to have organisms on ultrastructural study even though bacterial cultures of the valve were negative. The fourth heterograft, from a patient who died of coronary embolism secondary to dislodgment of vegetative material, contained structures resembling lysed bacteria. Observations in these 4 patients and review of published reports of infection involving 43 other patients with porcine valve heterografts indicates that infection in these valves: (1) develops in the fibrin layer that covers the cusps, (2) can involve the collagen in the leaflets, and (3) is uncommonly (three patients) associated with valve ring abscesses.

Infection of a valve prosthesis is a serious complication of cardiac valve replacement. Detailed descriptions have been made of the clinical and morphologic features of infections in rigid-framed prosthetic valves[1–18]; however, only a few reports have been published of infections in glutaraldehyde-preserved porcine valve heterografts,[19–32] and morphologic changes associated with these infections have received little attention. This communication describes gross, histologic and ultrastructural alterations associated with bacterial infection in four porcine valve heterografts, summarizes previous reports of infection in porcine heterografts and compares the features of infections in these valves and in other types of prosthetic heart valves.

Methods

Patients Studied

The study group consisted of four patients, three men and one woman, aged 28 to 68 years (average 50), who had bacterial infection in a glutaraldehyde-treated porcine valve heterograft. Evidence of infection was obtained from bacterial culture or morphologic examination of the prosthesis, or both. The clinical features of these four patients and the morphologic features of the heterografts are summarized in Tables I and II.

The porcine valve heterografts had been in place for 6 days to 28 months. In Patient 1, the heterograft was implanted in the aortic position. Patient 2 had two heterografts, one in the aortic and one in the mitral position; the latter heterograft did not become infected. Patient 3 also had two heterografts, one in the mitral and one in the tricuspid position; only the mitral heterograft became infected. In Patient 4, the heterograft was in the mitral position.

From the Pathology Branch, National Heart, Lung, and Blood Institute, National Institutes of Health, Bethesda, Maryland, and the Department of Pathology, Stanford University School of Medicine, Stanford, California. Manuscript received November 6, 1978; revised manuscript received January 2, 1979, accepted January 3, 1979.
Address for reprints: Victor J. Ferrans, MD, National Institutes of Health, Building 10, Room 7N-208, Bethesda, Maryland 20014.

TABLE I

Clinical Findings in Four Patients With Infected Porcine Valve Heterografts

Clinical Features	Patient 1	Patient 2	Patient 3	Patient 4
Age (yr)	66	68	28	44
Sex	F	M	M	M
Preop diagnosis	AR, aortic aneurysm	AR, MR	MR, TR	MR
Valve replaced with PVH	Aortic	Aortic and mitral	Mitral and tricuspid	Mitral
Factors predisposing to infection	0	0	Opiate addiction	0
Cultured organism	Mycobacterium chelonei cultured from tag	Enterobacter cloacae, α-Streptococcus, Citrobacter fuente	Staphylococcus aureus	None
Clinical evidence of PVH infection	0	Suggestive	+	Suggestive
Noncardiac infection	0	0	+	0
Antibiotic therapy before PVH excised	0	0	Nafcillin for 6 weeks	0
PVH dysfunction	0	+ (stenosis)	+ (stenosis)	+ (stenosis)
Interval between PVH implantation and removal	6 days	5 months	4.5 months	28 months
Outcome	Died of ascending aortic aneurysm	Died of coronary embolus	Alive; infected mitral PVH replaced with another PVH	Alive; PVH replaced with rigid-framed valve

+ = change present; 0 = change absent; α-Streptococcus = alpha-hemolytic streptococcus. AR = aortic regurgitation; MR = mitral regurgitation; preop = preoperative; PVH = porcine valve heterograft; TR = tricuspid regurgitation; TVR = tricuspid valve replacement.

Case Reports

Patient 1, who had a diagnosis of aortic regurgitation secondary to the Ehler-Danlos syndrome, died of complications of dissecting aneurysm 6 days after implantation of the aortic porcine valve heterograft. She had no clinical evidence of infection of the heterograft, but a tag of aortic tissue included in the heterograft container was cultured at the time of operation and eventually grew Mycobacterium chelonei.[33,34] At necropsy, the heterograft appeared grossly normal and was not cultured.

Patient 2, who had been hospitalized in 1974 for suspected (unproved, but treated) infective endocarditis, was admitted in August 1977 with congestive heart failure secondary to aortic and mitral regurgitation. The mitral and aortic valves were replaced by porcine valve heterografts. Two days after operation, the patient had an episode of atrial fibrillation, and expressive aphasia and right-sided hemiplegia developed. He was discharged several weeks later without further complications but, in January 1978, he died of a coronary embolus 1 day after admission for treatment of recurrent congestive heart failure. At necropsy, the cusps of the aortic heterograft were filled with abundant vegetations.

Patient 3, an opiate addict who had used drugs intravenously for about 10 years, had severe mitral and tricuspid valve regurgitation after three separate episodes of infective endocarditis (two with Staphylococcus aureus and one with alpha streptococcus). In August 1977, he underwent mitral and tricuspid valve replacement with porcine valve heterografts. The excised valves showed evidence of healed endocarditis, but no organisms were detected on culture or histologic study. One week after operation, complete heart block developed, requiring implantation of a permanent epicardial pacemaker. In November 1977, the patient was admitted with a Staphylococcus aureus infection involving the mitral valve heterograft and the site of implantation of the pacemaker batteries. The patient responded to removal (and replacement) of the pacemaker and to therapy with nafcillin; however, in January 1978, less than 2 weeks after discharge, he was again admitted with evidence of staphylococcal infection of the mitral valve heterograft. Because of the persistence of symptoms and echocardiographic findings suggestive of vegetations, this heterograft was replaced by another porcine valve. At operation the other cardiac valves, including the tricuspid porcine heterograft, were normal. The mitral valve

TABLE II

Morphologic Observations on Four Infected Porcine Valve Heterografts

		Microscopic Changes					
Case no.	Gross Appearance of Cusps	Fibrin	Inflammatory Cells	Disrupted Collagen	Calcific Deposits	Lipid Deposits	Organisms
1	Normal	+	0	+	0	0	Rods with flagella; located beneath thin fibrin layer covering surface
2	Friable tan-yellow vegetations narrowing valve orifice	+	+	++	0	0	Rounded "ghosts", not definitely identifiable as bacteria, in vegetations
3	Vegetations; valve orifice narrowed	+++	+	+++	+	++	Cocci in cusps and vegetations
4	Covered with thick shaggy material	++	+	+++	+	+++	Spore-forming, rod-like bacteria in cusps

0 = none; + = mild; ++ = moderate; +++ = severe.

heterograft contained multiple vegetations with gram-positive cocci. A small pocket of pus was present in the valve ring and grew Staphylococcus aureus in culture. The patient has done well since operation.

Patient 4 (Patient 10 in reference 35) had a history of an "autoimmune disease" characterized by vasculitis, arthritis and temporal arteritis. In 1974, because of mitral regurgitation caused by rupture of chordae tendineae, he underwent mitral valve replacement with a porcine valve heterograft. In June 1976, congestive heart failure developed; a mean diastolic pressure gradient of 34 mm Hg across the porcine mitral valve was recorded. The white blood cell count was 16,500/mm^3 of blood, but, no antibiotic treatment was given before reoperation because results of blood cultures were negative and there were no embolic signs or fever. At reoperation, the porcine valve appeared to be partially disintegrated and was covered with a large amount of shaggy gray friable material. The heterograft was replaced by a rigid-framed prosthesis, and the patient recovered uneventfully.

Preparation of Tissues

The porcine valve heterografts were removed either at operation (Patients 3 and 4) or at necropsy (Patients 1 and 2) and were fixed with cold 3 percent glutaraldehyde in 0.1 molar phosphate buffer, pH 7.2. Histologic sections were prepared according to techniques reported previously in detail.[35] Selected portions of the valves were cut, fixed with cold 1 percent osmium tetroxide in Millonig's phosphate buffer, and embedded in Maraglas®.[35] Sections, 0.5 μ thick, were stained with alkaline toluidine blue and examined with a light microscope to select areas for electron microscopic study. Ultrathin sections were stained with ethanolic uranyl acetate and Reynolds' lead citrate, and examined with a JEOL 100B electron microscope.

Results

The results of gross anatomic, histologic and ultrastructural examination of the four valves are summarized in Table II.

Patient 1: The porcine valve was grossly normal. Microscopically, it showed only minimal disruption of collagen and a few small (less than 20 μ in size) colonies of bacteria. The bacteria (Fig. 1) were located in a thin layer of fibrin that covered the heterograft and between this layer and the surface of the heterograft. They were not observed in deeper areas of tissue, were not associated with inflammatory cells and were not acid-fast. On ultrastructural examination (Fig. 2), the morphologic features of the bacteria corresponded to those of flagella-bearing gram-negative rods. These organisms appeared well preserved and could have been viable. The bacteria had thin cell walls and well defined trilaminar membranes. The cytoplasm of the bacteria contained abundant clusters of electron-dense granules scattered between clumps of nucleoid material. The bacteria had an average length of 2 μ and width of 0.5 μ.

Patient 2: The cusps of the porcine valve contained abundant friable yellow-tan vegetations that severely narrowed the valve orifice. Microscopically, the vegetations consisted of laminated masses of fibrin in which a few neutrophils and macrophages were present (Fig. 3, A to C). Special stains of histologic sections revealed no organisms; however, light and electron microscopic examination of plastic-embedded fragments of vegetations revealed the presence of rare foci of rounded or somewhat elongated structures that measured about 0.4 μ in diameter. These ghost-like structures had fragmented trilaminar membranes and dense, poorly defined contents (Fig. 3, D and E).

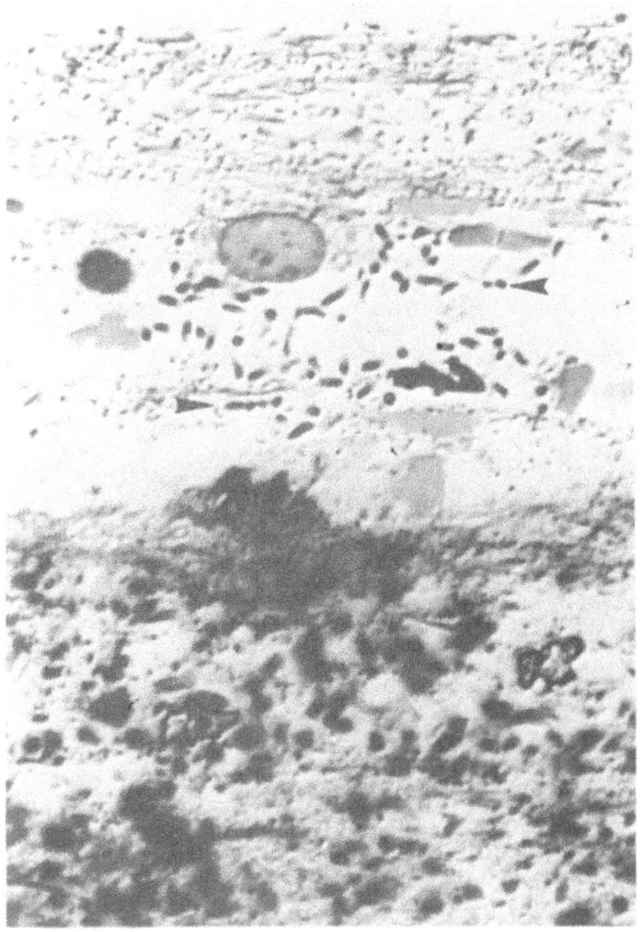

FIGURE 1. Patient 1. Light micrograph of section of the heterograft. A thin layer of fibrin overlies the surface of the heterograft, and a small cluster of bacteria (**arrowheads**) is located between the fibrin and the valve collagen. Section of plastic embedded tissue, 0.5 μ thick, stained with toluidine blue and viewed with Nomarski differential interference contrast optics (×1,600, reduced by 5 percent).

Patients 3 and 4: The valves from these two patients had extensive vegetations on the cusps. Although these valves demonstrated different organisms, they showed very similar ultrastructural changes, including severe disruption of the collagenous framework, lipid deposits and focal calcific deposits. The changes in collagen and the lipid deposits were similar to those previously described in deteriorating porcine valve heterografts.[35] The calcific deposits were present in fibrin-platelet thrombi. In addition, both valves had sites of deep penetration by bacteria into the substance of the leaflets. In contrast, polymorphonuclear leukocytes and macrophages were located mostly in the vegetations. In both valves, these cells were present only in small numbers on the surfaces of the leaflets and were essentially absent from the deep-seated areas of bacterial invasion.

In Patient 3 the bacteria in the porcine valve heterograft were readily identified as cocci on light microscopic study of histologic sections and plastic sections of tissue embedded for electron microscopy (Fig. 4). On ultrastructural study, these organisms appeared round in shape, measured up to 1.2 μ in diameter and had prominent cell walls, discrete plasma membranes, mesosomes and filamentous strands of nuclear material (Fig. 5). These ultrastructural features are known to

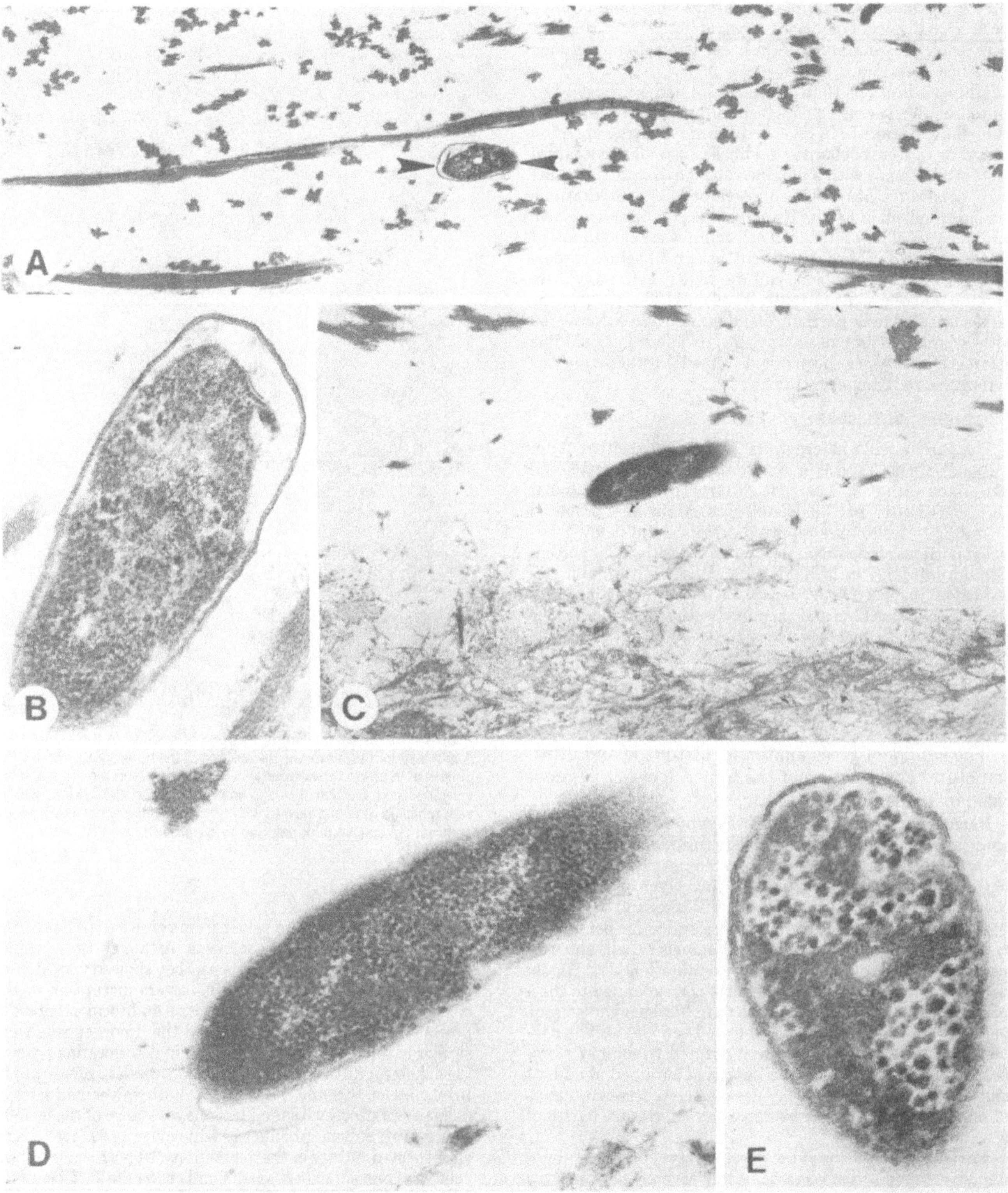

FIGURE 2. Patient 1. Electron micrographs showing the morphologic features of bacteria in the heterograft (all specified magnifications reduced by 2 percent). **A,** low magnification view of bacterium (**arrowheads**) surrounded by thin, elongated strands of fibrin (×14,600); **B,** bacterium from a section serial to that shown in **A** has trilaminar plasma membrane and a very thin cell wall of the type found in gram-negative bacteria (×66,500); **C,** another bacterium is immediately adjacent to layer of altered collagen at the surface of the heterograft (**bottom**). Fibrin strands are shown at **top** (×19,700); **D,** high magnification view of the same bacterium as in **C,** showing flagella (**lower left**) (×61,500); **E,** slightly oblique section through another bacterium showing the good preservation of its cytologic features. Note the plasma membrane and the thin cell wall (×75,000).

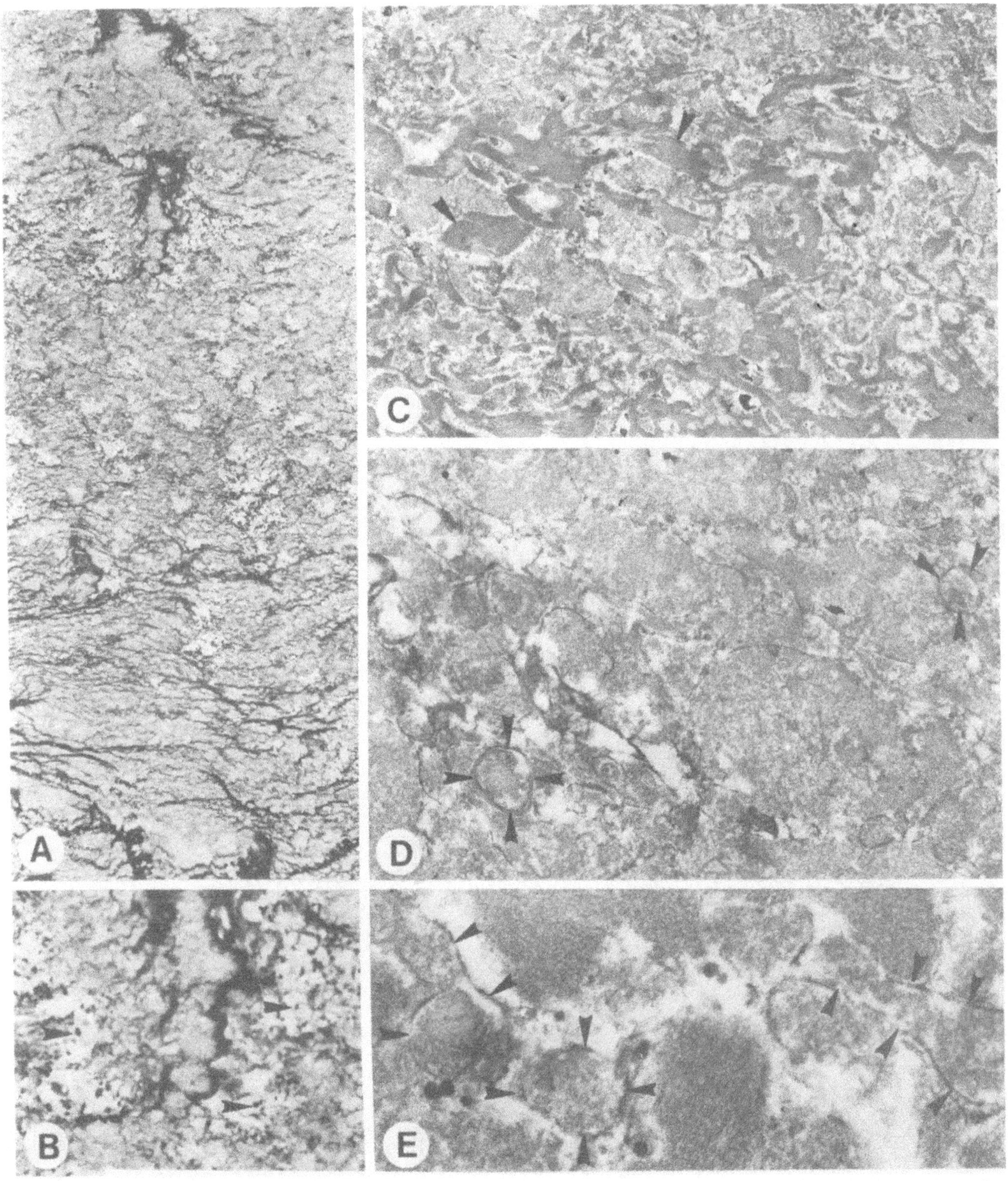

FIGURE 3. Patient 2. Light (**A** and **B**) and electron (**C, D** and **E**) micrographs of sections through large vegetation on cusp of heterograft. (all specified magnifications reduced by 2 percent). **A,** vegetation is composed of layered strands of fibrin. Section, 0.5 μ thick, toluidine blue stain (×250); **B,** Small rounded or slightly elongated particles (**arrowheads**) are present in close association with the fibrin. Section, 0.5 μ thick, toluidine blue stain (×800); **C,** low magnification electron micrograph of fibrin strands (**arrowheads**) in the vegetation (×12,000); **D,** "ghost-like" forms (**arrowheads**) resembling bacteria are present in an area similar to that shown in **B** (×34,000); **E,** high magnification view of structures (outlined by **arrowheads**) such as those shown in **D.** The gray material surrounding these structures is fibrin (×75,000).

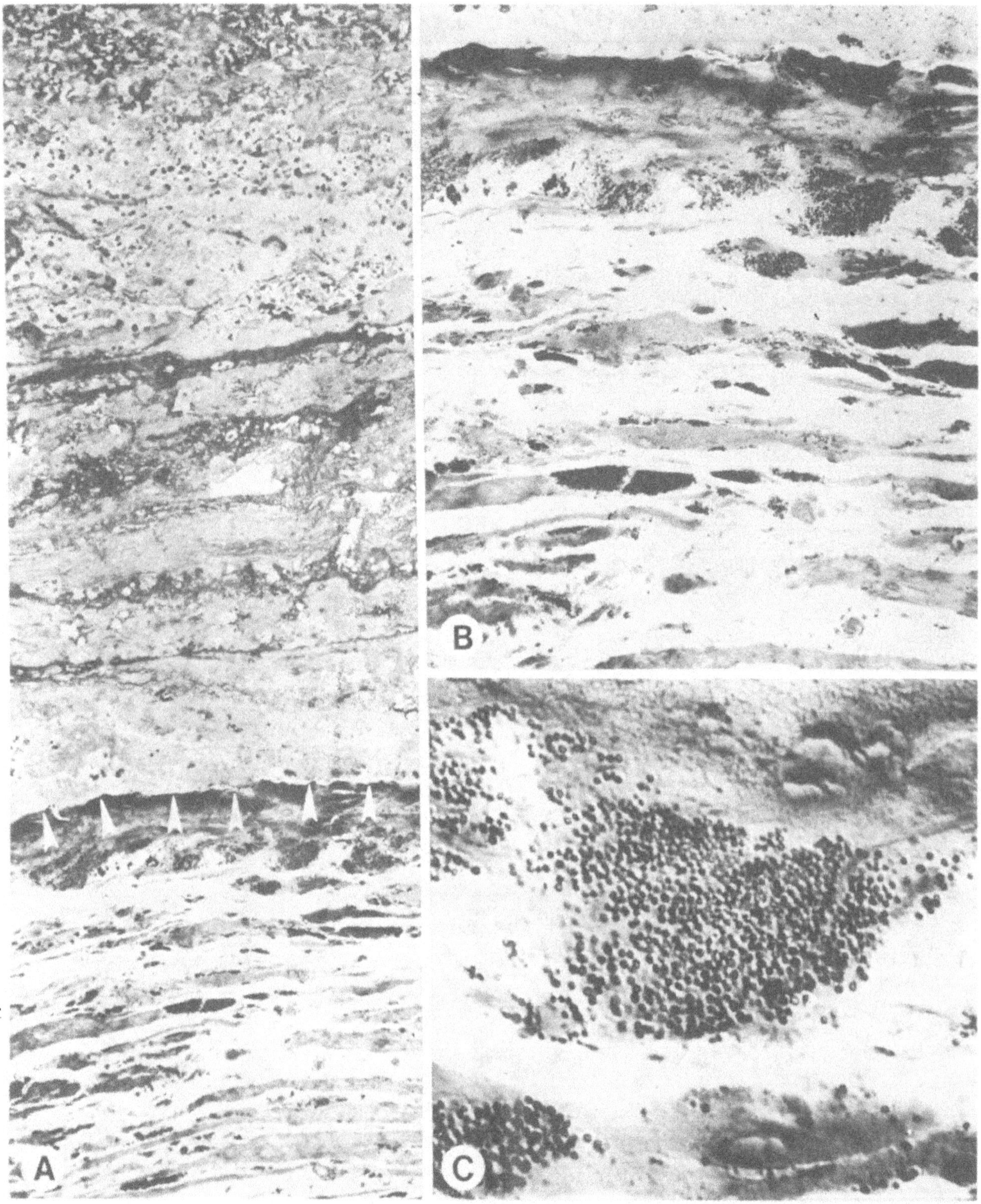

FIGURE 4. Patient 3. Light micrographs of sections, 0.5 μ thick, stained with toluidine blue, of valve heterograft (all specified magnifications reduced by 7 percent). **A,** low magnification view of large vegetation (**top** and **center**) overlying valve surface (indicated by **small white arrowheads**) and valve fibrosa. Vegetation contains layered fibrin and inflammatory cells (×200); (**B,** view of valve heterograft (corresponding to lower third of **A**) showing bacterial invasion of collagen bundles, which appear widely separated. Note the absence of inflammatory cells from this area of the heterograft (×400); **C,** high magnification micrograph (Nomarski differential interference contrast optics) of cluster of bacteria (same cluster as in upper right of **B**) having the typical morphologic features of cocci (compare with Fig. 5) (×1,600).

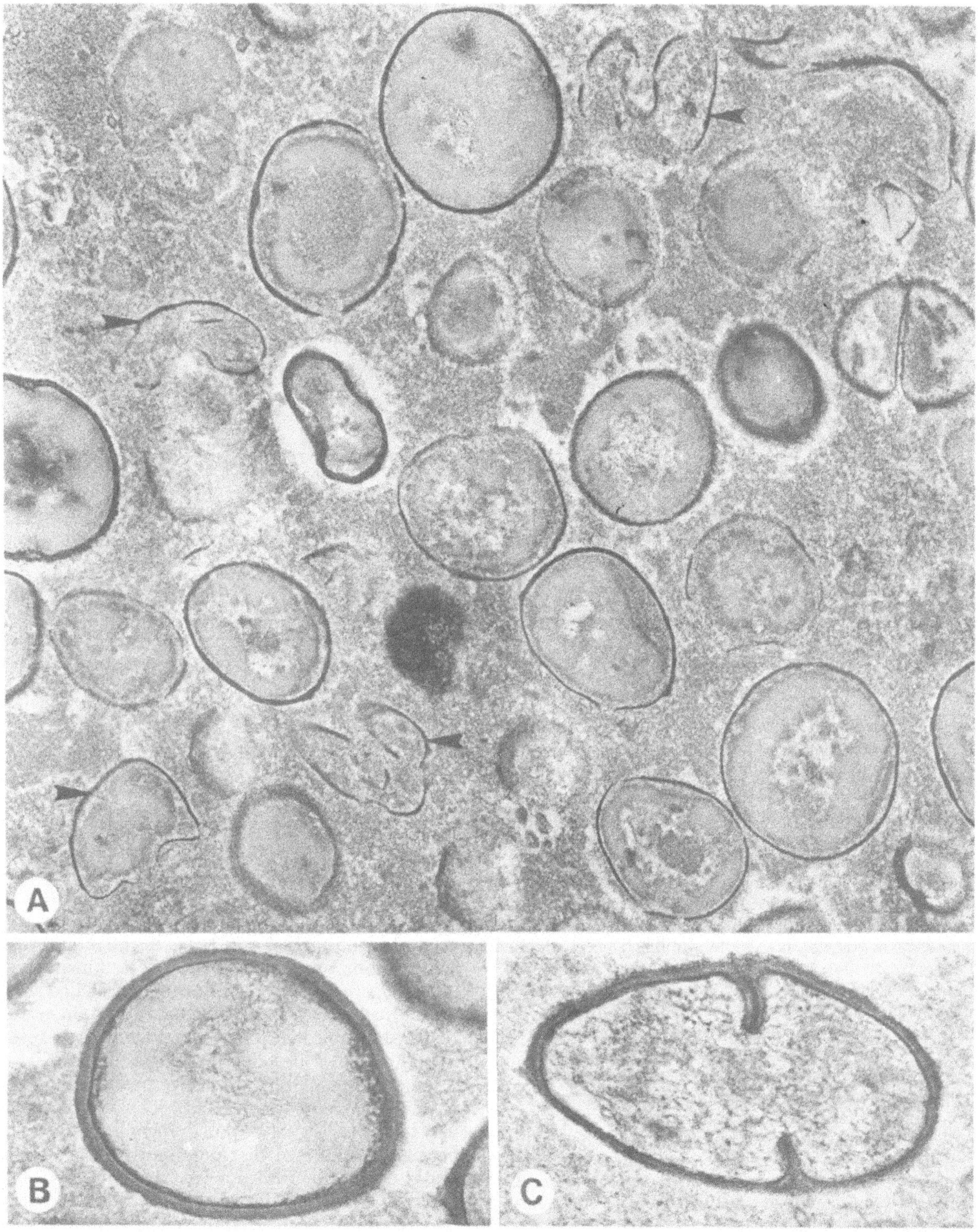

FIGURE 5. Patient 3. Electron micrographs of staphylococci in vegetations on the heterograft (all specified magnifications reduced by 9 percent). **A,** numerous closely packed organisms are embedded in amorphous material. Note that several of these bacteria have disrupted cell walls (**arrowheads**) and appear to have lysed (×35,400); **B,** intact bacterium with thick cell wall and pale-staining fibrillar nuclear material (×84,000); **C,** organism that is in process of dividing, as evidenced by partial formation of new septum composed of cell membrane and cell wall (×94,000).

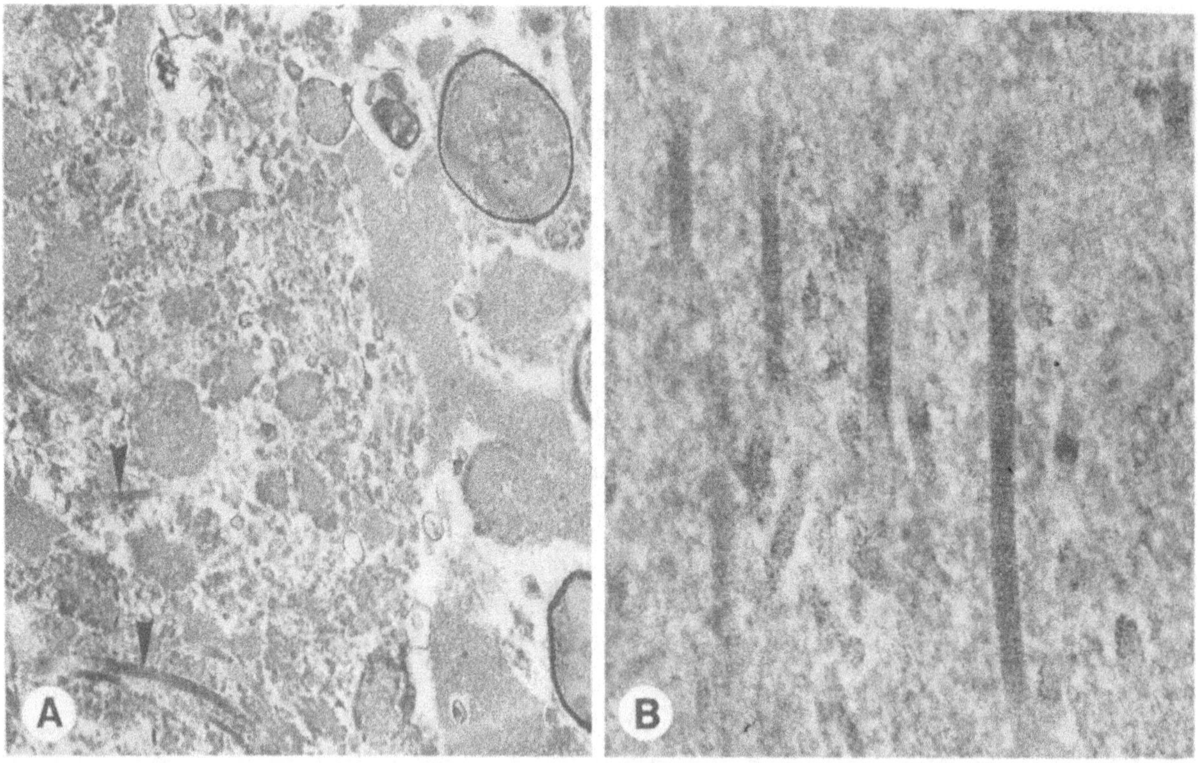

FIGURE 6. Patient 3. Electron micrographs of valve damage in heterograft (all specified in magnifications reduced by 10 percent). **A,** area of invasion of valve collagen by staphylococci (**upper right**). Note the severe disorganization of collagen structure (a few remaining collagen fibrils are indicated by **arrowheads**) and the accumulation of considerable amount of debris (×30,000); **B,** high magnification view of area similar to that in lower left of **A.** Only a few collagen fibrils are recognizable, and they are surrounded by gray material presumed to be necrotic collagen (×85,000).

be typical of staphylococci.[36–38] Many organisms appeared to be in different stages of lysis and nucleoid disintegration. Others showed evidence of continuing cell division, as manifested by the presence of partially developed cell walls. The cell walls in numerous bacteria were thinner than normal. Such cells were lysed and were in the process of extruding their content. The bacteria that had penetrated the deepest into the collagen framework of the cusps showed the least morphologic change. Many of these bacteria still had a normal cell wall structure, with outer and inner dense layers and an intervening less dense layer. Their cell walls also varied in thickness. The collagen bundles that had been invaded by bacteria were fragmented, disrupted and necrotic (Fig. 6).

In Patient 4 the valve was shaggy and necrotic. Bacteria in this valve were not identifiable on light microscopic study using special stains, but ultrastructural examination revealed a number of colonies of spore-forming rod-like bacilli measuring up to 1.5 μ in length and 0.3 μ in width. The appearance of these bacteria was variable (Fig. 7). Some organisms consisted mainly of empty shells and appeared dead; others were well preserved and could have been viable. The organisms present deep in the substance of the cusps were associated with severely necrotic connective tissue. As in the valve of Patient 3, inflammatory cells were present in the vegetations on the surface of the heterograft, but did not penetrate into the underlying collagen framework.

Discussion

Morphologic features of infection of porcine valve heterografts: The morphologic observations in these four patients illustrate the variety of clinical and morphologic changes associated with infection of porcine valve heterografts.

The findings in Patient 1 are compatible with a very early infection of a recently implanted (6 days) heterograft. This situation is complicated by the finding of two different organisms, one demonstrated morphologically in the valve itself and the other grown on culture of the aortic tissue tag. This infection was clinically inapparent, as would be expected in a valve that had only a few small colonies of bacteria. The excellent state of preservation of these organisms suggests that they were viable and probably had not been present at implantation of the valve (perhaps colonizing it before commercial processing) and then inactivated by treatment of the valve with glutaraldehyde before clinical use. However, the latter possibility cannot be excluded because it is known that porcine valves are collected under nonsterile conditions at the time when the animals are killed and that they are sterilized by the glutaraldehyde processing. In this respect, it must be noted that Ashraf and Bloor[39] reported the detection, using scanning electron microscopy, of elongated, rod-like bacteria on the surface of a porcine heterograft that had been in place in the aortic position for 2 months in a patient with a previous history of aortic regurgitation secondary to staphylococcal endocarditis. The clinical significance of the rod-like bacteria they found in this valve at necropsy is uncertain. The organisms found in our Patient 1 were located deep to the layer of fibrin

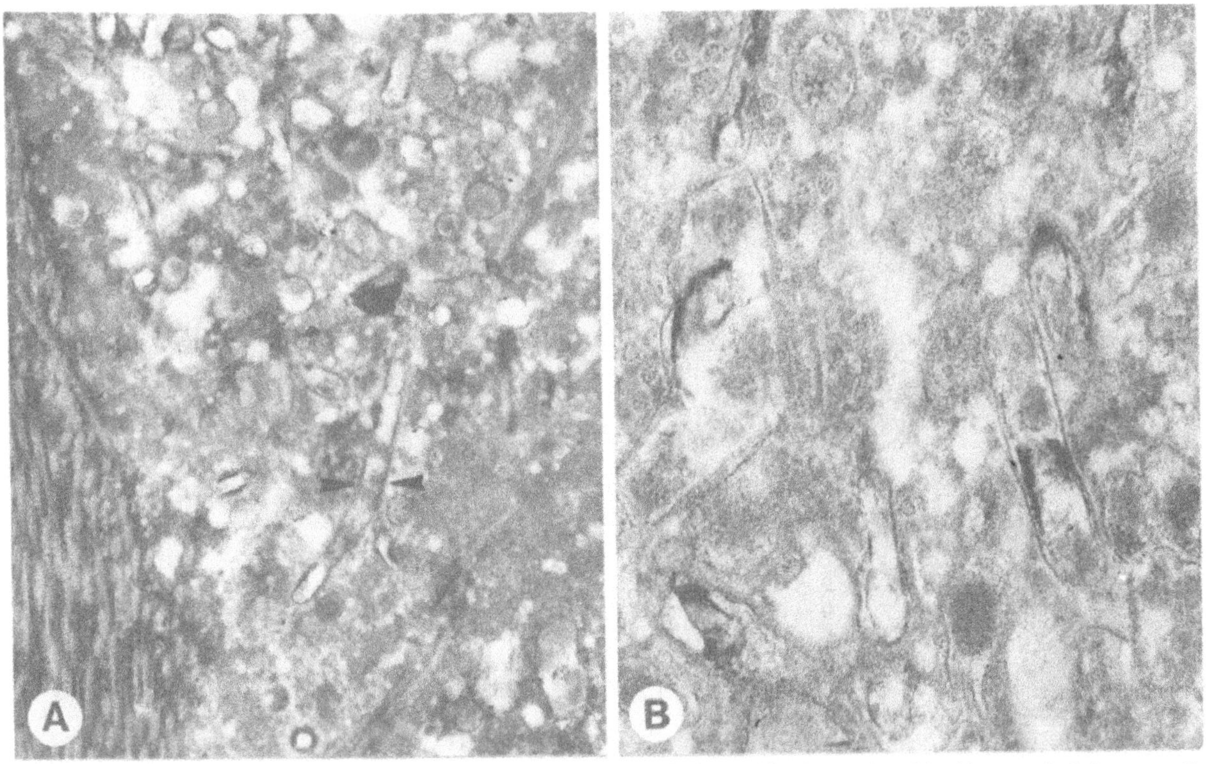

FIGURE 7. Patient 4. Electron micrographs of bacteria in heterograft (all specified magnifications reduced by 10 percent). **A,** low magnification view of colony of elongated, rod-like bacteria (**arrowheads**) deep in leaftlet of heterograft. Note the bundle of collagen fibrils at **lower left** and amorphous, dark gray material surrounding the bacteria. The round clear spaces represent lipid deposits (X22,500). **B,** the bacteria are surrounded in collagen and amorphous material. Some of the organisms have electron-dense lamellae in their cytoplasm (X45,000).

covering the surface of the heterograft, suggesting that they were not postmortem contaminants. Accordingly, we favor the possibility that these organisms represented an early stage of infection that would have become clinically manifest had the patient survived longer.

The species of the organism detected on ultrastructural study of the heterograft from Patient 1 could not be determined on the basis of morphologic study alone. Nevertheless, our observations show that the morphologic features of this organism differed from those of the Mycobacterium chelonei that grew on culture of an aortic tissue tag included in the container of the heterograft implanted in this patient.[33,34] The bacteria observed by us had flagella and thin cell walls. In contrast, mycobacteria are nonmobile and lack flagella; they have thick complex cell walls in which the mycobacterial waxes (responsible for acid-fastness) are present.[40–42] Thus, it is tempting to conclude that the heterograft from Patient 1 was infected with two different organisms. Among the patients reported to have received porcine valve heterografts from which the aortic tags grew Mycobacterium species in culture, only one[34] had clinical evidence of infection with this type of organism. This patient had pericardial effusion 2 months after valve implantation, and Mycobacterium chelonei was cultured from the pericardial fluid. We are aware of only one patient who had infection with Mycobacterium chelonei in a prosthetic heart valve.[43] This patient underwent aortic valve replacement with a Björk-Shiley valve because of endocarditis due to gram-positive cocci. Four and one-half months after operation, fever and aneurysmal dilatation of the ascending aorta developed. Blood cultures grew Mycobacterium chelonei. The patient died of rupture of the aneurysm, and at necropsy vegetations containing acid-fast bacilli (again shown by culture to be Mycobacterium chelonei) were found attached to the edge of the prosthesis and on the aortic incision line.

Patients 2 and 4 illustrate other problems encountered in the bacteriologic diagnosis of infections of porcine valve heterografts. Although Patient 2 had large florid vegetations filling the cusps and obstructing the orifice of this aortic porcine heterograft, and his death was caused by a coronary embolus, incontrovertible evidence of prosthetic infection could not be obtained. Culture of heart blood at necropsy grew three different organisms (alpha-streptococcus, Enterobacter cloacae, Citrobacter fuente), which were considered likely to be contaminants. Electron microscopic examination of the vegetations disclosed "ghost" forms that resembled bacteria but could not be unequivocally identified as such. These forms differed from the cell wall-deficient bacteria recently reported by Piepkorn and Reichenbach[44] to cause endocarditis involving native valves in four patients.

The nature of the infection in Patient 4 also remains uncertain because no growth was obtained on culture

TABLE III

Reports of Infection of Implanted Porcine Valve Heterografts

Author (Reference)	no. of PVH in Study	no. (%) of Inf. PVH (incidence)	Site of Inf. PVH	Time Bet. Impl. and Infection (mo)	Infecting Organism	Predisposing Factor	Total Patients With: PVH Sten.	PVH Reg.	Ring Abcess	PVH Leaf. Perf.	Perivalve Leak	Death Related to Infection
Zuhdi et al.[19]	137	1 (0.7)	A	>4.5	—	—	0	0	0	0	1	1
Carpentier et al.[20]	116	3 (2.6)	A	>12	—	—	—	—	—	—	—	1
			M	>2	—	—	—	—	—	—	—	1
			T	—	—	—	—	—	—	—	—	0
Horowitz et al.[21]	32	1* (3.1)	M	—	Strept	GU infection	0	0	0	0	0	0
McIntosh et al.[22]	136	5 (3.7)	A-V	2 valves <1	—	—	0	—	—	—	—	2
			A-V	3 valves >1	—	—	0	—	—	—	—	3
Buch et al.[23]	120	1 (0.8)	M	20	Enterococcus	Dental manipulation	—	0	—	—	—	0
Pipkin et al.[24]	75	1* (1.3)	A	39	—	—	—	1	—	—	—	1
Cohn et al.[25]	—	2 (—)	—	—	—	—	—	—	—	—	—	1
Stinson et al.[26]	218	1 (0.5)	A	—	—	—	—	1	—	—	—	1
	294	1 (0.3)	M	—	—	—	—	1	—	—	—	1
Gallucci[27]	387	3 (0.8)	—	—	—	—	—	—	—	—	—	—
Fishbein et al.[28]	363	4 (1.1)	A	31	α-Strept.	—	—	1	—	—	—	0
			M	12	Candida paropsilosis	—	—	1	—	—	—	0
			M	1.2	Pseudomonas aeruginosa	—	—	—	—	—	—	1
			A	0.5	Phycomyces	—	1	0	0	0	0	1
Moseley et al.[29]	1	1 (—)	P	0.5	Enterobacter Staph. epidermidis	—	0	0	0	0	0	0
Oyer et al.[30]	339	5 (1.5)	A	—	—	—	—	—	—	—	—	1
	426	1 (0.2)	M	—	—	—	—	—	—	—	—	1
Magilligan et al.[31]	470	11 (2.3)	A-V	32	Strept. faecalis	Opiate addict	—	0	—	—	—	0
			A	12	α-Strept.	—	0	1	1 (S)	0	0	1
			A	3	α-Strept.; Staph. epidermidis; H. influenzae	Opiate addict	0	0	0	0	0	0
			M	21	Enterobacter cloacae	—	—	0	—	—	—	0
			M	24	Strept. faecalis	—	0	0	0	0	0	0
			M	6	α-strept.	Opiate addict	—	0	—	—	—	0
			A	29	α-strept.	Dental extraction	0	1	1 (S)	0	0	1
			M	7	α-strept.	Opiate addict	0	0	0	0	0	0
			M	45	Strept. faecalis	—	—	0	—	—	—	0
			—	36	Strept. faecalis	—	2	0	0	0	0	1
			M	29	Candida	GI infection	0	0	0	0	0	0
Hatcher[32]	311	2 (0.6)	M	24	Candida	—	—	—	—	—	—	0
Present study	4	4 (—)	A	†	Mycobacterium chelonei† gram-neg. rod	—	0	0	0	0	0	0
			A	—	—	—	1	0	0	0	0	0
			M	2.5	Staph. aureus	Opiate addict	1	0	1	0	0	0
			M	‡	Spore-forming rod-like bacillus	—	1	0	0	0	0	0

TABLE III (continued)

Reports of Infection of Implanted Porcine Valve Heterografts

Author (Reference)	no. of PVH in Study	no. (%) of Inf. PVH (incidence)	Site of Inf. PVH	Time Bet. Impl. and Infection (mo)	Infecting Organism	Predisposing Factor	Total Patients With: PVH Sten.	PVH Reg.	Ring Abcess	PVH Leaf. Perf.	Perivalve Leak	Death Related to Infection
Totals		47	A = 16 (34%) M = 17 (36%) T = 1 (2%) P = 1(2%) A-V = 6 (13%) (−) = 6 (13%)				6 (13%)	7 (15%)	3 (6%)	0 (—)	1 (2%)	19 (40%)

* Infection suspected but not proved.
† Grown from aortic tag in culture taken at time of operation; valve itself not cultured.
— = data not available.
‡ Duration of infection could not be determined.
α-Strept. = alpha-hemolytic Streptococcus; A = aortic; A-V = atrioventricular (site not specified); Bet. = between; GI = gastrointestinal tract; GU = genitourinary tract; H = Hemophilus; Impl. = implantation; Inf. = infected; Leaf. = leaflet; M = mitral; neg. = negative; P = pulmonary; Perf. = perforation; PVH = porcine valve heterograft; Reg. = regurgitation; S = sterile; Staph. = Staphylococcus; Sten. = stenosis; T = tricuspid.

of the valve, even though bacterial colonies and necrotic leaflet tissue and vegetations were found when the heterograft was removed. The patient had not received antibiotic therapy before operation. Because the heterograft had been in place for 2 1/2 years, it seems likely that the infection was acquired after implantation rather than at the time of operation. Although it is possible that the infection was related to the cardiac catheterization performed before removal of the infected heterograft, the catheterization was undertaken because the patient already had evidence of obstruction to flow through the heterograft. Thus, ultrastructural study provided the only unequivocal evidence that the porcine valve heterograft in this patient was infected.

The histologic and ultrastructural findings on the porcine valve heterograft from Patients 2 and 3 show that severe destruction of the collagen framework can occur in infection of valve bioprostheses. In Patient 3, invasion and colonization by Staphylococcus aureus was observed not only within the vegetations filling the cusps of the heterograft but also deep in the leaflets. The severe destruction and necrosis of the collagen bundles in sites of deep penetration and colonization of the organisms can be attributed to proteolytic enzymes released by inflammatory cells and bacteria. Polymorphonuclear leukocytes and macrophages are known to produce a specific collagenase,[45,46] but Staphylococcus aureus is not. Nevertheless, the destructive effects of staphylococcal infections on native cardiac valves are well known. In the valve of Patient 2, inflammatory cells were localized only in the vegetations on the surface of the valve and not within the leaflets. This absence of inflammatory cells from deep areas of infected porcine valve heterografts is in keeping with previous observations[35] showing that inflammatory cells in noninfected porcine heterografts show no tendency to invade the leaflets but tend to remain localized on the surfaces.

Many of the staphylococci in the valve from Patient 3 had undergone morphologic changes, including increase in cell size and thinning of the cell walls, which probably resulted from treatment of the patient with nafcillin for 6 weeks before valve replacement. Such ultrastructural features have been described in penicillin-treated staphylococci.[38,47] However, not all of the bacteria were in a stage of lysis or degeneration. The colonies of bacteria situated in the collagen of the leaflet showed only slight morphologic changes, and a few of these bacteria appeared to be in the process of cell division. This would indicate that the antibiotic therapy was not effective against the deeper-penetrating bacteria and that some of the bacteria were still viable at the time of valve removal. This observation is consistent with the detection of Staphylococcus aureus on culture of the porcine valve heterograft at the time of removal.

Review of clinical and pathologic changes reported in infection of porcine valve heterografts: Including the 4 valves in the 4 patients in our study, infection in porcine valve heterografts has been reported in a total of 47 valves implanted in 47 patients.[18–32]

Because of the limited amount of information presented in many of these reports, the following data almost certainly underestimate the true incidence of the findings. Nevertheless, some useful generalizations can be derived from review of the observations in these patients (Table III). Two porcine valve heterografts had been implanted in at least 4 of the 47 patients; however, none of these 4 patients had infection in more than one heterograft, and the most downstream valve was the one always infected. Seventeen of the infected heterografts were in the mitral position, 16 in the aortic position, 1 in the tricuspid position and 1 in the pulmonary position; the site of implantation of the remaining 12 valves was not reported. In 6 patients, the infection occurred within 2 months after implantation; in 23 other patients, it became evident more than 2 months after implantation (maximal time 45 months), and in 18 patients the time at which infection developed was not specified.

Bacteriologic identification of a total of 24 infecting organisms was reported in 22 valves: Eleven of these organisms were streptococci, 3 staphylococci; 4 gram-negative rods and 4 fungi (including 3 candida species and 1 phycomyces). In two other valves (from two of our four patients) organisms were seen on morphologic study but were not identified bacteriologically.

The single factor most frequently identified as predisposing to infection of porcine valve heterografts was opiate addiction (five patients). All five patients had undergone implantation of a porcine valve heterograft as part of therapy for a separate episode of infective endocarditis involving the patient's own valve.

Dysfunction was reported to occur in 14 of the infected heterografts: 6 heterografts had stenosis due to vegetations interfering with cuspal motion; 7 had regurgitation, although perforation of the cusps was not specifically reported in any valve, and one had a perivalve leak. Valve ring abscesses were described in three patients, but were sterile in two of them. Of the 47 patients, 19 (40 percent) died of various complications of infection (Table III).

Comparison of features of infection involving porcine valve heterografts and other types of prosthetic heart valves: These observations show that infection of porcine valve heterografts differs in several respects from infection involving other types of prosthetic heart valves. There are several characteristics of infection of rigid-framed prosthetic valves[1-18]: (1) The infection does not involve the prosthetic material; instead, it involves biologic materials such as fibrin, organized thrombi and fibrous tissue that have covered the prosthetic valve; (2) the infection is characteristically located at the site of attachment of the sewing ring to host tissue; (3) valve ring abscesses are to be expected; and (4) the infection does not destroy the prosthesis itself although it may cause it to malfunction mechanically and to become detached from the valve ring.

In contrast to these characteristics of infection of rigid-framed prosthetic valves, infection of porcine valve heterografts has the following features: (1) It can involve the prosthetic material itself as well as fibrin, organized thrombi and fibrous tissue from the host; (2) it is localized in the cusps; (3) it can destroy the prosthesis itself and (4) it is uncommonly associated with valve ring abscesses. The destruction of bioprosthetic tissue is illustrated by our observations of invasion of the leaflet substance and severe breakdown of collagen in the heterografts from two or our patients (Patients 3 and 4). This pattern of localization of infection of porcine valve heterografts is similar to that reported in other types of bioprostheses, including homografts,[48-54] fascia lata valves[55-57] and pericardial valves.[57]

Perforation occurring in a cusp of a porcine valve as the result of infection has not been reported, in spite of the potential for destruction of infected bioprosthetic tissue, although prosthetic regurgitation due to unspecified anatomic lesions has been found in infected porcine valves (Table III). Perforations of the leaflets of porcine valves appear to be consequences of degenerative breakdown of their connective tissue.[35] Thus, the observations just reviewed suggest that, probably because of the glutaraldehyde treatment, porcine valve heterografts are less easily destroyed by infections than are native valves, homografts and fascia lata valves.

Prosthetic valve stenosis caused by infected vegetations appears to be a relatively common complication of porcine heterograft infection (Table III). This complication must be distinguished from obstruction to flow caused either by calcific deposits in the leaflets, with resulting loss of mobility, or by the presence of large noninfected thrombi within the cusps.

Valve ring abscesses and perivalve leaks (occurring in 3 and 1, respectively, of 47 patients) appear to be uncommon (Table III) when porcine valves become infected. The incidence rate of valve ring abscesses in patients with rigid-framed prosthetic valves is high. Arnett and Roberts and their co-workers[14,18] found valve ring abscesses in each of their 22 patients with fatal infection of rigid-framed prosthetic valves, and the entire circumference of the valve anulus was necrotic in two thirds of these patients.

The mortality rate of infection of porcine valve heterografts is high (40 percent) in spite of what appear to be more favorable characteristics of infection (Table III). Nevertheless, the data available are incomplete, and the number of patients whose exact cause of death was reported is too small for a meaningful analysis.

Possible mechanisms of infection of prosthetic heart valves: Although the site of infection might be expected to be similar in rigid-framed prostheses and in porcine valve heterografts, because the devices have similar sewing rings, this is not the case. In our Patient 1, fibrin deposits were the sites of localization of small bacterial colonies considered to represent early stages of infection. This observation is in accord with the results of ultrastructural studies of the early stages of infection in experimentally induced infective endocarditis in animals.[58-61] Those studies have shown that fibrin-platelet microthrombi are the sites of initial attachment and colonization of valves by bacteria and that denudation of valve endothelium (which exposes the highly thrombogenic connective tissue of the subendothelial region) is the factor leading to the formation of these microthrombi. It is known[35,62,63] that nonimplanted glutaraldehyde-stabilized porcine valve heterografts are denuded of endothelium and that after implantation they become covered with a layer of fibrin. This layer of fibrin, which does not become covered by endothelium or a fibrous sheath, appears to be the preferred site of bacterial invasion. It has been suggested that the sites of infection in rigid-framed prosthetic heart valves are small platelet-fibrin thrombi that become organized by undergoing fibroblastic invasion and grow to cover portions of the sewing cloth of the prosthesis.[64] A similar process of growth of host fibrous tissue occurs in implanted porcine valve heterografts. However, for reasons that may be related to the glutaraldehyde treatment of the porcine tissue, the ingrowth of host fibrous tissue does not extend into the cusps themselves.[35,62,63] Thus, bacteria appear to be more likely to colonize the fibrin on the cusps than the organizing fibrous tissue in the sewing ring.

In conclusion, our study shows that bacterial infections of porcine valve heterografts involve the valve cusps and can cause considerable destruction of prosthetic tissue. Such infections probably begin with the attachment of bacteria to the fibrin deposits that form on the cusp surfaces. Review of previous reports indicates that these infections have a high mortality rate, although they are not frequently associated with valve ring abscesses. Ultrastructural study can be of considerable value in assessing the extent of prosthetic tissue damage and in determining the nature of the bacterial infection.

References

1. **Roberts WC, Morrow AG:** Bacterial endocarditis involving prosthetic mitral valves. Clinical and pathologic observations. Arch Pathol Lab Med 82:164–169, 1966
2. **Stein PD, Harken DE, Dexter L:** The nature and prevention of prosthetic valve endocarditis. Am Heart J 71:393–407, 1966
3. **Amoury RA, Bowman FO Jr, Malm JR:** Endocarditis associated with intracardiac prostheses. Diagnosis, management, and prophylaxis. J Thorac Cardiovasc Surg 51:36–48, 1966
4. **Cohn LH, Roberts WC, Rockoff SD, Morrow AG:** Bacterial endocarditis following aortic valve replacement. Clinical and pathologic correlations. Circulation 33:209–217, 1966
5. **Block PC, DeSanctis, RW, Weinberg AN, Austen WG:** Prosthetic valve endocarditis. J Thorac Cardiovasc Surg 60:540–548, 1970
6. **Killen DA, Collins HA, Koenig MG, Goodman JS:** Prosthetic cardiac valves and bacterial endocarditis. Ann Thorac Surg 9:238–247, 1970
7. **Okies JE, Viroslav J, Williams TW Jr:** Endocarditis after cardiac valvular replacement. Chest 59:198–202, 1971
8. **Dismukes WE, Karchmer AW, Buckley MJ, Austen WG, Swartz MN:** Prosthetic valve endocarditis. Analysis of 38 cases. Circulation 48:365–377, 1973
9. **Slaughter L, Morris JE, Starr A:** Prosthetic valvular endocarditis. A 12-year review. Circulation 47:1319–1326, 1973
10. **Madison J, Wang K, Gobel FL, Edwards JE:** Prosthetic aortic valvular endocarditis. Circulation 51:940–949, 1975
11. **Wilson WR, Jaumin PM, Danielson GK, Giuliani ER, Washington JA II, Geraci JE:** Prosthetic valve endocarditis. Ann Intern Med 82:751–756, 1975
12. **Rubinstein E, Noriega ER, Simberkoff MS, Holzman R, Rahal JJ:** Fungal endocarditis: analysis of 24 cases and review of literature. Medicine 54:331–344, 1975
13. **Arnett EN, Roberts WC:** Prosthetic valve endocarditis. Clinicopathologic analysis of 22 necropsy patients with comparison of observations in 74 necropsy patients with active infective endocarditis involving natural left-sided cardiac valves. Am J Cardiol 38:281–292, 1976
14. **Arnett EN, Roberts WC:** Valve ring abscess in active infective endocarditis. Frequency, location, and clues to clinical diagnosis from the study of 95 necropsy patients. Circulation 54:140–145, 1976
15. **Quenzer RW, Edwards LD, Levin S:** A comparative study of 48 host valve and 24 prosthetic valve endocarditis cases. Am Heart J 92:15–22, 1976
16. **Sarma R, Roschke EJ, Harrison EC, Edmiston WA, Lau FYK:** Clinical experience with the Smeloff-Cutter aortic valve prosthesis: an 8-year follow-up study. Am J Cardiol 40:338–344, 1977
17. **Arnett EN, Roberts WC:** Clinicopathology of prosthetic valve endocarditis. In, Infections in Prosthetic Heart Valves and Vascular Grafts (Duma RJ, ed). Baltimore, University Park Press, 1977, p 17–41
18. **Arnett EN, Kastl DG, Garvin AJ, Roberts WC:** A conversation on prosthetic valve endocarditis. Am Heart J 93:510–517, 1977
19. **Zuhdi N, Hawley W, Voehl V, Hancock W, Carey J, Greer A:** Porcine aortic valves as replacements for human heart valves. Ann Thorac Surg 17:479–491, 1974
20. **Carpentier A, Deloche A, Relland J, Fabiani JN, Forman J, Camilleri JP, Soyer R, Dubost C:** Six-year follow-up of glutaraldehyde-preserved heterografts. With particular reference to the treatment of congenital valve malformations. J Thorac Cardiovasc Surg 68:771–782, 1974
21. **Horowitz MS, Goodman DJ, Fogarty TJ, Harrison DC:** Mitral valve replacement with the glutaraldehyde-preserved porcine heterograft. Clinical, hemodynamic, and pathological correlations. J Thorac Cardiovasc Surg 67:885–895, 1974
22. **McIntosh CL, Michaelis LL, Morrow AG, Itscoitz SB, Redwood DR, Epstein SE:** Atrioventricular valve replacement with the Hancock porcine xenograft: a five year clinical experience. Surgery 78:768–775, 1975
23. **Buch WS, Pipkin RD, Hancock WD, Fogarty TJ:** Mitral valve replacement with the Hancock stabilized glutaraldehyde valve. Clinical and laboratory evaluation. Arch Surg 110:1408–1415, 1975
24. **Pipkin RD, Buch WS, Fogarty TJ:** Evaluation of aortic valve replacement with a porcine xenograft without long-term anticoagulation. J Thorac Cardiovasc Surg 71:179–186, 1976
25. **Cohn LH, Sanders JH Jr, Collins JJ Jr:** Aortic valve replacement with the Hancock porcine xenograft. Ann Thorac Surg 22:221–227, 1976
26. **Stinson EB, Griepp RB, Oyer PE, Shumway NE:** Long-term experience with porcine aortic valve xenografts. J Thorac Cardiovasc Surg 73:54–63, 1977
27. **Gallucci V:** Discussion of presentation by Stinson et al.[26] J Thorac Cardiovasc Surg 73:62, 1977
28. **Fishbein MC, Gissen SA, Collins JJ Jr, Barsamian EM, Cohn LH:** Pathologic findings after cardiac valve replacement with glutaraldehyde-fixed porcine valves. Am J Cardiol 40:331–337, 1977
29. **Moseley PW, Ochsner JL, Mills NL, Chapman J:** Management of an infected Hancock prosthesis after repair of truncus arteriosus. J Thorac Cardiovasc Surg 73:306–308, 1977
30. **Oyer PE, Stinson EB, Griepp RB, Shumway NE:** Valve replacement with the Starr-Edwards and Hancock prostheses: comparative analysis of later morbidity and mortality. Ann Surg 186:301–309, 1977
31. **Magilligan DJ Jr, Quinn EL, Davila JC:** Bacteremia, endocarditis, and the Hancock valve. Ann Thorac Surg 24:508–518, 1977
32. **Hatcher C:** Discussion of presentation by Magilligan et al.[31] Ann Thorac Surg 24:517, 1977
33. Center for Disease Control: Isolation of mycobacteria species from porcine heart valve prostheses. Morbid Mortal Weekly Report

26:42–43, 1977
34. **Laskowski LF, Marr JJ, Spernoga JF, Frank NJ, Barner HB, Kaiser G, Tyras DH:** Fastidious mycobacteria grown from porcine prosthetic-heart-valve cultures. N Engl J Med 297:101–102, 1977
35. **Ferrans VJ, Spray TL, Billingham ME, Roberts WC:** Structural changes in glutaraldehyde-treated porcine heterografts used as substitute cardiac valves. Transmission and scanning electron microscopic observations in 12 patients. Am J Cardiol 41: 1159–1184, 1978
36. **Suganuma A:** Fine structure of Staphylococcus aureus. Ann NY Acad Sci 128:26–44, 1965
37. **Suganuma A:** Electron microscopic studies of staphylococci by serial sections. J Electron Microsc (Tokyo) 17:315–321, 1968
38. **Suganuma A:** Fine structure of staphylococci: electron microscopy. In, The Staphylococci (Cohen JO, ed). New York, John Wiley & Sons, 1972, p 21–40
39. **Ashraf M, Bloor CM:** Structural alterations of the porcine heterograft after various durations of implantation. Am J Cardiol 41: 1185–1190, 1978
40. **Imaeda T, Kanetsuna F, Galindo B:** Ultrastructure of cell walls of genus mycobacterium. J Ultrastruct Res 25:46–63, 1968
41. **Mohelska H, Holusa R, Kubin M, Smetana K:** Endocellular parasitism of Mycobacterium avium in rabbit liver. A morphological study. Exp Pathol (Jena) 10:122–131, 1975
42. **Levy L, Herman NG, Evans MJ, Krahenbuhl JL:** Susceptibility of thymectomized and irradiated mice to challenge with several organisms and the effect of dapsone on infection with Mycobacterium leprae. Infect Immun 11:1122–1132, 1975
43. **Altmann G, Horowitz A, Kaplinsky N, Frankl O:** Prosthetic valve endocarditis due to Mycobacterium chelonei. J Clin Microbiol 1: 531–533, 1975
44. **Piepkorn MW, Reichenbach DD:** Infective endocarditis associated with cell wall-deficient bacteria. Electron microscopic findings in four cases. Hum Pathol 9:163–173, 1978
45. **Horwitz AL, Hance AJ, Crystal RG:** Granulocyte collagenase: selective digestion of type I relative to type III collagen. Proc Natl Acad Sci USA 74:897–901, 1977
46. **Horwitz AL, Crystal RG:** Collagenase from rabbit pulmonary alveolar macrophages. Biochem Biophys Res Commun 69:296–303, 1976
47. **Murray RGE, Francombe WH, Mayall BH:** The effect of penicillin on the structure of staphylococcal cell walls. Can J Microbiol 5: 641–648, 1959
48. **Smith JC:** The pathology of human aortic valve homografts. Thorax 22:114–138, 1967
49. **Reichenbach DD, Mohri H, Merendino KA:** Pathological changes in human aortic valve homografts. Circulation 39, 40: Suppl I:I-47–I-56, 1969
50. **Clarkson PM, Barrat-Boyes BG:** Bacterial endocarditis following replacement of the aortic valve. Circulation 42:987–991, 1970
51. **Gonzalez-Lavin L, Al-Janabi N, Ross DN:** Long-term results after aortic valve replacement with preserved aortic homografts. Ann Thorac Surg 13:594–606, 1972
52. **Trimble AS:** Late results of homograft aortic valve replacement: a clinical and hemodynamic evaluation. In, Biologic Tissue in Heart Valve Replacement (Ionescu MI, Ross DN, Woller GH, ed). London, Butterworth, 1972, p 349
53. **Wallace RB, Londe SP, Titus JL:** Aortic valve replacement with preserved aortic homografts. J Thorac Cardiovasc Surg 67:44–50, 1974
54. **Anderson ET, Hancock EW:** Long-term follow-up of aortic valve replacement with the fresh aortic homograft. J Thorac Cardiovasc Surg 72:150–156, 1976
55. **Senning A, Rothlin M:** The late failure of autologous fascia lata valve grafts in the aortic position. In, Recent Trends in Cardiovascular and Thoracic Surgery (Borman JB, ed). Jerusalem, Alpha Press, 1975, p 81
56. **Ionescu MI, Abid A, Wooler H:** Experience with tissue heart valves. in Ref 55, p 105
57. **Yarbrough JW, Roberts WC, Reis RL:** Structural alterations in tissue cardiac valves implanted in patients and in calves. J Thorac Cardiovasc Surg 65: 364–375, 1973
58. **Geissinger H, Miniats O, Ruhnke H, Djurickovic D:** Experimental staphylococcal endocarditis in pigs. J Comp Pathol 83:323–335, 1973
59. **Mitomo Y:** Ultrastructural changes in the bacterial vegetative endocarditis. Bull Tokyo Med Dent Univ 21:79–105, 1974
60. **Durack D:** Experimental bacterial endocarditis. J Pathol 115:81–89, 1975
61. **Harasaki H:** Studies of the pathogenesis of bacterial endocarditis. Ryumachi 17:285–297, 1977
62. **Spray TL, Roberts WC:** Structural changes in porcine xenografts used as substitute cardiac valves. Gross and histologic observations in 51 glutaraldehyde-preserved Hancock valves in 41 patients. Am J Cardiol 40:319–330, 1977
63. **Spray TL, Roberts WC:** Structural changes in Hancock porcine xenograft cardiac valve bioprostheses. Adv Cardiol 22:241–251, 1978
64. **Robboy S, Kaiser J:** Pathogenesis of fungal infection on heart valve prostheses. Hum Pathol 6:711–715, 1975

Late failure of porcine valve heterografts in children

Heterograft porcine valves have gained wide acceptance in replacement of diseased cardiac valves, and their clinical performance in adults has been very satisfactory over follow-up periods of up to 8 years. Valve replacement in children is relatively infrequent and experience with porcine xenografts is necessarily small. Our combined experience at three university hospitals has been with 25 children, 17 months to 16 years of age, who have been followed for 10 to 54 months (mean follow-up 33 months). Porcine valves were used to replace the aortic valve in nine, the mitral valve in seven, both valves in two, the tricuspid valve in two, and the pulmonary valve in five patients. Severe bioprosthetic valve dysfunction has occurred in five (20%) of these patients so far and necessitated replacement because of severe stenosis in mitral (two) or aortic (three) valve prostheses at 18 to 45 months after implantation; one postoperative death occurred among the five reoperations. Pathological examination showed extensive fragmentation of collagen with focal heavy calcification and degeneration. In addition we have encountered deterioration and calcification of two porcine valves in 23 valved conduits followed for 12 to 70 months (mean 43 months), requiring removal and replacement of the valves 65 and 67 months after implantation. This experience indicates a disquietingly high incidence of relatively early failure of porcine xenograft valves in children. This is significantly higher than the failure rate observed in adult patients. The failure rate is not consistently related to the small size of an implanted valve which becomes relatively narrow with the growth of the patient, leading to excessive turbulence and trauma to the prosthesis. Other factors, including increased turnover of calcium and accelerated rejection in growing children, may contribute to these failures and should be examined in order to improve long-term results. A satisfactory performance would make heterografts the ideal valvular prosthesis in children, since anticoagulation is avoided.

Alexander S. Geha, M.D., M.S., Hillel Laks, M.D. (by invitation),
Horace C. Stansel, Jr., M.D., *New Haven, Conn.*, J. Fredrick Cornhill, Ph.D. (by invitation),
James W. Kilman, M.D., *Columbus, Ohio,* Mortimer J. Buckley, M.D., *Boston, Mass.*, and
William C. Roberts, M.D. (by invitation), *Bethesda, Md.*

The main advantage of biologic valve prostheses over mechanical valve prostheses is the low rate of thromboembolism without administration of anticoagulants. Biologic valves for cardiac valve replacement have been used since 1954 in various states of preservation of allografts or xenografts.[1] Varying problems with long-term durability, however, have characterized many of these valves in the past decade.[2-6] Subsequent improvements in the preservation, sterilization, and collagen stabilization of biologic valves by fixation with a diluted proprietary glutaraldehyde solution[7, 8] and utilization of flexible valve stents[9] have resulted in the availability of reasonably durable, relatively inert xenograft porcine valves for intracardiac valve replacement and for correction of congenital heart lesions through the use of valve-containing Dacron conduits.[10]

These glutaraldehyde-preserved porcine aortic valve xenografts have gained wide acceptance in replacement of diseased cardiac valves, and the advantages of their central flow characteristics, relatively low profile, and negligible embolization rate without anticoagulant therapy have been well documented in large clinical

From the Departments of Surgery, Yale University School of Medicine, New Haven, Conn., Ohio State University, Columbus, Ohio, and Harvard Medical School, Boston, Mass., and the Pathology Branch, National Heart, Lung and Blood Institute, Bethesda, Md.

Supported in part by research grant No. HL 19182, National Heart, Lung and Blood Institute, U. S. Public Health Service.

Read at the Fifty-ninth Annual Meeting of The American Association for Thoracic Surgery, Boston, Mass., April 30 to May 2, 1979.

Address for reprints: Alexander S. Geha, M.D., M.S., Professor of Surgery (Cardiothoracic), Room 136, FMB, Yale University School of Medicine, 333 Cedar St., New Haven, Conn. 06510.

Table I. *Late failure of porcine heterograft valves in children*

Type of operation	No. of patients: Operated	No. of patients: Late failure	Percent failure
AVR	9	3	33
MVR	7	2	29
AVR-MVR	2	–	–
PVR	5	–	–
TVR	2	–	–
Total operations for valve replacement	25	5	20

Legend: AVR, Aortic valve replacement. MVR, Mitral valve replacement. PVR, Pulmonary valve replacement. TVR, Tricuspid valve replacement.

Table II. *Anatomic location of late failing porcine heterograft valves in children**

Valve position	No. of valves implanted	Failing valves: No.	Failing valves: %
Aortic	11	3	27
Mitral	9	2	22
Tricuspid	2	–	–
Pulmonary	5	–	–
Total valves	27	5	19

*All patients under 16 years of age at time of operation, with a minimum follow-up of 10 months.

Table III. *Late failure of porcine valves in extracardiac conduits*

Type of conduit	No. of conduits implanted	No. of valves failed
LV apex to abdominal aorta	2	0*
Right ventricle to pulmonary artery	17	2
Fontan procedure	4	0
Total conduits	23	2 (9%)

Legend: Mean follow-up 43 months (12 to 70 months)

*One conduit removed at 10 months due to cause other than valve failure.

series.[11-13] Although their long-term durability has not been documented fully, and might be primarily a function of their ability to endure many millions of repeated mechanical loading events, their clinical performance has been very satisfactory over follow-up periods of up to 8 years in large series of adult patients.[14]

Valve replacement in children—in whom avoidance of anticoagulation is particularly desired—is relatively infrequent,[15, 16] and experience with porcine xenografts in the pediatric age group remains necessarily small. Our encounter of several cases of bioprosthetic dysfunction in children prompted our review of the results in this age group at three university hospitals. The purpose of this communication is to summarize the late postoperative results and to focus particularly upon long-term durability of this bioprosthesis in the pediatric age group.

Patients

Twenty-five children, 17 months to 16 years of age (mean 12.2 years), were long-term survivors of intracardiac valve replacement with glutaraldehyde-preserved porcine aortic valve xenografts.* The operations were performed between January, 1974, and June, 1978. Abnormal cardiac valves were replaced in 15 children at the Yale–New Haven Medical Center, in four children at Children's Hospital in Columbus, Ohio, and in six children at the Massachusetts General Hospital. Table I outlines the number of children receiving porcine xenograft intracardiac valves. Of the four children undergoing operation at Children's Hospital of Columbus, two had simultaneous aortic and mitral valve replacement, and one each had an aortic and a mitral valve replaced. Six children underwent operation at the Massachusetts General Hospital; five had mitral valve replacement and one had aortic valve replacement. The remaining operations, performed at the Yale–New Haven Medical Center, consisted of isolated replacement of the aortic valve in seven children, the mitral valve in one, the pulmonary valve in five, and the tricuspid valve in two. There were 12 boys and 13 girls in the total group.

Thus there were 27 valves at risk in 25 patients. Follow-up ranged from 10 to 54 months (mean 33). Complete follow-up was obtained in all patients.

Indications for valve replacement. Indications for replacement of the aortic valve with porcine xenografts included congenital lesions in seven children and rheumatic disease in two. Six of the seven children who underwent initial mitral valve replacement with a porcine xenograft valve had rheumatic mitral valve disease, and the seventh suffered injury to the mitral valve during surgical correction of congenital discrete subvalvular aortic stenosis. The two patients who had simultaneous mitral and aortic valve replacement with xenograft valves had rheumatic disease of both valves. Five children underwent pulmonary valve replacement for severe deformities of congenitally stenotic pulmonary valves, and two underwent tricuspid valve replacement for Ebstein's anomaly.

*Hancock Laboratories, Inc., Anaheim, Calif.

Extracardiac xenograft porcine valves. During the same period of time, 23 children operated upon by the Yale University surgical group* and ranging in age from 12 months to 16 years became long-term survivors after correction of complex congenital cardiac anomalies with the use of valve-containing conduits.† Two of these children had a shunt from the left ventricular apex to the abdominal aorta to circumvent severe congenital anomalies of the outflow tract of the left ventricle, 17 had a shunt from the right ventricle to the pulmonary artery (Rastelli procedure) for correction of truncus arteriosus and other lesions involving the outflow tract of the right ventricle, and four children had a right atrium–pulmonary artery shunt (Fontan procedure) for tricuspid atresia. These 23 children have been followed for 12 to 70 months (mean 43 months), with complete follow-up in all of them.

Results

Intracardiac valve replacement. Late bioprosthetic valve dysfunction, severe enough to require excision of the xenograft valve, developed in five (20%) of the 25 children who had undergone intracardiac valve replacement (Table I). There was no evidence of infection in any of these patients, and infection could not be identified in any of the five valves recovered from them. Late failure developed in three of the nine patients who had undergone isolated aortic valve replacement and in two of the seven with isolated mitral valve replacement. Table II outlines the anatomic location of the failing intracardiac bioprostheses. Three (27%) of the 11 valves in the aortic position and two (22%) of the nine valves in the mitral position have failed during the period of the study. Thus five (19%) of the 27 valves implanted have failed at periods varying between 18 and 45 months after implantation.

Late death occurred suddenly outside the hospital in two (8%) of the 25 patients owing to causes not clearly attributable to bioprosthetic valve dysfunction. These two deaths occurred 28 and 34 months after operation. Postmortem examination was not obtained in either case.

Valve-containing Dacron conduits. Two (9%) of the 23 valve-containing conduits malfunctioned severely enough to necessitate excision and replacement of the conduit during the period of follow-up (Table III). In both cases the right ventricle–pulmonary artery conduit was the dysfunctioning part. In one patient a 20 mm conduit had been inserted for repair of truncus arteriosus at 13 years of age. Because of recurrent stenosis this conduit was removed 65 months later and replaced with a 30 mm valved conduit. The truncal valve, which was regurgitant, was replaced with a 29 mm Björk-Shiley valve, and residual atrial and ventricular septal defects also were closed. In the second patient a 20 mm conduit had been inserted at the age of 5 years for the repair of truncus arteriosus. Because of stenosis of the porcine valve the patient underwent reoperation 67 months later with insertion of a 25 mm conduit, replacement of the truncal valve with a 29 mm Björk-Shiley prosthesis, and tricuspid valve annuloplasty. Both patients are doing well 6 and 8 months postoperatively. One patient with a conduit between the left ventricular apex and the abdominal aorta had the conduit removed at 10 months postoperatively because of infection. Two late deaths (9%) from causes other than xenograft valve dysfunction occurred in patients with conduits.

Clinical course of children with late xenograft valve failure. Table IV summarizes the clinical data in the five children who required reoperation for late bioprosthetic valve dysfunction. One death occurred after reoperation in an 11-year-old girl who, at the age of 9½ years, underwent replacement of the aortic valve with a 19 mm xenograft valve and replacement of the mitral valve with a Model M2 Starr-Edwards caged-ball valve for rheumatic aortic and mitral disease. Symptoms and signs of aortic stenosis developed about 18 months after the operation. These progressed to a severe degree, necessitating reoperation 26 months after the initial procedure. The failed aortic valve, which was heavily calcified, was excised (Fig. 1), the aortic anulus was closed with a prosthetic patch, and a conduit was established between the left ventricular apex and the abdominal aorta. Although her cardiac hemodynamic state was satisfactory after reoperation, she died of uncontrollable bleeding resulting from diffuse intravascular coagulation.

The other four patients survived reoperation and are doing well 2 to 30 months postoperatively. They include a 14-year-old white girl (Case 2) who, at the age of 3 years, had an aortic valvotomy which was followed by aortic and mitral regurgitation. A 19 mm aortic xenograft valve was inserted when she was 9 years old, but recurrent severe aortic stenosis and 2+ mitral regurgitation necessitated reoperation 45 months later. At reoperation, the aortic anulus was enlarged by extension of the aortic incision into the anterior mitral leaflet and a 21 mm Björk-Shiley valve was inserted. Following reoperation, mitral valve insufficiency wor-

*Seven of these operations were performed by one of the authors (H. L.) at St. Louis University, St. Louis, Mo.

†Hancock Laboratories, Inc., Anaheim, Calif.

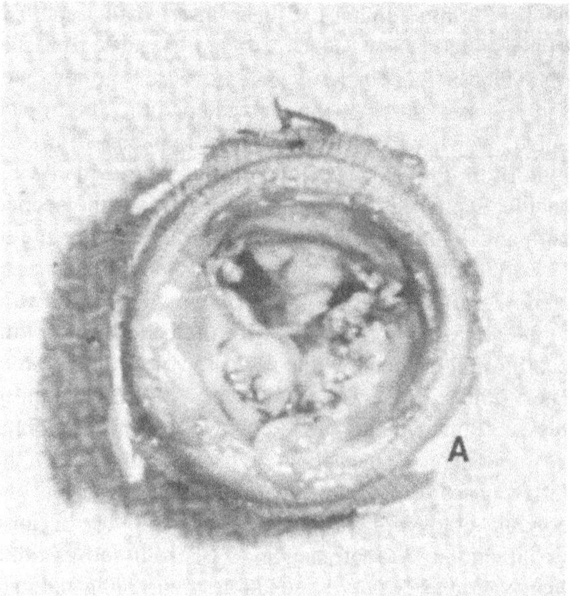

Fig. 1A. Aortic aspect of 19 mm porcine heterograft valve removed 26 months after implantation in the aortic position (Case 1).

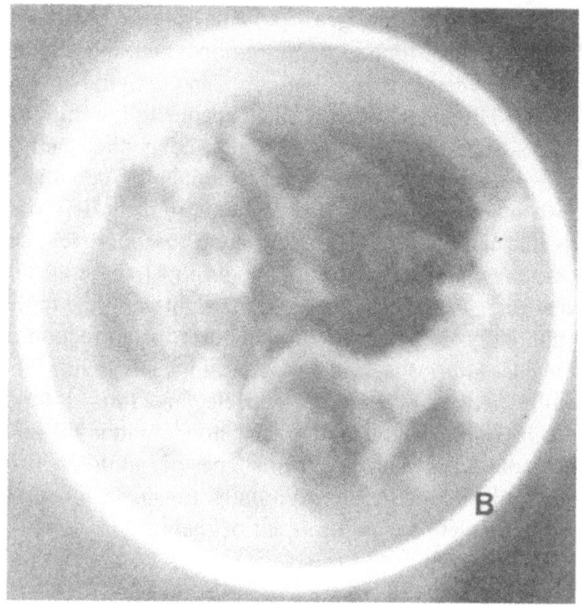

Fig. 1B. Radiograph of the same valve showing extensive calcification of the cusps and anulus of the valve.

Table IV. *Clinical data in patients with heterograft porcine valve failure*

Case	*Diagnosis*	*Sex, race*	*Age at operation (yr)*	*Hancock xenograft valve implanted*	*Internal to reoperation (mo)*	*Procedure at reoperation*	*Current status*
1	AR and MR, rheumatic	F, B	9½	Aortic, 19 mm (SE, M2 MV)	26	Excision AV; patch closure aortic anulus; LV apex–abdominal aortic conduit	Died after reoperation
2	AS, congenital	F, W	9	Aortic, 19 mm	45	AVR with 21 mm BS; annular enlargement; MVR 6 mo later with 33 mm Hancock valve for severe MR	Alive and well 12 mo after MVR
3	AS, rheumatic	M, B	16	Aortic, 25 mm	41	AVR with 27 mm BS	Alive and well 12 mo after second AVR
4	Subvalvular AS, congenital; MR injured during operation	M, W	5	Mitral, 27 mm	22	MVR with 29 mm BS	Alive and well 15 mo after MVR
5	MR, rheumatic	F, B	9½	Mitral, 29 mm	18	MVR with SE, M2	Alive and well 30 mo after MVR

Legend: AR, Aortic regurgitation. AS, Aortic stenosis. MR, Mitral regurgitation. SE, Starr-Edwards valve. BS, Björk-Shiley valve. AV, Aortic valve. AVR, Aortic valve replacement. MRV, Mitral valve replacement.

sened progressively and necessitated mitral valve replacement 6 months later. The anterior leaflet of the mitral valve had dehisced from the valve anulus at the site of the aortic annular enlargement procedure. The mitral valve was therefore replaced with a 33 mm Hancock xenograft 6 months after the insertion of the Björk-Shiley aortic valve. This xenograft was chosen to provide a prosthesis of adequate size and a bulky sewing ring to aid in closing the defect in the mitral valve anulus. She currently is doing well 12 months after the mitral valve replacement.

Pathologic changes in failing heterograft valves. The five valves recovered at reoperation exhibited strikingly similar findings. All five patients had had clinical

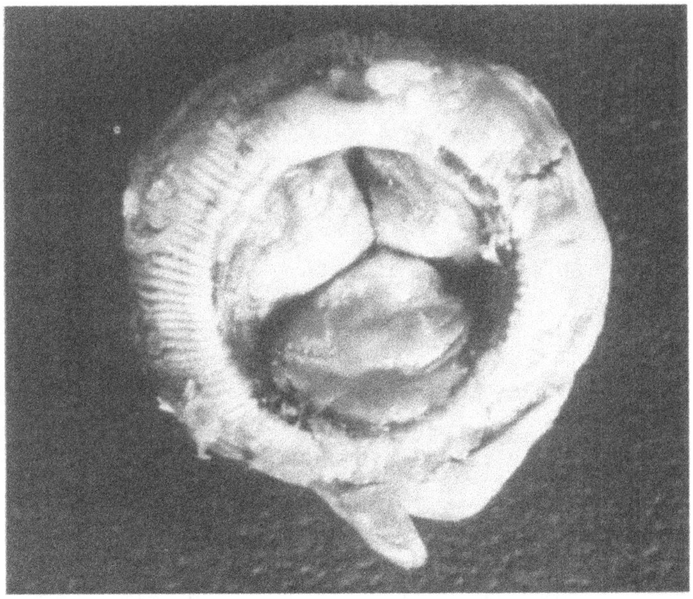

Fig. 2. Ventricular aspect of 29 mm porcine heterograft valve removed 18 months after implantation in the mitral position of a 9½-year-old girl (Case 5). The valve was grossly calcified with severe stenosis across it.

symptoms and signs indicative of stenosis through the heterograft valves, with varying degrees of insufficiency. On gross examination of each valve, the leaflets were found to be stiff and calcified, but without vegetations or thrombi (Figs. 1 and 2). Smooth, relatively flat plaques of calcified tissue also were found near the commissures and in adjacent regions of the aortic wall. Raised deposits of calcium of varying intensity were concentrated along the attached margins and the free margins close to the commissures (Fig. 1). Variable tears, ranging from 3 to 5 mm in length, were encountered through brittle, calcific areas in one or two leaflets of three of the five surgically recovered valves.

Histologic study confirmed the presence of plaque-like calcific deposits which disrupted portions of the leaflets, the aortic wall, and fibrous host tissue adjacent to the mineralized areas. The leaflets were covered by a layer of fibrin. Inflammatory cells were extremely scarce and were confined to the leaflet surfaces. In some areas, particularly in the spongiosa, the connective tissue structure of the valve showed considerable loosening and disruption (Fig. 3). In other areas, particularly in the fibrosa, the dense arrangement of the collagen had been maintained (Fig. 4). Most calcific deposits were located in the central layer of the leaflets, rather than near their surfaces (Fig. 4). These deposits occurred in close relation to the collagen and did not involve the fibrin layers. Calcific deposits in the aortic tissue adjacent to the leaflets involved the medial and adventitial layers; these deposits were not selectively localized in the aortic elastic tissue (Fig. 5).

Ultrastructural study confirmed the presence of a layer of fibrin and debris derived from blood cells on the surfaces of the leaflets (Fig. 6). The collagen in many areas of the valve had undergone considerable degeneration (Fig. 7). This degeneration led to the formation of finely granular deposits, which appeared to be derived from the breakdown of the collagen fibrils (Fig. 7). The plaque-like calcific deposits observed in histologic sections consisted of large numbers of aggregates of needle-shaped crystals of high electron density (Fig. 8). These aggregates were a few micra in diameter, tended to be spherical, and often contained highly dense cores. They seemed to have formed in the interstitium, with no apparent relationship to porcine or host cells or to elastic fibers. A relationship to collagen fibrils was sometimes evident; however, there was no preferential association between calcific deposits and degenerated collagen.

The pathological changes in the two conduit valve prostheses were similar to those in the intracardiac prostheses; the calcification had progressed to osseous/cartilaginous metaplasia of the valve leaflets in one of them.

Discussion

Bioprosthetic cardiac valves are associated with a low thromboembolic risk and obviate the need for anti-

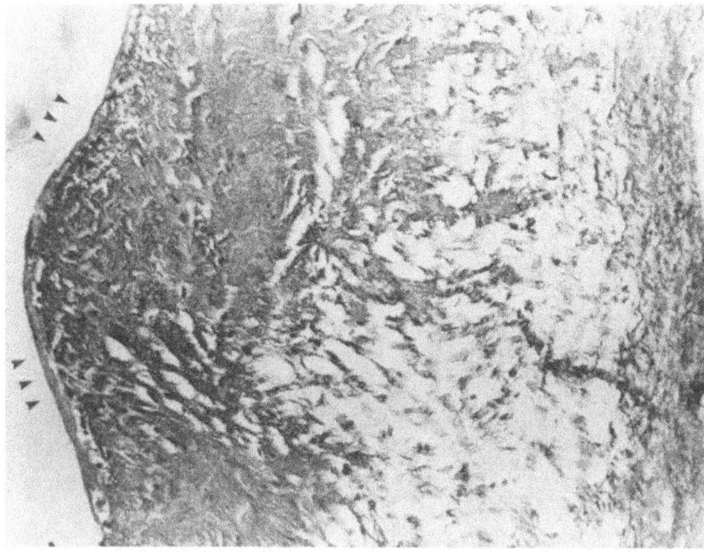

Fig. 3. Section through leaflet showing the fibrosa *(left)*, the ventricularis *(right)*, and the spongiosa, which is severely disrupted (lucent area at *right of center*). A thin layer of fibrin *(arrowheads)* covers the fibrosa. (Hematoxylin and eosin, original magnification ×250.)

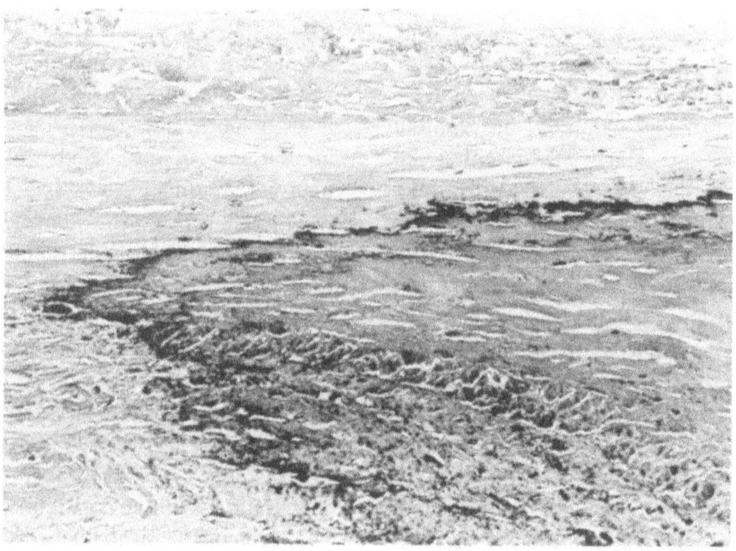

Fig. 4. Large calcific deposit (area with dark granules at *center* and *right*) in central areas of leaflet is separated by zone of compactly arranged collagen from layer of fibrin overlying valve surface. Note that arrangement of collagen is maintained in part of the calcific deposit. (Hematoxylin and eosin, original magnification ×250.)

coagulation in many patients. The heterograft tissue must be preserved, rendered immunologically acceptable, and sterilized. Mounting the valve on a support frame permits implantation by means of the same general techniques employed for insertion of mechanical prostheses.[2] Morphologic change in the tissue after implantation, however, limits durability and remains a significant long-term concern. Tissue fatigue and failure after relatively short periods discouraged the use of earlier heterograft heart valves fixed in formaldehyde and mounted on rigid support frames.[17] In 1968, Carpentier and associates[18] introduced glutaraldehyde as a

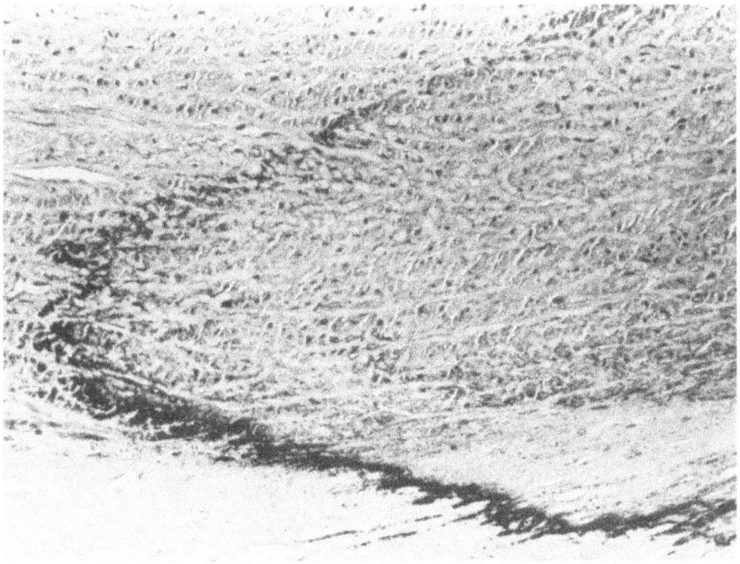

Fig. 5. Calcific deposit, similar to that shown in Fig. 4, involves medial (*top* and *center*) and adventitial layers (*bottom*) of aorta adjacent to base of cusp. (Hematoxylin and eosin, original magnification ×250.)

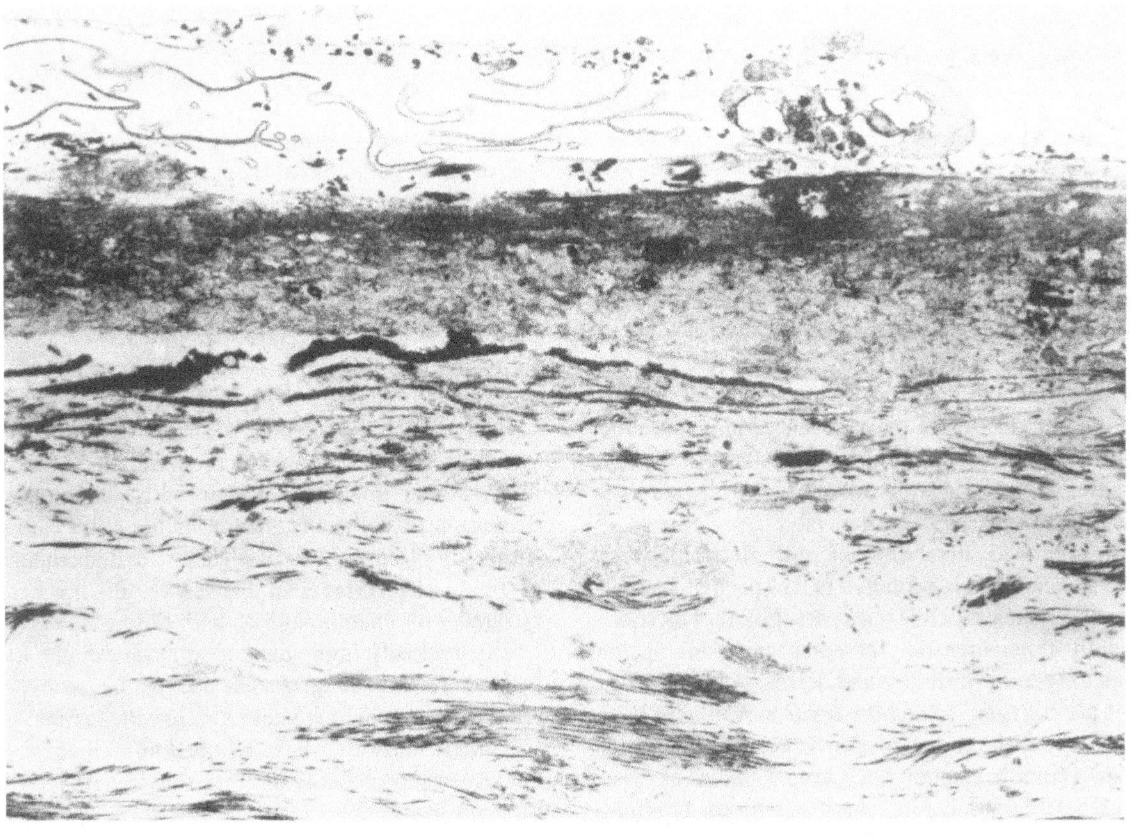

Fig. 6. Electron micrograph of surface of leaflet showing layer of debris composed of lysed erythrocytes and small strands of fibrin overlying a wide, electron-dense band of fibrin and partially disrupted collagen. (×9,750.)

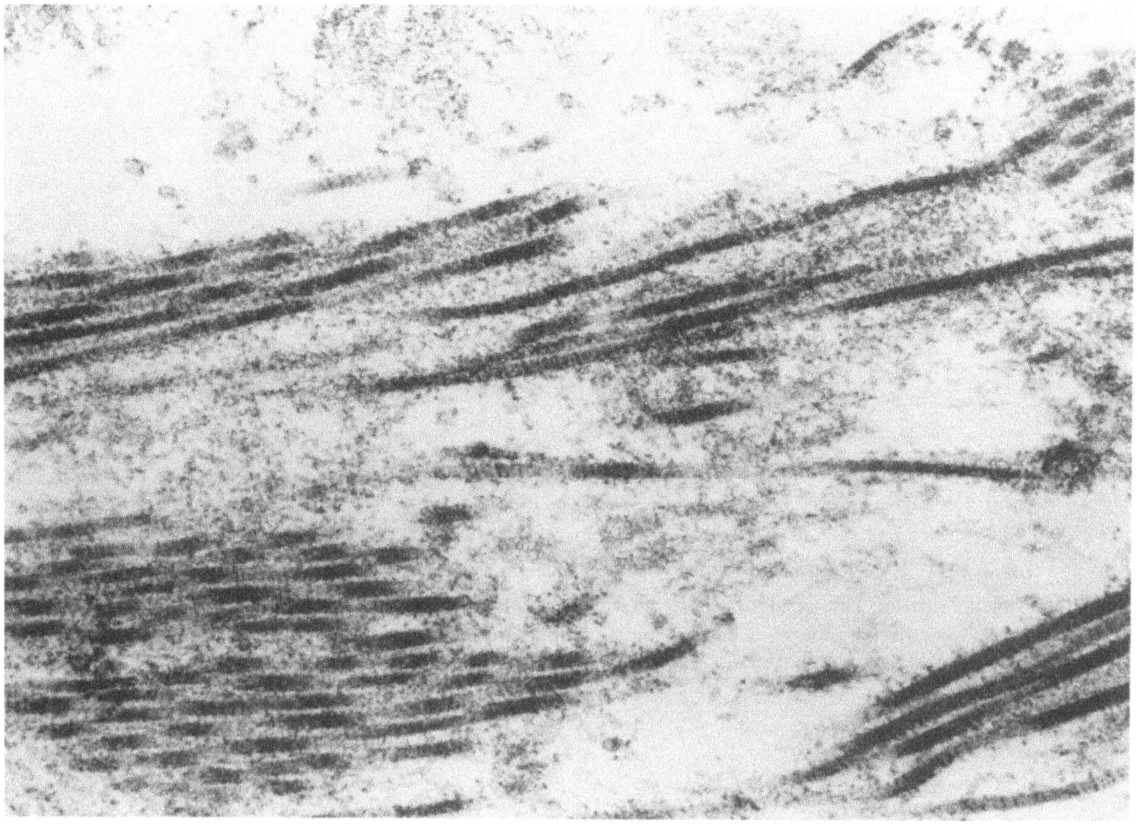

Fig. 7. Electron micrograph of collagen in valve fibrosa showing severely disrupted fibrils associated with granular material presumed to be derived from breakdown of collagen. (×53,000.)

compound for preparing the tissue, and this technique has provided a considerably more biologically stable heterograft valve. To increase further the durability of such valves, Reis and colleagues[9] developed a flexible stent which reduces the stress on the heterograft tissue. After the introduction of these advances in preparation and mounting of heterograft porcine valves, these bioprostheses achieved a wide acceptance in the surgical replacement of diseased cardiac valves.

The improved durability of the glutaraldehyde-preserved xenograft is attributed to the speed of fixation and to the increased collagen cross-linking which occurs with glutaraldehyde. Increased cross-linking increases long-term flexibility and decreases biodegradation of the collagen, so that the tissue is relatively inert with respect to the living host environment. Transmission and scanning electron microscopic studies of these porcine heterografts before and after various durations of implantation,[19, 20] however, show loss of endothelium and acid mucopolysaccharides during preimplantation processing. Within a few weeks of implantation, the valves show insudation of plasma proteins, penetration of erythrocytes into surface crevices, formation of a thin surface layer of fibrin, and deposition of microphages, giant cells, and a few platelets. Longer term (several months and longer) changes in valves free of infection are proportional to the time interval after implantation and consist of progressive disruption of collagen, erosion of the valve surfaces, formation of aggregates of platelets, and accumulation of lipid. The surfaces of the leaflets do not become covered with endothelium or with fibrous sheath.

The markedly improved durability of the glutaraldehyde-preserved xenografts has been borne out by many recent large clinical studies.[11–14] Excellent function of this bioprosthesis has been reported up to 8 years, with the actuarial probability of remaining free of valve dysfunction being 93% to 95% at 4 to 5 years for patients undergoing replacement of the aortic or mitral valve or both.[14] Our own experience with these bioprosthetic

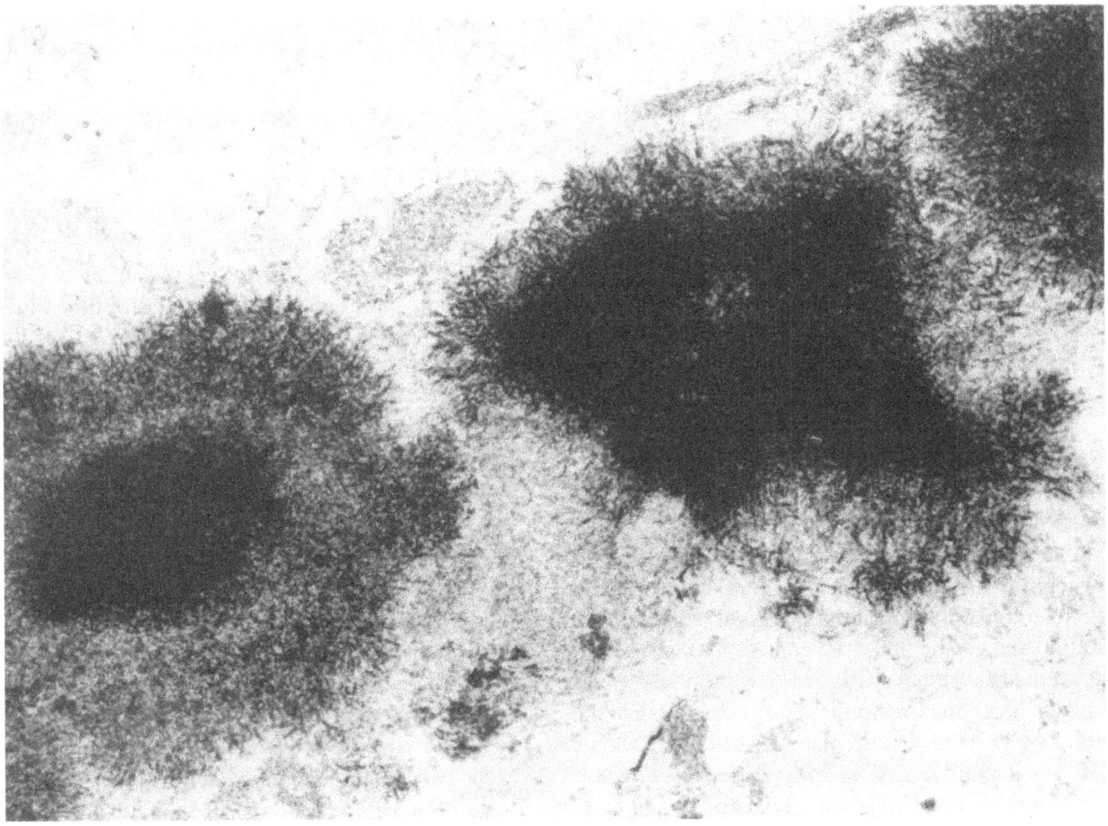

Fig. 8. High-magnification electron micrograph showing that calcific deposits in valve leaflets are composed of aggregates of fine, electron-dense, elongated crystals. (×132,500.)

valves in adults agrees with these reports, in that we have not observed primary dysfunction of a bioprosthetic valve in more than 300 adult patients followed for up to 6 years after implantation of heterograft porcine cardiac valves (unpublished data).

Relatively rare instances of primary tissue dysfunction to date have been reported with porcine aortic valve heterografts.[12–14, 21–29] Of 12 instances of primary bioprosthetic dysfunction in which the authors provided information about the age of the patients,[12, 22–26, 28] four occurred in children. These include patients reported by McIntosh,[12] Levitsky,[22] Brown,[23] and a patient of Reis cited by McIntosh.[12]

Valve replacement in children is somewhat infrequent,[15, 16] and long-term follow-up of porcine xenografts in the pediatric age group is relatively small. It is recognized that these bioprostheses have a smaller orifice-to-anulus ratio than some of the mechanical prostheses of the same size, especially the small valve sizes. However, should the performance of porcine heterograft valves in children be similar to that in adults, these bioprostheses would become an attractive choice when valve replacement is indicated in the pediatric population. This would be particularly true since avoidance of anticoagulation is highly desirable in children because of greater exposure to trauma and difficulties in administering drugs and drawing blood, especially in the first years of life. In addition, the prospect of childbearing poses another problem in anticoagulation of female adolescents. Our multi-institutional study which constitutes the first substantial series of porcine heterograft valves in children with long-term follow-up, however, raises serious doubts as to the advisability of indiscriminate use of porcine xenograft valves in pediatric patients before further elucidation and understanding of the causes of primary dysfunction.

In the absence of any bacteriologic or histopathological evidence of infection, speculation as to the possible causes of this high propensity for relatively early primary dysfunction of porcine heterograft valves in children include (1) perioperative technical factors, (2) a flaw in the initial prosthesis, (3) excessive wear and tear leading to mechanical fatigue, and (4) undetermined factors in the host.

Perioperative handling of the prostheses in each of our five patients with late failure was identical to the handling of other porcine heterograft valves in children as well as adults. Each of the surgical teams which performed these operations is involved with a large number of similar procedures in adults as well as children. Therefore, it appears extremely unlikely that faulty techniques of handling the valve account for this failure rate. In a similar vein, it is very unlikely that flaws in the initial prostheses are responsible for these failures, since the failed valves came from the same supply of stented porcine aortic xenograft valves used in adults and in children.

Fatigue-induced damage may well account for some of these failures. Carpentier[30] states that fatigue lesions which histologically appear as areas of collagen degeneration and elastic fiber fragmentation are inevitable owing to the basic nature of the bioprosthesis itself. He speculates that the currently available models of glutaraldehyde-fixed porcine heterograft valves should last 10 years, with a 15% to 20% incidence of valve failure. Broom[31] and Clark and associates[32] have demonstrated the vulnerability of glutaraldehyde-preserved porcine heart valves to compressive flexure in studies of in vitro accelerated fatigue testing. If an average heart rate of 72 beats per minute is assumed for normal adult human beings, each natural cardiac valve cycles 37.8 million times a year. It is recognized that children have a resting heart rate of 90 to 95 beats per minute, and since their level of activity is greater than that of most adults, their total number of cardiac cycles a day may approach twice that of adults. In addition, implantation of a valve with a relatively small orifice, such as in our two patients with 19 mm aortic prostheses, subjects these valves to a higher degree of fatigue in view of the substantial pressure gradient across them. This is probably true also of the two failures observed in the valves incorporated in extracardiac conduits. Both failed during the sixth year and had become relatively small for the size of the growing patients in whom they were implanted.

Although mechanical fatigue may account for the early appearance of failure in some of the heterograft valves in this report, it is difficult to implicate it in the failure of the valves in Cases 3 and 5, and even in Case 4. These patients had received relatively large heterograft valves, and there was no reason to expect an unusually high cardiac output in any of them. Although all the failing valves in this report were in the mitral or aortic position, one of us (W. C. R.) has observed a similar failure in a valve implanted at another medical center in the tricuspid position, where mechanical fatigue is much less likely. It is widely recognized that growing children have a higher rate of calcium turnover than adults. It is possible that this metabolic factor may be related to accelerated calcification of heterograft valves in children. Soft tissue calcification with normal serum calcium levels has been reported in adults with chronic renal failure,[33] and Fishbein and associates[26] reported calcification of both aortic and mitral porcine xenograft valves in patients maintained on chronic dialysis. Calcification of a normal mitral valve anulus also is encountered in patients with bone tumors who have a high calcium turnover. Therefore, it is possible that the foreign tissue of a porcine xenograft valve is more susceptible to calcification when implanted in children, whose calcium turnover is increased.

Although the glutaraldehyde-fixation treatment markedly decreases the antigenicity of porcine xenograft valves, it does not render them totally biologically inert. Therefore, it is possible that immunologic factors may have an effect in some children receiving such valve implants and eventually may lead to an accelerated rejection phenomenon, which results in relatively early degeneration of the bioprostheses.

Indications for the use of porcine xenograft valves in children thus remain controversial. In the individual case, the advantages of greater durability and bigger anulus-to-orifice ratio of mechanical prostheses must be weighed against the danger of anticoagulation. A porcine heterograft valve carries a high prospect of reoperation, possibly within 6 years. In the first years of life, when difficulties with anticoagulation are greater and the valves require changing within 3 to 4 years because of rapid growth, the porcine heterograft has distinct advantages. In the adolescent with borderline anulus size the decision is more difficult. In the patient who wishes to engage in vigorous sports or in girls contemplating childbearing, the porcine valve has distinct advantages which, for the individual patient, may even outweigh the disturbingly high incidence of early valve deterioration.

REFERENCES

1 Murray G: Homologous aortic valve segment transplants as surgical treatment for aortic and mitral insufficiency. Angiology **7**:446, 1956

2 Geha AS, Titus JL, McGoon DC: Fixation of aortic valve

homografts with metal rings. J THORAC CARDIOVASC SURG **54**:605, 1967

3 Ross D: Biologic valves. Their performance and prospects. Circulation **45**:1259, 1972

4 Angell WW, DeLameralle P, Shumway NE: Valve replacement. Present status of homograft valves. Prog Cardiovasc Dis **15**:589, 1973

5 Pacifico AD, Karp RB, Kirklin JW: Homografts for replacement of the aortic valve. Circulation **45, 46**:Suppl 1:36, 1972

6 O'Brien MF, Neilson GA, Galea EG: Heterograft valves. An analysis of clinical results of valve replacement. Circulation **41, 42**:Suppl 2:16, 1970

7 Carpentier A, Lemaigre G, Ladislas R: Biological factors affecting long-term results of valvular heterografts. J THORAC CARDIOVASC SURG **68**:771, 1974

8 Carpentier A, Dubost C: From xenograft to bioprosthesis. Evolution of concepts and techniques of valvular xenografts, Biological Tissue in Heart Valve Replacement, MI Ionescue, DN Ross, GH Wooler, eds., London 1972, Butterworth and Co., Ltd., p 515

9 Reis RL, Hancock WD, Yarbrough JW, Glancy DL, Morrow AG: The flexible stent. A new concept in the fabrication of tissue heart valve prostheses. J THORAC CARDIOVASC SURG **68**:771, 1974

10 Sade MR, Castaneda AR: The dispensable right ventricle. Surgery **77**:624, 1975

11 Cohn LH, Lambert JJ, Castaneda AR, Collins JJ: Cardiac valve replacement with the stabilized glutaraldehyde porcine aortic valve. Indications, operative results and followup. Chest **68**:162, 1975

12 McIntosh CL, Michaelis LL, Morrow AG: Atrioventricular valve replacement with the Hancock porcine xenograft. A five-year clinical experience. Surgery **78**:568, 1975

13 Stinson EB, Griepp RB, Oyer PE, Shumway NE: Long-term experience with porcine aortic valve xenografts. J THORAC CARDIOVASC SURG **73**:54, 1977

14 Oyer PE, Stinson EB, Reitz BA, Miller DC, Rossiter SJ, Shumway NE: Long-term evaluation of the porcine xenograft bioprosthesis. J THORAC CARDIOVASC SURG **78**:343, 1979

15 Stansel HC Jr, Nudel DB, Berman MA, Talner NS: Prosthetic valve replacement in children. Arch Surg **110**:1397, 1975

16 Chien S, Laks H, Fagan L, Terschluse BS, Kaiser G, Barner H, Willman VL: Valve replacement in children. Circulation **56**:Suppl 2:117, 1977

17 Gerbode F: Proceedings of the First International Works on Tissue Valves, October, 1969. Ann Surg **172**:Suppl 1:23, 1970

18 Carpentier A, Mancel P, Laurent D, Dubost C: Remplacement des valves mitrales et tricuspides par des heterogreffes. Ann Chir Thorac Cardiovasc **7**:33, 1968

19 Ferrans VJ, Spray TL, Billingham ME, Roberts WC: Structural changes in glutaraldehyde-treated porcine heterografts used as substitute cardiac valves. Am J Cardiol **41**:1159, 1978

20 Ashraf M, Bloor CM: Structural alterations of the porcine heterograft after various durations of implantation. Am J Cardiol **41**:1185, 1978

21 Zuhdi MN: The porcine aortic valve bioprosthesis. A significant alternative. Ann Thorac Surg **21**:573, 1976

22 Levitsky S: Discussion of Stinson et al[13]

23 Brown JW, Dunn JM, Spooner E, Kirsh MM: Late spontaneous disruption of a porcine xenograft mitral valve. J THORAC CARDIOVASC SURG **75**:606, 1978

24 Housman LB, Pitt WA, Mazur JH, Litchford B, and Gross SA: Mechanical failure (leaflet disruption) of a porcine aortic heterograft. J THORAC CARDIOVASC SURG **76**:212, 1978

25 Hetzer R, Hill JD, Kerth WJ: Thrombosis and degeneration of Hancock valves. Clinical and pathological findings. Ann Thorac Surg **26**:317, 1978

26 Fishbein MC, Gissen SA, Collins JJ: Pathology in patients with glutaraldehyde-fixed porcine cardiac valves. Am J Cardiol **40**:331, 1977

27 Davila JC, Magilligan DJ Jr, Lewis JW: Is the Hancock porcine valve the best cardiac valve substitute today? Ann Thorac Surg **26**:303, 1978

28 Platt MR: Discussion of Davila et al[27]

29 Hannah H, Reis RL: Current status of porcine heterograft prostheses. A 5-year appraisal. Circulation **54**:Suppl 3:27, 1976

30 Carpentier A: Discussion of Stinson et al[13]

31 Broom ND: Fatigue-induced damage in glutaraldehyde-preserved heart valve tissue. J THORAC CARDIOVASC SURG **76**:202, 1978

32 Clark RE, Swanson WM, Kardos JL: Durability of prosthetic heart valves. Ann Thorac Surg **26**:323, 1978

33 Kuzela DC, Huffer WE, Confer JD: Soft tissue calcification in chronic dialysis patients. Am J Pathol **86**:403, 1977

Discussion

(Papers by Oyer [page 343], Geha [page 351], and their associates)

DR. JEAN PAUL BINET

Paris, France

We introduced heterografts as a replacement for the aortic valve and then as a valved conduit in pulmonary stenosis in 1968. We have since inserted 43 heterografts in the pulmonary position in children for congenital disease. There were 17 cases of tetralogy of Fallot, 12 cases of persistent truncus arteriosus, 10 cases of pulmonary atresia with intact ventricular septum, and four cases of transposition of the great vessels with ventricular septal defect and pulmonary stenosis.

These valves were prepared by Claude Planché by means of the Carpentier technique and then by Hancock. There were 26 long-term survivors at 5 years, with no evidence of valve dysfunction. However, in the oldest patient, at 10 years, we have seen calcification and stenosis of the valve and have replaced three conduits.

I agree with Dr. Geha that the durability of the valves presents a problem for the long-term results in children.

DR. GEORGE A. TRUSLER
Toronto, Ontario, Canada

I would like to discuss Dr. Geha's paper specifically, focusing on the experience that the authors had in children.

[Slide] Our experience in Toronto is somewhat similar to theirs. From 1974 to 1979 we followed 36 children with porcine valves: 19 aortic, nine mitral, five pulmonary, and three tricuspid. Two of the 36 valves developed stenosis, calcification, and degeneration and had to be replaced. In addition, 57 children have valved conduits. We are not aware of calcification in any of these valved conduits at present, although many have been in place for only a short time. Four other children had Ionescu-Shiley bovine pericardial valves, three pulmonary and one mitral.

Recently a 3-year-old child with a 19 mm Ionescu-Shiley mitral valve returned with stenosis and regurgitation. The valve had been in place for only 13 months. Although the main problem was excessive tissue overgrowth of the valve commissures, there was also early calcification in the leaflets.

One of the two calcified porcine valves was a 27 mm mitral valve which had been implanted for 33 months in a boy who also had significant subaortic stenosis; thus the valve was subjected to relatively high left ventricular pressures. The other heavily calcified valve, a 23 mm Hancock valve, had been implanted in the aortic position for 21 months.

This experience supports the authors' premise that the incidence of failure of porcine and other xenograft valves is higher in children than in adults.

DR. RICHARD N. EDIE
New York, N. Y.

At Columbia-Presbyterian Medical Center in New York City we adopted the Hancock porcine valve prosthesis in 1974 and have used it since that time. Our results are consistent with those of the Stanford group.

Our over-all hospital mortality rate in all isolated aortic and mitral valve replacements from 1974 to 1978 is 4.5%, a figure comparable with that of the Stanford series. Our over-all late mortality rate for this same group of patients is 2.2%. We believe that these results are in large part due to the lack of thromboembolic complications of the porcine valve.

We performed an actuarial analysis of the projected survival comparing isolated porcine and mechanical valve replacement, both in the aortic and mitral positions. At 4 years, we found the predicted and projected survival of patients with porcine valves to be very stable, whereas the survival of those with mechanical valves continued to decrease.

We have performed 100 reoperations for excision of aortic valve homografts and Braunwald-Cutter aortic valve prostheses and in all have inserted a porcine valve. The hospital mortality rate is 2%. The early follow-up on these patients has been encouraging for the lack of valve-related complications.

Finally, we have been satisfied with the durability of the porcine valve in the 4 year period we have used it. We have had to reoperate in only three patients, one adult and two children, for primary valve failure, but we continue to share the concern of others regarding the use of porcine valves in children.

DR. PRAPHULLA K. BAJPAI
Dayton, Ohio

I wish to discuss the immunogenicity of tanned porcine heart valve heterografts.

In the first study, young rabbits were immunized with untreated or glutaraldehyde-treated porcine heart valve extracts in Freund's complete adjuvant. Sera obtained from rabbits in either group tested positive for the presence of antibodies against their corresponding antigens by capillary tube aggregation test and both tanned and untreated porcine heart valve antigens by complement fixation, hemagglutination, and double diffusion in gel precipitation tests. In the second study, untreated or glutaraldehyde-treated porcine heart valves were grafted subcutaneously in the abdominal region of young rabbits. Complement fixation test showed that sera obtained from rabbits of both groups reacted with both tanned and untreated porcine heart valve antigens. Intracutaneous injections of tanned or untreated porcine heart valve antigens gave positive skin reactions in rabbits grafted with either tanned or untreated porcine heart valve heterografts. Microscopic examination of graft sections retrieved from either group of rabbits at the end of 1, 2, or 3 months showed pathological changes similar to those shown by Dr. Geha in tanned porcine heart valve heterografts retrieved from children. These studies show that the tanned valve is immunogenic and not inert. Thus failure of tanned porcine heart valve heterografts in children could be due partially to their well-developed immune system.

DR. DENTON A. COOLEY
Houston, Texas

During the past 10 months we have implanted 344 Ionescu-Shiley bovine pericardial valves in 212 patients. These were equally divided between mitral and aortic replacements, with four being placed in the tricuspid and one in the pulmonary anulus. Some surgeons have been hesitant to use the new Ionescu valve because of unfavorable experience with the structurally similar prosthesis in which autologous fresh fascia lata was used. I believe the results with the glutaraldehyde-formalin–treated valve will be entirely different. Durability studies in the pulse duplicator or mock circulation demonstrate superior performance to the porcine tissue valve, and after a testing period equivalent to more than 10 years the pericardium remains intact.

In comparison to the porcine valves, and particularly in the smaller sizes, i.e., the 19 and 17 mm valves, the bovine pericardial valve has strikingly better hemodynamic function than the bovine grafts, which were obstructive in the smaller sizes even with the composite modification. In fact, at present the only disadvantage that I can see for the Ionescu valve is the rather high profile, which may make implantation into a narrow aortic anulus somewhat tedious; furthermore, if not inserted properly into the mitral anulus, the valve could impinge upon the intraventricular surfaces. May I ask if any one present has a longer period of follow-up to report on the Ionescu-Shiley bovine pericardial valve?

DR. JOSEPH W. LEWIS JR.

Detroit, Mich.

Since 1971 the Hancock porcine xenograft has been the valve of choice at Henry Ford Hospital. Xenograft valves of patients discharged from the hospital after operation (518 valves) during the period October, 1971, to December, 1978, were considered at risk. Sixteen patients required removal of the Hancock xenograft valves for spontaneous degeneration. This is defined as prosthetic stenosis or incompetence without a history of endocarditis or febrile illness when the explanted valves showed degenerative changes without evidence of bacterial infection or positive cultures. There were nine male and seven female subjects. Ages ranged from 10 to 67 years, with a mean of 43 years. The time from insertion to removal averaged 56 months, with a range of 14 to 76 months. Seven xenografts in the aortic and nine in the mitral positioned failed. A significant change in symptoms occurred on an average of 2½ months prior to reoperation.

With follow-up at 98.8% completeness, the actuarial incidence of failure owing to spontaneous degeneration was 4.6% of 127 valves at risk for 5 years, 9.6% of 68 valves at risk at 6 years, and 13.2% of 15 valves at risk for 7 years. The increased incidence of xenograft degeneration in our series seems to occur more than 4 years after implantation. This experience is somewhat different from that presented today. The reason for spontaneous degeneration remains obscure.

DR. ROBERT W. M. FRATER

Bronxville, N. Y.

Dr. Oyer's presentation was a model of what valve presentations should be. I wish to ask whether the incidence of thromboembolism was derived from a specific questionnaire being applied to each patient or from data available in the charts. I ask this because when we have subjected our patients with bioprostheses to a specific questionnaire to elicit evidence of transient cerebral ischemic attacks, we have found a significant difference between what we would have found had we not subjected them to that questionnaire and between the AVR patients and the MVR patients.

[Slide] The dotted line is the actuarial curve of MVR patients free from transient ischemic incidents, and the continuous line shows the same for the AVR patients. It is only because the aortic line is straight that we can be reasonably certain that we are uncovering something significant by subjecting the MVR patients to this questionnaire. The difference between these two groups at the 30 month mark is significant. My question, then, is whether the data on thromboembolism are derived from specific questions or merely from the records.

I would like to make one comment on the degeneration of porcine xenografts in children. Whether porcine, bovine, or human dura mater, when bioprostheses are placed in calves with artificial hearts, they show calcification within a few months. In addition, bioprostheses placed in adults with hyperparathyroidism and adults with renal failure also have shown premature calcification. Common to all of these conditions is a high rate of calcium turnover, which must be a contributing factor to the early failure in children.

DR. JOHN W. KIRKLIN

Birmingham, Ala.

I would like to ask Dr. Oyer whether he believes there is a difference between Dr. Lewis' data and his own, since in his own experience only 66 of approximately 1,200 patients have been followed more than 5 years.

DR. OYER *(Closing)*

Dr. Kirklin referred to the Henry Ford Hospital experience, from whence Dr. Lewis showed the actuarial valve-failure curve which, in contrast to our results, suggests increasing tissue failure beginning as early as 3½ years postoperatively. Experience with Hancock valves at Henry Ford Hospital began almost simultaneously with ours, so that the study period in our two series spanned the same time interval. It is thus intriguing that we note a rate of tissue failure so different from theirs. It is my understanding from Dr. Magilligan, also of that institution, that from 1971 through 1974 they were washing each valve at the time of operation with neomycin solution. It is now thought that neomycin may adversely affect the glutaraldehyde cross-linking interaction with the collagen within the valve leaflet in such a way as to alter the leaflet surfaces and thereby cause deposition of platelet aggregates and other cellular elements. These in turn may damage the leaflets directly or act as a nidus for late calcification. It would be of some interest if the Detroit group would break down their actuarial curves into two groups of patients, those in the early series treated with neomycin and those treated later; they now have 5 years of experience with valves not washed with neomycin, which should be enough follow-up to detect a difference between the two patient populations. That is the only explanation I have for the high late failure rate in the Hancock valve series from Detroit.

In response to Dr. Frater's question, our patients are followed by a telephone conversation personally with the patient and/or with the patient's referring doctor during the 3 month closing interval of the study. Data aides gather that information. They have a specific list of questions to ask of each patient.

In regard to calcification of these valves, we have noticed the same phenomenon in the artificial heart work that we have done using calves; in calves, tissue valves can become calcified as early as 1 month postoperatively. We also believe that the common denominator among all the groups of patients, as well as this animal model, is a high calcium turnover rate, which in some way establishes a propensity to deposit calcium within the "foreign" valvular tissue.

DR. GEHA *(Closing)*

I would like to thank the discussers for their comments. I am particularly interested in the several series mentioned by Drs. Binet, Trusler, Edie, and Lewis, who pointed out some failures in children, an experience not too different from ours. It is difficult to blame this early failure in children on one cause only. I think that we probably are dealing with a multifactorial picture. Some of the valves which have failed in our series definitely were subjected to accelerated wear and tear, whereas others were not. Dr. William Roberts has seen similar changes in a tricuspid valve porcine heterograft which, as far as I know, is the only one in this low-pressure location to exhibit such pathological changes.

We agree that an increased calcium turnover is included in the list of factors that may be incriminated. As Dr. Frater mentioned, there is an increased incidence of calcification in patients with renal dialysis and hyperthyroidism. Also, little children with bone tumors may exhibit calcification of the soft tissues and even of the mitral valves. Thus the increased calcium turnover of growing children probably plays an important role in the development of these bioprosthetic valvular calcifications.

I am sure there may be an immunologic process contributing to this calcification, as well. It is known that these valves are not totally immunologically inert despite the treatment with glutaraldehyde; thus it is probably a combination of factors which leads to this accelerated failure of heterograft valves in children.

In response to Dr. Cooley's question, we have not had any experience with the Ionescu-Shiley valves.

Ultrastructural alterations in porcine valvular heterografts

Summary

Light and electron microscopic studies were made of structural alterations in 30 porcine valvular heterografts removed from 28 patients either at necropsy (12 patients) or at reoperation for replacement of a malfunctioning heterograft (16 patients). Early (<2 months after implantation) morphological changes consisted of deposition of fibrin, macrophages and multinucleated giant cells on the valvular surfaces; insudation of plasma proteins into the valvular substance, and breakdown of collagen in superficial regions of the leaflets. Late (3 to 94 months after implantation) changes were characterized by progressively severe damage to the collagen, formation of aggregates of platelets on the valvular surfaces, lipid deposition, erosion of the surfaces, and development of calcific deposits.

Perforation of the leaflets, leading to prosthetic regurgitation, was a consequence of severe collagen breakdown. Conversely, prosthetic stenosis most frequently resulted from calcification of valvular collagen. Thus, alterations in collagen are of crucial importance in determining the long-term durability of porcine valvular heterografts.

It has been the experience of surgeons and clinicians that patients receiving glutaraldehyde-preserved porcine valvular heterografts generally follow satisfactory postoperative courses, with very low incidences of thromboembolic phenomena and without requiring long-term anticoagulant therapy (20, 22, 33). Nevertheless, relatively few of these patients have had these valves implanted for more than 5 years, and our knowledge of the anatomic changes that these valves undergo after implantation is limited. Concern has been expressed over the fact that the biological materials in these valves, especially the collagen, are subject to a number of processes of biodegradation and cannot be resynthesized because the glutaraldehyde processing results in death of the valvular connective tissue cells (8). Therefore, porcine valvular heterografts can be expected to undergo some degree of structural and functional deterioration after implantation. During the past three years, we have conducted a series of light and electron microscopic studies designed to define the nature and extent of pathologic changes that develop in porcine valvular heterografts that have been implanted in patients for various periods of time (8–10). This communication summarizes the results of these studies.

Materials and Methods

The morphologic studies to be described below were made on 30 porcine valvular heterografts obtained from 28 patients either at necropsy (12 patients) or at reoperation for replacement of a malfunctioning heterograft (16 patients). These patients, 14 men and 14 women, ranged in age from 2.5 to 65 years at the time of implantation of the heterograft. Twenty-two of the valves had been implanted in the mitral position, five in the aortic position, two in the tricuspid position, and one in the pulmonary position (in a pulmonary conduit). The period of time between implantation and removal of the heterograft ranged from 2 days to 94 months. Six of the valves had been implanted for less than one month; eight, between one month and one year; ten, between one and four years, and six, for longer than four years.

For purposes of comparison, light and electron microscopic studies were also made of: 1. two non-implanted porcine aortic valves (Hancock Laboratories) one mounted on a flexible stent, the other unmounted; 2. one non-implanted Carpentier-Edwards valve, also mounted on a stent; and 3. one normal porcine aortic valve, which was removed at thoracotomy from an adult animal and was not subjected to the glutaraldehyde processing by which these valves are prepared for implantation.

Immediately after removal, all valves were fixed with cold 3% glutaraldehyde in 0.1 M phosphate buffer, pH 7.2. After fixation, central strips extending from the anulus to the free margin of the leaflet were removed and processed for light microscopy and for transmission and scanning electron microscopy. For transmission electron microscopy, the strips of tissue were washed with buffered sucrose, postfixed with OsO_4, dehydrated and embedded in Maraglas. Sections of this tissue, 0.5μ thick, were examined with a light microscope to select areas for ultrathin sectioning. Ultrathin sections were stained either with uranyl acetate and lead citrate, or with the Kajikawa method (17) for demonstration of elastic tissue.

For scanning electron microscopy, the tissues were washed with buffered sucrose, rinsed with distilled water, dehydrated with acetone to the critical point of CO_2, coated with gold-palladium, and examined with a scanning electron microscope.

Results

Morphology of the Normal Porcine Aortic Valve

The two surfaces of the porcine aortic cusp will be referred to in this paper as inflow and outflow surfaces. When the valve is in its normal anatomical (semilunar) position, the inflow surface faces the ventricular cavity, and the outflow surface faces the aortic root. Each aortic valvular leaflet (Figures 1–5) consists of: 1. an endothelial cell layer that covers the outflow surface; 2. the fibrosa, a layer of dense fibrous connective tissue subjacent to the endothelium of the outflow surface; 3. the spongiosa, a layer that is adjacent to the fibrosa and contains loosely arranged fibrous connective tissue and abundant acid mucopolysaccharides; 4. the ventricularis, a thin layer of fibrous connective tissue that is subjacent to the inflow surface and tapers off gradually toward the free edge of the cusp; and 5. the endothelial cell layer that covers the inflow surface. Elastic fibers are considerably larger and more numerous in the ventricularis than in the fibrosa (Figures 2 and 3). This arrangement is similar to that in human aortic valves (15); however, in the pig aortic valve, the noncoronary leaflet is smaller than the other two leaflets, and the right coronary leaflet has a small shelf of cardiac muscle that extends into its base (4). It should be noted that porcine aortic valves sometimes exhibit small foci of accumulation of acid mucopolysaccharides (in the form of fine spicules) in subendothelial areas of the fibrosa (Figures 4 and 5); collagen fibrils are sparse in such areas.

Structure of Unimplanted Hancock and Carpentier-Edwards Porcine Valves
Morphologic studies did not reveal any significant differences between two unimplanted Hancock porcine valves (one mounted and one unmounted) and

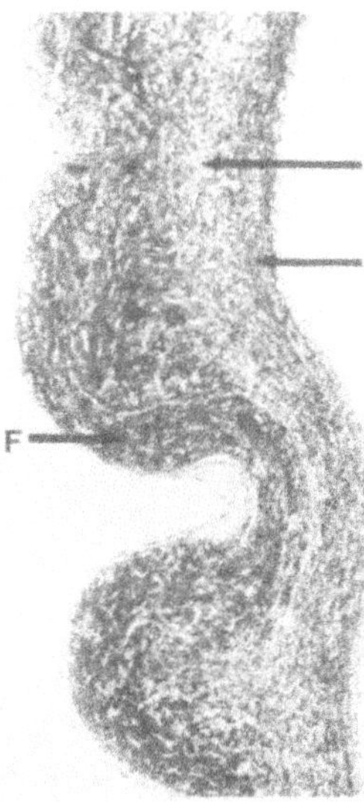

Figure 1

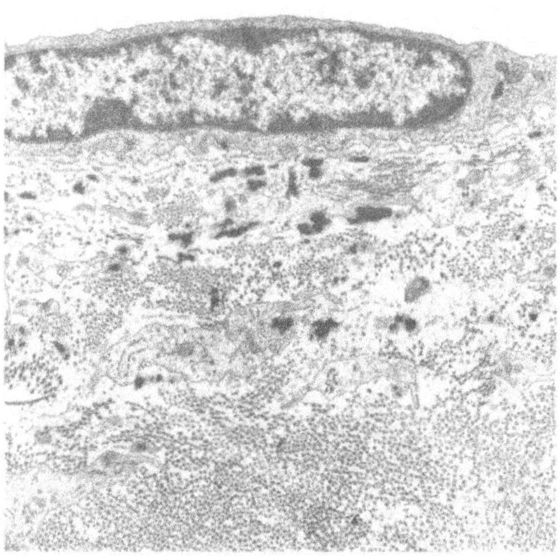

Figure 2

Figure 1: *Histology of normal porcine aortic valve leaflet. Inside of cusp is on left and central orifice of valve on right. Note layered arrangement of leaflet: the dense fibrosa (F), the loosely arranged spongiosa (S), and the ventricularis (V). Half-micron-thick section of plastic-embedded tissue, alkaline toluidine blue stain, X 125.*

Figure 2: *Electron micrograph showing ultrastructure of fibrosa in normal porcine aortic valve. Note: endothelial cell lining surface; densely packed collagen fibrils; valvular fibroblasts, and small, scanty elastic fibers that have been selectively stained black with the Kajikawa method. X 13,500.*

Figure 3

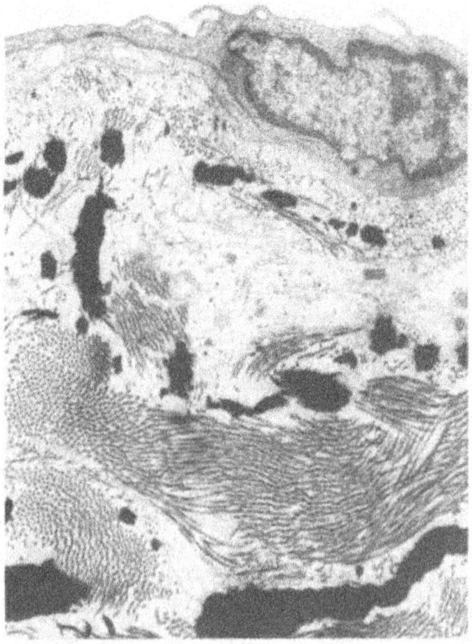

Figure 4

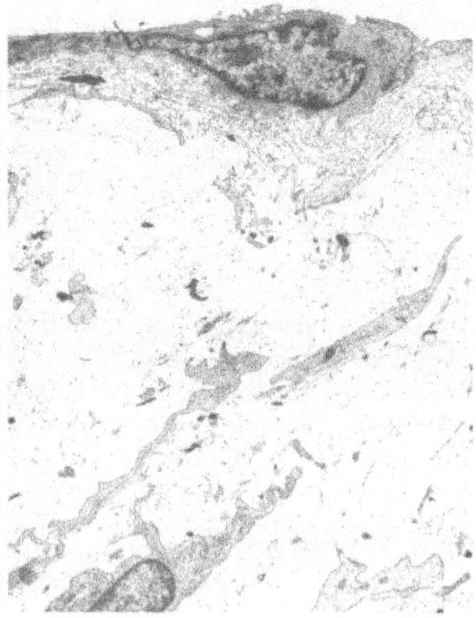

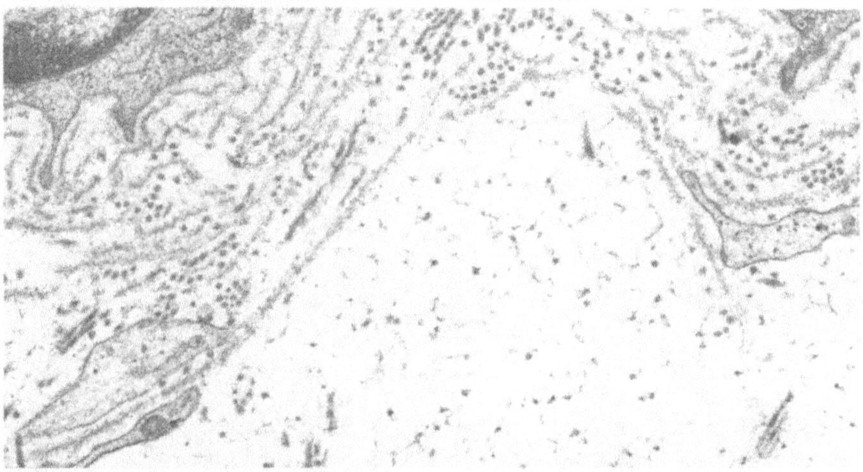

Figure 5

Figure 3: *Ultrastructure of ventricularis in normal porcine aortic valve. Comparison with Figure 2, shown at same magnification, indicates that elastic fibres in the ventricularis are much larger than in the fibrosa. X 13,500.*

Figure 4: *Electron micrograph of outflow surface of normal porcine aortic valve, showing unusual area in which collagen is very sparse and acid mucopolysaccharides (represented by minute spicules in otherwise clear subendothelial region) are abundant. Such areas eventually may become points of structural weakness after the acid mucopolysaccharide material is lost during preimplantation processing. X 9,000.*

Figure 5: *Higher magnification view of subendothelial region shown in Figure 4. The endothelial basal lamina is reduplicated, as is the case in the fibrosa. Collagen fibrils are few and small; fine filaments and spicules of acid mucopolysaccharide material are abundant. X 30,000.*

one mounted, unimplanted Carpentier-Edwards valve. All three valves showed disruption of the endothelial cell layer, with fairly complete loss of endothelial cells from the inflow surface and only partial loss from the outflow surface. On scanning electron microscopic examination, the inflow surfaces of each valve appeared much rougher than the corresponding outflow surfaces. The inflow surfaces were composed of small, cylindrical bundles of collagen fibrils and of larger bundles that represented either elastic fibers or large masses of collagen fibrils. In contrast, the outflow surfaces appeared smoother, more homogeneous, and composed of material resembling basement membrane; they did not exhibit large numbers of exposed collagen fibrils.

The unimplanted valves also showed loss of the ground substance of connective tissue, including the dense spicules of acid mucopolysaccharides and the network of fine filaments associated with the spicules, so that the collagen fibrils and elastic fibers (both of which remained structurally normal) appeared surrounded by a matrix of greatly increased electron lucency, with some "loosening" of their arrangement. Fibroblasts in these valves showed disruption of organelles and loss of integrity of cytoplasmic membranes. These alterations resembled autolytic changes.

Morphology of Short-Term (<2 Months) Implanted Porcine Valves

Structural alterations were evident in the surfaces and substances of the valves after implantation for short periods of time. Alterations involving the valvular surfaces (Figures 6 and 7) consisted of: 1. deposition of fibrin on both surfaces (more on the outflow than on the inflow surface), with formation of small thrombi; 2. entrapment of erythrocytes in a meshwork of fibrin; 3. adherence of erythrocytes, and occasionally of platelets, to the denuded surfaces of the valves; and 4. deposition of macrophages and giant cells on the surfaces, without penetration into the valvular substance. Changes involving the connective tissue components of the valves included: 1. insudation of plasma proteins into the substance of the leaflets (Figures 8 und 9); 2. penetration of erythrocytes and leukocytes into the spongiosa, presumably through crevices in the surfaces; 3. loosening of the arrangement of the bundles of collagen in the spongiosa and to a lesser extent in the fibrosa; and 4. evidence of mild disruption of collagen.

In three valves that had been implanted for less than one week, structural changes were minimal and consisted of deposition of a thin ($<10\mu$ in thickness) layer of fibrin (Figure 6) and occasional erythrocytes and platelets on the exposed collagen surfaces. Some insudation of plasma proteins, manifested by the finding of very finely fibrillar material between the collagen fibers, was already evident in superficial layers of the valves.

In the four valves that had been in place for one week to two months, the layers of fibrin were thicker, especially on the outflow surfaces; macrophages (Figure 10) and multinucleated giant cells (Figure 11) lined the surface of the leaflets. No phagocytosis of collagen by macrophages was observed. Multinucleated giant cells had organelles similar to those in macrophages. These giant cells showed greatly complex, interdigitating surface folds, and had from two to six irregularly arranged nuclei. Scanning electron microscopic examination

Figure 6

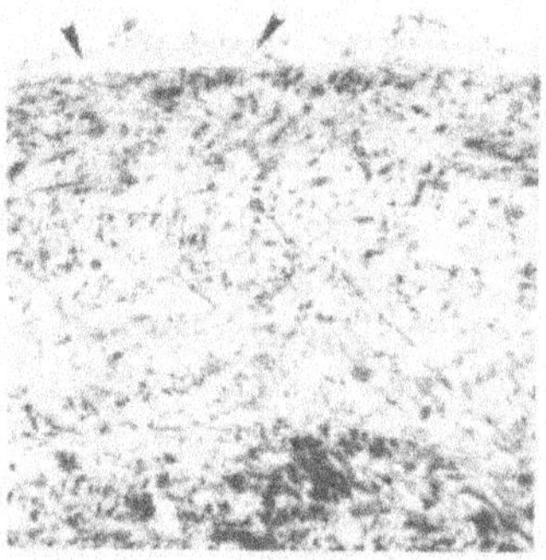

Figure 7

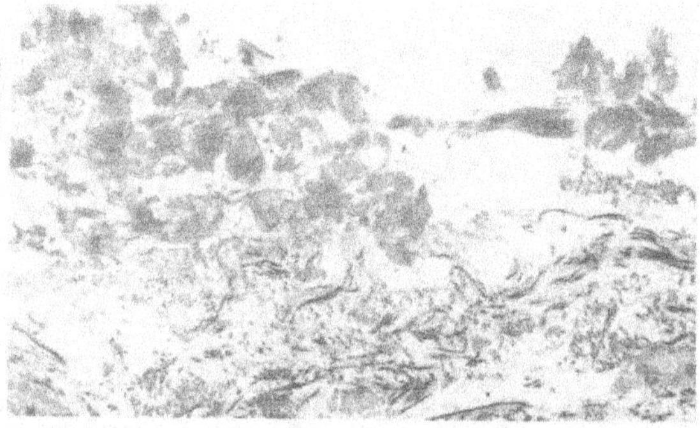

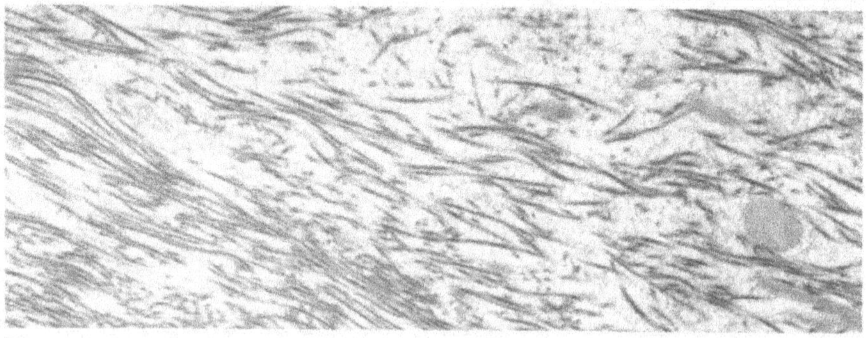

Figure 8

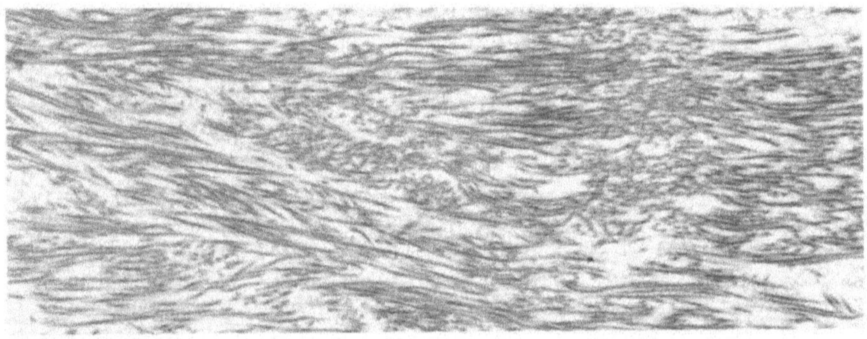

Figure 9

Figure 6: *Light micrograph of heterograft removed at necropsy three days after implantation in the mitral position. A thin layer of fibrin (arrowheads) covers the valvular surface. Alkaline toluidine blue stain. X 300.*

Figure 7: *Electron micrograph showing fibrin layer (arrowheads) on surface of same valve shown in Figure 6. X 11,000.*

Figure 8: *Superficial area of heterograft removed at necropsy 28 days after implantation. The collagen fibrils are widely separated by pale-staining deposits of finely fibrillar or amorphous material representing insudated plasma proteins. X 16,000.*

Figure 9: *Collagen located deeper in same valve as in figure 8 is more compactly arranged, although it also appears to be the site of mild insudation of plasma proteins. X 16,000.*

confirmed that the leaflets did not endothelialize but became covered with a discontinuous layer of fibrin, blood cells, and macrophages. The latter cells were more numerous in these valves than in valves that had been implanted for more than one year.

Figure 10

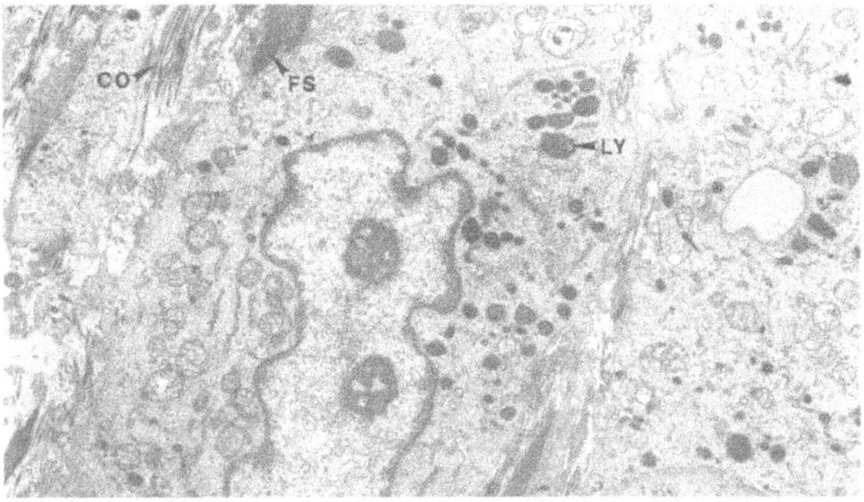

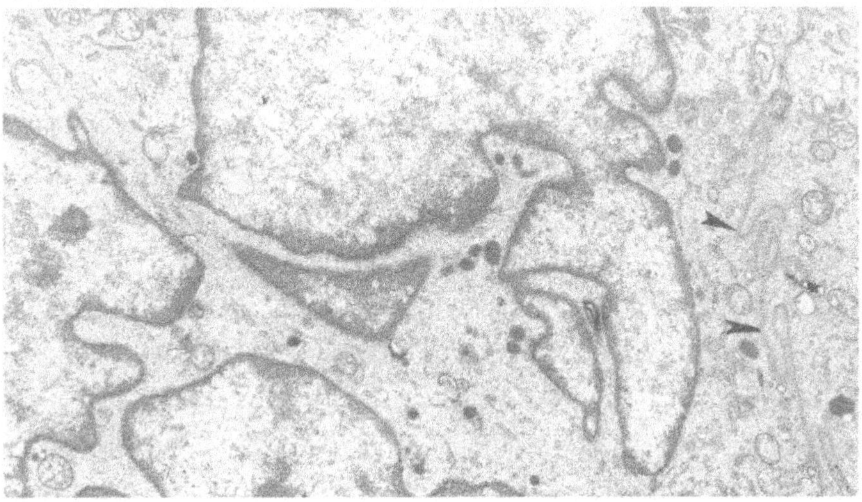

Figure 11

Figure 10: *Macrophages on surface of heterograft implanted for 28 days are adjacent to collagen fibrils (CO) and fibrin strands (FS). These cells contain abundant lysosomes (LY). X 14,000.*

Figure 11: *Part of multinucleated giant cell on surface of same valve shown in figure 10, showing several nuclei, lysosomes and interdigitations of the plasma membrane (arrowheads) with that of an adjacent cell. X 14,500.*

Alterations involving collagen fibrils consisted of increased granularity, irregularity of staining, and disruption of the fibrils. The latter change was associated with fraying or tufting of the ends of the collagen fibrils and with the appearance of finely fibrillar or granular material, which was presumed to be derived from disrupted collagen.

Morphology of Porcine Valves Implanted for 3 to 94 months

The most significant changes observed in porcine valves implanted for long periods of time (3 to 94 months) were disruption of collagen and formation of calcific deposits (Figures 12–15). The extent of collagen disruption correlated with the length of time the valve had been in place. By light microscopy, collagen breakdown was manifested by disappearance of the bundles of collagen fibrils and by the formation of a homogeneous, hyaline-appearing, pale-staining material (Figures 12, 13 and 15). By electron microscopy, areas of disrupted collagen were characterized by the presence of: 1. extremely fine granular material associated with short collagen fibrils (Figure 16) or 2. irregular clumps of coarsely granular material resembling fibrinoid (Figure 17). Electron-lucent particles ranging in size from 1,000 Å to 1 μ and resembling lipid droplets were present in all but two of the valves that had been implanted for 7 months or longer (Figures 18 and 19). Confirmation of the presence of lipid droplets in these valves was obtained by light microscopic study of frozen sections stained with oil red 0.

The surfaces of long-term implants also were associated with variable amounts of fibrin and variable numbers of erythrocytes, macrophages, and giant cells. Endothelial cells were found only in one valve (implanted for 21 months in the tricuspid position), in which they formed part of the surface of an incompletely organized thrombus. Valvular (porcine) fibroblasts, which appeared poorly preserved, were still present in all implanted valves. No evidence of fibroblastic ingrowth of host tissue (fibrous sheath) was observed in any valve leaflet. Platelet aggregates (as opposed to single platelets adhering to the surfaces) consisted of spherical masses of clumped platelets that were not associated with fibrin (Figure 20). The platelets at the base of the aggregates were in direct contact with valvular collagen and with finely fibrillar material presumed to be derived from disrupted collagen. Such aggregates were very frequent and large (up to 60 μ in diameter) in a valve that had been implanted for 76 months. This valve also showed several tears in the leaflets, extensive erosion of the valvular surfaces, and disruption and transformation of collagen in large areas of the fibrosa into finely fibrillar material.

Four valves showed evidence of infection. Morphologic observations related to these infections have been published in detail (10) and are reviewed by Dr. Billingham elsewhere in this symposium.

Severe disruption of collagen was observed in all valves that had been implanted for 4 years or longer (Figures 18 and 19). A total of 6 valves had perforated leaflets; these valves had been in place for periods of time ranging from 18 to 94 months (average 52.5 months). None of these valves showed evidence of infection; each had been implanted in the mitral position, and in each, the collagen was severely altered. Five of these 6 valves also showed calcific deposits; in 2 of

Figure 12

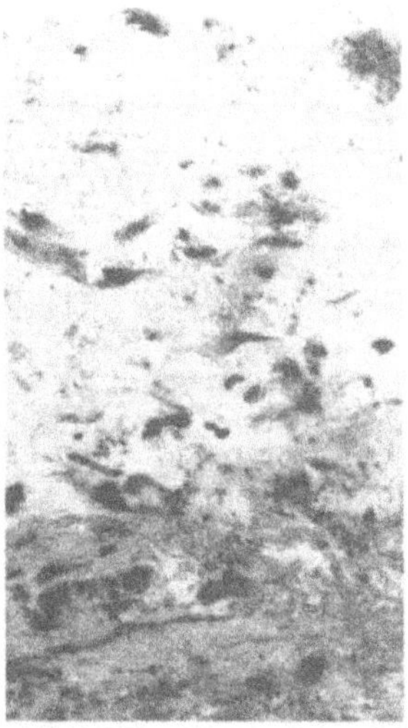

Figure 13

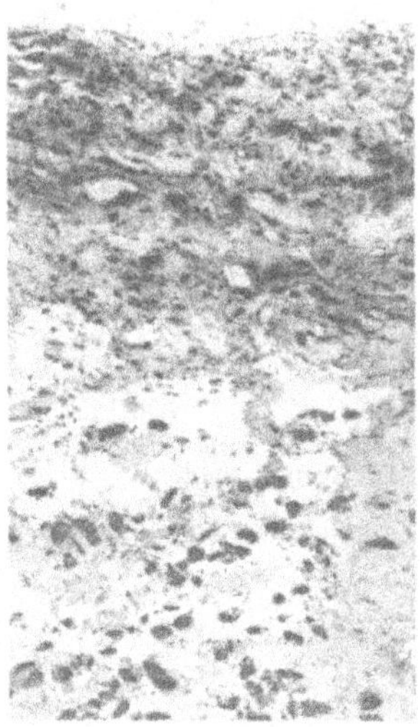

Figure 14

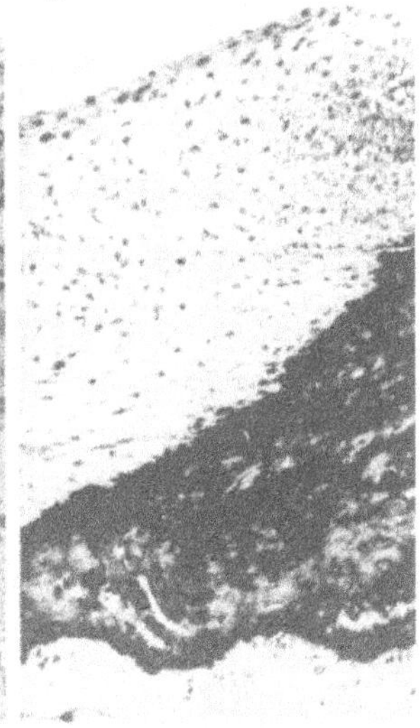

Figure 15

Figures 12–15: *Figures 12, 13 and 15 are light micrographs of plastic sections, stained with alkaline toluidine blue, of a heterograft removed because of regurgitation (torn leaflet) 76 months after implantation in the mitral position. Figure 14 is a histologic section, stained by the Movat pentachrome method, of a heterograft removed because of stenosis 30 months after implantation in the mitral position.*

Figure 12 *shows area of valvular surface in which most of the collagen is pale-staining and amorphous; only a few organized bundles of collagen remain. X 600.* Figure 13 *shows area in which collagen disruption has progressed to actual loss of valvular substance. X 600.* Figure 14 *illustrates calcific plaque that occupies the middle portion of the leaflet. Several of these plaques were present in each of the leaflets, severly limiting their mobility. X 300.* Figure 15 *shows the edge of an area of perforation of a leaflet. The perforation itself is at far right. The thickness of the leaflet tapers sharply toward the edge of the perforation, indicating that marked erosion of the leaflet has occurred. The collagen in this area is markedly disrupted and appears similar to that shown in Figure 13. Aggregates of platelets (arrowheads) are present on the surfaces. X 300.*

these, prosthetic valvular stenosis was considered to be the most significant lesion leading to replacement of the porcine valvular heterograft.

Calcific deposits (Figures 14 and 21–24) were found in a total of 14 valves. In 10 of these, the calcific deposits were visible grossly, and in 9 they were thought to be clinically significant in terms of producing prosthetic valvular stenosis. In

Figure 16

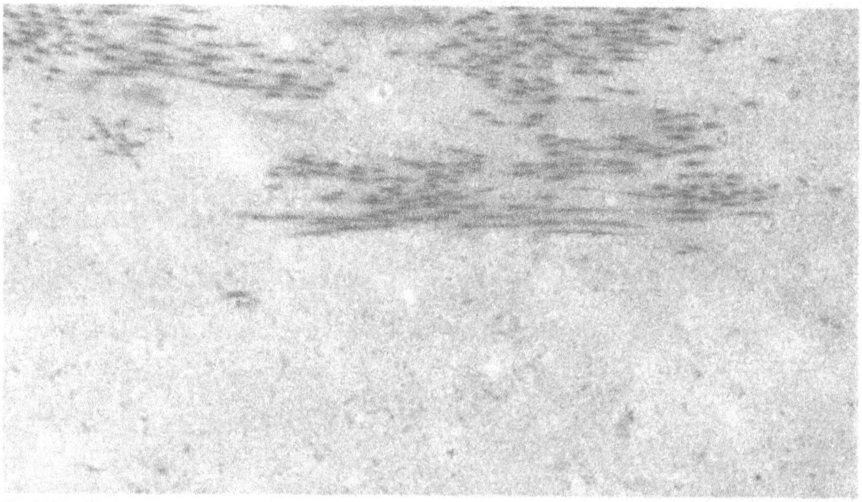

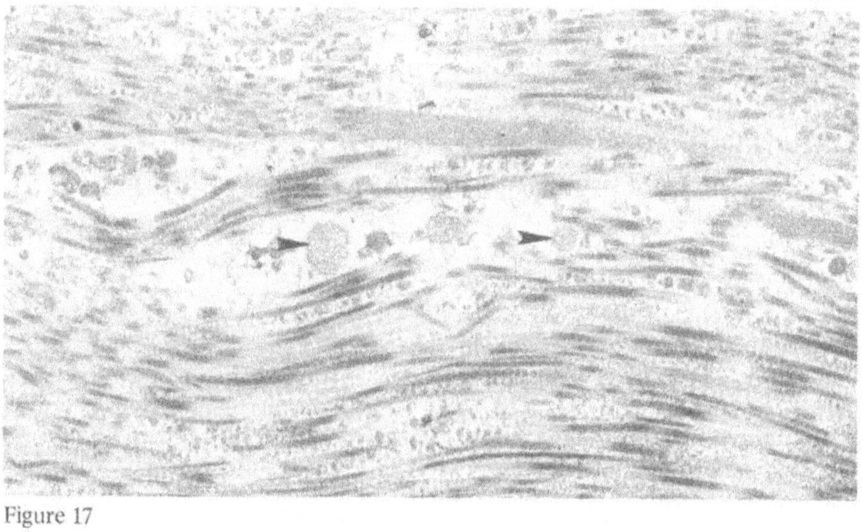

Figure 17

Figure 16: *Severe disruption of collagen in valve removed because of regurgitation 30 months after implantation in the aortic position. Most of the collagen has been replaced by finely granular material. X 22,500.*

Figure 17: *Rounded deposits of fibrinoid material (arrowheads) are located between collagen fibrils in normally functioning valve removed at necropsy 21 months after implantation in the mitral position. X 30,600.*

two patients, the calcific deposits were related to prosthetic valvular infection. Other factors predisposing to calcification were identified in only one patient, who died of renal failure three months after operation and was found to have small calcific deposits in his mitral heterograft. This valve, which was grossly normal, represented the earliest instance of calcification observed by us. The eight non-infected valves showing clinically significant calcification had been

Figure 18

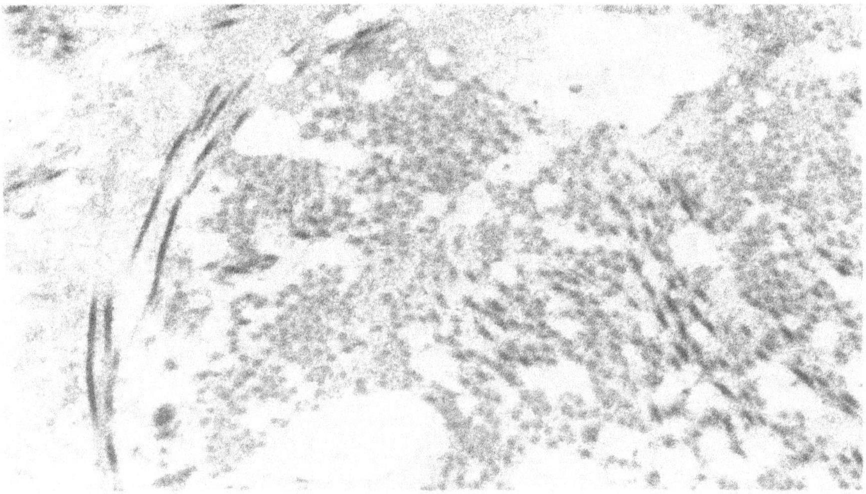

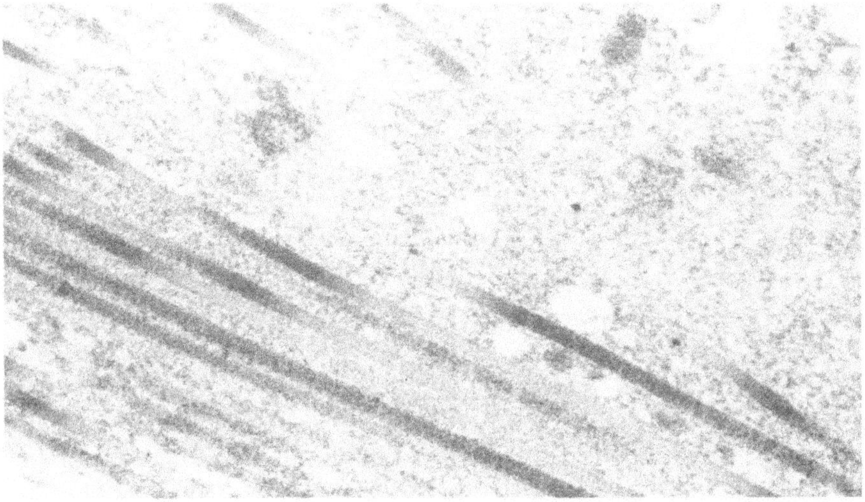

Figure 19

Figures 18 and 19: *Two views of collagen in valve removed at necropsy 94 months after implantation in the mitral position.* Figure 18 *shows extensive infiltration with electron-lucent lipid droplets. X 22,500.* Figure 19 *illustrates finely granular material, which is in various stages of being formed from collagen fibrils and which is associated with lipid droplets. X 66,000.*

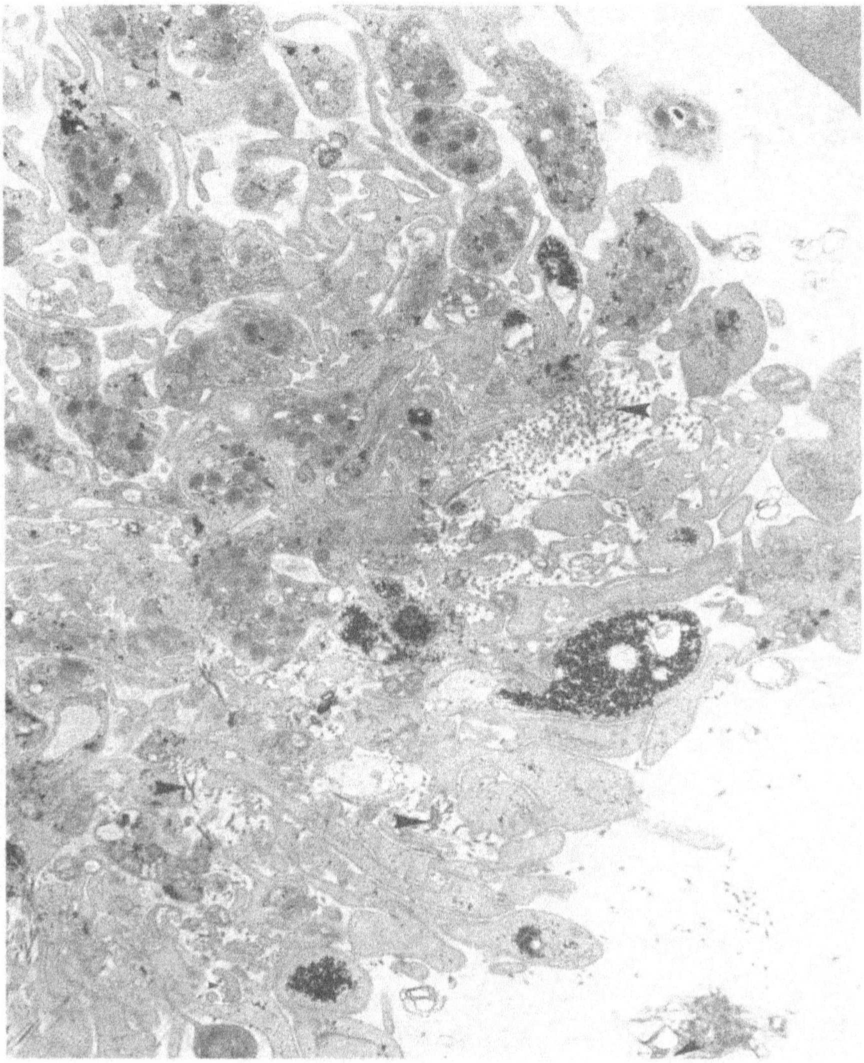

Figure 20: *Electron micrograph of platelet aggregate from valve shown in Figure 15. The platelets are well preserved, without degranulation, and are associated with small clusters of collagen fibrils (arrowheads). X 23,500.*

implanted for an average of 43 months (range, 10 to 60 months). The one infected valve with clinically significant calcification had been in place for 4.5 months and was the site of staphylococcal infection.

When minimal, calcific deposits tended to be localized near the commissures. When more severe, they involved the substance of the leaflets, especially near the apposing margins. Collagen fibrils were always the most important sites of formation of calcific deposits. Nevertheless, such deposits also involved:

organizing thrombi and vegetations; mitochondria of myocytes in the muscle shelf and of connective tissue cells in the leaflets; the porcine aortic wall, and adipose tissue cells at the junction of the leaflets and the aortic wall.

Three different patterns of ultrastructural organization were evident in calcific deposits associated with collagen fibrils (Figures 21–24). In the first of these

Figure 21

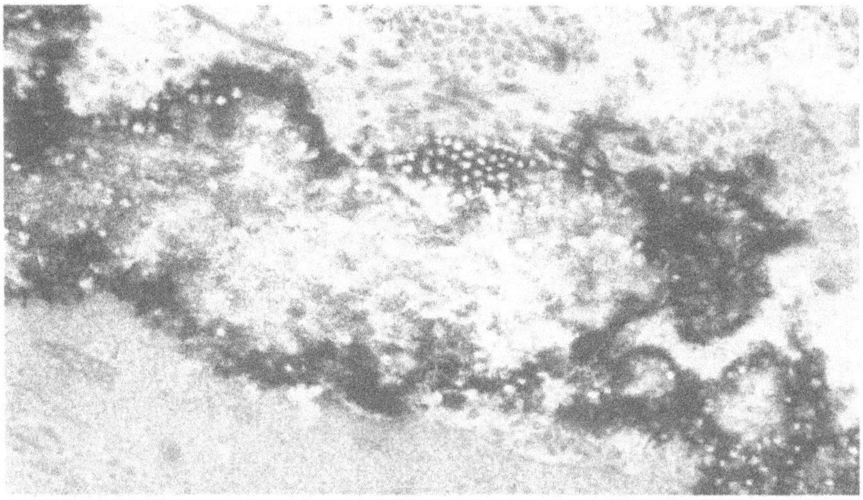

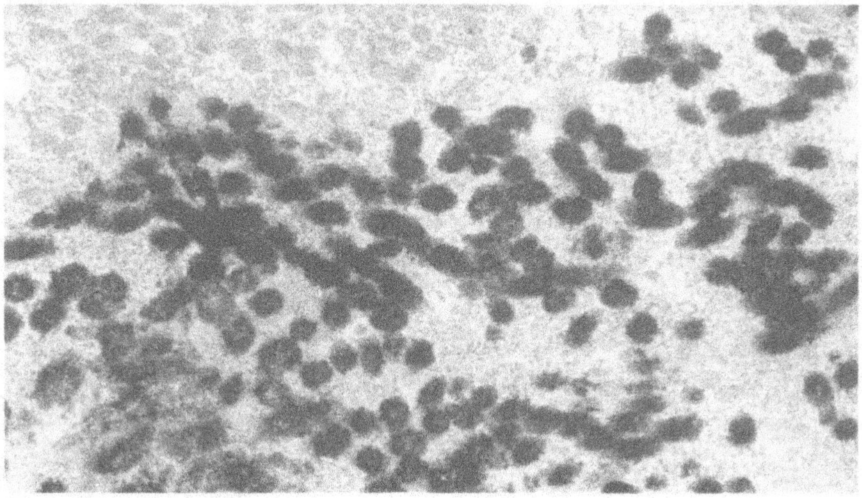

Figure 22

Figure 21: *View of small calcific plaque from valve shown in Figure 14. Most of the collagen at top appears normal, while that at bottom is severely disrupted. Some of the calcium deposits surround the collagen fibrils, which appear as round, lucent spaces (compare with figure 24). X 33,750.*

Figure 22: *Calcific deposits in this area of a valve, removed because of stenosis 41 months after implantation in the mitral position, overlie collagen fibrils and show very little tendency to spread into the interfibrillary spaces. X 77,500.*

(Figure 22), the calcific deposits seemed to overlie the collagen fibrils, but did not extend into the interfibrillary spaces. In the second, the calcific deposits were localized in the periphery of the collagen fibrils and in the interfibrillary spaces (Figures 21, 23 and 24), leaving clear, electron-lucent spaces in the centers of the fibrils. In the third pattern, the calcific deposits occupied both the

Figure 23

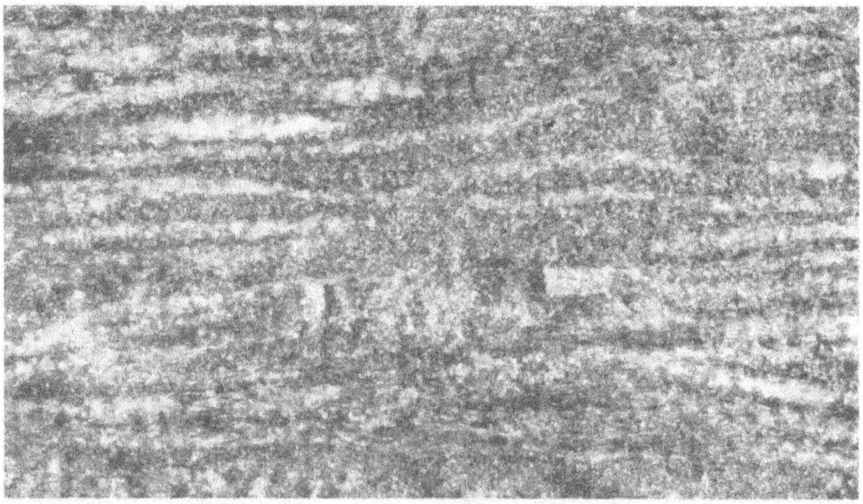

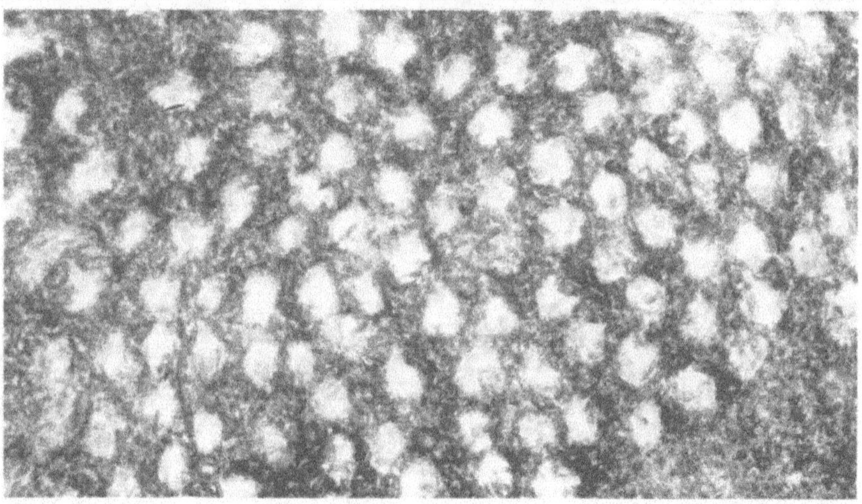

Figure 24

Figure 23: *Another area of same valve as in Figure 22, showing involvement of both the interfibrillary spaces and the collagen fibrils. X 75,000.*

Figure 24: *High magnification view of cross sections of calcified collagen fibrils in area similar to that shown in figure 22. Note the crystalline nature of the deposits and the lack of involvement of the central areas of the collagen fibrils, which appear lucent. X 125,000.*

interfibrillary spaces and the interior of the fibrils (Figure 23); this gave such deposits a relatively homogeneous appearance. The homogeneous pattern just described was characteristically present throughout central areas of large calcific masses. In contrast to this, the interfibrillary pattern was found either at the periphery of large calcific masses or throughout small calcific masses. Involvement of both the interior and the surfaces of collagen fibrils, with sparing of the interfibrillary space, was found only in small, scattered groups of collagen fibrils and not in association with large calcific deposits. A crystalline substructure (Figure 24) was found on high magnification study of most of the calcific masses. These crystals were either cylindrical, as in most of the deposits associated with collagen (280 to 330 Å in length and 65–80 Å in width) or plate-like, as in the deposits associated with organizing vegetations and in a few of the deposits associated with collagen. The calcific deposits appeared ultrastructurally similar in young and old patients. Severe degeneration of collagen usually was associated with the calcific deposits, but the most severely degenerated collagen was not necessarily the site of the heaviest calcification, and calcification sometimes was evident in areas in which the collagen showed mild or no change.

As mentioned previously, calcific deposits were sometimes found to overlie mitochondria and, rarely, nuclei of porcine cells in the leaflets; these, however, constituted only a very small fraction of the total of calcific deposits. No structures resembling the "matrix vesicles" described in other calcifying tissues (2, 12) were found in any valve.

Discussion

The observations in this study show that several morphologic changes develop in porcine aortic valves as a result of commercial processing before implantation, and that a number of other, more severe changes develop after implantation in patients. Preimplantation alterations include denudation of the endothelial cell layer, loss of acid mucopolysaccharides and loosening of the connective tissue framework. These changes appear to result from a combination of: 1. autolysis before the beginning of commercial processing; 2. the relatively poor tissue-fixing qualities of the low concentration (<1%) of glutaraldehyde used in commercial processing, and 3. handling before and during commercial processing.

Early Structural Changes

Structural changes found to occur early after implantation of porcine valvular heterografts consisted of: 1. deposition of a layer of fibrin on the valvular surfaces; 2. insudation of plasma proteins into the valvular substance; 3. breakdown of collagen in superficial areas of the leaflets; 4. formation of cracks in the surfaces, with penetration of blood elements into these spaces, and 5. the appearance of macrophages and multinucleated giant cells on the surfaces. The deposition of a layer of fibrin on the surfaces is a consequence of the loss of endothelium, which leaves the highly thrombogenic subendothelial connective tissue in direct contact with the blood. The fact that thromboembolic episodes are clinically uncommon (20, 22, 33) in patients with implanted porcine valvular heterografts is in accord with the concept that the glutaraldehyde processing markedly reduces the thrombogenic properties of the valvular connective tissue. Nevertheless, fibrin thrombi are common on the surfaces of porcine valvular heterografts, as shown by Spray and Roberts (28).

The insudation of plasma proteins is another consequence of the loss of the permeability barrier function of endothelium. Only one of the porcine valvular heterografts studied by us showed evidence of being reendothelialized, and this occurred only in an area overlying an organizing thrombus. The breakdown of collagen in superficial areas of the leaflets represents the onset of a process that subsequently involves deeper areas and eventually may result in perforation of the leaflets. The macrophages and multinucleated giant cells are regarded as indicating a foreign body type of reaction. For reasons that may be related to the glutaraldehyde processing, these cells show very little tendency to invade the substance of the leaflets. This is of importance in infections of heterografts, as bacteria can penetrate deeply into the leaflets while the inflammatory cells tend to remain in superficial layers (10). Surprisingly, macrophages and multinucleated giant cells were present in smaller numbers in valves that had been implanted for longer periods of time. Plasma cells and lymphocytes do not invade these valves, and it is reasonable to conclude that the glutaraldehyde fixation decreases the antigenicity of tissue components of porcine valvular heterografts.

Late Structural Changes

Some of the late structural changes in implanted porcine valvular heterografts represented progression of early changes. This was the case with the collagen breakdown, the extent of which increased with time after implantation; however, other changes, including the aggregates of platelets on the valvular surfaces, the lipid deposits and the calcific deposits, appeared to be **de novo** phenomena. The lipid deposits were associated with breakdown of collagen, and they probably formed as the result of insudation of plasma lipoproteins into the valvular tissue. The aggregates of platelets on the surfaces of the heterografts result from the well known tendency of collagen to induce aggregation of platelets. Such aggregates also have been detected on the surfaces of native aortic valves that have become stenotic (29); however, they also have been found on the surfaces of Silastic poppets in mechanical prostheses of the ball-valve type (1, 24). The ultrastructural observations in this report point to the possibility that small fibrin deposits and platelet aggregates form continuously on the surfaces of porcine valves and that, because of the mechanical forces to which they are subjected, the large majority of such deposits or aggregates are shed from the surfaces into the bloodstream before they have had an opportunity to grow to a large size. It appears unlikely that platelet aggregates would remain attached for a long time to the valvular surfaces, to which they are anchored only by a few strands of collagen fibrils.

The collagen breakdown in glutaraldehyde-preserved valvular heterografts is ultrastructurally similar to that described in other tissue valves, such as variously preserved homografts (13, 23), formalin- und glutaraldehyde-treated heterografts (21, 25, 31), and autologous fascia lata valves (14). These changes occur much more slowly in glutaraldehyde-treated valves than in other types of bioprostheses. Among the possible causes of damage to the collagen in porcine valvular heterografts are: 1. reversal of the glutaraldehyde-mediated cross-linking effect on proteins, with conversion of the collagen from the fibrillar to the soluble form; 2. binding of proteins to collagen, with formation of material resembling "fibrinoid"; 3. hydrolysis of collagen by specific collagenases present in inflammatory cells and by nonspecific proteolytic enzymes in inflammatory cells and blood plasma; 4. breakdown of collagen fibrils by mechanical forces of valvular motion (materials fatigue), and 5. erosion of superficial layers of valvular collagen by the forces of blood flow (shear stress). The work of Clark and collaborators (7) suggests that mechanical forces are of considerable importance in the pathogenesis of valve failure related to rupture of the leaflets. Detailed evaluation of these possible causes is of great importance because the breakdown of collagen is the factor leading to cuspal perforations and prosthetic valvular regurgitation.

Calcification

Several structural components of porcine valvular heterografts were found to be the sites of formation of calcific deposits; however, the deposits associated with collagen fibrils were the most important from the standpoint of clinical significance (i. e., producing valvular stenosis). Calcific deposits associated with vegetations or fibrin deposits were found in only 2 of the 14 valves in which calcification was present; only in one of these two valves were such deposits clinically significant. In contrast, calcification of valvular collagen appeared to be the mechanism producing porcine valvular stenosis in all other patients in whom this complication developed.

Recent reports have emphasized the occurrence of calcific stenosis in porcine valvular heterografts implanted in children and young adults (6, 11, 18, 19, 26). In the present study we found such calcification to occur not only in children and young adults but also in three elderly adults, each aged 65 years; in addition, we found clinically insignificant calcific deposits in several other adults. Hetzer et al. (16) also observed a calcified porcine valve in a 64 year-old woman. The statistical significance of these observations is very limited, because some of these heterografts were submitted to us for study specifically because they showed calcification. Nevertheless, it is clear from these observations that clinically significant calcific deposits can occur in porcine valvular heterografts implanted in adults as well as in children, and that detailed analysis of a large number of patients will be necessary to determine the true incidence of these changes in different age groups.

Severe degeneration of collagen was observed in each of the valves in which clinically significant calcific deposits occurred, suggesting that some alteration in valvular collagen is necessary in order for calcification to develop. Calcification is known to occur in other valvular bioprostheses, including fascia lata valves (14, 27) homografts (3, 23), dura mater valves (32) and pericardial valves (5, 30). It is presumed that calcific deposits in these valves do involve collagen in the leaflets, as suggested by published light micrographs; however, ultrastructural studies of calcific deposits have not been reported in any of these types of valves. In one homograft studied by us (unpublished observations), we have observed severe calcification of the collagen, with ultrastructural patterns of calcium deposition similar to those found in the porcine heterografts. The calcification of collagen in porcine valvular heterografts can be regarded as an example of the deposition of an inorganic matrix, composed of hydroxyapatite crystals, upon an organic matrix, composed of altered collagen fibrils. Thus, collagen fibrils are major sites of formation of nuclei of crystallization of hydroxyapatite, and this process appears similar to that which takes place (12) in other connective tissues that undergo calcification (i. e., bone, dentin, cementum and enamel). The deposition of calcium in connective tissues that normally undergo calcification is influenced by a number of chemicals, enzymes and hormones. It remains to be determined, however, whether such factors play a role in the formation of calcific deposits in porcine valvular heterografts. The unpredictability of the occurrence of such deposits in porcine valves (heavy calcific deposits requiring replacement of the porcine heterograft have been found as early as 19 (11) and 53 (16) days after implantation) suggests that it is not the degeneration of collagen (which is a widespread phenomenon) which by itself leads to calcification, but the interaction between this altered collagen and the chemical band hormonal milieu in which it is found.

References

1. Allwork S. P., Norton R.:
Surface ultrastructure of silicone rubber aortic valve poppets after long-term implantation. A scanning electron microscope study of four poppets.
Thorax **31**, 742 (1976)

2. Anderson H. C.:
Vesicles associated with calcification in the matrix of epiphyseal cartilage.
J. Cell Biol. **41**, 59 (1969)

3. Barratt-Boyes B. G., Roche A. H. G., Brandt P. W. T., Smith J. C., Lowe J. B.:
Aortic homograft valve replacement. A long-term follow-up of an initial series of 101 patients.
Circulation **40**, 763 (1969)

4. Binet J. P., Planche C., Weiss M.:
Heterograft replacement of the aortic valve.
In: Biological Tissue in Heart Valve Replacement, (Ionescu M. I., Ross D. N., Wooler G. H., editors), London, Butterworths, 409 (1972)

5. Björk V. O., Hulquist G.:
Teflon and pericardial aortic valve prostheses.
J. Thorac. Cardiovasc. Surg. **47**, 693 (1964)

6. Brown J. W., Dunn J. M., Spooner E., Kirsh M. M.:
Late spontaneous disruption of a porcine xenograft mitral valve. Clinical, hemodynamic, echocardiographic, and pathologic findings.
J. Thorac. Cardiovasc. Surg. **75**, 606 (1978)

7. Clark R. E., Swanson W. M., Kardos J. L., Hagen R. W., Beauchamp R. A.:
Durability of prosthetic heart valves.
Ann. Thorac. Surg. **26,** 323 (1978)
8. Ferrans V. J., Spray T. L., Billingham M. E., Roberts W. C.:
Structural changes in glutaraldehyde-treated porcine heterografts used as substitute cardiac valves. Transmission and scanning electron microscopic observations in 12 patients.
Am. J. Cardiol. **41,** 1159 (1978)
9. Ferrans V. J., Spray T. L., Billingham M. E., Roberts W. C.:
Ultrastructure of Hancock porcine valvular heterografts. Pre- and post-implantation changes.
Circulation **58,** Suppl. I, I–10 (1978)
10. Ferrans V. J., Boyce S. W., Billingham M. E., Spray T. L., Roberts W. C.:
Infection of glutaraldehyde-preserved porcine valvular heterografts.
Am. J. Cardiol., in press (1979)
11. Forfar J. C., Cotter L., Morritt G. N.:
Severe and early stenosis of porcine heterograft mitral valve.
Br. Heart J. **40,** 1184 (1978)
12. Frank R.-M., Voegel J.-C.:
Le cristal d'apatite biologique: son élaboration, son comportement physiologique et pathologique.
Biol. Cell. (Paris) **28,** 187 (1977)
13. Gavin J. B., Herdson P. B., Barratt-Boyes B. G.:
The pathology of chemically-sterilized human heart valve allografts.
Pathology **4,** 175 (1972)
14. Gersbach P., Wegmann W.:
Aorta valve replacement using autologous fascia lata transplants. Late morphological changes: an electron microscopic study.
Virchows Arch. (Pathol. Anat.) **364,** 235 (1974)
15. Gross L., Kugel M. A.:
Topographic anatomy and histology of the valves in the human heart.
Am. J. Pathol. **7,** 445 (1931)
16. Hetzer R., Hill J. D., Kerth W. J., Wilson A. J., Adappa M. G., Gerbode F.:
Thrombosis and degeneration of Hancock valves: clinical and pathological findings.
Ann. Thorac. Surg. **26,** 317 (1978)
17. Kajikawa K., Yamaguchi T., Katsuda S., Miwa A.:
An improved electron stain for elastic fibers using tannic acid.
J. Electron Microsc. (Tokyo) **24,** 287 (1975)
18. Kutsche L., Oyer P., Shumway N., Baum D.:
An important complication of Hancock mitral valve replacement in children.
Circulation **57** and **58,** Suppl. II, II–148 (1978)
19. Levitsky S.:
Discussion to paper by Stinson et al.
J. Thorac. Cardiovasc. Surg. **73,** 62 (1977)
20. McIntosh C. L., Michaelis L. L., Morrow A. G., Itscoitz S. B., Redwood D. R., Epstein S. E.:

Atrioventricular valve replacement with the Hancock porcine xenograft: a five year clinical experience.
Surgery **78**, 768 (1975)
21. Okamura K., Yuge I., Kawazoe K., Kitamura N., Koyanagi H., Konno S.:
A comparative study between glutaraldehyde-preserved aortic and pulmonary heterograft valves in the tricuspid position in dogs.
J. Cardiovasc. Surg. **17**, 178 (1976)
22. Pipkin R. D., Buch W. S., Fogarty T. J.:
Evaluation of aortic valve replacement with a porcine xenograft without long-term anticoagulation.
J. Thorac. Cardiovasc. Surg. **71**, 179 (1976)
23. Reichenbach D. D., Mohri H., Merendino K. A.:
Pathological changes in human aortic valve homografts.
Circulation **39**, Suppl. I, 47 (1969)
24. Rodman N. F., Doty D. B., Caughey R. C.:
Surface ultrastructural studies of mitral valve prosthetic devices. In:
Scanning Electron Microscopy 1974, part III. Proceedings of the Workshop on Advances in Biomedical Applications of the SEM, IIT Research Institute, Chicago, 729 (1974)
25. Rose A. G.:
Pathology of the formalin-treated heterograft porcine aortic valve in the mitral position.
Thorax **27**, 401 (1972)
26. Rose A. G., Forman R., Bowen R. M.:
Calcification of glutaraldehyde-fixed porcine xenograft.
Thorax **33**, 111 (1978)
27. Silver M. D., Hudson R. E. B., Trimble A. S.:
Morphologic observations on heart valve prostheses made of fascia lata.
J. Thorac. Cardiovasc. Surg. **70**, 360 (1975)
28. Spray T. L., Roberts W. C.:
Structural changes in porcine xenografts used as substitute cardiac valves. Gross and histologic observations in 51 glutaraldehyde-preserved Hancock valves in 41 patients.
Am. J. Cardiol. **40**, 319 (1977)
29. Stein P. D., Sabbah H. N., Pitha J. V.:
Continuing disease process of calcific aortic stenosis: role of microthrombi and turbulent flow.
Am. J. Cardiol. **39**, 159 (1977)
30. Yarbrough J. W., Roberts W. C., Reis R. L.:
Structural alterations in tissue cardiac valves implanted in patients and in calves.
J. Thorac. Cardiovasc. Surg. **65**, 364 (1973)
31. Yaroshinsky Y. N., Shekhter A. B., Artyukhina T. V., Glagoleva E. V., Fursov B. A.:
Electron microscopic study of the aortic valve allo- and xenotransplants following their prolonged functioning in the human heart.
Biull. Eksp. Biol. Med. **78**, 116 (1974)

32. Zerbini E. J., Puig L. B.:
Valvas cardiacas proteticas e biologicas. Especial referencia a valva de dura-mater.
Arch, Inst. Cardiol. México **47,** 650 (1977)
33. Zuhdi N., Hawley W., Voehl V., Hancock W. W., Carey J., Greer A.:
Porcine aortic valves as replacements for human heart valves.
Ann. Thorac. Surg. **17,** 479 (1974)

Postoperative Aortic Regurgitation From Incomplete Seating of Tilting-Disc Occluders Due to Overhanging Knots or Long Sutures*

Bruce F. Waller, M.D.; Michael Jones, M.D.; and William C. Roberts, M.D., F.C.C.P.

Certain clinical and morphologic features are described in three patients who developed severe aortic regurgitation after aortic valve replacement. The regurgitation, fatal in two of the three patients, resulted from long sutures or their knots or both overhanging the metallic ring of the prosthesis preventing complete seating of the occluder. In one patient, simply cutting the overhanging suture eliminated the aortic regurgitation. The problem of suture overhang appears more likely to occur when aortic valve replacement is carried out in patients with relatively small aortic roots. Before closing the aortotomy after aortic valve replacement, it is advisable to move the occluder back and forth to make sure its movement, and specifically, its ability to seat completely, is not limited by sutures which are too long.

Aortic regurgitation after aortic valve replacement usually results from incomplete seating of occluders due to thrombi, protruding calcific deposits or buckled aortic walls, or partial detachment of prosthetic rings from aortic "anuli" ("parabasilar leaks") due to suture break, infection, or insertion of an inadequate number of sutures to secure the prostheses.[1-6] In patients with both mitral and aortic valve prostheses, a strut of the mitral prosthesis has interfered with complete aortic poppet seating.[7] Another rare cause of aortic regurgitation after aortic valve replacement is long sutures or suture knots or both overhanging the orifice of the aortic prosthesis preventing complete seating of the occluder. This report describes three patients in whom the latter mechanism produced severe aortic regurgitation which was fatal and unrecognized in two patients.

*From the Pathology and Surgery Branches, National Heart, Lung, and Blood Institute, National Institutes of Health, Bethesda, MD.
Manuscript received October 18; revision accepted December 17.
Reprint requests: Dr. Roberts, National Institutes of Health, Bldg 10A, Room 3E30, Bethesda 20205

Case Reports

Pertinent observations in the three patients are summarized in Table 1. Each of the three patients was operated on by a different surgeon, and the operations were performed at two separate medical centers. Patient 1 died in the operating room; patient 2 died 29 hours after completion of operation, and patient 3 is living after reoperation 191 days after the first operation. The systemic arterial pressures and cardiac rates early after the first operation in patients 2 and 3 are

Table 1—*Clinical Observations in Three Patients with Severe Aortic Regurgitation Postoperatively from Overhanging Knots or Long Sutures Preventing Complete Seating of Prosthetic (Björk-Shiley [B-S]) Occluders***

	Patient 1: (26F)			Patient 2: (56F)			Patient 3: (49M)				
	BO	O	AO	BO	O	AO	BO	O_1	AO_1	O_2	AO_2
LV (s/d)†	143/12		. . .	128/8		. . .	190/16		135/28		. . .
SA (s/d)†	110/70		. . .	128/60		100/20	135/70		120/55		130/80
LV-SA (psg)†	33		. . .	0		. . .	55		15		. . .
AR (0-4+) by AAA	3+		. . .	3+		. . .	1+		3+		. . .
Size (mm) B-S inserted		21			19			21			
AR at O after AVR		+			. . .			+		0	
Days from O to death			0			1.2		|←	191	→|	

*Abbreviations are as follows: AAA indicates ascending aortic angiography; AO, after operation; AR, aortic regurgitation; AVR, aortic valve replacement; BO, before operation; d, diastolic; LV, left ventricular pressure; O, operation; psg, peak systolic gradient; s, systolic; and SA, systemic artery.
†Pressures in mm Hg.

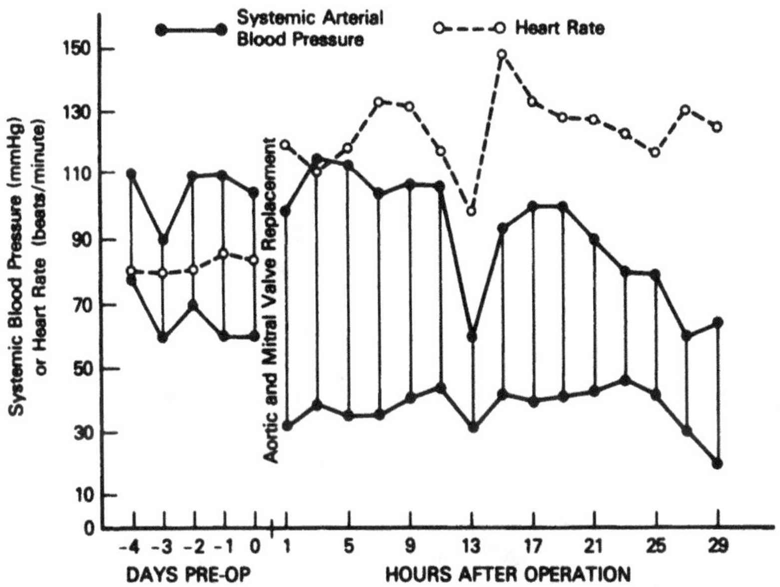

Figure 1. Systemic arterial blood pressures, and cardiac rates preoperatively and postoperatively in patient 2 who had both aortic and mitral valves replaced with prostheses. Appearance at autopsy of porcine bioprosthesis in mitral position indicated that this substitute valve had functioned normally during life so that lowered pressures and elevated heart rate could be attributed to altered function of the Björk-Shiley *aortic* prosthesis. Left ventricular myocardium also was free of foci or necrosis or fibrosis.

shown in Figures 1 and 2. In both, the systemic arterial diastolic pressures were lower; and the systemic arterial pulse pressures and the cardiac rates were higher than those recorded preoperatively. It was apparent that aortic regurgitation was present at operation in patients 1 and 3 after the aortic valve had been replaced, the aortotomy incision closed, and before the left ventricular drain had been removed but its mechanism was not learned in patient 1 until necropsy, and not until reoperation in patient 3 when sutures were found to overhang the orifice of the aortic-valve prosthesis. Simply cutting the single overhanging suture caused the aortic regurgitation to disappear in patient 3 (Fig 2). Patient 3 had had an uneventful early postoperative course after the first operation despite an unappreciated lower diastolic arterial blood pressure and sinus tachycardia (Fig 2). A murmur consistent with aortic regurgitation had not been heard in the first two weeks postoperatively, but one month after operation, a grade 1/6 diastolic blow was audible at the base of the heart. During the next four months, the diastolic murmur became more easily audible, and he had developed mild congestive heart failure. Repeat ascending aortic angiogram five months postoperatively had showed severe aortic regurgitation from incomplete diastolic closure of the tilting disc, and the second operation then was performed. Necropsies in both patients 1 and 2 showed similar overhanging sutures or knots or both (Fig 3 and 4).

Comments

Each of the three patients described herein had severe aortic regurgitation after aortic valve replacement because sutures or their knots or both over-

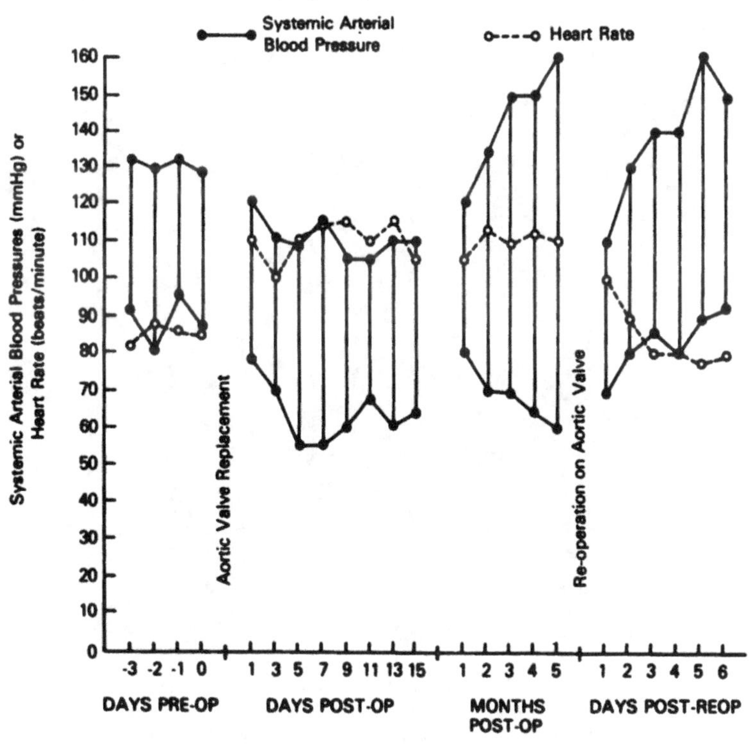

Figure 2. Systemic arterial blood pressures and heart rates preoperatively and postoperatively in patient 3 who had aortic valve replacement and reoperation five months after first aortic operation. Murmur of aortic regurgitation disappeared after second operation.

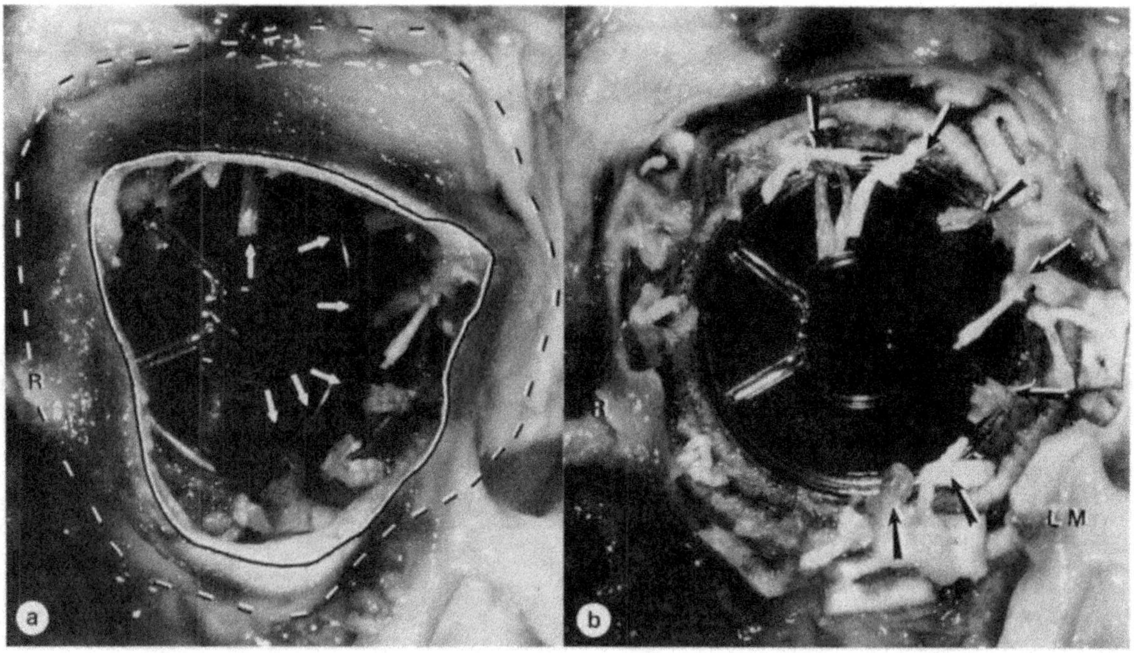

FIGURE 3. View from aorta at autopsy of Björk-Shiley tilting-disc prosthesis of patient showing long sutures (*a* and *b*) (*arrows*) which prevent complete seating of tilting-disc in ventricular diastole (*a*). Occluder has been made to seat completely in *b* and sutures which did overhang metallic ring bordering orifice are now laid over surface of metallic occluder. *Dashed line* outlines site of attachment of prosthesis to aortic "anulus." Circumference of aorta (*solid line*) above or cephalad to prosthesis is much smaller than circumference at site of attachment of prosthesis. Ideal is for both dashed and solid lines to coincide. Buckling inward of wall of aorta may be responsible in part at least for overhanging of the sutures.

hung the metallic rings of the tilting disc prostheses preventing complete seating of the occluders. Although recognized at operation, the aortic regurgitation was unrecognized in the early postoperative period in the two patients surviving operation, and recognized in one of them not until a month after operation.

The message of this report is obvious. Sutures placed to secure prosthetic valves should not be left so long that they could possibly overhang the prosthetic orifice rings and prevent the occluders from seating completely. Because the occluder of the Bjork-Shiley prosthesis is very light, much lighter than the poppet of the caged-ball prosthesis, items as small as sutures can prevent occluders from occluding. The aortotomy incision should not be closed

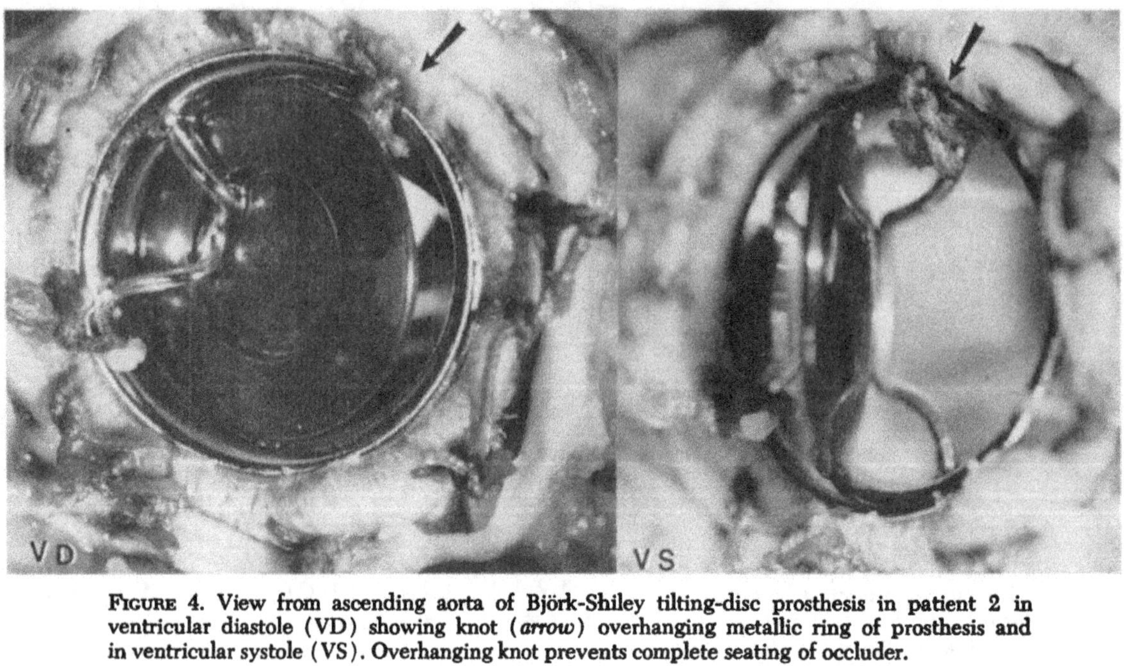

FIGURE 4. View from ascending aorta of Björk-Shiley tilting-disc prosthesis in patient 2 in ventricular diastole (VD) showing knot (*arrow*) overhanging metallic ring of prosthesis and in ventricular systole (VS). Overhanging knot prevents complete seating of occluder.

until it is certain that the occluder both opens and closes easily — without interference by sutures or other extraneous deposits such as calcium.[8]

Each patient described herein had small sized aortic prostheses inserted (Table 1) (Fig 4) despite severe aortic regurgitation preoperatively in two of them. Probably, the problem of "suture overhang" is more likely to occur in patients with small-sized aortic "roots" because the wall of aorta immediately above the site of attachment of the prosthetic sowing ring may "buckle-in" (see Fig 4) due to its outward protrusion at the site of prosthetic attachment. When the wall of aorta buckles toward the lumen just above or cephalad to the suture ring, the knots attaching the prosthesis to the aortic "anulus" have a greater chance of being pushed into the prosthetic orifice, thus overhanging the metallic ring of the orifice. Knotted 0 to 2-0 gauge sutures used for securing the prosthesis to the wall of aorta ("aortic-valve anulus") usually measure in vertical length about 3 to 4 mm and the suture tags at the ends of the knots usually about 2 to 3 mm. The width of the cloth portion of the sized 19-21 Bjork-Shiley prosthesis measures only about 3 mm. Therefore, if the aorta buckles toward the lumen just downstream from the site of prosthetic attachment, knots or sutures can readily be pushed into the prosthetic orifice and consequently overhang the metallic prosthetic ring. Obviously, the sutures should be placed toward the aortic wall rather than toward the metallic ring bordering the orifice of the prosthesis. It appears in our three patients that the sutures overhanging the orifice were those placed initially too close or immediately adjacent to the metallic rings of the prostheses. Thus, particular caution should be exerted in placing the sutures away from the metallic rings of the orifices and as close as possible to the wall of the aorta.

References

1 Roberts WC, Morrow AG. Causes of early postoperative death following cardiac valve replacement. J Thorac Cardiovasc Surg 1967; 54:422-437

2 Roberts WC, Morrow AG. Anatomic studies of hearts containing caged-ball prosthetic valves. Johns Hopkins Med J 1967; 121:271-295

3 Roberts WC, Morrow AG. Causes of death and other anatomic observations after cardiac valve replacement. In: Advances in cardiology: long-term prognosis following valve replacement: second conference on cardiovascular disease. Basel: S Karger, 1972:226-227

4 Roberts WC, Fishbein FC, Golden A. Cardiac pathology after replacement by disc prosthesis: a study of 61 necropsy patients. Am J Cardiol 1975; 35:740-760

5 Hammer WJ, Hearne MJ, Roberts WC. Cocking of a poppet-disc prosthesis in the aortic position: a cause of intermittent aortic regurgitation. J Thorac Cardiovasc Surg 1976; 71:259-261

6 Roberts WC, Hammer WJ. Cardiac pathology after valve replacement with a tilting disc prosthesis (Björk-Shiley type): a study of 46 necropsy patients and 49 Björk-Shiley prostheses. Am J Cardiol 1976; 37:1024-1033

7 Roberts WC, Lambird PA, Gott VL, Morrow AG. Fatal aortic regurgitation following replacement of the mitral and aortic valves: a mechanical complication of double valve replacement. J Thorac Cardiovasc Surg 1966; 52: 189-192

8 Jones AA, Otis JB, Fletcher GF, Roberts WC. A hitherto undescribed cause of prosthetic mitral valve obstruction. J Thorac Cardiovasc Surg 1977; 74:116-117

Prosthetic Cardiac Valves – A Comparison of the Four Basic Designs

W.C. Roberts and T.L. Spray

Since the first cardiac valve prosthesis was implanted in the normal anatomic position in 1960 (1), many different varieties of prostheses have been developed. In spite of the large number of types of prostheses used, none has been ideal to date. This report discusses the relative advantages and disadvantages of the various cardiac valve prostheses available today and the factors that should be taken into account in the selection of a prosthesis for a particular patient (2).

The multitude of types of prosthetic valves currently available can be divided into four basic designs. [1] caged ball, [2] caged disk, [3] tilting disk, and [4] tissue valve. These four basic types can be compared on the basis of the six ideal characteristics of a good prosthetic valve (Table 1): [1] good hemodynamics (competent and non-obstructive, or if so, to an insignificant degree), [2] nonthrombogenic, [3] does not degenerate, wear out, or vary, [4] does not alter blood components (hemolyze), [5] can be implanted without extraordinary technical skill, and (6) does not disturb the patient.

Analysis of each of the four types of substitute cardiac valves for the first four of these ideal characteristics should separate the good ones from the bad ones. The degree of difficulty or ease in inserting each of the four basic types of presently employed substitute valves is similar because all have rigid or semirigid frames and cloth-covered sewing rings. Furthermore, with the possible exception of the recent metal-track Starr-Edwards prosthesis, none of the presently used substitute valves make noise audible to the patient.

Caged Ball Prostheses

The caged ball (Table 2) was the first type of prosthesis used successfully for the treatment of valvular heart disease. Initially, it was used by Hufnagel in 1953 in the descending thoracic aorta for treatment of severe aortic regurgitation [3, 4]. In 1960, Starr

Table 1. Substitute cardiac valves: general characteristics

Type	Year introduced	Hemodynamics		Thrombotic	Hemolytic	Degenerates
		Obstructive	Incompetent			
Caged ball	1960	++	0	++	+	+
Caged disk	1965	+++	0	+++	+	+
Tilting disk	1967	+	0	+++	0	0
Tissue valve						
Homograft	1962	0	++	0	0	+
Xenograft	1965	++	0	0	0	++

Harken
Starr Edwards
McGovern
Smeloff-Cutter
Braunwald-Cutter
DeBakey

and Edwards successfully used the caged ball prosthesis in the mitral position [1] although Harken had earlier the same year utilized a similar prosthesis in the subcoronary (aortic) position [5, 6]. More information on this type of prosthesis is available than on any of the other prostheses because it has been more widely used and used for the longest times. Because the most information is available on this prosthesis and because it has been the one most widely employed, however, does not mean that it necessarily is the best prosthesis. This prosthesis, which has had a number of modifications (the word "modification" unfortunately is not synonymous with the word "improvement") during the past 20 years, in general, has adequate but not the best hemodynamic characteristics [7–10]. Although the introduction of cloth-covering on the struts and base has diminished the incidence of clinical events compatible with emboli, this prosthesis nevertheless continues to have a tendency to form thrombus, and anticoagulants are required [11]. It hemolyzes erythrocytes, more frequently and more severely after aortic than after mitral valve replacement and, also, more frequently and more severely after replacement with the cloth-covered models than with the non-cloth-covered models [12, 13]. Hemolysis, however, is rarely a major clinical problem with this prosthesis or with any of them because the bone marrow is capable of replacing the destroyed erythrocytes without development of anemia or thrombocytopenia.

Degeneration of the silicone rubber poppet was common in the caged ball prosthesis inserted before 1967 [14-19], but no degeneration or variance has been reported in the metallic (stellite-21) hollow poppet introduced at that time. The silicone rubber poppet models continue to be employed in some major centers, and it is likely that poppet degeneration eventually will occur in them. Such was the case with the Braunwald-Cutter aortic valve prosthesis, which has been withdrawn from the market [20]. Wear of cloth covering on both struts and orifice occurred in some of the completely cloth-covered caged ball prostheses, but strut cloth wear has not been observed since introduction of the metal track in the latest Starr-Edwards models.

A problem with the caged-ball prosthesis is that it may occupy too much space within either the cardiac ventricle or the aortic root, and because flow is entirely peripheral, there may not be adequate space between the surface of the poppet and the endocardium of the ventricle or the intima of the ascending aorta to adequately accommodate blood flow [21–24]. This situation accurs most frequently when mitral replacement is performed in a patient, usually a woman, with pure mitral stenosis and a normal aortic valve. In this circumstance, the left ventricle may not be of adequate size to accomodate the mitral prosthesis, and one or more struts of the prosthesis burrows into the myocardial wall, preventing adequate descent of the poppet, with resulting obstruction to left atrial emptying [21] (Fig. 1). This occurrence, obviously, is most likely when larger-sized prosthetics are utilized, but it may occur when even the smallest-sized caged ball prostheses are employed to replace purely stenotic mitral

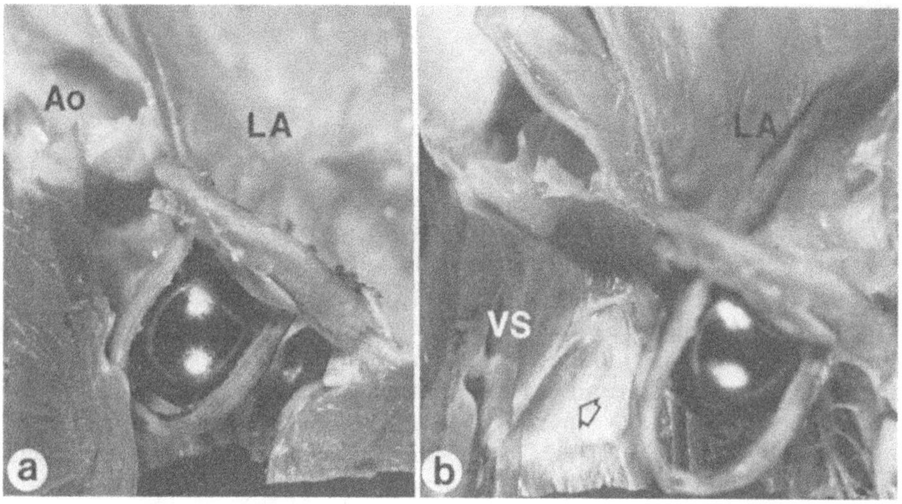

Fig. 1 a and b. Prosthetic disproportion with a size 2 M cloth-covered caged ball prosthesis in a woman with mitral stenosis (A75–257). Postoperatively, the mean diastolic gradient across the prosthetic valve was 7.8 mmHg. She remained in chronic congestive heart failure and died 5 years after valve replacement. At necropsy (**a**), struts of the prosthesis burrowed into the ventricular septum (*VS*), and the valve appeared to partially obstruct left ventricular outflow. **b** View with the prosthesis retraeted shows indentation (*arrow*) of the ventricular septum by one strut of the valve. *LA*, left atrium; *Ao*, aorta

valves. The most common circumstance in which fatal obstruction to left ventricular outflow occurs is in the patient with combined mitral and aortic valve disease. In most of these patients, irrespective of the type of aortic valve lesion, i.e., whether stenosis or pure regurgitation, the aortic root usually is not dilated, and consequently the space available in the aortic root to accomodate the caged ball may be limited. A particularly dangerous circumstance is combined mitral and aortic stenosis. In this circumstance, the left ventricular wall is hypertrophied, but its cavity is not dilated. Insertion of a mitral caged ball into a hypertrophied, nondilated left ventricle may obstruct left ventricular inflow or outflow. Ventricular inflow obstruction is probably even more common after replacement of the tricuspid valve than the mitral valve with a caged ball prosthesis, and utilization of this prosthesis in this position may therefore be unwise [25].

Although none of the various types of substitute cardiac valves are completely immune from it, prosthetic disproportion (prosthesis too large or ventricular cavity or aorta too small), both real and potential, is most frequent with the caged ball prosthesis. Therefore, it may be most wise to limit the use of this type of prosthesis to patients with purely incompetent or at least predominately incompetent valve lesions, i.e., to those patients in whom volume overload has produced large-sized left ventricular cavities or ascending aortas. Use of the caged ball prosthesis in patients with purely stenotic or predominately stenotic valve lesions appears unnecessary because of the availability of other excellent substitute cardiac valves. Because anticoagulants are required with the use of this valve and because prosthetic disproportion is a significant problem, use of this type of valve in children may not be preferred.

Caged Disk Prostheses

The caged disk prosthesis (Table 3), because of its "low profile" configuration, was introduced as an alternative to the caged ball prosthesis and believed initially to be particularly useful in the patient with the "small left ventricle," i.e., pure mitral stenosis. This initial hope, however, was ill-fated. This device has proved to be highly thrombogenic [26, 27] and the most obstructive of all the prosthetic valves presently in use [28-31]. In a recent study, although the pulmonary arterial pressures had decreased and the cardiac indexes increased, the mean diastolic pressure gradients across the mitral prosthesis (Beall type) was not significantly different postoperatively compared to the preoperative values [31]. In addition, the nonmetallic disks have shown evidence of degeneration [30, 32]. (Fig. 2), and strut fracture, of uncertain cause, with dislodgment of the disk occluder, has been reported [33, 34]. Hemolysis with this prosthesis is universal [30]. This device was utilized briefly in the aortic position [28, 30], but its use in this location was abandoned because of its obstructive, thrombogenic, and wear characteristics. More recently, a new type of caged disk, the Cooley-Cutter biconical disk, has been introduced for use in both atrioventricular and semilunar valve positions [35]. This newer prosthesis, which has a semi-diamond-shaped occluder rather than a flat one (like all other caged disks), nevertheless continues to have entirely peripheral flow characteristics, and therefore the hemodynamic features are unlikely to be ideal. Furthermore, intimal proliferation in the aortic root (where the coronary ostia are located) remains a potential problem with the peripheral flow type prostheses, probably most extensive with use of the caged disk [30]. Also very worrisome is disk cocking, a potential problem with all caged disks [26, 27, 32], including the newly introduced one, and its frequency of occurrence is entirely unknown. Possibly, nonfatal transient cocking is common, and fatal cocking of the caged disk may occur during life and be totally unrecognized at necropsy.

The presence of associated uncorrected valvular disease may be of considerable significance when a caged disk prosthesis is used [30]. Insertion of a caged disk in the mitral position in a patient with uncorrected (mild or moderate) aortic regurgitation may be dangerous since "cocking" or interference with the movement of the disk may occur from impingement on the disk by the regurgitant jet of blood. Hemodynamically insignificant mitral regurgitation may become significant when a caged disk (which is intrinsically obstructive) is used in the aortic position in a patient with combined aortic and mitral incompetence [30].

Table 3. Caged disk prostheses

Kay Shiley
Cross Jones
Hufnagel
Kay-Suzuki
Beall
Harken
Cooley-Bloodwell-Cutter
Cooley-Cutter

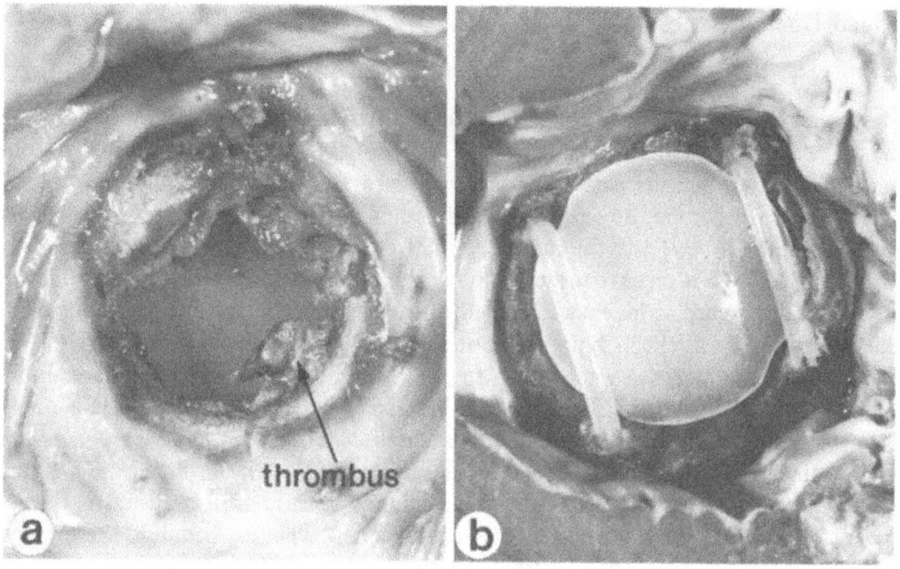

Fig. 2 a and b. Thrombosis and disk wear in a Hufnagel caged disk prosthesis implanted in the mitral position for 6 years (SH 75-124). a View of the prosthesis from the left atrium showing thrombus on the rim of the primary orifice. b View from the left ventricle showing notching of the disk by the struts

Tilting Disk Prostheses

The tilting disk (Table 4) has proved to be a good prosthesis for replacement of tricuspid, mitral, and aortic valves. Its semicentral flow usually allows minimal gradients [36, 37], its effect on red blood cell survival is minimal [38], and there has been no evidence of disk wear (variance) since the introduction of the carbon pyrolyte disk. This prosthesis, however, has a tendency to clot, and anticoagulants are required [38, 39]. Because movement of the disk is in close proximity to the sewing ring, the chances of interference to it by contact with adjacent mural endocardium or aortic intima is small, but it nevertheless, as with all prostheses, presents a potential problem if large-sized models are utilized in small-sized ventricles or aortas [38].

Uncorrected aortic regurgitation in patients who have had mitral valve replacement with a tilting disk prosthesis may interfere with the closure of the disk, especially if care is not taken to orient the valve such that the disk opens with the primary orifice directed posteriorly [40].

Table 4. Tilting disk prostheses

Wada-Cutter
Lillehei-Kastor
Björk-Shiley

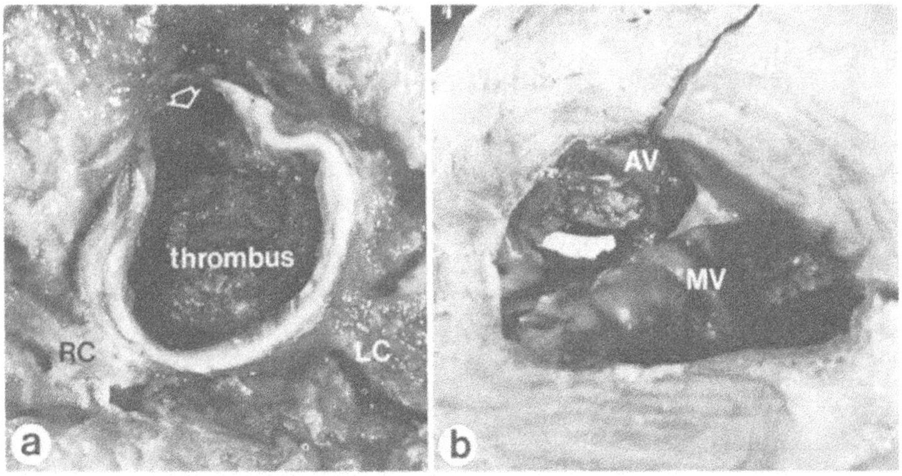

Fig. 3 a and b. Sudden thrombosis of a Bjölk-Shiley tilting disk prosthesis implanted for 6 months in the aortic position in a man with aortic stenosis (G75A–106). Chest pain occured suddenly, and he died in congestive heart failure. Anticoagulants had not been administered in the postoperative period. **a** View of the prosthesis from above, showing thrombus and fixation of the disk. Only a small orifice remains (*arrow*). *RC*, right coronary artery; *LC*, left coronary artery. **b** View of the prosthesis *(AV)* from the left ventricle, showing the thrombus and stenosis of the valve. *MV*, anterior mitral valve leaflet

The thrombogenicity of the tilting disk prosthesis, even in the presence of anticoagulation, remains a significant problem. Sudden thrombosis with stenosis and/ or regurgitation has been encountered [38, 39] (Fig. 3). The favorable hemodynamics in smaller-sized tilting disk prostheses makes their use desirable in children who require valve replacement at an early age. The absolute requirement for continuous anticoagulation with the use of these prostheses remains a significant disadvantage, however, in this group of patients.

Tissue Valves

Tissue valves (Table 5) in the form of aortic homografts, were first utilized for aortic valve replacement in 1962 [41, 42]. The initial results were gratifying: the valve lesions were usually ameliorated, and anticoagulants were not required. The problem, however, proved to be accelerated wear and tear with development of incompetency

Table 5. Tissue valves

Aortic valve homografts
Fascia lata
Parietal pericardium
Dura mater
Porcine xenograft

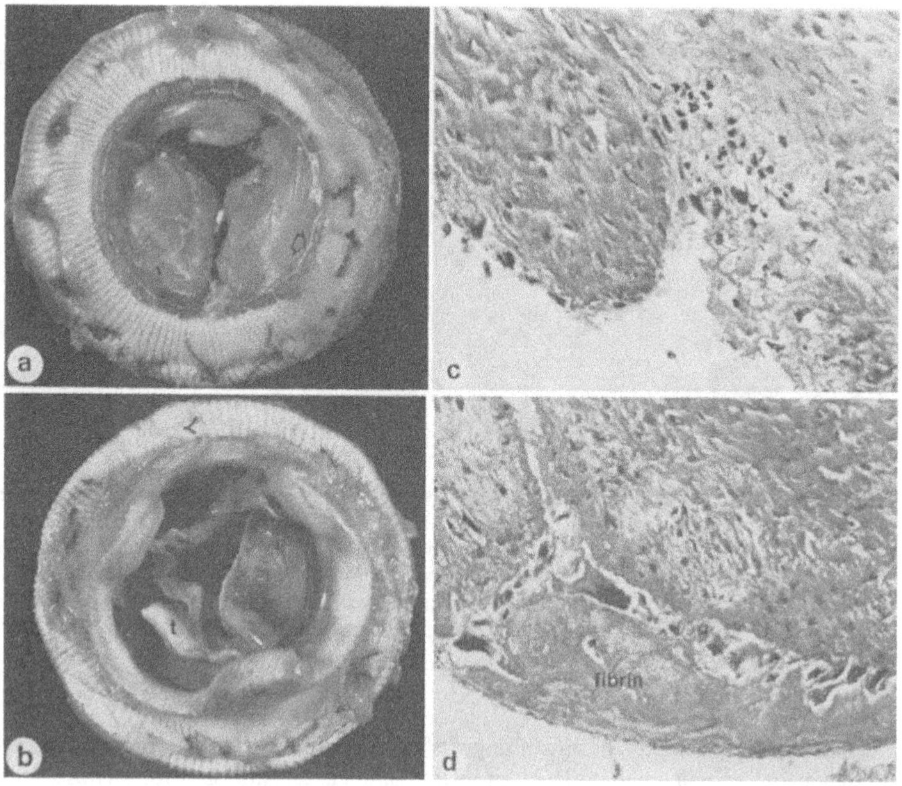

Fig. 4 a–d. Fibrin deposition and cellular reaction in a 66-day-old porcine tricuspid valve prosthesis (A75–242). The patient was receiving warfarin sodium throughout her postoperative course (due to the presence of a mechanical mitral valve prosthesis). She died 66 days after operation from prosthetic valve endocarditis (*Candida*) on her mechanical mitral prosthesis. **a** Porcine tricuspid bioprosthesis (PB) viewed from atrial aspect. Host tissue ingrowth is present over the sewing ring but stops at the junction with leaflet tissue (*arrow*). A thin coat of fibrin covers the leaflets. **b** View from right ventricular aspect showing organizing thrombus (*t*) in all three cusps. **c** Section of leaflet of the PB showing focal inflammatory cell infiltration into the leaflet. **d** Fibrin deposition and giant cell reaction on the ventricular surface of another leaflet. H E stain, x 350 (**c** and **d**)

[43, 44]. Other tissue valves followed, namely, fascia lata, dura mater, and parietal pericardium, but all proved to be poor valve substitutes because of their becoming stiff and relatively immobile [45-49]. At present, the fresh antibiotically sterilized homograft remains in use, but now the most commonly employed tissue valve is the porcine xenograft attached to a semiflexible stent and preserved by a glutaraldehyde process [50-52]. (It failed when preserved in formalin [45, 53].) This substitute valve is receiving increasingly greater enthusiasm. Although relatively few hemodynamic studies late postoperatively have been reported, pressure gradients across the porcine bioprosthesis have been recorded in all three valve positions despite its central flow. These gradients may in part be related to the presence of a "muscle shelf" on one leaflet of the valve, which limits its pliability. Of 56 patients studied late postoperatively after mitral replacement, the mean diastolic gradient averaged 6 mmHg [50, 51, 54], but of 37 patients studied at the National Heart and Lung Institute, no gradient

was recorded across the mitral porcine valve in 16 patients. Of 11 patients studied late postoperatively after tricuspid valve replacement with a porcine xenograft, the mean diastolic gradient averaged 4 mm Hg [51]. Hemodynamic data after aortic valce replacement with the porcine xenograft is virtually nonexistent: of five patients studied late postoperatively at the National Heart and Lung Institute, the peak systolic pressure gradients ranged 10 – 35 mmHg average: 18 mmHg [55]. Current modifications in the fabrication of these valves may improve the hemodynamic function (W.D. Hancock, 1976, personal communication).

With few exceptions [56], the porcine xenograft does not clot, and therefore, with few exceptions, anticoagulants are not required. This substitute valve does not damage blood elements [57]. The major concern with this substitute valve, of course, is its wear characteristics. The encouraging feature at this time is that there have been extremely few "valve failures" [50-52, 54-56]. Indeed, none of the other substitute valves cited have had so few problems in their first 5 years. Although results achieved with the porcine xenograft continue to be encouraging, relatively few patients, estimated to be less than 200, have had this substitute valve in place for longer than 5 years, and it will probably be after this period before signs of cuspal degeneration will appear.

In spite of the initial favorable results with the porcine xenograft valves, evidence is accumulating to suggest that the degenerative and inflammatory changes seen in formalin-fixed xenografts are present, but delayed, in the glutaraldehyde-fixed valves [56]. Histiocyte and giant cell accumulation along the surfaces of the cusps and focal inflammatory cell invasion of the structure of the cusps is a frequent finding in both early (< 2 months) and late (> 2 months) porcine xenografts [56] (Fig. 4). In addition, microscopic-sized deposits of fibrin are frequently present on the surfaces of the porcine valve leaflets, regardless of whether or not anticoagulation is used. In spite of the presence of these fibrin deposits, clinical evidence of thromboembolism is unusual with the use of the porcine xenograft [56].

It is likely that the cusps of the porcine valve will be subject to changes that affect all natural left-sided cardiac valves, namely, lipid deposition and calcification [58-60]. The changes occur in the native valves on the aortic aspects of the aortic valve cusps and on the ventricular aspects of the mitral valve cusps. It is likely that these changes will be accelerated in this substitute valve compared to the natural valve, but, at least by 5 years, calcific deposits in these cusps are infrequent and, when present, minimal in amount [56]. Small thrombi have been observed on the sinus aspects of the porcine cusps, and possibly it is the organization of these minute thrombi that has led to the calcific deposits, at this point, almost entirely microscopic in size [41, 56]. Prosthetic disproportion may be a problem with the use of porcine xenograft bioprostheses in spite of the fact that the leaflets are protected by a flexible stent. Implantation of a large porcine valve (to minimize the diastolic gradient) in the mitral position in a patient with a small left ventricle may result in inward pressure on the stent and undue stress on the cusps of the valve, leading to accelerated wear and valve failure (Fig. 5). The peripheral position of the struts of the porcine xenograft require care in placement of the valve in the aortic position so as to avoid interference with the coronary ostia.

The absence of a need for chronic anticoagulation, lack of hemolysis, and low embolic rate make the porcine xenograft desirable for use in cardiac valve replacement in younger patients. Unfortunately, this bioprothesis has shown rapid acceleration of

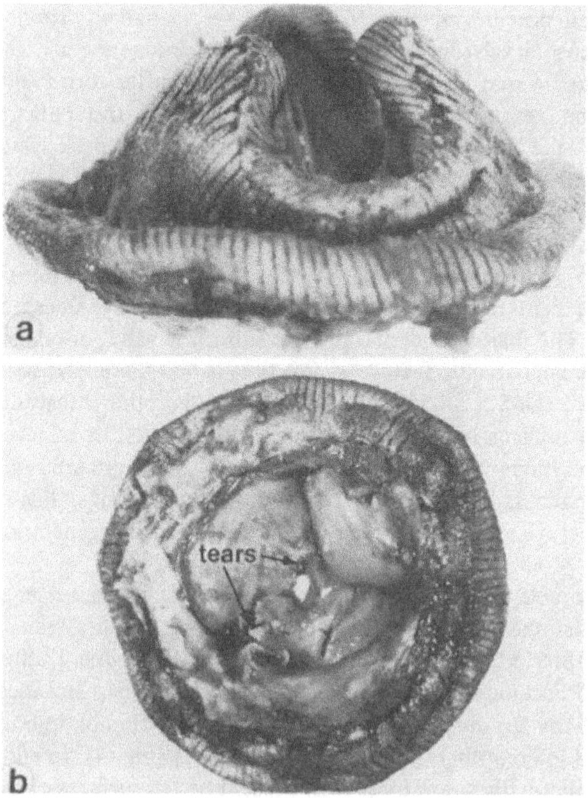

Fig. 5 a and b. Tissue degeneration and calcification in a 75-month-old porcine xenograft bioprosthesis that had been in the mitral position. The sudden occurrence of mitral regurgitation necessitated removal and replacement of the prosthesis. **a** Laterial view of the prosthesis showing bowing-in of all three struts due to compression by the left ventricular myocardium. **b** View of the prosthesis from the atrial aspect showing tears and fraying of two of the three leaflets and prolapse of the leaflets toward the left atrium

the degenerative process in children and therefore is not recommended for them. The potentially large gradients across the smaller prostheses and the undetermined long-term durability of the tissue valves, however, remain significant disadvantages for persons of all age groups.

After discussing the various types of prosthetic cardiac valves, a consideration of the factors that determine the outcome of valve replacement in a particular patient appears appropriate. At least six major factors appear to determine the result: (1) the type of substitute valve inserted, (2) the size of the prosthesis inserted, (3) the experience and technical skill of the surgeon, (4) the adequacy of the "pump team," anesthesiologists, surgeons, physicians, and nurses providing postoperative care, (5) the presence of associated (diagnosed or undiagnosed) or uncorrected cardiac disease or previous pericardiotomy, and (6) the preoperative status of the patient.

Assuming that the cardiac operation is to be performed in a large medical center where several cardiac operations are performed weekly by a surgeon or group of surgeons experienced in cardiac valve replacement, the most important factor at pre-

Table 6. Causes of prosthetic cardiac valve stenosis

1. Intrinsic stenosis of the prosthesis (design problem)
2. Inadequate space in left or right ventricle or in ascending aorta to freely accommodate prosthesis (prosthetic disproportion or tertiary orifice stenosis)
3. Thrombus formation on prosthesis
   - A) Prosthetic ring (primary orifice)
   - B) Prosthetic struts or lens causing sticking of poppet
   - C) Filling of cusps of tissue valves with decreased pliability of leaflets
4. Prosthetic variance
   - A) Swelling, due to lipid infiltration, of poppet causing it to stick either permanently or transiently in the cage
   - B) Grooving (notching) of the margins of the poppet also causing sticking or cocking (disk)

Table 7. Causes of prosthetic cardiac valve regurgitation

1. Slight regurgitation intrinsic to design of many prostheses
2. Peribasilar accessory communication
   - A) Inadequate number of sutures
   - B) Inadequate placement of sutures due to calcific deposits in or adjacent to annulus
   - C) Pulling loose of suture(s)
     - a) After replacement of anatomically normal or floppy valve
     - b) Infection at site of attachment of prosthesis
3. Thrombus formation on prosthetic struts preventing proper seating of poppet or causing it to stick in an open position
4. Prosthetic variance
   - A) Atrophy of poppet
     - a) Incomplete seating
     - b) Dislodgment
   - B) Fracture of poppet
     - a) Incomplete seating
     - b) Dislodgment
   - C) Fracture of strut
     - a) Dislodgment of poppet
   - D) Disruption of ring cloth
5. Mechanical interference to proper seating of poppet by
   - A) Unexcised calcific material or chordae tendeneae or suture between poppet and ring
   - B) Strut of a mitral prosthesis preventing proper seating of the poppet of an aortic prosthesis
   - C) An aortic regurgitant jet stream causing cocking with incomplete closure of a mitral poppet
6. Tissue degeneration with tears of cusps

sent determining the long-term outcome of valve replacement is probably the type of substitute valve inserted.

As described above, there are advantages and disadvantages to each of the types of cardiac prostheses currently available. The caged disk, however, would appear to be the least desirable: it clots, it sticks, it degenerates, and it has obstructive hemodynamic characteristics.

Since all cardiac valve prostheses currently available occupy space in the ventricle or aorta, prosthetic disproportion and resulting dysfunction remain a problem with each, especially if a prosthesis of too large a size is implanted. Because it has the largest structure, the caged ball might well be limited for use in patients with volume lesions (pure or predominant valvular regurgitation) who therefore have larger ventricles or aortas to accommodate the prosthesis. The result of prosthetic dysfunction or disproportion is either stenosis or regurgitation. The multiple causes of these complications of prosthetic valves are summarized in Tables 6 and 7.

In summary, a comparison of the features of each of the present designs of cardiac valve prosthesis shows that the ideal prosthesis is not currently available. The decision regarding which of the types of valve prostheses to use in any individual patient, therefore, is a value judgment. The relative durability of the valve, the hemodynamic demands of the patient, the need for anticoagulation, and the special anatomic features of the location in which the prosthesis is to be placed must all be considered in making the final decision.

References

1. Starr A, Edwards ML (1971) Mitral replacement: clinical experience with a ball-valve prosthesis. Ann Surg 154:726
2. Roberts WC (1976) Choosing a substitute cardiac valve: type, size, surgeon. Am J Cardiol 38: 633
3. Hufnagel CA, Harvey WP (1953) The surgical correction of aortic regurgitation. Preliminary Report. Bull Georgetown Univ Med Center 6:60
4. Hufnagel CA, Harvey WP, Rabil PJ, McDermott TF (1954) Surgical correction of aortic insufficiency. Surgery 35:673
5. Harken DE, Soroff HS, Taylor WJ, Lefemine AA, Gupta SK, Lunzer S (1960) Partial and complete prostheses in aortic insufficiency. J Thorac Cardiovasc Surg 40:744
6. Harken DE, Taylor WJ, Lefemine AA, Lunzer S, Low HBC, Cohen ML, Jacobey JA (1962) Aortic valve replacement with a caged ball valve. Am J Cardiol 9:292
7. Reis RL, Glancy DL, O'Brien K, Epstein SE, Morrow AG (1970) Clinical and hemodynamic assessments of fabric-covered Starr-Edwards prosthetic valves. J Thorac Cardiovasc Surg 59: 84, 104
8. Winter TO, Reis RL, Glancy DL, Roberts WC, Epstein SE, Morrow AG (1972) Current status of the Starr-Edwards cloth-covered prosthetic cardiac valves. Circulation (Suppl) 45/46:I-14
9. Levine FH, Copeland JG, Morrow AG (1973) Prosthetic replacement of the mitral valve. Continuing assessments of the 100 patients operated upon during 1961-1965. Circulation 47:518
10. Bonchek LI, Starr A (1975) Ball valve prostheses: current appraisal of late results. Am J Cardiol 35:843
11. Smithwick W, Kouchoukos NT, Karp RB, Pacifico AD, Kirklin JW (1975) Late stenosis of Starr-Edwards cloth-covered prostheses. Ann Thorac Surg 20:249
12. Roberts WC, Morrow AG (1966) Renal hemosiderosis in patients with prosthetic aortic valves. Circulation 36:390
13. Roberts WC, Morrow AG (1972) Causes of death and other anatomic observations after cardiac valve replacement. Adv Cardiol 7:226
14. Roberts WC, Morrow AG (1967) Late postoperative pathological findings after cardiac valve replacement. Circulation (Suppl) 35/36:I-48
15. Roberts WC, Morrow AG (1967) Anatomic studies of hearts containing caged-ball prosthetic valves. Johns Hopkins Med J 121:271
16. Roberts WC, Morrow AG (1968) Fatal degeneration of the silicone rubber ball of the Starr-Edwards prosthetic aortic valve. Am J Cardiol 22:614
17. Roberts WC, Morrow AG (1969) Late postoperative pathologic findings following cardiac valve replacement with Starr-Edwards prostheses. In: Proceedings of the Second National Conference of Prosthetic Heart Valves. Thomas, Springfield, Illinois, p 365

18. Roberts WC, Levinson GE, Morrow AG (1970) Lethal ball variance in the Starr-Edwards prosthetic mitral valve. Arch Intern Med 126:517
19. Roberts WC, Bulkley BH, Morrow AG (1973) Pathologic anatomy of cardiac valve replacement: a study of 224 necropsy patients. Prog Cardiovasc Dis 15:539
20. Pluth JR, Broadbent JC, Barnhorst DA, Danielson GK (1975) Aortic and mitral valve replacement with cloth-covered Braunwald-Cutter prosthesis. A three-year follow up. Ann Thorac Surg 20:239
21. Roberts WC, Morrow AG (1966) Mechanism of acute left arterial thrombosis after mitral valve replacement. Pathologic findings indicating obstruction to left atrial emptying. Am J Cardiol 18:497
22. Roberts WC, Lambird PA, Gott VL, Morrow AG (1966) Fatal aortic regurgitation following replacement of the mitral and aortic valves. A mechanical complication of double valve replacement. J Thorac Cardiovasc Surg 52:189
23. Roberts WC, Morrow AG (1967) Causes of early postoperative death following cardiac valve replacement. Clinico-pathologic correlations in 64 patients studied at necropsy. J Thorac Cardiovasc Surg 54:422
24. Seningen RP, Bulkley BH, Roberts WC (1974) Prosthetic aortic stenosis. A method to prevent its occurrence by measurement of aortic size from preoperative aortogram. Circulation 49: 921
25. Baxter RH, Bain WH, Rankin RJ, Turner MA, Escarous AE, Thomson RM, Lorimer AR, Lawrie DV (1975) Tricuspid valve replacement: a five-year appraisal. Thorax 30:158
26. Horsley HT, Rappoport, WJ, Vigoda PS. Vogel JHK (1970) Fatal malfunction of Edwards low-profile mitral valves. Circulation (Suppl) 41/42:II-39
27. Gunstensen J (1971) Acute dysfunction of Starr-Edwards mitral prostheses. Thorax 26:163
28. Olin C (1970) Evaluation of the Kay-Shiley disc valve prosthesis in the aortic position. Clinical and haemodynamic results, and experimental comparison with other prosthetic aortic valves. Scand J Thorac Cardiovasc Surg (Suppl) 7:1
29. Shepherd RL, Glancy DL, Reis RL, Epstein SE, Morrow AG (1973) Hemodynamic function of the Kay-Shiley prosthetic cardiac valve. Observations after mitral or tricuspid valve replacement. Chest 63:323
30. Roberts WC, Fishbein MC, Golden A (1975) Cardiac pathology after valve replacement by disc prosthesis. A study of 61 necropsy patients. Am J Cardiol 35:740
31. Fernandez J, Morse D, Spagna P, Lemole G, Gooch A, Yang SS, Maranhao V (1976) Results of mitral valve replacement with the Beall prosthesis in 209 patients. J Thorac Cardiovasc Surg 71:218
32. Hammer WJ, Hearne MJ, Roberts WC (1976) Cocking of a poppet disc prosthesis in the aortic position. A cause of intermittent aortic regurgitation. J Thorac Cardiovasc Surg 71: 259
33. Beall AC Jr, Morris GC Jr, Howell JF Jr, Guinn GA, Noon GP, Reul GJ Jr, Greenberg JJ, Ankeney JL (1973) Clinical experience with an improved mitral valve prosthesis. Ann Thorac Surg 15:601
34. Nathan MJ (1973) Strut fracture. A late complication of Beall mitral valve replacement. Ann Thorac Surg 16:610
35. Cooley DA, Sandiford FM, Wukasch DC, Reul GJ (1975) Mitral valve replacement with a new prosthesis. Experience with 366 patients. J Cardiovasc Surg Spec. No: 378
36. Böök K (1974) Mitral valve replacement with the Björk-Shiley tilting disc valve. A clinical and haemodynamic study in patients with isolated mitral valve lesions. Scand J Thorac Cardiovasc Surg (Suppl) 12:1
37. Björk VO, Henze A, Holmgren A (1974) Five years' experience with the Björk-Shiley tilting disc valve in isolated aortic valvular disease. J Thorac Cardiovasc Surg 68:393
38. Roberts WC, Hammer WJ (1976) Cardiac pathology after valve replacement with a tilting disc prosthesis (Björk-Shiley type): A study of 46 necropsy patients and 49 Björk-Shiley prostheses. Am J Cardiol 37:1024
39. Ben-Zvi J, Hildner FJ, Chandraratna PA, Samet P (1974) Thrombosis on Björk-Shiley aortic valve prosthesis. Clinical arteriographic, echocardiographic and therapeutic observations in seven cases. Am J Cardiol 34:538

40. Björk VO, Böök K, Holmgren A (1974) The Björk-Shiley mitral valve prosthesis. A comparative study with different prosthesis orientations. Ann Thorac Surg 18:379
41. Ross DN (1962) Homograft replacement of the aortic valve. Lancet II:487
42. Barratt-Boyes BG, Lowe JB, Cole DS, Kelly DT (1965) Homograft valve replacement for aortic valve disease. Thorax 20:495
43. Angell WW, Shumway NE, Kosek JC (1972) A five-year study of viable aortic valve homografts. J Thorac Cardiovasc Surg 64:329
44. Moore CH, Martelli V, Al-Janabi N, Ross DN (1975) Analysis of homograft valve failure in 311 patients followed up to 10 years. Ann Thorac Surg 20:274
45. Yarbrough JW, Roberts WC, Reis RL (1973) Structural alterations in tissue cardiac valves implanted in patients and in calves. J Thorac Cardiovasc Surg 65:364
46. Ionescu UI, Pakrashi BC, Mary DAS, Bartek IT, Wooler GH (1974) Replacement of heart valves with frame-mounted tissue grafts. Thorax 29:56
47. Nuno-Conceicao A, Puig LB, Verginelli G, Iryia K, Bittencourt D, Zerbini EJ, (1975) Homologous dura mater cardiac valves. Structural aspects of eight implanted valves. J Thorac Cardiovasc Surg 70:499
48. Mary DAS, Pakrashi, BC, Catchpole RW, Ionescu MI (1975) Tissue valves in the mitral position. Five years experience. Br Heart J 37:1123
49. Olsen EGJ, Al-Janabi N, Salamao CS, Ross DN (1975) Fascia lata valves: a clinicopathological study. Thorax 30:528
50. Horowitz MS, Goodman DJ, Fogarty TJ, Harrison DC (1974) Mitral valve replacement with the glutaraldehyde-preserved porcine heterograft. Clinical, hemodynamic, and pathological correlations J Thorac Cardiovasc Surg 67:885
51. McIntosh CL, Michaelis LL, Morrow AG, Itscoitz SB, Redwood DR, Epstein SE (1975) Atrioventricular valve replacement with the Hancock porcine xenograft: a five year clinical experience. Surgery 78:768
52. Pipkin RD, Buch WS, Fogarty TJ (1976) Evaluation of aortic valve replacement with a porcine xenograft without long-term anticoagulation. J Thorac Cardiovasc Surg 71:179
53. Zuhdi N, Hawley W, Voehl V, Hancock W, Carey J, Greer A (1974) Porcine aortic valves as replacement for human heart valves. Ann Thorac Surg 17:479
54. Johnson AD, Daily PO, Peterson KL, LeWinter M, DiDonna GT, Blair G, Niwayama G (1975) Functional evaluation of the porcine heterograft in the mitral position. Circulation (Suppl) 50/51:I–40
55. Reis RL, Hancock WD, Yarbrough JW. Glancy DL, Morrow AG (1971) The flexible stent. A new concept in the fabrication of tissue heart valve prostheses. J Thorac Cardiovasc Surg 62: 683
56. Spray TL, Roberts WC (1977) Structural changes in porcine xenografts used as substitute cardiac valves.Gross and histologic observations in 51 glutaraldehyde-preserved Hancock valves in 41 patients. Am J Cardiol 40:319
57. Rhoades GR, McIntosh CL (1977) Evaluation of hemolysis following replacement of atrioventricular valves with porcine xenograft (Hancock) valves. J Thorac Cardiovasc Surg 73:312
58. Roberts WC, Perloff JK, Constantino T (1971) Severe valvular aortic stenosis in patients over 65 years of age. A clinicopathologic study. Am J Cardiol 27:497
59. Roberts WC, Perloff JK (1972) Mitral valvular disease. A clinicopathologic survey of the conditions causing the mitral valve to function abnormally. Ann Intern Med 77:939
60. Roberts WC, Dangel JC, Bulkey BH (1973) Nonrheumatic valvular cardiac disease: a clinicopathologic survey of 27 different conditions causing valvular dysfunction. Cardiovasc Clin 5: 333

Calcific Deposits in Porcine Bioprostheses: Structure and Pathogenesis

VICTOR J. FERRANS, MD, PhD
STEVEN W. BOYCE
MARGARET E. BILLINGHAM, MD
MICHAEL JONES, MD
TOKUHIRO ISHIHARA, MD
WILLIAM C. ROBERTS, MD, FACC

Bethesda, Maryland
Stanford, California

Gross, histologic and ultrastructural studies were made of 14 porcine valve bioprostheses that were found to contain calcific deposits at the time of removal either at reoperation (13 patients) or at necropsy (1 patient). Eleven bioprostheses had been in the mitral position, 1 in the aortic, 1 in the tricuspid and 1 in a pulmonary conduit. The ages of the patients at the time of implantation ranged from 2.5 to 65 years (average 32), and the bioprostheses had been in place from 3 to 94 months (average 39). Analysis of these 14 bioprostheses and review of reports concerning 37 other calcified porcine bioprostheses suggest the following conclusions: (1) Calcific deposits occur commonly in bioprostheses implanted in patients of all ages, but are more likely to become severe and clinically significant in children and in young adults than in older patients. (2) Calcific deposits can lead to prosthetic valve stenosis, because they can limit the mobility of the cusps; however, they can also be associated with prosthetic valve regurgitation. (3) Metabolic disorders that could contribute to bioprosthetic calcification are not identifiable in most patients having calcified prosthetic tissue valves. (4) The two main sites of deposition of calcium phosphate in porcine valve bioprostheses are the connective tissue in the cusps, particularly in the spongiosa, and small thrombi on the surfaces. (5) Calcification of connective tissue first involves the collagen fibrils; calcification of thrombi involves the mitochondria in platelets and leukocytes trapped in the mesh of fibrin. From these two sites, calcific deposits can grow and spread into other areas of the cusps.

From the Pathology and Surgery Branches, National Heart, Lung, and Blood Institute, National Institutes of Health, Bethesda, Maryland, and the Department of Pathology, Stanford University School of Medicine, Stanford, California. Manuscript received January 21, 1980; revised manuscript received March 24, 1980, accepted April 3, 1980.

Address for reprints: Victor J. Ferrans, MD, Building 10, Room 7N208, National Institutes of Health, Bethesda, Maryland 20205.

A large majority of patients undergoing cardiac valve replacement with glutaraldehyde-treated porcine bioprostheses follow a clinically satisfactory course for the first 5 years after operation. Nevertheless, clinical and morphologic studies have documented certain complications leading to malfunction of porcine bioprostheses, mainly cuspal infection, perforation and calcification. Previous reports from our laboratory[1–3] have described gross, histologic and ultrastructural alterations developing in perforated or infected porcine bioprostheses. Calcification of porcine bioprostheses received little attention until recently, when isolated case reports[4–20] emphasized its occurrence, particularly in children and young adults. Although this complication may lead to a reduction in the mobility of the cusps and to bioprosthetic stenosis or regurgitation, detailed studies have not been made of the precise location, structure and pathogenesis of calcific deposits in porcine bioprostheses. This study presents morphologic observations on 14 porcine bioprostheses that were found to contain calcific deposits when removed after being in place from 3 to 94 months.

Methods

Patients (Table I)

The 14 patients had calcific deposits in the cusps of the porcine bioprostheses manifested on either gross or microscopic examination. Seven patients had been included in previous clinical reports.[1,2,16,19,21,22] The patients, six boys or men and eight girls or women, ranged in age from 2.5 to 65 years (mean 32) at the time of bioprosthetic implantation.

Six patients had rheumatic heart disease, six had congenital heart disease, one had infective endocarditis and one had pure mitral regurgitation of uncertain origin. Twelve patients underwent single valve replacement by a porcine bioprosthesis: nine had mitral valve replacement, one aortic valve replacement, one tricuspid valve replacement and one pulmonary valve replacement. The tricuspid valve was replaced in one patient with transposition of the great vessels; thus, it functioned as a systemic atrioventricular valve and hereafter will be considered as a "mitral" replacement. The pulmonary valve was replaced by a Hancock conduit in a patient with pulmonary valve atresia and ventricular septal defect. Two patients underwent replacement of both the mitral and the tricuspid valve: Patient 13 had severe stenosis of both natural valves; both implanted porcine bioprostheses eventually became regurgitant and had to be replaced; however, only the bioprosthesis in the tricuspid position became calcified. Therefore, the mitral bioprosthesis in this patient is not included in the study. Patient 8 had pure mitral and tricuspid regurgitation resulting from infective endocarditis; after double valve replacement, a new episode of infective endocarditis developed and the porcine bioprosthesis in the mitral position was removed. The bioprosthesis in the tricuspid position did not become infected and was not removed at reoperation.[1] The bioprosthesis in Patient 14, who died of mitral regurgitation of the bioprosthesis 94 months after its implantation, was recovered at necropsy. The 13 other bioprostheses were recovered at reoperation. The time interval between implantation and operative removal of the bioprostheses ranged from 3 to 94 months (average 39).

In 8 of the 13 patients who underwent reoperation, the procedure was performed because of prosthetic valve stenosis occurring 10 to 60 months (average 34) after implantation. Six of the eight stenosed bioprostheses had been placed in the mitral position, one in the aortic position and one in a pulmonary conduit. Another patient underwent reoperation because of a perivalvular leak 3 months after implantation; the bioprosthesis showed only minimal (clinically insignificant) calcific deposits. Three additional patients underwent reoperation because of prosthetic valve regurgitation caused by cuspal perforation or dehiscence. Patient 8 underwent reoperation because of prosthetic mitral infection causing both stenosis and regurgitation.

Examination after removal disclosed cuspal perforations in six bioprostheses that had been implanted for periods of 18 to 94 months (average 52). One patient had chronic renal insufficiency attributed to cephalothin toxicity; other metabolic diseases were not identified in any of the other patients.

Procedures

After removal, the bioprostheses were fixed with cold, 3 percent glutaraldehyde in 0.1 *M* phosphate buffer, pH 7.2, and processed for light and electron microscopic study. The bioprostheses were radiographed after fixation. For light microscopic examination, selected portions of the cusps were trimmed, decalcified with a mixture of sodium citrate and formic acid and embedded in paraffin. Histologic sections were stained according to the following methods: hematoxy-

TABLE I

Clinical and Morphologic Findings in 14 Patients With Calcific Deposits in Porcine Bioprostheses

Case	Age (yr) at PB Implantation	Sex	Valve Lesion	Site of PB	PB Size (mm)	PB Removal: Time (mo)	PB Removal: Cause	PB Cuspal Changes: Gross Ca^{++}	PB Cuspal Changes: Perf. Leaf.	PB Cuspal Changes: Red. Mob.	PB Cuspal Changes: Thr.	Previous Clinical Reports of Patients (reference)
1	2.5	M	MS (cong)	M	19	41	S	+	0	+	0	Pt. 6[16]
2	3.5	F	TGV-TR	M*	23	37	S	+	0	+	0	
3	5.5	F	MR (cong)	M	. . .	30	S	+	+	+	0	
4	8	F	MR (cong)	M	27	35	R	+	+	+	0	Pt.[22]
5	9	F	MR	M	29	18	S	+	+	+	0	Pt. 5[19]
6	11	M	PVA-VSD	PC	20	60	S	+	0	+	0	
7	23	F	AS	A	. . .	10	S	+	0	0	+	
8	28	M	IE,MV/TV	M	35	4.5	IE	+	0	+	+	Pt. 3[1]
9	42	M	MR	M	35	28	S,R,IE	0	0	0	0	Pt. 4[1]; Pt. 10[2]
10	55	F	MS	M	31	76	R	+	+	0	0	Pt. 12[2]; Pt.[21]
11	61	M	MS	M	29	3	PVL	0	0	0	+	Pt. 7[2]
12	65	F	MS	M	29	48	S	+	0	+	0	
13	65	F	MS,TR,TS	T	33	63	R	0	+	0	0	
14	65	M	MS	M	31	94	Death	+	+	+	0	

* Systemic atrioventricular valve.

A = aortic valve; AS = aortic stenosis; Ca^{++} = calcium; cong = congenital; IE = infective endocarditis; IE,MV/TV = infective endocarditis affecting the mitral and tricuspid valves; M = mitral valve; MR = mitral regurgitation; MS = mitral stenosis; PB = porcine bioprosthesis; PC = pulmonary conduit; Perf. Leaf. = perforated leaflet; Pt. = patient; PVA-VSD = pulmonary valve atresia-ventricular septal defect; PVL = perivalvular leak; R = regurgitation; Red. Mob. = reduced mobility of cusps; S = stenosis; T = tricuspid valve; TGV = transposition of the great vessels; Thr. = thrombus; TR = tricuspid regurgitation; TS = tricuspid stenosis; + = present; 0 = absent; . . . = information not available.

lin-eosin, Masson trichrome, Movat pentachrome, phosphotungstic acid-hematoxylin and von Kossa.

For study by transmission electron microscopy, tissues were processed as previously described.[2] For X-ray energy dispersive microanalysis of the calcific deposits, 1,000 Å thick sections of Maraglas®-embedded tissues were prepared, mounted on beryllium grids and examined with an ETEC scanning electron microscope equipped with an EDAX detector.

Results

Gross anatomic observations (Table I): Calcific deposits were grossly evident in 11 of the 14 recovered bioprostheses, and in 9 of these the flexibility and mobility of the cusps were reduced. In 10 of the 11 bioprostheses (from Patients 1 to 7, 10, 12 and 14) the calcific deposits were localized to the cusps; in the remaining bioprosthesis (from Patient 8), they involved infected vegetations.[1] Of the three bioprostheses without grossly evident calcific deposits (from Patients 9, 11 and 13), one (from Patient 9) was covered by thrombotic material, which was the site of infection and calcification evident only on microscopic examination[1,2]; another (from Patient 11) contained noncalcified thrombus, and the remaining one (from Patient 13) had a perforated cusp. The latter two bioprostheses (from Patients 11 and 13) had microscopic calcific deposits in the cuspal connective tissue. Thus, none of the 14 bioprostheses were normal on gross anatomic study.

Six of the 14 bioprostheses had one or more perforations in the cusps; 5 of these had grossly evident calcific deposits, which often were closely adjacent to the perforations. In each of the 10 bioprostheses with calcific deposits in the cusps, these deposits appeared similar and consisted of pale yellow, discrete, usually flat plaques that were raised and projected above both surfaces of the leaflets (Fig. 1 and 2). Less frequently, they formed irregularly shaped, conical or bulbous excrescences 1 to 2 mm in height. The calcific deposits tended to involve all three cusps to a similar extent. When minimal in amount, calcific deposits tended to be localized to areas of the cusps immediately adjacent to the commissures; when more extensive, they formed multiple foci including the areas of apposition of the cusps. The most extensive deposits involved the entire area of each cusp.

Histologic observations: The histologic appearance of the grossly visible calcific deposits (Fig. 3 and 4) was similar in each of the 10 bioprostheses with calcified cusps. The largest calcific deposits always involved the spongiosa (Fig. 3A) and sometimes they extended into immediately adjacent regions of the fibrosa and the ventricularis. Some small calcific deposits were confined entirely either to the fibrosa (Fig. 3B) or to the ventricularis. However, the large calcific deposits in the spongiosa more frequently displaced the other layers of the bioprosthesis, giving the appearance of raised plaques. These deposits often were multinodular, and adjacent nodules were separated from one another by fibrin deposits or by clear spaces (Fig. 4). Some of the latter spaces contained erythrocytes. Elastic fibers were devoid of calcium. The larger calcific deposits actually formed parts of the surfaces of the cusps, whose layered structure appeared to have been completely lost (by erosion of the superficial layers) in such areas. The basophilia of the calcific deposits in histologic sections stained with hematoxylin-eosin was much more pronounced in peripheral than in central regions (Fig. 3).

Calcific deposits also were recognized by electron microscopic study in: (1) the cardiac muscle shelf at the base of the right coronary cusp; (2) adipose tissue cells in the space between the aortic wall and the base of the cusps (Fig. 5A); (3) the aortic media at the level of, and just above, the base of the cusp (Fig. 5B); (4) organizing thrombi on the cuspal surfaces; and (5) infected vege-

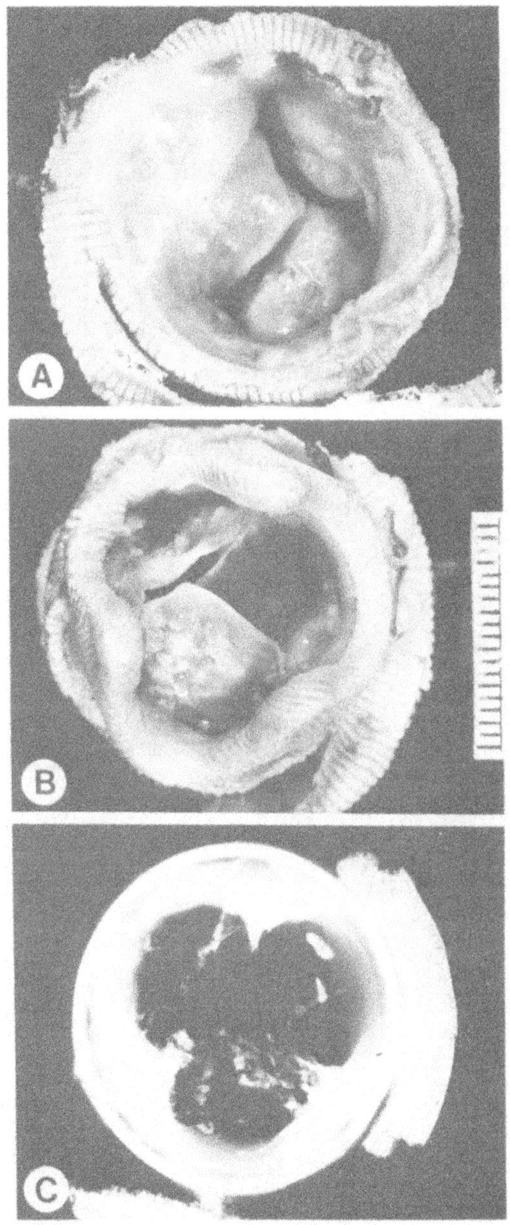

FIGURE 1. Case 12. Photographs of inflow surface (**A**), outflow surface (**B**) and roentgenogram (**C**) of bioprosthesis operatively removed, because of severe stenosis, 48 months after implantation in the mitral position. Calcific deposits are present in each cusp and are prominent in the commissural regions.

tations produced by staphylococci (Patient 8). In the first two of these sites, the calcific deposits were small. However, in the aortic wall the deposits were larger and formed plaques that extended throughout the media. Such deposits, which involved both the smooth muscle cells and the extracellular spaces, had strongly basophilic edges and much less basophilic cores (Fig. 5B). The deposits in the aortic wall were not continuous with those in the cusps, and therefore did not produce bioprosthetic dysfunction. The deposits in young and old patients were similar histologically.

Other histologic changes observed in the bioprostheses were (1) separation (delamination) of adjacent layers of connective tissue in the cusps, particularly in the spongiosa, leaving clear spaces that often were filled by proteinaceous material[2]; (2) loss of proteoglycan material from the spongiosa (best demonstrated with the Movat stain); (3) deposition of mononuclear cells, mostly macrophages, and multinucleated giant cells on the surfaces of the cusps, particularly in the outflow surfaces; and (4) focal thinning of the cusps, with fraying and erosion of the connective tissue. In Patients 3 to 5,

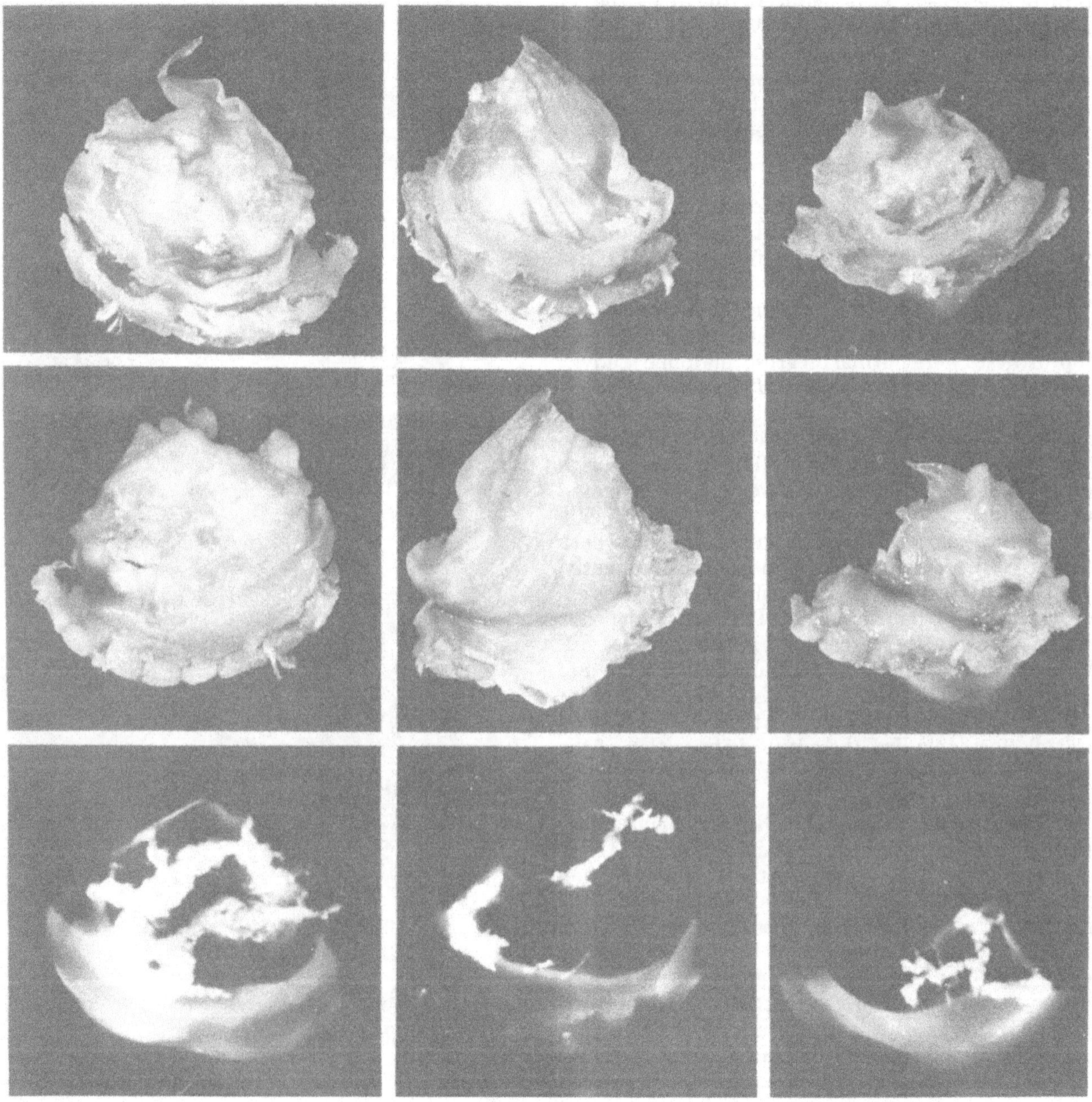

FIGURE 2. Case 1. Outflow surfaces **(top)**, inflow surfaces **(middle)** and roentgenograms **(bottom)** of the cusps of bioprosthesis removed at reoperation because of severe stenosis, 41 months after implantation in the mitral position. The true extent of the calcific deposits is difficult to assess from visual inspection, and the roentgenograms show that they consist of streaks that bear no relation to the normal anatomic features of the cusps.

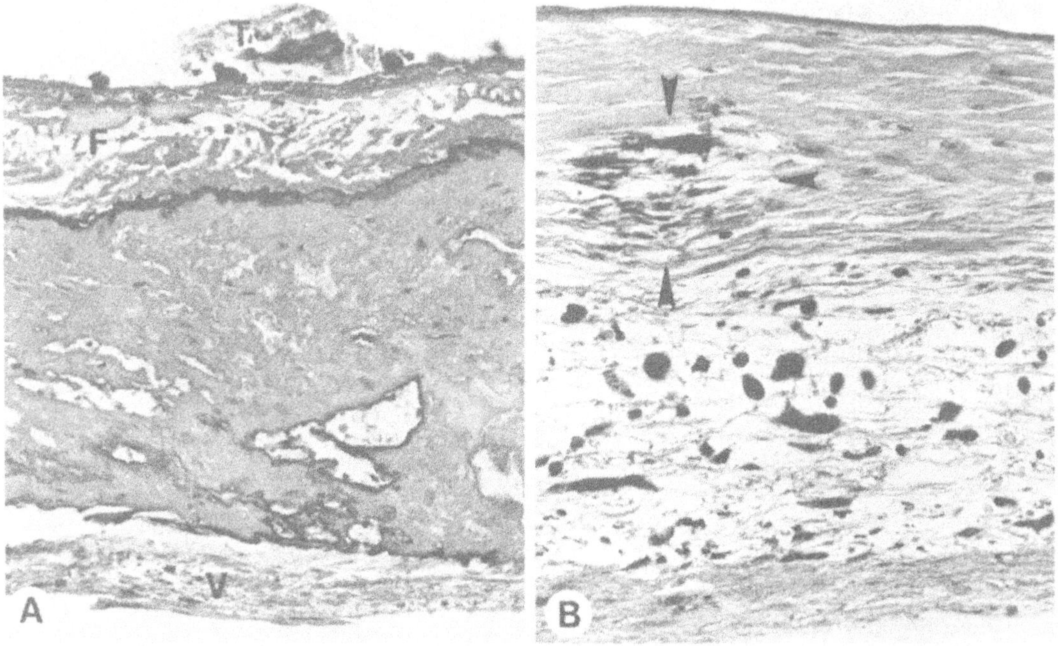

FIGURE 3. Case 3. Light micrographs of calcific deposits in the stenotic bioprosthesis operatively removed 30 months after implantation in the mitral position. **A,** deposit that fills area corresponding to spongiosa of normal cusp. The fibrosa (F) shown at **top** is partially disrupted; a small thrombus (T) is present on the outflow surface, and the ventricularis (V) is shown at **bottom.** Note the dark irregular borders of the calcific deposit and the empty spaces that it still contains (compare with the appearance of the spongiosa in **B. B,** small calcific deposit **(arrowheads)** is localized in fibrosa of bioprosthesis. Note the empty appearance of the spongiosa, which is delaminated and has lost its proteoglycan material. The dark material in the spongiosa probably represents precipitated plasma protein components. The ventricularis appears normal. (Hematoxylin-eosin ×250 [**A**] and Movat pentachrome ×250 [**B**], both reduced by 20 percent.)

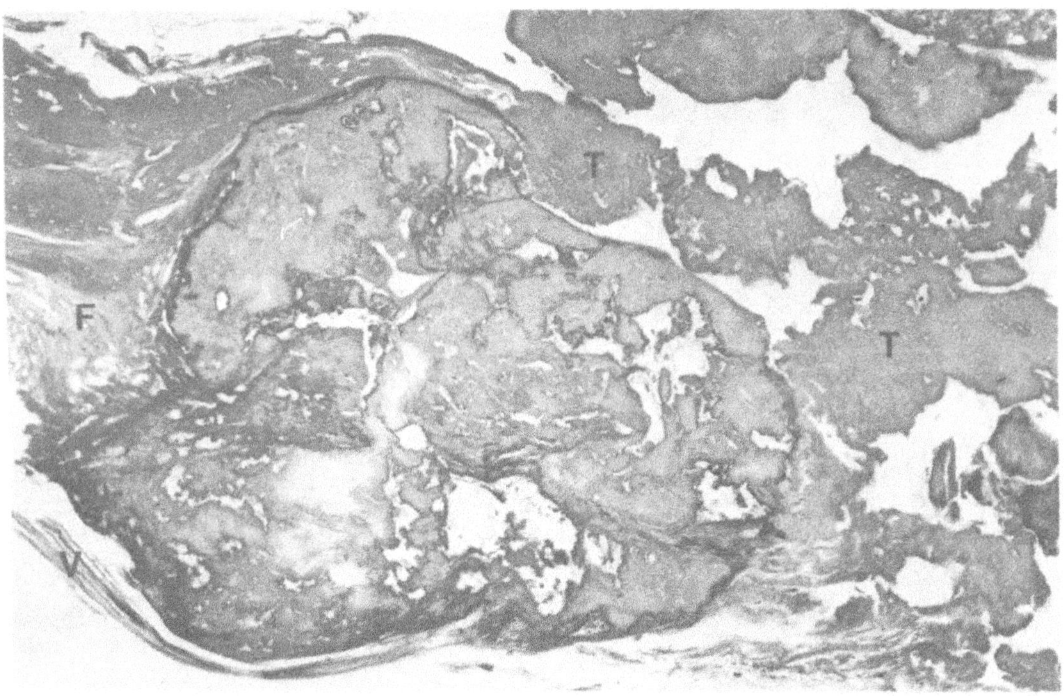

FIGURE 4. Case 3. Histologic appearance of large multinodular calcific deposit occupying practically the entire thickness of the cusp and associated with a large amount of thrombotic material (T), mostly fibrin. The structure of the cusp has been severely altered. Both the fibrosa (F) and the ventricularis (V) appear eroded on the **left** and completely disrupted on the **right.** (Movat pentachrome ×250, reduced by 20 percent.)

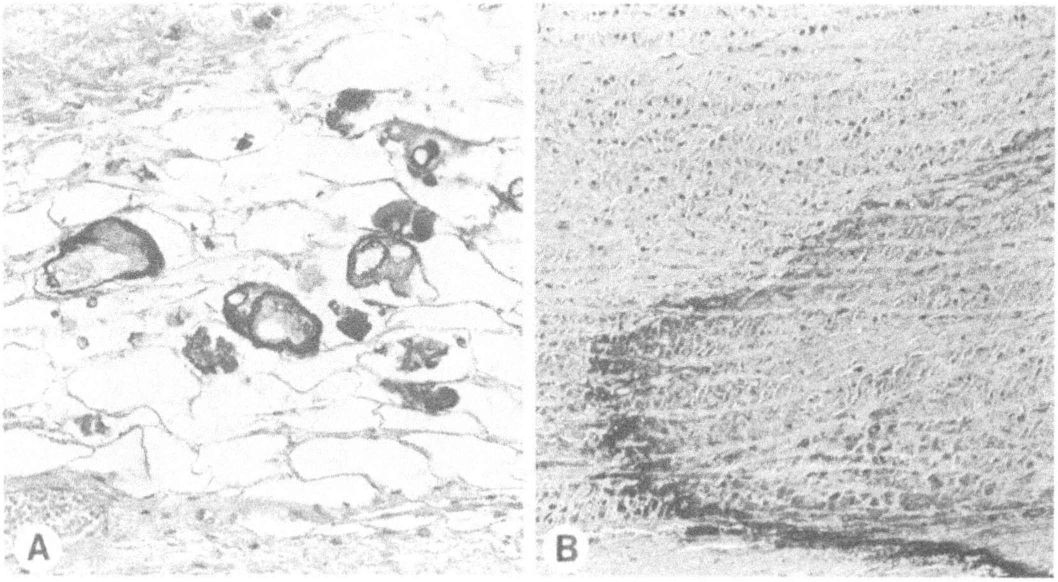

FIGURE 5. Case 8. Calcific deposits in adipose tissue cells at base of cusp (**A**) and in aortic wall (**B**). (Hematoxylin-eosin ×250 and ×150, respectively, reduced by 20 percent.)

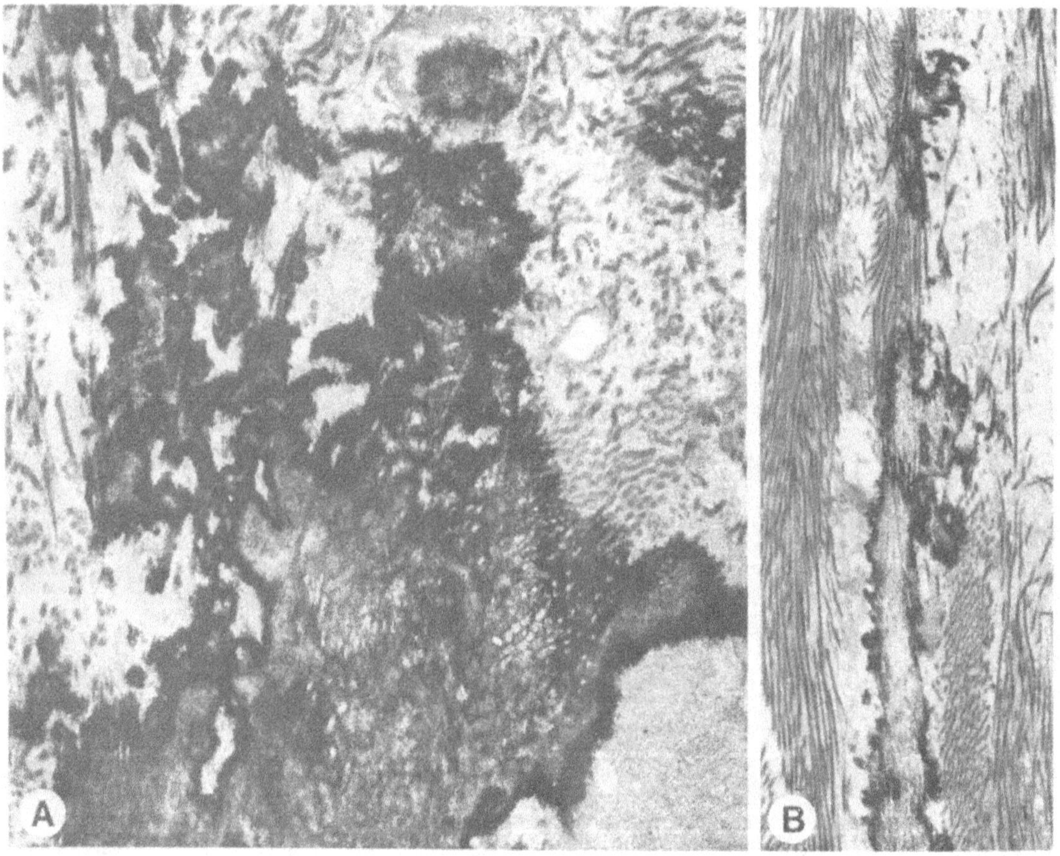

FIGURE 6. Case 3. Electron micrographs of calcific deposits associated with collagen fibrils. **A**, electron-dense crystals of calcium phosphate have completely surrounded several bundles of collagen fibrils at the periphery of a large calcific mass. **B**, small calcific deposit appears to be developing associated with a bundle of collagen fibrils. Note the characteristically dense border of the deposit (×22,000 [**A**] and ×15,000 [**B**], reduced by 20 percent.)

10, 13 and 14, the latter changes were associated with perforation of one or more of the cusps.

Ultrastructural observations: Certain early and late ultrastructural changes in porcine bioprostheses have been described in detail in previous publications from this laboratory.[2,3] Therefore, only changes related to calcification are described herein. Two types of calcific deposits were considered to be of significance in producing bioprosthetic stenosis: deposits related to calcification of cuspal connective tissue structures and deposits related to calcification of surface thrombi.

Calcification of cuspal connective tissue structures consistently involved collagen fibrils (Fig. 6 and 7) but seldom involved cell components of the cusps, and did not involve elastic fibers. Most deposits involved areas in which the collagen fibrils were relatively loosely arranged rather than tightly packed. Calcific deposits associated with collagen fibrils showed three different patterns of organization. In the first of these (Fig. 7, A and B), the calcific deposits directly involved the collagen fibrils but did not extend into the interfibrillary spaces. In the second (Fig. 6, A and B and 7, C and D), the calcific deposits were localized in the periphery of the collagen fibrils and in the interfibrillary spaces; however, the interior of the collagen fibrils was not involved, and the fibrils therefore appeared as electron-lucent cylinders surrounded by an extremely dense calcified matrix. In the third pattern (Fig. 7C), the cal-

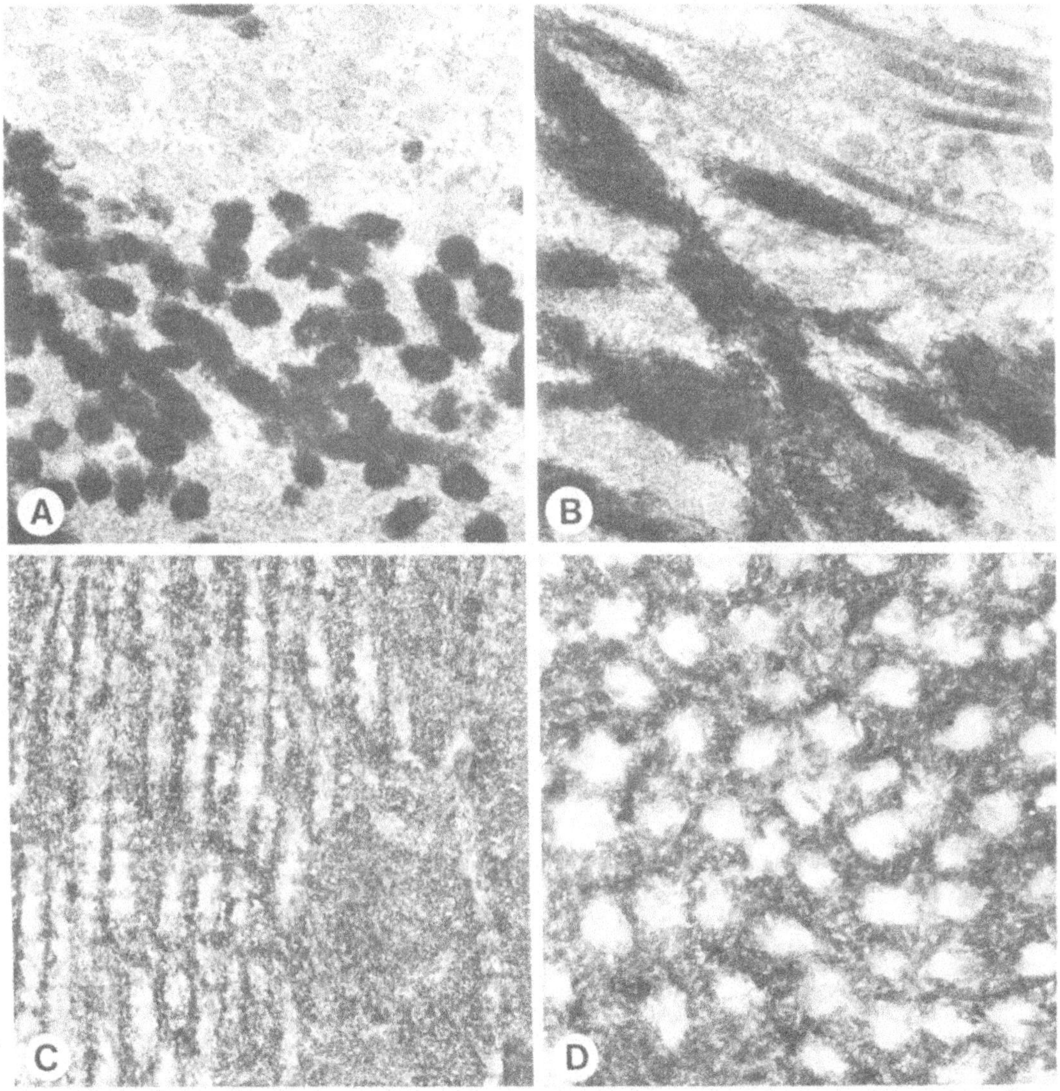

FIGURE 7. High magnification views of calcific deposits associated with collagen fibrils. Case 1, **A** and **C**; Case 3, **B**; Case 6, **D**. **A** and **B**, transverse (**A**) and longitudinal (**B**) views of deposits that involve the entire thickness of the collagen fibrils. In both views the calcified fibrils appear larger than adjacent uninvolved fibrils, suggesting spread of crystal growth into the interfibrillary spaces (×75,000 and ×60,000, respectively, reduced by 20 percent.) **C** and **D**, calcific deposits in both of these areas occupy interfibrillary spaces. In **C** the crystals are also present in the interior of the collagen fibrils, some of which (**upper right**) are barely discernible. In **D**, the crystalline nature of the calcific deposits is evident (×60,000 and ×127,000, respectively, reduced by 20 percent).

cific deposits occupied both the interfibrillary spaces and the interior of the fibrils, thus giving the deposits a relatively homogeneous appearance. This homogeneous pattern was characteristically present throughout the central areas of large calcific deposits. In contrast, the interfibrillary pattern was found either at the periphery of large masses or throughout small masses. Involvement of the collagen fibrils with sparing of the interfibrillary spaces was found only in small scattered groups of collagen fibrils, and not in association with large calcific deposits.

Most of the calcific deposits associated with connective tissue showed a crystalline substructure when examined at high magnifications, regardless of their pattern of organization with respect to the collagen fibrils. The crystals were cylindrical in shape and measured from 280 to 330 Å in length and from 65 to 80 Å in width. These crystals often were mixed with material that appeared amorphous even at very high magnification. Energy dispersive X-ray microanalysis revealed the presence of calcium and phosphorus in these crystals, and X-ray diffraction analysis disclosed patterns similar to that of apatite. Degeneration of the collagen (usually of severe degree) was often associated with the calcific deposits, but the most severely degenerated collagen was not necessarily the most calcified, and extensive calcific deposits sometimes were evident in areas where collagen showed little or no change.

Small calcific deposits were occasionally found to overlie mitochondria (Fig. 8A) and rarely, nuclei (Fig. 8B) of porcine cells in the cusps. They were located in areas in which other structures were severely calcified, and they constituted a small fraction of the total of calcific deposits. No structures resembling the "matrix vesicles" of other calcifying tissues[23,24] were found in any bioprosthetic cusp.

Calcific deposits associated with vegetations and thrombi were composed of plate- or needle-shaped crystals (Fig. 9), which measured up to 80 Å in maximal thickness and up to 1,000 Å in largest diameter. The smallest of these deposits were located within remnants or "ghosts" of platelets and leukocytes that appeared to have been trapped within a mesh of fibrin strands. These deposits usually were within mitochondria. The fibrin strands were not sites of deposition of calcific crystals.

Discussion

Features of Calcific Deposits in Porcine Bioprostheses:

Predisposing factors: This study reveals that calcification of porcine bioprostheses can occur in adults as well as in children, that the most important sites of formation of calcific deposits in both age groups are the connective tissue in the cusps and thrombi and vegetations on the surfaces, and that calcific deposits are an important cause of prosthetic valve dysfunction. Our findings are in accord with those of previous clinical studies[4–22] of calcification of porcine bioprostheses.

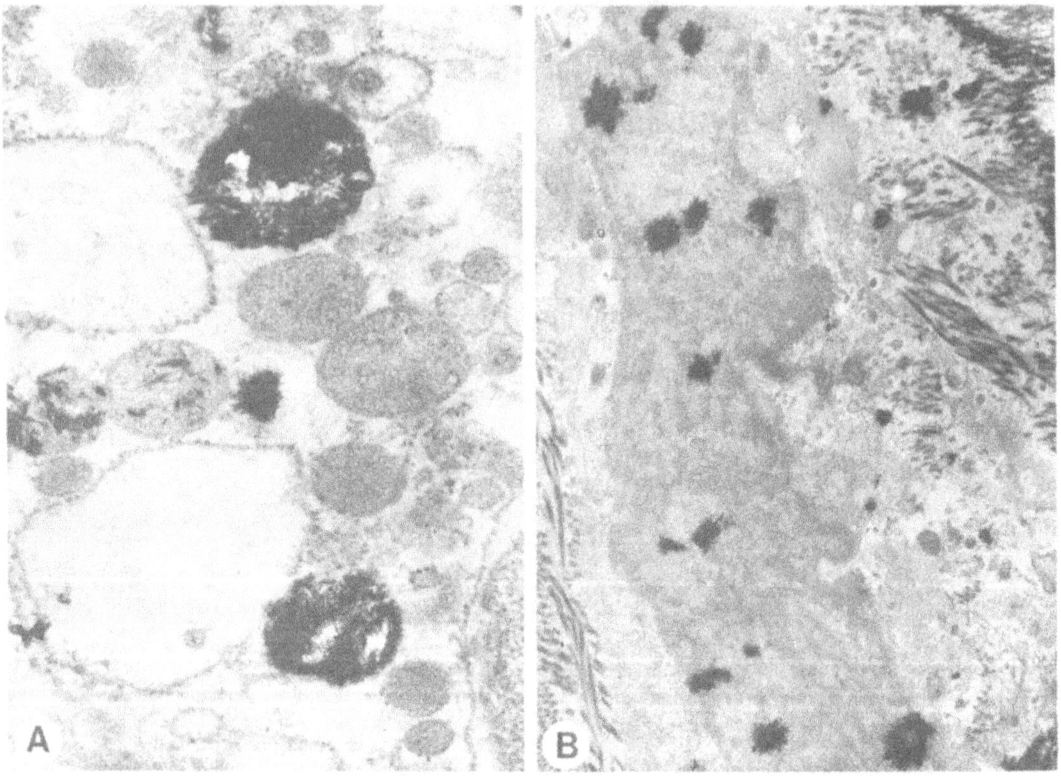

FIGURE 8. A, Case 1; **B,** Case 3. Intracellular calcific deposits in valvular connective tissue cells of porcine origin are few and small, and involved mitochondria (**A**) and nuclei (**B**), (×44,000 [**A**] and ×18,000 [**B**], reduced by 20 percent).

Those studies (Table II) have documented the occurrence of calcification in a total of 37 bioprostheses implanted in 34 patients. The time between implantation and removal of the bioprostheses averaged 28 months, which was less than the mean time of 39 months in our patients. This difference reflects the greater number of children in Table II than in our group of patients. The average age of our patients was 32 years; that of the patients in Table II was 23 years. Although these data indicate that calcification of porcine bioprostheses is more frequent and develops more rapidly in children and young adults than in older patients, our study shows that the gross anatomic, histologic and ultrastructural features of the calcific deposits are the same in both age groups, thus suggesting that the causative processes are similar. Evidence of infection was present in the calcified valves in two of our patients and in seven of the patients previously described (Table II). Metabolic factors that could have contributed to the formation of calcific deposits were identified in only one of our patients and in only three of the patients in Table II; in all four patients, the factor was chronic renal insufficiency.

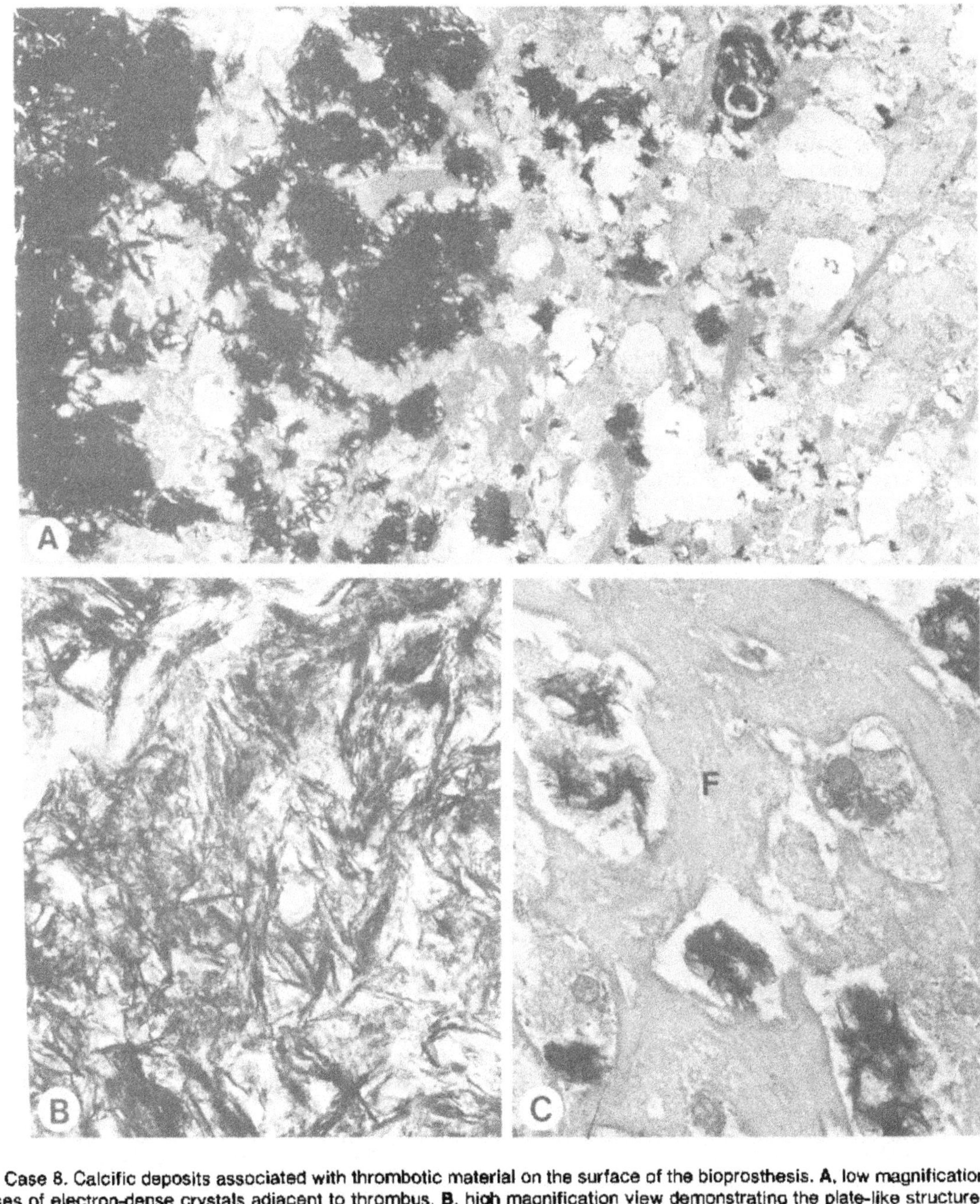

FIGURE 9. Case 8. Calcific deposits associated with thrombotic material on the surface of the bioprosthesis. **A**, low magnification view showing large masses of electron-dense crystals adjacent to thrombus. **B**, high magnification view demonstrating the plate-like structure of the crystals shown in **A**. **C**, remnants of platelets trapped in fibrin mesh (F) contain calcific deposits. (×13,000 [**A**], ×25,700 [**B**], ×37,000 [**C**], reduced by 20 percent.)

Thus, coexisting metabolic disorders are not recognizable in the majority of patients in whom calcific deposits develop in porcine bioprostheses.

Frequency: Such deposits are common. The 14 calcified bioprostheses reported in our study represent nearly 50 percent of all bioprostheses examined with electron microscopy in our laboratory. Because these bioprostheses were submitted for study for a variety of reasons, they do not constitute a representative sample of all implanted porcine bioprostheses. Nevertheless, in the only large institutional experience thus far reported, Billingham et al.[25] observed calcific deposits in 17 (34 percent) of 50 porcine bioprostheses recovered at Stanford University Hospital between 1974 and 1978. Failure to detect calcific deposits may be related to the fact that histologic sections of these bioprostheses usually are taken from the central portions of the cusps. Because the earliest deposits are most frequently located near the commissures, such deposits may be missed. In our experience, the most sensitive technique for detecting calcific deposits in porcine bioprostheses is X-ray examination of the entire explanted bioprosthesis.

Valve dysfunction: Factors such as size and location will determine whether the calcific deposits cause bioprosthetic dysfunction. Recent observations indicate that significant degrees of bioprosthetic stenosis related to calcification of porcine bioprostheses can occur in relatively asymptomatic patients.[26] This clinical situation parallels that which is well known to occur in stenosis affecting natural mitral values. Therefore, the lack of symptoms does not exclude the possibility of significant bioprosthetic stenosis.

Mechanisms of Calcific Deposits

Calcific deposits have been found in porcine bioprostheses implanted in experimental animals[27,28] as well as in other types of bioprostheses implanted in patients, including dura mater valves,[29] fascia lata valves,[28,30–33] porcine valves treated with formalin,[5] periodate[34] or mercuric salts,[5] fresh[28,35] or glutaraldehyde-treated[36] pericardial bioprostheses, and homografts preserved by antibiotics, beta-propriolactone, freeze-drying or irradiation.[37–42] In addition, calcific deposits involving thrombotic material deposited on the sewing ring[43] or on Teflon® cusps[35] also have occurred

TABLE II

Reports of Calcific Deposits in 37 Glutaraldehyde-Treated Porcine Bioprostheses Implanted in 34 Patients

Reference (first author)	PB (n) With Ca^{++}	Age (yr) at PB Implantation	Sex	Type of Heart Disease	Site of PB	PB Removal: Time (mo)	PB Removal: Cause	Factors Predisposing to Ca^{++}
Carpentier[4]	4	...	...	...	A	60	Death	...
		...	...	...	PC	16	Death	...
Zylberberg[5]	1	...	...	...	...	18	...	...
McIntosh[6]	1	...	...	...	m	56	...	...
Zuhdi[7]	6	...	...	...	...	...	IE	Infection
Magilligan[8]	2	...	...	...	A, m	36	Death	Infection
Levitsky[9]	1	8	...	...	...	19	Death	
Fishbein[10]; Cohn[17]	2	35	M	...	A, m	6	Death	Renal failure
Albert[11]	2	...	...	...	A	61	Stenosis	...
		...	...	...	m	12	Stenosis	...
Thiene[12]	3	...	...	...	...	...	...	...
Forfar[13]	1	26	M	Endocarditis	m	0.5	Stenosis	...
Rose[14]	1	13	F	...	m	12	Death	...
Hetzer[15]	1	64	F	...	m	2	Death	Renal failure
Kutsche[16]	3	8	F	MR (cong)	m	58	Stenosis	...
		12	M	MR (cong)	m	43	Stenosis	...
Platt[18]	1	50	M	...	...	33	Death	...
Geha[19]	5	9.5	F	AR	A	26	Stenosis	...
		9	F	AS (cong)	A	45	Stenosis	...
		16	M	AS	A	41	Stenosis	...
		5	M	MR	m	22	Stenosis	...
Lamberti[20]	3	18	F	MR	m	31	Stenosis	...
		45	F	MR, TR	m, T	16	Death	Renal failure
Total	37 (34 pts)	23 (average)	M 6; F 7		m 12; A 7; T 1; PC 1	28 (average)	Stenosis 10; IE 6; death 11	Renal failure 3; infection 7

A = aortic valve; AR = aortic regurgitation; AS = aortic stenosis; Ca^{++} = calcium; cong = congenital; IE = infective endocarditis; m = mitral valve; MR = mitral regurgitation; PB = porcine bioprosthesis; PC = pulmonary conduit; pts = patients; T = tricuspid valve; TR = tricuspid regurgitation; . . . = information not available.

in rigid-framed valves. The actual frequency of these changes has not been studied and the histologic features of calcific deposits in prosthetic heart valves have been the subject of few studies. The aortic wall in homografts has been reported to undergo much more severe calcification than the cusps.[40,44,45] The localization of calcific deposits in valve bioprostheses has not been studied in detail, although calcified collagen has been observed in variously prepared porcine bioprostheses.[5] In this study, several sites of calcification were identified in porcine bioprostheses. Among these were collagen, organized thrombi and vegetations, mitochondria and nuclei of cells of porcine origin, and the cytoplasm of adipose tissue cells. Of these sites, collagen and thrombotic material appeared to be the most important; the deposits at these sites represent the results of different mechanisms and therefore will be considered separately.

Calcification of collagen: The process of normal calcification of tissues such as bone, cartilage and teeth basically consists of the deposition of a crystalline inorganic phase, composed of a form of calcium phosphate known as hydroxyapatite, on a preexisting matrix of collagen fibrils that are associated with proteoglycans (complexes of proteins and acid mucopolysaccharides), noncollagen glycoproteins, peptides, lipids and other components of connective tissue ground substance.[46,47] The calcium and phosphate ions are derived from the circulating blood and can come into contact with the calcifying matrix either directly, by simple diffusion or after being absorbed and concentrated within connective tissue cells.[46]

The nature of the initial sites of formation of calcific deposits in the organic matrix of calcifying connective tissues is still the subject of controversy, although there is complete agreement that the end result, calcification of collagen, is similar regardless of the initial events. In early stages of development of bone, cartilage and dentine, the process of calcium deposition is initiated by structures known as matrix vesicles.[23,24] These vesicles are secreted by connective tissue cells, are limited by single trilaminar membranes and contain small needle-shaped crystals of calcium phosphate. These crystals grow in size as the membranes of the matrix vesicles rupture, and extension and coalescence of crystal growth lead to calcification of the collagen. In many instances other than early development, the process of calcification of collagenous structures occurs without participation of matrix vesicles, and in these instances the collagen itself becomes the site of formation and growth of nuclei of crystallization.[46,47] This mechanism appears to be responsible for calcification of connective tissue in porcine bioprostheses, in which we found no matrix vesicles. Porcine valve connective tissue cells cannot participate in a process of secretion of matrix vesicles, because these cells are killed by the commercial processing of glutaraldehyde. Direct involvement of collagen in the formation of calcific deposits also is suggested by our finding of small foci of calcium phosphate crystals overlying collagen fibrils. The morphologic features of calcified collagen in porcine bioprostheses are similar to those of calcific deposits occurring spontaneously and induced experimentally, both in vivo and in vitro, in collagen in tendons of animals[48–53] and in skeletal muscle of human beings with fibrositis (myositis) ossificans.[48]

The initial deposits of calcium in mineralizing connective tissues consist of amorphous calcium phosphate; this amorphous material is gradually transformed into crystalline hydroxyapatite.[52,53] The current concepts of the relation of the collagen to the calcific deposits are that (1) phosphate groups form covalent bonds that connect the organic and inorganic components in calcified tissues; (2) epsilon-amino groups present in lysine and hydroxylysine are of importance in forming the bonds between native collagen and phosphate groups; (3) many of the hydroxylysine residues normally are either linked (glycosylated) to noncollagen carbohydrate material or modified to form covalent cross-links; and (4) the three dimensional structure of the collagen fibril is also of importance in determining the availability of these groups for reacting with phosphate and serving as centers of nucleation.[46,53] Thus, all collagen appears to be theoretically capable of calcifying. The reason that many areas of collagen do not calcify in vivo has been attributed to the presence in the ground substance in such areas of proteoglycans and glycoproteins, which are associated with collagen[53,54] and which mask or block the sites that would react with phosphate and calcium to become nucleation centers.[53] This concept appears to be applicable to the calcification of collagen in porcine valve bioprostheses. This calcification is most marked in the spongiosa, the layer that in the native porcine valve is most abundant in proteoglycan material. We[2] have previously shown that this material is lost after commercial processing and implantation, and we believe that this loss of proteoglycan may predispose to calcification for two reasons. The first reason is the uncovering of phosphate-binding sites in the collagen, as previously mentioned. The second reason is the loss of proteoglycan, leaving empty spaces in the spongiosa; these spaces may become filled with deposits of plasma proteins and other blood constituents, which in turn may provide additional sites of calcification.

The possible participation of other proteins in calcification of collagen is suggested by the recent identification of several different classes of proteins that have a high binding affinity for calcium.[55–59] This binding affinity is related to their content of gamma-carboxyglutamic acid, an unusual amino acid that is formed by a reaction that requires vitamin K and bicarbonate. Some of these proteins (the vitamin K-dependent blood clotting proteins) are present in normal blood; others have been found in tissues undergoing normal (bone) or abnormal (renal calculi, atherosclerotic plaques, skin in scleroderma and dermatomyositis) calcification.[55–57] Levy et al.[58,59] found gamma-carboxyglutamic acid in hydrolysates of protein material extracted from porcine bioprostheses that had manifested calcific deposits after being implanted in patients, and from calcified native aortic valves, but not from noncalcified bioprostheses. The origin (from circulating blood or from in situ synthesis), the localization in the bioprosthetic tissue and the significance of this protein material in porcine valves have not yet been established. Nevertheless, these findings are important because they represent a new, incompletely understood aspect of biologic calcification.

The role of pretreatment with glutaraldehyde in modifying the tendency of porcine bioprostheses to undergo calcification is unclear. Such pretreatment introduces several additional cross-links in collagen, thus stabilizing the structure of the fibrils. This finding suggests that the inability of calcium and phosphate to penetrate into the highly cross-linked interior of the collagen fibrils may explain why calcific deposits often (Fig. 7, C and D) do not extend into the cores of collagen fibrils in porcine bioprostheses. Such penetration would result in complete calcification of the collagen fibrils (Fig. 7, A and B), which was a less frequent microscopic finding in our study. Glutaraldehyde reacts in a complex manner with free amino groups in lysine and hydroxylysine,[60] thus possibly preventing them from reacting with phosphate to initiate the formation of calcific deposits. However, it is probable that new lysine and hydroxylysine residues (or other reactive residues) are brought into the tissue after implantation through plasma proteins that penetrate between collagen fibers and permeate the connective tissue framework. A large incidence of calcification developed in porcine bioprostheses that had been prepared for clinical use by treatment first with sodium metaperiodate, a mild oxidizing agent,[61] and ethylene glycol and then with glutaraldehyde.[34] The exact relation between this oxidative process and the subsequent development of calcification has not been clarified. It is known from other observations[46,62] that the process of calcification of biologic materials is subject to considerable modifications by a wide variety of agents, including hormones (parathormone and calcitonin), vitamin D and alkaline phosphatase (an enzyme that hydrolyzes various phosphate esters and thus generates inorganic phosphate, which contributes to calcification). Thus, calcification of collagen in porcine bioprostheses tends to be most marked in children, in whom the balance of hormonal and metabolic factors clearly favors the deposition of calcium phosphate in collagen in other tissues such as bone. A predisposition to calcification of soft tissues is well known to occur in patients with chronic renal disease and secondary hyperparathyroidism.[63]

Calcification of thrombotic material: Thrombi in various sites are known to calcify, most notably in the left atrium of adults with mitral stenosis. The mechanisms of formation of calcific deposits in thrombi have not been studied ultrastructurally. Our observations show that the sites of initial calcification in thrombi and vegetations are platelets and leukocytes that become trapped in the fibrin mesh. The intracellular components that undergo calcification are the mitochondria, and crystal growth from these sites leads to the formation of large confluent and calcific masses. These masses in turn probably induce the formation of additional thrombi, and repeated episodes of thrombosis and calcification probably account for the layered or laminated appearance of calcific deposits of this type. As in the case of calcification of collagen, calcification of mitochondria represents a commonly occurring biologic phenomenon. Mitochondria are the sites of calcification in ischemic heart muscle cells[64,65] and in other cell types in many other conditions.[66] Thus, mitochondrial calcification constitutes a basic mechanism for the initiation of intracellular calcification, and from mitochondria the deposits can spread and fill the entire cell. This mechanism is important with respect to host cells in surface thrombi, but seems to be operational only to an extremely limited extent in the porcine cells in bioprostheses. Perhaps this is so because the accumulation of calcium in mitochondria, at least in its initial stages, is an active process that occurs in cells that may be injured but are still alive.[66] This process excludes porcine cells, which are killed by the glutaraldehyde processing.

Implications: Calcific deposits are commonly found in implanted porcine bioprostheses. In some of these prostheses, particularly in those implanted in children and young adults, they are the cause of important degrees of bioprosthetic dysfunction. They can be caused by calcification of cuspal collagen or of thrombotic material on the cuspal surfaces. An understanding of the mechanisms of formation of these two types of deposits is essential for the formulation of measures designed to prevent calcification of tissue valves.

Addendum

Four very recent reports[67–70] have provided additional documentation of the occurrence of early, severe calcification of porcine valve bioprostheses implanted in children and young adults without metabolic diseases or infective endocarditis. In some patients[68,69] the calcification was associated with degeneration of collagen. It was suggested[69] that this calcification may be promoted by host factors related to calcium homeostasis.

Acknowledgment

We express our appreciation for the skilled assistance of Esther Wilhoite (photography) and Dorothy Veigle (secretarial and editorial work).

References

1. **Ferrans VJ, Boyce SW, Billingham ME, Spray TL, Roberts WC.** Infection of glutaraldehyde-preserved porcine valve heterografts. Am J Cardiol 1979;43:1123–36.
2. **Ferrans VJ, Spray TL, Billingham ME, Roberts WC.** Structural changes in glutaraldehyde-treated porcine heterografts used as substitute cardiac valves. Transmission and scanning electron microscopic observations in 12 patients. Am J Cardiol 1978;41:1159–84.
3. **Ferrans VJ, Spray TL, Billingham ME, Roberts WC.** Ultrastructure of Hancock porcine valvular heterografts. Pre- and post-implantation changes. Circulation 1978;58:Suppl I:I-10–8.
4. **Carpentier A, Deloche A, Relland J, et al.** Six-year follow-up of

glutaraldehyde-preserved heterografts with particular reference to the treatment of congenital valve malformations. J Thorac Cardiovasc Surg 1974;68:771–82.
5. **Zylberberg L.** Contribution a l'étude des hétérogreffes aortiques par la microscopie électronique. Pathol Biol (Paris) 1975;23: 691–704.
6. **McIntosh CL, Michaelis LL, Morrow AG, Itscoitz SB, Redwood DR, Epstein SE.** Atrioventricular valve replacement with the Hancock porcine xenograft: a five year clinical experience. Surgery 1975;78:768–75.
7. **Zuhdi N.** The porcine aortic valve bioprosthesis: a significant alternative. Ann Thorac Surg 1976;21:573–5.
8. **Magilligan Jr DJ, Quinn EL, Davila JC.** Bacteremia, endocarditis, and the Hancock valve. Ann Thorac Surg 1977;24:508–18.
9. **Levitsky S.** Discussion of Stinson EB, Griepp RB, Oyer PE, Shumway NE. Long-term experience with porcine aortic valve xenografts. J Thorac Cardiovasc Surg 1977;73:54–62.
10. **Fishbein MC, Gissen SA, Collins JJ Jr, Barsamian EM, Cohn LH.** Pathologic findings after cardiac valve replacement with glutaraldehyde-fixed porcine valves. Am J Cardiol 1977;40:331–7.
11. **Albert HM, Bryant LR, Schechter FG.** Seven year experience with mounted porcine valves. Ann Surg 1977;185:717–23.
12. **Thiene G, Bortolotti U, Casarotto D, Gallucci V.** Pathology of porcine bioprostheses used as cardiac valve substitutes (abstr). XIIth Congress of the International Academy of Pathology and the 3rd World Congress of Academic and Environmental Pathology. Jerusalem, Israel 1978;Sept. 10–15:139.
13. **Forfar JC, Cotter L, Morritt GN.** Severe and early stenosis of porcine heterograft mitral valve. Br Heart J 1978;40:1184–7.
14. **Rose AG, Forman R, Bowen RM.** Calcification of glutaraldehyde-fixed porcine xenograft. Thorax 1978;33;111–4.
15. **Hetzer R, Hill JD, Kerth WJ, Wilson AJ, Adappa MG, Gerbode F.** Thrombosis and degeneration of Hancock valves: clinical and pathological findings. Ann Thorac Surg 1978;26:317–22.
16. **Kutsche LM, Oyer P, Shumway N, Baum D.** An important complication of Hancock mitral valve replacement in children. Circulation 1978;60:Suppl I:I-98–103.
17. **Cohn LH, Koster JK, Mee RBB, Collins JJ Jr.** Long-term follow-up of the Hancock bioprosthetic heart valve: a 6-year review. Circulation 1978;60:Suppl I:I-87–92.
18. **Platt MR.** Discussion of Davila JC, Magilligan DJ Jr, Lewis JW Jr. Is the Hancock porcine valve the best cardiac valve substitute today? Ann Thorac Surg 1978;26:303–16.
19. **Geha AS, Stansel HC Jr, Cornhill JF, Kilman JW, Buckley MJ, Roberts WC.** Late failure of porcine valve heterografts in children. J Thorac Cardiovasc Surg 1979;78:351–64.
20. **Lamberti JJ, Wainer BH, Fisher KA, Karunaratne HB, Al-Sadir J.** Calcific stenosis of the porcine heterograft. Ann Thorac Surg 1979;28:28–32.
21. **Spray TL, Roberts WC.** Structural changes in porcine xenografts used as substitute cardiac valves. Gross and histologic observations in 51 glutaraldehyde-preserved Hancock valves in 41 patients. Am J Cardiol 1977;40:319–30.
22. **Brown JW, Dunn JM, Spooner E, Kirsh MM.** Late spontaneous disruption of a porcine xenograft mitral valve. Clinical, hemodynamic, echocardiographic, and pathological findings. J Thorac Cardiovasc Surg 1978;75:606–11.
23. **Anderson HC.** Vesicles associated with calcification in the matrix of epiphyseal cartilage. J Cell Biol 1969;41:59–72.
24. **Yamada M.** Ultrastructural and cytochemical studies on the calcification of the tendon-bone joint. Arch Histol Jpn 1976;39: 347–78.
25. **Billingham ME, Ferrans VJ, Boyce SW, Spray TL, Roberts WC.** Bacterial infection in implanted porcine valve heterografts: a histopathologic and ultrastructural study. In: Sebening F, Klövekorn WP, Meisner H, Struck E, eds. Bioprosthetic Cardiac Valves. Munich: Deutsches Herzzentrum, 1979:281–94.
26. **Borkon AM, Isner JM, McIntosh CL, et al.** Late failures of Hancock porcine heterografts used for mitral valve replacement (abstr). Circulation 1979;59, 60:Suppl II:II-221.
27. **Okamura K, Yuge I, Kawazoe K, et al.** A comparative study between glutaraldehyde-preserved aortic and pulmonary heterograft valves in the tricuspid position in dogs. J Cardiovasc Surg 1976; 17:178–86.
28. **Yarbrough JW, Roberts WC, Reis RL.** Structural alterations in tissue cardiac valves implanted in patients and in calves. J Thorac Cardiovasc Surg 1973; 65:364–75.
29. **Zerbini EJ, Puig LB.** Valvas cardiacas proteticas e biologicas especial referencia a valva de dura-mater. Arch Inst Cardiol Mex 1977;47:650–7.
30. **Gersbach P, Wegmann W.** Aorta valve replacement using autologous fascia lata transplants. Late morphological changes. An electron microscopic study. Virchows Arch [Pathol Anat] 1974; 364:235–47.
31. **Senning A.** Discussion of Ionescu MI, Pakrashi BC, Mary DAS, Bartek IT, Wooler GH. Long-term evaluation of tissue valves. J Thorac Cardiovasc Surg 1974;68:361–79.
32. **Silver MD, Hudson REB, Trimble AS.** Morphologic observations on heart valve prostheses made of fascia lata. J Thorac Cardiovasc Surg 1975;70:360–6.
33. **Soorae AS, O'Kane H, Molloy PJ, Cleland J.** Comparative analysis of isolated aortic valve replacement with fascia lata and homograft valves. J Thorac Cardiovasc Surg 1978;76:46–55.
34. **Carpentier A.** From valvular xenograft to valvular bioprosthesis (1965–1977). Med Instrum 1977;11:98–101.
35. **Björk VO, Hultquist G.** Teflon and pericardial aortic valve prostheses. J Thorac Cardiovasc Surg 1964;47:693–701.
36. **Trusler GA.** Discussion of Geha AS, Stansel HC Jr, Cornhill JF, Kilman JW, Buckley MJ, Roberts WC. Late failure of porcine valve heterografts in children. J Thorac Cardiovasc Surg 1979;78: 351–64.
37. **Reichenbach DD, Mohri H, Merendino KA.** Pathological changes in human aortic valve homografts. Circulation 1969;39,40:Suppl I: I-47–56.
38. **Barratt-Boyes BG, Roche AHG, Brandt PWT, Smith JC, Lowe JB.** Aortic homograft valve replacement. A long-term follow-up of an initial series of 101 patients. Circulation 1969;40:763–75.
39. **Ross DN.** Aortic valvar replacements. Br Heart J 1971;33:39–41.
40. **Rocchini AP, Rosenthal A, Keane JF, Castaneda AR, Nadas AS.** Hemodynamics after surgical repair with right ventricle to pulmonary artery conduit. Circulation 1976;54:951–6.
41. **Moodie DS, Mair DD, Fulton RE, Wallace RB, Danielson GK, McGoon DC.** Aortic homograft obstruction. J Thorac Cardiovasc Surg 1976;72:553–61.
42. **Park SC, Neches WH, Lenox CC, Zuberbuhler JR, Bahnson HT.** Massive calcification and obstruction in a homograft after the Rastelli procedure for transposition of great arteries. Am J Cardiol 1973;32:860–4.
43. **Bulkley BH, Morrow AG, Roberts WC.** Calcification of prosthetic valve anuli: a late complication of cardiac valve replacement. Am Heart J 1974;87:129–33.
44. **Imamura ES, Konno S, Arai T, Sakakibara S.** Composite graft of heterologous pulmonary valve and prosthetic tube for the reconstruction of right ventricular outflow tract. Clinical application in four patients. J Thorac Cardiovasc Surg 1972;63:747–55.
45. **Behrendt DM, Kirsh MM, Stern A, Sigmann J, Perry B, Sloan H.** The surgical therapy for pulmonary artery-right ventricular discontinuity. Ann Thorac Surg 1974;18:122–37.
46. **Frank RM, Voegel JC.** Le crystal d'apatite biologique: son élaboration, son comportement physiologique et pathologique. Biol Cell (Paris) 1977;28:187–94.
47. **Montel G.** Constitutions et structure des Apatites biologiques: influence de ces facteurs sur leurs propriétés. Biol Cell (Paris) 1977;28:179–86.
48. **Gerlach U, Höhling HJ, Themann H.** Metabolism and structure of connective tissue during extraosseous calcification. Clin Orthop 1970;69:118–34.
49. **Höhling HJ, Ashton BA, Köster HD.** Quantitative electron microscopic investigations of mineral nucleation in collagen. Cell Tissue Res 1974;148:11–26.
50. **Höhling HJ, Barckhaus RH, Krefting ER, Schreiber J.** Electron microscopic microprobe analysis of mineralized collagen fibrils and extracollagenous regions in turkey leg tendon. Cell Tissue Res 1976;175:345–50.
51. **Bachra BN.** Calcification in vitro of collagenous model systems: chemical and electronmicroscopic aspects. Calcif Tissue Res 1970;Suppl 4:31–3.
52. **Termine JD.** Mineral chemistry and skeletal biology. Clin Orthop 1972;85:207–41.

53. **Glimcher MJ.** Composition, structure, and organization of bone and other mineralized tissues and the mechanism of calcification. In: Gleep RO, Astwood EB, Aurbach GD, Geiger SR, eds. Handbook of Physiology, Section 7, Endocrinology, Vol 7, Parathyroid Gland. Washington DC: American Physiological Society, 1976:25–116.
54. **Anderson JC.** Glycoproteins of the connective tissue matrix. Int Rev Connect Tissue Res 1976;7:251–322.
55. **Lian JB, Skinner M, Glimcher MJ, Gallop PM.** The presence of γ-carboxyglutamic acid in the proteins associated with ectopic calcification. Biochem Biophys Res Commun 1976;73:349–55.
56. **Lian JB, Prien El Jr, Glimcher MJ, Gallop PM.** The presence of protein-bound γ-carboxyglutamic acid in calcium-containing renal calculi. J Clin Invest 1977;59:1151–7.
57. **Levy RJ, Lian JB, Gallop PM.** Atherocalcin, a γ-carboxyglutamic acid containing protein from atherosclerotic plaque. Biochem Biophys Res Commun 1979;91:41–9.
58. **Levy RJ, Lian JB.** Studies on the etiology of calcific aortic valve disease: the role of the calcium binding amino acid, γ-carboxyglutamic acid (abstr). Circulation 1978;57,58: Suppl II:II-54.
59. **Levy RJ, Zenker JA, Lian JB.** Vitamin K-dependent calcium binding proteins in aortic valve calcification. J Clin Invest 1980;65: 563–6.
60. **Habeeb AFSA, Hiramoto R.** Reaction of proteins with glutaraldehyde. Arch Biochem Biophys 1968;126:16–26.
61. **Pearse AGE.** Histochemistry, Theoretical and Applied, Vol 1. 3rd ed. Boston: Little, Brown, 1968: 307–18.
62. **Fleish H, Neuman WF.** Mechanisms of calcification: role of collagen, polyphosphates, and phosphatase. Am J Physiol 1961; 200:1296–300.
63. **Kuzela DC, Huffer WE, Conger JD, Winter SD, Hammond WS.** Soft tissue calcification in chronic dialysis patients. Am J Pathol 1977;86:403–24.
64. **Buja LM, Dees JH, Harling DF, Willerson JT.** Analytical electron microscopic study of mitochondrial inclusions in canine myocardial infarcts. J Histochem Cytochem 1976;24:508–16.
65. **Hagler HK, Sherwin L, Buja LM.** Effects of different methods of tissue preparation on mitochondrial inclusions of ischemic and infarcted canine myocardium. Transmission and analytic electron microscopic study. Lab Invest 1979;40:529–44.
66. **Carafoli E, Crompton M.** Calcium ions and mitochondria. Symp Soc Exp Biol 1976;30:89–115.
67. **Bachet J, Bical O, Goudot B, et al.** Early structural failure of porcine xenografts in young patients. In Ref 25: 341–9.
68. **Thandroyen FT, Whitton IN, Pirie D, Rogers MA, Mitha AS.** Severe calcification of glutaraldehyde-preserved porcine xenografts in children. Am J Cardiol 1980;45:690–6.
69. **Silver MM, Pollock J, Silver MD, Williams WG, Trusler GA.** Calcification in porcine xenograft valves in children. Am J Cardiol 1980;45:685–9.
70. **Sanders SP, Freed MD, Norwood WI, Castaneda A, Nadas AS.** Early failure of porcine valves implanted in children (abstr). Am J Cardiol 1980;45:449.

Calcific Deposits Developing in a Bovine Pericardial Bioprosthetic Valve 3 Days After Implantation

TOKUHIRO ISHIHARA, M.D., VICTOR J. FERRANS, M.D., PH.D., MICHAEL JONES, M.D., HENRY S. CABIN, M.D., AND WILLIAM C. ROBERTS, M.D.

SUMMARY **Calcific deposits, localized in a thin layer of thrombus covering the cuspal surfaces, were present 3 days after implantation in a valved pulmonic conduit that contained an Ionescu-Shiley bovine pericardial valve and was placed in a 29-year-old man with double outlet right ventricle, valvular and infundibular pulmonic stenosis, and ventricular septal defect. Factors that may have contributed to such a rapid calcification were the relatively young age of the patient, the development of acute renal insufficiency postoperatively, and the administration of large amounts of calcium chloride intravenously during blood transfusions and during episodes of cardiac arrest.**

CALCIFICATION of bioprosthetic cardiac valves can lead to prosthetic stenosis, regurgitation or both.[1-10] Calcific deposits usually produce valvular dysfunction only after the bioprostheses have been in place for several years.[1] In some patients, however, calcific deposits have developed within a few months after implantation.[1-6, 10] In one exceptional patient,[4] a porcine bioprosthetic valve had to be removed because of calcification only 19 days after implantation. In this communication we describe anatomic findings in a pericardial bioprosthesis that developed calcific deposits within 3 days of implantation. Such rapid calcification of a valvular bioprosthesis has not been described previously.

Case Report

S. H. (CC. # 12-81-67-7), a 29-year old man, had double outlet right ventricle, valvular and infundibular pulmonic stenosis, ventricular septal defect and patent foramen ovale. At 4 years of age, he had had a left-sided Blalock-Taussig subclavian–pulmonary arterial anastomosis. At age 27 years (1978), this shunt was occluded. The blood hematocrit was 78%; studies of renal function and blood coagulation gave normal results, and the serum uric acid and bilirubin were slightly elevated. The peak systolic pressure gradient between the body of the right ventricle and the pulmonary trunk was 95 mm Hg. The systemic arterial oxygen saturation was 88%. A right-sided Blalock-Taussig subclavian–pulmonary arterial shunt was performed in October 1978. In November 1979, because he did not improve despite a functioning shun', he underwent closure of the ventricular septal defect and patent foramen ovale, and insertion of a valved conduit containing a size 22 Ionescu-Shiley bovine pericardial valve between the right ventricle and the pulmonary trunk. After operation, the patient was reexplored because of extensive bleeding. He had multiple areas of oozing, without a large source of bleeding and without a specific coagulation defect. He then developed a low cardiac output state, with a marked decrease in renal function and blood urea nitrogen and creatinine values of 54 and 5.2 mg/dl, respectively. Serum calcium was 4.2 mg/dl. Peritoneal dialysis was instituted. Hemodynamic evaluation revealed persistent right ventricular hypertension (104/4 mm Hg) and a pressure gradient of 80 mm Hg at the distal anastomosis between the conduit and the pulmonary artery. On the third day after operation, a revision of the distal anastomosis of the conduit was performed, but the patient died several hours later.

During the entire postoperative period, the serum calcium was never elevated. Because of bleeding, the patient received 65 units of whole blood, 18 units of fresh-frozen plasma and 39 units of platelets. He also received a total of 20 g of calcium chloride during the 3-day postoperative period, in association with the transfusions and during resuscitative efforts.

At necropsy, the pericardial tissue leaflets in the valved conduit were covered with a very thin layer of thrombus that did not interfere with leaflet mobility. Histologic study of right and left ventricular myocardium disclosed focal areas of necrosis, infiltration by polymorphonuclear leukocytes, and calcific deposits within necrotic myocardial cells.

Materials and Methods

Histologic and scanning and transmission electron microscopic studies were made of the pericardial tissue leaflets of the bioprosthesis implanted in the pulmonic conduit. For purposes of comparison, similar studies were made of three unimplanted Ionescu-Shiley valves obtained through courtesy of Ionescu-Shiley Laboratories, Inc., Irvine, California.

For histologic study, the tissues were fixed with buffered formalin, embedded in glycolmethacrylate plastic medium, sectioned at a thickness of 1 μ and

From the Pathology and Surgery Branches, National Heart, Lung, and Blood Institute, National Institutes of Health, Bethesda, Maryland.

Address for correspondence: Victor J. Ferrans, M.D., Ph.D., Building 10, Room 7N208, National Institutes of Health, Bethesda, Maryland 20205.

Received May 8, 1980; revision accepted June 30, 1980.

Circulation 63, No. 3, 1981.

stained using the hematoxylin-eosin, alkaline toluidine blue and von Kossa methods. For scanning electron microscopy, the tissues were fixed with phosphate-buffered glutaraldehyde, dehydrated, dried according to the critical point method, coated with gold-palladium, and examined with a JEOL-35C scanning electron microscope at an accelerating voltage of 20 kV.[11] For transmission electron microscopy, tissues were fixed with phosphate-buffered glutaraldehyde and prepared as described previously.[11]

Results

Histologic Observations

On histologic study, the pericardial connective tissue in the leaflets of the implanted valve appeared structurally comparable to that in unimplanted pericardial bioprostheses (figs. 1A and 1B). However, both the inflow and outflow surfaces and the free edge (tip) of each leaflet were covered by a continuous layer of thrombotic material that was 20–180 μ thick (figs. 1B–1D). These surface thrombi were composed of fibrin, erythrocytes and platelets. The thrombi showed basophilic staining in preparations stained with hematoxylin-eosin (fig. 1D) and gave a strongly positive reaction with the von Kossa method (fig. 1C). Pericardial mesothelial cells were not identified in any of the leaflets of the implanted valve or of the unimplanted valves. Small numbers of macrophages were present on the valvular surfaces. Giant cells were not found. A few strongly birefringent fibers that were about 15 μ in diameter were found on the valvular surfaces (figs. 1C–1E), where they had been incorporated into thrombi. These fibers were considered to be cotton fibers.

Scanning Electron Microscopic Observations

The outflow surfaces of the leaflets of unimplanted Ionescu-Shiley valves showed straight or curved grooves 10–20 μ wide (fig. 2A). The inflow surfaces of the same leaflets appeared much rougher in texture than the outflow surfaces, but did not show grooves (fig. 2B). Both the inflow and outflow surfaces of the leaflets of the valve that had been implanted in the patient were covered with thrombi that were directly superimposed on the most superficial layers of valvular collagen (figs. 2C–2F). Some of the grooves in the outflow surfaces of the explanted valve contained platelets, fibrin strands and erythrocytes (fig. 2E), even in areas where the surface adjacent to the grooves was free of thrombus. In areas of calcification of surface thrombi (fig. 2D), the fibrin strands were covered by clumps of finely granular material.

Transmission Electron Microscopic Observations

Observations on ultrathin sections examined by transmission electron microscopy revealed that the calcific deposits consisted of irregularly shaped masses (fig. 3A), usually 0.25–2.2 μ in diameter, composed of very fine needles or plate-like crystals of high electron density (fig. 3B). These crystals averaged 70 Å in thickness. These calcific masses were located between fibrin strands, which were not calcified. The calcific masses often appeared to be superimposed upon remnants of cells, which were identified as platelets, macrophages and leukocytes (fig. 3C). Most of these cells showed extensive degenerative and autolytic changes. The larger calcific masses were extremely dense, and structures associated with these masses were not discernible. A few calcific deposits were associated with the most superficial layers of valvular collagen (fig. 3D). Elastic fibers were not calcified, and there was no evidence of collagen degeneration. Deposits of fibrin were interspersed with the most superficial layers of collagen.

Discussion

Ionescu-Shiley pericardial valves have been used for several years with good clinical results;[12] however, anatomic studies have been made of limited numbers of valves of this type which have been removed after being implanted in patients,[12] and little information is available on the occurrence of calcific deposits in these valves. Calcific deposits are known to develop in other types of bioprostheses,[1] but the time of onset and the rate of deposition of calcium in bioprostheses are not known.

The host factors and tissue factors that cause calcification of bioprostheses are poorly understood. It is not known to what extent conclusions derived from studies of porcine bioprostheses will be applicable to pericardial bioprostheses. Porcine bioprostheses calcify more frequently and to a greater extent in patients who have one or more of the following predisposing conditions: younger than 35 years of age,[1, 3, 4, 7-10, 13-16] chronic renal disease,[1, 2, 10] and infection of the bioprosthesis.[1, 17, 18] Morphologic studies of Ionescu-Shiley valves have been too limited to determine the importance of these factors in predisposing to calcification of this type of bioprosthesis. Our patient was young and did have acute renal insufficiency, but had no evidence of infection in the bioprosthesis.

Ultrastructural studies have demonstrated that the two main anatomic sites of calcification of porcine valvular bioprostheses are collagen fibrils in the leaflets and surface thrombi and vegetations.[1] Evidence has been presented indicating that the initial deposits of calcium phosphate in thrombi and vegetations are localized in mitochondria of blood cells and platelets trapped in the fibrin mesh.[1] In the present study, calcific deposits were demonstrated in collagen and in surface thrombi, but almost all of the deposits were localized in thrombotic material. These deposits were structurally similar to those observed in porcine bioprostheses.[1] Studies in experimental animals have shown that a thin layer of fibrin is deposited on the leaflets of porcine bioprostheses within a few minutes after implantation.[19] In humans, such a layer of fibrin was observed in two Hancock bioprostheses that had been in place for only 2 and 3 days, respectively, but neither contained calcific

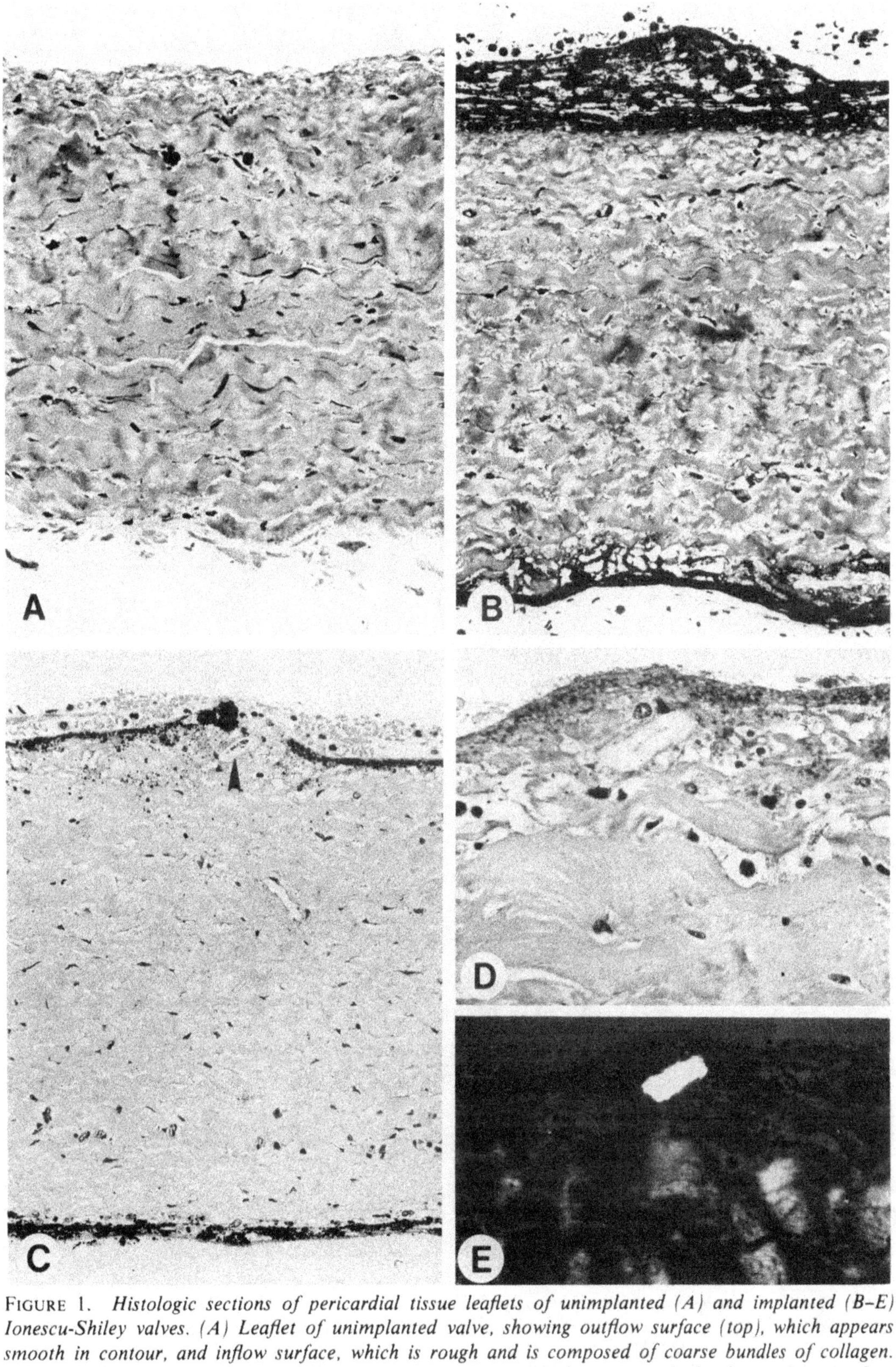

FIGURE 1. *Histologic sections of pericardial tissue leaflets of unimplanted (A) and implanted (B–E) Ionescu-Shiley valves. (A) Leaflet of unimplanted valve, showing outflow surface (top), which appears smooth in contour, and inflow surface, which is rough and is composed of coarse bundles of collagen. Alkaline toluidine blue stain; original magnification × 160. (B) Valve recovered after having been in place for 3 days, showing layer of thrombus covering both the outflow (top) and inflow (bottom) surfaces. Alkaline toluidine blue stain; original magnification × 160. (C) As in (B) but stained by the von Kossa method, to demonstrate calcific deposits (darkly stained) in layer of thrombus. A cotton fiber (arrowhead) is present in thrombus in outflow surface; original magnification × 160. (D) Higher magnification view of area similar to that in (C). The calcific deposits in the thrombus appear as small, dark granules (compare with figure 3A). Hematoxylin-eosin stain; original magnification × 400. (E) Polarization micrograph of area in (D), showing birefringence of cotton fiber; original magnification × 270.*

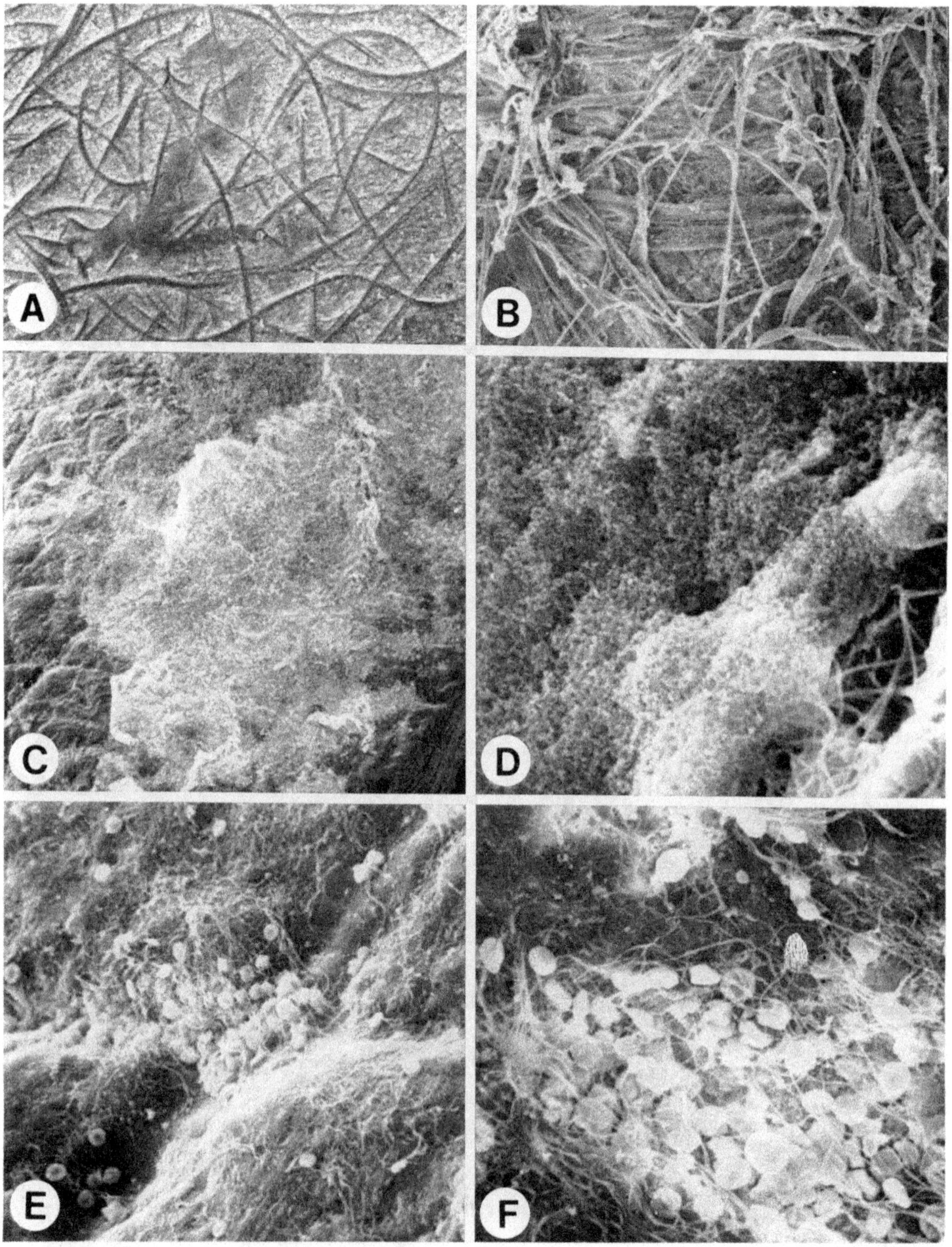

FIGURE 2. *Scanning electron micrographs of unimplanted Ionescu-Shiley valve (A and B) and of valve implanted for 3 days (C–F). (A) Outflow surface of unimplanted valve has numerous grooves that follow straight or curved paths. Magnification × 55. (B) Inflow surface of same leaflet as in (A) is composed of coarse bundles of collagen. No grooves are evident on this surface. Magnification × 55. (C) A thin layer of thrombotic material is present on outflow surface of implanted valve. Magnification × 55. (D) High-magnification view (× 2700) showing finely granular material in calcified thrombus. (E) Erythrocytes are located in two intersecting grooves (one groove runs from bottom left to upper right, and the other from mid-left to mid-right) in outflow surface of the valve. Magnification × 460. (F) High-magnification view (× 920) of small thrombus composed of erythrocytes enmeshed in fibrin.*

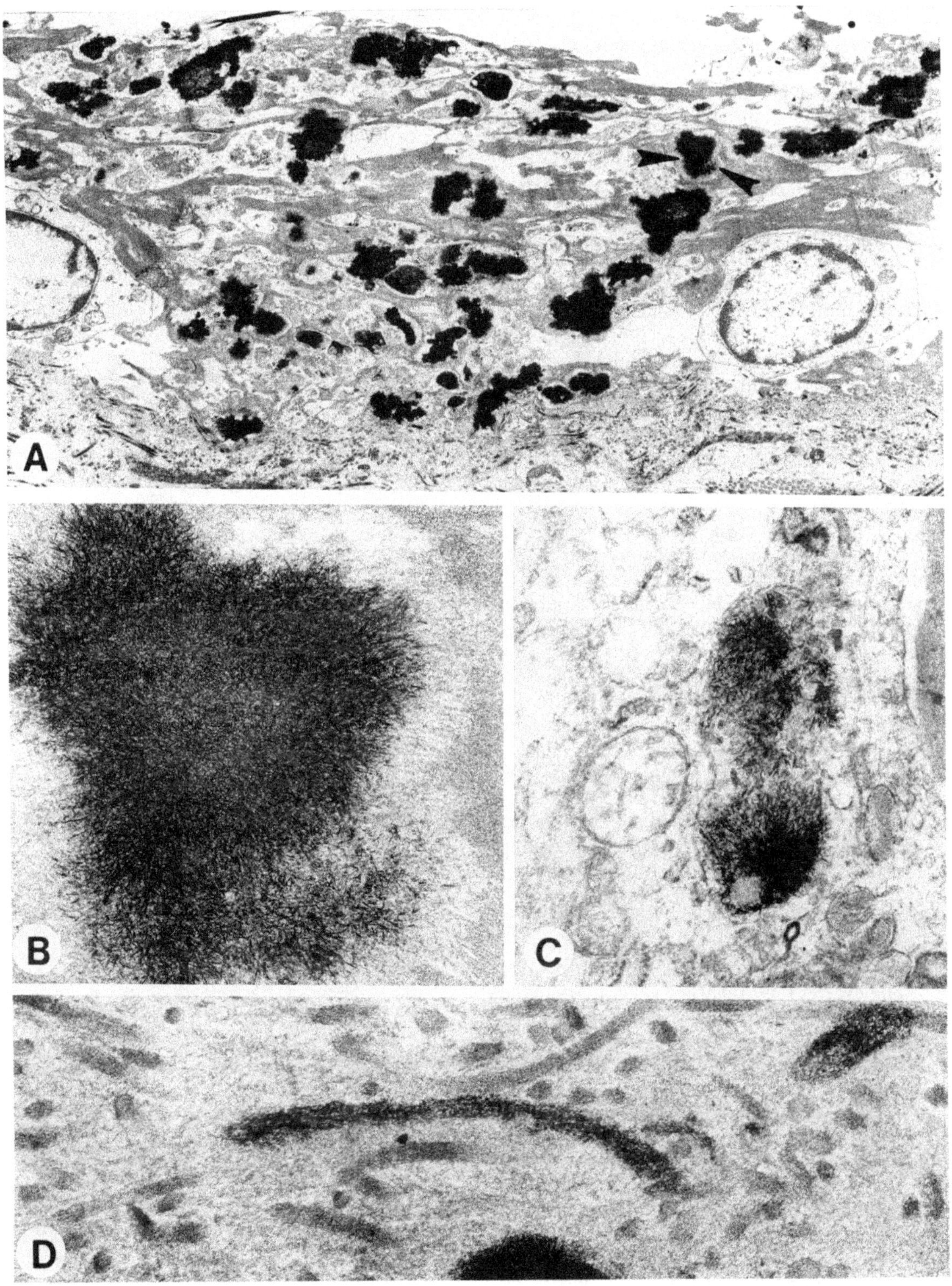

FIGURE 3. *Transmission electron micrographs of valve implanted for 3 days. (A) Low-magnification view of area near free edge of leaflet, showing calcific deposits, which appear black, and mononuclear cells within the mesh of fibrin in thrombus overlying the collagen at the leaflet surface. Arrowheads indicate calcific deposit shown at high magnification in (B). Magnification × 7000. (B) Calcific deposit in thrombus is composed of very fine needle-like crystals. Magnification × 58,500. (C) Calcific deposits are localized within cytoplasm of mononuclear cell. Magnification × 33,500. (D) Calcific deposits (black) overlie collagen fibrils in area near leaflet surface. Magnification × 56,250.*

deposits.[11] Thus, the changes we report apparently represent a very unusual phenomenon of early calcification of this surface layer. These calcific deposits probably would have become the cause of clinically significant bioprosthetic stenosis if our patient had survived longer.

Several factors may have contributed to the early calcification of the bioprosthesis in our patient: the low cardiac output syndrome, which led to renal insufficiency requiring peritoneal dialysis, and the large amounts of calcium chloride given intravenously because of the multiple blood transfusions and at times of resuscitative efforts. Another factor is the presence of proteins in the blood, which function in the coagulation process and which contain γ-carboxyglutamic acid, an unusual amino acid capable of avidly binding calcium.[20, 21] This amino acid has been extracted from calcified (but not from noncalcified) porcine bioprostheses.[20] Its association with calcification of pericardial bioprostheses has not been investigated.

Uptake of calcium by mitochondria of hypoxic or ischemic cells is known to occur not only in myocardium but also in other tissues,[22] and the availability of large amounts of calcium to blood cells incorporated into thrombi may have resulted in significant accumulation of calcium in these cells (thus initiating bioprosthetic calcification) under conditions of hypoxia associated with the low cardiac output state in our patient. The finding of calcific deposits in necrotic myocardial cells as in our patient is not unusual; it is frequently observed in patients who have the low cardiac output syndrome postoperatively.[23]

The cotton fibers on the surfaces of the cusps of the bioprosthesis may have been derived from the packing material in the valve container. Such fibers were not found in pulmonary or myocardial vessels. A fatal coronary embolus was produced by fragments of packing material in a porcine bioprosthesis.[24]

The morphologic observations on the unimplanted Ionescu-Shiley valves reveal marked asymmetry in the texture of the inflow and outflow surfaces of the pericardial tissue leaflets. The inflow surface is very rough and corresponds to the pericardial surface that faces the sternum. In contrast, the outflow surface is much smoother; it contains grooves that appear to have been made by a mechanical process and corresponds to the pericardial surface that faces the heart. These differences, which were consistently observed in the three unimplanted valves examined, provide a basis for the identification of the surfaces of Ionescu-Shiley valves; however, in animal experiments (unpublished observations) we found that the grooves tend to be obscured (as was the case in the valve from our patient) by the deposition of fibrin on the surfaces after the valves are implanted.

References

1. Ferrans VJ, Boyce SW, Billingham ME, Jones M, Ishihara T, Roberts WC: Calcific deposits in porcine bioprostheses: structure and pathogenesis. Am J Cardiol **46**: 721, 1980
2. Hetzer R, Hill JD, Kerth WJ, Wilson AJ, Adappa MG, Gerbode F: Thrombosis and degeneration of Hancock valves: clinical and pathological findings. Ann Thorac Surg **26**: 317, 1978
3. Rose AG, Forman R, Bowen RM: Calcification of glutaraldehyde-fixed porcine xenograft. Thorax **33**: 111, 1978
4. Forfar JC, Cotter L, Morritt GN: Severe and early stenosis of porcine heterograft mitral valve. Br Heart J **40**: 1184, 1978
5. Albert HM, Bryant LR, Schechter FG: Seven year experience with mounted porcine valves. Ann Surg **185**: 717, 1977
6. Bachet J, Bical O, Goudot B, Menu P, Richard T, Barbagelatta M, Guilmet D: Early structural failure of porcine xenografts in young patients. *In* Bioprosthetic Cardiac Valves, edited by Sebening F, Klövekorn WP, Meisner H, Struck E. München, Deutsches Herzzentrum, 1979, pp 341–349
7. Thandroyen FT, Whitton IN, Pirie D, Rogers MA, Mitha AS: Severe calcification of glutaraldehyde-preserved porcine xenografts in children. Am J Cardiol **45**: 690, 1980
8. Silver MM, Pollock J, Silver MD, Williams WG, Trusler GA: Calcification in porcine xenograft valves in children. Am J Cardiol **45**: 685, 1980
9. Sanders SP, Freed MD, Norwood WI, Castaneda A, Nadas AS: Early failure of porcine valves implanted in children. (abstr) Am J Cardiol **45**: 449, 1980
10. Fishbein MC, Gissen SA, Collins JJ Jr, Barsamian EM, Cohn LH: Pathologic findings after cardiac valve replacement with glutaraldehyde-fixed porcine valves. Am J Cardiol **40**: 331, 1977
11. Ferrans VJ, Spray TL, Billingham ME, Roberts WC: Structural changes in glutaraldehyde-treated porcine heterografts used as substitute cardiac valves. Transmission and scanning electron microscopic observations in 12 patients. Am J Cardiol **41**: 1159, 1978
12. Ionescu MI, Tandon AP, Mary DAS, Abid A: Heart valve replacement with the Ionescu-Shiley pericardial xenograft. J Thorac Cardiovasc Surg **73**: 31, 1977
13. Kutsche LM, Oyer P, Shumway N, Baum D: An important complication of Hancock mitral valve replacement in children. Circulation **60** (suppl I): I-98, 1978
14. Brown JW, Dunn JM, Spooner E, Kirsh MM: Late spontaneous disruption of a porcine xenograft mitral valve. Clinical, hemodynamic, echocardiographic, and pathological findings. J Thorac Cardiovasc Surg **75**: 606, 1978
15. Geha AS, Stansel HC Jr, Cornhill JF, Kilman JW, Buckley MJ, Roberts WC: Late failure of porcine valve heterografts in children. J Thorac Cardiovasc Surg **78**: 351, 1979
16. Magilligan DJ Jr, Lewis JW Jr, Jara FM, Stein PD, Riddle JM, Lee MW: Spontaneous degeneration of porcine bioprosthetic valves. Ann Thorac Surg **30**: 259, 1980
17. Zuhdi N: The porcine aortic valve bioprosthesis: a significant alternative. Ann Thorac Surg **21**: 573, 1976
18. Magilligan DJ Jr, Quinn EL, Davila JC: Bacteremia, endocarditis, and the Hancock valve. Ann Thorac Surg **24**: 508, 1977
19. Geroulanos S, Gossler W, Walpoth B, Turina M, Senning A: Frühe rasterelektronenoptische Oberflächenveränderungen nach orthotoper Pulmonalklappen-Xenotransplantation durch glutaraldehyd-konditionierte Schweineklappen. Eine experimentelle Studie an Hunden. Helv Chir Acta **46**: 91, 1979
20. Levy RJ, Lian JB: Studies on the etiology of calcific aortic valve disease: the role of the calcium binding amino acid, γ-carboxyglutamic acid. (abstr) Circulation **58** (suppl II): II-54, 1978
21. Levy RJ, Zenker JA, Lian JB: Vitamin K-dependent calcium binding proteins in aortic valve calcification. J Clin Invest **65**: 563, 1980
22. Trump BF, Berezesky IK, Laiho KU, Osornio AR, Mergner WJ, Smith MW: The role of calcium in cell injury. A review. Scan Electron Microsc 1980. In press
23. Reichenbach DD, Benditt EP: Catecholamines and cardiomyopathy: the pathogenesis and potential importance of myofibrillar degeneration. Hum Pathol **1**: 125, 1970
24. Tubbs RR, Picha GC, Levin HS, Groves L, Barenberg S: Cotton emboli (cellulose II polymorph, "rayon") of the coronary arteries. Hum Pathol **11**: 76, 1980

Structure of bovine parietal pericardium and of unimplanted Ionescu-Shiley pericardial valvular bioprostheses

To obtain a basis for the evaluation of postimplantation changes in bioprostheses made of parietal pericardium, we conducted comparative histologic, scanning and transmission electron microscopic studies of the structure of (1) normal bovine parietal pericardium, (2) glutaraldehyde-treated pericardial patches to be used for repair of cardiac defects, and (3) pericardial tissue cusps of unimplanted Ionescu-Shiley valves. Bovine parietal pericardium has three layers: (1) the serosa, or mesothelial cell layer; (2) the fibrosa, formed by diversely oriented, wavy bundles of collagen and by elastic fibers, and (3) the epipericardial connective tissue layer, which is partly continuous with the pericardiosternal ligaments. Pericardial patches and pericardial bioprosthetic cusps differ from normal pericardium by being denuded of mesothelium but they have normal degrees of waviness in their collagen. In Ionescu-Shiley valves, the inflow and outflow surfaces of each cusp correspond to the epipericardial and serosal surfaces of parietal pericardium, respectively. The inflow surfaces have a coarse texture, characterized by large bundles of collagen, and the outflow surfaces have numerous grooves, 10 to 30 μ in width and 20 μ in depth, which probably result from pressure exerted on the cuspidal surfaces by cotton material either during manufacturing or packing of the valves. Comparisons of the structure of bioprosthetic pericardial cusps and porcine aortic valve cusps show that the latter have reduced degrees of collagen waviness and a different layered structure: A layer similar to the spongiosa of aortic valve cusps is not present in pericardium. The functional implications of these observations are discussed in detail.

Tokuhiro Ishihara, M.D., Ph.D., Victor J. Ferrans, M.D., Ph.D., Michael Jones, M.D., Steven W. Boyce, B.A., and William C. Roberts, M.D., *Bethesda, Md.*

Detailed knowledge of the structural features of bioprosthetic cardiac valves is a prerequisite for evaluation of their performance under conditions of experimental testing and clinical use. Ultrastructural examination has been of value in assessing the changes that develop in porcine valvular bioprostheses after implantation in patients[1-3]; however, only very limited morphologic studies have been made of postimplantation changes in valvular bioprostheses made of bovine parietal pericardium.[4-8] Furthermore, porcine aortic valves differ structurally from parietal pericardium in a number of important respects, and it is not known to what extent the conclusions derived from studies of porcine bioprostheses are applicable to pericardial bioprostheses. To obtain a basis for evaluating postimplantation changes in these valves, we conducted the present studies, which characterized the structure of bovine parietal pericardium and unimplanted Ionescu-Shiley bovine pericardial valves.

From the Pathology Branch and the Surgery Branch, National Heart, Lung and Blood Institute, National Institutes of Health, Bethesda, Md. 20205.

Received for publication July 18, 1980.

Accepted for publication Oct. 27, 1980.

Address for reprints: Victor J. Ferrans, M.D., Ph.D., National Heart, Lung and Blood Institute, National Institutes of Health, Building 10, Room 7N208, Bethesda, Md. 20205.

Materials and methods

Comparative light and electron microscopic studies were made of the following: (1) normal bovine parietal pericardium obtained from the ventral (anterior) region of pericardium from three animals, each approximately 2 years of age; (2) bovine parietal pericardial cusps of three unimplanted Ionescu-Shiley valves (Shiley Laboratories, Inc., Irvine, Calif.); and (3) two unimplanted bovine pericardial patches (Edwards Laboratories, Inc., Santa Ana, Calif.). The pericardial tissue in the Ionescu-

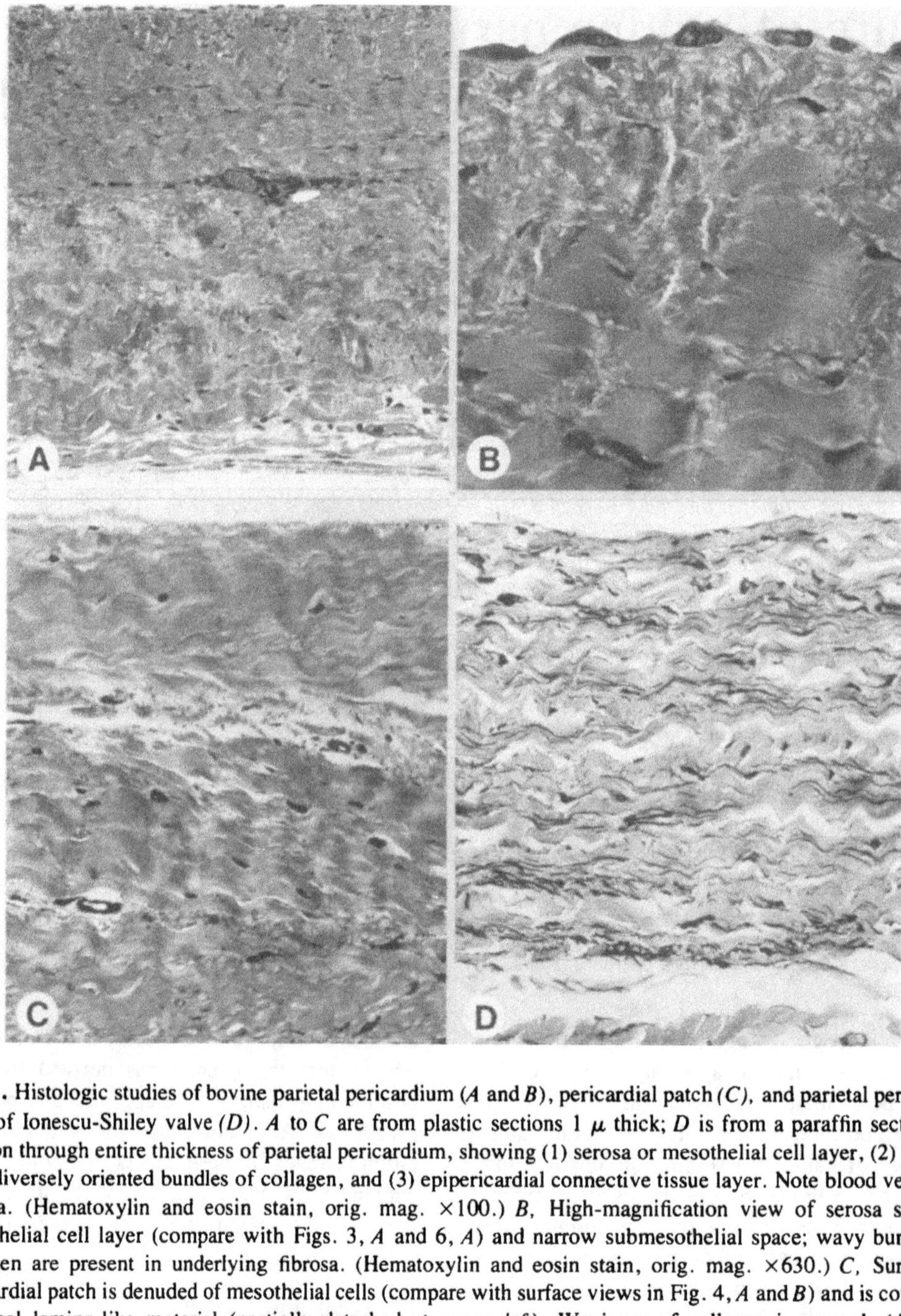

Fig. 1. Histologic studies of bovine parietal pericardium (*A* and *B*), pericardial patch (*C*), and parietal pericardial cusp of Ionescu-Shiley valve (*D*). *A* to *C* are from plastic sections 1 μ thick; *D* is from a paraffin section. *A*, Section through entire thickness of parietal pericardium, showing (1) serosa or mesothelial cell layer, (2) fibrosa, with diversely oriented bundles of collagen, and (3) epipericardial connective tissue layer. Note blood vessels in fibrosa. (Hematoxylin and eosin stain, orig. mag. ×100.) *B*, High-magnification view of serosa showing mesothelial cell layer (compare with Figs. 3, *A* and 6, *A*) and narrow submesothelial space; wavy bundles of collagen are present in underlying fibrosa. (Hematoxylin and eosin stain, orig. mag. ×630.) *C*, Surface of pericardial patch is denuded of mesothelial cells (compare with surface views in Fig. 4, *A* and *B*) and is composed of basal lamina-like material (partially detached at *upper left*). Waviness of collagen is normal. (Alkaline toluidine blue stain, orig. mag. ×250.) *D*, Elastic fibers (stained *black*) are distributed throughout pericardial cusp of Ionescu-Shiley valve. (Movat stain, orig. mag. ×160.)

Shiley valves is prepared by treatment with 0.5% glutaraldehyde, and the finished valves are stored in 4% formaldehyde.[4] The pericardial tissue patches are prepared by treatment with 0.625% glutaraldehyde, further sterilized with formalin, and are stored in 0.625% glutaraldehyde.

For light microscopic study, strips of parietal pericardium, pericardial valve cusps, and pericardial patches were fixed in buffered formalin, dehydrated, and embedded either in paraffin or in glycolmethacrylate. The fresh bovine parietal pericardium was maintained in its in vivo dimensions during fixation by being

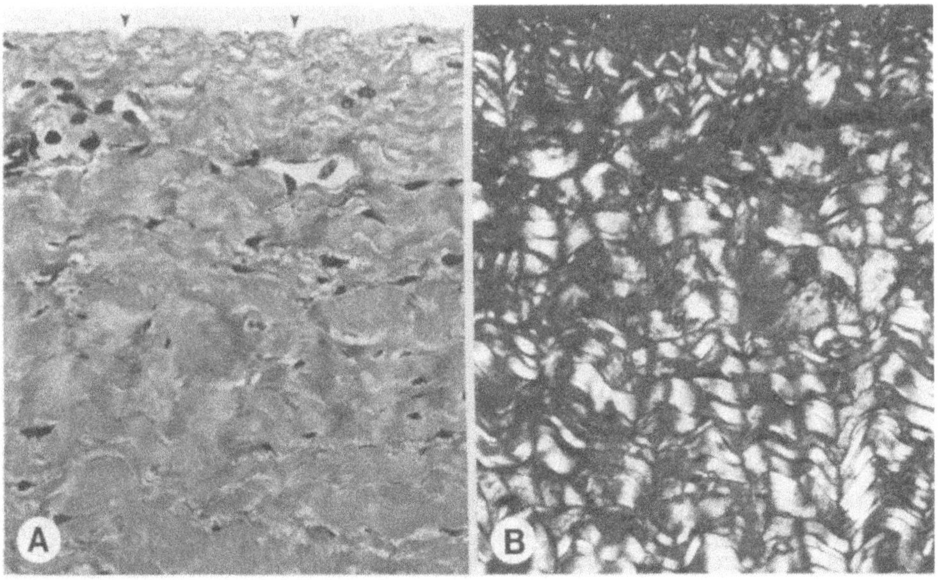

Fig. 2. Histologic studies of cusps of Ionescu-Shiley valve. *A*, Outflow (serosal) surface showing indentations *(arrowheads)* in surface (compare with surface views in Fig. 4, *B* and *D*), which is denuded of mesothelium. Collagen waviness is normal. *B*, Polarization photomicrograph of area similar to that in *A*, showing birefringence and waviness of collagen bundles. (*A* and *B*, Plastic sections stained with hematoxylin and eosin, orig. mag. ×250.)

pinned to a corkboard. Sections of paraffin blocks were stained with hematoxylin and eosin, Masson trichrome, and Movat pentachrome methods. Sections of glycolmethacrylate-embedded tissues were stained with hematoxylin and eosin and alkaline toluidine blue. It proved difficult to obtain completely artifact-free histologic sections of paraffin-embedded parietal pericardium (i.e., free of cracks, artifactual separation of collagen bundles, and artifactual loss of mesothelial cells); for this reason, glycolmethacrylate embedding was preferred for detailed study of this tissue. Nevertheless, since the variety of staining techniques (particularly connective tissue stains) that can be applied to glycolmethacrylate-embedded tissues is limited, both embedding techniques were necessary.

For scanning and transmission electron microscopic study, tissues were fixed with 3% glutaraldehyde in 0.1M phosphate buffer, pH 7.2, and washed with several changes of 5% sucrose in 0.1M phosphate buffer, pH 7.2. For scanning electron microscopy, the tissues were dehydrated, dried by the critical point method, coated with a layer of gold-palladium, and examined with a scanning electron microscope with accelerating voltages of 12 to 20 kV. For transmission electron microscopy, tissues were embedded in Maraglas resin and studied according to techniques previously described in detail.[1]

Results

Light microscopic observations.

Parietal pericardium. Normal bovine parietal pericardium varied in overall thickness from 0.3 to 0.7 mm and was composed of three well-defined layers: the serosa, the fibrosa, and the epipericardial connective tissue layer (Fig. 1, *A* and *B*). The serosa was formed by the surface layer of thin, flattened mesothelial cells facing the pericardial cavity and by a narrow submesothelial space. The fibrosa contained flattened, overlapping bundles of collagen which had a wavy appearance and were oriented in various directions. Elastic fibers also were present throughout the thickness of the fibrosa. The elastic fibers immediately subjacent to the mesothelium were smaller than those in deeper areas of the fibrosa. Scattered between the collagen bundles were connective tissue cells and vascular and neural elements. The connective tissue cells consisted mainly of greatly flattened, elongated fibroblasts and a few histiocytes and mast cells; adipose tissue cells were occasionally located in the fibrosa. The blood vessels coursed parallel to the surface and extended toward the serosa. The epipericardial connective tissue layer also contained collagen bundles, blood vessels, nerves, and variable numbers of adipose tissue cells. The adipose tissue cells tended to occur in clusters.

Pericardial patches. The most striking histologic

differences between native parietal pericardium (Fig. 1, *A* and *B*) and parietal pericardial patches (Fig. 1, *C*) were (1) complete loss of mesothelial cells from the serosal surface, which left exposed submesothelial connective tissue in the surface, and (2) loss of the clusters of adipose tissue cells present in the epipericardial surface. The patches ranged from 0.6 to 0.8 mm in overall thickness. Thus they were slightly thicker than native bovine parietal pericardium obtained for histologic studies. The serosal surfaces of pericardial patches were smooth; the epipericardial surfaces showed variable degrees of roughness.

Cusps of unimplanted Ionescu-Shiley valves. In the pericardial cusps of unimplanted Ionescu-Shiley valves, the serosal surface also was denuded of mesothelial cells and the epipericardial surface was free of adipose tissue cells (Figs. 1, *D* and 2, *A* and *B*). In each of the cusps, the serosal surface of the pericardium corresponded to the outflow surface of the bioprosthetic valve, and the epipericardial surface of the tissue corresponded to the inflow surface of the valve. As defined previously,[1] the outflow surface is that which faces the ventricle when the bioprosthesis is placed in the atrioventricular position, and that which faces either the aorta or the pulmonary trunk when the bioprosthesis is placed in the semilunar position. On gross anatomic inspection of Ionescu-Shiley valves, the outflow surfaces were much smoother than the inflow surfaces. This was a consequence of the coarseness of the collagen bundles in the epipericardial connective tissue layer, where they had been transected from their attachments to the dorsal surface of the sternum (pericardiosternal ligaments). The outflow surfaces of Ionescu-Shiley valves (Fig. 2, *A*) showed identations that measured from 10 to 30 μ in width and from 10 to 20 μ in depth. Cotton fibers were occasionally found on both surfaces. The collagen in the cuspal fibrosa (Fig. 2, *B*) showed a waviness comparable to that in normal bovine pericardium. The two surfaces of each cusp were parallel to each other, and the thickness of each cusp (range 0.4 to 0.6 mm) was comparable to that of normal bovine pericardium.

Scanning electron microscopic observations.

Normal bovine parietal pericardium. The serosal surface of parietal pericardium (Fig. 3, *A* to *D*) was completely covered by a continuous, single layer of mesothelial cells, which were polygonal and ranged from 10 to 15 μ in the largest dimension. The free surfaces of the mesothelial cells were characterized by the presence of numerous microvilli, which were 0.1 μ in width and 1 μ in length (Fig. 3, *A* and *B*). In addition, single cilia were encountered in most cells (Fig. 3, *C*). The cilia were 2 μ long and 0.2 μ wide. Thus they were larger than microvilli. In the majority of the cells, the microvilli tended to be more numerous in central than in peripheral areas (Fig. 3, *A*). In other cells, however, microvilli were very sparse in central areas (Fig. 3, *B*), and such areas were raised above the remainder of the surface. When parietal pericardium was subjected to excessive stretch (Fig. 3, *D*), the mesothelial cells became greatly elongated and appeared to be separated from adjacent cells by deep grooves. In areas in which the mesothelial cells had been denuded (Fig. 3, *E* and *F*), the pericardial surface was composed of fine, irregularly shaped fibrillar material, which was considered to represent basal lamina material and connective tissue microfibrils. At low magnification, the surface contour in these areas very much resembled a replica of the mesothelial surface, and discrete bundles of collagen did not form part of this surface. The epipericardial surface was composed of collagen bundles of variable size; however, as will be described later, this surface was smoother in normal pericardium than in the commercially processed pericardial patches and Ionescu-Shiley valves.

Pericardial patches. The surfaces of pericardial patches (Fig. 4, *A* to *C*) differed in several respects from the surfaces of Ionescu-Shiley valvular cusps (Fig. 4, *D* to *F*). The serosal surface of pericardial patches (Fig. 4, *A*) appeared relatively smooth, and in many areas it was morphologically similar to areas of parietal pericardium that had been denuded of mesothelial cells. At low magnification, the surface contour of these areas again resembled a replica of the mesothelial surface. These areas were covered by finely fibrillar basal lamina material. In other areas, this material had been lost, so that the bundles of collagen subjacent to the basal lamina were exposed (Fig. 4, *C*). Some of these bundles were well defined and had a wavy appearance; however, others showed considerable fraying and separation into smaller fibrils that followed tortuous courses. The epipericardial surfaces of the patches (Fig. 4, *E*) were composed of extremely rough bundles of collagen that coursed in various directions. These bundles were considerably larger and much less frayed than those in the serosal surface.

Cusps of unimplanted Ionescu-Shiley valves. The inflow surfaces of the cusps of unimplanted Ionescu-Shiley valves were morphologically indistinguishable from the epipericardial surfaces of the pericardial patches. Cotton fibers were occasionally found between the collagen bundles in the inflow surfaces of the cusps

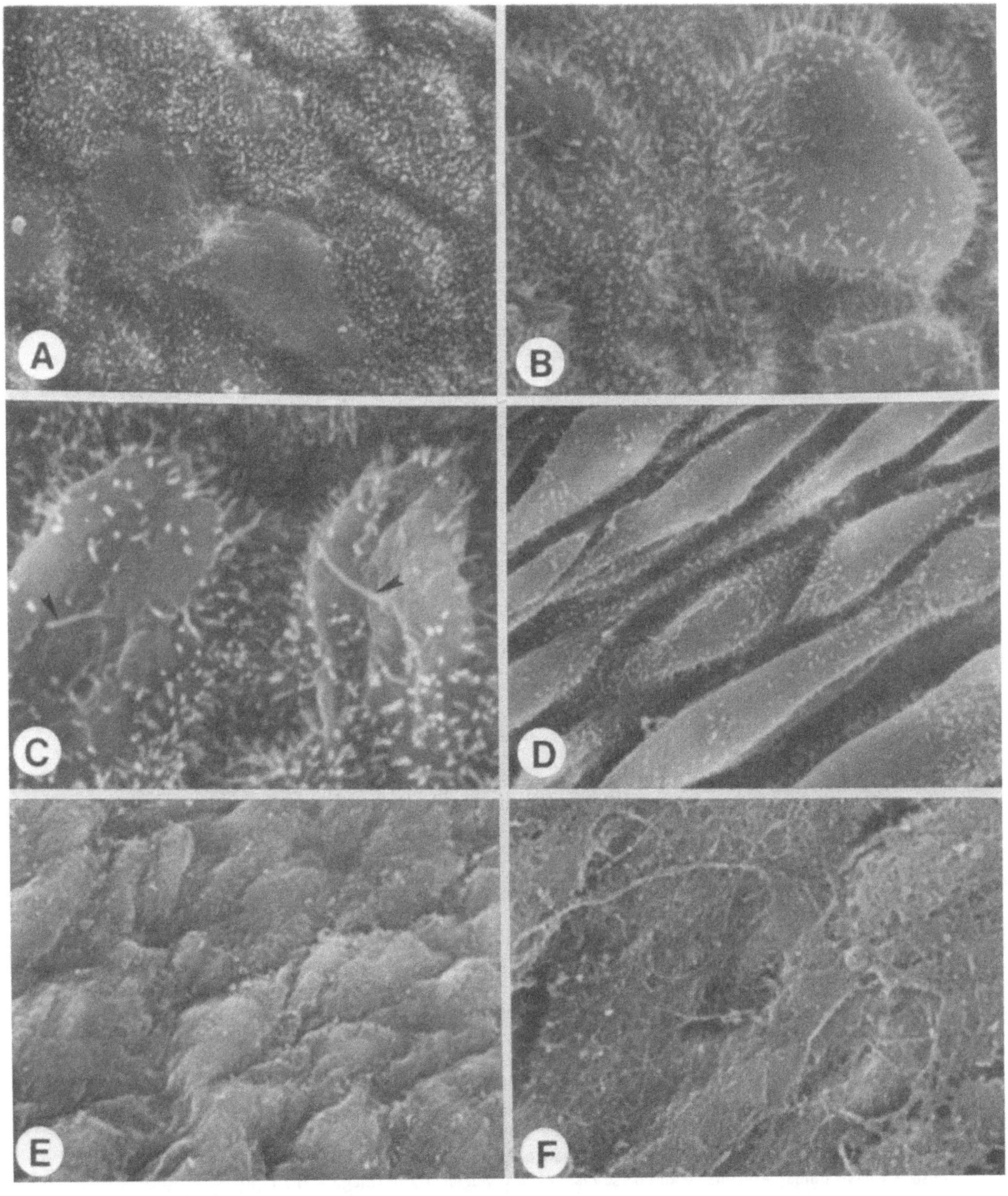

Fig. 3. Scanning electron micrographs of normal bovine parietal pericardium. *A*, Mesothelial cells are polygonal and have numerous surface microvilli. (×1,400.) *B*, Variations in distribution of surface microvilli (×3,750.) *C*, Cilia *(arrowheads)* are present in the surface of two mesothelial cells. (×5,500.) *D*, Mesothelial cells appear elongated in pericardium fixed under stretch. Compare with *A*. (×1,850.) *E*, Pericardial serosal surface in area denuded of mesothelial cells resembles replica of mesothelial cells. (×1,650.) *F*, Higher-magnification view of area similar to that in *E*, showing finely fibrillar material forming surface. (×3,700.)

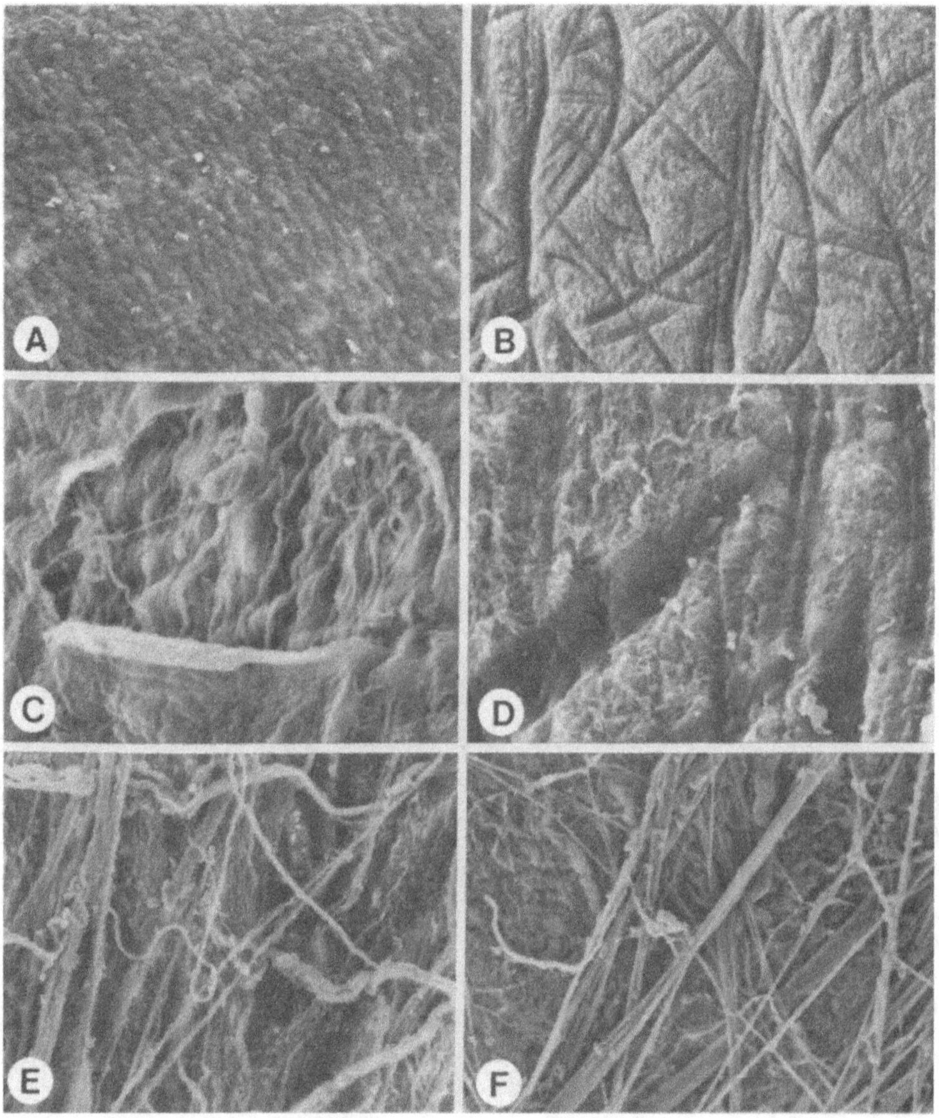

Fig. 4. Scanning electron micrographs of pericardial patch (*A*, *C* and *E*) and cusp of Ionescu-Shiley valve (*B*, *D* and *F*). *A*, Serosal surface of pericardial patch appears similar to that of parietal pericardium denuded of mesothelial cells (compare with Fig. 3, *E* and *F*). Surface ridges reflect the orientation of subjacent collagen bundles. (Orig. mag. ×130.) *B*, Outflow surface of Ionescu-Shiley valve cusp corresponds to serosal surface of pericardium but has completely different appearance because of presence of grooves. (Orig. mag. ×100.) *C*, High-magnification view of serosal surface of pericardial patch in area in which basal lamina has been torn and underlying collagen is exposed. (Orig. mag. ×520.) *D*, High-magnification view of outflow surface of Ionescu-Shiley valve cusp, showing ridges in grooves and fine, frayed collagen fibrils in surfaces between grooves. (Orig. mag. ×640.) *E* and *F*, Epipericardial surface of pericardial patch *(E)* and inflow surface of Ionescu-Shiley valve cusp *(F)* have similar structure, with coarse bundles of collagen. (Orig. mag. ×110.)

(Fig. 5, *A*). The outflow surfaces of the cusps of Ionescu-Shiley valves had a characteristic appearance, which was due to the presence of numerous grooves (Figs. 4, *B* and *D*). These grooves were shallow, usually not more than 20 μ in depth. They ranged from 10 to 30 μ in width and followed straight or curved paths. The bottom and sides of the grooves were considerably smoother than the surface areas between the grooves. Some of the grooves showed fine, longitudinally oriented striations. These striations resembled those present in the cotton fibers in the packing material used to maintain the shapes of the cusps (Fig. 5, *B*). The

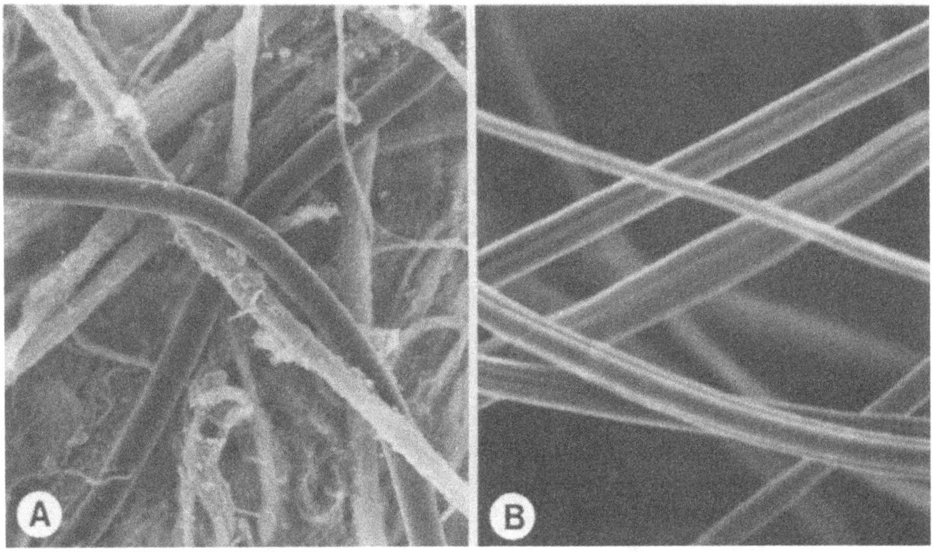

Fig. 5. Scanning electron micrographs of cotton fibers on inflow surface of Ionescu-Shiley valve cusp *(A)* and in packing material. Compare ridges *(B)* with those in valvular surfaces shown in Fig. 4, *B* and *D*. (Orig. mag.: *A*, ×330; *B*, ×280.)

outflow surface areas between the grooves had a very uniform appearance, and at low magnification they seemed very smooth. However, high-magnification study (Fig. 4, *E*) showed that they were constituted by very small, frayed, tangled collagen fibrils which followed irregular courses in different directions. No basal lamina-like material was observed in these surfaces.

Transmission electron microscopic observations. *Normal bovine pericardium.* The mesothelial cells forming the serosa had a flattened shape (Fig. 6, *A*) and were connected to one another by intercellular junctions (Fig. 6, *C* and *D*). The luminal surfaces had a finely filamentous glycocalyx or external lamina on the outer leaflet of the plasma membrane (Fig. 6, *D*). The microvilli contained a core of microfilaments 40 to 75 Å in diameter (Fig. 6, *B*). These filaments also extended into subjacent regions of the cytoplasm. The intercellular junctions were convoluted, often redundant, and consisted of zonulae occludentes (Fig. 6, *D*) (mainly located near the luminal and abluminal terminations of the areas of intercellular apposition) and of desmosomes (Fig. 6, *C*) (which were more irregularly distributed). The cytoplasm of mesothelial cells contained a few mitochondria, cisternae of rough-surfaced endoplasmic reticulum, lysosomes, coated and uncoated vesicles, Golgi complexes, free ribosomes, and two types of cytoplasmic filaments: actin-like filaments, similar to those in the cores of the microvilli, and cytoskeletal filaments (100 Å in diameter) (Fig. 6, *C* and *D*). The latter often formed bundles that were associated with desmosomes. The nuclei were flattened and were composed of the outer and inner nuclear membranes, the nuclear chromatin. Nucleoli were not prominent. The basal surfaces of the mesothelial cells varied from smooth to moderately irregular in contour. Finely fibrillar basal lamina material (Fig. 6, *D*) was present along the basal surfaces but did not form a discrete bandlike zone. Instead, this material merged into the immediately subjacent layer of connective tissue components, which consisted of connective tissue microfibrils and collagen fibrils. The microfibrils were oriented parallel to the basal surfaces of the cells, were 100 to 150 Å in diameter, and appeared morphologically similar to the microfibrils associated with elastic fibers. The collagen fibrils usually formed an interlacing network and, in general, they were also parallel to the basal surfaces of the cells. The following extracellular components of connective tissue were identified in the fibrosa: collagen fibrils, elastic fibers, connective tissue microfibrils, and proteoglycan granules. The collagen fibrils showed a considerable range of variation in size, from 300 to 1,400 Å. The elastic fibers were relatively large, 0.05 to 2 μ in diameter, and had their usual two components: amorphous (elastin) cores and peripherally located microfibrils. The latter were 100 to 150 Å in diameter, were similar to connective tissue microfibrils elsewhere, and were arranged parallel to the longitudinal axes of the elastic fibers. The proteoglycan granules and spicules were similar to those described in a variety of other tissues. In some areas, they

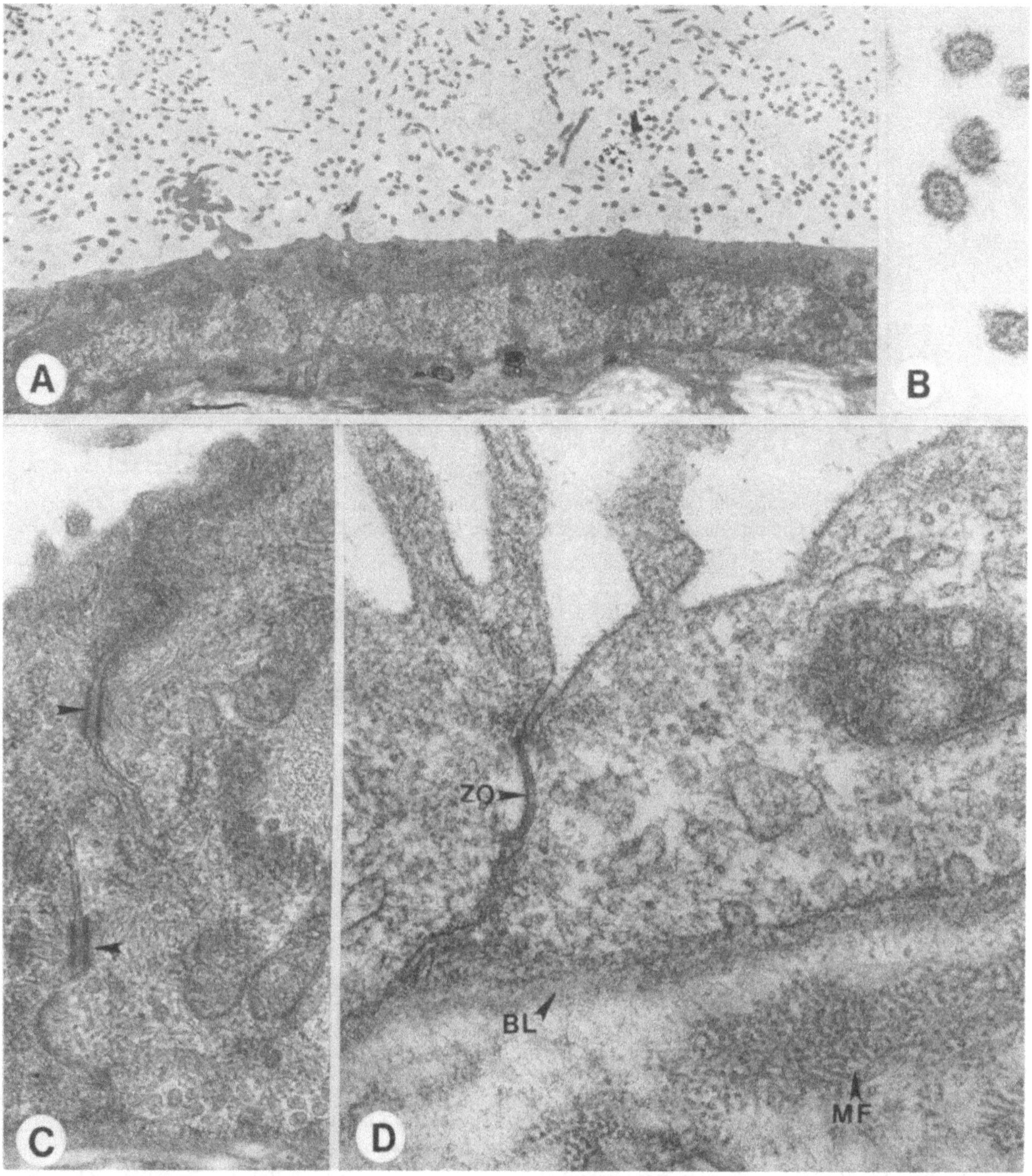

Fig. 6. Transmission electron micrographs of bovine parietal pericardium. *A,* Mesothelial cell has greatly flattened nucleus and numerous surface microvilli. (×12,000.) *B,* Cross-section of microvilli, showing their surface covering (glycocalyx) and their content of fine (actin-like) cytoplasmic filaments. (×80,000.) *C,* Two desmosomes *(arrowheads)* associated with 100 Å cytoplasmic filaments form part of junction between two adjacent mesothelial cells. (×36,800.) *D,* Area of junction between two cells, showing zonula occludens *(ZO),* longitudinally sectioned microvilli *(upper left),* mesothelial basal lamina *(BL),* and underlying bundles of connective tissue microfibrils *(MF).* (×74,200.)

formed a loosely arranged network that extended between collagen fibers. As mentioned previously, connective tissue cells found in parietal pericardium were fibroblasts, histiocytes, and mast cells; in addition, blood vessels and unmyelinated nerve fibers were encountered.

Pericardial patches. The serosal surfaces of pericardial patches (Fig. 7, *A*) were relatively smooth and were composed of collagen fibrils and connective tissue microfibrils. Mesothelial cells were completely absent, and some proteoglycan material appeared to have been lost from the tissue. The structure of the collagen fibrils and elastic fibers was similar to that in normal pericardium. However, adjacent bundles of collagen were more widely separated from one another. In addition, the quality of ultrastructural preservation of cellular elements was adequate only in certain areas; in others, the cells showed moderate autolytic changes.

Cusps of unimplanted Ionescu-Shiley valves. The outflow surfaces (i.e., serosal surfaces) of cusps of unimplanted Ionescu-Shiley valves differed ultrastructurally from the serosal surfaces of the pericardial patches in that the cusps lacked the layer of connective tissue microfibrils that formed the surface of the patches. This layer had been removed together with the mesothelial cells. The grooves observed on scanning electron microscopic study could not be identified. Some proteoglycan material appeared to have been lost. As in pericardial patches, collagen bundles were separated by clear spaces (Fig. 7, *B* and *C*). Preservation of other extracellular components of connective tissue was adequate, and cellular elements showed variable degrees of autolytic change.

Discussion

Structure of parietal pericardium. The structure of bovine parietal pericardium is basically similar to that in the human being.[9] The main difference between the two tissues is the greater thickness of bovine parietal pericardium. The mesothelial cells have shorter and less numerous microvilli in bovine pericardium than in human pericardium. Bovine pericardium also tends to have more numerous cells with flat surfaces containing very few microvilli. The microvilli on the pericardial surface are thought to function as friction-bearing structures and as a means of increasing the surface area available for fluid and solute transport.[9] The intercellular junctions provide specialized attachment devices for maintaining adhesion between adjacent cells and for providing permeability seals. The arrangement of the collagen in the pericardial fibrosa is characterized by two important features: (1) a multidirectional orientation of the bundles and (2) a waviness of the collagen fibrils within each bundle. This waviness and the multidirectionality of the collagen bundles are similar to those previously noted in human parietal pericardium. Both of these features are to be regarded as important determinants of the mechanical properties of parietal pericardial tissue. The orientation of the bundles permits multidirectional stretch. Since collagen fibrils are extremely inextensible, the degree to which parietal pericardium can be stretched would appear to be a function of three factors: (1) the amount of realignment that the variously oriented collagen bundles would undergo in response to unidirectional stretch; (2) the behavior of the elastic fibers in the tissue; and (3) the extent of waviness of the collagen, as this waviness disappears as the tissue is stretched.[9]

From their structural and engineering studies of porcine valves, Broom and Thomson[10] concluded that (1) the collagen in porcine valves fixed without pressure is wavy, (2) this waviness disappears when the valves are fixed under pressure, as is done during commercial processing of porcine bioprostheses, and (3) the waviness is important in equalizing the distribution of the mechanical forces that are applied to collagen during valvular opening and closure. Thus these studies suggest that preservation of the waviness of collagen in bioprosthetic valve cusps is highly desirable.

Comparison of cuspal structure in porcine valves and pericardial valves. The collagen in parietal pericardial cusps of Ionescu-Shiley valves has a waviness similar to that of parietal pericardium not subjected to commercial processing. This waviness is greater than that in collagen of cusps of porcine bioprostheses. The cuspal tissue in the latter bioprostheses also differs from that in pericardial bioprostheses in several other important respects. Pericardial tissue can be regarded as a single, relatively homogeneous sheet of multidirectional bundles of collagen and elastic fibers. In contrast, porcine aortic valve cusps are structurally very nonhomogeneous.[1] They have three well defined layers: (1) the ventricularis, which contains collagen and elastic fibers and faces the inflow surface; (2) the spongiosa, which is centrally located and contains loosely arranged collagen and large amounts of proteoglycans; and (3) the fibrosa, which contains very few, small elastic fibers and numerous, densely packed bundles of collagen oriented parallel to the free edge of the cusp (the preceding considerations concerning the waviness of collagen apply mainly to collagen in the fibrosa). Thus the arrangement of the collagen and the

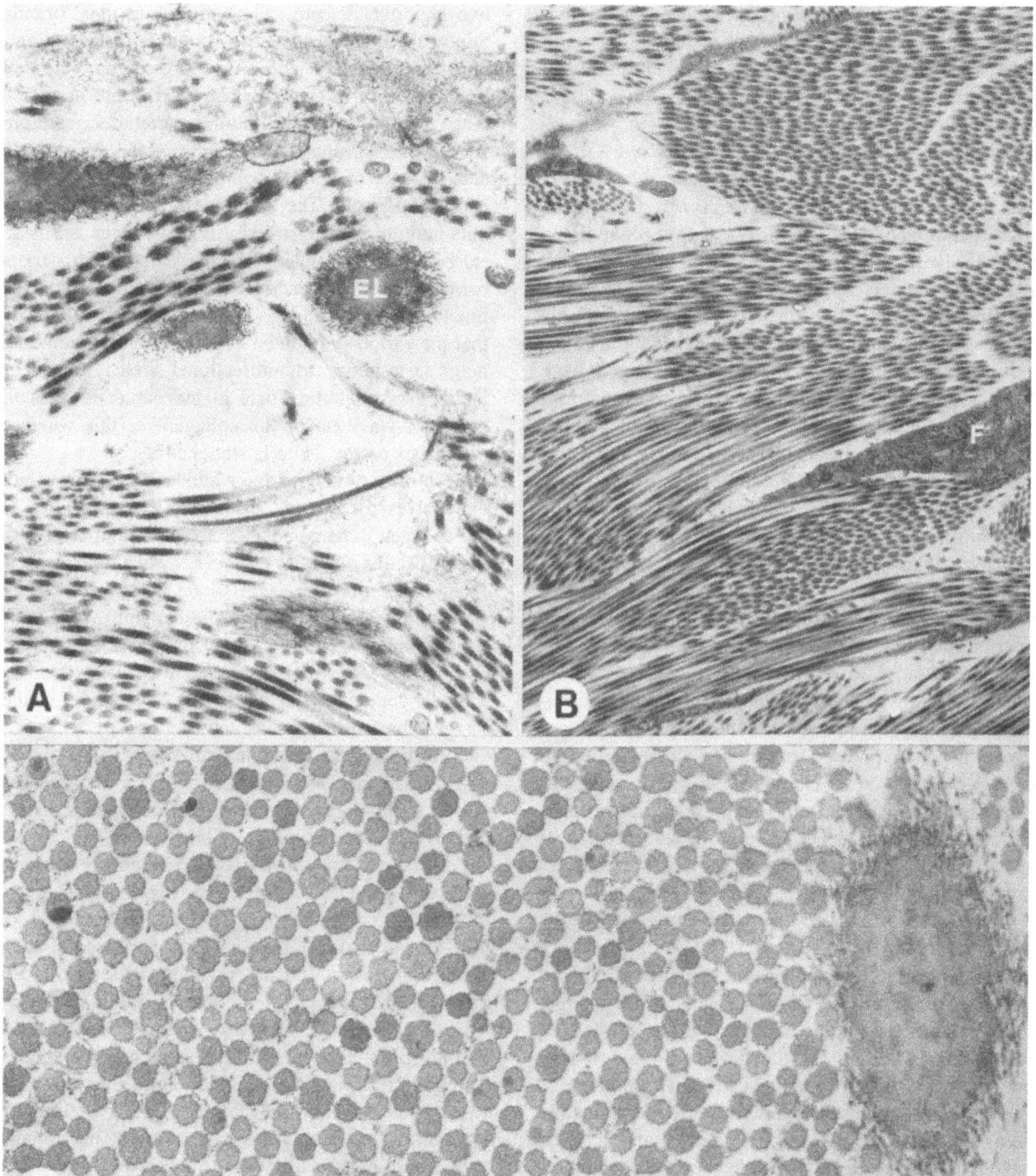

Fig. 7. Connective tissue structure in pericardial patch *(A)* and Ionescu-Shiley valve cusp (*B* and *C*). *A*, Serosal surface of patch *(top)* is composed of connective tissue microfibrils and collagen fibrils (compare with Fig. 6, *D*). Elastic fibers *(EL)* also are present near surface. (×18,700.) *B*, Multidirectional bundles of collagen in cuspal fibrosa. A pericardial fibroblast *(F)* is also shown. (×10,000.) *C*, High-magnification view of cross sections of collagen fibrils and elastic fiber *(right)* in cuspidal fibrosa. There is considerable variation in diameters of collagen fibrils. Elastic fiber shows normal elastin core and peripherally located microfibrils. (×52,600.)

distribution of the elastic fibers are entirely different in parietal pericardium and in aortic valve cusps. In addition, parietal pericardium lacks the central layer (spongiosa) of proteoglycan material, which would appear to dampen friction between the two outer layers of porcine valves. Nevertheless, much of the proteoglycan material is lost from the spongiosa of porcine valves during commercial processing and after implantation so that there are empty spaces into which plasma proteins and blood elements can penetrate.[1] In addition, these spaces can become sites of "delamination" and calcification.[3] These spaces are not present in parietal pericardial cusps; however, these cusps do not have any barriers to the penetration of plasma proteins or blood elements, and their bundles of collagen are more widely separated from one another than is the case in unprocessed pericardium. Pericardial cusps contain small blood vessels, which course between the bundles of collagen without disrupting their continuity; however, it remains to be determined whether, after they are stiffened by fixation, these vessels can withstand repeated cycles of bending without breaking and becoming sites of structural weakness. In porcine valves, blood vessels are smaller, very few in number, and limited in distribution to the basal regions of the cusps.

Comparison of surface structure in porcine valves and pericardial valves. Each of the surfaces of the cusps of pericardial and porcine bioprostheses lacks a cellular lining layer. Nevertheless, both the inflow and outflow surfaces of pericardial cusps differ from the corresponding surfaces of porcine aortic valve cusps. The inflow surfaces of pericardial cusps are extremely rough, much more so than the inflow surfaces of porcine aortic valve cusps. Some of this roughness is inherent to the epipericardial surface, and some is acquired during processing, perhaps in the course of the mechanical cleaning and removal of adipose tissue. It remains to be determined whether platelets and fibrin will tend to accumulate in the interstices of this rough surface after implantation. It seems preferable to place this rough surface on the inflow side of the valve (as has been done by the manufacturer), where the forces of flow would tend to minimize these accumulations.

The outflow surfaces of Ionescu-Shiley pericardial cusps have a unique appearance, which is due to the presence of numerous shallow grooves. These are not evident in the inflow surfaces of these valves or in either of the surfaces of unprocessed pericardium or pericardial patches. The scanning electron microscopic structure of these grooves suggests that they are produced by pressure rather than by abrasion or by gouging. Nevertheless, our observations show that the outflow surfaces of Ionescu-Shiley pericardial cusps are more heavily abraded than are the corresponding surfaces of pericardial patches. Because of the similarity of these grooves to those produced by prolonged pressure applied to pericardial patches (even after fixation) with the cotton packing of the Ionescu-Shiley valves, we conclude that the grooves on the outflow surfaces of the cusps of these valves are produced by the cotton during some step(s) of the manufacturing and packing process. It is not known whether these grooves have any functional significance, although they are areas of potential accumulation of platelets and other blood elements.

REFERENCES

1 Ferrans VJ, Spray TL, Billingham ME, Roberts WC: Structural changes in glutaraldehyde-treated porcine heterografts used as substitute cardiac valves. Transmission and scanning electron microscopic observations in 12 patients. Am J Cardiol **41:**1159-1184, 1978

2 Ferrans VJ, Boyce SW, Billingham ME, Spray TL, Roberts WC: Infection of glutaraldehyde-preserved porcine valve heterografts. Am J Cardiol **43:**1123-1136, 1979

3 Ferrans VJ, Boyce SW, Billingham ME, Jones M, Ishihara T, Roberts WC: Calcific deposits in porcine bioprostheses. Structure and pathogenesis. Am J Cardiol **46:** 721-734, 1980

4 Ionescu MI, Tandon AP: The Ionescu-Shiley pericardial xenograft heart valve, Tissue Heart Valves, Chap 6, M Ionescu, ed., London, 1979, Butterworth & Co., Ltd., p 201

5 Ionescu MI, Tandon AP: Long term clinical and haemodynamic evaluation of the Ionescu-Shiley pericardial xenograft heart valve, Bioprosthetic Cardiac Valves, Chap 5, F Sebening, WP Klövekorn, H Meisner, E Struck, eds., Munich, 1979, Deutsches Herzzentrum München, Publisher, p 199

6 Björk VO, Hultquist G: Teflon and pericardial aortic valve prostheses. J THORAC CARDIOVASC SURG **47:**693-701, 1964

7 Yarbrough JW, Roberts WC, Reis RL: Structural alterations in tissue cardiac valves implanted in patients and in calves. J THORAC CARDIOVASC SURG **65:**364-375, 1973

8 Trusler GA: Discussion of Geha AS, Laks H, Stansel HC Jr, Cornhill JF, Kilman JW, Buckley MJ, Roberts WC: Late failure of porcine valve heterografts in children. J THORAC CARDIOVASC SURG **78:**351-364, 1979

9 Ishihara T, Ferrans VJ, Jones M, Boyce SW, Kawanami O, Roberts WC: Histologic and ultrastructural features of normal human parietal pericardium. Am J Cardiol **46:** 744-753, 1980

10 Broom ND, Thomson FJ: Influence of fixation conditions on the performance of glutaraldehyde-treated porcine aortic valves. Towards a more scientific basis. Thorax **34:**166-176, 1979

Occurrence and Significance of Endothelial Cells in Implanted Porcine Bioprosthetic Valves

TOKUHIRO ISHIHARA, MD, PhD
VICTOR J. FERRANS, MD, PhD
MICHAEL JONES, MD
STEVEN W. BOYCE, MD
WILLIAM C. ROBERTS, MD

Bethesda, Maryland

Histologic and scanning and transmission electron microscopic studies were made to determine the frequency of occurrence of endothelial cells in 49 porcine valve bioprostheses removed from 43 patients 2 days to 113 months (average 35 months) after implantation. Endothelial cells were found in none of 17 bioprostheses in place for less than 1 year, in 5 (23 percent) of 22 in place for 1 to 5 years and in 7 (70 percent) of 10 in place for longer than 5 years.

The 12 bioprostheses in which endothelial cells were present had been implanted in the atrioventricular position (7 of 32 in the mitral position and 5 of 6 in the tricuspid position) for 21 to 113 months (average 71). Endothelial cells were not found in any of 11 bioprostheses implanted in the semilunar position (9 in the aortic position and 2 in pulmonary conduits); however, all but one of these bioprostheses had been in place for less than 5 years. Endothelial cells were concentrated along the basal regions of the cusps. These cells did not grow in direct contact with valve collagen, but were attached to fibrin, thrombi or fibroelastic host tissue (fibrous sheath) on the valve surfaces. The growth of endothelial cells and associated fibrous tissue may serve to increase the structural stability of bioprosthetic valve cusps, which may be of functional importance several years after implantation when the porcine connective tissue may have undergone significant deterioration.

Among the important blood-tissue interactions that occur at the surfaces of implanted bioprosthetic heart valves are: (1) the deposition of a layer of fibrin on the surface; (2) the adherence of macrophages, platelets and leukocytes; (3) the development of thrombi; and (4) the covering of the bioprosthetic cusps by endothelial cells.[1] The investment of the surfaces of bioprostheses by a protective layer of endothelial cells of host origin would appear to be a desirable event. Endothelial cells have been reported in only two porcine bioprostheses,[1-3] both implanted in the tricuspid position. Nevertheless, the actual frequency of occurrence of endothelial cells in implanted porcine bioprostheses has not been investigated systematically, and the following reservations apply to the results of previous histologic studies of these bioprostheses: (1) Endothelial cells are easily detached and lost during cutting and staining of paraffin sections, and (2) by light microscopy, it is difficult to distinguish endothelial cells from macrophages that have attached to the surfaces of the bioprostheses and have become flattened. We therefore undertook a detailed investigation of the occurrence of endothelial cells on the surfaces of 49 porcine valve bioprostheses that had been in place from 2 days to 113 months.

From the Pathology Branch and the Surgery Branch, National Heart, Lung, and Blood Institute, National Institutes of Health, Bethesda, Maryland.
Manuscript received December 8, 1980; revised manuscript received February 24, 1981, accepted March 10, 1981.
Address for reprints: Victor J. Ferrans, MD, National Institutes of Health, Building 10, Room 7N208, Bethesda, Maryland 20205.

Methods

Patients studied: The morphologic studies that follow were made on 49 porcine valve bioprostheses implanted in 43 patients (24 men and 19 women) aged 2 to 68 years (average 42) at the time of the implantation. Thirty-two valves had been implanted in the mitral position, 9 in the aortic position, 6 in the tricuspid position and 2 as valved conduits in the pulmonary position. The period of time between implantation and removal varied from 2 days to 113 months (average 35 months). Pertinent clinical and anatomic data on these patients are summarized in Table I.

The patients were classified into three groups according to the time the bioprosthesis had been in place: Group I consisted of 15 patients (8 men and 7 women) with 17 bioprosthetic valves (12 in the mitral position, 4 in the aortic position and 1 in the tricuspid position) implanted for less than 1 year (average 3.5 months).

Group II was composed of 20 patients (13 men and 7 women) with 22 bioprosthetic valves (14 in the mitral position, 5 in the aortic position, 2 in the tricuspid position and 1 in a pulmonary conduit) implanted for 1 to 5 years (average 33 months).

Group III consisted of eight patients (three men and five women) with 10 bioprosthetic valves (6 in the mitral position, 3 in the tricuspid position and 1 in a pulmonary conduit) implanted for more than 5 years (average 90 months).

Preparation of tissues: All valves were fixed with cold 3 percent glutaraldehyde in 0.1 *M* phosphate buffer (pH 7.2). After fixation, two cusps of each valve were removed from the stent and processed for histologic examination and for scanning and transmission electron microscopic study. The methods utilized in these studies have been described in detail.[1]

Results

The pathologic changes that develop in porcine valve bioprostheses after implantation have been described in detail in several reports from our laboratory.[1,2,4,5] Therefore, this communication describes only those alterations that pertain to endothelial cells and related surface structures of the bioprostheses. Observations on the occurrence of endothelial cells in the bioprostheses from each of the three groups of patients are presented first and are followed by a description of the light and electron microscopic characteristics of these endothelial cells and related components.

Occurrence of Endothelial Cells in Explanted Bioprostheses

Group I (prostheses implanted for less than 1 year): None of the bioprostheses implanted in patients in group I contained endothelial cells of host origin. Two valves did contain very small numbers of endothelial cells; however, because of their morphologic features on scanning electron microscopic study, which were similar to those of endothelial cells found in commercially processed but unimplanted bioprostheses,[1] these cells were identified as porcine endothelial cells that had remained attached to the valve surfaces.

Group II (prostheses implanted for 1 to 5 years): Endothelial cells were identified in 5 (23 percent) of the 22 valves from patients in group II, including 3 of the 14 valves placed in the mitral position and each of the 2 valves placed in the tricuspid position, but none of the 5 valves placed in the aortic position or the 1 valve in a pulmonary conduit. In none of these valves were the surfaces completely covered by endothelial cells. In each valve, the endothelial cells formed patches in both the inflow and the outflow surfaces, usually in greater numbers in the latter. They were also more frequent in the proximal than in the middle third of the cusp, and were seldom found in the distal third.

Group III (prostheses implanted for more than 5 years): Endothelial cells were present in 7 (70 percent) of the 10 valves from patients in group III, including 4 of 6 valves implanted in the mitral position and each of the 3 valves implanted in the tricuspid position. These cells were not present in the valved conduit implanted in the pulmonary position. As in the case of endothelium-lined valves from patients in Group II, those from patients in group III were only partially covered by endothelial cells.

Correlation with clinical or anatomic features: Thus, 12 of the 49 bioprostheses examined were partially covered by endothelial cells. Included among these

TABLE I

Clinical and Morphologic Observations in 10 Patients With 12 Endothelialized Bioprostheses*

Case	Age at Implantation (yr)	Sex	Valve Replaced by BP	Time BP in Place (mo)	Reason for Removal	Thrombus or Fibrous Sheath	Ca++	Infection	Perforation
1	57	F	TV	21	N	+	0	0	0
2	49	F	MV	27	S	+	+	0	0
3	55	M	TV	40	R	+	+	+	0
4	36	M	MV	42	S	+	+	+	0
5	2	M	MV	50	S	+	+	0	+
6	65	F	TV	63	R	+	+	0	0
			MV	63	R	+	+	0	+
7	47	F	TV	100	S; R	+	+	0	0
8	50	F	MV	107	S; R	+	+	0	+
9	59	M	MV	107	R	+	0	0	0
10	31	F	MV	113	R	+	+	0	0
			TV	113	—	+	+	0	0
Mean	45			70.5					
Totals		M = 4; F = 6	MV = 7; TV = 5		R = 7; S = 5	12	9	2	3

BP = bioprosthesis; Ca++ = calcification; MV = mitral valve; N = necropsy; R = regurgitation; S = stenosis; TV = tricuspid valve. + = present; 0 = absent.

* The bioprosthesis from Patient 2 was a Carpentier-Edwards valve; all others were Hancock valves. Patients 1, 7, 9 and 10 had received anticoagulant therapy after implantation of the bioprosthesis.

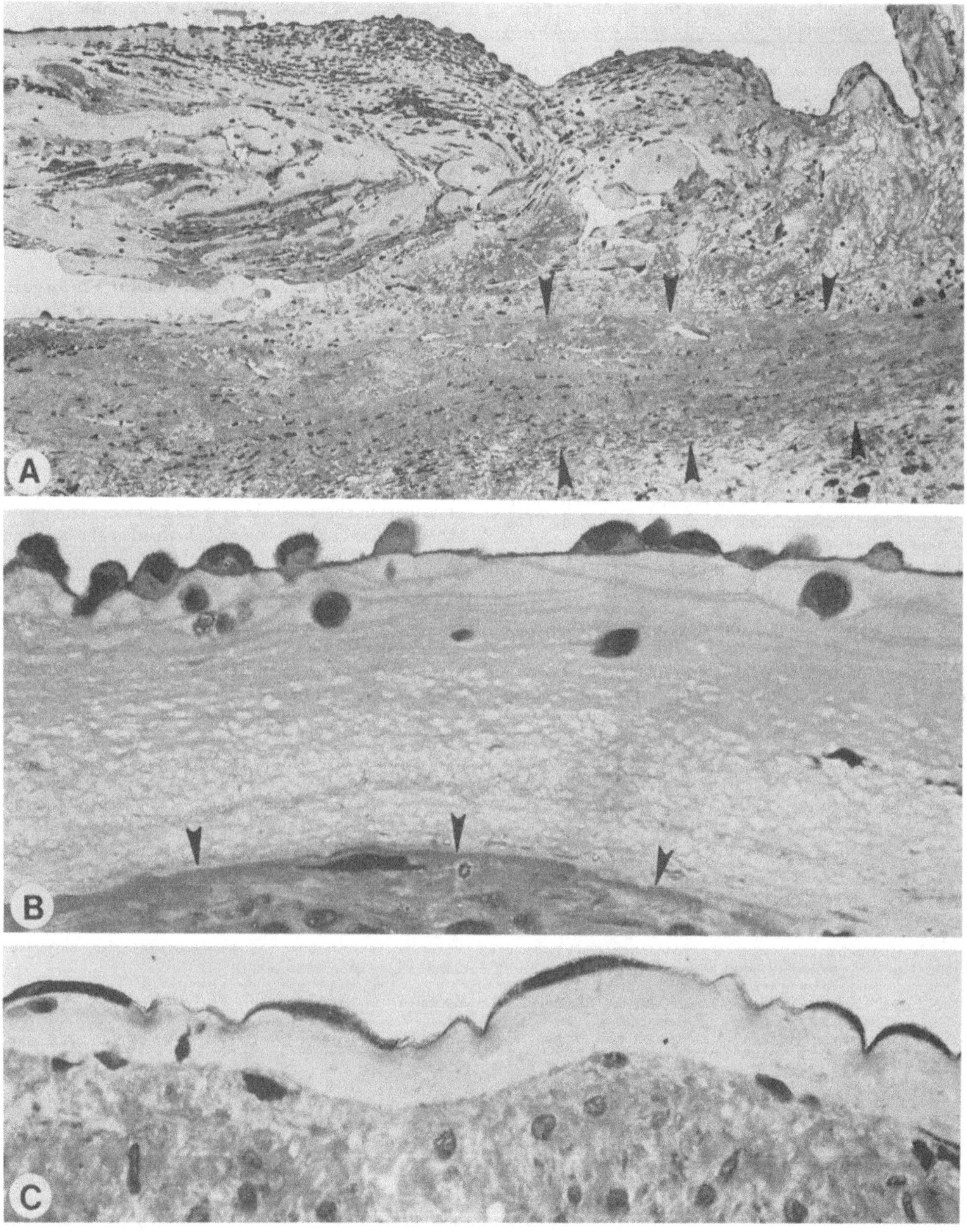

FIGURE 1. Histologic features of endothelial cells in bioprostheses. **A**, endothelial cells line the surface of layered, partially organized thrombus on the outflow surface of the cusp of a bioprosthesis removed 107 months after implantation in the mitral position. The valve fibrosa is outlined by **arrowheads**. **B**, plump endothelial cells cover the surface of the fibrous sheath that has extended over the outflow surface (**arrowheads** indicate boundary of porcine valve collagen in fibrosa) of a bioprosthesis removed 113 months after implantation in the tricuspid position. **C**, attenuated endothelial cells are present in another area of the bioprosthesis shown in **B**. (Alkaline toluidine blue stain ×100 [**A**] and ×630 [**B** and **C**].)

were 7 of 32 valves implanted in the mitral position and 5 of 6 valves implanted in the tricuspid position. Endothelial cells were not found in any of the valves implanted in the semilunar position (that is, 9 valves in the aortic position and 2 valved conduits implanted in the pulmonary position). Endothelial cells were not present in the regions of perforations in the three valves in which this complication was found, although these cells were found in other regions of each of the three valves. Other than these relations, review of the patient data failed to yield any correlations between the presence of endothelial cells and other clinical or anatomic features, including (1) age of the patient; (2) presence of infection, thrombus, calcific deposits or collagen degeneration in the bioprosthesis, and (3) occurrence of bioprosthetic stenosis or regurgitation.

Histologic Observations

Considerable numbers of blood-derived elements, including red blood cells, platelets, macrophages and strands of fibrin, were attached to the surfaces of each of the valves from patients in group I. These surfaces lacked a cell lining and consisted of bundles of collagen fibrils. Accumulations of red blood cells, fibrin and platelets were defined as "new thrombi" and were found in 16 valves from patients in group I. Partially organized thrombi that frequently contained calcific deposits were found in two valves in group I and in practically all of the valves in groups II and III. Most of these thrombi were of microscopic size.

The endothelial cells found in the valves from patients in groups II and III varied considerably in size, morphologic features and population density (Fig. 1). They measured up to 30 μ in length and 10 μ in thickness. Some endothelial cells were extremely thin and attenuated, especially those in sparsely populated areas; others, particularly those in the most densely populated areas, were much thicker and had more pronounced, centrally located nuclear bulges. Most areas of the valve surfaces that were not invested by endothelium were covered by a layer of fibrin, to which platelets, macrophages and a few leukocytes were attached. Some of these cells appeared to be directly attached to the surfaces of the valves (rather than to the fibrin). Macrophages and leukocytes were also occasionally found within thrombi or connective tissue beneath the endothelial cells. Fibroblastic growth in areas beneath endothelial cells was very sparse, and smooth muscle cells were seldom found in these areas.

In some valves, the endothelial cells had grown over an organizing thrombus; in others, they were superimposed on a layer of fibroelastic tissue (fibrous sheath) that had extended from the sewing ring into the cusp proper. Endothelial cells seldom were found directly overlying the porcine connective tissue at the surfaces of the cusps. In some valves it proved difficult to distinguish organizing thrombi from the fibrous sheaths. Intermediate forms seemed to exist between a thrombus and a fibrous sheath at the base of the cusps, even though the fibroelastic structure of the sheath was evident in areas over the stent. The elastic fibers in the fibrous sheath appeared much finer than those in the cusp, and the thickness of the fibrous sheath was less than that of the cusp itself.

Scanning Electron Microscopic Observations

Microvilli and cilia (Fig. 2): Some of the endothelial cells appeared polygonal in shape; others appeared elongated, with their long axes oriented parallel to the free edge of the cusp (Fig. 2, B to D). Their surfaces had variable numbers of microvilli, which measured up to 1 μ in length and 0.1 μ in width. Microvilli differed clearly from the cytoplasmic folds and ruffles of macrophages, and tended to be concentrated in the central regions of the cells. Some cells also had elongated or bleb-like cytoplasmic processes (Fig. 2E). Single cilia, which measured 0.2 μ in diameter and 4 μ in length, were found in some endothelial cells (Fig. 2E). These cilia differed in size and length from microvilli. The junctions between adjacent endothelial cells were very conspicuous in some areas, in which they were visualized as zones of obvious cellular overlapping. In other areas, particularly those in which the endothelial cells were more flattened, the intercellular junctions were much less prominent.

Platelets: Platelets were not adherent to the endothelial surfaces, although they frequently were found in large numbers in the immediate vicinity of the lateral edges of sheets of endothelial cells (Fig. 2F). Most platelets adherent to the surfaces of the bioprostheses had elongated processes that extended from their main oval-shaped cytoplasmic mass. Some platelets appeared to have undergone an additional process of spreading and flattening. This process was associated with the formation of layers of these altered platelets (Fig. 3, A and B). When viewed at low magnification with the scanning electron microscope, such layered platelets resembled endothelial cells; however, the two types of cells were easily distinguished at higher magnification.

Macrophages: Macrophages varied in morphology (Fig. 3, C and D). Many of these cells had a characteristic appearance, with a spherical shape and numerous cytoplasmic ruffles (filopodia). Certain macrophages appeared flattened and spindle-shaped, with cytoplasmic processes in contact with those of adjacent cells. Although these macrophages resembled endothelial cells, they did not contain microvilli and their cytoplasmic processes interdigitated loosely, without forming junctional complexes such as those connecting adjacent endothelial cells.

Transmission Electron Microscopic Observations

Endothelial cells: In spite of their variations in size and shape, endothelial cells exhibited a number of consistent ultrastructural features (Fig. 4, A to E). The nuclei were single, flattened and centrally located. The cytoplasm contained variable numbers of ribosomes; cisterns of rough-surfaced endoplasmic reticulum and lysosomes; Golgi zones located close to the nuclei; occasional coated vesicles and multivesicular bodies; few uncoated plasmalemmal vesicles; extremely numerous

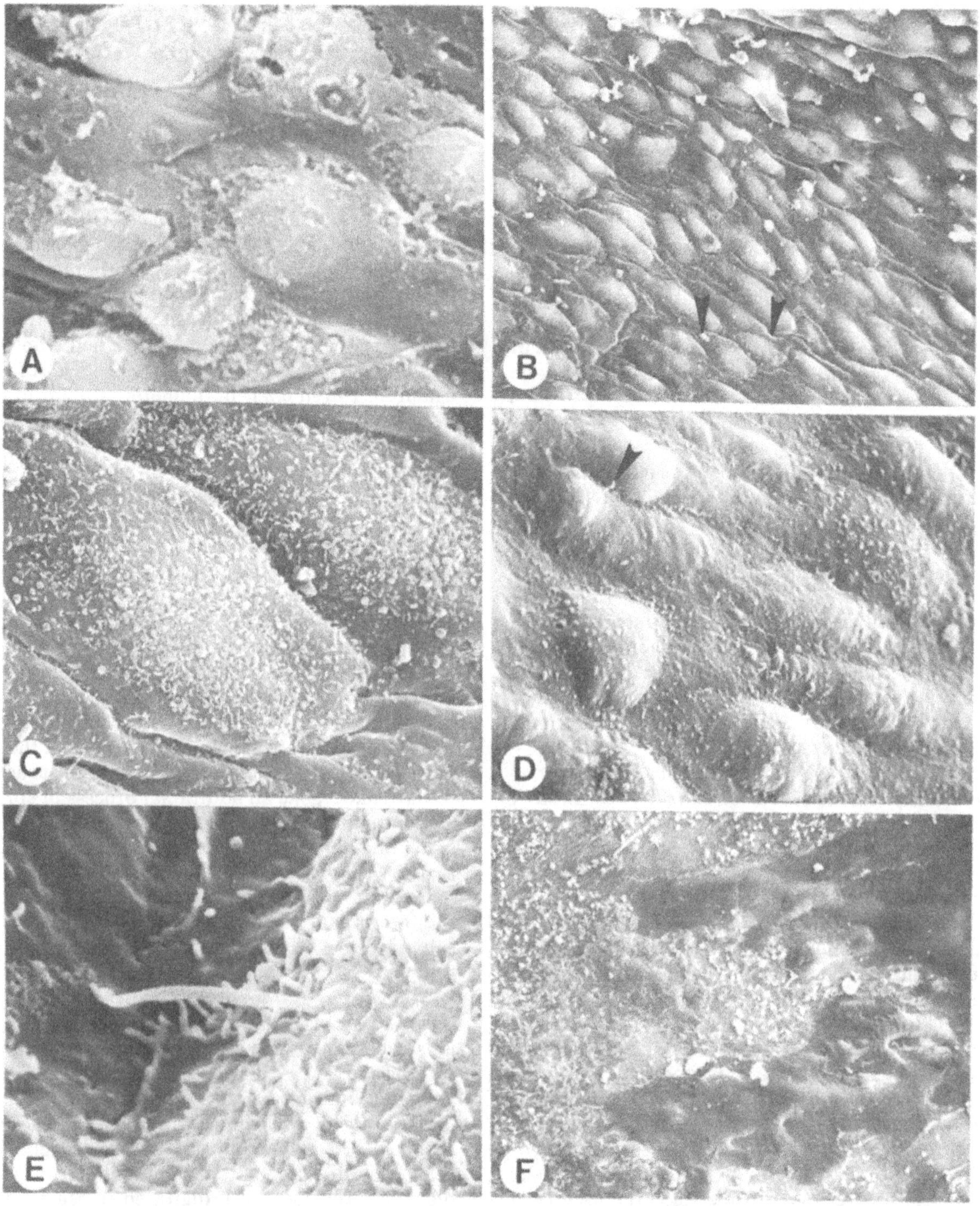

FIGURE 2. Scanning electron micrographs of endothelial cells in bioprostheses. **A**, severely disrupted endothelial cells are present on outflow surface of a bioprosthesis removed because of a perivalve leak 3 months after implantation in the mitral position. These cells are considered to be porcine endothelial cells that remained attached to the cusps after commercial processing and implantation of the bioprosthesis. (×2,300.) **B**, low magnification view of host endothelial cells present on the outflow surface of the bioprosthesis shown in Figure 1, B and C. The cells indicated by **arrowheads** are shown at higher magnification in **C**. (×380.) **C**, higher magnification of cells shown in **B**, showing details of surface morphology. The endothelial cells are covered by microvillous projections and their cell boundaries appear as deep clefts. (×3,200.) **D**, endothelial cells on outflow surface of the bioprosthesis shown in Figure 1A. The nuclei form bulges and intercellular junctions are inconspicuous. Note cilium (**arrowhead**) in one of the cells. (×1,700.) **E**, high magnification view of cilium and microvillous processes on luminal surface of endothelial cell in the bioprosthesis shown in **B** and **C**. (×11,500.) **F**, low magnification view of edge of area covered by endothelial cells in the bioprosthesis shown in Figure 1A. These endothelial cells have smooth surfaces, in contrast to adjacent areas in which platelets and red blood cells are attached to fibrin and collagen. (×380.)

cytoskeletal filaments, which were arranged in bundles in the perinuclear areas (Fig. 4C), and small, discrete bundles of actin-like filaments (Fig. 4D). In some cells, the actin filaments were associated with accumulations of electron-dense material. Unequivocally identifiable Weibel-Palade bodies were not found.

Adjacent endothelial cells interdigitated and overlapped to a variable extent, and their lateral surfaces were connected by junctional complexes (Fig. 4E). These consisted of zonulae adherentes (tight junctions) and occupied only a small fraction of the total area of intercellular contact. Wide gaps were apparent between some of these areas of specialized contact. The luminal surfaces of endothelial cells had microvilli, and their basal surfaces were invested by external lamina or basement membrane material. In some cells, this material formed a single layer; in others, it showed a considerable degree of multilayering, with electron-lucent spaces between adjacent layers (Fig. 4A). Macrophages and platelets observed in this study were ultrastructurally similar to those previously described by us in implanted porcine bioprostheses.[1]

Adjacent cellular and extracellular components: The nature of the cellular and extracellular components subjacent to the endothelial cells was variable. In areas in which the endothelial cells were overlying a thrombus (Fig. 5, A to D), the fibrin and the cells in the thrombus usually were layered, and the endothelial cells were separated from the most superficial layer of fibrin by one or more layers of basal lamina material. Sometimes the fibrin and the basal lamina material were closely intermixed with one another and with amorphous material of unknown origin. A few macrophages, platelets and polymorphonuclear leukocytes were found beneath the layer of endothelial cells. Connective tissue cells were found in these thrombi only in very small numbers, and consisted of elongated fibroblast-like cells that lacked an external lamina. These cells contained small

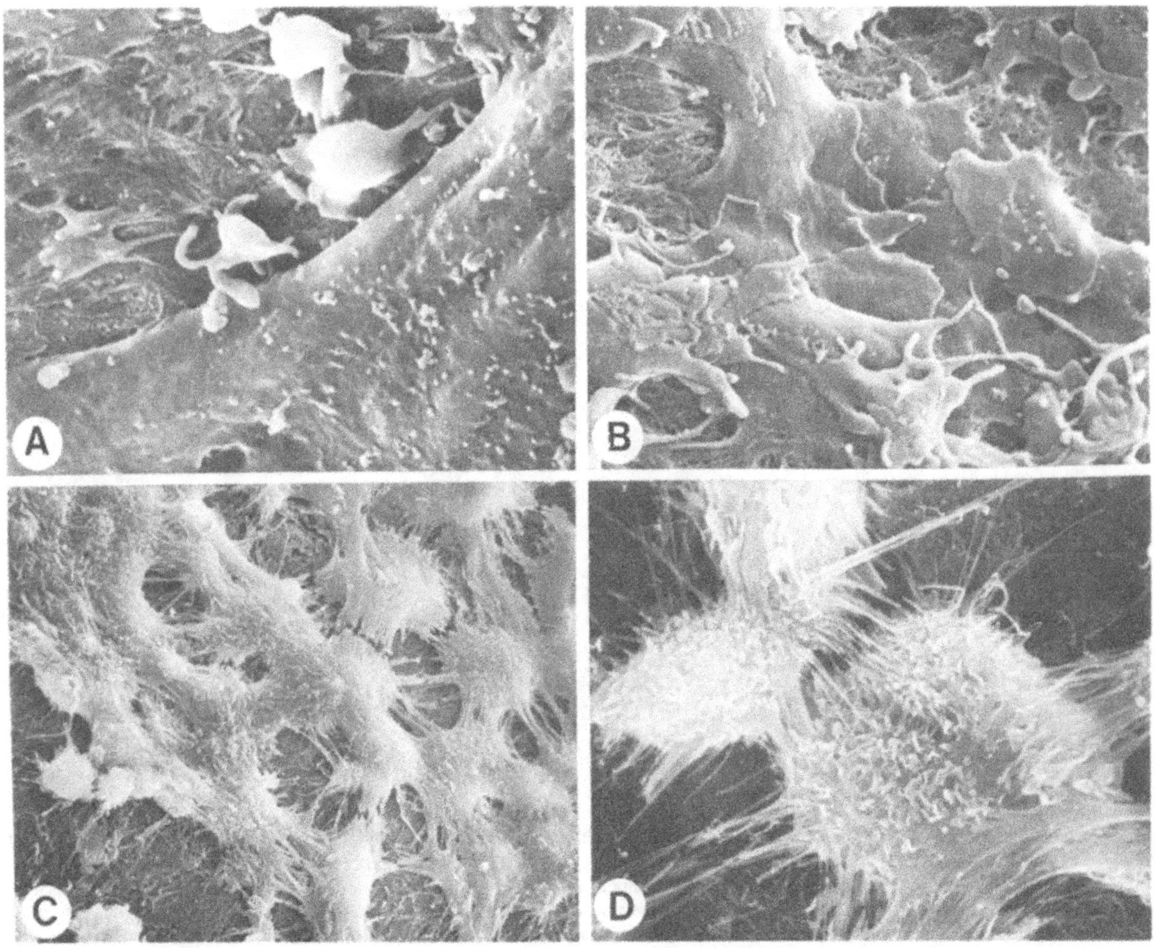

FIGURE 3. Scanning electron micrographs of endothelial cells (**A**), platelets (**A** and **B**) and macrophages (**C** and **D**) on the surfaces of bioprostheses. **A** and **B** are from the bioprosthesis shown in Figure 1A; **C** and **D** are from a bioprosthesis removed because of calcific stenosis 27 months after implantation in the mitral position. **A**, high magnification view of an area at the edge of a sheet of endothelial cells showing platelets adherent to the denuded surface (**upper left**) immediately adjacent to an endothelial cell (**lower right**). Note the elongated processes of the platelet at **center.** (×5,900.) **B**, aggregated, flattened platelets cover this area of the surface of the bioprosthesis. (×5,800.) **C**, at low magnification, these clustered macrophages resemble endothelial cells. (×1,000.) **D**, higher magnification view of the specimen shown in **C**. Macrophages have abundant, fine cytoplasmic ruffles and elongated processes. (×2,500.)

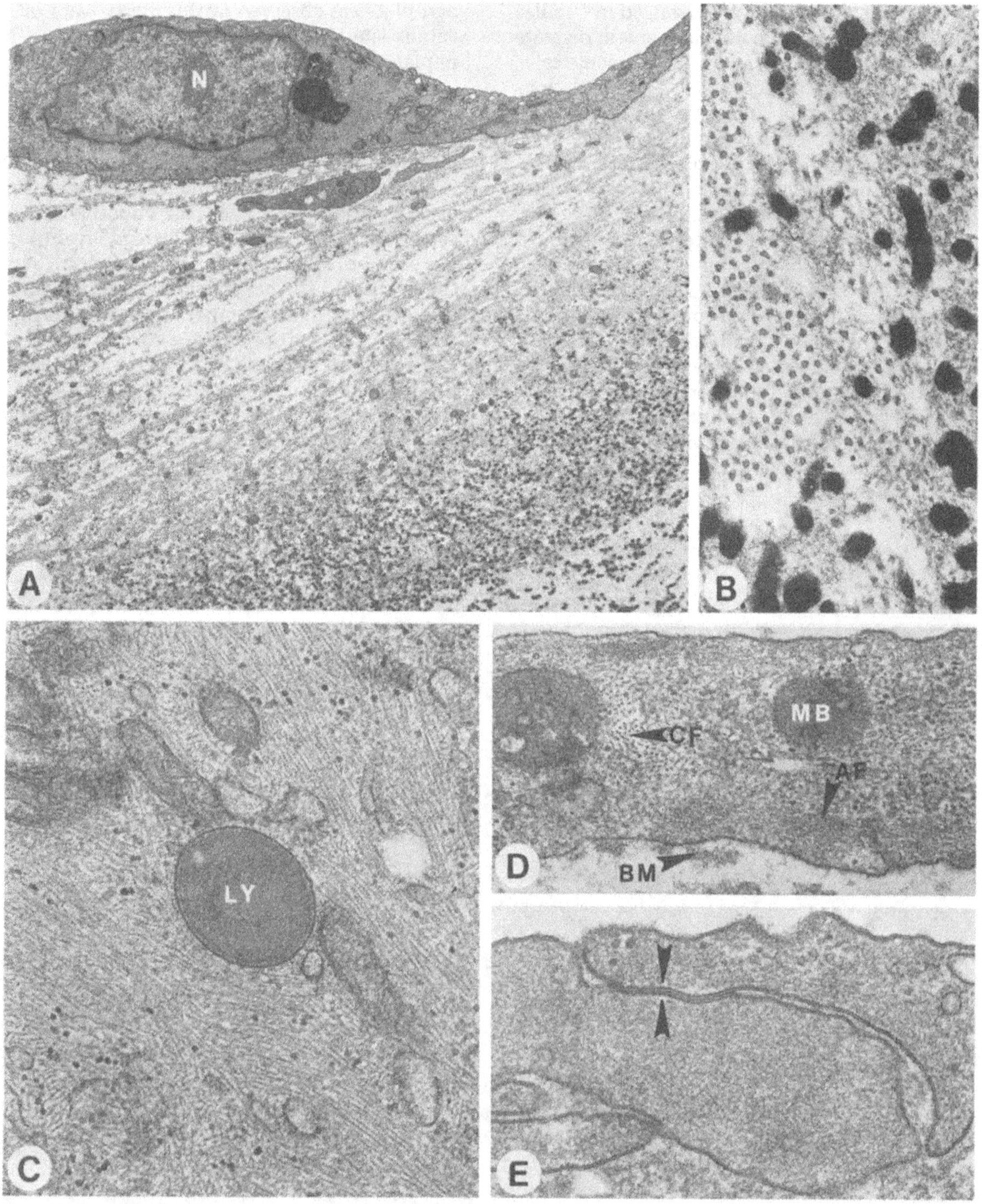

FIGURE 4. Transmission electron micrographs of endothelial cells on a bioprosthesis removed 113 months after implantation in the tricuspid position. Compare with Figures 1, B and C, taken from the same bioprosthesis. **A**, low magnification view of the central area of an endothelial cell growing on a fibrous sheath covering a cusp of bioprosthetic valve. Note the nucleus (N), small mitochondria and numerous cytoskeletal filaments in cytoplasm. The cell overlies multiple, loosely arranged layers of basement membrane-like material. These layers are superimposed on a layer of fine elastic fibers (shown in **black**) and collagen fibrils. (Kajikawa stain for elastic tissue ×9,400, reduced by 12 percent.) **B**, high magnification view of connective tissue in the fibrous sheath shown in **A**. Collagen fibrils are small and irregular in cross-sectional outline; elastic fibers, stained **black**, also are of small diameter (less than 0.2 μ). (Kajikawa stain for elastic tissue ×47,000, reduced by 12 percent.) **C**, portion of cytoplasm of an endothelial cell, showing a lysosome (LY) and numerous cytoplasmic filaments of the cytoskeletal type. (×41,000.) **D**, Cytoskeletal filaments (CF), actin filaments (AF) and multivesicular bodies (MB) are present in the cytoplasm of an endothelial cell. Irregularly distributed patches of basement membrane-like material (BM) are found along the basal surface of the cell. (×41,000.) **E**, zonula occludens (tight junction), outlined by **arrowheads**, connects two adjacent endothelial cells. (×59,000.)

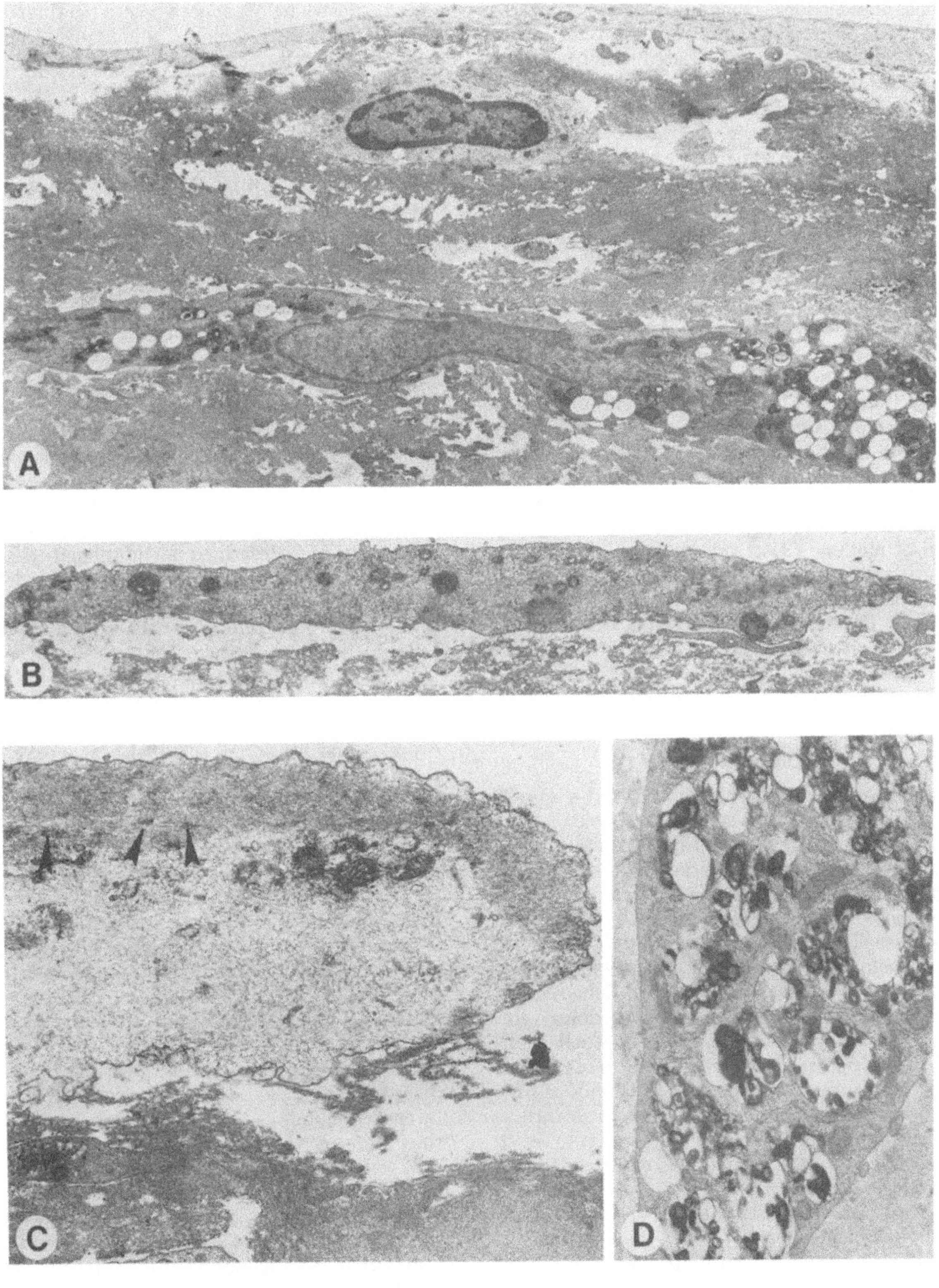

FIGURE 5. Transmission electron micrographs of endothelial cells lining the surface of thrombus in another cusp of the bioprosthesis (implanted for 113 months in the tricuspid position) shown in Figure 4. **A,** low magnification view showing the very thin, attenuated cytoplasm of an endothelial cell overlying thrombus composed of darkly stained masses of fibrin. A poorly differentiated mesenchymal cell and an elongated macrophage containing numerous lipid droplets and dense bodies are present within the thrombus. (×7,000, reduced by 15 percent.) **B,** higher magnification view of an endothelial cell such as that shown in **A**. The cell contains abundant cytoplasmic filaments and overlies loosely arranged strands of fibrin. (×14,000, reduced by 15 percent.) **C,** cytoplasm of an endothelial cell at the edge of a layer lining thrombus. This cell rests on a mass of fibrin and contains numerous cytoplasmic filaments. In the most superficial portion of the cytoplasm, these filaments are of the actin type; they are tightly packed and are associated with small accumulations of dense material (**arrowheads**). Such filaments probably mediate the motility of endothelial cells. (×24,000, reduced by 15 percent.) **D,** cytoplasm of macrophage that contains numerous dense bodies composed of dark lamellae and lucent spaces. The lamellae are presumed to represent lipid material derived from platelets and plasma lipoproteins. (×19,000, reduced by 15 percent.)

numbers of mitochondria, moderate numbers of cisterns of rough-surfaced endoplasmic reticulum and a few lysosomes. These cells were associated with irregularly coursing collagen fibrils that had a normal, distinct periodicity but were unusually slender (300 Å in diameter) and often appeared irregular rather than circular in transverse sections. A similar type of slender collagen fibril was prevalent in the fibrous connective tissue that had grown into the lumens of pulmonary conduits.

Fibrous sheaths: The fibrous sheaths (Fig. 6, A to D) differed ultrastructurally from thrombi in that they contained an abundance of elastic fibers in addition to the type of slender collagen fibril mentioned. These elastic fibers (Fig. 6, A and B) were also small (0.5 to 1.5 μ in diameter), and their size served to distinguish them from the larger and less numerous elastic fibers (of porcine origin) present in the various layers of the cusps of porcine bioprostheses. Elastic fibers in fibrous sheaths were difficult to identify in routinely stained preparations for electron microscopy and were best visualized in sections stained according to the method of Kajikawa et al.[6] A considerable amount of amorphous material of moderate electron density and unknown composition was closely associated with other connective tissue components in fibrous sheaths. Fibroblast-like cells, similar to those just described, were found in the connective tissue in the fibrous sheaths (neointima), whether or not they were covered by endothelium (Fig. 6C). Smooth muscle cells were found in areas in which the fibrous sheaths were well developed (Fig. 6D).

Discussion

The results of this study show that endothelial cells partially covered the surfaces of 12 (24 percent) of 49 porcine valve bioprostheses that had been implanted in 43 patients. The frequency of this finding was much higher than had been expected on the basis of previous descriptions[1,2,4,5,7] of the morphology of implanted bioprostheses. This apparent discrepancy is accounted for by two factors: (1) the inclusion in this report of large numbers of bioprostheses implanted for long periods of time, and (2) the more sensitive methodology employed in this study. The presence of endothelial cells showed definite correlations with the sites of implantation of the bioprostheses and with the period of time they had been in place. These two factors seemed to have a considerable influence upon the extent to which host tissue grew over the sewing ring and extended into the area of the porcine cusps.

Identification of endothelial cells: In each of the 12 valves in which they were found, endothelial cells were identified on the basis of their histologic and ultrastructural characteristics. They formed continuous monolayers, and they had surface microvilli, single cilia, coated and uncoated vesicles, intercellular junctions of the zonula occludens type and numerous cytoplasmic filaments. The latter were of two types: actin-like filaments and cytoskeletal filaments. Both of these are known to occur[8–10] in endothelial cells and in a variety of other cell types and are therefore not useful markers for identifying a given cell type. Weibel-Palade bodies, which constitute a specific morphologic marker for endothelial cells,[11] were not observed in this study. The function of these organelles is unknown; they are not present in all endothelial cells[12] and they are uncommon in endocardial endothelium.[13] The presence of microvilli, single cilia and zonulae occludentes provides a basis for distinguishing endothelial cells from smooth muscle cells, macrophages and fibroblasts.

Modified smooth muscle cells have been found to form an endothelial-like lining layer in the early stages of healing in experimentally denuded aortic intima.[14–16] However, these smooth muscle cells differ from endothelial cells in several respects: Their scanning electron microscopic appearance is different, because they have prominent surface blebs but lack microvillous projections; they have peripherally located dense bodies, which constitute myofilament insertion sites; they often have basal lamina material covering their luminal surfaces, and they do not form extensively interdigitating junctional complexes with zonulae occludentes such as those found in endothelial cells. Such junctions also are absent in macrophages and fibroblasts. The association of electron-dense material with actin filaments has previously been described in endothelial cells in coronary arteries and in other sites (see references 10 and 17 for reviews). The characteristics just cited serve to differentiate smooth muscle cells from the endothelial cells observed in this study. The latter cells also differed from macrophages in their surface morphology, which was characterized by filopodia rather than by microvilli, and in their internal structure, in which numerous lipid droplets and lysosomes filled with phagocytosed material were prominent.[1] Thus, the endothelial cells observed in this study had morphologic features that allowed them to be distinguished from other cell types. Such features were similar to those of endothelial cells found previously[1,3] in porcine bioprostheses and in other types of bioprosthetic heart valves.

Relation of the presence of endothelial cells to site of implantation of the bioprosthesis and to time elapsed between implantation and retrieval. All 12 bioprostheses in which endothelial cells were present had been implanted in the atrioventricular position, and the incidence of endothelialization was greater in the valves placed in the tricuspid position than in those placed in the mitral position. The covering of the cusps by endothelium was a slow process, as demonstrated by the findings in the three groups of patients. Endothelial cells were not found in any of the valves implanted for less than 1 year but were present in 23 percent of valves retrieved 1 to 5 years after implantation and in 70 percent of valves implanted for longer than 5 years. The two pulmonary conduits and the nine aortic bioprostheses had been in place for considerably less time than the valves that became endothelialized in the mitral or tricuspid position (mean 73 and 67 months, respectively). Therefore, additional studies will be necessary to determine whether bioprostheses implanted in the semilunar position can become endothelialized after being in place for very long periods of time.

The lower pressures in the right atrium and right ventricle must be considered important contributory factors to the large incidence of endothelialization of

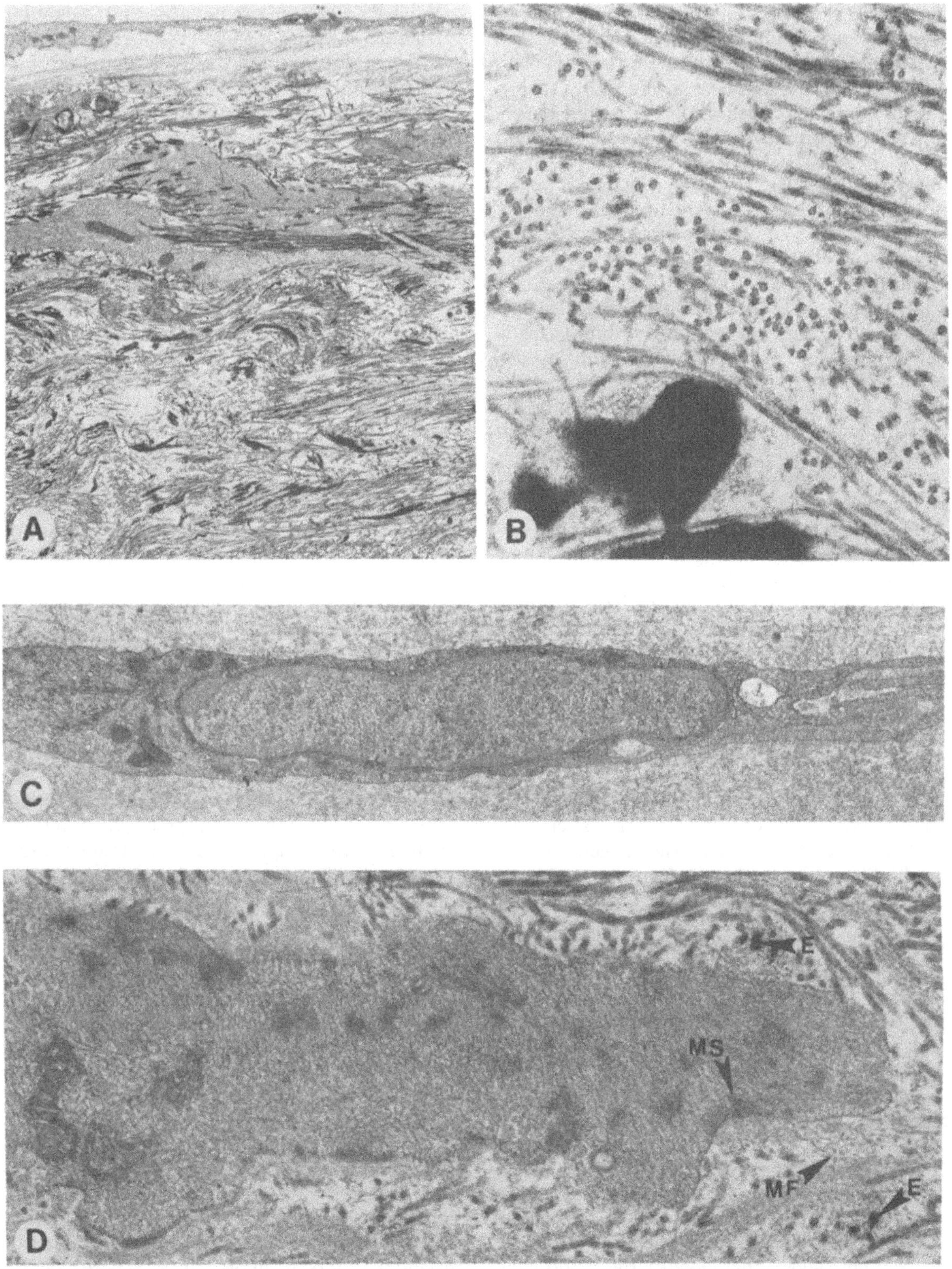

FIGURE 6. Ultrastructure of fibrous sheaths covering bioprosthetic cusps. **A** and **D** are from mitral bioprosthesis removed 107 months after implantation; **B** is from a tricuspid bioprosthesis removed 113 months after implantation, and **C** is from a mitral bioprosthesis removed 113 months after implantation. **A**, low magnification view showing endothelial cell (**top**) overlying well organized bundles of collagen and small elastic fibers (stained **black**). This fibrous sheath is much better developed than that shown in Figure 4A. (Kajikawa stain for elastic tissue ×9,000, reduced by 15 percent.) **B**, in this well developed sheath, the elastic fibers are larger than in the less developed sheath shown in Figure 4B, but the collagen fibrils are similar and probably represent type III collagen. (Kajikawa stain for elastic tissue ×50,000, reduced by 15 percent.) **C**, view of fibroblast in sheath. The cell is thin and elongated, lacks a basement membrane and is surrounded by unorganized, finely filamentous material. (×17,000.) **D**, part of cytoplasm of typical smooth muscle cell in well developed fibrous sheath. Cell contains filaments and myofilament insertion sites (MS) and it is surrounded by basement membrane material, collagen, elastic fibers (E) and connective tissue microfibrils (MF). (×33,000.)

porcine bioprostheses implanted in the tricuspid position.[3] Hemodynamic studies in five of our six patients with a tricuspid bioprosthesis indicated that they had normal or nearly normal right atrial and right ventricular pressures after their initial operation but before failure of their left-sided bioprosthesis (four patients) or shortly before death from arrhythmias and myocardial failure (one patient). The sixth patient, who died of bioprosthetic infection, did not undergo hemodynamic studies. These findings support the concept that hemodynamic forces in the right side of the heart allow endothelial cells to spread over the bioprosthetic cusps. It would seem that the shear stress exerted by the flow of blood across the surfaces of bioprosthetic cusps is lowest in the tricuspid position, thus minimizing the tendency of these forces to detach endothelial cells from the surfaces of the cusps.This shear stress would be expected to be lower in the outflow surfaces than in the inflow surfaces.

The detachment of endothelial cells from vascular surfaces appears to depend on two factors: (1) the magnitude of the shear stress forces exerted on the endothelial cells, and (2) the strength of the adhesion of the endothelial cells to the underlying connective tissue. It is known that high shear stress causes detachment of endothelial cells from the surfaces of arteries,[18,19] and measurements have been made of the magnitude (400 dynes/cm^2) of such forces (critical yield stress) in the canine thoracic aorta.[18,19] Shear stress forces well in excess of the critical yield stress do occur in the vicinity of the surfaces of mechanical valve prostheses implanted in the aortic position[20]; in bioprosthetic heart valves such forces are of lesser magnitude[21] but still in excess of the acute yield stress of endothelial cells in arteries. The attachment of endothelial cells to the surfaces of porcine bioprostheses often was mediated by one or more layers of fibrin or by poorly organized, multilayered basement membrane material. For these reasons, it would seem that endothelial cells do grow on porcine bioprostheses but are detached because their adhesion to the surfaces is poor and because they are subjected to excessive mechanical forces.

Growth of endothelial cells over thrombi and fibrous sheaths: Our observations show that endothelial cells do not grow directly on the surface collagen of porcine bioprosthetic cusps, but require host material (fibrin, thrombus or fibrous sheath) superimposed on this collagen. The cells involved in this process probably originate from endocardial endothelium that first grows into the area of the stent. Nevertheless, the possibility that they are blood-borne cannot be excluded, because other studies[22] have shown that blood-borne endothelial cells can populate vessel segments suspended in midstream in thoracic aorta.

The occurrence of fibrous sheaths covered by endothelium has been noted in porcine bioprostheses[2,3] *as well as in other types of bioprostheses,*[23-29] but the fine structure of these sheaths has not previously been described. Only limited growth of fibrous sheaths has been found in the great majority of porcine bioprostheses.[30] Valve dysfunction can be caused by thickening or contraction of a fibrous sheath covering a cusp of a porcine bioprosthesis,[30,31] but this is uncommon. This complication appears to be more frequent in other bioprostheses, such as fascia lata valves[29] and homografts,[28] in which fibrous sheaths seem to grow more rapidly. Thus, the slow and limited growth of fibrous sheaths in porcine bioprostheses is advantageous in this respect.

The ultrastructural morphology of the elastic fibers and collagen fibrils in the fibrous sheaths of porcine bioprostheses was distinctive. The small size of the elastic fibers in the sheath served to distinguish them from the elastic fibers in the fibrosa and ventricularis layers of the cusps.[1] The collagen fibrils were structurally similar to type III collagen, which is known to occur normally in blood vessels and cardiac valves.[32,33] The cellular sources responsible for the synthesis of these components in implanted porcine bioprostheses were not specifically identified in this study; however, fibroblasts, smooth muscle cells and endothelial cells are capable of synthesizing type III collagen, and smooth muscle cells and endothelial cells are known to synthesize elastic fibers.[33,34] The presence of smooth muscle cells in fibrous sheaths is explained on the basis of transformation of fibroblasts, first into myofibroblasts and then into smooth muscle cells, as fibrous scar tissue undergoes maturation. Such a phenomenon is well known to occur in other organs.[35-38]

The covering of the surfaces of porcine valve bioprostheses by endothelium could have the following functional consequences: (1) preventing the formation of fibrin deposits and the attachment of platelets and macrophages to the surfaces of the cusps; (2) decreasing the tendency for the development of thrombi; (3) providing a defense against valve infection; (4) reinforcing the mechanical strength of the basal regions of the cusps, where perforations tend to occur; and (5) presenting a barrier to the penetration of plasma proteins and other components that may contribute to the formation of calcific deposits.

Conclusions: Endothelial cells grow to a limited extent, as a function of time, over the surfaces of cusps of porcine bioprostheses implanted in the atrioventricular position. Such growth is more frequent and prominent in tricuspid than in mitral bioprostheses, in the proximal third than in the other two thirds of the cusps, and in bioprostheses implanted for longer than 5 years. Endothelial cells were not observed in aortic or pulmonary bioprostheses, but the number of these valve prostheses studied was too small to exclude completely the possibility that they also can be covered by endothelium after being in place for long periods of time. The growth of endothelial cells may increase the functional stability of bioprosthetic cusps; however, considerable structural deterioration of these cusps may occur before structural reinforcement by endothelial cell growth becomes evident. This structural reinforcement may be of particular importance several years after implantation when the connective tissue in the cusps may be greatly deteriorated.

References

1. **Ferrans VJ, Spray TL, Billingham ME, Roberts WC.** Structural changes in glutaraldehyde-treated porcine heterografts used as substitute cardiac valves. Transmission and scanning electron microscopic observations in 12 patients. Am J Cardiol 1978;41: 1159–84.
2. **Spray TL, Roberts WC.** Structural changes in porcine xenografts used as substitute cardiac valves. Gross and histologic observations in 51 glutaraldehyde-preserved Hancock valves in 41 patients. Am J Cardiol 1977;40:319–30.
3. **Sade RM, Greene WB, Kurtz SM.** Structural changes in a porcine xenograft after implantation for 105 months. Am J Cardiol 1979; 44:761–6.
4. **Ferrans VJ, Boyce SW, Billingham ME, Spray TL, Roberts WC.** Infection of glutaraldehyde-preserved porcine valve heterografts. Am J Cardiol 1979;43:1123–36.
5. **Ferrans VJ, Boyce SW, Billingham ME, Jones M, Ishihara T, Roberts WC.** Calcific deposits in porcine bioprostheses: structure and pathogenesis. Am J Cardiol 1980;46:721–34.
6. **Kajikawa K, Yamaguchi T, Katsuda S, et al.** An improved electron stain for elastic fibers using tannic acid. J Electron Microsc (Tokyo) 1975;24:287–9.
7. **Fishbein MC, Gissen SA, Collins JJ Jr, et al.** Pathology in patients with glutaraldehyde-fixed porcine cardiac valves. Am J Cardiol 1977;40:331–7.
8. **Korn ED.** Biochemistry of actomyosin-dependent cell motility: a review. Proc Natl Acad Sci USA 1978;75:588–99.
9. **Lazarides E.** Intermediate filaments as mechanical integrators of cellular space. Nature 1980;283:249–56.
10. **Ferrans VJ.** Vascular structure. In: Patel DJ, Vaishnav RN, eds. Basic Hemodynamics and Its Role in Disease Processes. Baltimore: University Park Press, 1980:105–54.
11. **Weibel ER, Palade GE.** New cytoplasmic components in arterial endothelia. J Cell Biol 1964;23:101–12.
12. **Davison PM, Bensch K, Karasek MA.** Growth and morphology of rabbit marginal vessel endothelium in tissue culture. J Cell Biol 1980;85:187–98.
13. **Haust MD, Wyllie JC, More RH.** Electron microscopic observations on certain dense bodies in fibroblasts, synovial and endocardial cells. Rev Can Biol 1966;25:117–27.
14. **Stemerman MB, Spaet TH, Pitlick F, Cintron J, Lejnieks I, Tiell ML.** Intimal healing. The pattern of reendothelialization and intimal thickening. Am J Pathol 1977;87:125–42.
15. **Haudenschild CC, Schwartz SM.** Endothelial regeneration. II. Restitution of endothelial continuity. Lab Invest 1979;41:407–18.
16. **Schwartz SM, Stemerman MB, Benditt EP.** The aortic intima. II. Repair of the aortic lining after mechanical denudation. Am J Pathol 1975;81:15–41.
17. **Ferrans VJ, Roberts WC.** Structural features of cardiac myxomas. Histology, histochemistry and electron microscopy. Hum Pathol 1973;4:111–46.
18. **Fry DL.** Acute vascular endothelial changes associated with increased blood velocity gradients. Circ Res 1968;22:165–97.
19. **Fry DL.** Certain histological and chemical responses of the vascular interface to acutely induced mechanical stress in the aorta of the dog. Circ Res 1969;24:93–108.
20. **Yoganathan AP, Corcoran WH, Harrison EC.** Wall shear stress measurements in the near vicinity of prosthetic aortic heart valves. J Bioeng 1978;2:369–79.
21. **Yoganathan AP, Corcoran WH, Harrison EC.** *In vitro* fluid dynamics of the St. Jude, Ionescu-Shiley and Carpentier-Edwards aortic heart valve prostheses. In: Schneck DJ, ed. Biofluid Mechanics, Vol 2. New York: Plenum Press, 1980:295–316.
22. **Stump MM, Jordan GL Jr, DeBakey ME, Halpert B.** Endothelium grown from circulating blood on isolated intravascular dacron hub. Am J Pathol 1963;43:361–7.
23. **Mohri H, Reichenbach DD, Barnes RW, Merendino KA.** A biologic study of the homologous aortic valve in dogs. J Thorac Cardiovasc Surg 1967;54:622–9.
24. **Suzuki A, Mackrell J, Kay EB.** Mitral valve replacement with transplant valves. J Thorac Cardiovasc Surg 1970;60:13–25.
25. **Gavin JB, Herdson PB, Barratt-Boyes BG.** The pathology of chemically-sterilized human heart valve allografts. Pathology 1972;4:175–83.
26. **Gavin JB, Herdson PB, Monro JL, Barratt-Boyes BG.** Pathology of antibiotic-treated human heart valve allografts. Thorax 1973; 28:473–81.
27. **Bernhard A, Thiede A, Müller-Hermelink H-K, Krug A, Fischer K, Yankah AC.** Mitral valve replacement with autologous fascia lata. Results of morphologic examinations. J Thorac Cardiovasc Surg 1973;65:94–102.
28. **Gavin JB, Monro JL.** The pathology of pulmonary and aortic valve allografts used as mitral valve replacements in dogs. Pathology 1974;6:119–27.
29. **Willen R, Dubiel WT, Johansson L.** Viability and surface properties of autologous fascia lata heart valve grafts. A radioautographic and scanning electron microscopical study. Ann Thorac Surg 1974; 18:597–607.
30. **Angell WW, Angell JD.** Porcine valves. Prog Cardiovasc Dis 1980;23:141–66.
31. **Bortolotti U, Gallucci V, Casarotto D, Thiene G.** Fibrous tissue overgrowth on Hancock mitral xenografts: a cause of late prosthetic stenosis. Thorac Cardiovasc Surg 1979;27:316–8.
32. **Mannschott P, Herbage D, Weiss M, Buffevant C.** Collagen heterogeneity in pig heart valves. Biochim Biophys Acta 1976;434: 177–83.
33. **Miller EJ.** Biochemical characteristics and biological significance of the genetically-distinct collagens. Mol Cell Biochem 1976;13: 165–92.
34. **Rennard SI, Ferrans VJ, Bradley KH, Crystal RG.** Lung connective tissue. In: Witschi H, ed. Pulmonary Toxicology. Boca Raton, Fl: CRC Press, in press.
35. **Madden JW, Carlson EC, Hines J.** Presence of modified fibroblasts in ischemic contracture of the intrinsic musculature of the hand. Surg Gynecol Obstet 1975;140:509–16.
36. **Gabbiani G, Hirschel BJ, Ryan GB, et al.** Granulation tissue as a contractile organ. A study of structure and function. J Exp Med 1972;135:719–34.
37. **Gabbiani G, Majno G.** Dupuytren's contracture. Fibroblast contraction? An ultrastructural study. Am J Pathol 1972;66:131–46.
38. **Majno G, Gabbiani G, Hirschel BJ, et al.** Contraction of granulation tissue in vitro, similarity to smooth muscle. Science 1971;173: 548–50.

Structure and Classification of Cuspal Tears and Perforations in Porcine Bioprosthetic Cardiac Valves Implanted in Patients

TOKUHIRO ISHIHARA, MD, PhD
VICTOR J. FERRANS, MD, PhD
STEVEN W. BOYCE, MD
MICHAEL JONES, MD
WILLIAM C. ROBERTS, MD, FACC

Bethesda, Maryland

Morphologic studies were made of cuspal tears and perforations in 16 porcine valve bioprostheses that had been implanted in 14 patients (9 male and 5 female) ranging in age from 2 to 65 years. Eleven bioprostheses had been in the mitral position for 30 to 123 months, four in the aortic position for 15 to 40 months and one in a valved pulmonary conduit for 96 months. The cuspal lesions were classified into four types. Type I lesions, which involved the free edges of the cusps, were the most common of all lesions and occurred with equal frequency in mitral and aortic bioprostheses. Regardless of position of implantation, type I lesions were more frequent in the right coronary cusp than in the other cusps. Ultrastructural study showed that these lesions develop as consequences of breakdown of collagen at the free edges of the cusps, usually near the commissures. Type II lesions consisted of linear perforations that extended along the basal regions of the cusps, forming an arc parallel to the sewing ring. These lesions were uncommon and resulted from separation of bundles of collagen. Type III lesions, which were large, round or oval perforations that occupied central regions of the cusps, were more common in aortic than in mitral bioprostheses. They were characterized by marked destruction of cuspal tissue and were most frequently associated with infection. Type IV lesions were small pinhole-like perforations; they usually were multiple, localized in central regions of the cusps and associated with calcific deposits. Type IV lesions were more common in mitral than in aortic bioprostheses. Regardless of position, they were more frequent in the left and noncoronary cusps than in the right coronary cusp (which may be protected by its muscle shelf against this type of perforation). It is concluded that cuspal tears and perforations develop in implanted bioprostheses as consequences of structural failure of connective tissue components.

Infection, calcific deposits and cuspal disruption are the most important complications that develop in implanted porcine valve bioprostheses. The anatomic features of degenerative changes, infection and calcific deposits in bioprostheses have been reported in detail.[1–7] However, cuspal disruption, characterized by tears and perforations, has been described only briefly in follow-up series and in individual case reports,[1–31] and systematic studies have not been made to determine the patterns of anatomic distribution and the relative frequency of occurrence of these lesions in the different cusps of the bioprostheses. These questions are examined in detail in this communication, which presents a detailed description of morphologic observations in 16 porcine valve

From the Pathology Branch and the Surgery Branch, National Heart, Lung, and Blood Institute, National Institutes of Health, Bethesda, Maryland. Manuscript received March 6, 1981; revised manuscript received May 12, 1981, accepted May 21, 1981.
Address for reprints: Victor J. Ferrans, MD, Building 10, Room 7N208, National Institutes of Health, Bethesda, Maryland 20205.

bioprostheses that were found to have cuspal tears or perforations when recovered after implantation in 14 patients.

Methods

Patients and bioprostheses: The 16 bioprostheses in the study were recovered from 14 patients (9 male and 5 female), who ranged in age from 2 to 65 years. Clinical findings on these patients and morphologic observations on their bioprostheses are summarized in Table I. Eleven bioprostheses had been in place in the mitral position for 30 to 123 months, four others had been in the aortic position for 15 to 40 months and one had been in a valved pulmonary conduit for 96 months. Twelve bioprostheses were recovered at operation and four at necropsy. Four bioprostheses had clinical and morphologic evidence of bacterial infection.

Techniques of examination: Immediately after removal, each bioprosthesis was fixed with cold 3 percent glutaraldehyde in phosphate buffer. A roentgenogram of the entire bioprosthesis was taken to determine the pattern of distribution of calcific deposits, and photographs were then taken of the inflow and outflow surfaces. Selected portions of the cusps were taken for histologic study and for scanning and transmission electron microscopic examination. Techniques used for these studies have been described in detail previously.[1,3] When the amount of tissue available for study of a lesion was very limited, the preferred procedure was first to process the tissue sample for scanning electron microscopic study (which yielded the most useful information) and then to embed it in glycolmethacrylate resin for obtaining sections, 1 μ thick, to be stained by a variety of histologic methods, including hematoxylin-eosin and the von Kossa stain for calcium.

Classification of tears and perforations: Detailed observations were made of the incidence and characteristics of the tears and perforations in each of the three cusps (anatomic left, right and noncoronary) of each bioprosthesis. These le-

TABLE I

Clinical and Morphologic Observations on 16 Perforated Bioprostheses in 14 Patients

Case	Age (yr) (at Implant.) & Sex	Valve Replaced by BP	Time BP in Place (mo)	Reason for BP Removal	Ca++ in BP	Ca++ Assoc. With Perf.	Infect. of BP	Fibrous Sheath	Type and Location of Perforation: RC	LC	NC	Perf. (total n)
A. Mitral Position												
1	5 F	MV	30	S	+	+	0	0	IV	—	IV	
2	— M	MV	33	IE	+	0	+	0	—	—	IV	
3	8 F	MV	35	R	+	+	0	0	III	IV	—	
4	57 M	MV	36	S	+	+	0	0	I	IV	I, IV	
5	55 M	MV	40	N	+	0	0	0	I	I	I	
6	2 M	MV	50	S + R	+	+	0	+	—	IV	IV	
7	65 F	MV	63	R	+	+	0	+	—	II	—	
8	55 F	MV	76	N	+	+	0	0	I	I	—	
9	65 M	MV	94	N	+	+	0	0	I	I	—	
10	50 F	MV	107	S	+	+	0	+	—	IV	—	
11	53 M	MV	123	R	+	+	0	0	I	—	—	
Subtotals	Avg 41 M 6 F 5	11	Avg 62	S 3 R 3 S + R 1 N 3 IE 1	11	9	1	3	I 5 II 0 III 1 IV 1 7	I 3 II 1 III 0 IV 4 8	I 2 II 0 III 0 IV 4 6	10 1 1 9 21
B. Aortic Position												
12	30 M	AV	15	R	0	0	0	0	—	I	—	
13	35 M	AV	27	IE	+	0	+	0	I	III	I	
2	— M	AV	33	IE	+	0	+	0	III	—	—	
5	55 M	AV	40	N	+	0	+	0	I	III	I	
Subtotals	Avg 40 M 4 F 0	4	Avg 29	R 1 N 1 IE 2	3	0	3	0	I 2 II 0 III 1 IV 0 3	I 1 II 0 III 2 IV 0 3	I 2 II 0 III 0 IV 0 2	5 0 3 0 8
C. Valved Pulmonary Conduit												
14	6 M	PV	96	S	+	+	0	0	I 1	—	—	1
Totals for all BP	Avg 37 M 9 F 5	MV 11 AV 4 PV 1	Avg 56	S 4 R 4 S + R 1 N 4 IE 3	15	10	4	3	I 8 II 0 III 2 IV 1 11	I 4 II 1 III 2 IV 4 11	I 4 II 0 III 0 IV 4 8	16 1 4 9 30

Assoc. = associated; AV = aortic valve; Avg = average; BP = bioprosthesis; Ca++ = calcific deposits; Implant. = implantation; IE = infective endocarditis; Infect. = infection; LC = left coronary cusp; MV = mitral valve; N = necropsy; NC = noncoronary cusp; Perf. = perforation; PV = pulmonary valve; R = regurgitation; RC = right coronary cusp; S = stenosis; + = present; 0 = absent.

sions were classified into four types, according to the diagrams shown in Figure 1. Type I lesions were defined as tears involving the free edges of the cusps. Type II, III and IV perforations did not involve the free edges of the cusps. Type II lesions consisted of linear perforations that extended along the basal regions of the cusps forming an arc parallel to the sewing ring. Type III lesions were large, round or oval perforations that occupied the central regions of the cusps, often in association with extensive destruction of cuspal tissue. Type IV lesions were small, pinhole-like and rounded perforations; they usually were multiple and localized in central regions of the cusps, often in association with multiple calcific deposits. Examples of the four types of lesions are shown in Figure 2.

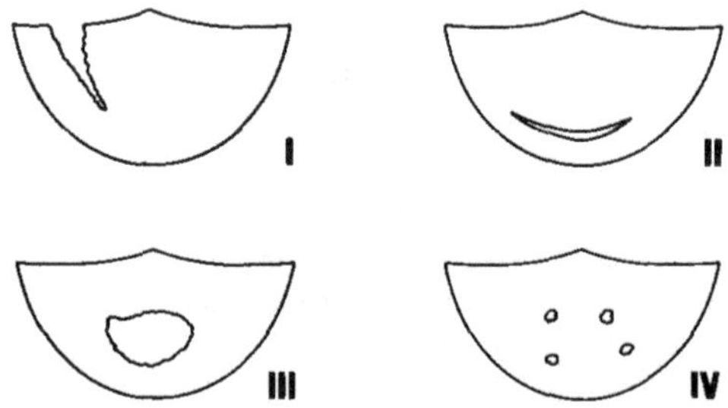

FIGURE 1. Diagram showing the four types of tears and perforations in porcine valve bioprostheses according to their localization and to the presence or absence of involvement of the cuspal free edge.

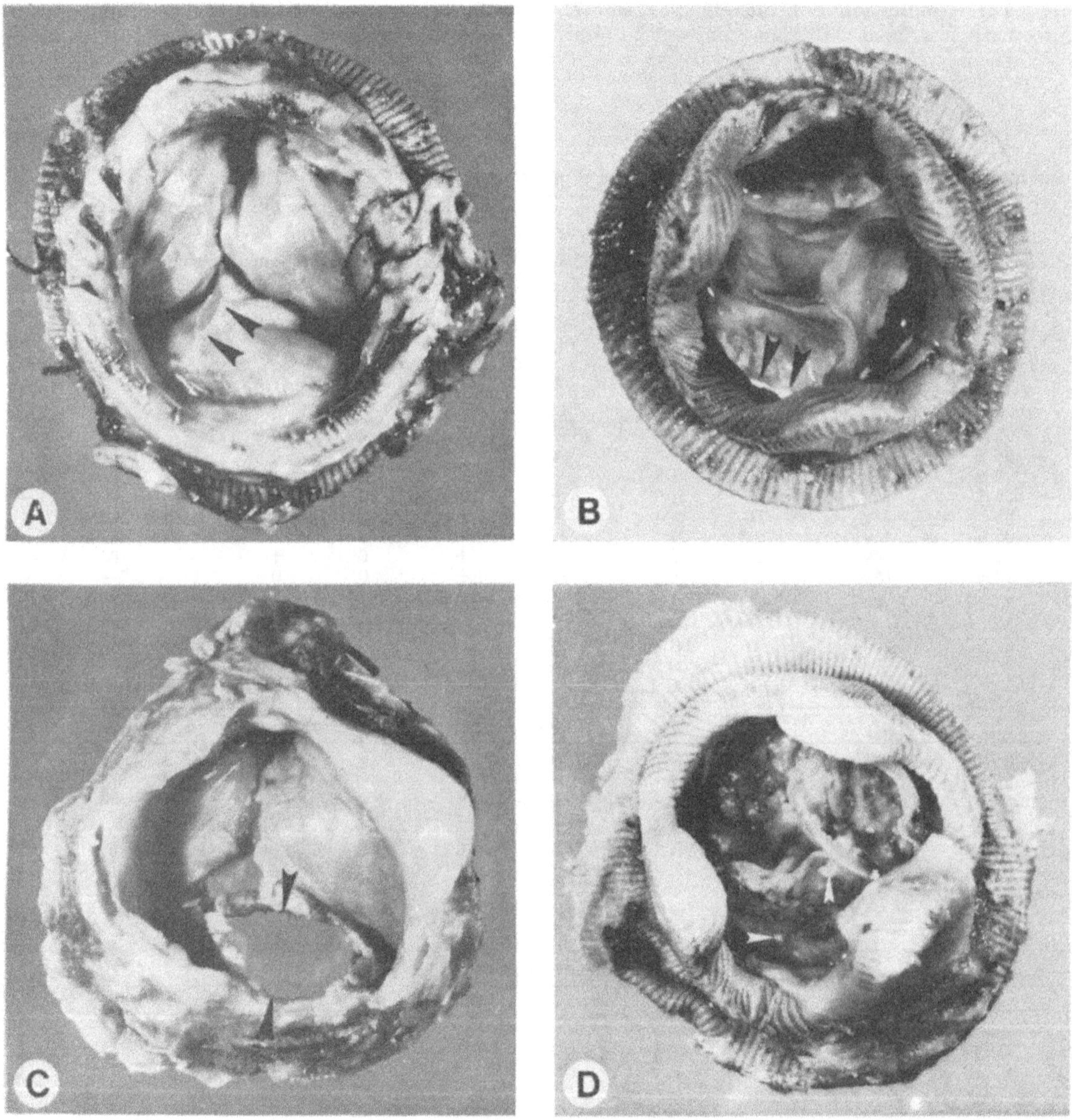

FIGURE 2. Photographs (**A** and **C** = inflow surface; **B** and **D** = outflow surface) showing examples, indicated by **arrowheads,** of the four types of cuspal lesions outlined in Figure 1. **A,** type I lesion in aortic bioprosthesis from Patient 12; **B,** type II lesion in mitral bioprosthesis from Patient 7; **C,** type III lesion in infected aortic bioprosthesis from Patient 13; and **D,** multiple, small type IV lesions in heavily calcified mitral bioprosthesis from Patient 6.

Results

Gross Anatomic Observations

Overall incidence of the four types of lesions: A total of 30 tears and perforations were identified in the 48 cusps of the 16 bioprostheses (Table I). Of the four types (Fig. 2) of cuspal lesions, type I lesions were the most common, accounting for more than 50 percent of the total number. Type II lesions were rare, occurring but once. Type III lesions also were uncommon, accounting for four perforations; three of these lesions were associated with infection of the bioprosthesis. Type IV lesions involved a total of nine cusps and in each of these they were multiple.

Two thirds of the total number of perforations, including 10 of type I, 1 of type II, 1 of type III and 9 of type IV, occurred in the 11 bioprostheses that had been implanted in the mitral position. Eight perforations, five of type I and three of type III, were found in the four bioprostheses that had been implanted in the aortic position. The bioprosthesis that had been implanted as part of a valved pulmonary conduit had a type I tear in the right coronary cusp.

Relation of lesion types to position in which the bioprostheses had been implanted: Type I lesions (Fig. 2A) were observed with equal frequency in the cusps of bioprostheses implanted in the mitral and in the aortic position. The only type II lesion (Fig. 2B) was found in a mitral bioprosthesis. Type III lesions (Fig. 2C) were more frequently found in bioprostheses implanted in the aortic (3 of 8 lesions) than in the mitral (1 of 21 lesions) position. This difference was statistically significant ($p = 0.03$) according to the two-tailed Student's t test. However, three of the four bioprostheses that had been implanted in the aortic position were infected at the time of removal, and it was found to be more likely ($p = 0.02$), according to the two-tailed Student's t test, that a type III perforation would occur in an infected than in a noninfected bioprosthesis. Nevertheless, a type III lesion did not occur in the only mitral bioprosthesis that was infected. Type IV perforations (Fig. 2D), which accounted for nearly half of all the lesions observed in the 11 bioprostheses implanted in the mitral position, occurred much more frequently ($p = 0.02$ according to the two-tailed Student's t test) in mitral than in aortic bioprostheses.

Incidence of lesions in the three cusps of the bioprostheses: The total numbers of tears and perforations were distributed with near equality in the right coronary, left coronary and noncoronary cusps of the 16 bioprostheses. However, the frequency of occurrence of the different types of lesions varied in each cusp. In the right coronary cusp, type I tears occurred more frequently ($p < 0.05$) according to the chi-square test than did type II, III or IV perforations, regardless of the position of valve implantation. Type IV perforations were very uncommon in the right coronary cusp. In contrast, the left coronary cusp and the noncoronary cusp demonstrated an equal proclivity for type I and type IV lesions, with type II and type III lesions being uncommon.

Other correlations between types of perforations and clinical and anatomic changes: Fifteen of the 16 perforated bioprostheses had been implanted for longer than 2 years. The exception to this was one noninfected aortic bioprosthesis in which regurgitation due to a type I tear developed 15 months after implantation. The average time in place for the 16 bioprostheses was 56 months. The four perforated bioprostheses that had been implanted in the aortic position had been in place for less than half of the time of those that had been implanted in the mitral position (mean 29 versus mean 62 months). However, because three of the four aortic bioprostheses were infected, it was not possible to establish a definite correlation between position of implantation and average time in place before removal for malfunction. Similarly, there was no relation between the patients' ages at the time of implantation and the type of cuspal lesions that developed subsequently.

Calcific deposits were present in 15 of the 16 bioprostheses. In 10 of the 15 the calcific deposits were immediately adjacent to the areas of perforation; of the remaining 6 perforated bioprostheses, 4 were infected and the other 2 had only type I tears.

Histologic Observations

The following types of changes (Fig. 3) were observed on histologic examination of the perforated bioprostheses: (1) alterations in connective tissue components, (2) calcific deposits, and (3) changes related to infection. The general features of these changes have been described in previous communications from this laboratory[1-3] and are illustrated in Figure 3. The four types of lesions were consistently characterized by fragmentation or loss of connective tissue components, or both, from the cusps. Type I lesions (Fig. 3, A and B) were associated with fragmentation of collagen and with loss of its normal staining properties, so that the affected areas of collagen appeared less intensely stained with toluidine blue and with eosin than was normal collagen (Fig. 3B). On examination with polarized light microscopy, these areas also appeared less intensely birefringent than did normal collagen. Similar changes were evident in the type II lesion examined. The type III lesions associated with infection had considerable amounts of disorganized necrotic collagen along their edges, together with fibrin deposits, platelets, and inflammatory cells (Fig. 3, C and D). The infecting organisms were easily identifiable in each of these lesions (Fig. 3D). The noninfected type III lesion had extensive calcific deposits around its edges; thus, it resembled a large type IV lesion.

The edges of type IV lesions consisted of various combinations of damaged, fragmented collagen and large, nodular calcific deposits (Fig. 3E). The calcific deposits in areas of perforations occupied parts of the spongiosa, from which zone they extended toward the surfaces, most often projecting into the cuspal pockets. The overall thickness of the cusps was appreciably in-

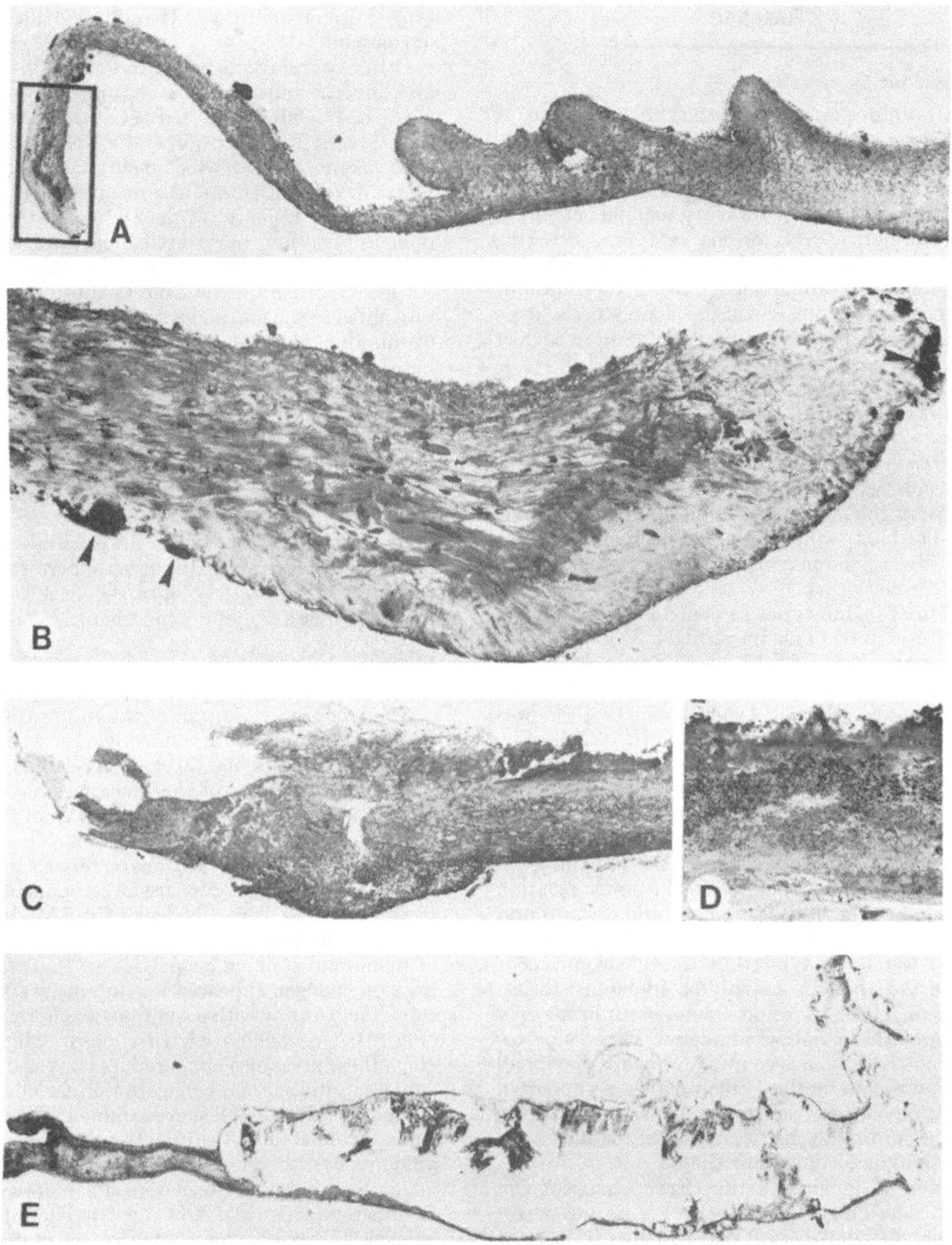

FIGURE 3. Histologic appearance of tears and perforations in porcine bioprostheses (1 μ thick sections of glycolmethacrylate-embedded tissues, alkaline toluidine blue stain). **A,** low magnification view of cuspal tissue in area of type I tear in aortic bioprosthesis shown in Figure 2A. The inflow surface is at **bottom,** the outflow surface at **top.** The edge of the tear is enclosed within the **rectangle** at **left;** the ridges inside the cusp pocket are seen at the **upper center** and **right. B,** higher magnification view of cuspal tissue forming the edge of the tear shown in **A.** This edge is constituted by a zone of lightly stained, damaged collagen that is distinguishable from the darker, more normal-staining collagen elsewhere in the cusp. Aggregates of platelets (**arrowheads**) are present on the surfaces. **C,** edge of type III perforation associated with bacterial infection in the aortic bioprosthesis from Patient 2. The edge of the perforation is shown at the **far left;** necrotic, infected cuspal tissue undergoing disruption is seen at **center** and **right. D,** higher magnification view of area on right side of **C,** showing fibrin deposits and numerous cocci. **E,** edge of type IV perforation associated with calcification of cuspal connective tissue in the bioprosthesis shown in Figure 2D. Normal tissue is shown at **left;** a large calcific deposit (partially lost during tissue preparation) occupies the area at **center** and **right.** The perforation edge is at the **far right.** Note the increase in cuspal thickness and almost complete loss of normal cuspal connective tissue in the area of calcification. (**A** and **C** ×40, **B** and **D** ×250, **E** ×25, all reduced by 17 percent.)

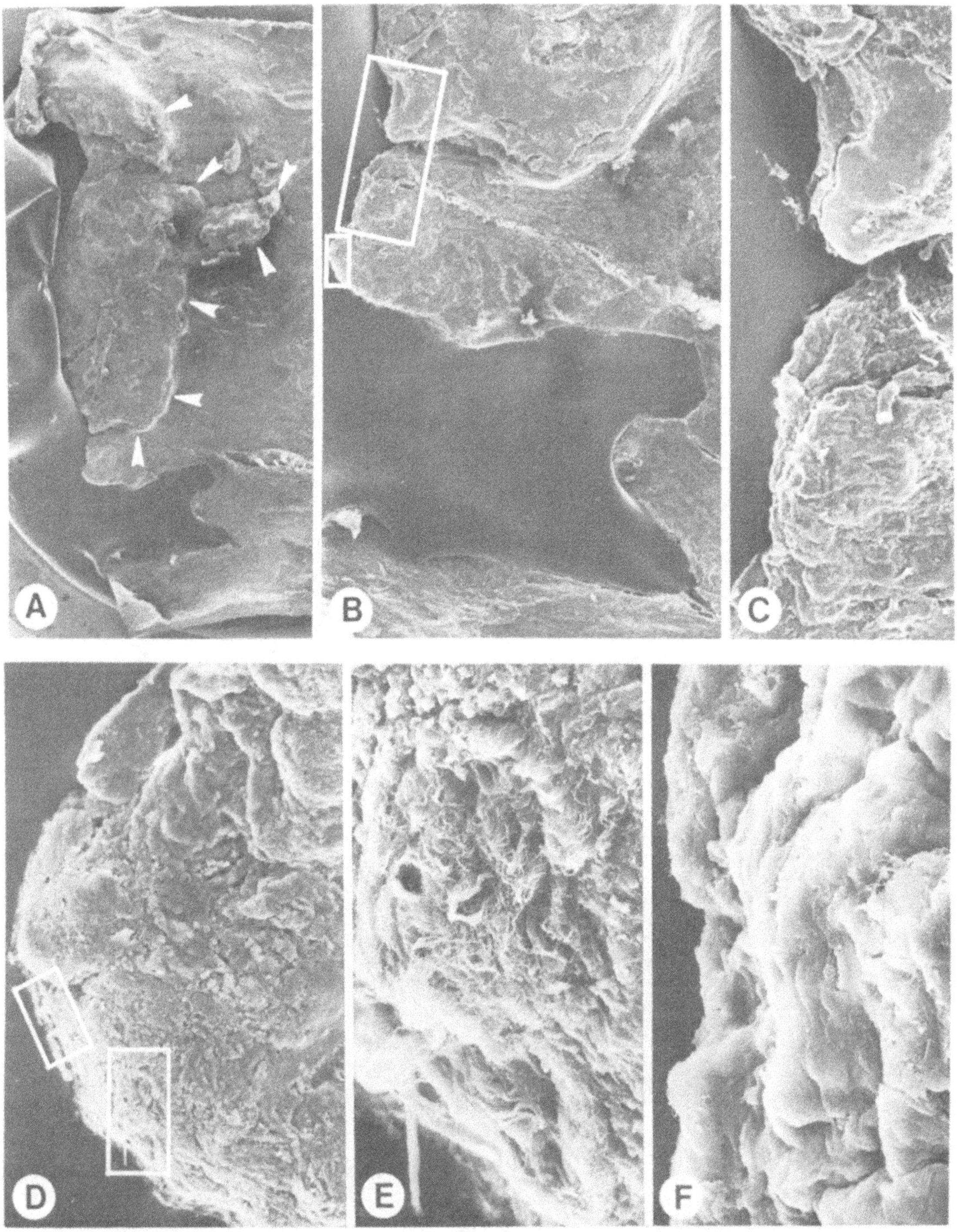

FIGURE 4. Scanning electron micrographs of edges of type I tear in mitral bioprosthesis from Patient 11. **A,** low magnification view of one side of the tear, which extends from the free edge (**top**) to the base (**bottom**) of the cusp. The outflow surface of cusp is shown. The raised areas at **center** and **upper right** are calcific deposits (**arrowheads**). The smooth area at **center left** and the arc-like structure at **lower left** are parts of the metal stub in which the specimen was mounted for scanning electron microscopic observation. **B,** higher magnification view of the area in which the tear widens and extends toward the base and the center of cusp. Note the erosion of tissue at edge and fragmentation of tissue layers at the boundary between raised and flat areas of tissue. The area within the **large rectangle** is shown at higher magnification in **C;** the area within the **small rectangle,** in **D. C,** area of fragmentation and erosion of connective tissue at the lower edge of the calcific deposit. **D,** view of the area within the **small rectangle** in **B.** Although this area appears smooth at low magnification, higher magnification reveals that it consists of terrace-like zones of progressively more fragmented and eroded tissue. The areas indicated by the **large** and the **small rectangle** are shown at higher magnification in **E** and **F,** respectively. **E,** fraying of collagen fibrils is demonstrated. **F,** bundles of collagen in this region are separated but appear smooth and nonfrayed. (**A** ×12, **B** ×36, **C** ×120, **D** ×300, **E** ×1,200, **F** ×1,500, all reduced by 17 percent.)

creased in regions of calcification. The layers of cuspal connective tissue immediately overlying the calcific deposits had been displaced from their normal position and often had been almost completely eroded.

Scanning Electron Microscopic Observations

Type I lesions (*Fig. 4*) extended irregularly from the free edges toward central regions of the cusps. The edges of these lesions appeared irregular, showing evidence of erosion, fragmentation, separation and breakage of connective tissue components. The erosion was manifested by marked thinning of the cuspal tissue. This thinning progressed toward the lesion edges, in which successive layers of connective tissue showed increasing degrees of damage. Although many of these areas appeared smooth at low magnification, study at high

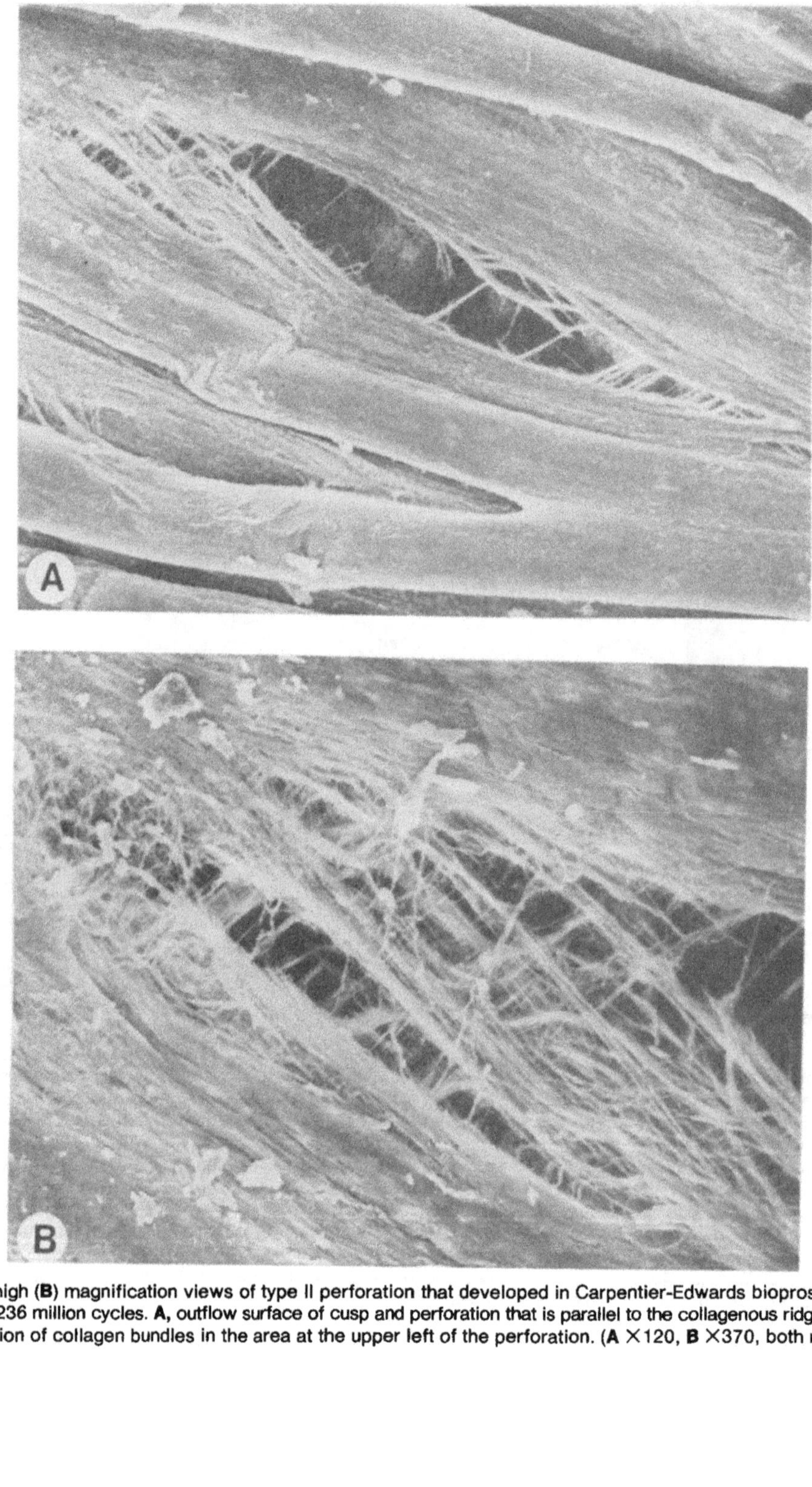

FIGURE 5. Low (**A**) and high (**B**) magnification views of type II perforation that developed in Carpentier-Edwards bioprosthesis after accelerated fatigue testing in vitro for 236 million cycles. **A,** outflow surface of cusp and perforation that is parallel to the collagenous ridges on the cuspal surface. **B,** separation and disruption of collagen bundles in the area at the upper left of the perforation. (**A** ×120, **B** ×370, both reduced by 18 percent.)

magnification revealed that they contained frayed ends of collagen fibrils and elastic fibers.

The type II lesion differed from the other types in that it showed a considerable amount of separation of bundles of collagen that were oriented parallel to the free edge of the cusps. This lesion type was reproduced easily in bioprostheses subjected to accelerated fatigue testing in vitro (Fig. 5).

The edges of type III lesions (*Fig. 6*) appeared very irregular and had strands of fibrin and necrotic collagen that projected into the lumen of the perforation. In infected type III lesions, inflammatory cells were abundant and microorganisms were unequivocally identified along the edges.

Type IV lesions (*Fig. 7*) often were associated with nodular calcific deposits. Some of these were raised but had smooth surfaces composed of collagen and fibrin, whereas others had irregular surfaces composed of partially eroded calcific deposits and damaged collagen. Platelets were frequently adherent to collagen in these areas.

Transmission Electron Microscopic Observations

Study by transmission electron microscopy revealed basically similar connective tissue changes along the edges of perforations not associated with infection. These changes (Fig. 8, A and B) consisted of the following: (1) fragmentation of collagen fibrils; (2) marked decrease in the numbers of collagen fibrils; (3) presence of large amounts of amorphous to finely granular material between the remaining collagen fibrils; (4) irregular stainability of the collagen; (5) infiltration by numerous lipid droplets that measured up to 1 μ in di-

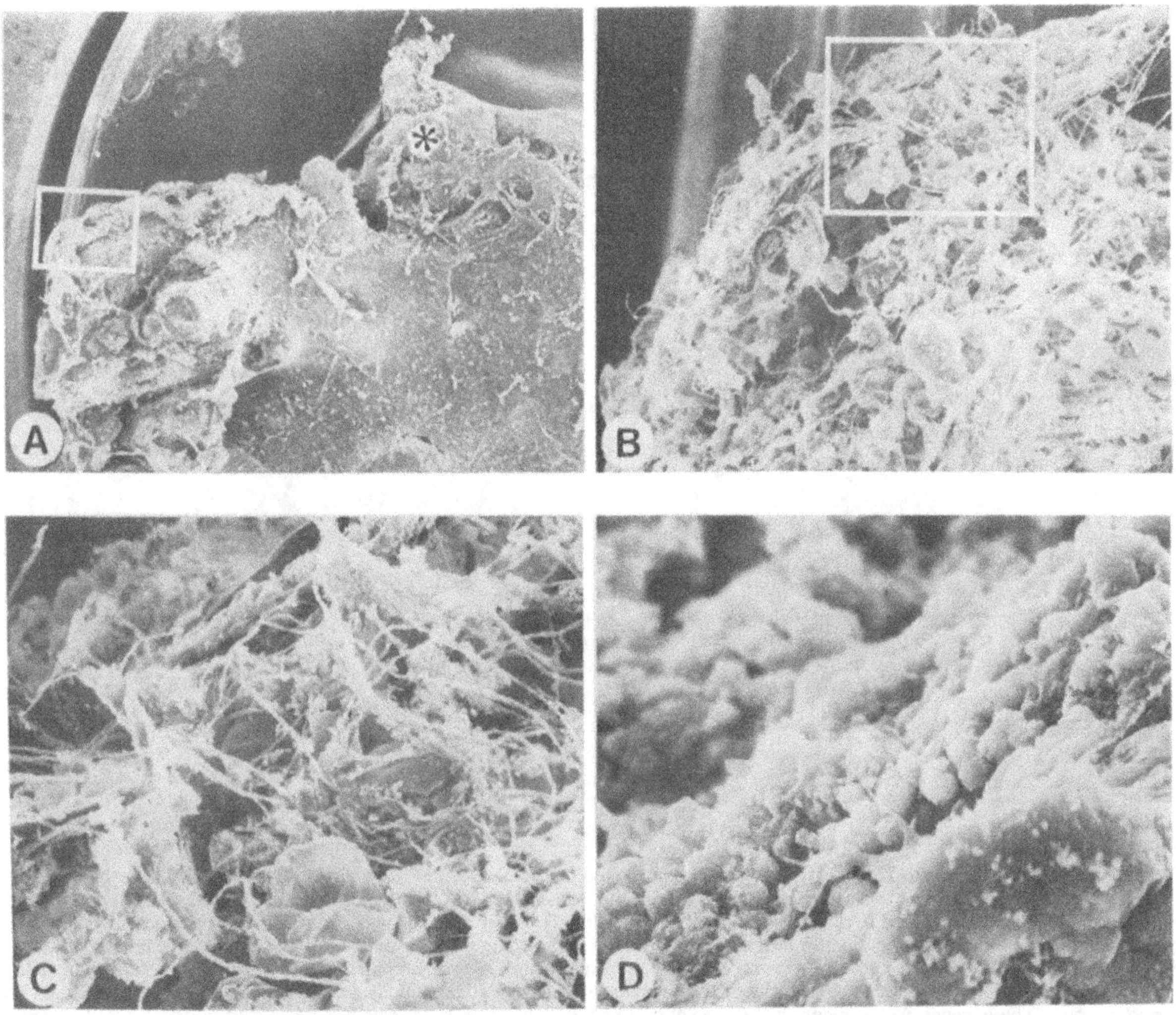

FIGURE 6. Scanning electron micrographs of edge of type III perforation in infected aortic bioprosthesis from Patient 13 (compare with gross photo of bioprosthesis in Fig. 2C). **A,** low magnification view of part of edge, showing highly irregular borders. The **rectangle** indicates the area shown at higher magnifications in **B** and **C.** The area indicated by the asterisk is shown at higher magnification in **D.** The arcs at **left** in **A** and **B** are parts of the specimen mounting stub. **B** and **C,** areas in which the surface is composed of fibrin strands and amorphous debris. The area enclosed within the **rectangle** in **B** is shown at higher magnification in **C. D,** a colony of rounded bacteria responsible for bioprosthetic infection is seen near the edge of the perforation. (**A** ×19, **B** ×250, **C** ×780, **D** ×4,500, all reduced by 17 percent.)

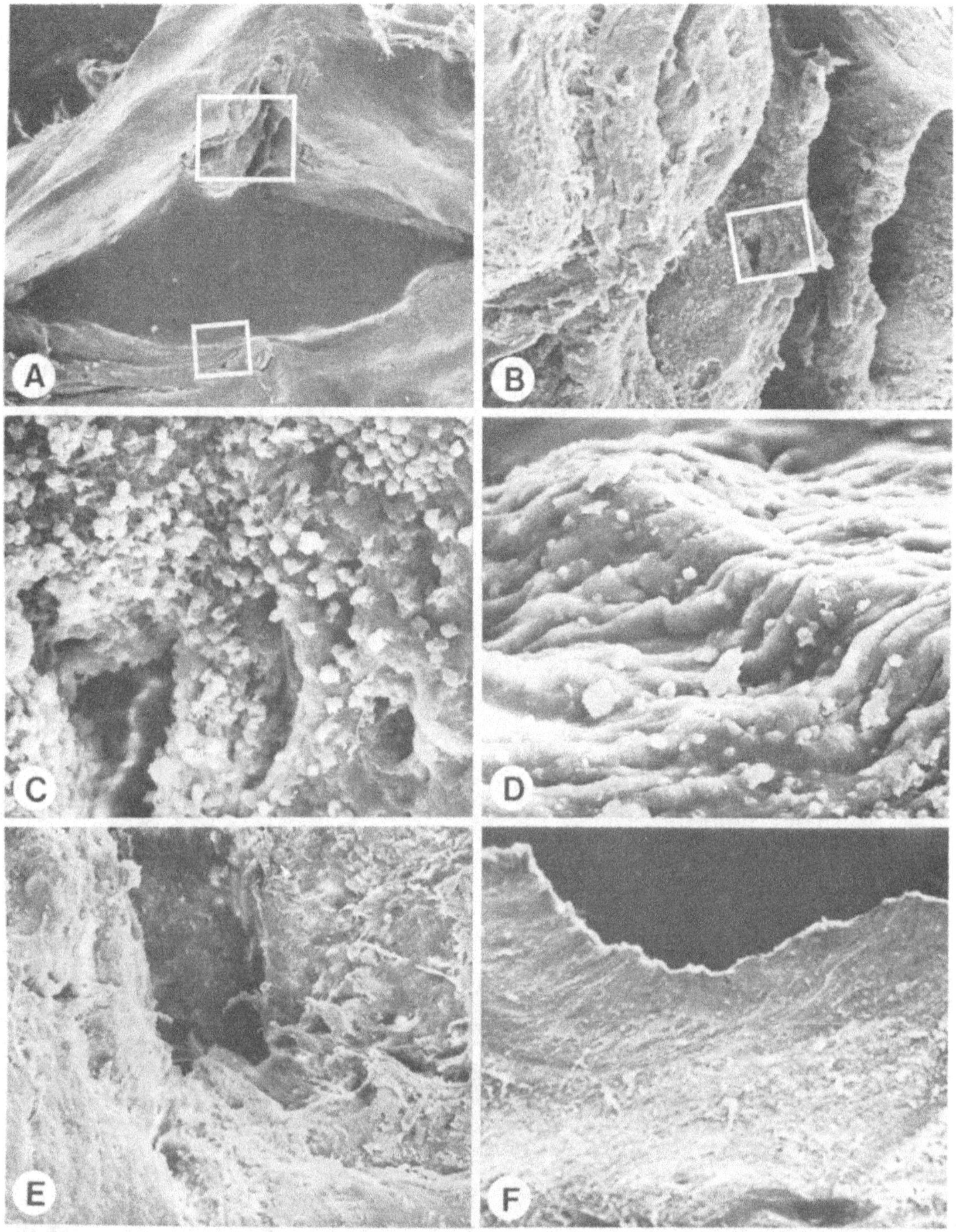

FIGURE 7. Scanning electron micrographs of type IV perforations in the bioprostheses of Patient 6 (**A** to **D**), Patient 10 (**E**) and Patient 2 (**F**). **A,** an oblong perforation appears to be extending (**upper center**) toward the free edge of the cusp. Areas within the **large** and the **small rectangle** are shown at higher magnification in **B** and **D,** respectively. **B,** higher magnification view of the area of extension of the perforation, showing breakage and separation of adjacent layers of connective tissue. The area within the **rectangle** is shown again in **C. C,** eroded surface of the bioprosthesis is covered with platelets. **D,** area from the **small rectangle** in **A,** showing platelets overlying a surface composed of collagen bundles arranged in parallel. **E,** the edge of this perforation appears as a crater with highly irregular sides composed of frayed collagen bundles. **F,** tissue at the edge of this perforation has been considerably thinned by erosion of cuspal connective tissue. (**A** ×40, **B** ×240, **C** ×1,800, **D** ×1,200, **E** ×66, **F** ×110, all reduced by 17 percent.)

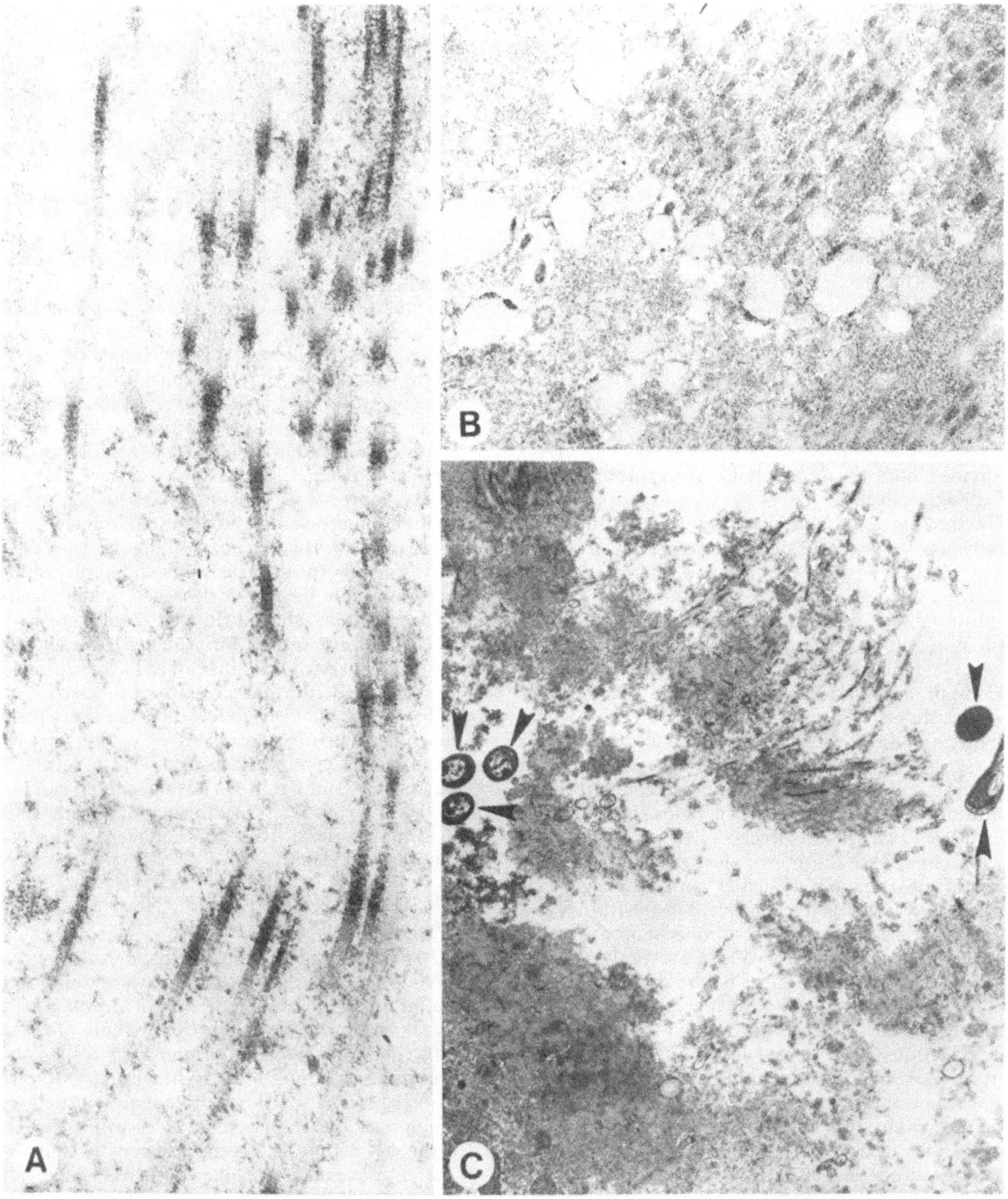

FIGURE 8. Transmission electron micrographs of cuspal connective tissue at edges of perforations in mitral bioprostheses from Patient 10 (**A** and **B**) and Patient 2 (**C**). **A,** disrupted collagen fibrils end in tufts of finely granular material. Considerable amounts of similar material are scattered in interstitium. Compare with the scanning electron micrograph of the same perforation shown in Figure 7E. **B,** lipid droplets (L) are associated with damaged collagen and granular material. **C,** bacteria (**arrowheads**) are adjacent to damaged collagen at the edge of the perforation. (**A** ×45,000, **B** ×43,000, **C** ×13,000, all reduced by 18 percent.)

ameter and often were associated with the amorphous material described previously; (6) evidence of calcification of collagen fibrils; and (7) few or no alterations involving elastic tissue. In addition to these alterations, areas of infection had marked necrotic changes and contained bacteria (Fig. 8C). The calcific deposits were ultrastructurally similar to those described in detail from this laboratory.[3]

Discussion

Connective tissue failure: The observations in this study show that cuspal tears and perforations develop in bioprostheses as the final consequences of tissue failure. These observations also suggest that connective tissue failure develops in areas in which mechanical forces are exerted in a highly localized manner either because of the patterns of opening and closure of the bioprosthetic cusps or because of the presence of calcific deposits. The three main connective tissue components of porcine bioprostheses are elastic fibers, proteoglycans and collagen fibrils.

Elastic fibers: Elastic fibers in implanted bioprostheses show few structural alterations. They are small in size, relatively few in number and mainly localized in the ventricularis layer. Their functional role in maintaining the integrity of glutaraldehyde-treated bioprostheses is uncertain. In contrast to this, both the proteoglycan material and the collagen fibrils play important but different roles with respect to the durability of bioprostheses.

Proteoglycans: Proteoglycans are major components of the spongiosa, from which they are largely extracted during preimplantation processing and soon after implantation.[1] Their loss from the spongiosa is thought to have at least two critical effects. The first of these is a marked change in the mechanical properties of the matrix of the spongiosa. Proteoglycans form a gel that dampens and cushions the movement of the fibrosa and the ventricularis with respect to one another during valve opening and closure. When proteoglycans are extracted, this damping effect is lost and "delamination" or separation of adjacent layers of cuspal connective tissue develops.[1,3,4] The second consequence of the extraction of proteoglycans is the formation of empty spaces in the spongiosa. Such spaces become filled with plasma proteins and formed elements of the blood, and eventually become sites of calcification.[3] It is clear from our observations that type IV cuspal perforations tend to develop in close association with calcific deposits.

Collagen: Because collagen is the most important structural component of bioprosthetic heart valves, tissue failure in these devices must be regarded mainly as collagen failure. It is evident that tissue failure (that is, breakdown of collagen) can be mediated by different mechanisms (infection, poorly understood biochemical factors, purely mechanical factors) and can be localized in different areas of the cusps, thus resulting in the four types of tears and perforations observed in this study.

Role of infection: Our observations also show that the frequency distributions of some of these lesions vary in the three cusps and according to the sites of implantation of the bioprostheses. The contribution of bioprosthetic infection to cuspal perforations was evident in four of the bioprostheses, and in these the resulting lesions had a characteristic morphology. It has been postulated that subclinical infection can contribute to bioprosthetic failure.[4] However, we have encountered only one example of this, and the infecting organisms were demonstrated in this bioprosthesis by transmission electron microscopy.[2]

Role of biochemical changes: The contribution of biochemical changes to the breakdown of collagen remains to be defined. It is known that treatment with aldehyde fixatives increases considerably the extent of collagen cross-linking and the resistance of collagen to attack by collagenases.[32,33] However, it is not known whether these modified properties are altered by severe degrees of mechanical disruption of the collagen fibrils. Furthermore, it is possible that the glutaraldehyde treatment increases the brittleness of collagen. Although the reasons for this are not completely clear, the cuspal areas forming the edges of tears and perforations show a considerable degree of decrease in the numbers of collagen fibrils; those fibrils that remain are associated with large amounts of amorphous to finely granular material and with lipid droplets. These alterations indicate that the normal mechanical properties of these areas of tissue have been lost, because these properties depend on the integrity of the collagen. As discussed in detail later, the morphologic patterns of localization of the cuspal lesions that we have observed can be interpreted in terms of the localization of mechanical forces of compressive flexure of collagen[34] during valve opening and closure.

Pathogenesis of Different Types of Tears and Perforations

Type I lesions: These lesions, defined as tears involving the free edge of the cusp, were found to have a similar incidence in bioprostheses implanted in the mitral and in the aortic position. In both of these positions they were the most common type of lesion. They were more common in the right coronary cusp than in the other two cusps. They did not appear to be related to bioprosthetic infection or calcification. Our concept of the pathogenesis of type I lesions is that they are caused by breakage of collagen fibrils located along the free edge of the cusp. Such tears did not involve the central third of the free edge; instead, they were found in the lateral thirds, in which the edge of the cusp is thinner than in the central third (the latter is reinforced by the nodulus Arantii). The collagen along the free edge of the cusp is arranged parallel to this edge, extending from one commissure to the other. The mechanical forces of compressive flexure to which this collagen is subjected during valve opening and closure[34] are considered to be the main factors responsible for the development of type I tears. Such flexure-induced breakage of collagen would appear to be increased (over that in normal valves in situ) by two factors: treatment of the tissue with glutaraldehyde under pressure, and the mounting of the bioprosthesis on a stent. Fixation under pressure decreases the collagen waviness or "crimping."[34] This collagen waviness serves the purpose of distributing the bending stresses more evenly than is the case with collagen that has been straightened out.[34]

The use of a flexible stent and the technique of placement of sutures anchoring the aortic wall to the dacron covering of the stent have been considered to diminish the likelihood of cuspal tears.[4] These are thought to occur with greater frequency in bioprostheses with rigid stents than in those with flexible stents. Nevertheless, the contribution of the flexible stent in this regard has been questioned,[35] and we found type I tears to be the most common type of lesions in porcine aortic valve bioprostheses mounted in flexible stents. The nonexpanding nature of the bioprosthetic stent contrasts with the normal aortic valve ring, which undergoes expansion as the valve opens in vivo and in situ. This expansion allows the cusps to move to the open position, without bending in the radial direction, during isovolumetric contraction.[36,37] During aortic valve closure, the contraction of the ring to its minimal perimeter displaces the cusps inward, thus reducing the distance that the cusps must travel to close the valve.[36,37] In contrast, the cusps of porcine bioprostheses with nonexpansile stents do not open before the end of isovolumetric systole; instead, the cusps are opened by the rapid ventricular ejection, creating increased bending stresses. In addition, valve closure is delayed until reverse flow is established; then the cusps have to arrest the momentum of blood, causing further mechanical stresses upon the cusps.[38]

The pattern of uneven opening of the cusps of porcine bioprostheses is also thought to contribute to the development of localized bending stresses. These cusps open unevenly, with the right coronary cusp tending to open less than the other two cusps (because of the cardiac muscle shelf that it contains). The degree to which the three cusps open is related to the characteristics of the flow through the valve.[39] Under circumstances of low flow, the shape of the orifice created by the opening of these cusps tends to be triangular, under which conditions the free edges of the cusps undergo maximal bending not at the commissures but, instead, at points between the commissures and the junctions of the central and the lateral thirds of the free edges (particularly in the right coronary cusp). Thus, it seems reasonable to conclude that the patterns of opening and closure of the cusps of porcine bioprostheses, together with the straightening of the waviness of the collagen fibrils, tend to result in bending stresses which become localized at certain points along the free edges. Therefore, tears that develop along the free edges of the cusps can be regarded as flexure lesions analogous to those that are related to "hinging" of the basal regions of the cusps.

Type II lesions: These lesions, defined as perforations parallel to the basal attachment of the cusp, were more uncommon than had been anticipated in light of (1) the relatively minimal thicknesses of the basal regions of the cusps, and (2) the "hinging" motion reported to occur in these regions during cuspal opening and closure.[4] Nevertheless, the possibility must be considered that type II lesions, particularly those that develop in bioprostheses implanted in the aortic position, may progress to type III lesions before the bioprosthesis fails clinically. Evidence presented in this study suggests that separation of adjacent, parallel bundles of collagen plays an important role in the pathogenesis of type II lesions. This concept is based on scanning electron microscopic observations made on porcine bioprostheses failing in vitro during the course of extended durability testing. Such a separation of collagen bundles was not a feature of the other three types of lesions. The relatively high frequency of type II lesions in bioprostheses subjected to accelerated fatigue testing is probably related to the high speed of valve motion, which tends to maximize the "hinging" and to keep it more sharply localized to a given region. Other observations suggest that formation of a fibrous sheath and covering of basal portions of bioprosthetic cusps by endothelial cells of host origin also protect against development of type II lesions.[40]

Tears and perforations have been reported in bioprostheses subjected to accelerated fatigue testing.[41,42] The relation between these lesions and those observed in our study is difficult to evaluate because the hemodynamics and the pattern of bioprosthetic cuspal motion are different in vivo and in conditions of in vitro testing. Furthermore, the analysis of lesion types presented in our study has not been applied to valve failure in vitro. The very few reports published of perforations developing under conditions of accelerated fatigue testing have described type I, II and III lesions that appear similar on gross anatomic study to those described in this communication.

Type III lesions: These lesions, consisting of rounded or oval perforations involving central areas of the cusps, were more common in bioprostheses implanted in the aortic position than in those implanted in the mitral position. The considerable loss of cuspal tissue found in these lesions was associated either with infection or with severe degenerative changes, including fragmentation and breakdown of collagen, lipid infiltration and calcific deposits.

Type IV lesions: These lesions were related to calcific deposits, and we believe that they develop as a consequence of bending stresses at the boundaries between highly rigid calcific deposits and adjacent areas of soft, degenerated collagen. Type IV lesions may progress to type III lesions, particularly in bioprostheses implanted in the aortic position. This possibility is suggested by the paucity of type IV lesions in aortic bioprostheses, a finding that could be interpreted as meaning that a small (type IV) perforation could expand and become a large (type III) perforation. Type

IV lesions tended to be multiple and occurred more frequently in the noncoronary and left coronary cusps than in the right coronary cusp. The muscle shelf that extends into the proximal third of the right coronary cusp may have exerted a protective effect against the development of these lesions, possibly by providing additional structural support, by undergoing less calcification and by minimizing bending stresses in this cusp. In contrast, type I lesions were more common in the right coronary cusp than in the other two cusps, a finding that again seems to reflect the anatomic and functional asymmetry of the porcine aortic valve.

In conclusion, the results of our study show that cuspal tears and perforations develop as consequences of structural failure of connective tissue components. Four different types of these lesions can be recognized according to their anatomic features. These features reflect different pathogenetic mechanisms, including mechanical factors, biochemical alterations and infection.

References

1. **Ferrans VJ, Spray TL, Billingham ME, Roberts WC.** Structural changes in glutaraldehyde-treated porcine heterografts used as substitute cardiac valves. Transmission and scanning electron microscopic observations in 12 patients. Am J Cardiol 1978;41: 1159–84.
2. **Ferrans VJ, Boyce SW, Billingham ME, Spray TL, Roberts WC.** Infection of glutaraldehyde-preserved porcine valve heterografts. Am J Cardiol 1979;43:1123–36.
3. **Ferrans VJ, Boyce SW, Billingham ME, Jones M, Ishihara T, Roberts WC.** Calcific deposits in porcine bioprostheses: structure and pathogenesis. Am J Cardiol 1980;46:721–34.
4. **Angell WW, Angell JD.** Porcine valves. Prog Cardiovasc Dis 1980;23:141–66.
5. **Spray TL, Roberts WC.** Structural changes in porcine xenografts used as substitute cardiac valves. Gross and histologic observations in 51 glutaraldehyde-preserved Hancock valves in 41 patients. Am J Cardiol 1977;40:319–30.
6. **Fishbein MC, Gissen SA, Collins JJ Jr, Barsamian EM, Cohn LH.** Pathologic findings after cardiac valve replacement with glutaraldehyde-fixed porcine valves. Am J Cardiol 1977;40:331–7.
7. **Magilligan DJ Jr, Lewis JW Jr, Jara FM, et al.** Spontaneous degeneration of porcine bioprosthetic valves. Ann Thorac Surg 1980;30:259–66.
8. **Carpentier A, Deloche A, Relland J, et al.** Six-year follow-up of glutaraldehyde-preserved heterografts. With particular reference to the treatment of congenital valve malformation. J Thorac Cardiovasc Surg 1974;68:771–81.
9. **Gallucci V.** Discussion of Carpentier et al.[8] J Thorac Cardiovasc Surg 1974;68:782.
10. **McIntosh CL, Michaelis LL, Morrow AG, Itscoitz SB, Redwood DR, Epstein SE.** Atrioventricular valve replacement with the Hancock porcine xenograft: a five year clinical experience. Surgery 1975;78:768–75.
11. **Hannah H, Reis RL.** Current status of porcine heterograft prostheses. A 5- year appraisal. Circulation 1976;54:Suppl III:III-27–31.
12. **Cevèse PG, Gallucci V, Morea M, Volta SD, Fasoli G, Casarotto D.** Heart valve replacement with the Hancock bioprosthesis. Analysis of long-term results (abstr). Circulation 1977;56:Suppl II:II-16.
13. **Zuhdi N.** The porcine aortic valve bioprosthesis: a significant alternative. Ann Thorac Surg 1976;21:573–5.
14. **Stinson EB, Griepp RB, Oyer PE, Shumway NE.** Long-term experience with porcine aortic valve xenografts. J Thorac Cardiovasc Surg 1977;73:54–63.
15. **Housman LB, Pitt WA, Mazur JH, Litchford B, Gross SA.** Mechanical failure (leaflet disruption) of a porcine aortic heterograft. Rare cause of acute aortic insufficiency. J Thorac Cardiovasc Surg 1978;76:212–3.
16. **Hetzer R, Hill JD, Kerth WJ, Wilson AJ, Adappa MG, Gerbode F.** Thrombosis and degeneration of Hancock valves: clinical and pathological findings. Ann Thorac Surg 1978;26:317–22.
17. **Brown JW, Dunn JM, Spooner E, Kirsh MM.** Late spontaneous disruption of a porcine xenograft mitral valve. Clinical, hemodynamic, echocardiographic, and pathological findings. J Thorac Cardiovasc Surg 1978;75:606–11.
18. **Bloch WN Jr, Karcioglu Z, Felner JM, Miller JS, Symbas PN, Schlant RC.** Idiopathic perforation of a porcine aortic bioprosthesis in the aortic position. Chest 1978;74:579–81.
19. **Oyer PE, Stinson EB, Reitz BA, Miller DC, Rossiter SJ, Shumway NE.** Long-term evaluation of the porcine xenograft bioprosthesis. J Thorac Cardiovasc Surg 1979;78:343–50.
20. **Geha AS, Laks H, Stansel HC Jr, et al.** Late failure of porcine valve heterografts in children. J Thorac Cardiovasc Surg 1979;78: 351–64.
21. **Magilligan DJ, Lewis JW, Jara FM, Lakier JB, Davila JC.** Indications for reoperation after bioprosthetic valve implantation. Experience with the porcine xenograft valve. In: Sebening F, Klövekorn WP, Meisner H, Struck E, eds. Bioprosthetic Cardiac Valves. Munich: Deutsches Herzzentrum München 1979:319–33.
22. **Oyer PE, Stinson EB, Rossiter SJ, Miller DC, Reitz BA, Shumway NE.** Extended experience with the Hancock xenograft bioprosthesis. In Ref 21:47–59.
23. **Bachet J, Bical O, Goudot B, Menu P, Richard T, Barbagelatta M, Guilmet D.** Early structural failure of porcine xenografts in young patients. In Ref 21:341–9.
24. **Le Clerc JL, Deuvaert FE, Wellens F, Goffin Y, Primo G.** A four year experience of bioprosthetic cardiac valve replacement. Early and late results. In Ref 21:27–38.
25. **Myerowitz PD, Lamberti JJ, Replogle RL, Schwarz D, Anagnostopoulos E.** Delayed complications following heterograft valve replacement. In Ref 21:335–40.
26. **Angell WW.** A nine year experience with the Angell-Shiley xenograft and a comparative literature review of the porcine bioprosthesis versus the mechanical prosthesis. In Ref 21: 81–104.
27. **Monties JR, Goudard A, Blin D, et al.** 481 bioprosthetic valves. Early and middle term results. In Ref 21:39–46.
28. **Casarotto D, Bortolotti U, Thiene G, Gallucci V, Cevèse PG.** Long-term results (from 5 to 7 years) with the Hancock S-G-P bioprosthesis. J Cardiovasc Surg (Torino) 1979;20:399–406.
29. **Williams JB, Karp RB, Kirklin JW, et al.** Considerations in selection and management of patients undergoing valve replacement with glutaraldehyde-fixed porcine bioprostheses. Ann Thorac Surg 1980;30:247–58.
30. **Sanders SP, Levy RJ, Freed MD, Norwood WI, Castaneda AR.** Use of Hancock porcine xenografts in children and adolescents. Am J Cardiol 1980;46:429–38.
31. **Crupi G, Gibson D, Heard B, Lincoln C.** Severe late failure of a porcine xenograft mitral valve: clinical, echocardiographic, and pathological findings. Thorax 1980;35:210–2.
32. **Woodroof E.** The chemistry and biology of aldehyde treated tissue heart valve xenografts. In: Ionescu MI, ed. Tissue Heart Valves. London: Butterworths, 1979:347–62.
33. **Harris ED Jr, Farrell ME.** Resistance to collagenase: a characteristic of collagen fibrils cross-linked by formaldehyde. Biochim Biophys Acta 1972;278:133–41.
34. **Broom ND.** Fatigue-induced damage in glutaraldehyde-preserved heart valve tissue. J Thorac Cardiovasc Surg 1978;76:202–11.
35. **Thomson FJ, Barratt-Boyes BG.** The glutaraldehyde-treated heterograft valve. Some engineering observations. J Thorac Cardiovasc Surg 1977;74:317–21.

36. **Thubrikar M, Bosher LP, Nolan SP.** The mechanism of opening of the aortic valve. J Thorac Cardiovasc Surg 1979;77:863–70.
37. **Thubrikar M, Nolan SP, Bosher LP, Deck JD.** The cyclic changes and structure of the base of the aortic valve. Am Heart J 1980; 99:217–24.
38. **Thubrikar M, Piepgrass WC, Deck JD, Nolan SP.** Stresses of natural versus prosthetic aortic valve leaflets in vivo. Ann Thorac Surg 1980;30:230–9.
39. **Wright JTM.** Hydrodynamic evaluation of tissue valves. In Ref 32:29–87.
40. **Ishihara T, Ferrans VJ, Jones M, Boyce SW, Roberts WC.** Occurrence and significance of endothelial cells in implanted porcine bioprosthetic valves. Am J Cardiol 1981;48:443–54.
41. **Clark RE, Swanson WM.** In vitro durability of Hancock model 242 porcine heart valve. J Thorac Cardiovasc Surg 1979;78:277–80.
42. **Estes MS, Komatsu SK, Nashef A, Lane E.** In-vitro testing of bioprostheses. In Ref 21:271–7.

Complications of cardiac valve replacement: Characteristic abnormalities of prostheses pertaining to any or specific site

William C. Roberts, M.D. *Bethesda, Md.*

It has been over 21 years since successful replacement of one or more cardiac valves became a reality, and since then many thousands of patients with severely symptomatic valvular heart disease have had valve replacement with complete loss or sharp decrease in their symptoms of cardiac dysfunction. Although the chance of successful valve replacement in most patients is very high, occasional, often predictable, complications are recognized to occur both early and late in some patients in whom this precedure is carried out. Since 1960, I have examined at necropsy over 600 hearts, submitted from around the U.S.A., containing one or more prosthetic valves, and certain complications of cardiac valve replacement observed in them are delineated in this presentation.

COMPLICATIONS COMMON TO ANY VALVE SITE AND MOST OR ALL PRESENTLY AVAILABLE MECHANICAL OR BIOPROSTHETIC VALVES

1. Prosthetic size disproportion. The normal cardiac valves consist of thin, very pliable leaflet-like structures which allow central flow of blood and occupy very little space within the ventricles or great arteries in which they reside. Mechanical valves and even tissue valves attached to rigid or semirigid stents and rings, in contrast, are rigid except for movement of the occluder or cusps; they often prevent central flow, and they occupy noncompressible space. Early in the history of cardiac valve replacement, there appeared to be a tendency to insert as large a prosthesis as possible because of its tendency to be less inherently obstructive than the smaller sized prosthesis. Experience taught, however, that if a mechanical prosthesis was too big for the ventricle or ascending aorta into which it was to reside, that movement of the occluder could be limited, with the potential for varying degrees of obstruction to flow.[1-15] At one time, a common view was that this disproportion problem was mainly one produced by caged-ball prostheses because they were larger than most subsequently utilized mechanical prostheses. This view, however, is incorrect. No mechanical valve and no tissue valve (Fig. 1) attached to a frame is immune to the problem of prosthetic disproportion.

The usual consequence in the mitral position is interference to left atrial (LA) emptying (or to left ventricular filling) and, rarely, in my experience, despite beliefs to the contrary, interference with left ventricular (LV) emptying (LV outflow obstruction).[1] The usual consequence in the aortic position is interference to LV emptying. Prosthetic disproportion is most likely to occur in the mitral position when valve replacement is carried out for pure mitral stenosis (MS) (or in combined MS and aortic valve stenosis), and in aortic position when the aorta is small because of aortic stenosis (AS) associated with mitral valve disease or because of acute aortic regurgitation (AR) when the aorta has not had adequate time to dilate. Large-sized prostheses, whether caged-ball (Starr-Edwards), tilting disc (Björk-Shiley or St. Jude), or nontilting disc (Kay-Shiley) must be avoided in small-sized patients with purely stenotic valvular lesions. Determining proper prosthetic size only in the operating room without consideration of the hemodynamic lesion and the lean weight of the patient can lead to prosthetic disproportion, a major problem in the early years of valve replacement, but even today an occasional problem.[15]

2. Prosthetic thrombosis. It took years before all clinicians dealing with patients who had mechanical prosthetic valves became convinced that anticoagulation (warfarin sodium) was essential. After that principle was established, mechanical valve thrombosis became less of problem. Nevertheless, of

From the Pathology Branch, National Heart, Lung and Blood Institute, National Institutes of Health.

Received for publication Aug. 31, 1981; accepted Sept. 14, 1981.

Reprint requests: William C. Roberts, M.D., Pathology Branch, NHLBI—NIH, Bldg. 10A, Room 3E-30, Bethesda, MD 20205.

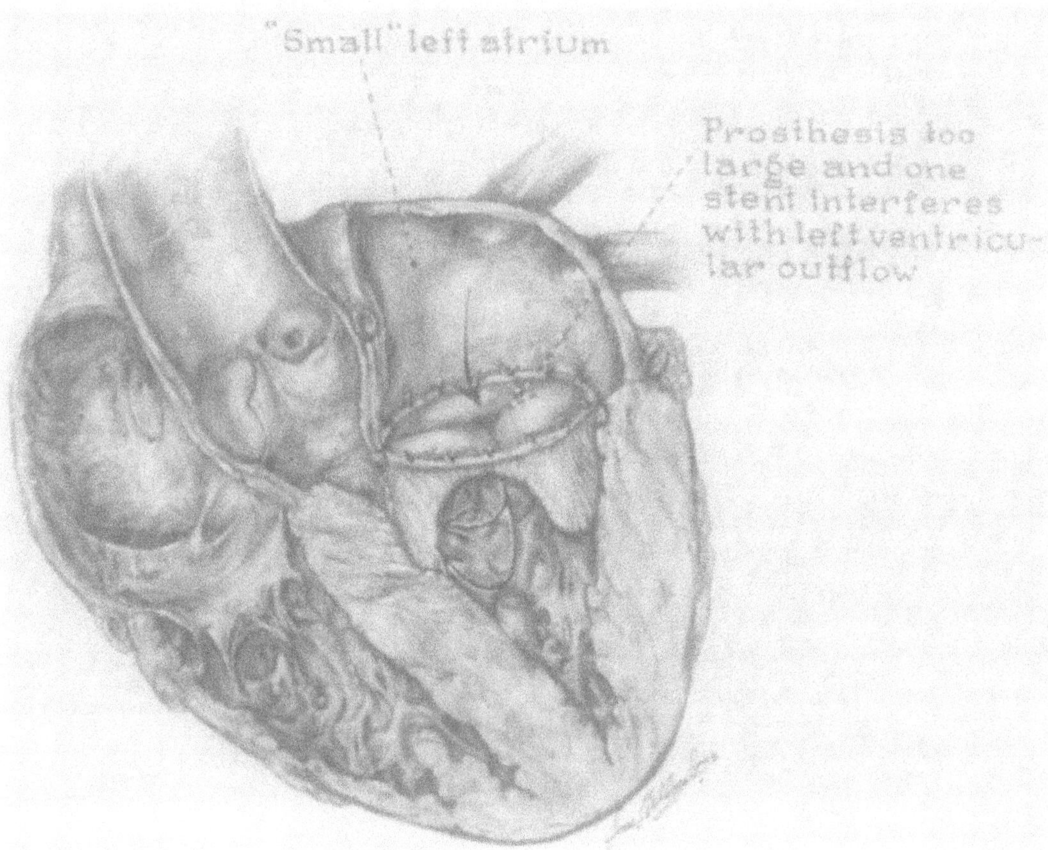

Fig. 1. Obstruction to left ventricular outflow by stent of mitral prosthesis. The porcine bioprosthesis (33 mm) appears to be too large for the left ventricle in this woman (GW No. 79A-73) with severe acute mitral regurgitation from sudden rupture of several chordae tendineae. Despite the volume lesion, the left ventricle had not had adequate time to dilate and the large-sized prosthesis was oriented so that one of its large stents partially obstructed left ventricular outflow (and, additionally, contacted the ventricular septum).

patients with mechanical valves, prosthetic thrombus occurs in some patients who are well anticoagulated, and occasionally it does *not* occur in patients who have never received anticoagulants. Thrombus is often observed in porcine bioprostheses which have been in place for over 2 months, but usually the thrombi are so small that functioning of the prosthesis is not altered.[15-17]

3. Para-anular prosthetic ring discontinuity (peribasilar leak). Parabasilar communications appear to result from placement of an inadequate number of sutures in the sewing ring (because of anular calcific deposits for example) or the pulling loose of one or more sutures; primarily after replacement of anatomically normal (as in papillary muscle dysfunction) or floppy mitral valves, or in AR secondary to a disease of the wall of aorta (as in the Marfan syndrome) rather than of aortic valve cusp, or in infection (prosthetic endocarditis) at the site of attachment of a prosthesis.[4]

4. Prosthetic degeneration or wear. Amost all of the initial models of presently utilized mechanical prostheses had evidence of wear or variance of one or more parts. The silicone rubber poppet utilized in the initial models of the caged-ball prosthesis took in lipids, which resulted in their swelling (with impaction in the cage) or in large cracks which allowed some of them to dislodge from the cage.[4, 8, 12, 18-20] Hopefully, the change (about 1966) in the processing of the silicone rubber has alleviated this problem. The utilization of cloth around the struts of the cage led to "cloth-wear" (Fig. 2), and the disastrous introduction by the manufacturer of the "close-clearance" cage which led to sticking of the poppet in the midportion of the cage and often to sudden death. In the latest model Starr-Edwards valve, wear of the metallic studs on the inner lining of the ring has led to contact of the metallic poppet with the cloth of the ring with subsequent disruption of the cloth. Fracture of the strut or occluder (Delrin) also occurred in a few of the earlier models of the tilting and nontilting discs.

Much evidence has accumulated to indicate that the cusps of the porcine bioprosthesis will eventually

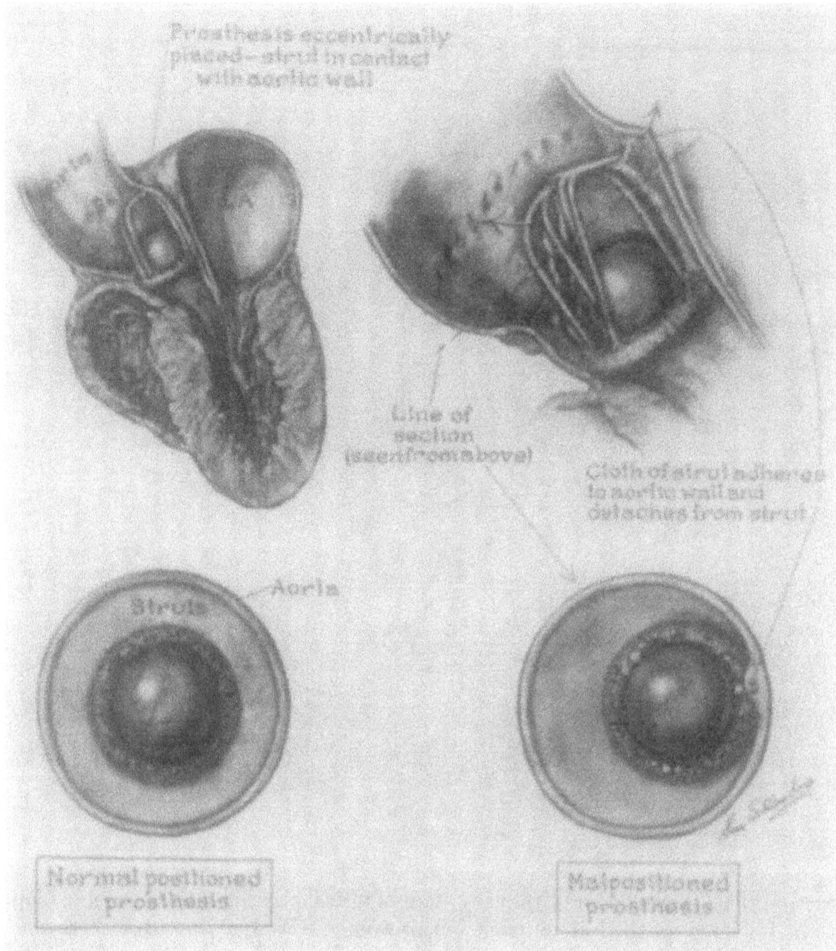

Fig. 2. Cloth-wear on stents of a caged-ball prosthesis in a 76-year-old man (NWH No. A80-233) who died of carcinoma many years after aortic valve replacement and an asymptomatic postoperative course. At necropsy, one of the three stents contacted the intimal lining of the aorta and eventually the aortic wall completely encircled the one stent and the cloth became detached from the other two stents. Although a rather striking finding at necropsy, the cloth degeneration and aortic-wall overgrowth did not cause symptoms during life.

degenerate,[15-17, 21-24] and the same fate may be in store for the bovine parietal pericardial bioprosthesis. This prosthesis has had the best first 5-year record of any of the presently commonly employed prostheses but its 6- to 10-year record may not be good. Numerous reports have described heavy calcification and cuspal disruption of the porcine bioprosthesis after the first 5-year period—enough evidence to convince me that this prosthesis should not be the prosthesis of choice for persons who can tolerate antiocoagulants and are over age 20 and under age 60 or 65 years.

5. Suture overhang of prosthetic orifice. If a suture or knots overhang the metallic ring of a caged-disc or tilting disc prosthesis, the consequence might be prosthetic regurgitation.[25] Such was the case in three patients reported earlier from this laboratory: fatal AR was the consequence in two, and the AR in the third was relieved simply by cutting one overhanging suture. More recently, the same mechanism caused mitral regurgitation (MR) after replacement with a tilting disc prosthesis. This mechanism is less likely to occur with caged-ball prostheses because the margin of error is simply greater than with the more delicate tilting-disc type prostheses.

6. Prosthetic endocarditis. With mechanical prostheses, the infection is always beneath the site of attachment of the prosthesis, i.e., ring abscess is inevitable[26-31] (Fig. 3). With tissue valves mounted on frames, the infection may be limited to the cusps. Thus if one has a substitute cardiac valve which is infected, it is better that the infection involve a bioprosthesis rather than a mechanical valve. If endocarditis occurs in a patient in whom more than one mechanical or bioprosthetic valves is in place, the infection nearly always involves only the most downstream prosthetic valve.

7. Entanglement of sutures beneath the occluder.

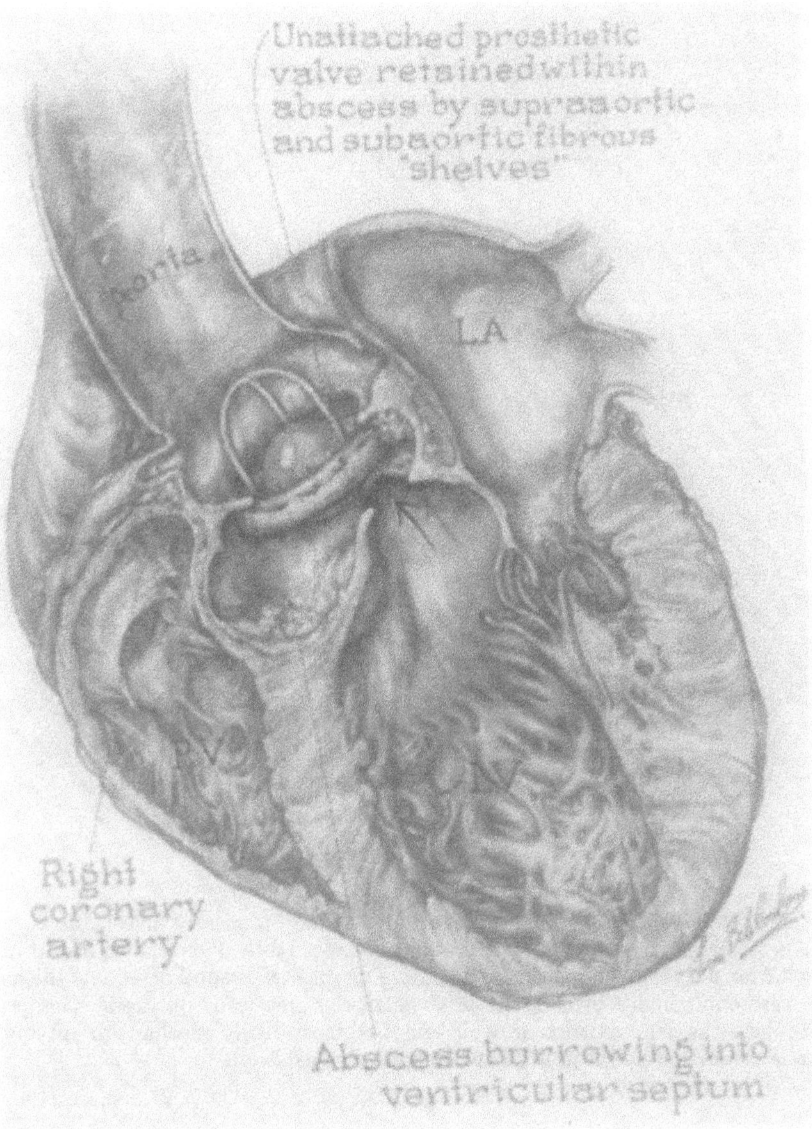

Fig. 3. Prosthetic valve endocarditis. Shown is the heart of a 39-year-old woman (HGH No. A80-29) who underwent aortic valve replacement 8 years earlier because of severe aortic regurgitation secondary to intravenous heroin-induced infective endocarditis. She was asymptomatic thereafter, however, except for occasional ventricular arrhythmias, until 26 hours before death when she had the sudden development of unconsciousness and was found to have an intracerebral bleed. At necropsy, the caged-ball prosthesis was completely detached due to infection beneath the prosthetic ring. The prosthesis was prevented from dislodging by a "constricting" fibrous ring just cephalad to the prosthetic anulus. During her last 8 years of life, there was never clinical evidence of infective endocarditis.

Suture entanglement beneath the occluder during insertion of a mitral prosthesis may prevent descent of the occluder during ventricular diastole.[32] Simply making certain by manual manipulation that the mitral occluder descends freely before closing the left atriotomy incision might prevent this technical problem from being fatal.

8. Incomplete removal of native valve or its calcific deposits preventing complete occluding of the prosthetic orifice by the occluder. If calcific deposits involve the attachment of a valve leaflet to its "anulus," complete débridement of the calcium may not be possible. If a rather sizable calcific nodule remains after valvular excision, the residual calcific debris, on rare occasion, may interfere with complete closure of the occluder.[3]

9. Dislodgment of portion of native cardiac valve during its excision. It is preferable to remove a calcified cardiac valve intact rather than in multiple fragments to prevent the possiblity of embolism.[33]

10. Development of calcific deposits beneath site of attachment of a prosthetic valve ring. During both

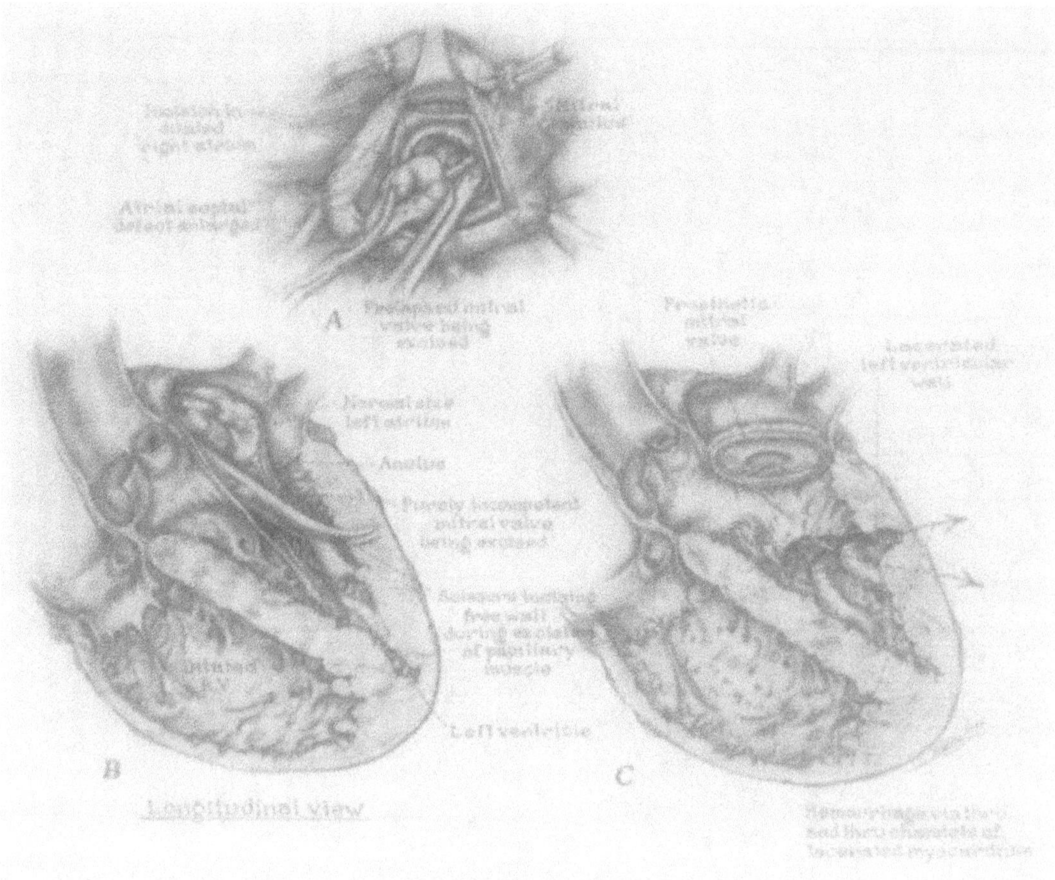

Fig. 4. Incision of left ventricular free wall during excision of mitral valve. This 50-year-old woman (WAH No. A78-28) had an atrial septal defect and a prolapsed mitral valve. The mitral valve was excised when viewing it from a right atrial incision after enlarging the atrial septal defect. As the patient was being weaned from cardiopulmonary bypass, the left ventricular free wall ruptured. Necropsy disclosed the linear incision into the left ventricular wall and the most likely mechanism (in my view) for the catastrophe was scissor incision into it during mitral valve excision.

phases of the cardiac cycle, a rigid-framed prosthesis moves. This back-and-forth "rocking" motion over many years may stimulate the development of calcific deposits beneath the prosthetic anulus.[34] As long as the deposits are small, significant functional consequences are unlikely but larger ones theorically could disrupt a suture which holds the prosthetic ring in place. This "anular calcium" is most likely to develop > 5 years after mitral replacement with a "heavy" prosthesis (caged-ball), but to date I am aware of no functional consequences of its development.

11. Hemolysis of blood elements. Most mechanical cardiac valves decrease the half-life of erythrocytes, leukocytes, and even platelets, but in all but a few patients the bone marrow accelerates its production and anemia or leukopenia or thrombocytopenia is rarely a consequence. On occasion, however, hemolysis is a problem, most frequently in patients with caged-ball prostheses (particularly with the fully cloth-covered models), in patients with aortic valve prostheses as opposed to other replaced valves, and in patients with parabasilar leaks as opposed to patients with intract parabasilar regions.[35]

COMPLICATIONS LIMITED TO A PARTICULAR VALVE SITE IRRESPECTIVE OF TYPE OF PROSTHESIS UTILIZED

1. Disruption of connection between LA and LV at mitral anulus with extravasation of blood into atrioventricular sulcus. When calcific deposits are located in the mitral anular region in addition to their being located in the mitral leaflets, excision of the mitral valve including one or more anular calcific deposits may lead to loss of continuity between the walls of LA and LV with extravasation of blood into the left atrioventricular sulcus with or without fatal bleeding into the pericardial sac.[3]

2. Excision of portion of LV free wall beneath papillary muscle during excision of papillary muscle with

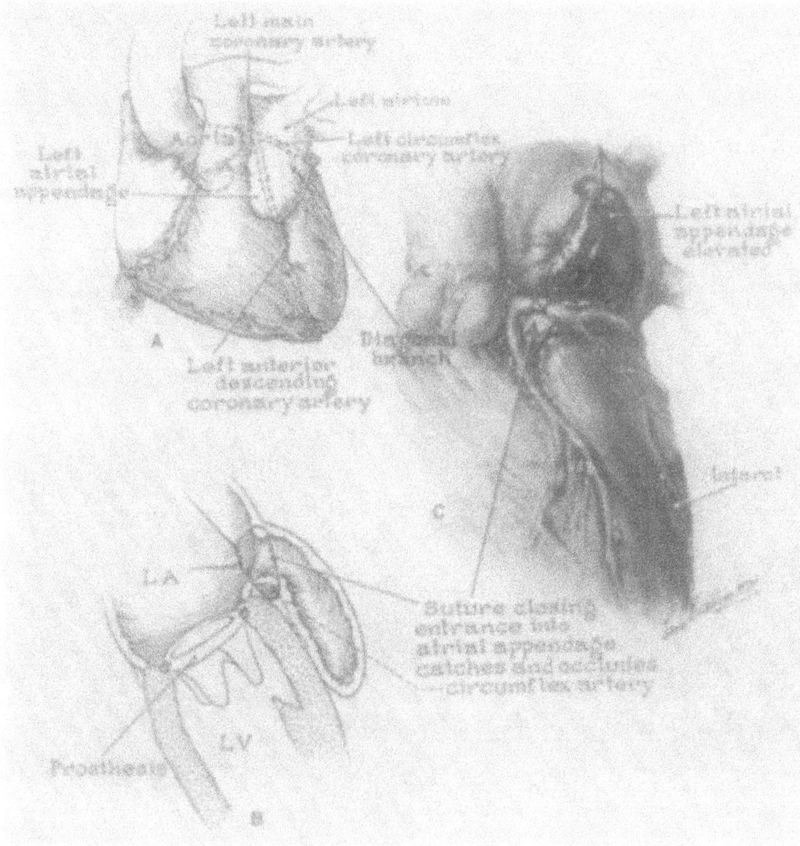

Fig. 5. Occlusion of left circumflex coronary artery by sutures utilized to close the mouth of the left atrial appendage in a 62-year-old man (No. A78-59) who died with a lateral wall left ventricular acute infarct 5 days after mitral valve replacement.

resulting rupture or aneurysmal formation. If during mitral valve excision a LV papillary muscle, grasped with a clamp, is pulled toward LA before the papillary muscle incision is made, a portion of LV free wall in addition to papillary muscle may be excised.[3] Depending on how much LV free wall is excised, the results may be through-and-through rupture or aneurysmal formation.[4]

3. **Incision of LV free wall midway between mitral anulus and stump of LV papillary muscle during mitral valve excision.** A number of reports have described rupture of the LV wall after mitral valve replacement, and most often the rupture was attributed to a stent of either a mechanical or a porcine valve's burrowing through the free wall.[36] Its mechanism has never been precisely determined, in my view, but the rupture or aneurysm site in the LV free wall is midway between the mitral anulus and stump of the papillary muscle. This complication unfortunately is not rare. At one major medical center this complication was reported in 1980 to be the most common cause of early death after mitral valve replacement.[36] I believe its cause is inadvertent incision of the LV free wall during the incision of the chordae tendineae, for the "tear" into LV free wall is linear and often involves the entire free wall of the LV.[37] (Fig. 4). Furthermore, it may be a considerable distance from a prosthetic stent. I have seen this complication in about 10 patients at necropsy. All have had relatively small hearts with normal sized LA and LV cavities. The mitral hemodynamic lesion in each was either chronic MS or acute MR. The atrium was entered in all but one (Fig. 4) by an interatrial groove incision and this incision was relatively short in length due to the small size of the heart. The distance from the interatrial groove incision to the inadvertent LV circular incision was about 8 to 9 cm, exposure of the mitral valve was poor, visualization of the tips of the incising or excising mitral valve scissors had to be poor or inadequate, and during either the opening or closing maneuver or both the scissors' tips incised a portion of LV free wall while the mitral valve was being excised.

4. **Damage to left circumflex coronary artery or coronary sinus during insertion of mitral prosthesis or**

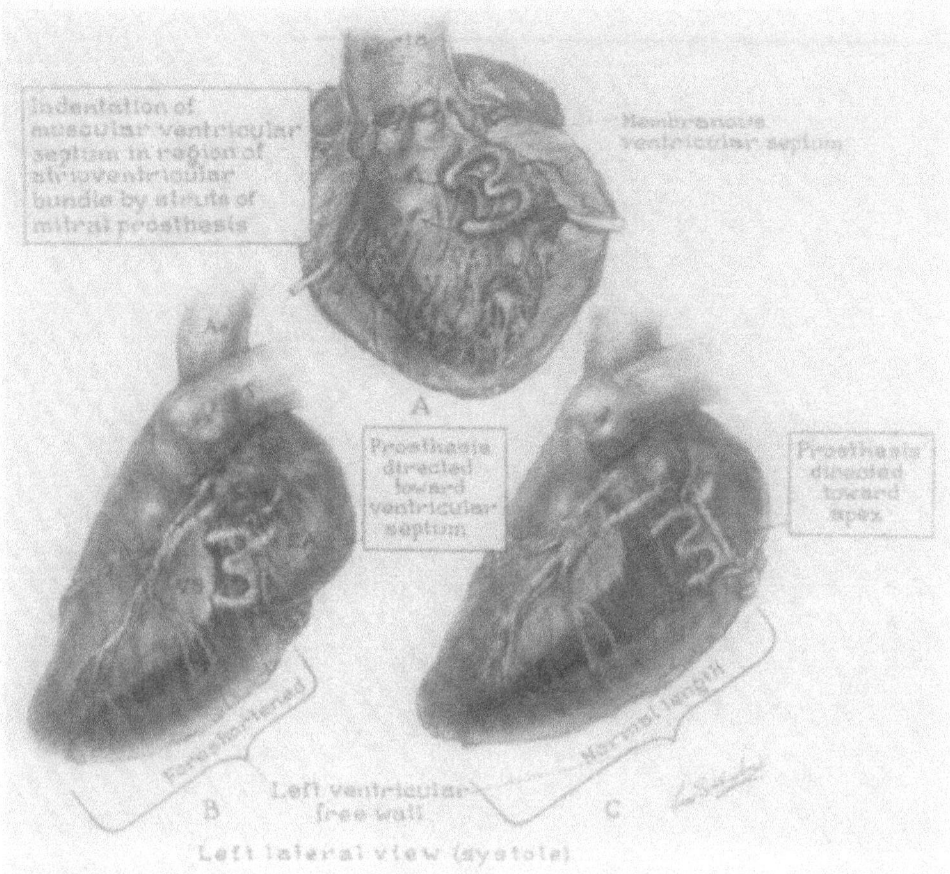

Fig. 6. Contact of stents of porcine bioprosthesis in the mitral position with the ventricular septum probably during ventricular systole only. This 71-year-old woman (WHC No. A80-5) underwent mitral replacement 38 days before death because of severe mitral regurgitation associated with idiopathic dilated cardiomyopathy. Although no definite consequence of this contact between prosthesis and ventricular septum was apparent, this type contact has been recognized to produce ventricular arrhythmias and possibly even sudden death.

during suture obliteration of entrance into LA appendage. Although I have not seen this complication personally, damage to the left circumflex coronary artery (LC) or coronary sinus or both during mitral replacement has been observed by others. Both of these vessels are located in the left atrioventricular sulcus which is less than a centimeter from where sutures are placed into the most basal portion of mitral leaflet during insertion of the prosthesis. Occlusion of the LC by a suture may result in a ventricular arrhythmia or acute myocardial infarction or both, whereas occlusion of the coronary sinus usually does not produce a clinically recognized functional consequence. During suture obliteration of the mouth of a LA appendage, complete obliteration by a suture of the lumen of the LC which courses just beneath the entrance into the appendage may occur (Fig. 5).

5. Contact of cage or stent of mitral prosthesis with ventricular septum or LV free wall producing ventricular arrhythmia. Contact of the cage or stent of a mitral or tricuspid valve prosthesis with the ventricular septum or even LV free wall not only may result in LV inflow or outflow obstruction, but the "tickling" of the myocardium by the prosthesis may produce a ventricular arrhythmia which may be fatal (Fig. 6). This mechanism has been documented by echocardiography during life and indentations of the ventricular septum, particularly by the cage of a caged-ball prosthesis or by a stent of a porcine bioprosthesis, may be observed at necropsy (Fig. 6). This situation is most liable to occur when relatively large-sized prostheses are employed in relatively small-sized ventricles.

6. Diffuse or extensive LV fibrosis post-mitral replacement. Whenever the LV papillary muscles are excised, their "raw" stumps are eventually covered by dense fibrous tissue. Thus mural endocardial fibrosis over the stumps of the papillary muscles is an expected late finding after mitral valve replacement. On rare occasion, not only is the endocardial covering over the papillary muscles thickened by

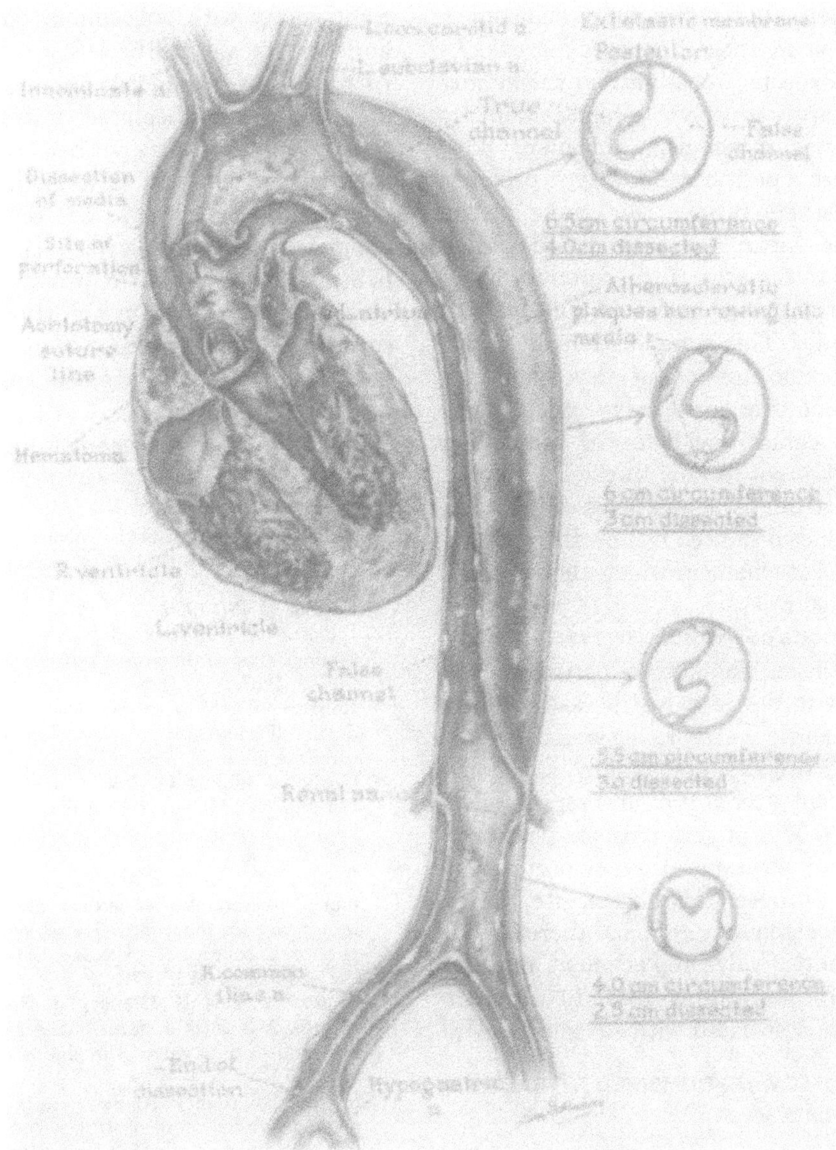

Fig. 7. Aortic dissection after aortic valve replacement. This 50-year-old man (No. A76-125) had his stenotic congenitally bicuspid aortic valve replaced with a caged-ball prosthesis 10 years before death. At operation the ascending aorta was normal. He died suddenly after asymptomatic 10-year period and necropsy disclosed a healed dissection involving the entire aorta. His systemic arterial pressure had always been normal (100/75 mm Hg). Histologically the media of the aorta were normal. The dissection appears to have started in the vicinity of the aortotomy incision.

fibrous tissue, but the same process may involve most of the remaining portion of LV.[38] The mechanism of this diffuse or extensive endocardial fibrosis is unclear. Initially, the concept was presented that the ball-in-a-cage prosthesis "stirred up" the blood in the LV cavity and the anatomic consequence of the "churning" up and down movement was endocardial thickening. Another view has been that the extensive endocardial thickening was the consequence of poor myocardial protection at the time of valve replacement, but the endocardial thickening to my knowledge has been observed only after mitral valve replacement, not post-aortic valve replacement.

7. Obstruction of coronary ostium by aortic prosthetic ring or stent. This complication of aortic valve replacement is rare but it may result in fatal acute myocardial infarction or ventricular arrhythmia. Utilization of a porcine valve, which has relatively large stents in a small aorta with improper positioning of the stents, is the most likely situation where this complication may occur today.

8. Intimal thickening in aortic root post-aortic valve replacement. Whenever the intimal surface of aorta is touched, the endothelial cells are immediately removed and the underlying media is exposed. Usually healing occurs simply by proliferation of new endothelial cells, but occasionally collagen is deposited in excess in these "exposed" areas. In addition to some expected focal intimal thickening in the aortic root after aortic valve replacement by the above-mentioned mechanism, turbulent flow, particularly through a peripheral flow type prosthesis, may lead to severe intimal thickening in the aortic root. If the aortic root intimal thickening involves the aorta in the area of the coronary ostia, the latter may be narrowed and this may lead to myocardial ischemia.[2] This complication, however, has proved to be uncommon but nevertheless a well-documented one after aortic valve replacement. In patients with clinical evidence of red blood hemolysis, the aortic root intimal thickening can be predicted to be particularly severe because its origin is primarly turbulence produced by flow through the prothesis, the same mechanism which shortens the half-life of red blood cells.[8]

9. Dissection of aorta post-aortic valve replacement. Aortic dissection is a well-known occurrence in certain patients with aortic valve disease, but its occurrence *after* aortic valve replacement is not widely appreciated (Fig. 7). Fortunately, this complication is infrequent after aortic valve replacement (described in only 0.07% of such patients postoperatively[39]). Dissection, however, also may occur after aortotomy for any purpose (cannulation site, aortocoronary conduit anastomosis, etc.) and therefore its occurrence after aortic valve replacement may be more related to the aortotomy than to inherent disease of the aorta associated with AS and/or AR.

COMPLICATIONS FOLLOWING COMBINED MITRAL AND AORTIC VALVE REPLACEMENT

1. Contact of aortic valve poppet with stent or ring of mitral prosthesis causing AR. The basal attachment of the anterior mitral leaflet is about 1 cm caudal to the bases of the aortic valve cusps, and after replacement of both valves the fixation rings of the two prostheses are in close proximity. Ordinarily this juxtaposition produces no hemodynamic disturbance. If the mitral prosthesis is particularly large, however, one of its stents or even its ring may lie directly beneath the orifice of the aortic prosthesis, and during ventricular diastole the poppet of the aortic prosthesis may contact the stent or ring of the mitral prosthesis, the aortic proppet may be prevented from seating, and AR, which may be fatal, may result.[40] This complication has been observed only when the mitral valve has been replaced with a very large-sized prosthesis.

2. Compression of anomalous LC by mitral and aortic prosthetic fixation rings. The most common important coronary anomaly is origin of the LC from the right artery with subsequent coursing behind the aorta on its way to the left atrioventricular sulcus. Although potentially this anomalous artery could be damaged during isolated mitral or aortic valve replacement, such has not been reported. Damage to this artery, however, is a distinct danger if both mitral and aortic valves are replaced, because the anomalous coronary artery courses between the fixation rings of these two prosthesis and thus it may be compressed by them.[41] Fortunately, because this coronary anomaly occurs about once in 300 human hearts and combined replacement of both mitral and aortic valves is even less frequent, this complication of valve replacement is extremely rare.[41]

REFERENCES

1. Roberts WC, Morrow AG: Mechanisms of acute left atrial thrombosis after mitral valve replacement. Pathologic findings indicating obstruction to left atrial emptying. Am J Cardiol **18**:497, 1966.
2. Roberts WC, Morrow AG: Late postoperative pathologic findings after cardiac valve replacement. Circulation (suppl) **36**:I48, 1967.
3. Roberts WC, Morrow AG: Causes of early postoperative death following cardiac valve replacement. Clinico-pathologic correlations in 64 patients studied at necropsy. J Thorac Cardiovas Surg **54**:422, 1967.
4. Roberts WC, Morrow AG: Anatomic studies of hearts containing caged-ball prosthetic valves. Johns Hopkins Med J **121**:271, 1967.
5. Roberts, WC, Morrow AG: Causes of death and other anatomic observations after cardiac valve replacement. *In* Long-term prognosis following valve replacement. Second Conference on Cardiovascular Disease. Basel, S. Karger, Advances in Cardiology **7**:226, 1972.
6. Winter TQ, Reis RL, Glancy, DL, Roberts WC, Epstein SE, Morrow AG: Current status of Starr-Edwards cloth-covered prosthetic cardiac valves. Circulation (Suppl) **45** and **46**:I-14, 1972.
7. Shepard RL, Glancy DL, Stinson EB, Roberts WC: Hemodynamic confirmation of obstruction to left ventricular inflow by a caged-ball prosthetic mitral valve. Case report. J Thorac Cardiovas Surg **65**:252, 1973.
8. Roberts WC, Bulkley BH, Morrow AG: Pathologic anatomy of cardiac valve replacement: A study of 224 necropsy patients. Progr Cardiovasc Dis **15**:539, 1973.
9. Roberts WC: Operative treatment of hypertrophic obstructive cardiomyopathy. The case against mitral valve replacement. Am J Cardiol **32**:377, 1973.
10. Seningen RP, Bulkley BH, Roberts WC: Prosthetic aortic stenosis. A method to prevent its occurrence by measurement of aortic size from preoperative aortogram. Circulation **49**:921, 1974.
11. Fishbein MC, Roberts WC, Golden A, Hufnagel CA: Cardiac pathology after aortic valve replacement using Hufnagel trileaflet prostheses: A study of 20 necropsy patients. Am Heart J **89**:443, 1975.
12. Roberts WC, Fishbein MC, Golden A: Cardiac pathology after valve replacement by disc prosthesis. A study of 61 necropsy patients, Am J Cardiol **35**:740, 1975.
13. Roberts WC, Hammer WJ: Cardiac pathology after valve replacement with a tilting disc prosthesis (Björk-Shiley type). A study of 46 necropsy patients and 49 Björk-Shiley prostheses. Am J Cardiol **37**:1024, 1976.
14. Roberts WC: Choosing a substitute cardiac valve: Type, size, surgeon. Am J Cardiol **38**:633, 1976.
15. Spray TL, Robert WC: Structural changes in porcine xenografts used as substitute cardiac valves. Gross and histologic

observations in 51 glutaraldehyde-preserved Hancock valves in 41 patients. Am J Cardiol **40**:319, 1977.

16. Ferrans VJ, Spray TL, Billingham ME, Roberts WC: Structural changes in glutaraldehyde-treated porcine heterografts used as substitute cardiac valves. Transmission and scanning electron microscopic observations in 12 patients. Am J Cardiol **41**:1159, 1978.
17. Ferrans VJ, Boyce SW, Billingham ME, Jones M, Ishihara T, Roberts WC: Calcific deposits in porcine bioprosthesis: Structure and pathogensis. Am J Cardiol **46**:721, 1980.
18. Roberts WC, Morrow AG: Fatal degeneration of the silicone rubber ball of the Starr-Edwards prosthetic aortic valve. Am J Cardiol **22**:614, 1968.
19. Roberts WC, Levinson GE, Morrow AG: Lethal ball variance in the Starr-Edwards prosthetic mitral valve. Arch Intern Med **126**:517, 1970.
20. Fishbein MC, Roberts WC: Late postoperative anatomic observations after insertion of Hufnagel caged-ball prostheses in descending thoracic aorta. Chest **68**:6, 1975.
21. Yarbrough JW, Roberts WC, Reis, RL: Structural alterations in tissue cardiac valves implanted in patients and in calves. J Thorac Cardiovasc Surg **65**:364, 1973.
22. Geha AS, Laks H, Stansel HC Jr., Cornhill JF, Kilman JW, Buckley MJ, Roberts WC: Late failure of porcine valve heterografts in children. J Thorac Cardiovasc Surg **78**:351, 1979.
23. Ishihara T, Ferrans VJ, Jones M, Cabin HS, Roberts WC: Calcific deposits developing in a bovine pericardial bioprosthetic valve 3 days after implantation. Circulation **63**:718, 1981.
24. Ishihara T, Ferrans VJ, Jones M, Boyce SW, Roberts WC: Structure of bovine parietal pericardium and of unimplanted Ionescu-Shiley pericardial valvular bioprostheses. J Thorac Cardiovasc Surg **81**:747, 1981.
25. Waller BF, Jones M, Roberts WC: Postoperative aortic regurgitation from incomplete seating of tilting-disc occluders due to overhandling knots or long sutures. Chest **78**:565, 1980.
26. Cohn LH, Roberts WC, Rockoff SD, Morrow AG: Bacterial endocarditis following aortic valve replacement. Clinical and pathologic correlations. Circulation **33**:209, 1966.
27. Archard HO, Roberts WC: Bacterial endocarditis after dental procedures in patients with aortic valve prostheses. J Am Dental Assoc **72**:648, 1966.
28. Roberts WC, Morrow AG: Bacterial endocarditis involving prosthetic mitral valves. Clinical and pathologic observations. Arch Pathol **82**:164, 1966.
29. Arnett EA, Roberts WC: Prosthetic valve endocarditis. Clinico-pathologic analysis of 22 necropsy patients with comparison of observations in 74 necropsy patients with active infective endocarditis involving natural left-sided cardiac valves. Am J Cardiol **38**:281, 1976.
30. Arnett EN, Kastl DG, Garvin AJ, Roberts WC: A conversation on prosthetic valve endocarditis. Am Heart J **93**:510, 1977.
31. Ferrans VJ, Boyce SW, Billingham ME, Spray TL, Roberts WC: Infection of glutaraldehyde-preserved porcine valve heterografts. Am J Cardiol **43**:1123, 1979.
32. Jones AA, Otis JB, Fletcher GF, Roberts WC: A hitherto undescribed cause of prosthetic mitral valve obstruction. J Thorac Cardiovasc Surg **74**:116, 1977.
33. Roberts WC, Morrow AG: Cardiac valves and the surgical pathologist. Arch Pathol **82**:309, 1966.
34. Bulkley BH, Morrow AG, Roberts WC: Calcification of prosthetic valve anuli: A late complication of cardiac valve replacement. Am Heart J **87**:129, 1974.
35. Roberts WC, Morrow AG: Renal hemosiderosis in patients with prosthetic aortic valves. Circulation **33**:390, 1966.
36. Cobbs BW Jr, Hatcher CR Jr, Craver JM, Jones EL, Sewell CW: Transverse midventricular disruption after mitral valve replacement. Am Heart J **99**:33, 1980.
37. Roberts WC, Mason DT, Engle MA, Cohn LH: Cardiology 1981. New York, 1981, Yorke Medical Books, p 364.
38. Roberts WC, Morrow AG: Secondary left ventricular endocardial fibroelastosis following mitral valve replacement. Cause of cardiac failure in the late postoperative period. Circulation **37** and **38**(suppl II):101, 1968.
39. Muna WF, Spray TL, Morrow AG, Roberts WC: Aortic dissection after aortic valve replacement in patients with valvular aortic stenosis. J Thorac Cardiovasc Surg **74**:65, 1977.
40. Roberts WC, Lambird PA, Gott VL, Morrow AG: Fatal aortic regurgitation following replacement of the mitral and aortic valves. A mechanical complication of double valve replacement. J Thorac Cardiovasc Surg **52**:189, 1966.
41. Roberts WC, Morrow AG: Compression of anomalous left circumflex coronary arteries by prosthetic valve fixation rings. J Thorac Cardiovasc Surg **57**:834, 1969.

Inward stent-post bending of a porcine bioprosthesis in the mitral position

Cause of bioprosthetic dysfunction

Certain clinical and morphologic features are described in a patient with severe bioprosthetic obstruction 9 years after mitral valve replacement. At reoperation, severe inward bending of the stent-posts was found without significant bioprosthetic cuspal abnormalities. "Polymer creep" is considered responsible for the stent-post deformity.

A. Michael Borkon, M.D., Charles L. McIntosh, M.D., Ph.D., Michael Jones, M.D., William C. Roberts, M.D., and Andrew G. Morrow, M.D., *Bethesda, Md.*

The morphologic features of late bioprosthetic valve failure have been well described.[1-5] In most patients, bioprosthetic failure was the result of cuspal calcification and collagen disruption. Deterioration of the other components of the bioprosthesis infrequently has been responsible for failure. Recently, permanent inward stent-post deformity producing secondary valvular orifice obstruction and valvular failure has been reported after aortic valve replacement with Hancock bioprostheses and is believed to have resulted from stent-post compression from a narrow aortic root.[6, 7] Experimental studies have shown that stent-post deformity may result also from "polymer creep," an aging characteristic of polypropylene.[8] Stent-post deformity has not been described previously in the mitral position. Such was the case, however, in the case described herein.

Case report

A 50-year-old white woman underwent closed mitral commissurotomy in September, 1960, and was well thereafter until November, 1969, when congestive heart failure reappeared and repeat cardiac catheterization was performed (Table I). On Nov. 3, 1970, she underwent aortic valve replacement with a No. 8 Starr-Edwards Model 2310 prosthesis and mitral replacement with a No. 29 Hancock bioprosthesis. The postoperative course was uncomplicated, and she was discharged receiving warfarin sodium. Cardiac catheterization (Table I), 7 months after operation, disclosed a residual mean gradient across the Hancock mitral bioprosthesis of 7 mm Hg and a calculated mitral valve orifice area of 2.4 cm². She was symptomatically improved (New York Heart Association Functional Class II). In September, 1979, she began to have increasing symptoms of congestive heart failure. A Grade 2/6 systolic ejection murmur was heard at the right upper sternal border and a Grade 2/6 holosystolic murmur at the apex and axilla. These murmurs were unchanged from prior examinations. No diastolic murmur was heard. Repeat

Table I. *Hemodynamic data*

	Immediately preoperatively	*Months preoperatively*	
		7	*106*
Rhythm	Atrial fibrillation	Sinus	Atrial fibrillation
Pressures (mm Hg):			
Right atrium (mean)	5	2	11
Right ventricle (s/d)*	53/5	38/6	108/10
Pulmonary artery (s/d)	53/25	38/18	108/10
Pulmonary artery wedge (PAW)	m = 26 v = 36	m = 15 a = 16 v = 22	m = 32 v = 46
Left ventricle (LV) (s/d)	170/8	170/12	190/14
Aorta (s/d)	160/80	155/77	190/86
PAW/LV mdg = mean diastolic gradient	8	7	11
Cardiac output (L/min)	3.4	5.4	3.3
Mitral valve area (cm²)	—	2.4	1.0

*s/d = systolic/diastolic.

From the Clinic of Surgery and the Pathology Branch, National Heart, Lung and Blood Institute, Bethesda, Md.

Received for publication March 2, 1981.

Accepted for publication May 19, 1981.

Address for reprints: Andrew G. Morrow, M.D., National Heart, Lung and Blood Institute, Bethesda, Md. 20205.

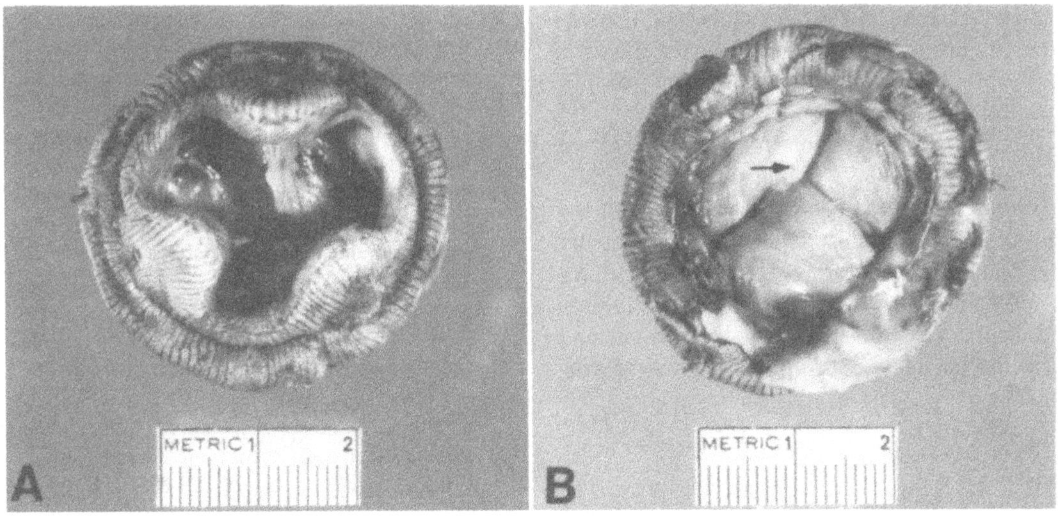

Fig. 1. Mitral bioprostheses removed from the patient 107 months after implantation. *A*, Ventricular aspect. The stent-posts are bent inward, producing secondary valve orifice obstruction. Valve leaflets are thin and pliable. *B*, Atrial aspect. There is a pinhole leaflet perforation *(arrow)*.

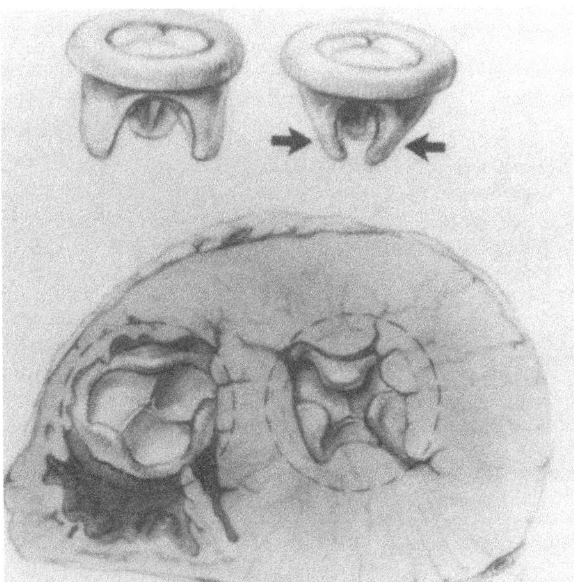

Fig. 2. Mechanism of stent-post deformity due to left ventricular compression from bioprosthesis-ventricular disproportion.

cardiac catheterization (Table I) on Sept. 19, 1979, demonstrated severe stenosis of the bioprosthetic mitral valve (mean mitral gradient 11 mm Hg and calculated orifice area 1.0 cm^2). The mitral Hancock bioprosthesis was replaced with a Starr-Edwards valve. The postoperative course was uneventful, and she remains well.

The cusps of the bioprosthesis removed at operation were thin and delicate and a small tear was present adjacent to one commissure. The stent-posts were indented inward and appeared to result in bioprosthetic obstruction (Fig. 1).

Comments

The flexible stent was developed in 1970 by Reis and associates[9] to improve Hancock valve durability by diminishing stress on the bioprosthetic cusps. In most instances leaflet calcification and collagen disruption result in bioprosthetic dysfunction. Deterioration of the Stellite ring, polypropylene stent, or Dacron cloth covering has seldom been implicated as a primary mechanism of bioprosthetic valve failure. In two recently reported cases there was permanent inward stent-post deformity causing significant valve orifice obstruction after aortic valve replacement with Hancock bioprostheses. In both cases, the bioprosthesis was compressed by a small aortic root and was associated with bioprosthetic thrombosis[6] or severe hemolysis.[7]

Stent-post deformity producing obstruction and requiring reoperation has not previously been reported after mitral valve replacement. Spray and Roberts[1] observed stent-post deformity associated with bioprosthetic failure due to leaflet degeneration, but they did not discuss its significance. Pohlner et al[8] demonstrated that polypropylene may be subject to "polymer creep" from persistent cyclic fatigue, producing permanent inward stent-post migration and bioprosthetic failure. Possibly, "polymer creep" may have been responsible for the secondary valve orifice obstruction in our patients, as cardiac catheterization documented worsening of the bioprosthetic stenosis and no cuspal abnormalities were identified that could account for this degree of obstruction.

Left ventricular compression may also result in stent-post deformity owing to bioprosthesis-ventricular disproportion if proper care is not taken in sizing not only the mitral valve anulus, but also the ventricular cavity, as demonstrated in Fig. 2. It is unlikely that this was the mechanism of stent-post deformity in the patient presented because obstruction developed late and the ventricular cavity at both operations was of adequate size.

REFERENCES

1 Spray TL, Roberts WC: Structural changes in porcine xenografts. Am J Cardiol **40:**319-330, 1977

2 Ferrans VJ, Spray TL, Billingham ME, Roberts WC: Structural changes in glutaraldehyde-treated porcine heterografts used as substitute cardiac valves. Am J Cardiol **41:**1159-1184, 1978

3 Ferrans VJ, Spray TL, Billingham ME, Roberts WC: Ultrastructure of Hancock porcine valvular heterografts. Pre-and postimplantation changes. Circulation **58:**Suppl 1:10-18, 1978

4 Hezter R, Hill JD, Kerth WJ, Wilson AJ, Adappa MG, Gerbode F: Thrombosis and degeneration of Hancock valve. Clinical and pathological findings. Ann Thorac Surg **26:**317-322, 1978

5 Fishbein MC, Gissen SA, Collin JT, Barsamian EM, Cohn LH: Pathologic findings after cardiac valve replacement with glutaraldehyde-fixed porcine valves. Am J Cardiol **40:**331-337, 1977

6 Salomon NW, Copeland JG, Goldman S, Larson DF: Unusual complication of the Hancock porcine heterograft. Strut compression in the aortic root. J THORAC CARDIOVASC SURG **77:**294-296, 1979

7 Magilligan DJ, Fisher E, Alam M: Hemolytic anemia with porcine xenograft aortic and mitral valves. J THORAC CARDIOVASC SURG **79:**628-631, 1980

8 Pohlner PG, Thompson FJ, Hjelm E, Barratt-Boyes BG: Experimental evaluation of aortic hemograft valves mounted on flexible support frames and comparison with glutaraldehyde-treated porcine valves. J THORAC CARDIOVASC SURG **77:**287-293, 1979

9 Reis RL, Hancock WD, Yarbrough JW, Glancy DL, Morrow AG: The flexible stent. J THORAC CARDIOVASC SURG **62:**683-689, 1971

Intracuspal hematomas in implanted porcine valvular bioprostheses

Clinical and experimental studies

Intracuspal hematomas were found in three of 57 porcine valvular bioprostheses implanted as substitute cardiac valves in 50 patients and in 11 of 29 similar bioprostheses implanted in sheep. The three valves implanted in patients had been in the mitral position for 27, 65, and 107 months. Of the valves implanted in sheep, six had been in the mitral position and five in the tricuspid position for periods of time ranging from 20 minutes to 7 months. In each patient and in four of 11 sheep, the hematomas involved more than one cusp. These lesions were localized in the spongiosa, extended from the basal region toward the free edge of the cusp, and formed a plane of dissection which involved the spaces left in the spongiosa by the removal of proteoglycan material during preimplantation commercial processing. In one patient, the hematomas limited the mobility of the cusps and appeared to have been the cause of clinically significant prosthetic mitral stenosis; in the other two patients and in the experimental animals, the hematomas were smaller and of uncertain hemodynamic significance. Intracuspal hematomas may become sites of eventual formation of calcific deposits. The pathogenesis of intracuspal hematomas is related to the entry of blood into the space between the sewing ring and the most basilar region of the bioprosthetic tissue. This space extends throughout the circumference of the bioprosthesis and is continuous with the spongiosa, the layer in which the hematoma develops. The blood penetrates into this space through the suture line between bioprosthetic tissue and sewing ring on the inflow surface of porcine valvular bioprostheses which have been mounted on atrioventricular type stents. Intracuspal hematomas were not found in bioprostheses mounted on aortic type stents, in which these sutures are more protected and more closely spaced, or in pericardial bioprostheses, which do not have a spongiosa.

Tokuhiro Ishihara, M.D., Ph.D., Victor J. Ferrans, M.D., Ph.D., Glenn R. Barnhart, M.D., Michael Jones, M.D., Charles L. McIntosh, M.D., Ph.D., and William C. Roberts, M.D., *Bethesda, Md.*

The presence of erythrocytes in cuspal connective tissue is a relatively common finding in implanted porcine valvular bioprostheses. The extent to which this occurs is variable and is more pronounced in valves that have been in place for long periods of time.[1] Nevertheless, this problem has not been studied systematically, and large accumulations of erythrocytes leading to grossly visible intracuspal hematomas have not been reported in implanted porcine valvular bioprostheses.

From the Pathology Branch and the Surgery Branch, National Heart, Lung, and Blood Institute, National Institutes of Health, Bethesda, Md.

Received for publication April 28, 1981.

Accepted for publication June 15, 1981.

Address for reprints: Dr. Victor J. Ferrans, Building 10, Room 7N208, National Institutes of Health, Bethesda, Md. 20205.

The present communication describes the morphologic characteristics of intracuspal hematomas found in porcine valvular bioprostheses that had been implanted as substitute cardiac valves in patients (three of 57 valves) and in experimental animals (11 of 29 valves).

Materials and methods

Gross anatomic, histologic, and transmission and scanning electron microscopic studies were made of a total of 86 porcine valvular bioprostheses that had been implanted in patients (57 valves, Group I) or in young sheep (29 valves, Group II).

Group I valves had been implanted in a total of 50 patients, who ranged in age from 2 to 68 years (mean 42 years) at the time of operation. Thirty-five of the valves had been implanted in the mitral position, 13 in the aortic position, six in the tricuspid position, and

Table I. *Clinical and morphological findings in three patients with intracuspal hematomas in cardiac valvular bioprostheses*

Pt. No.	Age (at impl.) and sex	Valve replaced, BP type	Time BP in place (mo)	Reason for BP removal	Hematomas in cusps R	L	N	Macrophages in hematomas	Fibrous sheath on BP	Ca^{++} in BP	Perf. in cusp
1	59, M	MV-H	107	Abn. color*	+	+	+	+	+	0	0
2	49, F	MV-CE	27	Stenosis	+	+	+	+	+	+	0
3	65, F	MV-H†	65	Reg.	+	+	+	+	+	+	L

Legend: 0, Absent. +, Present. Abn., Abnormal. BP, Bioprosthesis. Ca^{++}, Calcific deposits. CE, Carpentier-Edwards valve. H, Hancock valve. impl., Implantation. L, Left coronary cusp. MV, Mitral valve. N, Noncoronary cusp. perf., Perforation. R, Right coronary cusp. Reg., Regurgitation.

*At time of aorta-coronary bypass the bioprosthesis was inspected (because of the long time it had been in place), found to be abnormal in color, and replaced.

†Tricuspid valve also was replaced by a bioprosthesis, in which hematoma did not develop.

Table II. *Clinical and morphological findings in 11 sheep with intracuspal hematomas in cardiac valvular bioprostheses*

Sheep No.	Valve replaced, BP type	Time BP in place	Reason for BP removal	Cause of death	Hematomas in cusps R	L	N	Macrophages in hematomas	Fibrous sheath on BP	Ca^{++} in BP
1	MV-H	20 min	D	CAE	+	+	0	0	0	0
2	MV-X	20 min	D	CHF, CHB	+	+	0	0	0	0
3	MV-X	12 hr	D	RF	+	+	+	0	0	0
4	MV-H	20 hr	D	RF	+	0	0	0	0	0
5	MV-X	1 day	D	RF	+	0	+	0	0	0
6	TV-H	4 days	D	RF	+	0	0	0	0	0
7	TV-H	4 days	D	RF	+	0	0	+	0	0
8	MV-X	3 wk	D	RF	+	0	0	0	0	+
9	TV-H	5 mo	E	–	0	+	0	+	+	+
10	TV-H	6 mo	E	–	+	0	0	0	+	+
11	TV-H	7 mo	E	–	0	+	0	+	+	+
Totals	MV = 6 TV = 5		D = 8 E = 3		R = 9; L = 5; N = 2			3	3	4

Legend: 0, Absent. +, Present. BP, Bioprosthesis. Ca^{++}, Calcific deposits. CAE, Coronary air embolism. CHB, Complete heart block. CHF, Congestive heart failure. D, Death. E, Elective sacrifice. H, Hancock valve. L, Left coronary cusp. MV, Mitral valve. N, Noncoronary cusp. R, Right coronary cusp. RF, Respiratory failure. X, Xenotech valve. TV, Tricuspid valve.

three as valved pulmonic conduits. The period of time between implantation and removal of the bioprostheses varied from 2 days to 123 months (mean 37 months). This group of valves constitutes the total number of porcine valvular bioprostheses (removed for a variety of reasons) that have been examined by light and electron microscopy in our laboratory. Intracuspal hematomas were found in three of these 57 valves (Table I).

Group II valves (Table II) consisted of 13 Hancock valves (Hancock Laboratories, Anaheim, Calif.), eight Carpentier-Edwards valves (American Edwards Laboratories, Santa Ana, Calif.), and eight Xenotech valves (Xenotech Laboratories, Inc., Irvine, Calif.) which had been implanted in sheep with an average age of 5 months, either in the tricuspid position (21 valves) or in the mitral position (eight valves), for periods of time ranging from 20 minutes to 7 months.[2] These experiments were undertaken for studying the processes of calcification and degeneration of bioprosthetic valves in young animals. The Hancock and Xenotech valves used for implantation in the mitral (size 21) and tricuspid (size 25) positions were mounted in stents of the type employed for use in the atrioventricular position; however, size 21 Carpentier-Edwards valves were available to us only in stents of the type used for the aortic position. These stents differ in some important respects from those used in the atrioventricular position. Of the 11 animals observed to have intracuspal hematomas, three were killed electively and eight died (six of respiratory failure, one of coronary air em-

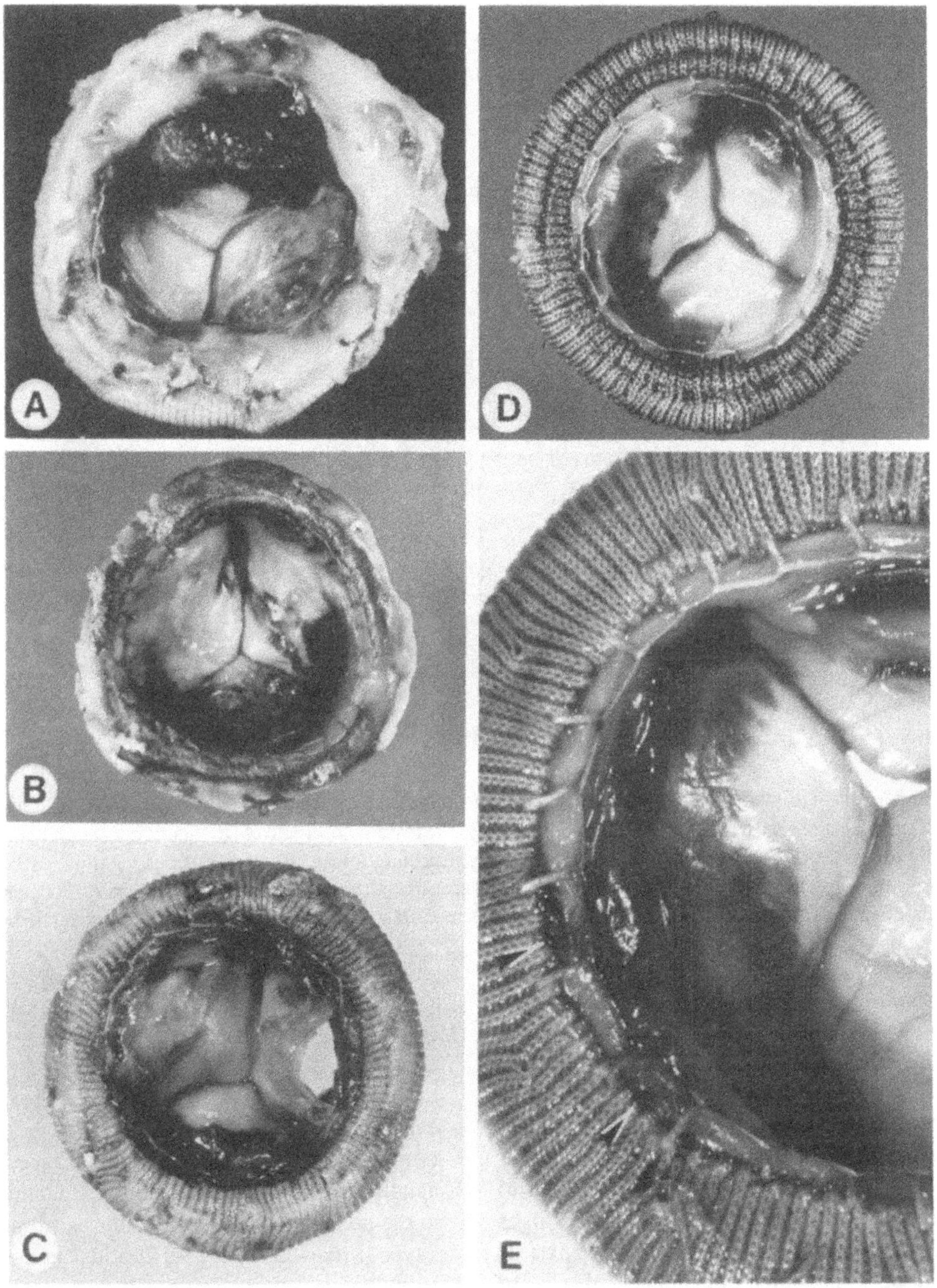

Fig. 1. Gross photographs of inflow surfaces of porcine valvular bioprostheses that developed intracuspal hematomas after implantation in patients *(A* to *C)* and sheep *(D* and *E)*. *A*, Bioprosthesis from Patient 1, showing large hematoma in the right coronary cusp *(top)* and smaller ones in the noncoronary cusp *(lower left)* and the left coronary cusp *(lower right)*. *B*, Bioprosthesis from Patient 2 has large hematoma in the noncoronary cusp *(lower center)*. Smaller hematomas are seen in the right coronary cusp *(upper left)* and the left coronary cusp *(upper right)*. *C*, Bioprosthesis from Patient 3, showing hematoma in the noncoronary cusp *(lower center)*. Hematomas also are present in the other two cusps, and a perforation is seen in the left coronary cusp. *D*, Bioprosthesis from sheep No. 3 demonstrates presence of hematoma involving each cusp 12 hours after implantation in the mitral position. *E*, Bioprosthesis from sheep No. 1, which died of coronary air embolism 20 minutes after implantation in the mitral position. Note apparent points of entry *(arrowheads)* of blood into space between bioprosthetic tissue and sewing ring.

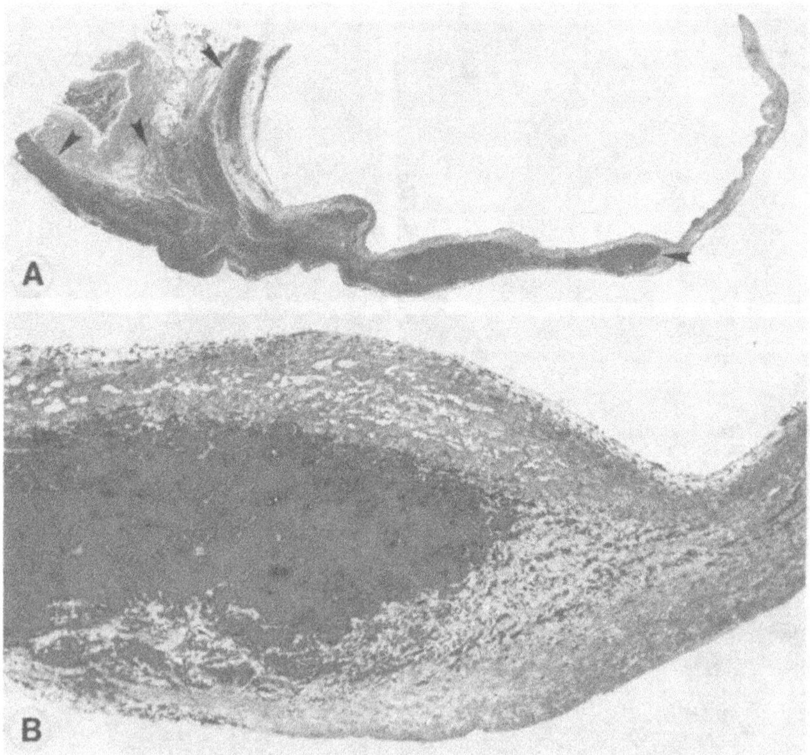

Fig. 2. Microscopic study of right coronary cusp of bioprosthesis from Patient 1. Sections, 1 μ thick, of plastic-embedded tissue. (Alkaline toluidine blue stain.) Compare with Fig. 1, *A*. *A*, Section through entire cusp, showing extension of hematoma *(arrowheads)* from basal portion toward free edge of cusp. Inflow surface is at *bottom;* outflow surface, at *top*. (Orig. mag. ×15.) *B*, Terminal portion of hematoma shown in *A*. The hematoma is localized in the spongiosa. Note degenerative changes in collagen in fibrosa *(top center)* and moderate numbers of macrophages *(far right)*. (Orig. mag. ×100.)

bolism, and one of congestive heart failure and complete heart block). Techniques used for histologic and ultrastructural study of the tissues have been described in detail elsewhere.[1-4]

Gross anatomic observations.

Group I valves. Intracuspal hematomas (Fig 1, *A* to *C*) were observed in each of the cusps in three valves (two Hancock valves and one Carpentier-Edwards valve) that had been implanted in patients (Table I). In all but one of these cusps, the hematomas were single and extended from the sewing ring toward the free edge of the cusp, occupying its basal one third to one half; however, the hematoma extended through the basal three fourths of the right coronary cusp of the bioprosthesis from Patient 1. This cusp also contained a small, apparently separate hematoma near its tip. The hematomas appeared as areas of reddish-black discoloration of the cusps. However, this discoloration was not clearly evident in areas in which the cuspal surfaces were covered by a thick fibrous sheath.

Grossly evident, nodular, calcific deposits were observed only in the valve from Patient 2; a break in the continuity of the inflow surface of the right coronary cusp was also found in this valve. This defect, however, was not located immediately over the main portion of the hematoma and it could have resulted from handling of the specimen after explantation. In addition to the hematomas, the bioprosthesis from Patient 3 had a type II (basilar linear) perforation[3] in the left coronary cusp.

The junction between the sewing ring and the bioprosthetic tissue in the inflow surface was completely covered by fibrous tissue in the bioprosthesis from Patient 1; in the bioprostheses from Patients 2 and 3, it was partially covered by fibrous tissue. In the bioprosthesis from patient 2, this fibrous tissue was partially disputed in the area adjacent to the hematoma; however, this disruption could have been caused by operative removal of the bioprosthesis. In two of the three bioprostheses (from Patients 1 and 3), all the continuous suture lines between the bioprosthetic tissue and the mounting frame were intact, but some of the sutures were looser and more irregularly placed than is normally the case. In the bioprosthesis from Patient 2, part of the suture line was buried in fibrous tissue, and some of the sutures that remained visible also appeared looser and more irregular than normal.

Group II valves. Intracuspal hematomas (Fig. 1, *D* and *E*) were found in a total of 11 of the 29 bioprostheses that had been implanted in sheep, including seven of the eight that had been implanted for less than 1 week and four of the 21 that had been implanted for 3 weeks to 7 months. The 11 intracuspal hematomas occurred in five of the 21 bioprostheses that had been implanted in the tricuspid position and in six of the 10 implanted in the mitral position.

Of the seven bioprostheses (four Hancock valves and three Xenotech valves) which were implanted for less than 1 week and which developed intracuspal hematomas, five had been in the mitral position and two in the tricuspid position. The hematomas involved one cusp in seven valves and more than one cusp in the other four valves. They were more frequent in the right coronary cusp (seven valves) than in the left coronary cusp (three valves) and the noncoronary cusp (two valves).

Of the four bioprostheses (three Hancock valves and one Xenotech valve) that had been implanted for longer than 3 weeks and developed intracuspal hematomas, three had been in the tricuspid position and one in the mitral position. In these four bioprostheses, the hematomas involved the right coronary cusp in two and the left coronary cusp in the other two; the noncoronary cusp was not involved in any of these four valves.

Grossly, these hematomas resembled those observed in the bioprostheses implanted in patients, but differed from the latter in the appearance of certain areas of the inflow surface at the junction between the base of the cusp and the sewing ring. Such areas were sites of dark red, linear thrombi (Fig. 1, *B*), and when the sutures securing the cuspal tissue to the sewing ring were cut, it could be seen that thrombi extended from these areas into either the spongiosa or (in the case of the right coronary cusp) the muscular shelf. The suture lines in these areas were not disrupted, but in some instances the apposition of bioprosthetic tissue to sewing ring was less than optimal, and the free edge of the tissue (i.e., left ventricular outflow tract endocardium just beneath the lower edge of the cusp) had been unevenly or incompletely folded under before suturing the leaflet tissue to the sewing ring.

Histologic observations.

Group I valves. Microscopically (Figs. 2 and 3), the intracuspal hematomas in Group I valves consisted of accumulations of large numbers of erythrocytes in areas

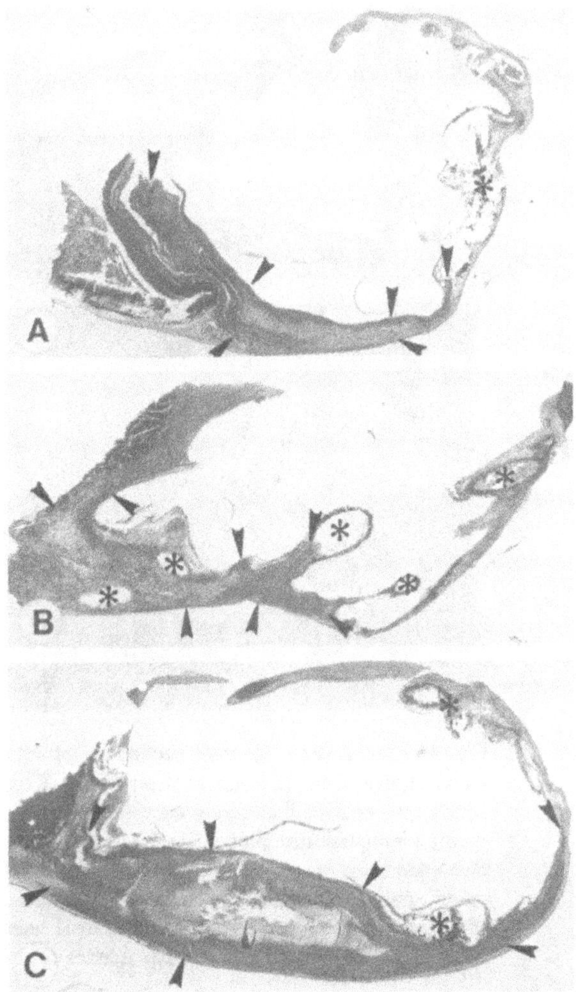

Fig. 3. Histologic sections of left *(A)*, right *(B)*, and noncoronary *(C)* cusps of bioprosthesis from Patient 2. Nodular calcific deposits *(asterisks)* and hematomas *(arrowheads)* are present in each cusp. The noncoronary cusp is greatly thickened by the hematoma. Compare with Fig. 1, *B*. Sections, 1 μ thick, of plastic-embedded tissue. (Alkaline toluidine blue; orig. mag. ×11.)

of the valvular spongiosa in which delamination of the connective tissue had occurred. The erythrocytes in these areas were associated with smaller numbers of leukocytes, macrophages, and platelets, and with fibrin strands. The relative sizes of these lesions, the numbers of macrophages that they contained, and the degree of valvular thickening that they produced varied considerably from one cusp to another in each of these three valves. Morphologic observations in these valves are summarized in Table I.

In the bioprosthesis from Patient 1 (Fig. 2), erythrocytes were present within delaminated areas of the spongiosa of each cusp. In the right coronary cusp,

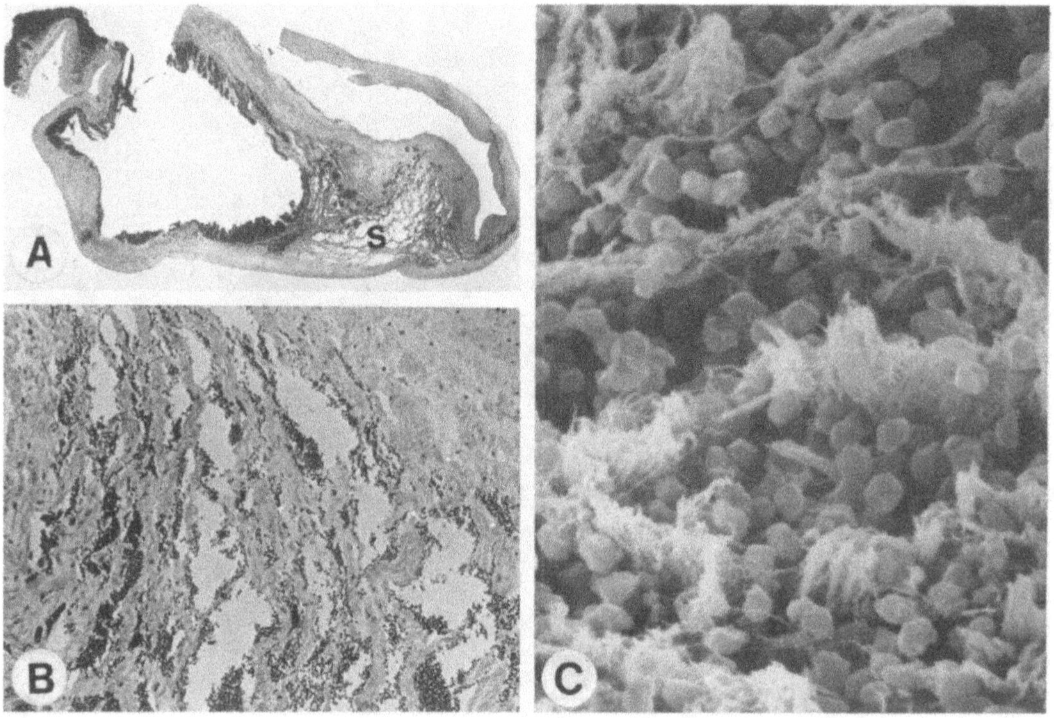

Fig. 4. *A* and *B* show 1 μ thick sections of plastic-embedded tissue, showing intracuspal hematoma in bioprosthesis implanted for 12 hours in sheep No. 3. Compare with Fig. 1, *D*. *A*, View of entire right coronary cusp, which was removed intact from the sewing ring. A portion of the muscle shelf had been removed from this cusp during preimplantation processing, leaving a space that is continuous with the spongiosa *(S)* (Alkaline toluidine blue stain; orig. mag. ×9.) *B*, Part of widened basal portion of spongiosa, with numerous erythrocytes filling empty spaces. (Hematoxylin-eosin stain; orig. mag. ×100.) *C*, Scanning electron micrograph of the cut surface of a cusp showing morphology of intracuspal hematoma in bioprosthesis implanted in sheep No. 1. Layers of collagen fibrils in spongiosa separate masses of erythrocytes. (Orig. mag. ×1,660.)

which was the most heavily involved, the hematoma had caused considerable thickening of the spongiosa and marked thinning of the fibrosa and the ventricularis. In some areas of this cusp, the hematoma extended almost to the surface of the ventricularis. This hematoma was largest at the base of the cusp and tapered off gradually toward the free edge. In the basal and middle thirds of the right coronary cusp, the hematoma contained lacunar spaces that resembled recanalizing thrombi. The erythrocytes in less severely involved portions of the cusp often formed rows, which were arranged parallel to the surfaces of the cusp and were separated from one another by thin layers of connective tissue. The erythrocytes in this cusp were well "hemoglobinized." Macrophages were relatively few in number and contained only moderate quantities of cytoplasmic granules (indicative of phagocytosis). The other two cusps in this valve contained smaller hematomas, which also were located in the spongiosa.

In addition to the hematomas just described, each cusp of the bioprosthesis from Patient 1 contained multiple, small areas of accumulations of small numbers of erythrocytes. Some of these were located in the spongiosa; others, in the fibrosa and ventricularis, and even between the cusp itself and the fibrous sheath[4] that extended from the sewing ring and covered the surfaces of the basal regions of the cusps. Calcific deposits were not present in any of the cusps, but surface microthrombi and areas of degeneration of connective tissue were evident in each cusp.

Histologic study of the bioprosthesis from Patient 2 (Fig. 3) demonstrated very severe thickening of the noncoronary cusp by a large hematoma. Very few macrophages were present in this large hematoma; however, these cells were abundant in microscopic-sized hematomas present in the other two cusps of this bioprosthesis. Degenerative changes and calcific deposits were present in each cusp and often were immediately adjacent to the microscopic-sized hematomas. The bioprosthesis from Patient 3 was minimally calcified, showed moderate degenerative changes, contained relatively small hematomas, and had abundant macrophages on its surfaces.

Group II valves. In the valves that had been implanted in sheep for less than 1 week (Fig. 4), the hematomas filled the space between the sewing ring and the basal portion of the spongiosa. In each right coronary cusp, the hematoma also extended into the region of the muscle shelf. From the basal regions the hematomas appeared to have spread into more distal portions of the valves by forming a plane of dissection through the spongiosa. Areas of spongiosa adjacent to the hematomas often were filled with material that was considered to represent accumulation of serum proteins. The fibrosa and the ventricularis in these valves appeared similar to those in unimplanted valves,[1] without degeneration, calcification, or infection. The valvular surfaces were not covered by fibrous sheaths. Most of the erythrocytes in the hematomas in these valves appeared well "hemoglobinized" and were associated with only a few leukocytes. Macrophages filled with phagocytosed material were not found in these hematomas.

Of the four valves that had been implanted in sheep for more than 3 weeks, three were partially covered by fibrous sheaths, and all four had calcific deposits. The latter were localized in the muscle shelf in two valves, in a thrombus in one valve, and within cuspal connective tissue in two valves (Table II). As in the other valves included in this study, the hematomas extended from the basal regions of the cusps toward the free edges, forming a plane of dissection through the spongiosa. In each of these valves, the fibrosa and the ventricularis were reduced in thickness, and small, focal areas of infiltration of erythrocytes were present in both of these layers with no apparent relationship to the large hematomas in the spongiosa.

Scanning electron microscopic observations.

Group I valves. Scanning electron microscopic studies revealed that the surfaces of the bioprostheses from Patients 1 and 2 were covered by large numbers of platelets and smaller numbers of macrophages showing features similar to those described elsewhere.[1, 4] Small cracks were found in the most superficial layers of valvular connective tissue in the bioprosthesis from Patient 1, but no large breaks in the continuity of the surfaces were detected. The bioprosthesis from Patient 2 also contained calcific deposits that protruded above the cuspal surfaces. The basal regions of both bioprostheses were partially covered by an incomplete layer of endothelial cells. Examination of the cut surfaces of the cusps clearly showed the localization of the hematomas in the spongiosa, the presence of erythrocytes between adjacent layers of collagenous fibers, and the altered shapes of the erythrocytes in these areas.

Group II valves. Group II valves did not have any large surface openings that could have allowed the entry of large amounts of blood into the spongiosa. In the valves implanted for more than 1 month, both surfaces of each cusp were partially covered by a fibrous sheath lined by a layer of endothelial cells. Denuded areas of the valve surfaces were associated with variable numbers of platelets, macrophages, and small surface thrombi. Examination of the cut surfaces of the cusps showed that the hematomas (Fig. 4, *C*) were localized in the spongiosa, the appearance of which was similar to that in Group I valves.

Transmission electron microscopic observations. Transmission electron microscopic observations on all three bioprostheses that had been implanted in patients demonstrated calcific deposits and degenerative changes, similar to those described previously,[1, 5] in the cuspal connective tissue. Of relevance to the present study were the findings in areas of hematomas of (1) phagocytosis of erythrocytes by macrophages and (2) accumulations of material, considered to be old fibrin deposits, around erythrocytes. Similar findings were noted in hematomas in valves implanted in sheep.

Discussion

The observations in this communication show that intracuspal hematomas occur in porcine valvular bioprostheses implanted as substitute cardiac valves either in patients or in experimenal animals, and that they can develop both early and late after implantation. These observations also document the morphology, consequences, and pathogenesis of intracuspal hematomas.

Morphology and consequences of intracuspal hematomas. All intracuspal hematomas occupied the spongiosa, a layer that in unimplanted valves contains empty spaces left by the loss of proteoglycan material during commercial processing. The hematomas extended from the basal region toward the free edge of the cusp, forming a plane of dissection through the spongiosa. The separation of layers of connective tissue in these areas was reminiscent of that seen in dissecting arterial aneurysms. The importance of the plane of dissection through the spongiosa is emphasized by the fact that we have not found intracuspal hematomas in bovine pericardial bioprostheses, which do not have[6] a layer of tissue corresponding to the spongiosa of porcine valvular bioprostheses.

The two main potential consequences of intracuspal hematomas lead to bioprosthetic stenosis and consist of reduction in the mobility of the affected cusps and calcification of the hematoma. The first of these consequences was demonstrated in Patient 2, in whom prosthetic mitral stenosis necessitated reoperation 27 months after implantation of the bioprosthesis. The explanted bioprosthesis contained calcific deposits; however, these were relatively small and its seems likely (compare Fig. 3, *A* to *C*) that the marked thickening of the bioprosthetic cusps (particularly the noncoronary cusp) by intracuspal hematomas played a major role in the pathogenesis of the stenosis in Patient 2. The valves removed from Patients 1 and 3 had smaller hematomas and these were associated with less severe cuspal thickening. Thus it seems less likely that these hematomas were the cause of severe bioprosthetic dysfunction. In Patient 3, the main cause of bioprosthetic dysfunction was regurgitation related to a large basilar linear perforation[3] near the base of the left coronary cusp. In the presence of this lesion, the contribution of intracuspal hematomas to prosthetic stenosis could not be evaluated. A significant end-diastolic gradient was found in only one of the three animals that were studied hemodynamically 1 month or longer after implantation of the bioprostheses in which hematomas were found. The gradient in this animal, however, probably was largely due to severe ingrowth of fibrous tissue over both surfaces of the cusps. Thus it would appear that intracuspal hematomas are a cause of bioprosthetic stenosis only when they are large and interfere with the mobility of the affected cusps.

A relationship of intracuspal hematomas to the subsequent development of calcific deposits was suggested by the fact that both of these changes were localized in the spongiosa. In addition, accumulations of erythrocytes often were found immediately adjacent to calcific deposits, particularly of those which were large and nodular. Nevertheless, intermediate stages in the transformation of hematomas into calcific deposits were not observed and, for this reason, it remains uncertain that hematomas contribute directly to the formation of calcific deposits. An effort was made, based on the recognition of macrophages ingesting erythrocytes, to estimate the amount of time elapsed between the occurrence of the hematoma and the removal of the bioprosthesis. Macrophages were not associated with hematomas in Group II valves that had been implanted for 1 week or less; however, macrophages were infrequent in the hematomas in Group II valves implanted for 3 weeks or longer, and the hematomas in valves implanted for up to 6 months showed no tendency to become organized by ingrowth of fibrous tissue. Thus the time course of invasion by macrophages appears to be much slower in intracuspal hematomas than in other types of hematomas, such as those induced by intramuscular or subcutaneous injections of blood in experimental animals.[7, 8] At least one major reason for this would appear to be the difficulty that macrophages and other inflammatory cells have in penetrating through the surfaces into the spongiosa of glutaraldehyde-treated porcine valvular bioprostheses.[1] Similarly, the usual absence of organization of the intracuspal hematomas is attributable to the lack of penetration of fibroblasts and other connective tissue cells into the spongiosa of the glutaraldehyde-treated valves.

It is not known for what period of time erythrocytes can remain within an intracuspal hematoma while maintaining relatively normal shapes and hemoglobin content. It seems highly unlikely that such a period would exceed a few months, even under circumstances of very limited attack by macrophages and organization by fibroblasts. Thus it seems unavoidable to conclude that the hematomas found in the bioprostheses from each of the three patients 27 to 107 months after implantation had been of recent origin. This suggests the possibility that such hematomas can be recurrent and can resolve by lysis or liquefaction rather than by organization.

Pathogenesis of intracuspal hematomas. The two possibilities that must be considered to account for the entry of blood into the spongiosa are (1) a direct communication with the cuspal surface through a hole or defect either in the ventricularis or the fibrosa and (2) penetration through the junction between bioprosthetic tissue and sewing ring in either the inflow or outflow surfaces. The first of these possibilities is considered unlikely because surface defects found by scanning electron microscopy in the bioprostheses in the present study were very small and shallow. Only in Patient 2 was a larger defect observed, and this may have been produced after removal of the bioprosthesis. Furthermore, we have observed intracuspal hematomas in only one bioprosthetic cusp (in the bioprosthesis from Patient 3) in which development of a perforation had caused obvious exposure of spongiosa tissue to the blood. In fact, the hematoma in this cusp did not extend to the vicinity of the perforation, and we have not observed intracuspal hematomas in other bioprostheses in which cuspal perforations occurred.[3] It would seem that blood that penetrated into the spongiosa through a free two-way communication would be expressed from this layer by the mechanical forces associated with cardiac pumping and valvular motion. Thus it appears necessary to postulate a mechanism by which blood becomes trapped within the spongiosa.

The evidence presented in this report strongly indicates that the junction of the sewing ring and the bioprosthetic tissue on the inflow surface is the site of entry of blood into the spongiosa. The sewing ring–outflow surface junction always appeared normal, tightly sutured, and microscopically free of involvement by the hematomas. In contrast to this, the hematomas always involved the space between the inflow surface of the sewing ring and the most peripheral region of the spongiosa. This space is continuous throughout the circumference of the bioprosthesis, a fact which explains the involvement of more than one cusp in most of the affected valves. When blood penetrates into this space, it can extend into the entire periphery of the bioprosthesis, involving the spongiosa and gradually progressing into more distal areas of the cusp. Our observations also suggest that blood gains access into this space through gaps between the edge of the bioprosthetic tissue and the sewing ring at the inflow surface. In porcine valvular bioprostheses mounted in stents for use in the atrioventricular position, the suture line on the inflow surface is completely exposed, although it tends to be covered by a fibrous tissue sheath in valves that have been implanted for long periods of time. We believe that when small gaps are present in this junction, they are enlarged when the bioprosthesis is in the open position, so that blood can enter into the space just described; that these gaps tend to close, trapping the blood that has penetrated into the space, when the bioprosthesis is in the closed position. The pressure exerted on the closed cusps of the bioprosthesis would then tend to force the trapped blood into the path of least resistance, which would be into the empty spaces of the spongiosa. Our observations indicate that hematomas also can develop rather late after implantation, perhaps because of delayed alterations in the suture line, contraction of fibrous tissue near the suture line, or degeneration and disruption of bioprosthetic tissue in this area. Nevertheless, these hematomas are microscopically similar to those developing early after implantation. The infrequency of hematomas in bioprostheses implanted for long periods of time appears to be due to the fact that access to the space between the bioprosthetic tissue and the sewing ring of these valves tends to be sealed by ingrowth of a fibrous sheath of host origin. The higher incidence of hematomas in the right coronary cusp probably is related to the fact that some of the cardiac muscle tissue that extends into the base of the right coronary cusp is removed during preparation of the bioprosthesis, so that there is a larger space, into which blood can penetrate, at the base of this cusp.

We did not observe hematomas in 16 Ionescu-Shiley pericardial bioprostheses (which do not have a spongiosa) or in eight Carpentier-Edwards bioprostheses (which had been mounted in aortic type stents) implanted in the atrioventricular position in experimental animals. The suture line securing bioprosthetic tissue to sewing ring on the inflow surface is much less exposed, and the sutures are much closer together (as is also the case in Ionescu-Shiley pericardial bioprostheses) in commercially available porcine valvular bioprostheses mounted in aortic type stents than in those mounted in atrioventricular type stents. These differences appear to be responsible for the absence of hematomas in Ionescu-Shiley valves and in the Carpentier-Edwards valves with aortic type stents used in the present study, as well as in bioprostheses implanted in the aortic position in patients. In conclusion, the evidence presented in this study strongly suggests that the occurrence of intracuspal hematomas in porcine valvular bioprostheses is basically related to the technique employed to attach the bioprosthetic tissue to the sewing ring, and to the type of mounting stent used for bioprostheses to be implanted in the atrioventricular position.

We appreciate the skilled assistance of Mrs. Dorothy Veigle (secretarial and editorial work), Miss Margaret M. M. Moore, and Mrs. Esther Wilhoite (photography).

REFERENCES

1 Ferrans VJ, Spray TL, Billingham, ME, Roberts WC: Structural changes in glutaraldehyde-treated porcine heterografts used as substitute cardiac valves. Transmission and scanning electron microscopic observations in 12 patients. Am J Cardiol **41:**1159-184, 1978

2 Barnhart GR, Jones M, Ishihara T, et al: Degeneration and calcification of bioprosthetic cardiac valves. Animal model: bioprosthetic tricuspid valve implantation in sheep. Am J Pathol **106:**136-139, 1982

3 Ishihara T, Ferrans VJ, Boyse SW, et al: Structure and classification of cuspal tears and perforations in porcine bioprosthetic cardiac valves implanted in patients. Am J Cardiol **48:**665-678, 1981

4 Ishihara T, Ferrans VJ, Jones M, et al: Occurrence and significance of endothelial cells in implanted porcine bioprosthetic valves. Am J Cardiol **48:**443-454, 1981

5 Ferrans VJ, Boyce SW, Billingham ME, Jones M, Ishihara T, Roberts WC: Calcific deposits in porcine bioprostheses. Structure and pathogenesis. Am J Cardiol **46:**721-734, 1980

6 Ishihara T, Ferrans VJ, Jones M, Boyce SW, Roberts WC: Structure of bovine parietal pericardium and of unimplanted Ionescu-Shiley pericardial valvular bioprostheses. J Thorac Cardiovasc Surg **81:**747-757, 1981

7 Lalonde J-MA, Ghadially FN, Massey KL: Ultrastructure of intramuscular haematomas and electron-probe X-ray analysis of extracellular and intracellular iron deposits. J Pathol **125:**17-23, 1978

8 Lalonde J-MA, Ghadially FN: Ultrastructure of experimentally produced subcutaneous haematomas in the rabbit. Virchows Arch [Cell Pathol] **25:**221-232, 1977

Intracuspal Hematomas in Bioprosthetic Valves: Pathologic Findings and Clinical Implications

GLENN R. BARNHART, M.D., TOKUHIRO ISHIHARA, M.D., PH.D., VICTOR J. FERRANS, M.D., PH.D., MICHAEL JONES, M.D., CHARLES L. MCINTOSH, M.D., PH.D., AND WILLIAM C. ROBERTS, M.D.

SUMMARY The presence of intracuspal hematomas (ICHs) was investigated in 156 valvular bioprostheses, including 57 (all porcine aortic valvular bioprostheses) that had been implanted in patients and 99 (64 porcine aortic valvular bioprostheses, 29 bovine pericardial bioprostheses and six human dura mater bioprostheses) that had been implanted in sheep. ICHs were found in three mitral bioprostheses in patients and in 14 porcine aortic valvular bioprostheses (nine mitral and five tricuspid) in sheep. Hematomas were not found in the dura mater or pericardial bioprostheses. In each patient and in six of the 14 sheep, the hematomas involved more than one cusp and consisted of erythrocyte accumulations in the spongiosa. They extended from the basal region toward the free edge of the cusp and formed a plane of dissection that involved the spaces left in the spongiosa by removal of proteoglycan material during commercial processing. ICHs may become sites of formation of calcific deposits. ICHs result from entry of blood into the space between the sewing ring and the most basilar region of the bioprosthetic tissue. This space extends throughout the circumference of the bioprosthesis and is continuous with the spongiosa, the layer in which the hematoma develops. The blood penetrates this space through the suture line between bioprosthetic tissue and sewing ring on the inflow surface of porcine valvular bioprostheses mounted on atrioventricular-type stents. ICHs were not found in porcine valvular bioprostheses mounted on aortic-type stents, in which the sutures are more protected and more closely spaced, or in bioprostheses constructed of tissues (parietal pericardium and dura mater), which lack a spongiosa.

ERYTHROCYTES are commonly found in the cuspal connective tissue of implanted porcine valvular bioprostheses,[1] but reports of large accumulations of erythrocytes leading to grossly visible intracuspal hematomas in implanted porcine valvular bioprostheses are rare.[2] In this report, we describe the pathologic findings and clinical implications of intracuspal hematomas in three of 57 patients and 14 of 99 sheep.

Materials and Methods

Gross anatomic, histologic, and scanning and transmission electron microscopic studies were made of 156 valvular bioprostheses implanted in patients (57 valves) or in young sheep (99 valves).

Valves had been implanted in 50 patients, ages 2–68 years (mean 42 years) at operation. Thirty-five valves were implanted in the mitral position, 13 in the aortic position, six in the tricuspid position and three in valved pulmonic conduits. The time between implantation and removal of the bioprostheses ranged from 2 days to 123 months (mean 37 months). Intracuspal hematomas were found in three of these 57 valves.

The valves implanted in sheep included 25 Hancock porcine aortic valves, 14 Carpentier-Edwards porcine aortic valves, 25 Xenotech porcine aortic valves, 29 Ionescu-Shiley bovine pericardial valves, and six human dura mater valves (Barone Laboratories). The valves were implanted in the tricuspid (44 valves) or mitral position (55 valves), for periods ranging from 20 minutes to 7 months. These investigations were performed to study the degeneration of bioprosthetic valves.[2] The Hancock and Xenotech valves were mounted on stents of the type used in the atrioventricular position, and the Carpentier-Edwards valves were mounted on stents of the type used in the aortic position. The Ionescu-Shiley valves had the single-type stent manufactured for the semilunar and atrioventricular position. Fourteen sheep had valves with intracuspal hematomas; three were killed for elective studies and 11 died (nine of cardiopulmonary failure, one of coronary air embolism and one of refractory ventricular fibrillation). The techniques we used for histologic and ultrastructural study of the tissues have been described.[1–4]

Gross Anatomic Observations

Intracuspal hematomas were found in all cusps of three valves in patients, (two Hancock valves and one Carpentier-Edwards valve). In two of these valves, the hematomas were single and extended from the sewing ring to the free edge of the cusp; the right coronary cusp of one valve also contained a small, apparently separate hematoma at the cuspal tip. The hematomas appeared as areas of reddish-black discoloration of the cusps.

Calcific deposits were grossly evident only in a valve from one patient; a break in continuity of the inflow surface of the right coronary cusp was also found in this valve. This defect was not located immediately over the main portion of the hematoma. In addition to a hematoma, the bioprosthesis from another patient had a basilar linear perforation in the left coronary cusp.

The junction between the sewing ring and the bioprosthetic tissue on the inflow surface was completely covered by fibrous tissue in the bioprosthesis from one patient; in the bioprostheses from the other two patients, it was partially covered by fibrous tissue. In the bioprosthesis from one of the latter two patients, this fibrous tissue was partially disrupted in the area adjacent to the hematoma. This disruption could have been

From the Surgery and Pathology Branches, National Heart, Lung, and Blood Institute, National Institutes of Health, Bethesda, Maryland.

Address for correspondence: Michael Jones, M.D., Building 10, Room 2N242, National Institutes of Health, Bethesda, Maryland 20205.

Circulation 66 (suppl I), 1982.

caused by operative handling. In these three bioprostheses, some of the sutures in the continuous suture line between the bioprosthetic tissue and the mounting frame were loose and irregularly placed.

Intracuspal hematomas (fig. 1) were found in 14 of the 99 bioprostheses in sheep, including 10 of the 24 that had been implanted for less than 1 week and four of the 75 that had been implanted for 3 weeks to 7 months. The 14 intracuspal hematomas (nine in Hancock valves and five in Xenotech valves) occurred in five of the 44 tricuspid bioprostheses and in nine of the 55 mitral prostheses. Hematomas were not found in Carpentier-Edwards, Ionescu-Shiley or dura mater valves.

Of the 10 bioprostheses (six Hancock and four Xenotech) that were implanted for less than 1 week and developed intracuspal hematomas, eight had been in the mitral position and two in the tricuspid position. The hematomas involved one cusp in eight valves and more than one cusp in the other six valves. They were more frequent in the right coronary cusp (10 valves) than in the left coronary cusp (four valves) and the noncoronary cusp (three valves).

Of the four bioprostheses (three Hancock and one Xenotech) that had been implanted for longer than 3 weeks and developed intracuspal hematomas, three had been in the tricuspid position and one in the mitral position. In these four bioprostheses, the hematomas involved the right coronary cusp in two and the left coronary cusp in the other two; the noncoronary cusp was not involved in these four valves.

The hematomas in valves implanted in sheep differed from those in the bioprostheses in patients in the appearance of certain areas of the inflow surface at the junction between the base of the cusp and the sewing ring. Such areas were the sites of dark red, linear thrombi that extended into the spongiosa or (in the right coronary cusp) the muscular shelf. The suture lines in these areas were not disrupted, but in some instances the apposition of the bioprosthetic cuspal tissue to the sewing ring was less than optimal, and the free edge of the tissue (i.e., the left ventricular outflow tract endocardium just beneath the lower edge of the cusp) had been unevenly or incompletely folded under before the leaflet tissue was sutured to the sewing ring (fig. 1).

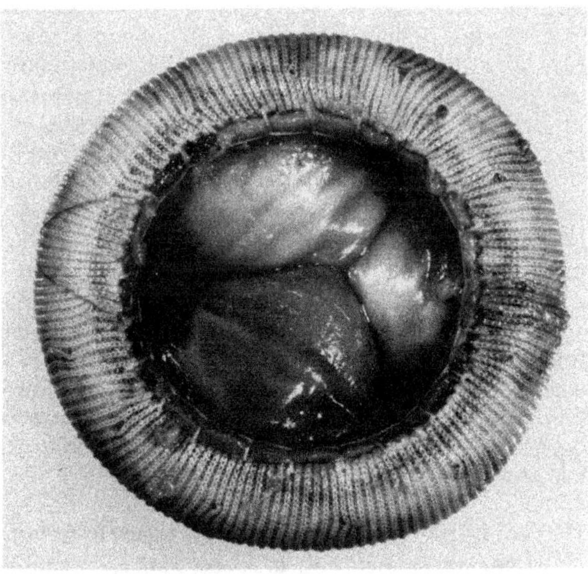

Figure 1. *Intracuspal hematoma (dark areas) is present in porcine aortic bioprosthetic valve implanted in the mitral position in a sheep that died of cardiopulmonary failure 2 hours after operation.*

Histologic Observations

The intracuspal hematomas in the valves from the three patients consisted of accumulations of large numbers of erythrocytes in areas of the valvular spongiosa in which the connective tissue had delaminated (fig. 2). The erythrocytes in these areas were associated with smaller numbers of leukocytes, macrophages and platelets and with fibrin strands. The relative sizes of these lesions, the numbers of macrophages that they contained, and the degree of valvular thickening that they produced varied considerably from one cusp to another in these three valves.

The hematoma in the right coronary cusp of the bioprosthesis from one patient had caused considerable thickening of the spongiosa and marked thinning of the fibrosa and the ventricularis. This hematoma was largest at the base of the cusp and tapered gradually toward the free edge. The erythrocytes in less se-

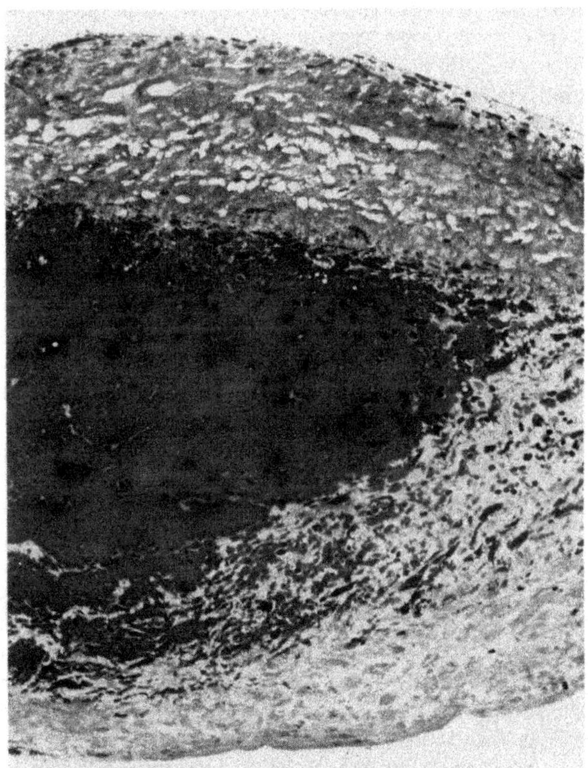

Figure 2. *Photomicrograph of section of porcine aortic bioprosthetic valve removed from a patient 107 months after implantation in the mitral position. Erythrocytes from a large mass that occupies the spongiosa and extends from the basilar region toward the tip of the cusp (i.e., from left to right). The fibrosa is at the top and the ventricularis at the bottom of the figure. Hematoxylin-eosin stain; magnification × 160.*

verely involved portions of the cusp often formed rows arranged parallel to the surface of the cusp and separated from one another by thin layers of connective tissue. Macrophages were relatively few in number and contained only moderate quantities of phagocytosed cytoplasmic granules. The other two cusps in this valve contained smaller hematomas, also located in the spongiosa. Each cusp of the bioprosthesis from this patient also contained multiple small areas of erythrocyte accumulation, some in the spongiosa and others in the fibrosa and ventricularis, and even between the cusp itself and the fibrous sheath[4] that extended from the sewing ring and covered the surfaces of the basal regions of the cusps. Calcific deposits were not present in any of the cusps, but surface microthrombi and areas of degeneration of connective tissue were evident in each cusp.

In the bioprosthesis from another patient, the noncoronary cusp was markedly thickened by a large hematoma, and microscopic hematomas were present in the other two cusps. Degenerative changes and calcific deposits were present in each cusp, often immediately adjacent to the microscopic hematomas. The bioprosthesis from the third patient was minimally calcified, showed moderate degenerative changes, contained relatively small hematomas, and had abundant macrophages on its surface.

In the valves that had been implanted in sheep for less than 1 week, the hematomas filled the space between the sewing ring and the basal portion of the spongiosa. In each right coronary cusp, the hematoma also extended into the region of the muscle shelf. From the basal regions the hematomas appeared to have spread into the more distal portions of the valves by dissecting through the spongiosa. Areas of spongiosa adjacent to the hematomas often were filled with material we thought represented accumulations of serum proteins. The fibrosa and the ventricularis in these valves appeared similar to those in unimplanted valves,[1] without degeneration, calcification, infection or fibrous sheaths. Most of the erythrocytes in the hematomas in these valves appeared morphologically to contain normal amounts of hemoglobin and were associated with only a few leukocytes. Macrophages filled with phagocytosed material were not found in these hematomas.

Of the four valves that had been implanted in sheep for more than 3 weeks, three were partially covered by fibrous sheaths, and all four had calcific deposits. As in the other valves, the hematomas in these valves extended from the basal regions of the cusps toward the free edges, forming a plane of dissection through the spongiosa. The fibrosa and the ventricularis were thinned, and small, focal areas of erythrocyte infiltration were presesnt in both layers, but were not apparently related to the large hematomas in the spongiosa.

Transmission and Scanning Electron Microscopic Observations

Transmission electron microscopic observations of all three bioprostheses in patients showed calcific deposits and degenerative changes in the cuspal connective tissue, similar to those described previously.[1,5] In areas of hematomas we found phagocytosis of erythrocytes by macrophages and accumulations of material considered to be old fibrin deposits around the erythrocytes. Our findings in hematomas in valves implanted in sheep were similar. Scanning electron microscopic examination of the cut surfaces of the cusps clearly showed the localization of hematomas in the spongiosa and the presence of erythrocytes between adjacent layers of collagenous fibers (figs. 3 and 4).

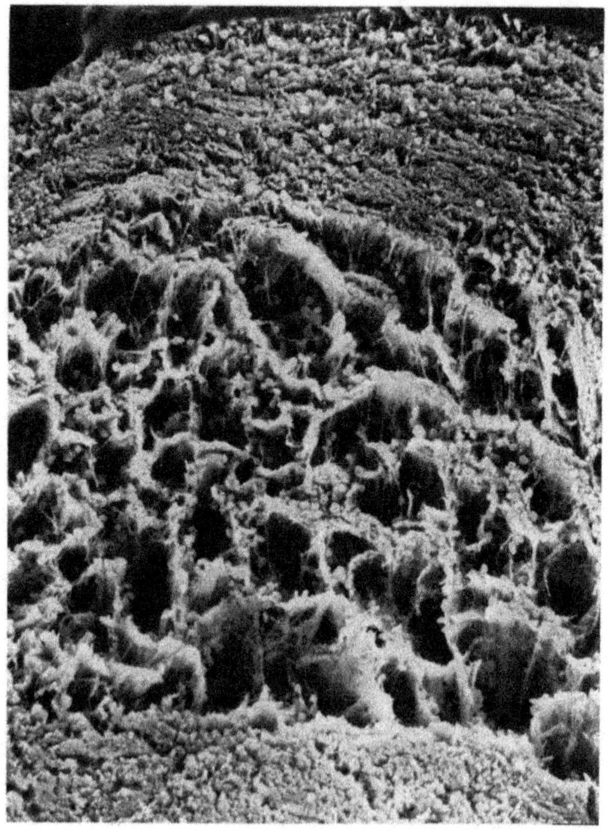

FIGURE 3. *Scanning electron micrograph of the cut surface of a porcine aortic valvular bioprosthesis implanted in the mitral position in a sheep that died of a coronary air embolus at operation. The fibrosa is at the top, the spongiosa in the center and the ventricularis at the bottom. The empty spaces in the spongiosa were left by removal of proteoglycans during preimplantation processing. Magnification × 320.*

Discussion

Our study shows that intracuspal hematomas can be found early and late after implantation of porcine cardiac bioprosthetic valves in patients and in sheep. Our observations also document the morphology, consequences, incidence and pathogenesis of intracuspal hematomas.

Morphology and Consequences of Intracuspal Hematomas

All intracuspal hematomas occupied the spongiosa, a layer that in unimplanted valves contains empty spaces left by the loss of proteoglycan material during commercial processing. The hematomas extended from the basal region toward the free edge of the cusp

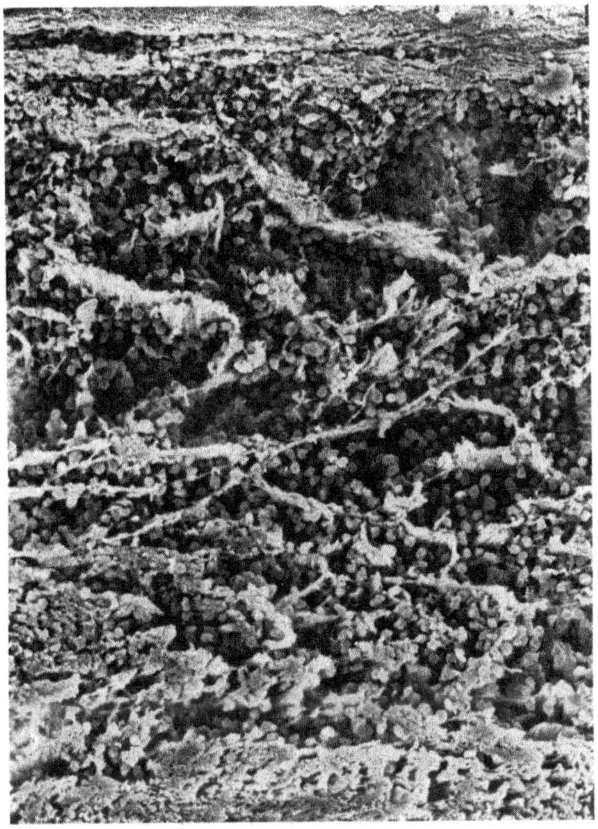

FIGURE 4. *Photomicrograph from a more proximal region of the valve shown in figure 2. The empty spaces in the spongiosa have been filled with erythrocytes. Magnification × 420.*

by dissecting through the spongiosa. This separation of layers of connective tissue is similar to that in dissecting arterial aneurysms. The plane of dissection through the spongiosa is significant in that we have not found intracuspal hematomas in dura mater or in bovine pericardial bioprostheses, which do not have a layer of tissue corresponding to the spongiosa of porcine valvular bioprostheses.[6]

The two principal potential consequences of intracuspal hematomas — reduction in the mobility of the affected cusps and calcification of the hematoma — led to stenosis of the bioprosthesis. One patient had reduced cusp mobility that led to prosthetic mitral stenosis, which necessitated reoperation 27 months after implantation of the valves. When removed, this bioprosthesis contained calcific deposits, but they were small and it seemed likely that marked cuspal thickening by intracuspal hematomas played a major role in the pathogenesis of the stenosis. The valves removed from the other two patients had smaller hematomas, which were associated with less severe cuspal thickening. A significant end-diastolic gradient was found in only one of the three sheep studied hemodynamically 1 month or longer after implantation of the bioprostheses in which the hematomas were found. The gradient was probably largely due to severe ingrowth of fibrous tissue over both surfaces of the cusps. Thus, it would appear that intracuspal hematomas cause bioprosthetic stenosis only when they are large and interfere with the mobility of the affected cusps.

A relationship of intracuspal hematomas and calcific deposits was suggested by the fact that both of these changes were localized in the spongiosa. In addition, erythrocyte accumulations were often found adjacent to calcific deposits, particularly those that were large and nodular. Nevertheless, intermediate stages in the transformation of hematomas into calcific deposits were not observed, and for this reason, it remains uncertain that hematomas contribute directly to the formation of calcific deposits. Macrophages were not associated with hematomas in the valves that had been implanted in the sheep for 1 week or less; however, macrophages were infrequent in the hematomas in the valves implanted in sheep for 1 month or longer, and the hematomas in valves implanted for up to 6 months showed no tendency to become organized by ingrowth of fibrous tissue into the affected areas. Thus, the time course of invasion by macrophages and organization by fibroblasts appears to be much slower in intracuspal hematomas than in other types of hematomas, such as those induced by intramuscular or subcutaneous injections of blood in experimental animals.[7, 8] One major reason for this would appear to be the difficulty that macrophages, other inflammatory cells and fibroblasts have in penetrating into the spongiosa of glutaraldehyde-treated porcine valvular bioprostheses.[1]

It is not known how long erythrocytes can maintain relatively normal shapes and hemoglobin contents within intracuspal hematomas. It seems highly unlikely that such a period would exceed a few months, even under circumstances of very limited attack by macrophages and organization by fibroblasts. Thus, the hematomas found in the bioprostheses of the three patients 27–107 months after implantation were probably of recent origin. Such hematomas may recur, and resolve by lysis or liquefaction rather than by organization.

Pathogenesis of Intracuspal Hematomas

The entry of blood into the spongiosa could be due to a direct communication with the cuspal surface through a hole or defect either in the ventricularis or the fibrosa or to penetration through the junction between bioprosthetic tissue and sewing ring either in the inflow or outflow surfaces. The first possibility is unlikely because the surface defects found by scanning electron microscopy were very small and shallow. Blood penetrating into the spongiosa through a free two-way communication would be expelled from this layer by mechanical forces associated with cardiac pumping and valvular motion. Thus, it appears necessary to postulate a mechanism by which blood becomes trapped in the spongiosa.

The junction of the sewing ring and the bioprosthetic tissue on the inflow surface is a likely site of entry of blood into the spongiosa. The junction of the sewing ring and the outflow surface always appeared normal, tightly sutured, and microscopically free of involvement by hematoma. In contrast, hematomas always involved the space between the inflow surface of the sewing ring and the most peripheral region of the spongiosa. The continuity of this space throughout the circumference of the bioprosthesis accounts for the involvement of more than one cusp in most of the affected valves and for the gradual progression into more distal areas of the cusps. In porcine valvular bioprostheses mounted on atrioventricular-type stents, the suture line on the inflow surface is completely exposed. Small gaps in this junction would become enlarged when the bioprosthesis is in the open position, which would allow entry of blood into the space just described. When the bioprosthesis is closed, these gaps would tend to close, forcing the trapped blood into the empty spaces of the spongiosa. Hematomas also can develop late after implantation, perhaps because of delayed alterations in the suture ring, contraction of fibrous tissue near the suture line, or degeneration and disruption of bioprosthetic tissue in this area; these hematomas are microscopically similar to those developing early after implantation. Hematomas are infrequent in bioprostheses implanted for long periods of time because access to the space between the bioprosthetic tissue and the sewing ring of these valves is eventually sealed by ingrowth of a fibrous sheath of host origin. The higher incidence of hematomas in the right coronary cusp is probably related to the fact that some of the cardiac muscle tissue that extends into the base of the right coronary cusp is removed during preparation of the bioprosthesis, leaving a larger space into which blood can penetrate at the base of this cusp.

We did not observe hematomas in Ionescu-Shiley pericardial bioprostheses (which do not have a spongiosa), in Carpentier-Edwards bioprostheses (which had been mounted on aortic-type stents) or in human dura mater valves implanted in the atrioventricular position in the sheep. The suture line securing the bioprosthetic cuspal tissue to the sewing ring on the inflow surface is much less exposed, and the sutures are much closer together (as in the Ionescu-Shiley pericardial bioprostheses) in porcine valvular bioprostheses mounted on aortic-type stents than in those mounted on atrioventricular-type stents. These differences appear to be responsible for the absence of hematomas in the Carpentier-Edwards valves with aortic-type stents implanted in the sheep as well as in aortic bioprostheses implanted in the patients. Dura mater and parietal pericardium do not have a tissue layer that corresponds to the spongiosa of porcine valves, and for this reason hematomas are not likely to develop in valves manufactured of these materials.

In conclusion, the occurrence of intracuspal hematomas in porcine valvular bioprostheses is related to the presence of a space in the spongiosa, to the technique used to attach the bioprosthetic tissue to the sewing ring, and to the type of stent used to mount the bioprosthesis for implantation in the atrioventricular position.

References

1. Ferrans VJ, Spray TL, Billingham ME, Roberts WC: Structural changes in glutaraldehyde-treated porcine heterografts used as substitute cardiac valves. Transmission and scanning electron microscopic observations in 12 patients. Am J Cardiol **41:** 1159, 1978
2. Barnhart GR, Jones M, Ishihara I, Chavez AM, Rose DM, Ferrans VJ: Degeneration and calcification of bioprosthetic cardiac valves. Animal model: bioprosthetic tricuspid valve implantation in sheep. Am J Pathol **106:** 136, 1982
3. Ishihara T, Ferrans VJ, Boyce SE, Jones M, Roberts WC: Structure and classification of cuspal tears and perforations in porcine bioprosthetic cardiac valves implanted in patients. Am J Cardiol **48:** 665, 1981
4. Ishihara T, Ferrans VJ, Jones M, Boyce SE, Roberts WC: Occurrence and significance of endothelial cells in implanted porcine bioprosthetic valves. Am J Cardiol **48:** 443, 1981
5. Ferrans VJ, Boyce SW, Billingham ME, Jones M, Ishihara T, Roberts WC: Calcific deposits in porcine bioprostheses: structure and pathogenesis. Am J Cardiol **46:** 721, 1980
6. Ishihara T, Ferrans VJ, Jones M, Boyce SE, Roberts WC: Structure of bovine parietal pericardium and of unimplanted Ionescu-Shiley pericardial valvular bioprostheses. J Thorac Cardiovasc Surg **81:** 747, 1981
7. Lalonde JMA, Ghadially FN, Massey KL: Ultrastructure of intramuscular haematomas and electron-probe x-ray analysis of extracellular and intracellular iron deposits. J Pathol **125:** 17, 1978
8. Lalonde JMA, Ghadially FN: Ultrastructure of experimentally produced subcutaneous haematomas in the rabbit. Virchows Arch [Cell Pathol] **25:** 221, 1977

Complications of Cardiac Valve Replacement

William C. Roberts

It has been over 21 years since successful replacement of one or more cardiac valves became a reality, and since then, many thousands of patients with severely symptomatic valvular heart disease have had valve replacement, with complete loss or sharp decrease in their symptoms of cardiac dysfunction. Although the chance of successful valve replacement in most patients is very high, occasional, often predictable, complications are recognized to occur both early and late in some patients in whom this procedure is carried out. Since 1960, I have examined at necropsy over 600 hearts, submitted from around the USA, containing one or more prosthetic valves, and certain complications of cardiac valve replacement observed in them will be summarized in this chapter.

COMPLICATIONS COMMON TO ANY VALVE SITE AND TO MOST OR ALL VALVES

Prosthetic Size Disproportion. The normal cardiac valves consist of thin, very pliable, leaflet-like structures that allow central flow of blood and occupy very little space within the ventricles or great arteries in which they reside. Mechanical valves and even tissue valves attached to rigid or semirigid stents and rings, in contrast, are rigid except for movement of the occluder or cusps. They often prevent central flow, and they occupy noncompressible space. Early in the history of cardiac valve replacement, there appeared to be a tendency to insert as large a prosthetic valve as possible because the large ones were prone to be less obstructive than the smaller sized ones. Experience taught, however, that if a mechanical prosthesis was too big for the ventricle or ascending aorta in which it was to reside, movement of the occluder could be limited, with the potential for varying degrees of obstruction to flow.[1-15] At one time, a common view was that this disproportion problem was one produced mainly by caged ball prostheses because they were larger than most subsequently utilized mechanical prostheses. This view, however, proved incorrect. No mechanical valve and no tissue valve (Fig. 96-1) attached to a frame is immune to the problem of prosthetic disproportion.

The consequence of placement in the mitral position is, usually, interference with left atrial emptying or with left ventricular filling and, seldom, in my view despite others' beliefs to the contrary, interference with left ventricular emptying (left ventricular outflow obstruction).[1] The usual consequence of placement in the aortic position is interference with left ventricular emptying. Prosthetic disproportion is most likely to occur in the mitral position when valve replacement is carried out for pure mitral stenosis (or combined mitral and aortic valve stenosis) and in the aortic position when the aorta is small when there is aortic stenosis associated with mitral valve disease or there is acute aortic regurgitation when the aorta has not had adequate time to dilate. Large-sized prostheses, whether caged ball (Starr-Edwards), tilting disc (Björk-Shiley or St. Jude), or nontilting disc (Kay-Shiley) must be avoided in small patients with purely stenotic valvular lesions. Determining proper prosthetic size only in the operating room without consideration of the hemodynamic lesion and the lean weight of the patient can lead to prosthetic disproportion, a major problem in the early years of valve replacement, but even today an occasional problem.[15]

Prosthetic Thrombosis. It was years before all doctors dealing with patients who had mechanical prosthetic valves became convinced that anticoagulation (warfarin sodium) was essential. When anticoagulation became accepted ther-

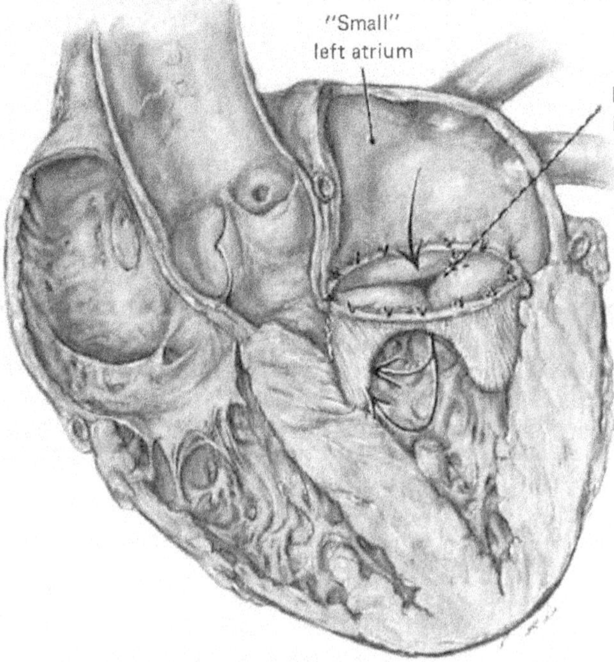

FIG. 96-1. Obstruction to left ventricular outflow by stent of mitral prosthesis. The porcine bioprosthesis (33 mm) appears to be too large for the left ventricle in this woman with severe acute mitral regurgitation from sudden rupture of several chordae tendineae. Despite the volume lesion, the left ventricle had not had adequate time to dilate, and the large-sized prosthesis was oriented so that one of its large stents partially obstructed left ventricular outflow and, additionally, contacted the ventricular septum.

apy, mechanical valve thrombosis became less of a problem. Nevertheless, prosthetic thrombus occurs in some patients who are well anticoagulated, and, occasionally, it does *not* occur in patients who have never received anticoagulants. Thrombus is often observed in porcine bioprostheses that have been in place for over two months, but usually the thrombi are so small that function of the prosthesis is not altered.[15-17]

Para-anular Prosthetic Ring Discontinuity (Parabasilar Leak). Parabasilar communications appear to result from placement of an inadequate number of sutures in the sewing ring (because of anular calcific deposits, for example) or from the pulling loose of one or more sutures after replacement of anatomically normal (as in papillary muscle dysfunction) or floppy mitral valves, in aortic regurgitation secondary to a disease of the wall of aorta (as in Marfan's syndrome) rather than of aortic valve cusp, or in infection (prosthetic endocarditis) at the site of attachment of a prosthesis.[4]

Prosthetic Degeneration or Wear. Almost all of the initial models of presently utilized mechanical prostheses had evidence of wear or variance of one or more parts. The silicone rubber poppets utilized in the initial models of the caged ball prosthesis took in lipids, which resulted in their swelling and impacting in the cage (see Chapter 94, Fig. 94-1) or developing large cracks that allowed some to dislodge from the cage.[4,8,12,18-20] Hopefully, the change, about 1966, in the processing of the silicone rubber has alleviated this problem. The utilization of cloth around the struts of the cage led to cloth fragmentation (Fig. 96-2) and to the introduction by the manufacturer of the close-clearance cage, a disastrous modification in which the poppet sometimes stuck in the midportion causing sudden death. In the latest model Starr-Edwards valve, wear of the metallic studs on the inner lining of the ring has led to contact of the metallic poppet with the cloth of the ring, with subsequent disruption of the cloth. Fracture of the strut or occluder (Delrin) also occurred in a few

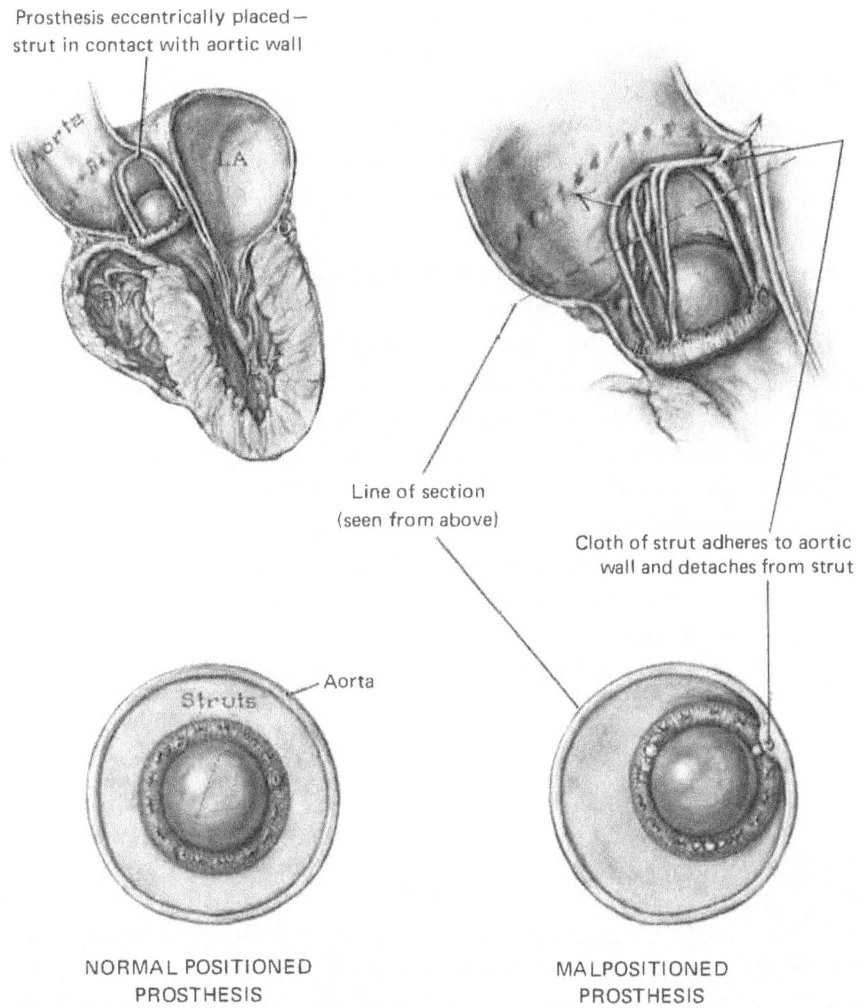

FIG. 96-2. Cloth wear on stents of a caged ball prosthesis in a 76-year-old man who died of carcinoma many years after aortic valve replacement and an asymptomatic postoperative course. At necropsy one of the three stents contacted the intimal lining of the aorta, and eventually the aortic wall completely encircled the one stent and the cloth became detached from the other two stents. Although a rather striking finding at necropsy, the cloth degeneration and aortic wall overgrowth did not cause symptoms during life.

of the earlier models of the tilting and nontilting discs.

Much evidence has accumulated to indicate that the cusps of the porcine bioprosthesis will eventually degenerate,[15-17,21-24] and the same fate may be in store for the bovine parietal pericardial bioprosthesis. This prosthesis has had the best first 5-year record of any of the commonly employed prostheses, but its 6-to-10-year record may not be good. Numerous reports have described heavy calcification and cuspal disruption of the porcine bioprosthesis after the first 5-year period, enough evidence to convince me that this prosthesis should not be the prosthesis of choice for persons who can tolerate anticoagulants and are under age 60 or 65 years.

Suture Overhang of Prosthetic Orifice. If a suture or knot overhangs the metallic ring of a caged disc or tilting disc prosthesis, the consequence might be prosthetic regurgitation.[25] Such was the case in three patients reported earlier from this laboratory: fatal aortic regurgitation was the consequence in two, and the aortic regurgitation in the third was relieved simply by cutting one overhanging suture. More recently, the same mechanism caused mitral regurgitation after replacement with a tilting disc prosthesis. This mechanism is less likely to occur with the caged ball prosthesis because the margin of error is greater than with the more delicate tilting disc type prosthesis.

Prosthetic Endocarditis. With mechanical prostheses, the infection always occurs beneath the site of attachment of the prosthesis, thus, ring abscess is inevitable[26-31] (Fig. 96-3). With tissue valves mounted on frames, the infection may be limited to the cusps. Therefore, if one has a substitute cardiac valve that is infected, it is better that it be a bioprosthesis rather than a mechanical valve. If endocarditis occurs in a patient in whom more than one mechanical or bioprosthetic valve is in place, the infection nearly always involves only the most downstream valvular prosthesis.

Entanglement of Sutures Beneath the Occluder. Suture entanglement beneath the occluder during insertion of a mitral prosthesis may prevent descent of the occluder during ventricular diastole.[32] Simply making certain by manual manipulation that the mitral occluder descends freely before closing the left atriotomy incision might prevent this technical problem and thus a fatality. (See Chapter 89.)

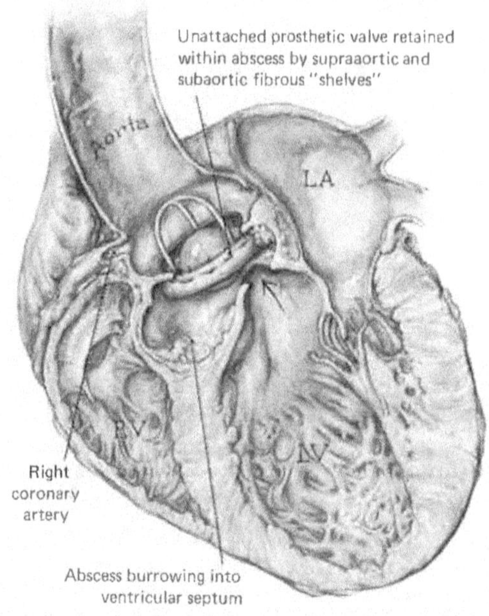

FIG. 96-3. Prosthetic valve endocarditis. Heart of a 39-year-old woman who underwent aortic valve replacement eight years earlier because of severe aortic regurgitation secondary to intravenous heroin-induced infective endocarditis. She was asymptomatic thereafter, however, except for occasional ventricular arrhythmias, until 26 hours before death when she suddenly became unconscious and was found to have an intracerebral bleed. At necropsy, the caged ball prosthesis was completely detached due to infection beneath the prosthetic ring. The prosthesis was prevented from dislodging by a constricting fibrous ring just cephalad to the prosthetic anulus. During her last eight years of life, there was never clinical evidence of infective endocarditis.

Incomplete Removal of Native Valve or Calcific Deposits Preventing Occlusion. If calcific deposits involve the attachment of a valve leaflet to its anulus, complete debridement of the calcium may not be possible. If a rather sizable calcific nodule remains after valvular excision, the residual calcific debris, on rare occasion, may interfere with complete closure of the occluder.[3]

Dislodgment of Portion of Native Cardiac Valve during Excision. It is preferable to remove a calcified cardiac valve intact rather than in multiple fragments to prevent the possibility of embolism.[33]

Development of Calcific Deposits beneath Site of Attachment of Prosthetic Valve Ring. During both phases of the cardiac cycle, a rigid-framed prosthesis moves. This back-and-forth rocking motion over many years may stimulate the development of calcific deposits beneath the prosthetic anulus.[34] As long as the deposits are small, significant functional consequences are unlikely, but larger ones theoretically could disrupt a suture that holds the prosthetic ring in place. This anular calcium is most likely to develop 5 years or more after mitral replacement with a heavy prosthesis (caged ball), though to date I am aware of no functional consequences of its presence.

Hemolysis of Blood Elements. Most mechanical cardiac valves shorten the half-life of erythrocytes, leukocytes, and even platelets, but in all but a few patients, bone marrow production of these is accelerated, and anemia, leukopenia, or thrombocytopenia is rarely a consequence. On occasion, however, hemolysis is a problem, most frequently in patients with caged ball prostheses (particularly with the fully cloth-covered models), in patients with aortic valve prostheses as opposed to other replaced valves, and in patients with parabasilar leaks as opposed to patients with intact parabasilar regions.[35]

COMPLICATIONS LIMITED TO PARTICULAR VALVE SITE

MITRAL VALVE POSITION

Disruption of Connection between Left Atrium and Left Ventricle at Mitral Anulus. When calcific deposits are located in the mitral anular region in addition to the mitral leaflets, excision of the mitral valve, including one or more anular calcific deposits, may cause a loss of continuity between the walls of the left atrium and left ventricle, with extravasation of blood into the left atrio-ventricular sulcus with or without fatal bleeding into the pericardial sac.[3]

Excision of Portion of Left Ventricular Free Wall beneath Papillary Muscle. If during mitral valve excision a left ventricular papillary muscle, grasped with a clamp, is pulled toward the left atrium before the papillary muscle incision is made, a portion of left ventricular free wall in addition to papillary muscle may be excised.[3] Depending on how much left ventricular free wall is excised, the result may be through-and-through rupture or aneurysmal formation.[4]

Incision of Left Ventricular Free Wall. A number of reports have described rupture of the left ventricular wall after mitral valve replacement. This complication is not rare. At one major medical center, this complication was reported in 1980 to be the most common cause of early death after mitral valve replacement.[36] Most often the rupture was attributed to the burrowing through the free wall of a stent of either a mechanical or a porcine valve.[36] In my view the mechanism has never been precisely determined. I believe the cause may, on the basis that the rupture or aneurysm site in the left ventricular free wall is midway between the mitral anulus and stump of the papillary muscle, be inadvertent incision of the left ventricular free wall during the incision of the chordae tendineae. The tear into the left ventricular free wall is linear, often involves the entire free wall of the left ventricle,[37] (Fig. 96-4) and, furthermore, can be a considerable distance from a prosthetic stent. I have seen this complication in about 10 patients at necropsy. All have had relatively small hearts, with normal-sized left atrial and left ventricular cavities. The mitral hemodynamic lesion in each was either chronic mitral stenosis or acute mitral regurgitation. At operation the atrium had been entered in all but one patient (Fig. 96-4) by incision in the interatrial groove. The incision was relatively short because of the small size of the heart. The distance from the interatrial groove incision to the inadvertent left ventricular circular incision was as much as 8 to 9 cm, exposure of the mitral valve was poor, visualization of the tips of the incising or excising mitral valve scissors was unquestionably poor or inadequate, and during the scissors' opening or closing, or both, while excising the mitral valve their tips incised a portion of left ventricular free wall.

Damage to the Left Circumflex Coronary Artery or Coronary Sinus. Although I have not seen this complication personally, damage to the left circumflex coronary artery or coronary sinus or both during mitral replacement has been observed by others. Since both of these vessels are located in the left atrio-ventricular sulcus, they lie less than 1 cm from where sutures are placed into the most basal portion of mitral leaflet during insertion of the prosthesis. Occlusion of the left circumflex coronary artery by a suture may result in a ventricular arrhythmia or acute myocardial infarction or both, whereas occlusion of the coronary sinus usually does not produce clinically recognized dysfunction. Also during suture obliteration of the mouth of the left atrial appendage, there may be a complete obliteration by a suture of the lumen of the left circumflex coronary artery, which courses just beneath the entrance into the appendage (Fig. 96-5).

Contact of Cage or Stent of Mitral Prosthesis with Ventricular Septum or Left Ventricular Free Wall. Contact of the cage or stent of a mitral or tricuspid valve prosthesis with the ventricular septum or even the ventricular free wall not only may result in ventricular inflow or outflow obstruction, but the tickling of the myocardium by the prosthesis may produce a ventricular arrhythmia that may be fatal (Fig. 96-6). This mechanism has been documented by echocardiography during life, and indentations of the ventricular septum, particularly by the cage of a caged ball prosthesis or by a stent of a porcine bioprosthesis, may be observed at necropsy (Fig. 96-6). This situation, of course, is most liable to occur when relatively large sized prostheses are employed in relatively small sized ventricles.

Diffuse or Extensive Left Ventricular Endocardial Fibrosis. Whenever the left ventricular papillary muscles are excised, their raw stumps are eventually covered by dense fibrous tissue. Thus, mural endocardial fibrosis over the stumps of the papillary muscles is an expected late finding after mitral valve replacement. On rare occasion, not only is the endocardial covering over the papillary muscles thickened by fibrous tissue but the same process may involve most of the remaining portion of left ventricle.[38] The mechanism of this diffuse or extensive endocardial fibrosis is unclear. Initially, the concept was presented that the ball-in-a-cage prosthesis stirred up the blood in the left ventricular cavity, and the anatomic consequence of the churning up and down movement was intimal thickening. Another view has been that the extensive endocardial thickening was the consequence of poor

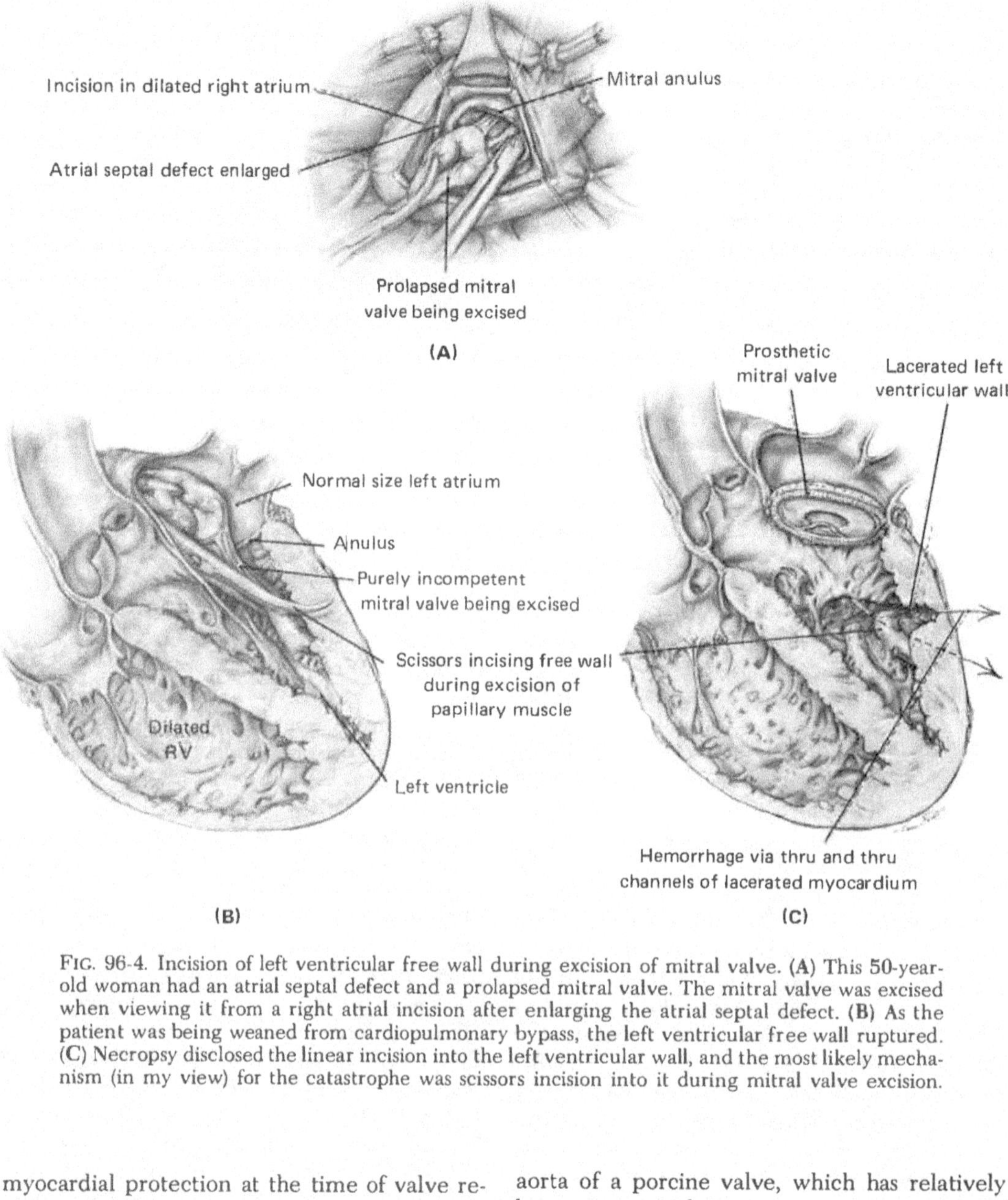

FIG. 96-4. Incision of left ventricular free wall during excision of mitral valve. (**A**) This 50-year-old woman had an atrial septal defect and a prolapsed mitral valve. The mitral valve was excised when viewing it from a right atrial incision after enlarging the atrial septal defect. (**B**) As the patient was being weaned from cardiopulmonary bypass, the left ventricular free wall ruptured. (**C**) Necropsy disclosed the linear incision into the left ventricular wall, and the most likely mechanism (in my view) for the catastrophe was scissors incision into it during mitral valve excision.

myocardial protection at the time of valve replacement; but to my knowledge, the endocardial thickening has been observed only after mitral valve replacement, not aortic valve replacement. This lesion is not the same as the constrictive endocarditis of unknown etiology described by Löffler[39] and treated by surgical excision by Dubost.[40]

Aortic Valve Position

Obstruction of Coronary Ostium by Prosthetic Ring or Stent. This complication, which is rare, may result in a fatal acute myocardial infarction or ventricular arrhythmia. Utilization in a small aorta of a porcine valve, which has relatively large stents, with improper positioning of the stents is the most likely cause of this complication today.

Intimal Thickening in Aortic Root. Wherever the intimal surface of the aorta is touched, the endothelial cells are immediately removed, and the underlying media is exposed. Usually, healing occurs simply by proliferation of new endothelial cells, but occasionally collagen is deposited in excess in these exposed areas. Thus, some focal intimal thickening in the aortic root is expected after aortic valve replacement. Turbulent flow, particularly that through a peripheral

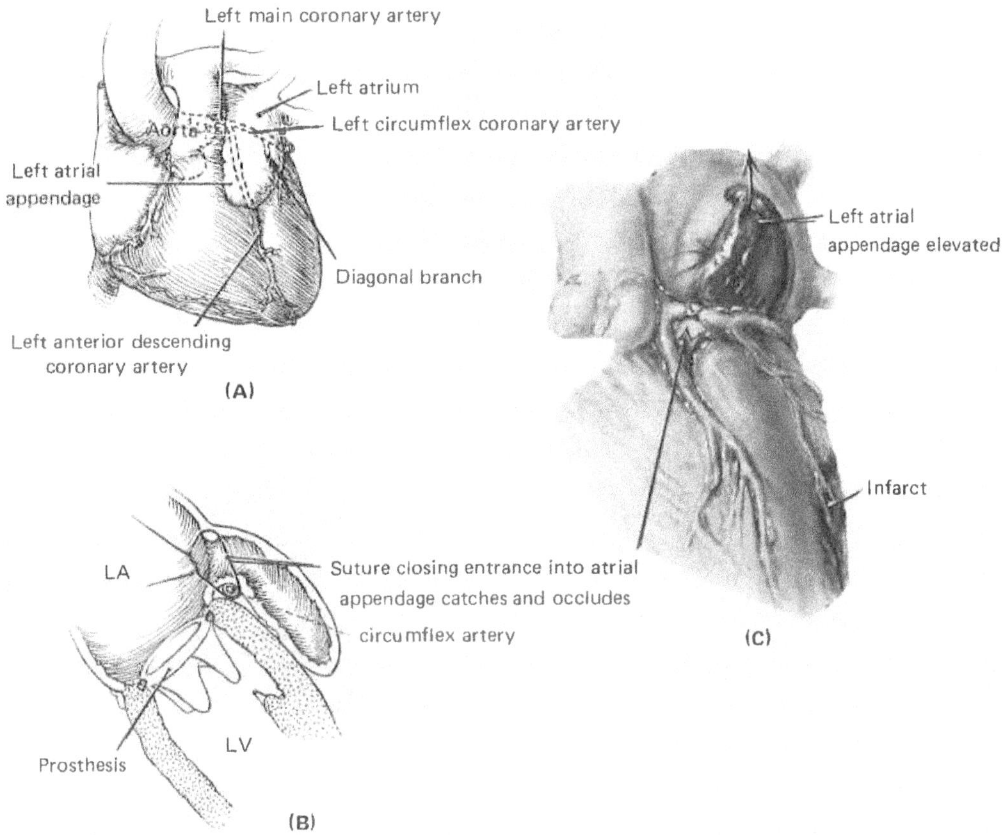

FIG. 96-5. **(A, B)** Occlusion of left circumflex coronary artery by sutures utilized to close the mouth of the left atrial appendage in a 62-year-old man who died with a lateral wall left ventricular acute infarct **(C)** five days after mitral valve replacement.

flow type prosthesis, may lead to severe intimal thickening. If the intimal thickening involves the aorta in the area of the coronary ostia, the latter may be narrowed, and this may lead to myocardial ischemia.[2] This complication, however, has proved to be uncommon but, nevertheless, a well-documented one after aortic valve replacement. In patients with clinical evidence of red blood cell hemolysis, the aortic root intimal thickening can be predicted to be particularly severe because its origin is primarily turbulence produced by flow through the prosthesis, the same mechanism that shortens the half-life of the red blood cells.[8]

Dissection of Aorta. Aortic dissection is a well-known occurrence in certain patients with aortic valve disease, but its occurrence *after* aortic valve replacement is not widely appreciated (Fig. 96-7). Fortunately, this complication is infrequent after aortic valve replacement (described in only 0.07 percent of such patients postoperatively[41]). Dissection also may occur after aortotomy for any purpose (cannulation site, aortocoronary conduit anastomosis, and so on), and, therefore, its occurrence after aortic valve replacement may be more related to the aortotomy than to inherent disease of the aorta associated with aortic valve stenosis or regurgitation.

COMBINED MITRAL AND AORTIC VALVE POSITIONS

Contact of Aortic Valve Poppet with Stent or Ring of Mitral Prosthesis. The basal attachment of the anterior mitral leaflet is about 1 cm caudal to the bases of the aortic valve cusps, and after replacement of both valves, the fixation rings of the two prostheses are in close proximity. Ordinarily, this juxtaposition produces no hemodynamic disturbance, but if the mitral prosthesis is particularly large, one of its stents

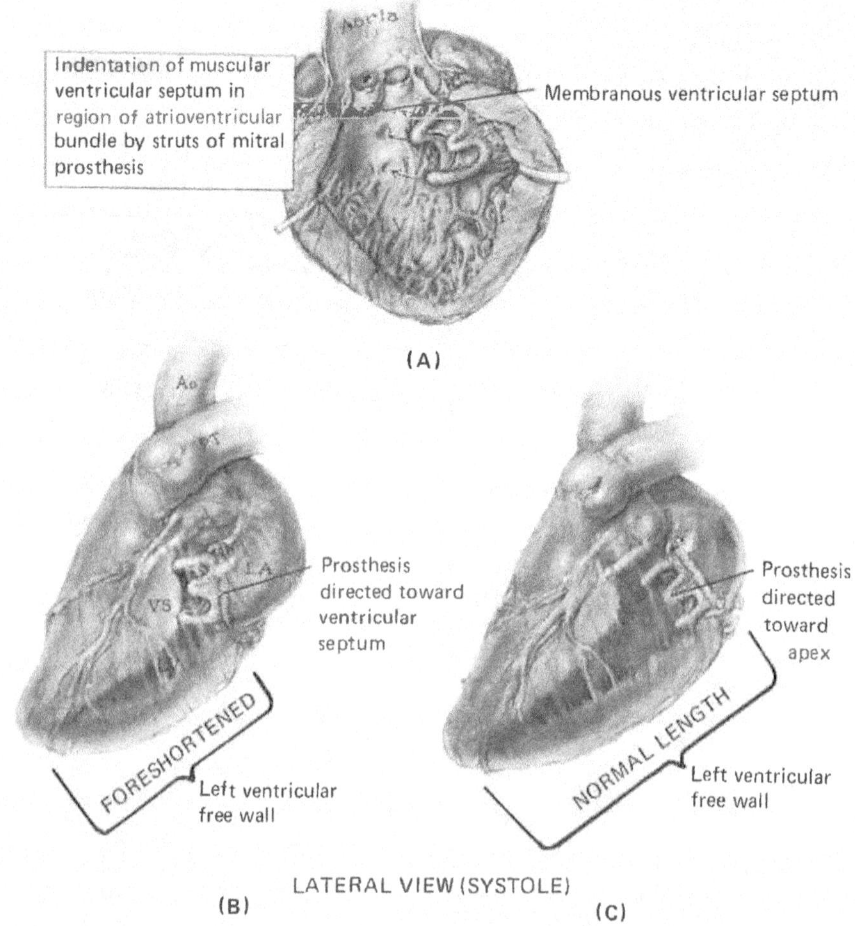

FIG. 96-6. Contact of stents of porcine bioprosthesis in the mitral position with the ventricular septum, probably during ventricular systole only. (A, B) A 71-year-old woman underwent mitral replacement 38 days before death because of severe mitral regurgitation associated with idiopathic dilated cardiomyopathy. Although no definite consequence of this contact between prosthesis and ventricular septum was apparent, this type of contact has been recognized to produce ventricular arrhythmias and possibly even sudden death. (C) Illustration of the ideal fixation of a porcine prosthesis in the mitral position.

or even its ring may lie directly beneath the orifice of the aortic prosthesis, and during ventricular diastole, the poppet of the aortic prosthesis may contact the stent or ring of the mitral prosthesis, the aortic poppet may be prevented from seating, and aortic regurgitation, which may be fatal, may result.[42] This complication has been observed only when the mitral valve has been replaced with a very large sized prosthesis.

Compression of Anomalous Left Circumflex Coronary Artery. The most common important coronary anomaly is origin of the left circumflex coronary artery from the right coronary artery with subsequent coursing behind the aorta on its way to the left atrio-ventricular sulcus. Although potentially this anomalous artery could be damaged during isolated mitral or aortic valve replacement, such has not been reported. Damage to this artery, however, is a distinct possibility if both mitral and aortic valves are replaced: the anomalous coronary artery courses between the fixation rings of these two prosthesis and thus may be compressed by them.[43] Fortunately, because this coronary anomaly occurs about once in 300 human hearts and combined replacement of both mitral and aortic valves is even less frequent, this complication of valve replacement is extremely rare.[43]

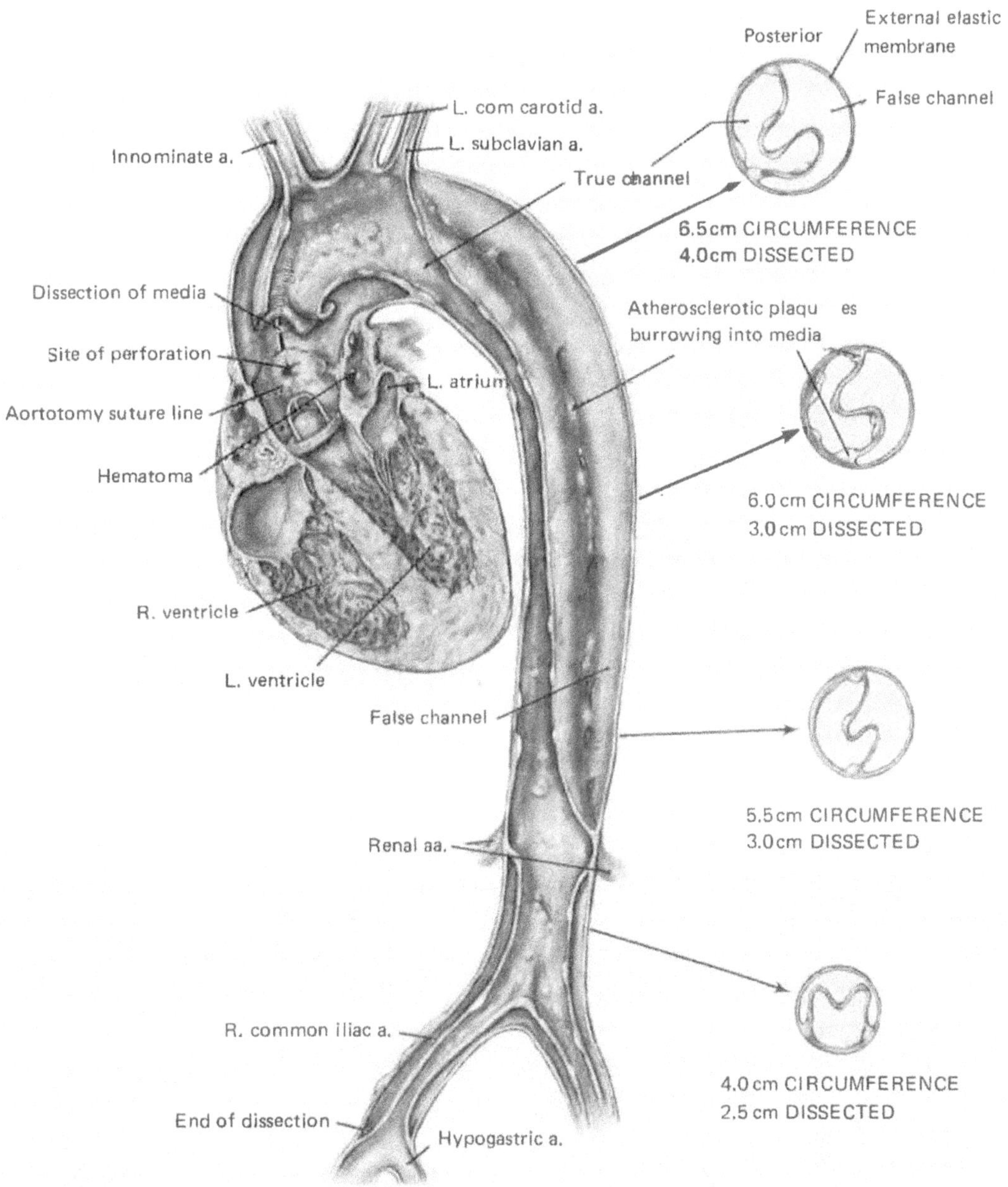

FIG. 96-7. Aortic dissection after aortic valve replacement. This 50-year-old man had his stenotic, congenitally bicuspid aortic valve replaced with a caged ball prosthesis 10 years before death. At operation, the ascending aorta was normal. He died suddenly after an asymptomatic 10-year period, and necropsy disclosed a healed dissection involving the entire aorta. His systemic arterial pressure had always been normal (100/75 mm Hg). Histologically, the media of the aorta was normal. The dissection appears to have started in the vicinity of the aortotomy incision.

TRICUSPIC VALVE POSITION

Contact of Cage or Stent of Tricuspid Prosthesis with Ventricular Septum or Right Ventricular Free Wall. This contact is a potential cause of ventricular arrhythmias and partial obstruction to right ventricular outflow, or inflow, or both.

Damage to Right Coronary Artery or Coronary Sinus During Valve Insertion. This is a theoretical, or potential, complication only as no reports of this damage have come to my attention.

Damage to A-V Node or Bundle During Valve Insertion. Conduction system injury is most likely to occur when sutures are placed in the anulus attached to the septal leaflet. (See Chapter 92.)

References

1. Roberts WC, Morrow AG: Mechanisms of acute left atrial thrombosis after mitral valve replacement. Pathologic findings indicating obstruction to left atrial emptying. Am J Cardiol 18:497, 1966
2. Roberts WC, Morrow AG: Late postoperative pathologic findings after cardiac valve replacement. Circulation 36 (Suppl):48, 1967
3. Roberts WC, Morrow AG: Causes of early postoperative death following cardiac valve replacement. Clinico-pathologic correlations in 64 patients studied at necropsy. J Thorac Cardiovasc Surg 54:422, 1967
4. Roberts WC, Morrow AG: Anatomic studies of hearts containing caged-ball prosthetic valves. Johns Hopkins Med J 121:271, 1967.
5. Roberts WC, Morrow AG: Causes of death and other anatomic observations after cardiac valve replacement. Long-Term Prognosis Following Valve Replacement, Second Conference on Cardiovascular Disease. Adv Cardiol 7:226, 1972
6. Winter TQ, Reis RL, Glancy DL, et al.: Current status of Starr-Edwards cloth-covered prosthetic cardiac valves. Circulation 45 (Suppl I):14, 1972
7. Shepard RL, Glancy DL, Stinson EB, et al.: Hemodynamic confirmation of obstruction to left ventricular inflow by a caged-ball prosthetic mitral valve. Case report. J Thorac Cardiovasc Surg 65:252, 1973
8. Roberts WC, Bulkley BH, Morrow AG: Pathologic anatomy of cardiac valve replacement: a study of 224 necropsy patients. Prog Cardiovasc Dis 15:539, 1973
9. Roberts WC: Operative treatment of hypertrophic obstructive cardiomyopathy. The case against mitral valve replacement. Am J Cardiol 32:377, 1973
10. Seningen RP, Bulkley BH, Roberts WC: Prosthetic aortic stenosis. A method to prevent its occurrence by measurement of aortic size from preoperative aortogram. Circulation 49:921, 1974
11. Fishbein MC, Roberts WC, Golden A, et al.: Cardiac pathology after aortic valve replacement using Hufnagel trileaflet prostheses: a study of 20 necropsy patients. Am Heart J 89:443, 1975
12. Roberts WC, Fishbein MC, Golden A: Cardiac pathology after valve replacement by disc prosthesis. A study of 61 necropsy patients. Am J Cardiol 35:740, 1975
13. Roberts WC, Hammer WJ: Cardiac pathology after valve replacement with a tilting disc prosthesis (Björk-Shiley type). A study of 46 necropsy patients and 49 Björk-Shiley prostheses. Am J Cardiol 37:1024, 1976
14. Roberts WC: Choosing a substitute cardiac valve: type, size, surgeon. Am J Cardiol 38:633, 1976
15. Spray TL, Roberts WC: Structural changes in porcine xenografts used as substitute cardiac valves. Gross and histologic observations in 51 glutaraldehyde-preserved Hancock valves in 41 patients. Am J Cardiol 40:319, 1977
16. Ferrans VJ, Spray TL, Billingham ME, et al.: Structural changes in glutaraldehyde-treated porcine heterografts used as substitute cardiac valves. Transmission and scanning electron microscopic observations in 12 patients. Am J Cardiol 41:1159, 1978
17. Ferrans VJ, Boyce SW, Billingham ME, et al.: Calcific deposits in porcine bioprosthesis: structure and pathogenesis. Am J Cardiol 46:721, 1980
18. Roberts WC, Morrow AG: Fatal degeneration of the silicone rubber ball of the Starr-Edwards prosthetic aortic valve. Am J Cardiol 22:614, 1968
19. Roberts WC, Levinson GE, Morrow AG: Lethal ball variance in the Starr-Edwards prosthetic mitral valve. Arch Intern Med 126:517, 1970
20. Fishbein MC, Roberts WC: Late postoperative anatomic observations after insertion of Hufnagel caged-ball prostheses in descending thoracic aorta. Chest 68:6, 1975
21. Yarbrough JW, Roberts WC, Reis RL: Structural alterations in tissue cardiac valves implanted in patients and in calves. J Thorac Cardiovasc Surg 65:364, 1973
22. Geha AS, Laks H, Stansel HC Jr, et al.: Late failure of porcine valve heterografts in children. J Thorac Cardiovasc Surg 78:351, 1979
23. Ishihara T, Ferrans VJ, Jones M, et al.: Calcific deposits developing in a bovine pericardial bioprosthetic valve three days after implantation. Circulation 63:718, 1981
24. Ishihara T, Ferrans VJ, Jones M, et al.: Structure of bovine parietal pericardium and of unimplanted Ionescu-Shiley pericardial valvular bioprostheses. J Thorac Cardiovasc Surg 81:747, 1981
25. Waller BF, Jones M, Roberts WC: Postoperative aortic regurgitation from incomplete seating of tilting-disc occluders due to overhanging knots or long sutures. Chest 78:565, 1980
26. Cohn LH, Roberts WC, Rockoff SD, et al.: Bacterial endocarditis following aortic valve replacement. Clinical and pathologic correlations. Circulation 33:209, 1966
27. Archard HO, Roberts WC: Bacterial endocarditis after dental procedures in patients with aortic valve prostheses. J Am Dent Assoc 72:648, 1966
28. Roberts WC, Morrow AG: Bacterial endocarditis involving prosthetic mitral valves. Clinical and pathologic observations. Arch Pathol 82:164, 1966
29. Arnett EA, Roberts WC: Prosthetic valve endocarditis. Clinico-pathologic analysis of 22 necropsy patients with comparison of observations in 74 necropsy patients with active infective endocarditis involving natural left-sided cardiac valves. Am J Cardiol 38:281, 1976
30. Arnett EN, Kastl DG, Garvin AJ, et al.: A conversation on prosthetic valve endocarditis. Am Heart J 93:510, 1977
31. Ferrans VJ, Boyce SW, Billingham ME, et al.: Infection of glutaraldehyde-preserved porcine valve heterografts. Am J Cardiol 43:1123, 1979
32. Jones AA, Otis JB, Fletcher GF, et al.: A hitherto undescribed cause of prosthetic mitral valve obstruction. J Thorac Cardiovasc Surg 74:116, 1977

33. Roberts WC, Morrow AG: Cardiac valves and the surgical pathologist. Arch Pathol 82:309, 1966
34. Bulkley BH, Morrow AG, Roberts WC: Calcification of prosthetic valve anuli: a late complication of cardiac valve replacement. Am Heart J 87:129, 1974
35. Roberts WC, Morrow AG: Renal hemosiderosis in patients with prosthetic aortic valves. Circulation 33:390, 1966
36. Cobbs BW Jr, Hatcher CR Jr, Craver JM, et al.: Transverse midventricular disruption after mitral valve replacement. Am Heart J 99:33, 1980
37. Roberts WC, Mason DT, Engle MA, et al.: Cardiology 1981. New York, Yorke Medical Books, 1981, p 364
38. Roberts WC, Morrow AG: Secondary left ventricular endocardial fibroelastosis following mitral valve replacement. Cause of cardiac failure in the late postoperative period. Circulation 37, 38 (Suppl II):101, 1968
39. Löffler W: Endocarditis parietalis fibroplastica mit Bluteosinophile. Schweiz Med Wochenschr 6:817, 1936
40. Dubost C: The surgical treatment of constrictive fibrous endocarditis. J Cardiovasc Surg 19:581, 1978
41. Muna WF, Spray TL, Morrow AG, et al.: Aortic dissection after aortic valve replacement in patients with valvular aortic stenosis. J Thorac Cardiovasc Surg 74:65, 1977
42. Roberts WC, Lambird PA, Gott VL, et al.: Fatal aortic regurgitation following replacement of the mitral and aortic valves. A mechanical complication of double valve replacement. J Thorac Cardiovasc Surg 52:189, 1966
43. Roberts WC, Morrow AG: Compression of anomalous left circumflex coronary arteries by prosthetic valve fixation rings. J Thorac Cardiovasc Surg 57:834, 1969

Comparison of Late Degenerative Changes in Porcine Bioprostheses in the Mitral and Aortic Valve Position in the Same Patient

CAROLE A. WARNES, MB, BS, MRCP, MEREDITH L. SCOTT, MD, GARY M. SILVER, MD, CLAUDE W. SMITH, MD, VICTOR J. FERRANS, MD, PhD, and WILLIAM C. ROBERTS, MD

Porcine bioprostheses implanted in both the mitral and aortic valve positions simultaneously in 5 patients aged 20 to 61 years (mean 45) were reexamined 18 to 107 months (mean 51) later. In 4 patients, the degenerative changes were distinctly more severe in the bioprostheses in the mitral than in the aortic valve position.

Many reports have described degenerative changes in porcine bioprostheses implanted in either the mitral or aortic valve position.[1–5] None, however, have described morphologic alterations in bioprostheses in both positions in the same patient. The latter situation, of course, allows one bioprosthesis to serve as a control for the other. This report summarizes clinicopathologic findings in 5 patients in whom porcine aortic bioprostheses had been implanted 18 to 107 months earlier in both mitral and aortic valve positions.

Patients Studied

Clinical findings: Clinical and morphologic findings in the 5 patients are summarized in Table I. At the time of initial double valve replacement, the 5 patients (4 men) ranged in age from 20 to 61 years (mean 45). Late postoperatively, chronic congestive heart failure developed in 4 (all but Patient 1), and 3 of them (Patients 2, 3, and 5 [Table I]) had their malfunctioning bioprostheses in both the mitral and aortic valve positions excised, and replaced with mechanical prostheses. The remaining patient (Case 4), who had chronic congestive heart failure, died from complications of primary biliary cirrhosis before her malfunctioning bioprosthesis in the mitral position could be replaced. The 1 patient (Case 1) without clinical evidence of congestive cardiac failure or prosthetic valve dysfunction died from complications of habitual alcoholism.

Morphologic findings: The 10 bioprostheses are illustrated in Figures 1 to 5. Each cusp was thicker than normal, and *cuspal mobility* appeared distinctly diminished in 5 bioprostheses (3 mitral and 2 aortic). Each of these 5 bioprostheses appeared on visual inspection to have some degree of obstruction, and catheterization in 2 patients (Cases 2 and 3) confirmed bioprosthetic stenosis in both mitral and aortic positions.

Calcific deposits were present in 1 or more cusps in all 10 bioprostheses. In 4 of the 5 patients, the calcific deposits were clearly larger on the cusps of the bioprostheses in the mitral position than on the cusps in the aortic position. In 2 patients (Cases 3 and 5) *cuspal tears* were present, and they also involved only the bioprostheses in the mitral position. Bioprosthetic *thrombus* was present only in the patient (Case 2) with infective endocarditis.

Of the 2 patients in whom the bioprostheses had been in place for <2 years, 1 (Patient 1) had mild degenerative changes in both valves, those in the aortic position being slightly more marked. The other patient (Case 2) whose bioprosthetic valves deteriorated rapidly had clinical and morphologic evidence of infective endocarditis; vegetations, present on both bioprostheses, contained fungi and bacteria, but no inflammatory cells, cuspal tears, or perforations.

Discussion

Examination of the bioprostheses located in both mitral and aortic valve positions clearly demonstrated in 4 of the 5 patients greater degeneration of the bioprosthetic cusps located in the mitral valve position than in those in the aortic valve position. The reasons

From the Pathology Branch, National Heart, Lung, and Blood Institute, National Institutes of Health, Bethesda, Maryland; the Departments of Surgery, Florida Hospital, Florida Heart Institute, Orlando, Florida, O'Connor Hospital, San Jose, California; and Providence Hospital, Columbia, South Carolina. Manuscript received and accepted December 3, 1982.

Address for reprints: Carole A. Warnes, MB, BS, MRCP, Building 10A, Room 3E30, National Institutes of Health, Bethesda, Maryland 20205.

TABLE I Clinical and Morphologic Data in the 5 Patients With Porcine Bioprostheses in Both the Mitral and Aortic Valve Positions

Case	Age Bioprosthesis Implanted (yr)	Duration (mo) Bioprosthesis in Place	Sex	AF	TC (mg/dl)	Bioprosthetic Dysfunction by Auscultation				Hemodynamic Data* (mm Hg)				Died	Ca^{++} (0–4+) on Bioprosthesis	
						MS	MR (0–4+)	AS	AR (0–4+)	LV (s/d)	SA s/d	LV-Ao (psg)	PAW-LV (mdg)		MV	AV
1	40	18	M	+	98	0	0	0	0	—	100/70†	—	—	+	1+	2+
2	61	20	M	+	149	+	4+	+	2+	118/8	80/55	38	6	0	3+	2+
3	20	48	M	0	183	+	4+	+	0	130/15	96/70	34	15	0	3+	1+
4	54	60	F	+	259	+	+	0	0	—	100/90†	—	—	+	4+	2+
5	48	107	M	0	160	0	4+	0	0	107/12	96/57	11	0	0	2+	1+

* Obtained just before replacement of the bioprostheses.
† Indirect.
AF = atrial fibrillation; Ao = aorta; AR = aortic regurgitation; AS = aortic stenosis; AV = aortic valve; Ca^{++} = calcium; CHF = congestive heart failure; LV = left ventricular pressure; mdg = mean diastolic gradient; MR = mitral regurgitation; MS = mitral stenosis; MV = mitral valve; PAW = pulmonary arterial wedge; psg = peak systolic gradient; s/d = peak systole/end-diastole; TC = total serum cholesterol; — = not done; 0 = absent; + = present.

for the more extensive degeneration of the bioprostheses in the mitral position are unclear but at least 4 factors need consideration.

1. *The closing pressure on the bioprosthesis in the mitral position is higher than that on the bioprosthesis in the aortic position.*

2. *The pressure difference across the closed bioprosthesis in the mitral position is far higher than that across the closed bioprosthesis in the aortic position.* The higher the pressure difference across the closed bioprosthesis, the greater the tensile stress on the cusps.[6]

3. *The presence of a bioprosthesis composed of a semilunar valve in the atrioventricular valve position*

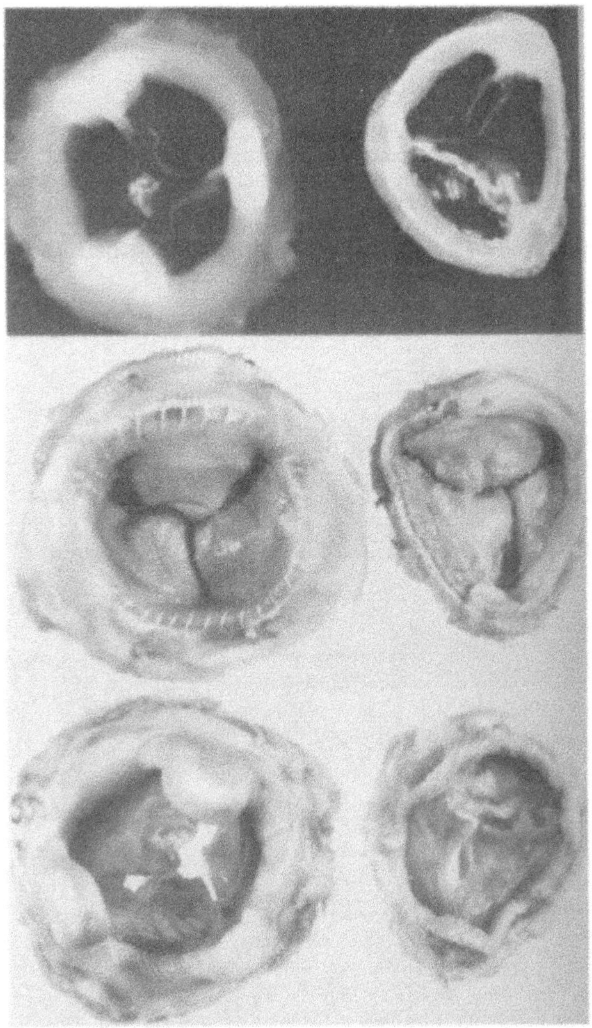

FIGURE 1. Patient 1 (Table I). Excised porcine bioprostheses from the mitral (**left**) and aortic (**right**) valve positions. **Top,** radiographs showing a minute calcific deposit in 1 of 3 cusps of the bioprosthesis in the mitral position and more calcium in 1 of the 3 cusps in the bioprosthesis in the aortic position. **Middle,** views of mitral-position bioprosthesis from the atrial aspect and of the aortic-position bioprosthesis from the ventricular position. **Bottom,** view of the mitral-position bioprosthesis from the ventricular aspect and of the aortic-position bioprosthesis from the aortic aspect.

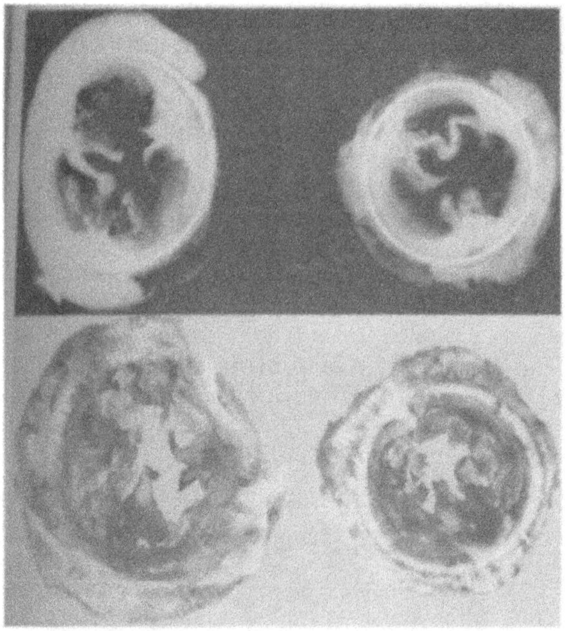

FIGURE 2. Patient 2. **Top,** radiographs showing extensive calcific deposits in all 3 cusps of the bioprostheses in both mitral (**left**) and aortic (**right**) valve positions. **Bottom,** view of the mitral-position bioprosthesis from the atrial aspect and of the aortic-position bioprosthesis from the ventricular aspect. There is considerable destruction of cusps of both bioprostheses caused at least in part by infective endocarditis. Sections had been removed previously for histologic studies.

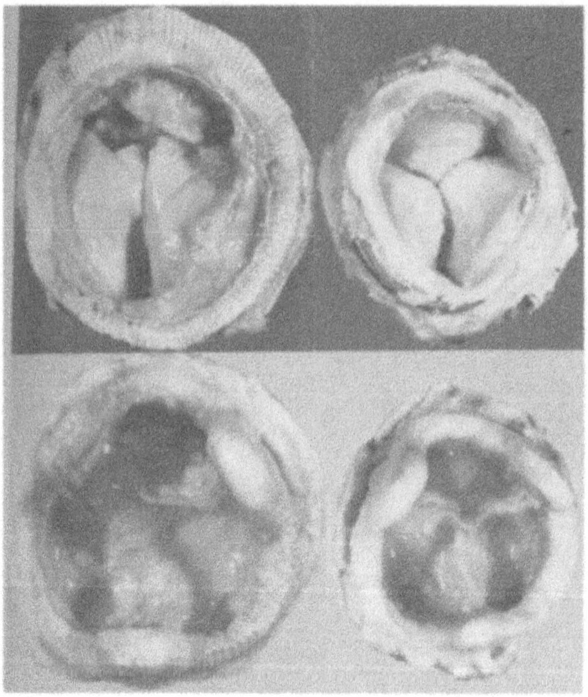

FIGURE 3. Patient 3. **Top,** view of the mitral-position bioprosthesis (**left**) from the atrial aspect and the aortic-position bioprosthesis (**right**) from the ventricular position. **Bottom,** view of the mitral-position bioprosthesis (**left**) from the ventricular aspect showing extensive calcific deposits in all 3 cusps. The aortic-position bioprosthesis viewed from the aortic aspect is on the right.

may prevent equal distribution of the left ventricular systolic pressure on each of the 3 bioprosthetic cusps (Fig. 6), whereas the aortic diastolic pressure is probably equally distributed on each of the 3 aortic valve cusps.

4. *Sinus rhythm theoretically causes more work for the cusps of a mitral valve than for the cusps of an aortic valve*, as atrial contraction partly reopens the valve. In contrast, the aortic valve opens only once during each cardiac cycle. The "double movement" of mitral opening when the mitral valve consists of an

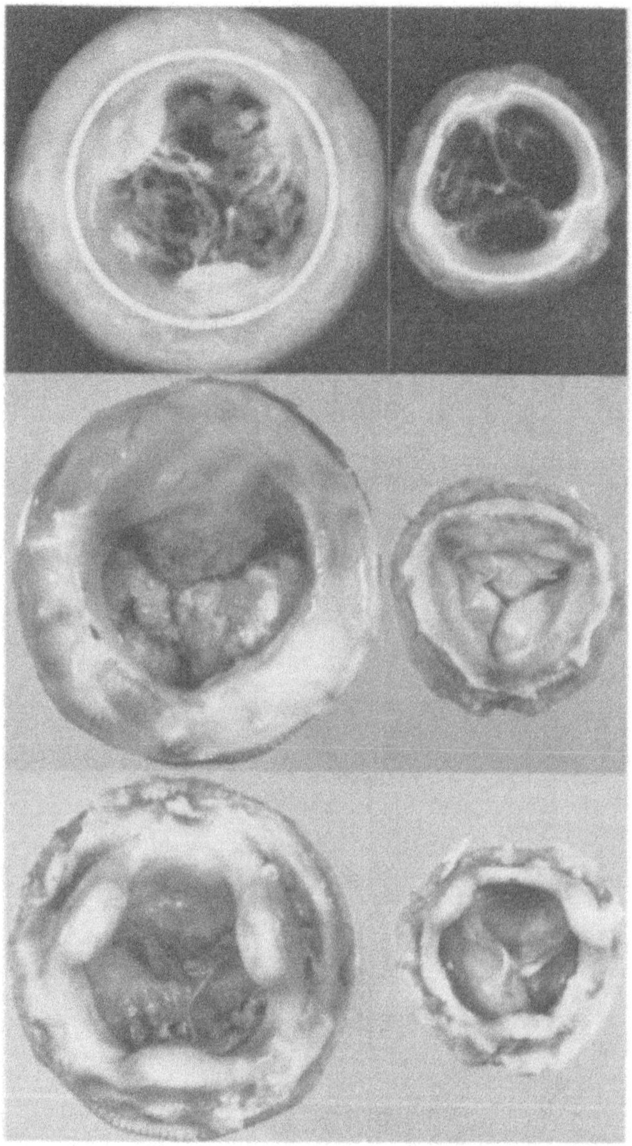

FIGURE 4. Patient 4. **Top,** radiographs showing extensive calcific deposits in all 3 cusps of the bioprosthesis in the mitral position (**left**) and much smaller amounts of calcium in the aortic-position bioprosthesis (**right**). **Middle,** view of the mitral-position bioprosthesis (**left**) from the atrial aspect and of the aortic-position bioprosthesis (**right**) from the ventricular aspect. **Bottom,** view of the mitral-position bioprosthesis (**left**) from the ventricular aspect and of the aortic-position bioprosthesis (**right**) from the aortic aspect.

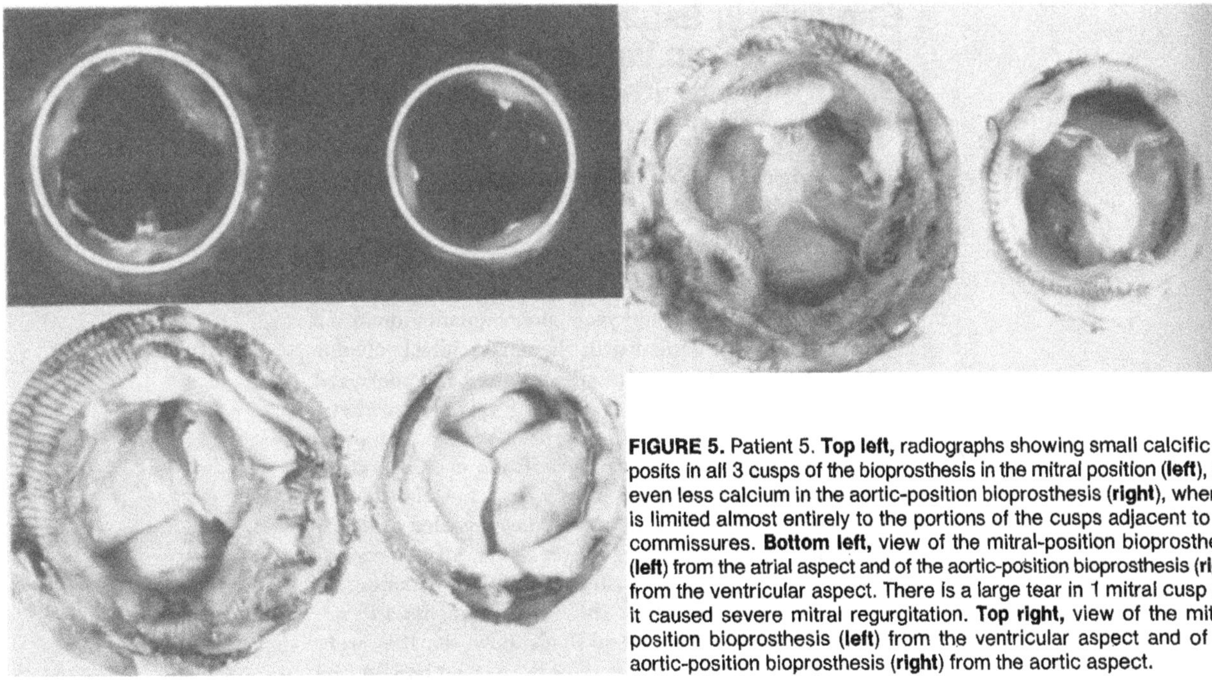

FIGURE 5. Patient 5. **Top left,** radiographs showing small calcific deposits in all 3 cusps of the bioprosthesis in the mitral position (**left**), and even less calcium in the aortic-position bioprosthesis (**right**), where it is limited almost entirely to the portions of the cusps adjacent to the commissures. **Bottom left,** view of the mitral-position bioprosthesis (**left**) from the atrial aspect and of the aortic-position bioprosthesis (**right**) from the ventricular aspect. There is a large tear in 1 mitral cusp and it caused severe mitral regurgitation. **Top right,** view of the mitral-position bioprosthesis (**left**) from the ventricular aspect and of the aortic-position bioprosthesis (**right**) from the aortic aspect.

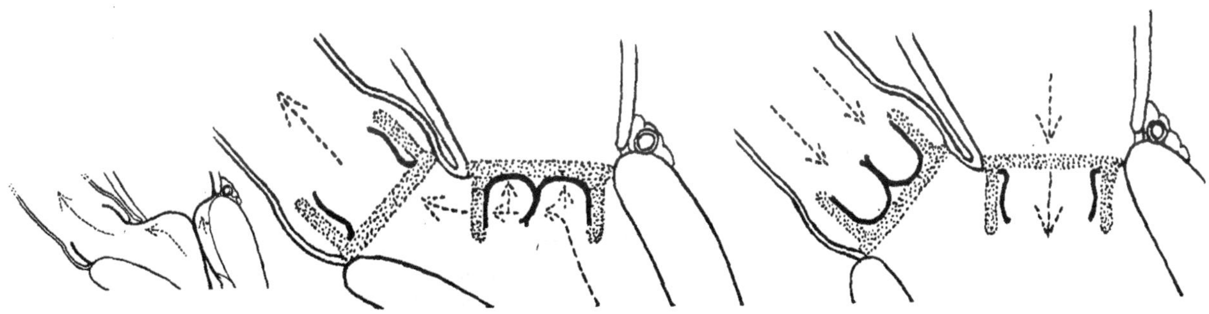

FIGURE 6. Diagrams of normal mitral valve (**left**) as it might appear during ventricular systole, and of a heart containing bioprostheses in both the mitral and aortic valve positions (**center and right**). With a semilunar valve in the mitral position, left ventricular systolic pressure does not easily "glide" from the ventricular aspect of the cusps to the aorta as it does with the native anterior mitral leaflet (**left**).

aortic valve bioprosthesis, theoretically causes additional bending of the cusps near the commissures. This local concentration of deformation on the cusps near the commissures may accelerate fatigue fractures of the collagen bundles.[7]

Acknowledgment: We thank Margaret M. M. Moore, who photographed the bioprostheses and Mary McMahon, who typed the manuscript.

References

1. **Spray TL, Roberts WC.** Structural changes in porcine xenografts used as substitute cardiac valves. Gross and histologic observations in 51 glutaraldehyde-preserved Hancock valves in 41 patients. Am J Cardiol 1977;40: 319–330.
2. **Ferrans VJ, Boyce SW, Billingham ME, Jones M, Ishihara T, Roberts WC.** Calcific deposits in porcine bioprostheses: structure and pathogenesis. Am J Cardiol 1980;46:721–734.
3. **Fishbein MC, Gisson SA, Collins JJ Jr, Barsamian EM, Cohn LH.** Pathologic findings after cardiac valve replacement with glutaraldehyde-fixed porcine valves. Am J Cardiol 1977;40:331–337.
4. **Ferrans VJ, Spray TL, Billingham ME, Roberts WC.** Structural changes in glutaraldehyde-treated porcine heterografts used as substitute cardiac valves. Transmission and scanning electron microscopic observations in 12 patients. Am J Cardiol 1978;41:1159–1184.
5. **Cipriano PR, Billingham ME, Oyer PE, Kutsche LM, Stinson EB.** Calcification of porcine prosthetic heart valves. A radiographic and light microscopic study. Circulation 1982;66:1100–1104.
6. **Thubrikar M, Piepgrass WC, Deck JD, Nolan SP.** Stress of natural versus prosthetic aortic valve leaflets in vivo. Ann Thorac Surg 1980;30:230–239.
7. **Broom ND.** Fatigue-induced damage in glutaraldehyde-preserved heart valve tissue. J Thorac Cardiovasc Surg 1978;76:202–211.

Cholesteryl Ester Crystals in a Porcine Aortic Valvular Bioprosthesis Implanted for Eight Years*

Victor J. Ferrans, M.D., Ph.D.; Bruce McManus, M.D., Ph.D.; and William C. Roberts, M.D., F.C.C.P.

Masses of crystals, which were largely composed of cholesteryl esters, were found in a porcine aortic valvular bioprosthesis removed eight years after implantation in the mitral position in a patient with rheumatic mitral valvular stenosis. Histologic sections of grossly raised and nonraised yellow lesions in the three cusps of this bioprosthesis revealed large clefts, which on frozen section contained lipid-positive, birefringent crystals. These crystals gave a positive reaction with the Schultz test for cholesterol. Biochemical analyses of isolated nodules revealed a cholesterol content of 40 nmole/mg of wet tissue. Of this cholesterol, 88 percent was esterified, and the remaining 12 percent was free cholesterol. These cholesterol deposits are most likely derived from blood lipids; however, they were not related to hyperlipidemia, since the patient had normal blood levels of cholesterol and triglycerides.

Small lipid droplets are found relatively frequently in connective tissue of the leaflets of implanted cardiac valvular bioprostheses, as documented by previous electron microscopic observations from this laboratory;[1] however, crystalline deposits of cholesterol have not been reported previously in implanted bioprostheses. Such a finding forms the basis of the present report.

Case Report

A 76-year-old woman with a history of rheumatic mitral valvular stenosis, previous closed mitral commissurotomy (1966), and replacement of the mitral valve with a Hancock porcine aortic valvular bioprosthesis (1973) died in December 1981 in intractable chronic congestive heart failure. She had marked pulmonary arterial hypertension (100/10 mm Hg before mitral replacement and 75/15 mm Hg six months after operation) and elevation of left ventricular end-diastolic pressure (20 mm Hg in 1974); her systemic arterial blood pressure ranged up to 170/90 mm Hg. The bioprosthetic heart valve was considered to have functioned normally until the patient's death. Blood lipids had been within normal limits; cholesterol was 189 ± 36 mg/dl (mean ± SD of nine values), and triglycerides were 107 mg/dl (mean of three values).

Anatomic Findings

At autopsy, the heart weighed 820 g. The coronary arteries were free of atherosclerotic plaques. Atherosclerotic changes in aorta, cerebral vessels, and peripheral systematic arteries were mild. The left atrium was markedly dilated and contained a small mural thrombus. Both ventricles were hypertrophied, and the left was dilated. Focal fibrous intimal thickening was present in the main left and right pulmonary arteries. The mitral prosthesis was well-secured, without perivalvular leaks. The atrial and ventricular aspects of the prosthetic valve ring were covered by fibrous tissue;

*From the Pathology Branch, National Heart, Lung, and Blood Institute, National Institutes of Health, Bethesda, Maryland.
Reprint requests: Dr. Ferrans, National Institutes of Health, Bldg 10, Rm 7N208, Bethesda 20205

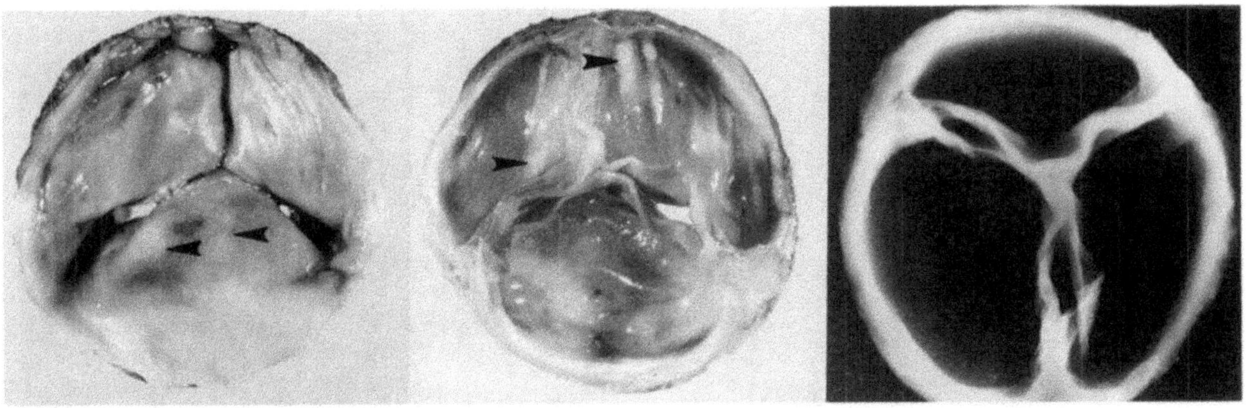

FIGURE 1. Views of the porcine bioprosthesis after removal from the mitral position and detachment from the stents. A, *left:* Inflow surface, showing light areas (*arrowheads*) corresponding to large crystalline deposits. The cusps appear otherwise normal. B, *center:* Outflow (left ventricular) surface, showing raised crystalline deposits (arrowheads). C, *right:* Radiograph of the bioprosthesis, confirming the absence of calcific deposits in the cusps.

this tissue, however, did not impinge on the bioprosthetic cusps. No tears or perforations were present in the cusps. Tiny, elevated, yellow nodules, up to 2 mm in diameter, were evident grossly in each of the cusps, particularly on their outflow surfaces (Fig 1A and B). Calcific deposits were not found on roentgenographic examination of the bioprosthesis (Fig 1C). Study of histologic sections revealed that the yellow nodules on the leaflets were composed of masses of crystals embedded in a coarsely granular, eosinophilic matrix (Fig 2 to 5). In sections of plastic-embedded tissues these crystals appeared as empty, rectangular clefts that measured up to several hundred μ in length. No cellular reaction (macrophages, foam cells, giant cells, or other inflammatory cells) was associated with these nodules of crystals. Smaller, nonraised masses of crystals were also present within the leaflet connective tissue. Sections stained by the von Kossa method did not show calcific deposits either in association with the crystals or elsewhere in the bioprosthetic tissue. Frozen sections stained with oil red O or with Sudan black B revealed multiple, small, nonbirefringent, darkly stained lipid droplets; the crystals described above were much less intensely stained than the lipid droplets. The crystals were markedly birefringent (Fig 4 and 5) and gave a positive reaction with the Schultz method for the histochemical demonstration of cholesterol.

In addition to the lipid infiltration described above, the connective tissue in the bioprosthetic leaflets showed moderate degrees of delamination (separation of the connective tissue layers) and degeneration, with the formation of many empty spaces within the substance of the leaflets. Fibrous sheaths or thrombi were not present over the cusps, and few cells (mostly macrophages) were present on the cuspal surfaces.

In order to further investigate the composition of the crystalline material, two nodules were excised from the leaflets with the aid of a dissecting microscope and submitted for biochemical analysis. The results, expressed in nanomoles per mg of wet tissue weight (mean ± SE of quadruplicate determinations), were as follows: total cholesterol, 40.25 ± 2.72, of which 5.18 ± 0.75 was in the form of free cholesterol and 34.07 ± 2.82 in the form of cholesteryl esters.

DISCUSSION

The observations in the present study document the presence of crystals, composed mainly of cholesteryl esters, in a bioprosthesis which had been implanted in the mitral position for eight years, during which time it had functioned well. Deposits of lipid droplets, presumed to be composed of triglycerides, have been observed in other bioprostheses,[1] but such large, crystalline masses have not been reported previously, to our knowledge, in implanted bioprostheses. Various types of lipid deposits are known to occur in native cardiac valves in a number of metabolic disorders. Most notable among the latter is homozygous type 2 hyperlipoproteinemia, in which the aortic valve is the site of formation of large intracellular (foam cells) and extracellular deposits of cholesteryl esters; other valves are involved to a much lesser extent.[2-6] Other diseases in which lipid deposits have been found in cardiac valves include Fabry's disease,[7,8] Farber's

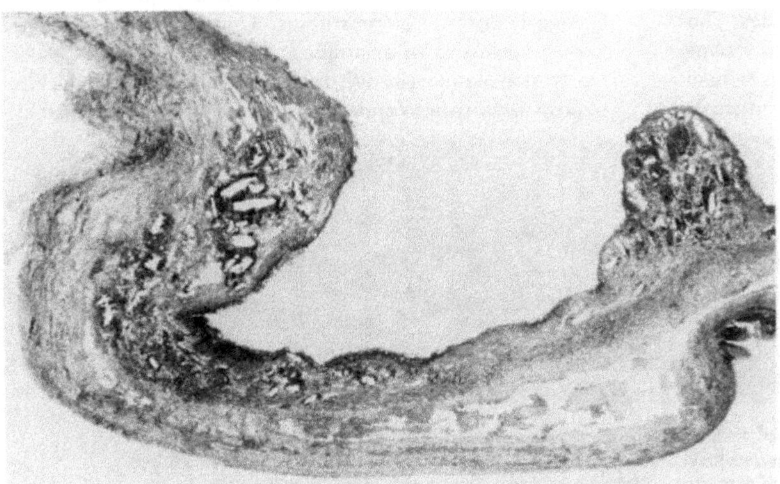

FIGURE 2. Section of cusp, showing numerous, large clefts within the connective tissue matrix of the cusp and nodular excrescence on the outflow surface. Areas of delamination of cuspal connective tissue are also noted. Alkaline toluidine blue stain, ×50.

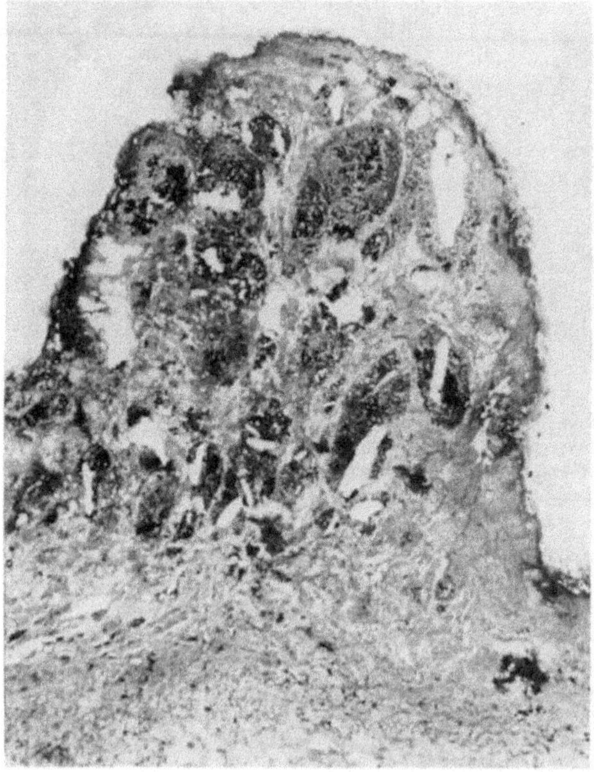

FIGURE 3. High-power view of lesion shown in Figure 2. The supporting stroma is predominantly collagenous; however, a rather deeply staining, granular material is associated with the clefts remaining after lipid removal. Alkaline toluidine blue stain, ×160.

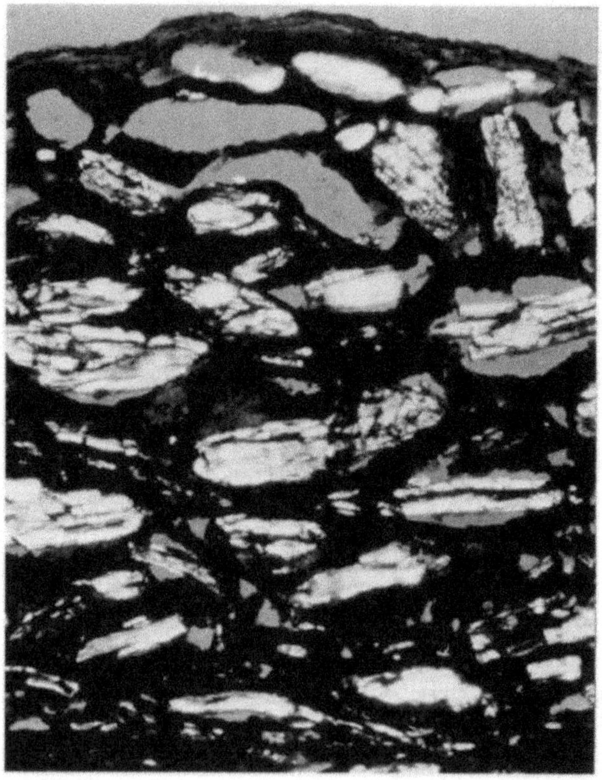

FIGURE 5. High-power polarized light micrograph showing the birefringent crystals in cuspal tissue. Sudan black B stain, ×400.

disease,[9] generalized GM_1 gangliosidosis,[10,11] and Sandhoff's disease,[12] in which glycolipids are stored in valvular connective tissue cells, and cholesteryl ester storage disease,[13] in which cholesteryl ester deposits have been detected in aortic valve. Lipid deposits also occur in association with the lesions of calcific aortic stenosis and mitral annular calcification.[14,15] The silicone rubber balls in certain mechanical prosthetic valves have been reported[16] to undergo infiltration with lipids derived from plasma lipoproteins; consequent swelling and deformation of the ball may cause mechanical dysfunction of the prosthesis.

The reason for the accumulation of cholesterol in the bioprosthesis from our patient remains unclear. This patient did not have hyperlipidemia, as demonstrated by multiple measurements of serum cholesterol and triglycerides. Thus, these deposits cannot be regarded as consequences of hypercholesterolemia. The deposits in the bioprosthesis from our patient were localized mainly on the outflow (ventricular) surface of the bioprosthesis, the site receiving the highest ventricular pressure. It was surprising to find that these deposits were not in association with a foreign body reaction or any other type of inflammatory infiltrate, such as occurs with cholesterol deposits in other areas of the body. This lack of inflammatory reaction probably was due to the fact that the cholesterol crystals were localized within the glutaraldehyde-fixed porcine valvular tissue, which usually is not invaded by inflammatory cells.[1] These deposits probably are derived from circulating plasma lipoproteins, since there were no cells identified in adjacent areas of valvular tissue which could have synthesized these large amounts of cholesterol *in situ*. Morphologic observations on valvular bioprostheses implanted for eight years or longer have been few, and it remains to be determined how prevalent this change is in these bioprostheses. This is difficult to judge from review of gross anatomic and histologic observations. On gross anatomic study, these deposits can resemble calcific deposits, which also appear as pale nodules. It is possible

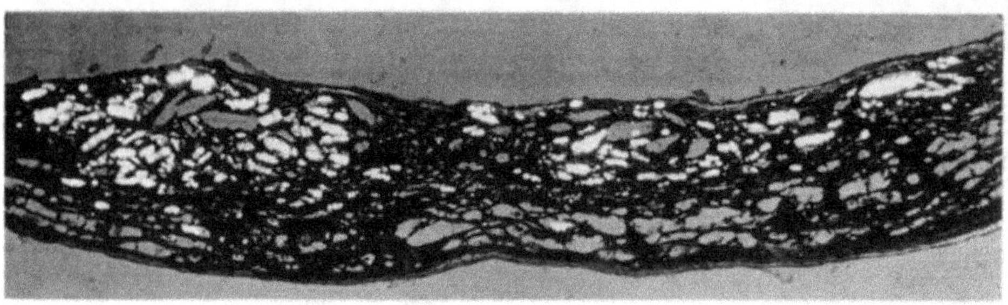

FIGURE 4. Polarized light micrograph of portion of a cusp, showing diffuse infiltration of the cuspal tissue by birefringent crystals, which tend to be localized on the outflow side of the cusp. Additional clefts without birefringent material represent areas of extensive delamination of collagen. (Sudan black B stain, ×40).

that mild degrees of this alteration are relatively frequent, but are not detected by study of routine histologic sections, from which the cholesterol is removed during tissue processing. Polarized light microscopy of frozen sections is the method of choice for the demonstration of these cholesterol deposits.

ACKNOWLEDGMENT: We are grateful to Dr. Jeffrey M. Hoeg of the Molecular Disease Branch, National Heart, Lung, and Blood Institute, for performing the cholesterol analyses.

References

1 Ferrans VJ, Spray TL, Billingham ME, Roberts WC. Structural changes in glutaraldehyde-treated porcine heterografts used as substitute cardiac valves: Transmission and scanning electron microscopic observations in 12 patients. Am J Cardiol 1978; 41:1159-1184

2 Stanley P, Chartrand C, Davignon A. Acquired aortic stenosis in a twelve-year-old girl with xanthomatosis. N Engl J Med 1965; 273:1378-1380

3 Rothbard S, Hagstrom JWC, Smith JP. Aortic stenosis and myocardial infarction in hypercholesterolemic xanthomatosis. Am Heart J 1967; 73:687-692

4 Wennevold A, Jacobsen JG. Acquired supravalvular aortic stenosis in familial hypercholesterolemia: a hemodynamic and angiographic study. Am J Med 1971; 50:823-827

5 Barr DP, Rothbard S, Eder HA. Atherosclerosis and aortic stenosis in hypercholesteremic xanthomatosis. JAMA 1954; 156:943-947

6 McCleary JE, Brunsting LA, Kennedy RLJ. Primary xanthoma tuberosum in children; with classification of xanthomas. Pediatrics 1959; 23:67-75

7 Desnick RJ, Blieden LC, Sharp HL, Hofschire PJ, Moller JH. Cardiac valvular anomalies in Fabry disease: clinical, morphologic, and biochemical studies. Circulation 1976; 54:818-825

8 Ferrans VJ, Hibbs RG, Burda CD. The heart in Fabry's disease: a histochemical and electron microscopic study. Am J Cardiol 1969; 24:95-110

9 Farber S, Cohen J, Uzman LL. Lipogranulomatosis. A new lipoglycoprotein "storage" disease. Mt Sinai J Med (NY) 1957; 24:816-837

10 Gonatas NK, Gonatas J. Ultrastructural and biochemical observations on a case of systemic late infantile lipidosis and its relationship to Tay-Sachs disease and gargoylism. J Neuropathol Exp Neurol 1965; 24:318-340

11 Hadley RN, Hagstrom JWC. Cardiac lesions in a patient with familial neurovisceral lipidosis (generalized gangliosidosis). Am J Clin Pathol 1971; 55:237-240

12 Blieden LC, Desnick RJ, Carter JB, Krivit W, Moller JH, Sharp HL. Cardiac involvement in Sandhoff's disease: inborn error of glycosphingolipid metabolism. Am J Cardiol 1974; 34:83-88

13 Fredrickson DS, Ferrans VJ. Acid cholesteryl ester hydrolase deficiency. (Wolman's disease and cholesteryl ester storage disease). In: Stanbury JB, et al, eds. The metabolic basis of inherited disease, 4th ed. New York: McGraw-Hill, 1978:670-687

14 Kim KM, Valigorsky JM, Mergner WJ, et al. Aging changes in the human aortic valve in relation to dystrophic calcification. Hum Pathol 1976; 7:47-60

15 Roberts WC, Perloff JK. Mitral valvular disease: a clinicopathologic survey of the conditions causing the mitral valve to function abnormally. Ann Intern Med 1972; 77:939-975

16 Carmen R, Mutha SC. Lipid absorption by silicone rubber heart valve poppets—in vivo and in vitro results. J Biomed Material Res 1972; 6:327-346

Severe Mitral Regurgitation Immediately After Mitral Valve Replacement With a Parietal Pericardial Bovine Bioprosthesis

Marc A. Silver, MD
Philip R. Oranburg, MD
William C. Roberts, MD

From the Pathology Branch, National Heart, Lung, and Blood Institute, National Institutes of Health, Bethesda, Maryland. Manuscript received and accepted April 5, 1983.

The occurrence of severe mitral regurgitation (MR) immediately after mitral valve replacement (MVR) is exceedingly rare. One cause is interference with closure of a prosthetic occluder by the left ventricular wall, calcific deposits, or residual unexcised mitral leaflet or chordae tendineae.[1] Another cause is incomplete obliteration by suture of the space between the prosthetic or bioprosthetic ring and the native anulus, resulting in a paraanular communication.[1] A third and hitherto unreported cause of severe MR immediately after MVR by a bioprosthesis is described in the patient below.

A 64-year-old man who had had a precordial systolic murmur for many years had been asymptomatic until 25 days before MVR, when signs of active infective endocarditis appeared; severe congestive heart failure followed shortly thereafter. Group B beta hemolytic streptococcus was grown on blood cultures. A grade 3/6 precordial apical systolic blowing murmur consistent with MR was audible. The pulmonary arterial wedge mean pressure was 35, V-wave 50, and pulmonary arterial pressure 57/20 mm Hg. At MVR, a vegetation was present on the posterior mitral leaflet to which several chordae had ruptured; the leaflet appeared to prolapse toward left atrium. The purely regurgitant valve was replaced with a 25-mm Ionescu-Shiley bioprosthesis. The patient's early postoperative course was characterized by systemic hypotension and coma. A murmur consistent with MR was heard on precordial examination 2 days after operation. He died 8 days after operation, never having regained consciousness. At necropsy, the heart weighed 690 g. Sutures surrounded 2 of the 3 stents of the mitral bioprosthesis, causing a straight-line stretching of the margins of the bioprosthetic cusps between the 3 commissures. The result was a triangular-shaped severely incompetent bioprosthetic orifice (Fig. 1).

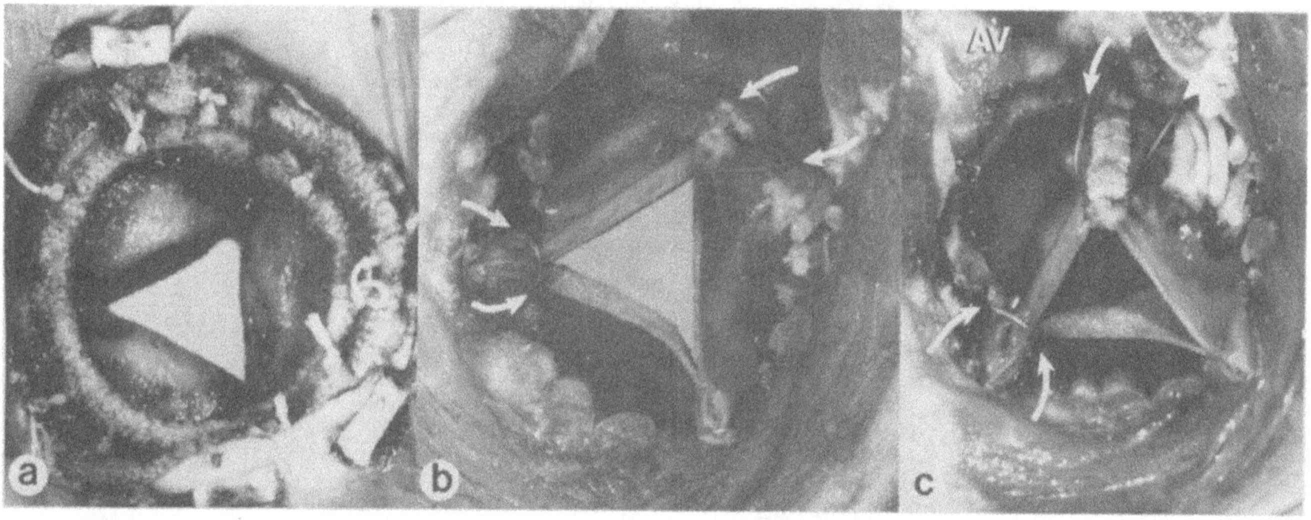

FIGURE 1. Mitral bioprosthesis in the patient described. **a,** view from left atrium showing a triangular orifice. **b and c,** 2 views from the left ventricular aspect. The **arrows** point to the 2 sutures which encircled the stents, causing tautness of the cusps and preventing them from coapting during ventricular systole.

Thus, sutures encircling 2 of the 3 bioprosthetic stents tautened the cusps, producing severe MR. The left atrium should not be closed after MVR until it is clear that the cusps of a tissue valve or the occluder of a mechanical valve[2] are freely mobile.

References

1. **Roberts WC.** Complications of cardiac valve replacement: characteristic abnormalities of prostheses pertaining to any or specific site. Am Heart J 1982;103:113–122.
2. **Jones AA, Otis JB, Fletcher GF, Roberts WC.** A hitherto undescribed cause of prosthetic mitral valve obstruction. J Thorac Cardiovasc Surg 1977;74: 116–117.

Wear of the Metallic Studs on the Composite Seat of the 2320 Starr-Edwards Aortic Valve and Its Clinical Consequences

CAROLE A. WARNES, MB, BS, MRCP, CHARLES L. McINTOSH, MD, PhD, and WILLIAM C. ROBERTS, MD

The 2320 Starr-Edwards aortic valve has a composite seat with metallic studs that protrude through the cloth. Certain clinical and morphologic findings are described in 6 patients who had this prosthesis in situ for 50 to 144 months (mean 92). Considerable disruption of the cloth covering both struts and base, and varying degrees of wear of the metallic studs that line the luminal side of the prosthetic ring occurred in each. Excessive stud wear resulted in severe disruption of the cloth lining the interior of the prosthetic ring. Cloth disruption may be associated with hemolytic anemia, embolic consequences, or both. Of our 6 patients, 4 had severe hemolytic anemia, 4 had neurologic events compatible with emboli and 1 died suddenly. Stud wear as observed in the 2320 series Starr-Edwards prosthesis also may occur in the models 2310 and 2400 prostheses, which have the same composite seat.

(Am J Cardiol 1983;52:1062–1065)

The 2320 Starr-Edwards aortic valve prosthesis, introduced in 1971, consists of a cloth-covered metallic cage with a metallic poppet (Stellite 21). Metal studs (pins), which project toward the lumen beyond the orifice cloth, are the only portions of the ring or struts not covered by cloth (Fig. 1). Wear of the cloth that covers the seat and struts has been well described and may cause intravascular hemolysis and systemic emboli.[1–4] Wear of the metallic studs that protrude into the interior from the metallic ring of this prosthesis, however, has not been described. This report describes findings in 6 patients in whom stud wear was observed late after aortic valve replacement (AVR) with a 2320 Starr-Edwards prosthesis.

Patients

Certain clinical features of the 6 patients are summarized in Table I. At the time of AVR, Patient 4 also had a mitral commissurotomy, Patient 6 a mitral valve replacement (porcine bioprosthesis) and Patient 1 both mitral and tricuspid valve replacements (porcine bioprostheses). At catheterization 6 months postoperatively, the peak systolic pressure gradients between left ventricle and aorta (at the level of the prosthesis) ranged from 13 to 40 mm Hg (mean 20). Four patients later had repeated neurologic events compatible with emboli; the initial episode occurred 7 to 48 months after AVR. In 3 of the 4 patients (Patients 1, 3 and 4), warfarin sodium was discontinued 6 months after AVR, as was the policy at the time. After the first neurologic event, Patients 3 and 4 again received warfarin, but Patient 3 had 3 further embolic events while fully anticoagulated. Patient 1, who had severe hepatic disease, was treated with aspirin and dipyridamole, and had no further embolic events.

Four patients had profound hemolytic anemia and, despite oral iron and folic acid, became transfusion-dependent. The hemolytic nature of the anemia in these cases was established by the presence of high reticulocyte counts, increased lactate dehydrogenase levels, urobilinogen in the urine and low haptoglobin levels. The mechanical origin of the hemolysis was suggested by the presence of schistocytes (fragmented red cells). The Coombs' tests were repeatedly negative in all cases except Patient 1, who also had chronic active hepatitis and an intermittently positive Coombs' test. Hemoglobin electrophoresis and glucose-6 dehydrogenase levels were normal in all. Patients 1 and 2 had red-blood cell survivals of only 12 and 9 days, respectively (normal 28 to 30 days). No drug taken by any patient could be incriminated in the hemolytic process.

Patient 5, who had neither hemolytic anemia nor peripheral emboli, died suddenly and unexpectedly 112 months after AVR. The other 5 patients underwent reoperation 50 to 144 months after the initial AVR. The indication for operation in each was either severe hemolytic anemia, recurrent emboli or both. Three patients also had mild (grade 1 to 2/6 diastolic basal murmur) aortic regurgitation, confirmed in Patient 1 by aortography.

No perivalvular communication involved any aortic prosthesis at reoperation or necropsy. Although all 6 patients had wear of the cloth around the 3 struts, the most striking cloth

From the Pathology and Surgery Branches, National Heart, Lung, and Blood Institute, National Institutes of Health, Bethesda, Maryland.
Manuscript received and accepted August 1, 1983.

TABLE I Clinicopathologic Features of 6 Patients with 2320 Starr-Edwards Prostheses and Stud Wear

Pt	Age (yr) at AVR	Sex	Size AVP	Pressures (mm Hg) 6 mo After AVR: LV	SA	LV-SA Psg	Duration (mo) AVP In Situ	AR Murmur After AVR	Clinical Embolic Events	HA	(Peak) Reticulocyte count (%)	Lowest Hematocrit (%) Before 2320 AVP Removed	Follow-up (mo) After AVP Removed	Present Blood Hematocrit (%)	Stud Wear (1–3+)
1	62	F	9A	145/8	130/60	15	50	+	+	+	5	21	22	†	+
2	61	M	9A	—	—	40	63	0	0	+	9	12	30	43	+
3	35	M	10A	145/8	132/70	13	90	+	+	0	—	33	40	50	+
4	54	F	8A	140/8	125/80	15	94	0	+	+	4	26	7	38	+++
5	42	M	12A	115/3	100/70	15	112	0	0	0	—	—	†	†	+++
6	50	F	8A	165/12	145/70	20	144	+	+	+	5	24	†	†	++

AR = aortic regurgitation; AVP = aortic valve prosthesis; AVR = aortic valve replacement; HA = hemolytic anemia; LV = left ventricle; Psg = peak systolic gradient; SA = systemic artery; † = died; + = present; 0 = absent; — = not applicable or not available.

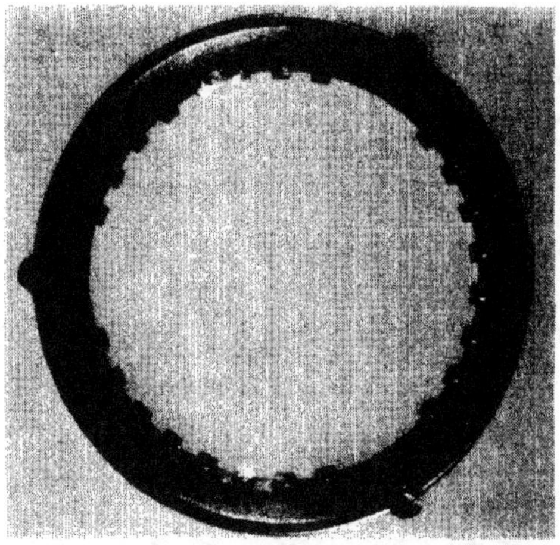

FIGURE 1. Metallic seat of a 2320 Starr-Edwards prosthesis that had been in place for 30 days. The cloth covering the ring has been removed to demonstrate normal stud height.

wear occurred at the interior of the primary valve orifice. In each case, the studs had been eroded to varying degrees by contact with the metallic ball, with subsequent fragmentation of the cloth covering of the primary orifice (Fig. 2). The stud height was reduced circumferentially, but stud erosion was not symmetric around the ring, suggesting that the poppet had been seating eccentrically. In 2 patients (Patients 4 and 5), the studs in 1 area had been eroded completely flush with the metallic ring; the resultant eccentric seating of the ball had burnished the rim of the valve ring (Fig. 3 and 4).

In the 5 patients who underwent reoperation, the prosthesis in the aortic position was replaced with a bioprosthesis; an additional mitral bioprosthesis was implanted in Patient 4. Patient 6, who had severe pulmonary hypertension, also had tricuspid annuloplasty, but died several days postoperatively with sepsis. Patient 1 died 22 months after reoperation from gastrointestinal bleeding and hepatic failure. Patients 2, 3 and 4 have done well, with no further embolic episodes or intravascular hemolysis.

Discussion

The 3 struts of the 2320 Starr-Edwards aortic valve initially are completely covered with 2 layers of cloth. The inner layer is Teflon, and the outer layer is polypropylene so that even if the inner cloth is torn, the polypropylene maintains its tubular configuration around the strut. The metal studs of the composite seat project at regular intervals through the knitted cloth, and therefore provide the seat for the poppet. The resulting increase in orifice-to-ball ratio was devised to improve the hemodynamic profile of the valve. The metal studs are initially machined to a spherical radius slightly larger than the radius of the poppet to minimize ball contact with the sharp edges of the studs (Fig. 5). The studs were designed so that they protruded slightly above the cloth to enable them to be burnished by the poppet for a short time after implantation, so the surfaces of the studs precisely match the spherical surface of the poppet.[5] The burnishing of the studs continues until the seat becomes a continuous plane of metal studs and compressed cloth. The manufacturer anticipated that after this initial period of burnishing, no other significant change would occur to the studs.

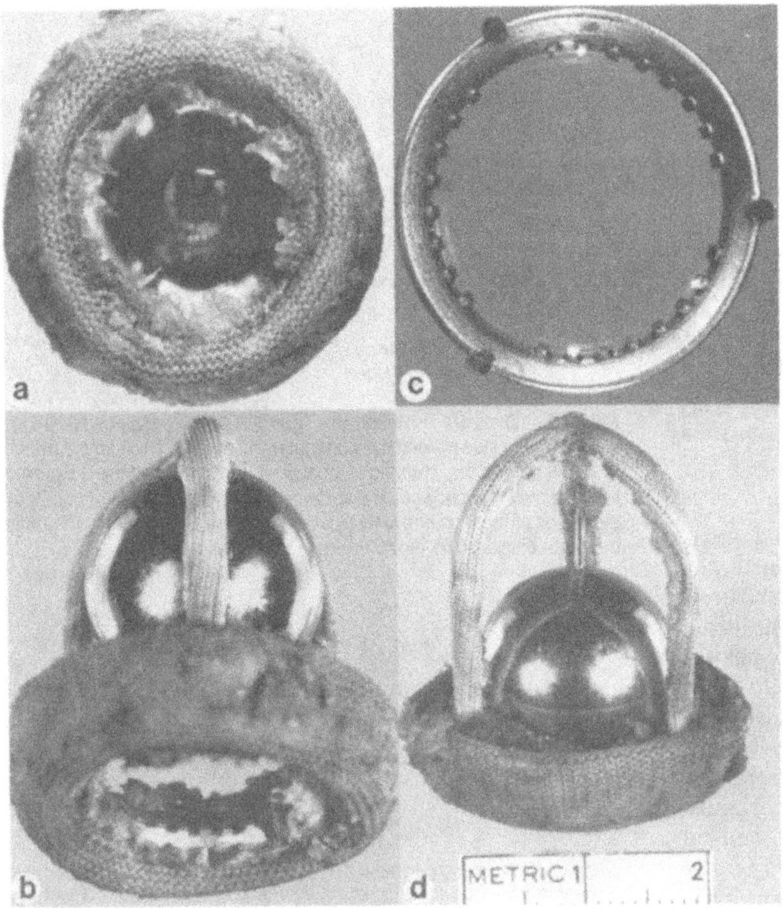

FIGURE 2. Prosthesis from Patient 3. **a,** view from left ventricular aspect showing disrupted cloth on the ring. **b,** view of interior of ring, which had been denuded of cloth. **c,** metallic ring in which all cloth has been removed and the 3 metallic stents severed. The studs are mildly eroded. **d,** view of prosthesis from the side showing exposed metal on 1 stent due to disruption of cloth.

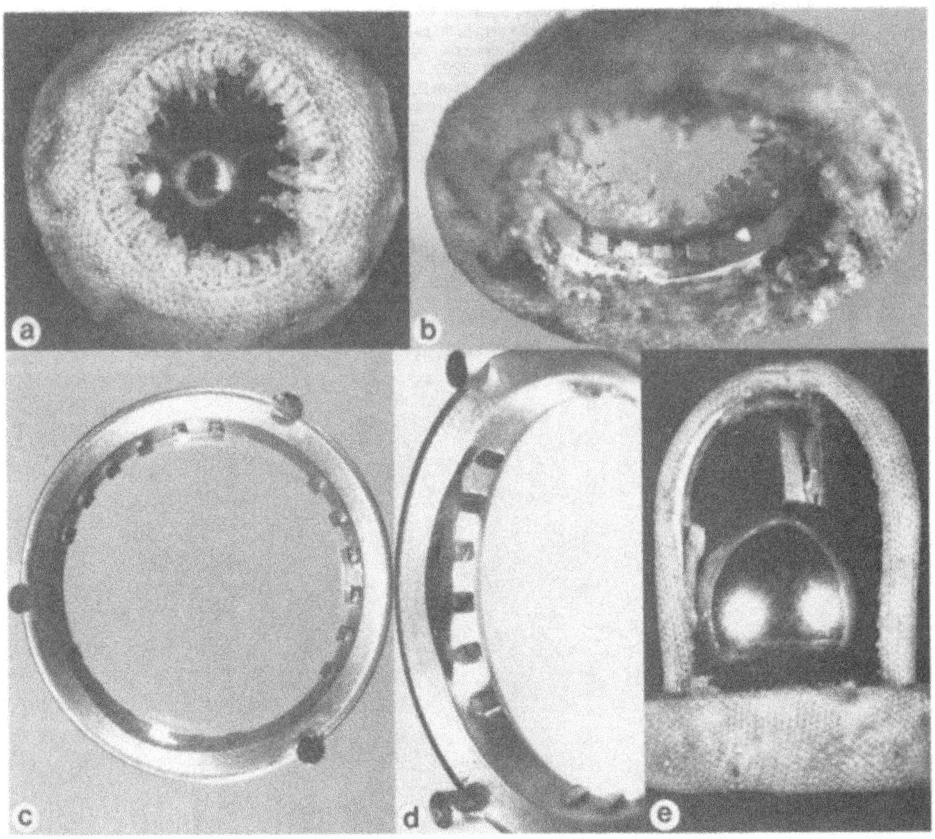

FIGURE 3. Prosthesis from Patient 4. **a,** view from left ventricular aspect showing disrupted cloth protruding toward the lumen. **b,** view of ring showing exposed metal due to disruption of cloth. **c,** metallic ring after the cloth was removed showing severe degrees of stud erosion and also erosion of the metallic ring itself. **d,** close-up of portion of ring disclosing the completely eroded studs and adjacent burnished ring. **e,** side view showing exposed metal of stents due to cloth disruption.

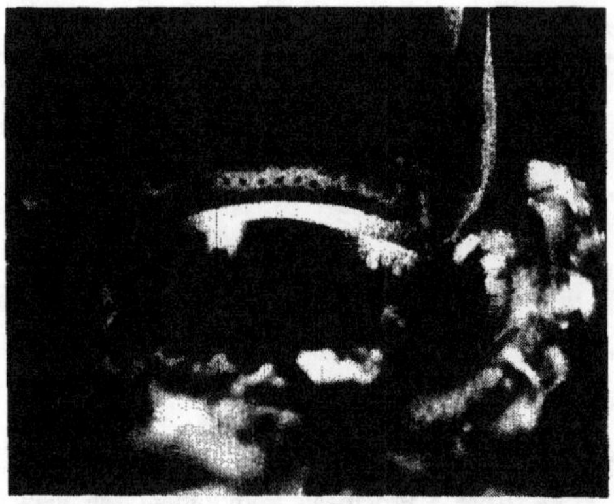

FIGURE 4. Prosthesis from Patient 5 showing severe erosion of the studs and some burnishing of the adjacent metallic ring. All cloth on the interior of the ring was disrupted.

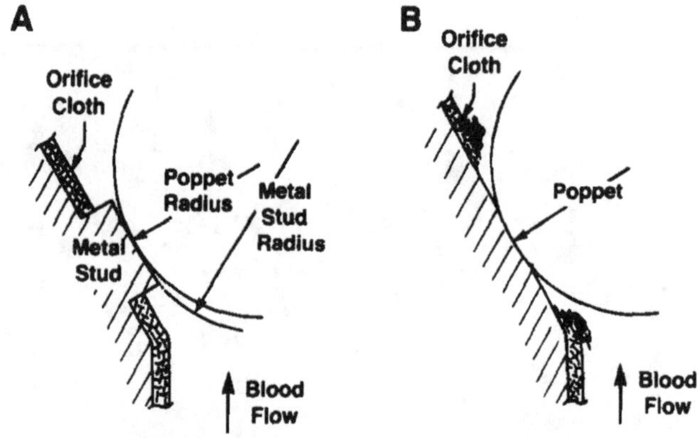

FIGURE 5. Diagram demonstrating contact of the poppet with the unworn metallic stud (A) and the completely worn stud (B). A small amount of burnishing of the metallic stud occurs normally until the surface of the stud matches perfectly the surface of the poppet (A). Cloth contacts the bases of the stud normally (A), but when the stud wears sufficiently, the cloth disrupts (B). Adapted from Hodam et al.[5]

Examination of the excised prostheses of our 6 patients, however, clearly demonstrates greater-than-anticipated burnishing—indeed erosion—of the studs of the seat, with disintegration of the surrounding cloth. The resultant eccentric seating of the poppet may cause aortic regurgitation and contribute to increased turbulence and hemolysis. These results suggest that when 2320 aortic Starr-Edwards valves have been in situ for >4 years, the metallic studs have eroded abnormally and considerable disruption of the ring cloth can be anticipated. The consequence, as demonstrated by the findings in our 6 patients, may be severe hemolytic anemia, embolic episodes, or aortic regurgitation. Approximately 14,000 of this model prostheses were issued for implantation between 1971 and 1976, but they are no longer manufactured. The number of these prostheses explanted to date is unknown. The same composite seat design also is used for the models 2310 and 2400 aortic prostheses, which therefore may be susceptible to the same degenerative change and clinical sequelae. Production of both models 2310 and 2400 also has been discontinued.

Acknowledgment: The photographs were taken by Margaret M. Moore.

References

1. **Crawford FA, Sethi GK, Scott SM, Takaro T.** Systemic emboli due to cloth wear in a Starr-Edwards Model 2320 aortic prosthesis. Ann Thoracic Surg 1973;16:614–619.
2. **Bonchek LI, Starr A.** Ball valve prostheses: current appraisal of late results. Am J Cardiol 1975;35:843–854.
3. **Reis RL, Glancy DL, O'Brien KO, Epstein SE, Morrow AG.** Clinical and hemodynamic assessments of fabric-covered Starr-Edwards prosthetic valves. J Thorac Cardiovasc Surg 1970;59:84–91.
4. **Isom OW, Spencer FC, Glassman E, Teiko P, Boyd AD, Cunningham JN, Reed GE.** Long term results in 1375 patients undergoing valve replacement with the Starr-Edwards cloth-covered steel ball prosthesis. Ann Surg 1977;186:310–322.
5. **Hodam R, Anderson R, Starr A, Wood J, Dobbs J, Raible D.** Further evaluation of the composite seat cloth-covered aortic prosthesis. Ann Thoracic Surg 1971;12:621–638.

A Precaution When Using the St. Jude Medical Prosthesis in the Aortic Valve Position

ELIZABETH M. ROSS, MD,
WILLIAM C. ROBERTS, MD

The St. Jude Medical (SJM) prosthesis is increasingly being used for cardiac valve replacement. In 1980, the manufacturer supplied 9,000 SJM prostheses to surgeons, and in 1983 this number had increased to 18,500. From 1977 through 1983, 45,000 SJM prostheses were supplied to surgeons. The SJM prosthesis appears to be durable,[1,2] its orifice area is larger for its size than any other mechanical prosthesis or for any tissue valve mounted on a frame,[3–8] its low profile prevents interference to leaflet movement by adjacent tissues, and it appears to be less destructive to blood elements than any other mechanical prosthesis.[9] Its major disadvantage is its delicate hinge mechanism, which could be interfered with more easily than other mechanical prostheses by thrombus or suture or a calcific deposit.[10–12] Additionally, like all mechanical prosthetic valves, anticoagulants are required.[13] The SJM prosthesis is a bit more expensive than other available mechanical prostheses or bioprostheses.

Recently, we examined the hearts of 2 patients who died early after replacement of the aortic valve with a SJM prosthesis. In each patient, it appeared that movement of 1 of the 2 SJM prosthetic leaflets was interfered with by underlying severe hypertrophy and leftward positioning of the ventricular septum in 1 patient (who died 6 days after aortic valve replacement) and by underlying severely thickened anterior mitral leaflet in the other patient (who could not be separated from cardiopulmonary bypass).

To better understand the real or potential interference to movement of 1 or both leaflets of a SJM prosthesis in the aortic valve position, an appreciation of the normal opening and closing of these leaflets of the SJM prosthesis is essential. The 2 leaflets are suspended on parallel pivots, which allows each leaflet to open to 85° from the closed position (Fig. 1 and 2). This allows an orifice area of 1.6 to 5.1 cm^2 for valve sizes 18 to 33. The valve in the open position has 3 approximately equal-sized orifices. The leaflets are contained within a pyrolyte ring, and this results in a low-profile configuration. In the closed position, the leaflets fall entirely within the orifice ring and the leaflets meet the valve housing at a 30° to 35° angle. The seamless sewing cuff is made of double velour Dacron and is attached to the pyrolyte valve ring such that the leaflets do not contact the cuff. In the aortic valve position, the "v" formed by the 2 leaflets of the SJM prosthesis when the valve is closed points "upstream," i.e., toward the left ventricle. The key element to proper opening of the SJM valve in the aortic valve position during ventricular systole is the application of a greater pressure to the leaflet peripheral to the pivot compared to that applied central to the pivot. If either the ventricular septum or anterior mitral leaflet prevents adequate pressure from contacting the leaflet peripheral to the pivot, leaflet opening could be incomplete or prevented (Fig. 3).

The most likely circumstance in which the ventricular septum could prevent the application of adequate pressure's being applied to the undersurface of a SJM leaflet in the aortic valve position is in the older patient with aortic valve stenosis. In the normal aging process, the ascending aorta moves toward the right (presumably because the elasticity of the aortic wall diminishes and blood ejected from the left ventricle contacts the right wall of the aorta) and the left ventricular cavity gets smaller (presumably because the cardiac output and stroke volume decrease). The combination of the rightward movement of the aorta and the decreasing size of the left ventricular cavity results in the most cephalad portion of the muscular ventricular septum being located directly beneath the aortic valve, rather than to the right of it as in younger persons. When this normal occurrence of aging is complicated by aortic valve stenosis, the movement of the ascending aorta to the right is exaggerated (presumably because of the poststenotic jet effect) and the severe hypertrophy of the left ventricular walls allows even more of the ventricular septum to be located directly beneath the aortic valve (Fig. 4). The result, as we believe occurred in 1 of our 2 patients mentioned earlier, may be incomplete or total lack of opening of 1 of the SJM prosthetic leaflets as a result of inadequate application of left ventricular systolic pressure's being applied to the ventricular as-

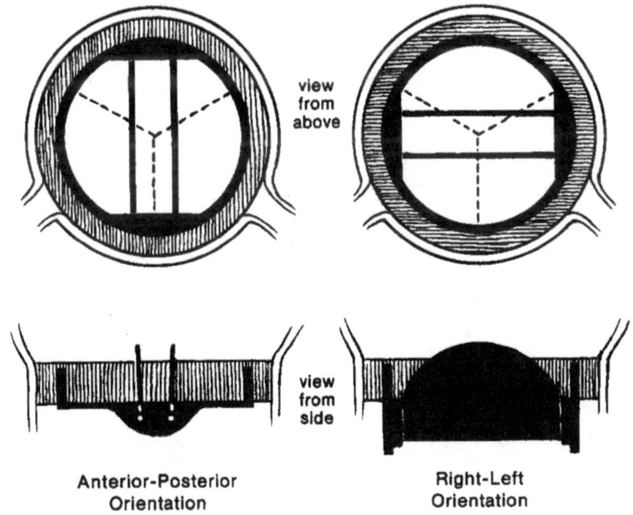

FIGURE 1. Two orientations of a St. Jude prosthesis in the aortic valve position during ventricular systole.

From the Pathology Branch, National Heart, Lung, and Blood Institute, National Institutes of Health, Bethesda, Maryland. Manuscript received and accepted March 21, 1984.

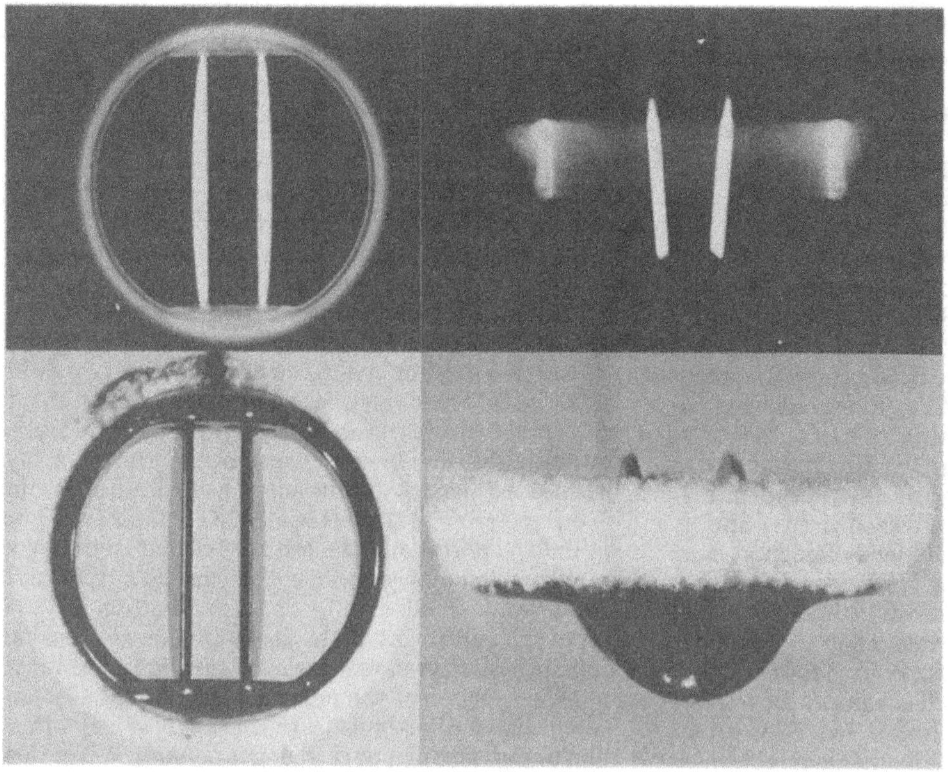

FIGURE 2. Views of the St. Jude's Medical prosthesis from below (**left**) and from the side (**right**). Radiographs are shown in the **upper panel.**

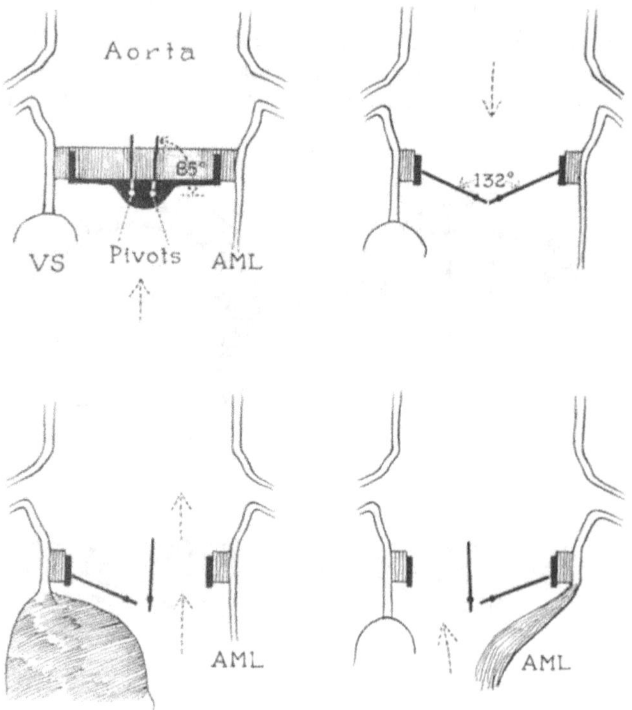

FIGURE 3. Diagram showing a St. Jude Medical prosthesis in the aortic valve position and how the 2 leaflets normally open and close (**upper panel**). **Lower left,** diagram showing how a thickened ventricular septum (VS) could prevent opening of 1 of the 2 prosthetic disc. **Lower right,** diagram showing how a very thickened anterior mitral leaflet (AML) may prevent opening 1 of the 2 prosthetic leaflets.

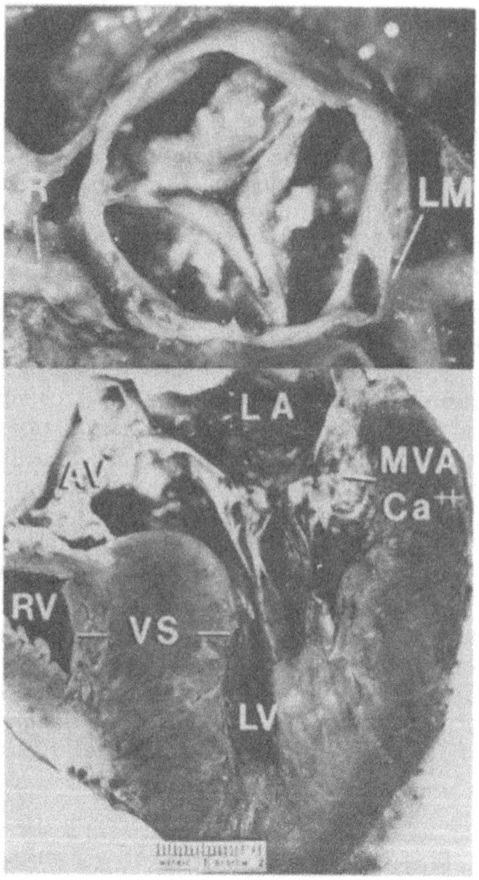

FIGURE 4. Severely stenotic aortic valve from above (**top**) and longitudinal view of heart (**bottom**) showing a very thick ventricular septum (VS) with its crest pointing toward the left atrium (LA) and the aortic valve (AV) located almost to the right of the VS. Blood exiting the left ventricle (LV) must take a very sigmoid route. LM = left main coronary artery; MVA Ca++ = mitral valve anular calcium; R = right coronary artery; RV = right ventricular cavity.

pect of the leaflets. Awareness of the hazard of a thick ventricular septum directly beneath an excised aortic valve should caution the operator that a prosthesis (or bioprosthesis) other than a SJM might be preferred or that the orientation of the SJM prosthesis should be such that the septum could not prevent one of the SJM leaflets from receiving properly applied left ventricular systolic pressure. The orientation judgment with a SJM prosthesis must be made before insertion of the first prosthetic securing suture because rotation of the pyrolyte ring is not advised after the prosthesis has been sewn to the aortic wall.

References

1. **Nicoloff DM, Emery RW, Arom KV, Northrup WF, Jorgensen CR, Wang Y, Lindsay WG.** Clinical and hemodynamic results with the St. Jude Medical cardiac valve prosthesis. J Thorac Cardiovasc Surg 1981;82:674–683.
2. **Horstkotte D, Korfer R, Seipie L, Bircks W, Loogen F.** Late complications in patients with Bjork-Shiley and St. Jude Medical heart valve replacement. Circulation 1983;68:suppl II:II-175–II-184.
3. **Emery RW, Nicoloff DM.** St. Jude Medical cardiac valve prosthesis in vitro studies. J Thorac Cardiovasc Surg 1979;78:269–276.
4. **Wortham DC, Tri TB, Bowen TE.** Hemodynamic evaluation of the St. Jude Medical valve prosthesis in the small aortic anulus. J Thorac Cardiovasc Surg 1981;81:615–620.
5. **Gill CC, King HC, Lytle BW, Cosgrove DM, Golding LA, Loop FD.** Early clinical evaluation after aortic valve replacement with the St. Jude Medical valve in patients with a small aortic root. Circulation 1982;66:147–149.
6. **Yoganathan AP, Chaux A, Gray RJ, DeRobertis M, Matloff JM.** Flow characteristics of the St. Jude prosthetic valve: An in vitro and in vivo study. Artificial Organs 1982;6:289–294.
7. **Horstkotte D, Haerten K, Seipel L, Korfer R, Budde T, Bircks W, Loogen F.** Central hemodynamics at rest and during exercise after mitral valve replacement with different prostheses. Circulation 1983;68:161–168.
8. **Yoganatham AP, Chauz A, Gray RJ, Woo YR, DeRobertis M, Williams FP, Matloff JM.** Bileaflet tilting disc and porcine aortic valve substitutes: In vivo hydrodynamic characteristics. J Am Coll Cardiol 1984;3:321–327.
9. **Lillehei CW.** Worldwide experience with the St. Jude valve prosthesis: clinical and hemodynamic results. Contemp Surg 1982;20:87.
10. **Nunez L, Iglesias A, Sotillo J.** Entrapment of leaflet of St. Jude Medical cardiac valve prosthesis by miniscule thrombus: report of two cases. Ann Thorac Surg 1979;29:567–569.
11. **Commerford PJ, Lloyd EA, DeNobrega JA.** Thrombosis of St. Jude Medical cardiac valve in the mitral position. Chest 1981;80:326–327.
12. **Ziemer G, Luhmer I, Oelert H, Borst HG.** Malfunction of a St. Jude Medical heart valve in mitral position. Ann Thorac Surg 1981;33:391–395.
13. **Chaux A, Gray RJ, Matloff JM, Feldman H, Sustaita H.** An application of the new St. Jude valvular prosthesis. J Thorac Cardiovasc Surg 1981;81:202–211.

Fatal Bioprosthetic Regurgitation *Immediately After* Mitral and Tricuspid Valve Replacements with Ionescu-Shiley Bioprostheses

WANDA M. LESTER, MD
WILLIAM C. ROBERTS, MD

Significant cardiac valve regurgitation *immediately after* cardiac valve replacement is rare. Silver et al[1] described a patient who had severe bioprosthetic regurgitation immediately after replacement of the mitral valve with an Ionescu-Shiley bioprosthesis. The

From the Pathology Branch, National Heart, Lung, and Blood Institute, National Institutes of Health, Bethesda, Maryland 20205. Dr. Lester was a fellowship from the Canadian Heart Foundation. Manuscript received and accepted November 5, 1984.

regurgitation resulted from inadvertent encircling of 2 of the 3 stents of the bioprosthesis by sutures, which prevented mobility of the cusps and closure of the bioprosthetic orifice. In this report we describe another patient in whom a similar mechanism caused severe bioprosthetic regurgitation in both mitral and tricuspid valve positions. Because this mechanism of development of severe bioprosthetic regurgitation is apparently not well appreciated, we describe this second patient in hopes of preventing this fatal complication in others.

E.R., a 55-year-old woman, died shortly after her fifth cardiac operation. She had had mitral commissurotomies when 26 and 35 years old, aortic (Björk-Shiley) and mitral (Hancock) valve replacements when 46 years old, and tricuspid valve replacement (Hancock) 1 month later. Apart from an intracranial hemorrhage later in the same year (1976), which led to cessation of warfarin therapy and the use of aspirin and dipyridamole, she did well until about 4 months before death, when exertional dyspnea, easy fatigability, abdominal swelling and leg edema developed. Because of worsening symptoms and signs, she was hospitalized 2 months later. The neck veins were distended while she was sitting up and v waves were visible. Rales were present over both lower lung fields. The liver was large and pulsatile. Electrocardiogram showed atrial fibrillation and right bundle branch block. At cardiac catheterization, the pressures (in mm Hg) were: right atrial mean 14, v wave 18; right ventricle, 70/16; pulmonary artery, 70/25 (mean 35); pulmonary arterial wedge mean 13, v wave 16; left ventricle, 110/12, and aorta, 110/60. The mean diastolic gradient between pulmonary artery wedge position and left ventricle was 5 mm Hg and the mean gradient between right atrium and right ventricle was 2 mm Hg. On left ventricular angiogram, the bioprosthesis in the mitral position was competent. The ejection fraction was 44%. Selective coronary angiograms showed no abnormalities. Aortogram disclosed 1+/4+ aortic regurgitation. The cardiac index was 2.1 liters/min/m^2.

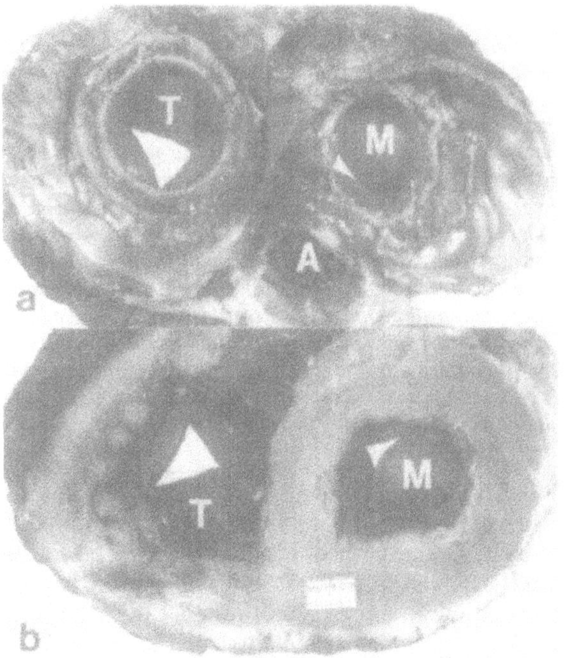

FIGURE 1. a, heart after removal of the atrial walls showing the bioprostheses in the tricuspid (T) and mitral (M) valve positions. The orifices of both bioprostheses are open and triangular in shape. The Björk-Shiley mechanical prosthesis in the aortic (A) valve position appeared to have functioned well. **b,** view from the ventricular aspect.

Pulmonary function tests were consistent with moderate to severe pulmonary obstructive disease.

The Hancock bioprosthesis in the mitral position was replaced with a size 27 and the Hancock bioprosthesis in the tricuspid position was replaced with a size 29 Ionescu-Shiley

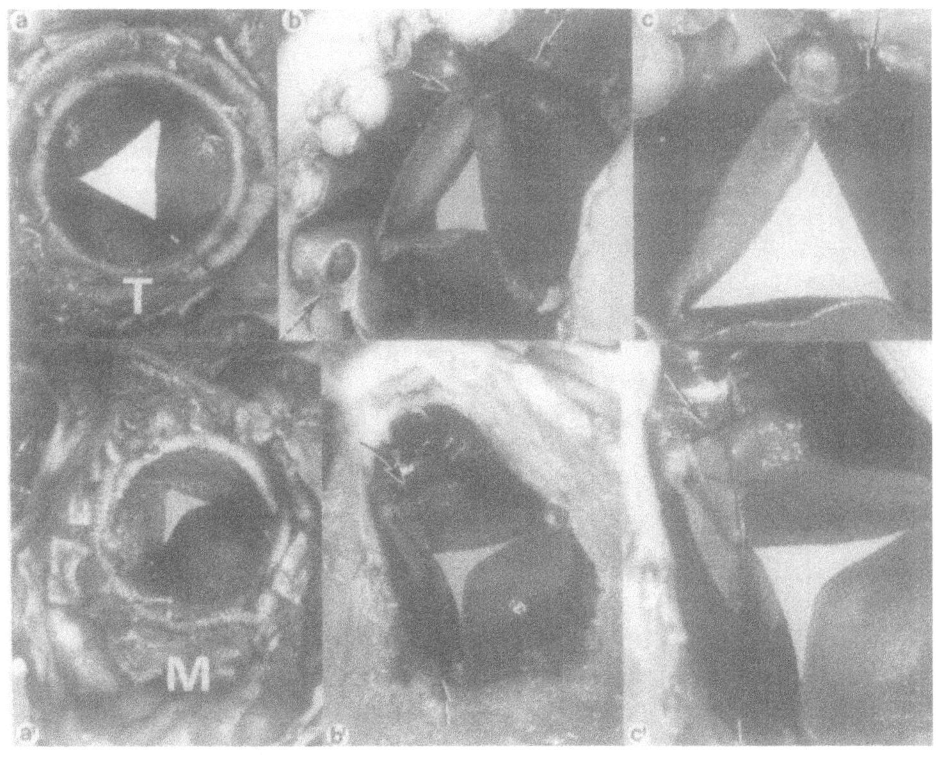

FIGURE 2. Close-up views of the Ionescu-Shiley bioprostheses in the tricuspid (T) and mitral (M) valve positions. **a** and **a′,** from the atrial aspects, the orifices of each are fixed in a triangular shape. **b,** 1 stent (**dashed arrow**) has burrowed into the right ventricular free wall. One stent is encircled by a suture (**curved solid arrows**). **b′,** 1 suture (**arrows**) crosses 2 bioprosthetic cusps holding each rigidly in place. The Björk-Shiley prosthesis is visible at the **upper left. c,** another view of the suture encircling the stent. **c′,** close-up of the suture inadvertently holding down 2 bioprosthetic cusps. (Photographs by M.M.M. Moore.)

bioprosthesis. Evident of poor cardiac output with some excessive bleeding was evident immediately after discontinuing bypass. The patient died about 8 hours after beginning the operation. Each cusp of the excised Hancock bioprostheses was intact and both valve orifices were competent. At necropsy, 1 stent of the bioprosthesis in the tricuspid valve position had burrowed into the right ventricular myocardium, and 1 stent of this bioprosthesis was surrounded by a suture (Fig. 1 and 2). The consequence of these 2 misadventures was a straightening of the free margins of 2 of the 3 cusps so that this bioprosthetic orifice was fixed in an open triangular-shaped position. One suture used to insert the bioprosthesis in the mitral position crossed 2 of the 3 bioprosthetic cusps, making each immobile and preventing closure of the bioprosthetic orifices (Fig. 1 and 2). The occluder of the Björk-Shiley prosthesis in the aortic valve position moved normally.

The fifth and last operation in the patient was done because of distended neck veins, subcutaneous edema and ascites, findings believed to have resulted from regurgitation of the bioprosthetic valve in the tricuspid valve position. The presence or absence of regurgitation was not confirmed by right ventricular angiography. At operation, no peribasilar bioprosthetic communications were present, each of the 3 cusps of both bioprostheses was intact, and both orifices appeared to close satisfactorily. After replacement of the bioprostheses in both tricuspid and mitral valve positions with "new"—and larger—bioprostheses, the patient had evidence of severe low cardiac output. Necropsy disclosed that at least 2 of the 3 cusps of each of the 2 newly inserted bioprostheses were immobile because either inadvertent suture on the ventricular aspects of the bioprosthetic orifices or burrowing of a stent into the myocardial wall had caused straightening of the distal margins of the bioprosthetic cusps and prevented cuspal movements so that the bioprosthetic orifices could not close during ventricular systole. Had smaller bioprostheses been used in this 81-pound, 61-inch-tall woman, possibly inadvertent anchoring of the sutures over the margins of the cusps and the burrowing of 1 stent into a myocardial wall would have been prevented. It is, of course, unwise to close an atriotomy incision until the operator has satisfactorily shown that each cusp of the bioprosthesis is freely mobile, a requirement to prevent bioprosthetic regurgitation.

References

1. **Silver MA, Oranburg PR, Roberts WC.** Severe mitral regurgitation after mitral valve replacement with a parietal pericardial bovine bioprosthesis. Am J Cardiol 1983;52:218–219.

Complication After Replacement of the Mitral Valve with either Mechanical or Bioprosthetic Heart Valves

William C. Roberts

It has been 25 years since successful replacement of one or more cardiac valves became a reality, and since then many thousands of patients with severely symptomatic valvular heart disease have had valve replacement with complete loss or sharp decrease in their symptoms of cardiac dysfunction. Although the chance of successful valve replacement in most patients is very high, occasional, often predictable, complications are recognized to occur both early and late in some patients in whom this procedure is carried out. Since 1960, I have examined at necropsy nearly 900 hearts, submitted from centers scattered over the USA, containing one or more prosthetic or bioprosthetic valves. Certain complications of mitral valve replacement are summarized in this chapter.

Classification of complications

Complications of mitral valve replacement can be classified, of course, in several ways. A common means is division of the complications into those occurring *early*, i.e. during the first 60 days after valve replacement, and into those occurring *late*, i.e. over 60 days after valve replacement. Another basis of subdivision involves analysis of complications common to any valve site and to most or all presently available mechanical or bioprosthetic valves and complications limited to a particular valve site, in this case those limited to mitral valve replacement and to a particular type of substitute valve. The latter classification will be utilized in this presentation. Complications occurring early versus those occurring late will be obvious from consideration of each complication separately.

Complications common to any valve site and to most or all presently available mechanical or bioprosthetic valves

Prosthetic size disproportion

The normal cardiac valve consists of thin, pliable leaflet-like structures which allow central flow of blood and occupy little space within the ventricles or great arteries in which they reside. Mechanical valves and even tissue valves attached to rigid or semirigid stents and rings, in contrast, are rigid except for movement of the occluder or cusps; they often prevent central flow, and they occupy non-compressible space. Early in the history of cardiac valve replacement, there appeared to be a tendency to insert as large a prosthesis as possible because of its tendency to be less inherently obstructive than the smaller-sized prosthesis. Experience taught, however, that, if a mechanical prosthesis was too big for the ventricle into which it was to reside, that movement of the occluder could be limited, with the potential for varying degrees of obstruction to flow[13,19,20,22–24,29,31,32,35,36,38,39,41,45,46]. At one time, a common view was that this disproportion problem was mainly one produced by caged-ball prostheses because they were larger than most subsequently utilized mechanical prostheses. This view, however, is incorrect. No mechanical valve and no tissue valve attached to a frame is immune to the problem of prosthetic disproportion.

The usual consequence in the mitral position is interference to left atrial emptying (or to left ventricular filling) and, rarely, in my experience, despite beliefs to the contrary, interference to left ventricular emptying (left ventricular outflow obstruction)[29].

Prosthetic disproportion is most likely to occur in the mitral position when valve replacement is carried out for pure mitral stenosis (or in combined mitral stenosis and aortic valve stenosis). Large-sized prostheses, whether caged-ball (Starr–Edwards), tilting disc (Björk–Shiley), or non-tilting disc (Kay–Shiley) must be avoided in small-sized patients with purely stenotic valvular lesions. Insertion of too large a prosthesis or bioprosthesis in the mitral position can also lead to severe mitral regurgitation. If a too large tilting disc type prosthesis is used, for example, a portion of the margin of the occluder (Björk–Shiley prosthesis) may contact the ventricular septum or left ventricular free wall during ventricular systole preventing the occluder from returning to the closed position (*Figure 23.1*). If a too large tissue valve mounted on stents is inserted, the stents can be bent inward causing redundancy of the bioprosthetic cusps and at least the potential for mitral regurgitation (*Figures 23.2* and *23.3*). A mitral bioprosthesis must be oriented in such a way that one stent does not interfere with left ventricular outflow (*Figure 23.4*). A mitral prosthesis or bioprosthesis, if too large, may cause the mitral annulus to be pushed too close to the aortic valve and set the stage for a mitral-valve's inserting suture to tear an aortic valve cusp with resulting aortic regurgitation (*Figure 23.5*). Determining proper prosthetic size only in the operating room without consideration of the hemodynamic lesion and the lean weight of the patient can lead to prosthetic disproportion, a major problem in the early years of valve replacement, but even today an occasional problem[19].

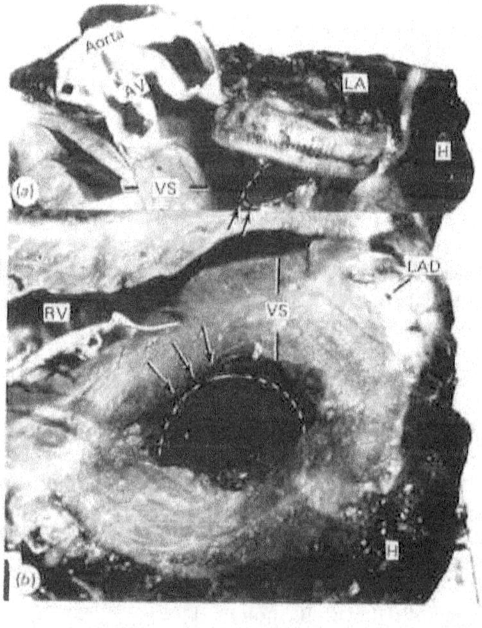

Figure 23.1. Prosthetic regurgitation after mitral valve replacement with a large-sized Björk–Shiley prosthesis (31 mm) in a 54-year-old man (NNMC no. A75–110) with isolated mitral stenosis. Although the occluder appeared to have opened well, i.e. without lateral interference from the ventricular septum (VS), the occluder (disc) was prevented from seating by the ventricular septum which 'moved inward' during ventricular systole. The patient could not be separated from cardiopulmonary by-pass. (*a*) View after longitudinal cut of the left ventricular outflow tract showing the mitral prosthesis, left atrium (LA), aortic valve (AV) and aorta. The margins (dashed lines) of the descended disc contact the ventricular septum. (*b*) View after transverse cut of the cardiac ventricles again showing the disc's margin (dashed white line) contacting the ventricular septum. LAD = left anterior descending coronary artery; RV = right ventricular cavity; H = hemorrhage into atrio-ventricular sulcus and other subepicardial adipose tissue.

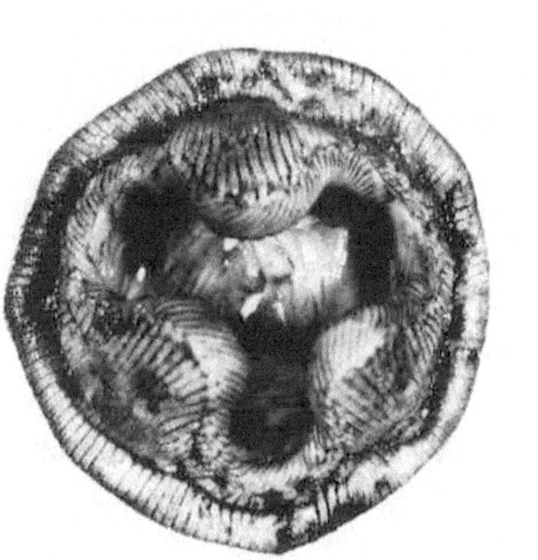

Figure 23.2. Porcine bioprosthesis explanted from the mitral position. The stents are bent inward apparently because the bioprosthesis was too large for the mitral area into which it was inserted. This bioprosthesis had been in place for 75 months.

Prosthetic thrombosis

It took years before all clinicians dealing with patients who had mechanical prosthetic valves became convinced that anticoagulation (warfarin sodium) was essential. After that principle was established, mechanical valve thrombosis became less of a problem. Nevertheless, of patients with mechanical

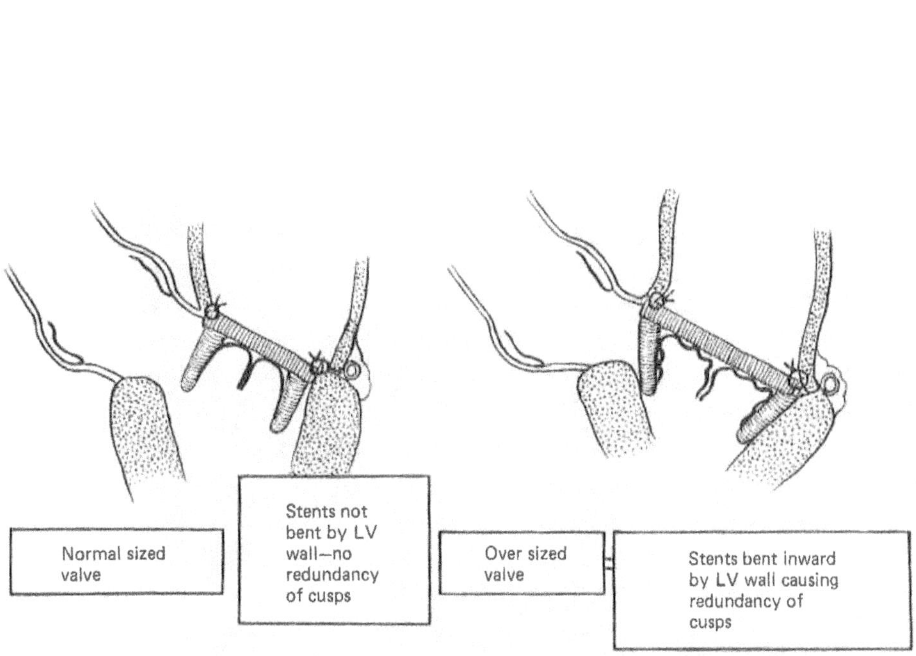

Figure 23.3. Diagram showing possible consequence of inserting a tissue valve (mounted on stents) which is too large for the mitral position. The stents may be bent inwards and then the cuspal margin length can be proportionally increased.

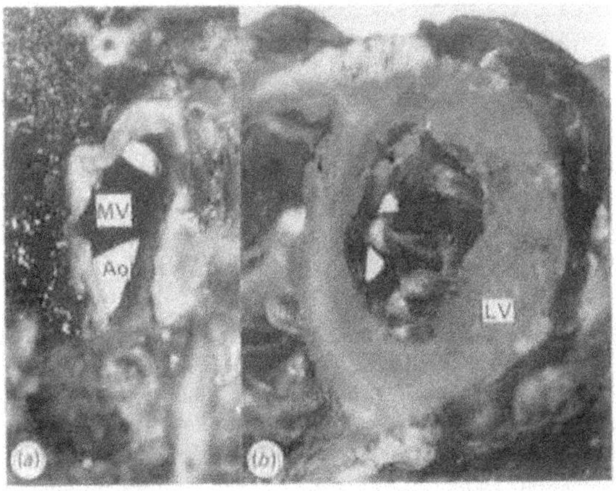

Figure 23.4. Strut of porcine bioprosthesis in the mitral position partially obstructing left ventricular (LV) outflow in a 54-year-old woman who had undergone tricuspid and mitral valve (MV) replacement with mechanical prostheses for valve stenosis 3 days before death. She had low cardiac output requiring pressor agents post-operatively. The prosthetic valve sounds were poorly heard and re-exploration performed on the third post-operative day revealed that the mechanical tricuspid prosthesis had thrombosed. Both mechanical prostheses in the tricuspid and mitral positions were replaced with porcine bioprostheses, but the patient could not be separated from cardio-pulmonary by-pass. At necropsy, one strut of the mitral prosthesis partially obstructed left ventricular outflow (*a*). (*b*) Ventricular aspect, showing placement of the porcine bioprosthesis in the outflow tract. (Reproduced from Spray and Roberts[11] with permission of the Publishers.)

valves, prosthetic thrombus occurs in some patients who are well anticoagulated, and occasionally it does not occur in patients who have never received anticoagulants. Thrombus is often observed in porcine bioprostheses which have been in place for over 2 months, but usually the thrombi are so small that functioning of the prosthesis is not altered[9,11,41].

Para-annular prosthetic ring discontinuity (parabasilar leak)

Parabasilar communications appear to result from placement of an inadequate number of sutures in the sewing ring (because of annular calcific deposits for example) or the pulling loose of one or more sutures, primarily after replacement of anatomically normal (as in papillary muscle dysfunction) or floppy mitral valves or in infection (prosthetic endocarditis) at the site of attachment of a prosthesis[27].

Prosthetic and bioprosthetic degeneration or wear

Almost all of the initial models of presently utilized mechanical prostheses had evidence of wear or variance of one or more parts. The silicone rubber poppet utilized in the initial models of the caged-ball prosthesis took in lipids (turned from white to yellow), which resulted in their swelling (with impaction in the cage) or in large cracks which allowed some of them to

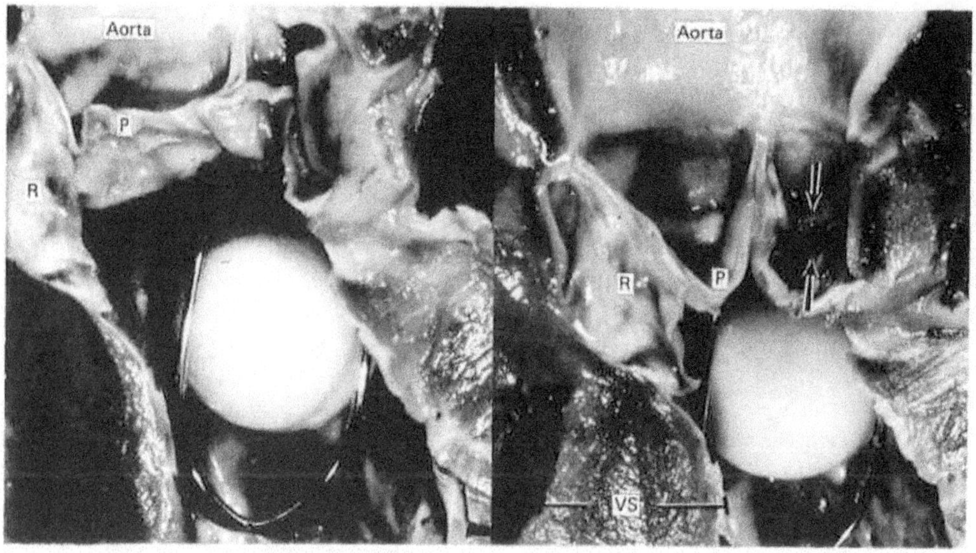

Figure 23.5. Two views of the opened left ventricular outflow tract exposing a Starr–Edwards prosthesis in the mitral position of a 50-year-old man (82A–8) who died several hours after mitral valve replacement from excessive bleeding. The mitral prosthesis is a size 4M, the largest one presently available, and the patient's pre-operative hemodynamic lesion was pure mitral stenosis. The left ventricular cavity was not dilated. The ring of the mitral prosthesis contacts the bases of 2 aortic valve cusps and a suture to secure the mitral prosthetic annulus pierced both the left aortic valve cusp (visible between the arrows in the right view) and posterior aortic valve cusps. The mitral prosthesis is obviously too large for this particular patient's left ventricular cavity. VS = ventricular septum.

dislodge from the cage[12,22,23,26,31,34,43]. In a few patients, the silicone rubber poppets deceased in size without turning yellow and this occurrence also allowed for dislodgement of the poppet from the cage. Hopefully, the change (about 1966) in the processing of the silicone rubber has alleviated this problem. The utilization of cloth around the struts of the cage led to 'cloth-wear', and the disastrous introduction by the manufacture of the 'close-clearance' cage which led to sticking of the poppet in the mid-portion of the cage and often to sudden death. In the latest model Starr–Edwards valve, wear of the metallic studs on the inner lining of the ring has led to contact of the metallic poppet with the cloth of the ring with subsequent disruption of the cloth. Fracture of the strut or occluder (Delrin) also occurred in a few of the earlier models of the tilting and non-tilting discs.

Much evidence has accumulated to indicate that the cusps of the porcine bioprosthesis will eventually degenerate[7,9,15–17,24,26,41,44] (*Figure 23.6*), and the same fate probably is in store for the bovine parietal pericardial bioprosthesis. This bioprosthesis has had the best first 5-year record of any of the presently employed prostheses or bioprostheses but its 6 to 10-year record may not be so good. Numerous reports have described heavy calcific deposits and cuspal disruption of the porcine bioprosthesis after the first 5-year period – enough evidence to convince me that this prosthesis should not be the prosthesis of choice for persons who can tolerate anticoagulants and are over 30 years and under 60 or 65 years old.

Tissue valves in the mitral position do less well than similar type bioprostheses in either the aortic or tricuspid-valve positions[7,44]. My colleagues and I have re-examined porcine bioprostheses in both the mitral and aortic valve positions implanted simultaneously in 5 patients aged 20–61 years (mean 45) 18–107 months (mean 51) earlier[44]. In 4 of the 5 patients, the degenerative changes were distinctly more severe in the bioprostheses in the mitral than in the aortic valve position. Similarly, my associates and I have examined porcine bioprostheses implanted into and explanted from both mitral and tricuspid valve positions simultaneously in 6 patients aged 30–64 years (mean 45) 62–128 months (mean 100) earlier[17]. In all 6 patients, the degenerative changes were distinctly more severe in the bioprostheses in the mitral than in the tricuspid-valve position.

The reasons for the more extensive degeneration of the bioprostheses in the mitral position are unclear but at least 3 factors need consideration. *The closing pressure on the bioprosthesis in the mitral position is higher than that on the bioprosthesis in either the aortic or tricuspid-valve position. The pressure difference across the closed bioprosthesis*

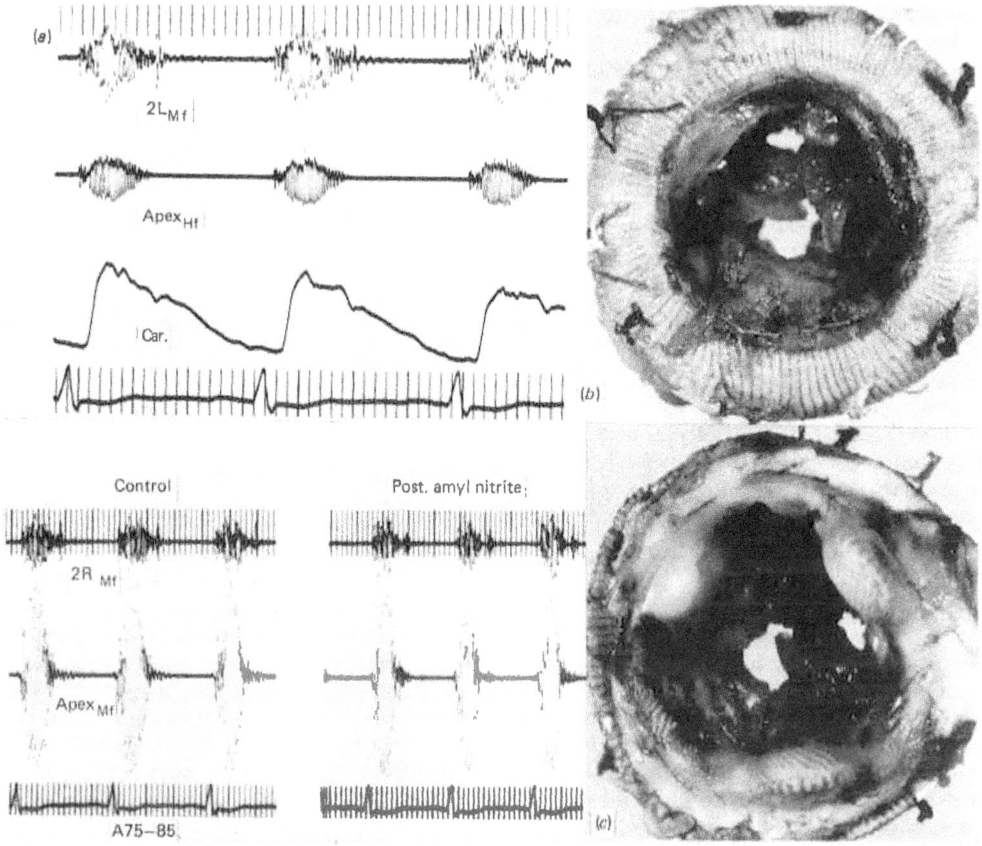

Figure 23.6. Cuspal degeneration in a 56-month-old porcine bioprosthesis in the mitral position. The patient had undergone mitral valve replacement and aortic and tricuspid-valve commissurotomy for mitral, aortic and tricuspid stenosis. She did well for 56 months (without anticoagulant therapy) when she had the sudden onset of left-sided chest pain and dyspnea, and a murmur of mitral regurgitation was heard for the first time post-operatively. At no time was evidence for infective endocarditis present. Phonocardiograms (*a*) now showed a systolic precordial murmur consistent with mitral regurgitation (no increase with amyl nitrite). Cardiac catheterization revealed 4+/4+ mitral regurgitation, and at re-operation the cusps of the 29-mm porcine mitral bioprosthesis (*b, c*) were disrupted and thrombus was adherent to them. At re-operation, the porcine mitral valve was replaced with a new porcine bioprosthesis. The tricuspid valve, which was stenotic, was also replaced with a porcine bioprosthesis, and the aortic valve, which was both stenotic and regurgitant, was replaced with a size 7A, model 2320 Starr–Edwards prosthesis. The patient did well for the first 2 weeks post-operatively but experienced sudden chest pain on the fourteenth post-operative day and died. (Reproduced from Spray and Roberts[41] with permission of the Publishers.)

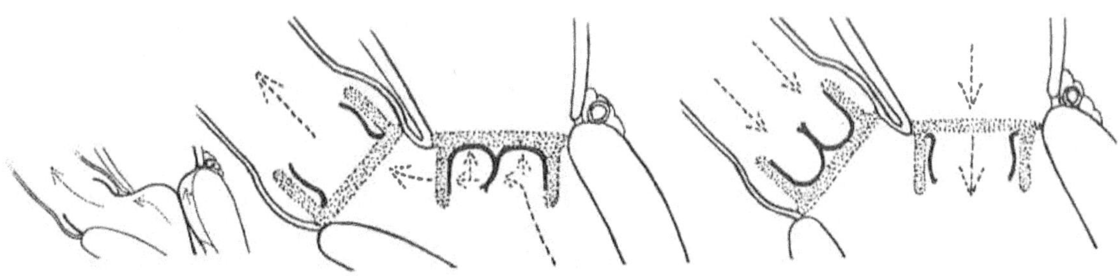

Figure 23.7. Diagrams of normal mitral valve (left) as it might appear during ventricular systole, and of a heart containing bioprostheses in both the mitral and aortic valve positions (center and right). With a semilunar valve in the mitral position, left ventricular systolic pressure does not easily 'glide' from the ventricular aspect of the cusps to the aorta as it does with the native anterior mitral leaflet (left). (Reproduced from Warnes *et al.*[44] with permission of the Publishers.)

in the mitral position is far higher than that across the closed bioprosthesis in either the aortic or tricuspid-valve positions. The higher the pressure difference across the closed bioprosthesis, the greater the tensile stress on the cusps. *The presence of a bioprosthesis composed of a semilunar valve in the atrio-ventricular valve position may prevent equal distribution of the left ventricular systolic pressure on each of the 3 bioprosthesis cusps,* whereas the aortic diastolic pressure (at least) is probably equally distributed on each of the 3 aortic valve cusps (*Figure 23.7*).

Suture overhang of prosthetic orifice

If a suture or knots overhang the metallic ring of a caged-disc or tilting disc prosthesis, the consequence might be prosthetic regurgitation[42]. This problem is more common after aortic valve replacement than after mitral replacement and has been observed only with use of mechanical prostheses containing tilting or non-tilting discs.

Prosthetic endocarditis

With mechanical prostheses, the infection is always beneath the site of attachment of the prosthesis, i.e. ring abscess is inevitable[1–3,8,10,27,32]. With tissue valves mounted on frames, the infection may be limited to the cusps, but it also may involve the site of attachment of the prosthesis. Thus, if one has a substitute cardiac valve which is infected, it is better that the infection involve a bioprosthesis rather than a mechanical valve. If endocarditis occurs in a patient in whom more than one mechanical or bioprosthetic valve is in place, the infection nearly always involves only the most downstream prosthetic or bioprosthetic valve.

Incomplete removal of native valve or its calcific deposits preventing complete occluding of a prosthetic orifice by the occluder

If calcific deposits involve the attachment of a valve leaflet to its 'annulus', complete debridement of the calcium may not be possible. If a rather sizable calcific nodule remains after valvular excision, the residual calcific debris, on rare occasion, may interfere with complete closure of the occluder[32].

Dislodgment of portion of native cardiac valve during its excision

It is preferable to remove a calcified cardiac valve intact rather than in multiple fragments to prevent the possibility of embolism[28].

Development of calcific deposits beneath site of attachment of a prosthetic valve ring

During both phases of the cardiac cycle, a rigid-framed prosthesis moves. This back-and-forth 'rocking' motion over many years may stimulate the development of calcific deposits beneath the prosthetic annulus[4]. As long as the deposits are small, significant functional consequences are unlikely, but larger ones theoretically could disrupt a suture which holds the prosthetic ring in place. This 'annular calcium' is most likely to develop more than 5 years after mitral replacement with a 'heavy' prosthesis (caged-ball), but to date I am aware of no functional consequences of its development.

Hemolysis of blood elements

Most mechanical cardiac valves decrease the half-life of erythocytes, leukocytes, and even platelets, but in all but a few patients the bone marrow accelerates its production and anemia or leukopenia or thrombocytopenia is rarely a consequence. On occasion, however, hemolysis is a problem, most frequently in patients with caged-ball prostheses (particularly with the fully cloth-covered models), in patients with aortic valve prostheses as opposed to other replaced valves, and in patients with parabasilar leaks as opposed to patients with intact parabasilar regions[30].

Complications limited to mitral (or tricuspid) valve replacement irrespective of type of prosthesis or bioprosthesis utilized

Disruption of connection between left atrium and left ventricle at mitral annulus with extravasation of blood into atrio-ventricular sulcus

When calcific deposits are located in the mitral leaflets, excision of the mitral valve including one or more annular calcific deposits may lead to loss of continuity between the walls of left atrium and left ventricle with extravasation of blood into the left atrio-ventricular sulcus with or without fatal bleeding into the pericardial sac[32]. If a prosthesis or bioprosthesis with an annulus much larger than the native mitral annulus is inserted, disruption of the native annulus may occur and the result is extravasation of blood into the left atrio-ventricular sulcus with or without subsequent rupture into the pericardial sac (*Figures 23.1,23.5,23.8–23.11*).

Excision of portion of left ventricular free wall beneath papillary muscle during excision of papillary muscle with resulting rupture or aneurysmal formation

If during mitral valve excision a left ventricular papillary muscle, grasped with a clamp, is pulled toward left atrium before the papillary muscle incision if made, a portion of left ventricular free wall in addition to papillary muscle may be excised[32] (*Figures 23.8* and *23.9*). Depending on how much left ventricular free wall is excised, the results may be through-and-through rupture or aneurysmal formation.

Incision of left ventricular free wall midway between mitral annulus and stump of left ventricle papillary muscle during mitral valve excision

A number of reports have described rupture of the left ventricular free wall about midway between the stump of the papillary muscle and mitral annulus after mitral valve replacement, and most often the rupture was attributed to a stent of either a mechanical or a bioprosthetic valve's burrowing through the free wall. Its mechanism has never been precisely determined. This complication unfortunately is not rare. At one major medical center this complication was reported in 1980 to be the most common cause of early death after mitral valve replacement[6]. I believe its cause is inadvertent incision of the left ventricular free wall during the incision of the chordae tendineae, for the 'tear' into left ventricular free wall is linear and often involves the entire free wall of the left ventricle[25] (*Figures 23.8, 23.9, 23.12–23.14*). Furthermore, it may be a considerable distance from a prosthetic stent. I have seen this complication in 10 patients at necropsy[25]. In 5 patients the laceration led to ventricular free wall rupture, with immediate hemopericardium in 2 and delayed (2 to 4 days) rupture in the other 3. Of the other 5 patients, 3 developed aneurysm of the left ventricular free wall, the mouth of which was located midway between mitral annulus and papillary muscle stump, the sites of the lacerations observed in the other 7 patients. The remaining 2 patients had midway lacerations which produced neither rupture nor aneurysmal formation. The midway left ventricular lacerations are considered the result of left ventricular incisions made at the time of mitral valve excision, generally in a setting where the left-sided cardiac chambers were only mildly dilated or normal and the tips of the blades of the scissors may have been inadequately visualized during mitral excision. This complication can be prevented by leaving the posterior mitral leaflet and its attached chordae intact or by applying exquisite care during the mitral excision procedure, or both. Thus, left ventricular midway rupture may be the most common cause of death early after mitral valve replacement and operatively induced left ventricular lacerations may lead to left ventricular aneurysm late post-operatively.

Damage to left circumflex coronary artery or to coronary sinus during insertion of mitral prosthesis or during suture obliteration of entrance into left atrium appendage

Although I have not seen this complication personally, damage to the left circumflex coronary artery or coronary sinus or both during mitral replacement has been observed by others. Both of these vessels are located in the left atrio-ventricular sulcus which is less than a centimeter from where sutures are placed into the most basal portion of mitral leaflet during insertion of the prosthesis. Occlusion of the left circumflex by a suture may result in a ventricular arrhythmia or acute myocardial infarction or both, whereas occlusion of the coronary sinus usually does not produce a clinically recognized functional consequence. During suture obliteration of the mouth of a left atrium appendage, complete obliteration by a suture of the lumen of the left circumflex, which courses just beneath the entrance into the appendage, may occur[21] (*Figure 23.15*).

Contact of cage or stent of mitral prosthesis with ventricular septum or left ventricular free wall producing ventricular arrhythmia

Contact of the cage or stent of a mitral valve prosthesis or bioprosthesis with the ventricular septum or even left ventricular free wall not only may result in left ventricular inflow or outflow obstruction, but the 'tickling' of the myocardium by the prosthesis or bioprosthesis may produce a ventricular arrhythmia which may be fatal[21] (*Figure 23.16*). This mechanism has been documented by echocardiography during life and indentations of the ventricular septum, particularly by the cage of a caged-ball prosthesis or by a stent of a porcine bioprosthesis, may be observed at necropsy.

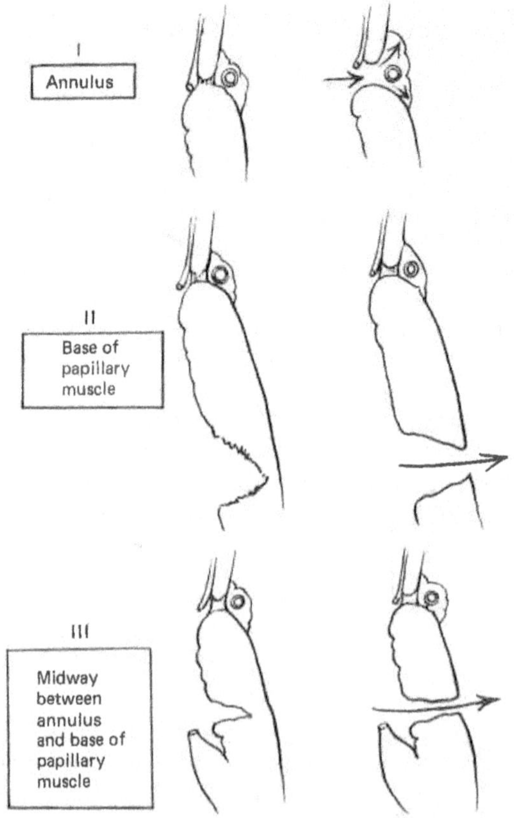

Figure 28.8. Diagram showing left-sided cardiac rupture sites during or following mitral valve replacement.

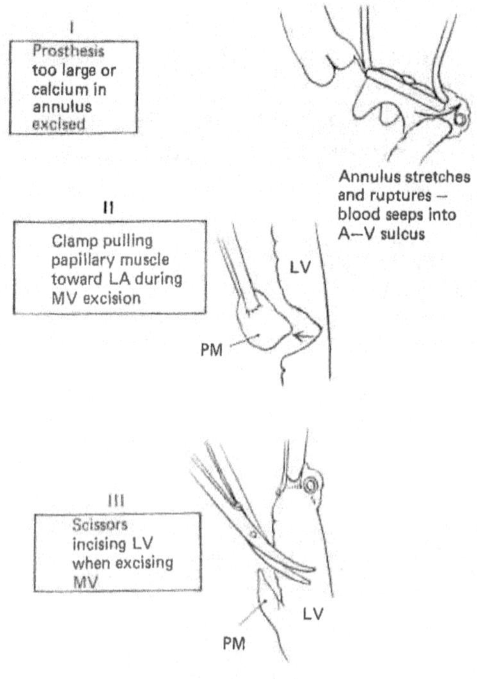

Figure 28.9. Mechanisms of left-sided cardiac rupture during or following mitral valve replacement.

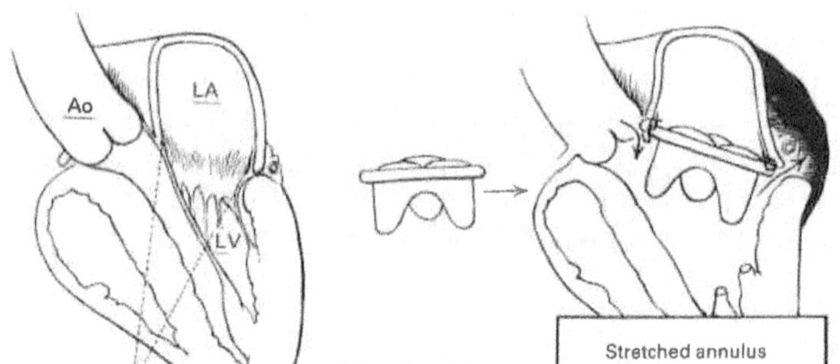

Figure 28.10. A mechanism of rupture at the mitral annular region during mitral valve replacement.

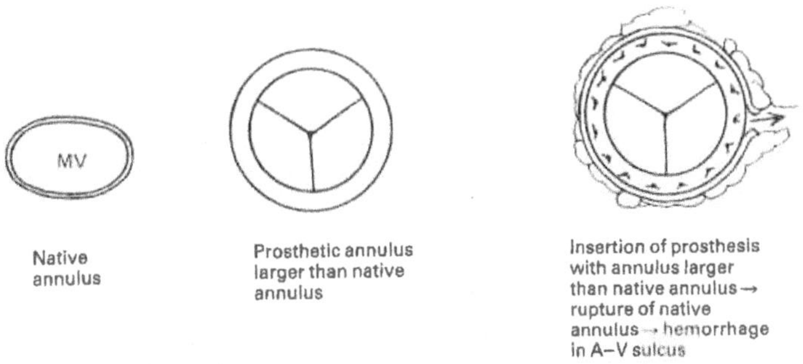

Figure 23.11. Diagram illustrating a mechanism by which mitral annular disruption can occur at the site of attachment of a mitral prosthesis or bioprosthesis.

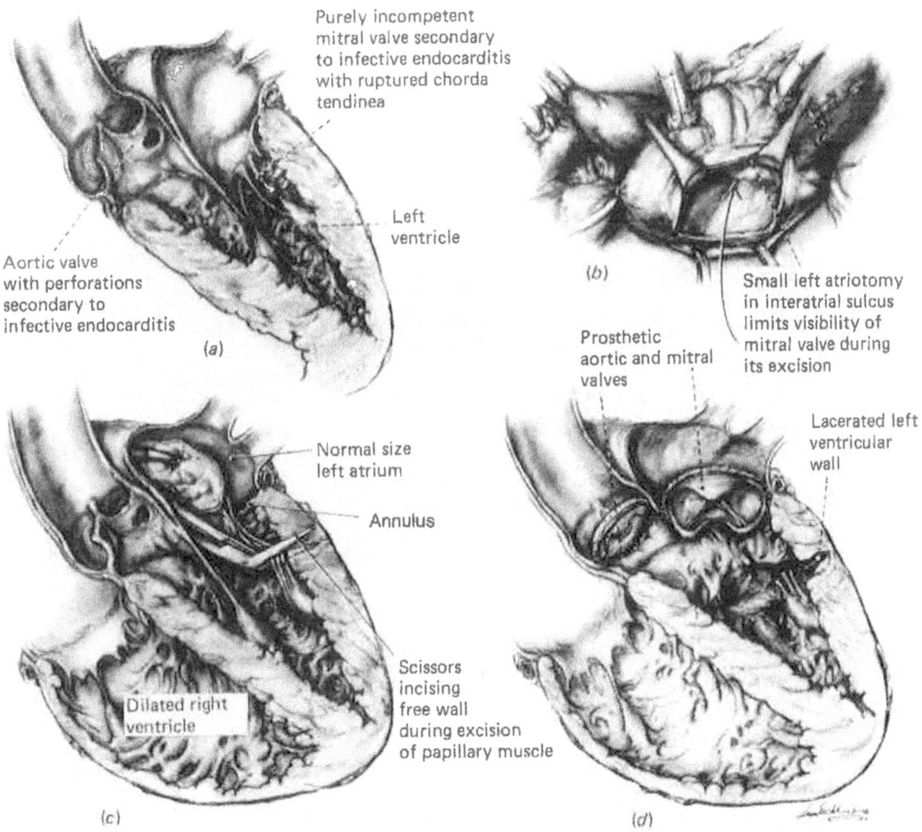

Figure 23.12. Drawing depicting the likely mechanism of left ventricular free wall rupture about midway between the stumps of a left ventricular papillary muscle and the mitral valve annulus in a 44-year-old man (78A–81) who died 4 days after mitral valve replacement. (Reproduced from Roberts *et al.*[25] with permission of the Publishers.)

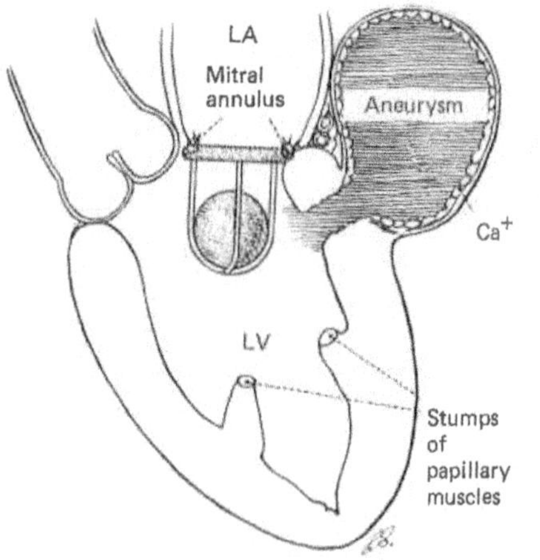

Figure 23.13. Drawing showing a large submitral left ventricular aneurysm, the mouth of which is located about midway between the mitral annulus and the papillary muscle stumps, in a 68-year-old woman (78A–105) who died 2464 days after mitral replacement. The wall of the aneurysm was heavily calcified and its egg-shaped calcific wall was readily visible on chest radiograph during the last few years of life. (Reproduced from Roberts *et al.*[25] with permission of the Publishers.)

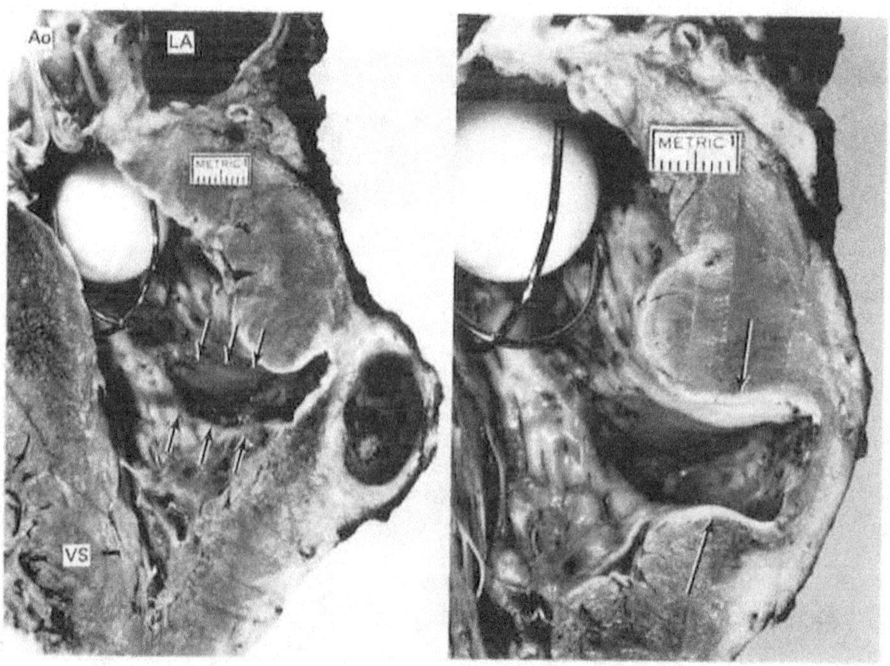

Figure 23.14. View of the left ventricle disclosing a free wall aneurysm (between the arrows) in the patient briefly described in *Figure 23.5*. This 50-year-old man (82A–8) underwent replacement of the mitral valve at 37 with a non-tilting disc, and at re-operation shortly before death the free wall aneurysm shown here was found. It is likely that the aneurysm resulted from inadvertent left ventricular free wall incision at the time of mitral valve excision 13 years earlier. The wall of the aneurysm (left) is heavily calcified and most of the lumen is filled with thrombus. Ao = aorta; LA = left atrium; VS = ventricular septum.

This situation is most liable to occur when relatively large-sized prostheses are employed in relatively small-sized ventricles.

Diffuse or extensive left ventricular fibrosis after mitral replacement

Whenever the left ventricular papillary muscles are excised, their 'raw' stumps are eventually covered by dense fibrous tissue. Thus, mural endocardial fibrosis over the stumps of the papillary muscles is an expected late finding after mitral valve replacement. On rare occasion, not only is the endocardial covering over the papillary muscles thickened by fibrous tissue, but the same process may involve most of the remaining portion of left ventricle[35]. The mechanism of this diffuse or extensive endocardial fibrosis is unclear. Initially, the concept was presented that the ball-in-a-cage prosthesis 'stirred up' the blood in the left ventricular cavity and the anatomic consequence of the 'churning' up-and-down movement was endocardial thickening. Another view has been that the extensive endocardial thickening was the consequence of poor myocardial protection at the time of valve replacement, but the endocardial thickening, to my knowledge, has been observed only after mitral valve replacement, not after isolated aortic valve replacement.

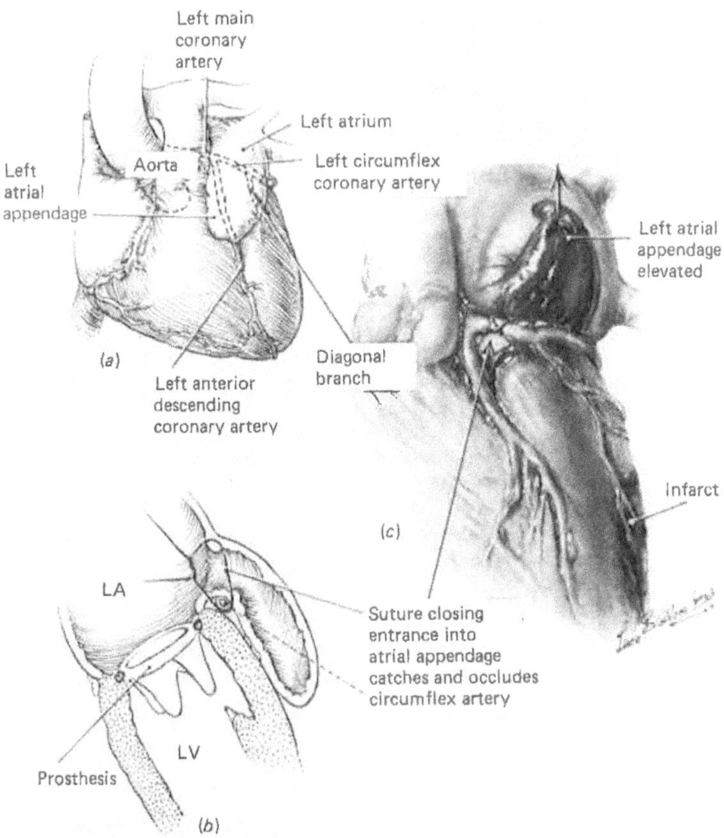

Figure 28.15. Drawing demonstrating occlusion of the left circumflex coronary artery by sutures used to close the mouth of the left atrial appendage in a 62-year-old man (A78–59) who died with a lateral wall left ventricular acute myocardial infarct 5 days after mitral valve replacement. (Reproduced from Roberts[21] with permission of the Publishers.)

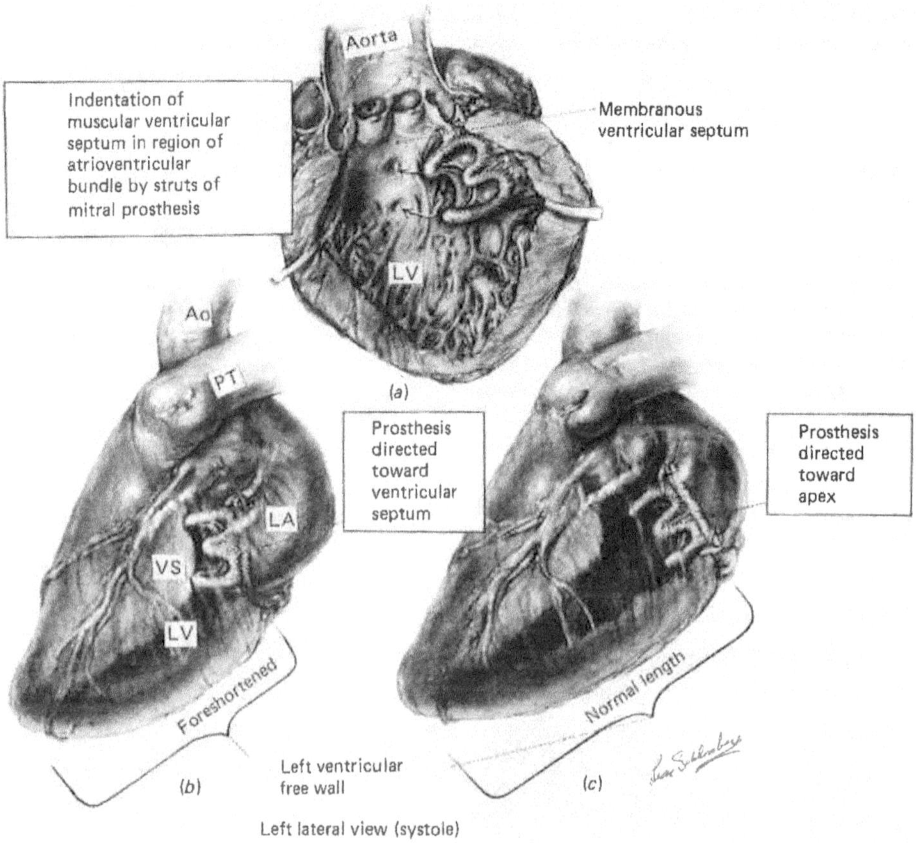

Figure 23.16. Drawing showing contact of stents or porcine bioprosthesis in the mitral position with the ventricular septum probably during ventricular systole only. This 71-year-old woman (A80–5) underwent mitral replacement 38 days before death because of severe mitral regurgitation associated with idiopathic dilated cardiomyopathy. Although no definite consequence of this contact between prosthesis and ventricular septum was apparent, this type of contact has been recognized to produce ventricular arrhythmias and possibly even sudden death. (Reproduced from Roberts[21] with permission of the Publishers.)

Tear or perforation of aortic valve cusp by suture during insertion of a mitral valve prosthesis or bioprosthesis

Normally the site of attachment of a mitral prosthesis or bioprosthesis to the most basal portion of the anterior mitral leaflet is only about 1 cm below the most caudal attachment of 2 aortic valve cusps. If the mitral prosthesis is too large for the area of the mitral orifice (after excision of the mitral leaflets and chordae), the ring of the prosthesis or bioprosthesis at the site of excision of the anterior mitral leaflet may be pushed cephalad so that the circumstance is produced whereby one or more sutures utilized to attach the cloth ring of the prosthesis or bioprosthesis to the base of the anterior mitral leaflet inadvertently tears an aortic valve cusp because of the proximity of the 2 structures (*Figure 23.6*). This circumstance has been observed by me only when a very large (too large) mitral prosthesis or bioprosthesis has been employed for mitral replacement.

Dislodgment of a fragment of left ventricular papillary muscle with resulting systemic embolism during papillary muscle excision for mitral valve replacement

In 1965, Friedman and I[14] described a patient who had a cerebral arterial embolus during mitral valve commissurotomy. Recently, Isner and associates[5] described a patient in whom a fatal embolus to a major coronary artery occurred during or shortly after mitral valve replacement. The embolus consisted of a fragment of myocardium, presumably previously a part of the left ventricular papillary muscle.

Entanglement of sutures beneath the mitral occluder causing prosthetic mitral stenosis

Suture entanglement beneath the occluder during insertion of a mitral prosthesis may prevent descent of the occluder during ventricular diastole[18] (*Figure 23.17*). Simply making certain by manual manipulation that the mitral occluder descends freely before closing the left atriotomy incision might prevent this technical problem from being fatal.

Mitral regurgitation due to entanglement of sutures on bioprosthetic stents

Silver and associates[40] described a patient who had severe mitral regurgitation immediately after replacement of the mitral valve with a bovine parietal pericardial bioprosthesis. Two sutures had inadvertently caught a bioprosthetic stent and when each was tightened, the margins of the bioprosthetic cusps were made taut producing an incompetent bioprosthetic orifice (*Figure 23.18*). Obviously, it is important to be certain that the bioprosthetic cusps are freely mobile before the left atriotomy is closed.

Acute mitral regurgitation after mitral replacement with a porcine bioprosthesis has also been observed early post-operatively and re-operation has disclosed that 1 of the 3 aortic valve bioprosthetic cusps was in a fixed open position[37]. The reason for the failure of 1 of the 3 bioprosthetic cusps to close properly was not determined in the 2 reported patients in whom this complication was described[37].

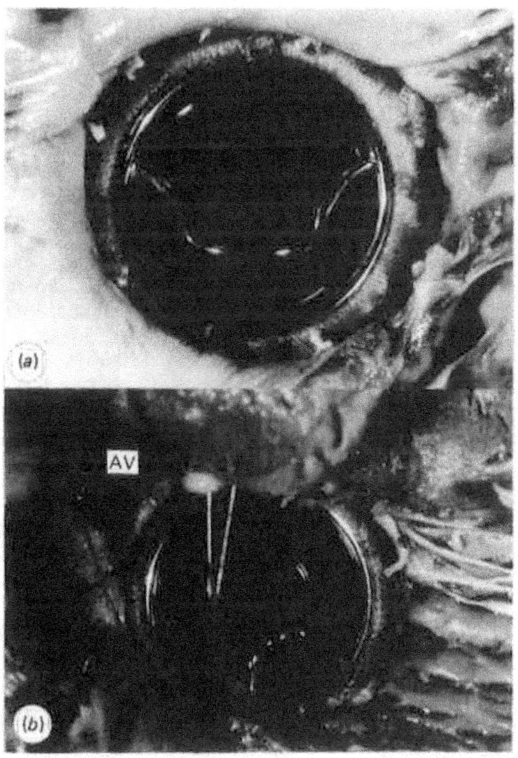

Figure 23.17. Björk–Shiley prosthesis in the mitral position in a 36-year-old woman who underwent mitral and aortic valve replacements because of pure mitral and aortic regurgitation resulting from active beta-hemolytic *Streptococcus*, Group B, endocarditis. After replacement of the mitral valve with a size 29 mm and the aortic valve with a size 25 mm Björk–Shiley prosthesis, she was weaned from cardio-pulmonary by-pass with difficulty, and a counterpulsation aortic balloon was inserted. Although she manifested features of the low cardiac output syndrome, she lived nearly 12 hours after leaving the operating room. At necropsy, the occluder of the mitral prosthesis was unable to descend more than 2 mm toward the left ventricular cavity because of 3 sutures which had become entangled across its central axis resulting in severe prosthetic obstruction (*b*). The mitral prosthesis as viewed from the left atrium is shown in (*a*). AV = aortic valve prosthesis. (Reproduced from Jones *et al.*[18] with permission of the Publishers.)

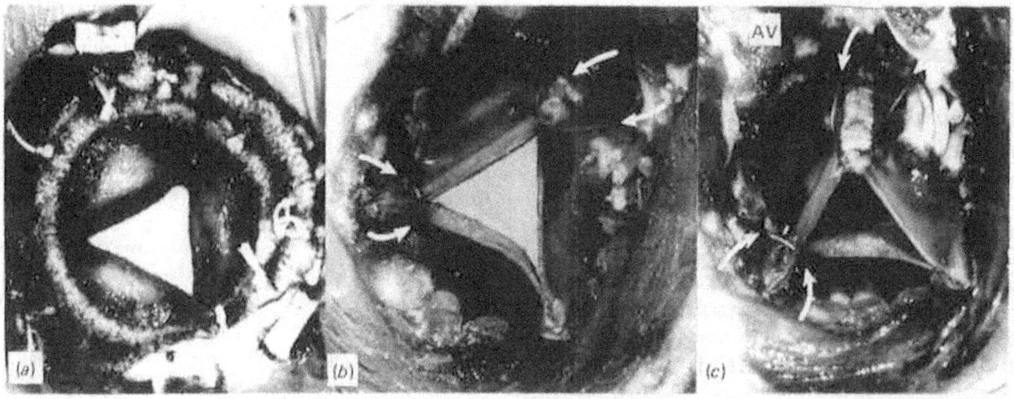

Figure 23.18. Ionescu–Shiley bioprosthesis in the mitral position in a 64-year-old man who underwent mitral valve replacement because of severe pure mitral regurgitation due to active Group B beta-hemolytic *Streptococcus* endocarditis. The native valve was replaced with a 25-mm bovine parietal pericardial bioprosthesis and he lived 8 days thereafter during which time a murmur consistent with mitral regurgitation was audible. At necropsy, sutures surrounded 2 of the 3 stents of the bioprosthesis, causing a straight-line stretching of the margins of the bioprosthetic cusps between the 3 commissures. The result was triangular-shaped severely incompetent bioprosthetic orifice. (*a*) From left atrial view. (*b*) and (*c*) from left ventricle. The arrows point to the 2 sutures which encircled the stents, causing tautness of the cusps and preventing them from coapting during ventricular systole.

Summary

Described in this chapter are 10 complications common to any valve site and to most or all presently available mechanical or bioprosthetic cardiac valves and 10 other complications limited to mitral (or tricuspid) valve replacement irrespective of the type of prosthesis or bioprosthesis utilized.

References

1. ARCHARD, H.O. and ROBERTS, W.C. Bacterial endocarditis after dental procedures in patients with aortic valve prosthesis. *Am. Dental Assoc.*, 72, 648 (1966).
2. ARNETT, E.N., KASTL, D.G., GARVIN, A.J. and ROBERTS, W.C. A conversation on prosthetic valve endocarditis. *Am. Heart J.*, 93, 510 (1977).
3. ARNETT, E.N. and ROBERTS, W.C. Prosthetic valve endocarditis: clinico-pathologic analysis of 22 necropsy patients with comparison of observations in 74 necropsy patients with active infective endocarditis involving natural left-sided cardiac valves. *Am. J. Cardiol.*, 38, 281 (1976).
4. BULKLEY, B.H., MORROW, A.G. and ROBERTS, W.C. Calcification of prosthetic valve annuli: a late complication of cardiac valve replacement. *Am. Heart J.*, 87, 129 (1974).
5. CASE RECORDS OF THE MASSACHUSETTS GENERAL HOSPITAL (CASE no. 46–1983). Discussions by J.M. Isner and S.S. Lee. *N. Engl. J. Med.*, 309, 1283 (1983).
6. COBBS, B.W. Jr, HATCHER, C.R. Jr, CRAVER, J.M., JONES, E.L. and SEWELL, C.W. Transverse mid ventricular disruption after mitral valve replacement. *Am. Heart J.*, **99**, 33 (1980).
7. COHEN, S.R., SILVER, M.A., McINTOSH, C.L., and ROBERTS, W.C. Comparison of late (62–140 months) degenerative changes in simultaneously implanted and explanted porcine (Hancock) bioprostheses in the tricuspid and mitral valve positions in 6 patients. *Am. J. Cardiol.*, **53**, 1468 (1984).
8. COHN, L.H., ROBERTS, W.C., ROCKOFF, S.D. and MORROW, A.G. Bacterial endocarditis following aortic valve replacement. Clinical and pathologic correlations. *Circulation*, **33**, 209 (1956).
9. FERRANS, V.J., BOYCE, S.W., BILLINGHAM, M.E., JONES, M., ISHIHARA, T. and ROBERTS, W.C. Calcific deposits in porcine bioprosthesis: structure and pathogenesis. *Am. J. Cardiol.*, **46**, 721 (1980).
10. FERRANS, V.J., BOYCE, S.W., BILLINGHAM, M.E., SPRAY, T.L. and ROBERTS, W.C. Infection of glutaraldehyde-preserved porcine valve heterografts. *Am. J. Cardiol.*, **43**, 1123 (1979).
11. FERRANS, F.J., SPRAY, T.L., BILLINGHAM, M.E. and ROBERTS, W.C. Structural changes in glutaraldehyde-treated porcine heterografts used as substitute cardiac valves. Transmission and scanning electron microscopic observations in 12 patients. *Am. J. Cardiol.*, **41**, 1159 (1978).
12. FISHBEIN, M.C. and ROBERTS, W.C. Late postoperative anatomic observations after insertion of Hufnagel caged-ball prostheses in descending thoracic aorta. *Chest*, **68**, 6 (1975).
13. FISHBEIN, M.C., ROBERTS, W.C., GOLDEN, A. and HUFNAGEL, C.A. Cardiac pathology after aortic valve replacement using Hufnagel trileaflet prostheses: a study of 20 necropsy patients. *Am. Heart J.*, **89**, 443 (1975).

14. FRIEDMAN, R.M. and ROBERTS, W.C. Myocardial embolus – a complication of mitral valvulotomy. *N. Engl. J. Med.*, **272**, 251 (1965).
15. GEHA, A.S., LAKS, H., STANSEL, H.C. Jr, CORNHILL, J.F., KILMAN, J.W., BUCKLEY, M.J. *et al.* Late failure of porcine valve heterografts in children. *J. Thorac. Cardiovasc. Surg.*, **78**, 351 (1979).
16. ISHIHARA, T., FERRANS, V.J., JONES, M., BOYCE, S.W. and ROBERTS, W.C. Structure of bovine parietal pericardium and of unimplanted Ionescu–Shiley pericardial valvular bioprostheses. *J. Thorac. Cardiovasc. Surg.*, **81**, 747 (1981).
17. ISHIHARA, T., FERRANS, V.J., JONES, M., CABIN, H.S. and ROBERTS, W.C. Calcific deposits developing in a bovine pericardial bioprosthetic valve 3 days after implantation. *Circulation*, **63**, 718 (1981).
18. JONES, A.A., OTIS, J.B., FLETCHER, G.F. and ROBERTS, W.C. A hitherto undescribed cause of prosthetic mitral valve obstruction. *J. Thorac. Cardiovasc. Surg.*, **74**, 116 (1977).
19. ROBERTS, W.C. Choosing a substitute cardiac valve: type, size, surgeon. *Am. J. Cardiol.*, **38**, 633 (1976).
20. ROBERTS, W.C. Operative treatment of hypertrophic obstructive cardiomyopathy. The case against mitral valve replacement. *Am. J. Cardiol.*, **32**, 377 (1973).
21. ROBERTS, W.C. Complications of cardiac valve replacement: characteristic abnormalities of prostheses pertaining to any or specific site. *Am. Heart J.*, **103**, 113 (1982).
22. ROBERTS, W.C., BULKLEY, B.H. and MORROW, A.G. Pathologic anatomy of cardiac valve replacement: a study of 224 necropsy patients. *Prog. Cardiovasc. Dis.*, **15**, 539 (1973).
23. ROBERTS, W.C., FISHBEIN, M.C. and GOLDEN, A. Cardiac pathology after valve replacement by disc prosthesis: a study of 61 necropsy patients. *Am. J. Cardiol.*, **35**, 740 (1975).
24. ROBERTS, W.C. and HAMMER, W.J. Cardiac pathology after valve replacement with a tilting disc prosthesis (Björk–Shiley type). A study of 46 necropsy patients and 49 Björk–Shiley prostheses. *Am. J. Cardiol.*, **37**, 1024 (1976).
25. ROBERTS, W.C., ISNER, J.M. and VIRMANI, R. Left ventricular incision midway between the mitral annulus and the stumps of the papillary muscles during mitral valve excision with or without rupture or aneurysmal formation: analysis of 10 necropsy patients. *Am. Heart J.*, **104**, 1278 (1982).
26. ROBERTS, W.C., LEVINSON, G.E. and MORROW, A.G. Lethal ball variance in the Starr–Edwards prosthetic mitral valve. *Arch. Intern. Med.*, **126**, 517 (1970).
27. ROBERTS, W.C. and MORROW, A.G. Bacterial endocarditis involving prosthetic mitral valves. Clinical and pathologic observations. *Arch. Pathol.*, **82**, 164 (1966).
28. ROBERTS, W.C. and MORROW, A.G. Cardiac valves and the surgical pathologist. *Arch. Pathol.*, **82**, 309 (1966).
29. ROBERTS, W.C. and MORROW, A.G. Mechanisms of acute left atrial thrombosis after mitral valve replacement. Pathologic findings indicating obstruction to left atrial emptying. *Am. J. Cardiol.*, **8**, 497 (1966).
30. ROBERTS, W.C and MORROW, A.G. Renal hemosiderosis in patients with prosthetic aortic valves. *Circulation*, **33**, 390 (1966).
31. ROBERTS, W.C. and MORROW, A.G. Anatomic studies of hearts containing caged-ball prosthetic valves. *Johns Hopkins Med. J.*, **121**, 271 (1967).
32. ROBERTS, W.C. and MORROW, A.G. Causes of early postoperative death following cardiac valve replacement. Clinico-pathologic correlations in 64 patients studied at necropsy. *J. Thorac. Cardiovasc. Surg.* **54**, 422 (1967).
33. ROBERTS, W.C. and MORROW, A.G. Late postoperative pathologic findings after cardiac valve replacement. *Circulation*, **36** and **37**, Suppl., I, 48 (1967).
34. ROBERTS, W.C. and MORROW, A.G. Fatal degeneration of the silicone rubber ball of the Starr–Edwards prosthetic aortic valve. *Am. J. Cardiol.*, **22**, 614 (1968).
35. ROBERTS, W.C. and MORROW, A.G. Secondary left ventricular endocardial fibroelastosis following mitral valve replacement. Cause of cardiac failure in the late postoperative period. *Circulation*, **37** and **37**, Suppl., II, 101 (1968).
36. ROBERTS, W.C. and MORROW, A.G. Causes of death and other anatomic observations after cardiac valve replacement. In *Long-Term Prognosis Following Valve Replacement*, Second Conference on Disease, S. Karger, Basel. *Adv. Cardiol.*, **7**, 226 (1972).
37. SARABU, M.R. and PARKER, F.B. Jr. Unusual complication of porcine heterograft. *Ann. Thorac.Surg.*, **35**, 553 (1983).
38. SENINGEN, R.P., BULKLEY, B.H. and ROBERTS, W.C. Prosthetic aortic stenosis. A method to prevent its occurrence by measurement of aortic size from preoperative aortogram. *Circulation*, **49**, 921 (1974).
39. SHEPARD, R.L., GLANCY, D.L., STINSON, E.B. and ROBERTS, W.C. Hemodynamic confirmation of obstruction to left ventricular inflow by a caged-ball prosthetic mitral valve. Case report. *J. Thorac. Cardiovasc. Surg.*, **65**, 252 (1973).
40. SILVER, M.A., ORANBURG, P.R. and ROBERTS, W.C. Severe mitral regurgitation immediately after mitral valve replacement with a parietal pericardial bovine bioprosthesis. *Am. J. Cardiol.*, **52**, 218 (1983).
41. SPRAY, T.L. and ROBERTS, W.C. Structural changes in porcine xenografts used as substitute cardiac valves. Gross and histologic observations in 51 glutaraldehyde-preserved Hancock valves in 41 patients. *Am J. Cardiol.*, **40**, 319 (1977).
42. WALLER, B.F., JONES, M. and ROBERTS, W.C. Postoperative aortic regurgitation from incomplete seating of tilting-disc occluders due to overhanding knots or long sutures. *Chest*, **78**, 565 (1980).
43. WARNES, C.A., McINTOSH, C.L. and ROBERTS, W.C. Wear of the metallic studs on the composite seat of the 2320 Starr–Edwards aortic valve and its clinical consequences. *Am. J. Cardiol.*, **52**, 1062 (1983).
44. WARNES, C.A., SCOTT, M.L., SILVER, G.M., SMITH, C.W., FERRANS, V.J. and ROBERTS, W.C. Comparison of late degenerative changes in porcine bioprostheses in the mitral and aortic valve position in the same patient. *Am. J. Cardiol.*, **51**, 965 (1983).
45. WINTER, T.Q., REIS, R.L., GLANCY, D.L., ROBERTS, W.C., EPSTEIN, S.E. and MORROW, A.G. Current status of Starr–Edwards cloth-covered prosthetic cardiac valves. *Circulation*, **45** and **46**, Suppl., I, 14 (1972).
46. YARBROUGH, J.W., ROBERTS, W.C. and REIS, R.L. Structural alterations in tissue cardiac valves implanted in patients and in calves. *J. Thorac. Cardiovasc. Surg.*, **65**, 364 (1973).

Valve Excision Only Versus *Valve Excision Plus Replacement* for Active Infective Endocarditis Involving the Tricuspid Valve

DEBORAH J. BARBOUR, MD, and WILLIAM C. ROBERTS, MD

M.B., a 28-year-old intravenous (i.v.) drug user, had Group D alpha Streptococcus *endocarditis and underwent tricuspid valve excision without replacement. Late postoperatively, he was asymptomatic, but died from a heroin overdose 11 months after operation (Fig. 1).*

Y.W., a 30-year-old i.v. drug user, had Staphylococcus aureus *endocarditis with severe right-sided congestive heart failure (CHF) and underwent tricuspid valve excision and replacement with a porcine bioprosthesis. Nearly 5 months later the bioprosthesis became infected and it was excised without being replaced (Fig. 2). Shortly thereafter, however, severe right-sided CHF reappeared and, as a consequence, a porcine bioprosthesis was reinserted into the tricuspid valve position. Six weeks after this third operation she was asymptomatic.*

From the Pathology Branch, National Heart, Lung, and Blood Institute, National Institutes of Health, Bethesda, Maryland 20205. Manuscript received May 31, 1985, accepted August 13, 1985.

Infective endocarditis involving the tricuspid valve is fairly common in i.v. drug users. The infection on this valve, when bacterial in nature, can usually be eradicated by antibiotic therapy. In an occasional patient, however, persistence of positive blood cultures, repeated pulmonary emboli or development of intractable CHF despite appropriate antibiotic therapy without associated left-sided cardiac valve involvement necessitates operative intervention. But what type of operative intervention should be performed? Excision of the tricuspid valve only or excision plus concurrent replacement (Fig. 3)? This article will examine the arguments for each of these 2 therapeutic options.

Review of previous published reports yielded at least 15 patients who had isolated excision of their infected native tricuspid valves with concurrent placement of either a mechanical prosthesis or a bioprosthesis in the tricuspid valve position.[1-5] Of the 5 patients

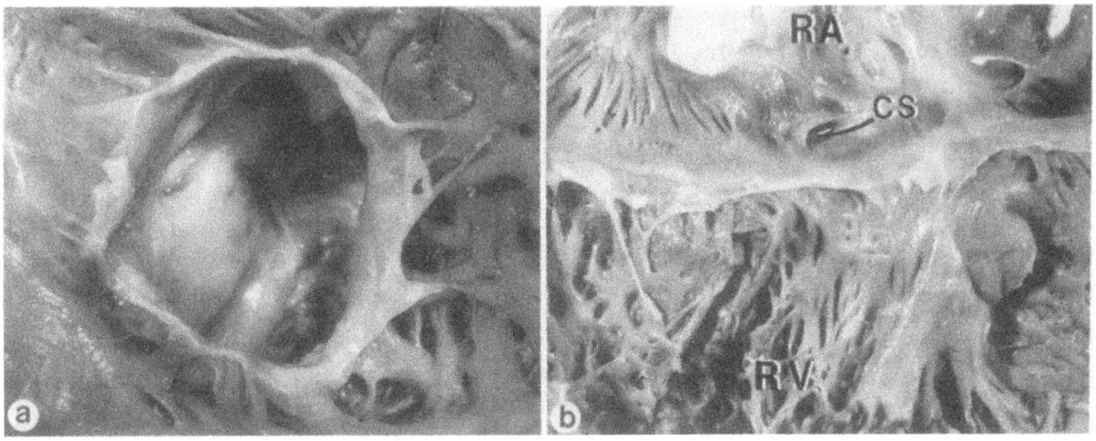

FIGURE 1. Patient M.B. *a,* **intact tricuspid valve anulus viewed from the ventricular side 11 months after excision of most of the leaflets and chordae tendineae.** *b,* **opened tricuspid valve anulus, right atrium (RA) and right ventricle (RV). The tricuspid valve anulus measured 16.5 cm in circumference (normal <12.0 cm). (His mitral valve anulus measured 11.0 cm in circumference [normal <11.0 cm]).**

with mechanical prostheses,[1–4] 2 died in the early postoperative period; 1 patient, who underwent excision of the prosthesis 6 weeks after the initial operation because of prosthetic valve endocarditis, had moderate CHF but no sign of infection 9 months later; and 2 were asymptomatic 12 and 21 months, respectively, after operation. Each of the other 10 patients had tricuspid valve replacement with a porcine bioprosthesis, all since 1980; none died early and 3 died late (1 at 6 months postoperatively from a perforated ulcer and sepsis, and 2 after prosthetic valve endocarditis developed).

In 1971, Arbulu et al[3] reported excision of infected tricuspid valves without replacement in 4 i.v. drug abusers: 1 died of infection 7 weeks later and the other 3 were alive at 1 month, 8 months and 11 years, respectively. In 1981, Arbulu and Asfaw[6] described results of tricuspid valve excision without replacement for tricuspid valve endocarditis (2 patients also concurrently had their infected pulmonic valves excised without replacement) in 61 patients, 29 of whom were operated on by the authors and the other 32 by other surgeons. Of the 61 patients, 6 died within 60 days of operation and 5 died later (2 from "recurrent endocarditis"). Of the remaining 50 patients, 11 subsequently had a prosthesis or bioprosthesis inserted into the tricuspid valve position. Of the 61 patients described by Arbulu and Asfaw,[6] 45 patients between 1970 and 1981 had tricuspid valve excision without replacement, 37 of whom (61%) were reported to have "good" results ("eradication of the infection and absence of hemodynamic problems") and 4 (7%), "fair" results ("eradication of the endocarditis but presence of hemodynamic problems such as tachycardia, mild symptoms and signs of right or left ventricular failure, or biventricular failure"). Actuarial analysis of these patients who underwent tricuspid valve excision without replacement predicted 86% survival at 10 years.

No postoperative hemodynamic data is available in the 13 patients who survived the early postoperative period after isolated replacement of the tricuspid valve for active infective endocarditis.[1,2,4,5] Robin et al[7]

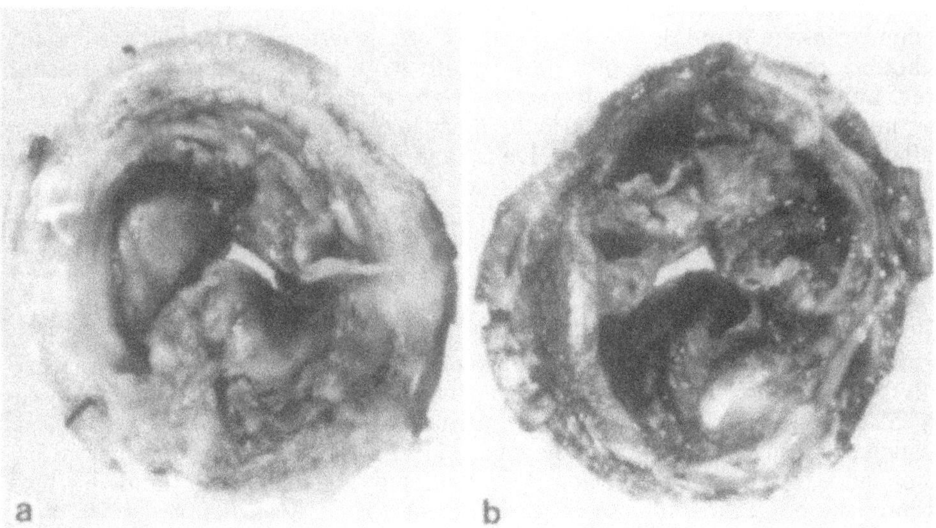

FIGURE 2. Patient Y.W. Operatively excised porcine bioprosthesis from the tricuspid valve position. The bioprosthesis was excised nearly 5 months after its implantation because it became infected. *a,* **right atrial aspect.** *b,* **right ventricular aspect. Infected thrombus (vegetation) is present on both aspects of the cusps.**

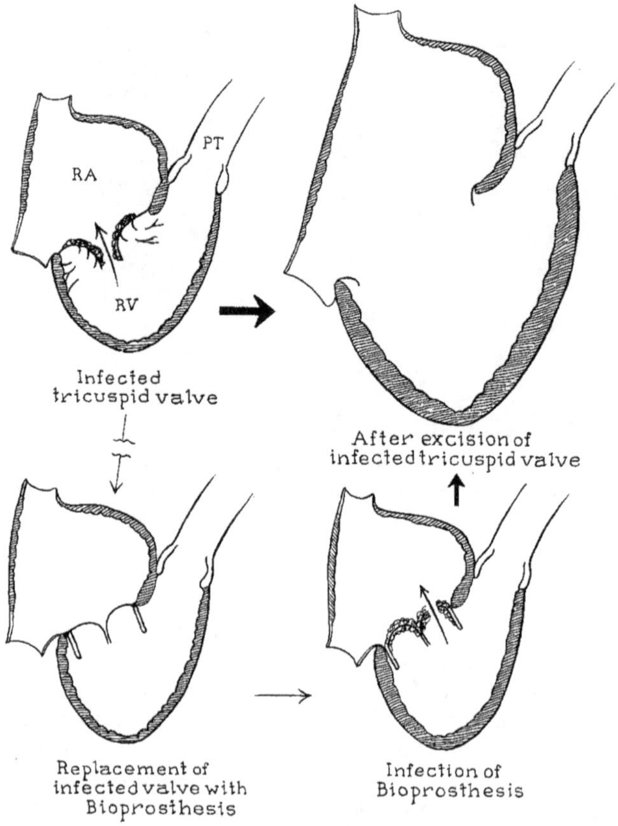

FIGURE 3. Diagram showing the possible operative interventions for resistant infective endocarditis involving the tricuspid valve. *Top panel* shows the expected late consequences of tricuspid valve excision without replacement as occurred in our patient M.B. *Lower panel* shows what happened in our patient Y.W. who initially had replacement of the infected native tricuspid valve with a bioprosthesis, which in turn became infected, necessitating its excision without concurrent replacement.

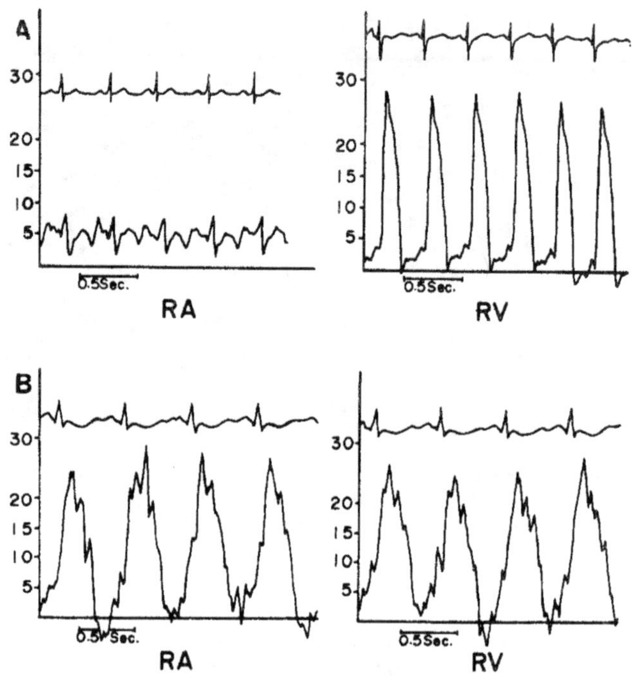

FIGURE 4. Preoperative (*upper panel*) and postoperative (*lower panel*) pressure tracings from right atrium (RA) and right ventricle (RV) in a patient with active tricuspid valve endocarditis reported in 1975 by Robin et al.[7] Postoperatively, the pressure tracing of the right atrium and right ventricle are identical. The numbers in the *vertical columns* in all 4 diagrams are mm Hg. (Reproduced with permission of Robin et al and *The American Journal of Cardiology*.)

described both pre- and postoperative hemodynamic data in 10 patients who had tricuspid valve excision without replacement for active infective endocarditis. Postoperatively, the right atrial and right ventricular pressure tracings were similar, indeed virtually identical (Fig. 4). In their 10 patients, the mean right atrial pressure preoperatively was 4.4 mm Hg (range 3 to 6) and postoperatively it was 13.3 mm Hg (range 10 to 17). The average values of the right and left ventricular systolic and diastolic pressures, pulmonary arterial systolic and diastolic pressures, and the mean aortic pressures were normal and similar preoperatively and postoperatively, whether the patients were free of evidence of right-sided cardiac failure (7 patients) or had right-sided cardiac failure (3 patients). The precise interval between tricuspid valve excision without replacement and postoperative cardiac catheterization was not stated by Robin et al, but the maximal interval was only 48 months, and probably much less.

It is clear that tricuspid valve excision for active infective endocarditis involving this valve removes the source of pulmonary emboli, which occur in virtually all such patients and is the major cause of symptoms. Furthermore, from the aforementioned data, an asymptomatic state can be achieved for varying periods in most patients, in the absence of a tricuspid valve, as long as the right ventricular systolic pressure is normal or near normal. Because most patients with infective endocarditis involving the tricuspid valve are i.v. drug users and their habit usually is not discontinued following a tricuspid valve operation, it appears most reasonable to perform tricuspid valve excision without accompanying valve replacement to prevent the introduction of a "foreign body" which, of course, would be exquisitely sensitive to infection. The insertion of a bioprosthesis or prosthesis provides a nidus more prone to infection than the native tricuspid valve. Furthermore, insertion of the bioprosthesis or prosthesis usually leads to some degree of obstruction between the right atrium and right ventricle during ventricular diastole. Additionally, if the substitute cardiac valve is a bioprosthesis, replacement of it will be indicated some years later because of expected degeneration with long-term wear.[8,9] For these reasons, tricuspid valve excision without replacement appears, in our view, preferable to tricuspid valve excision with concurrent replacement for life-threatening active infective endocarditis involving this valve. It is likely, however, that most patients having tricuspid valve excision without replacement will eventually require the insertion of a prosthesis or a bioprosthesis into the tricuspid valve position, but the interval between operations may be many years and this time may be sufficient to allow cessation of i.v. drug use.

References

1. Kennedy JH, Sabga GA, Fisk AA, Sancetta SM. *Isolated tricuspid valvular insufficiency due to subacute bacterial endocarditis. J Thorac Cardiovasc Surg 1966;51:498–506.*
2. Jimenez-Martinez M, Lopez-Cuellar M, Quinones-Morales R. *Isolated tricuspid endocarditis with ventricular septal defect. J Thorac Cardiovasc Surg 1971;61:665–669.*
3. Arbulu A, Thoms NW, Chiscano A, Wilson RF. *Total tricuspid valvulectomy without replacement in the treatment of Pseudomonas endocarditis. Surg Forum 1971;22:162–164.*
4. Michl L, Shumacker HB Jr, Hobbs D. *Tricuspid valvulectomy. Surg Gynecol Obstet 1973;137:590–592.*
5. Stern HJ, Sisto DA, Strom JA, Soeiro R, Jones SR, Frater RWM. *Immediate tricuspid valve replacement for endocarditis: indications and results (abstr). Am Assoc Thorac Surg, Program of Annual Meeting, 1985: 44.*
6. Arbulu A, Asfaw I. *Tricuspid valvulectomy without prosthetic replacement. Ten years of clinical experience. J Thorac Cardiovasc Surg 1981; 82:684–691.*
7. Robin E, Thoms NW, Arbulu A, Ganguly SN, Magnisalis K. *Hemodynamic consequences of total removal of the tricuspid valve without prosthetic replacement. Am J Cardiol 1975;35:481–486.*
8. Cohen SR, Silver MA, McIntosh CL, Roberts WC. *Comparison of late (62 to 140 months) degenerative changes in simultaneously implanted and explanted porcine (Hancock) bioprostheses in the tricuspid and mitral valve positions in six patients. Am J Cardiol 1984;53:1599–1602.*
9. Silver MA, Cohen SR, McIntosh CL, Cannon RO III, Roberts WC. *Late (5 to 132 months) clinical and hemodynamic results after either tricuspid valve replacement or anuloplasty for Ebstein's anomaly of the tricuspid valve. Am J Cardiol 1984;54:627–632.*

Extensive Multifocal Myocardial Infarcts from Cloth Emboli After Replacement of Mitral and Aortic Valves with Cloth-Covered, Caged-Ball Prostheses

Allen L. Dollar, MD, Marie-Lydie Pierre-Louis, MD,
Charles L. McIntosh, MD, PhD, and William C. Roberts, MD

The early Starr-Edwards prosthetic heart valve models (series 1000, 1200 and 1260) contained no cloth on the inner aspects of the ring or on the struts. In an attempt to reduce the frequency of thrombus on the prostheses, a cloth covering was later added to cover the inside portion of the ring and the struts. Almost simultaneously, a stellite poppet was substituted for the silicone rubber poppet in many prostheses. Although these modifications did reduce the frequency of embolic events, a new problem was introduced, namely cloth wear. Cloth wear led in some patients to dysfunction of prostheses, hemolytic anemia and systemic emboli.[1-7] As the cloth on these prosthetic valves wore, cloth occasionally embolized to 1 or more systemic organs. Such resulting organ infarcts

From the Pathology and Surgery Branches, National Heart, Lung, and Blood Institute, National Institutes of Health, Bethesda, Maryland 20892, and the District of Columbia Medical Examiner's Office, District of Columbia, Washington, DC. Manuscript received April 19, 1989; revised manuscript received and accepted May 11, 1989.

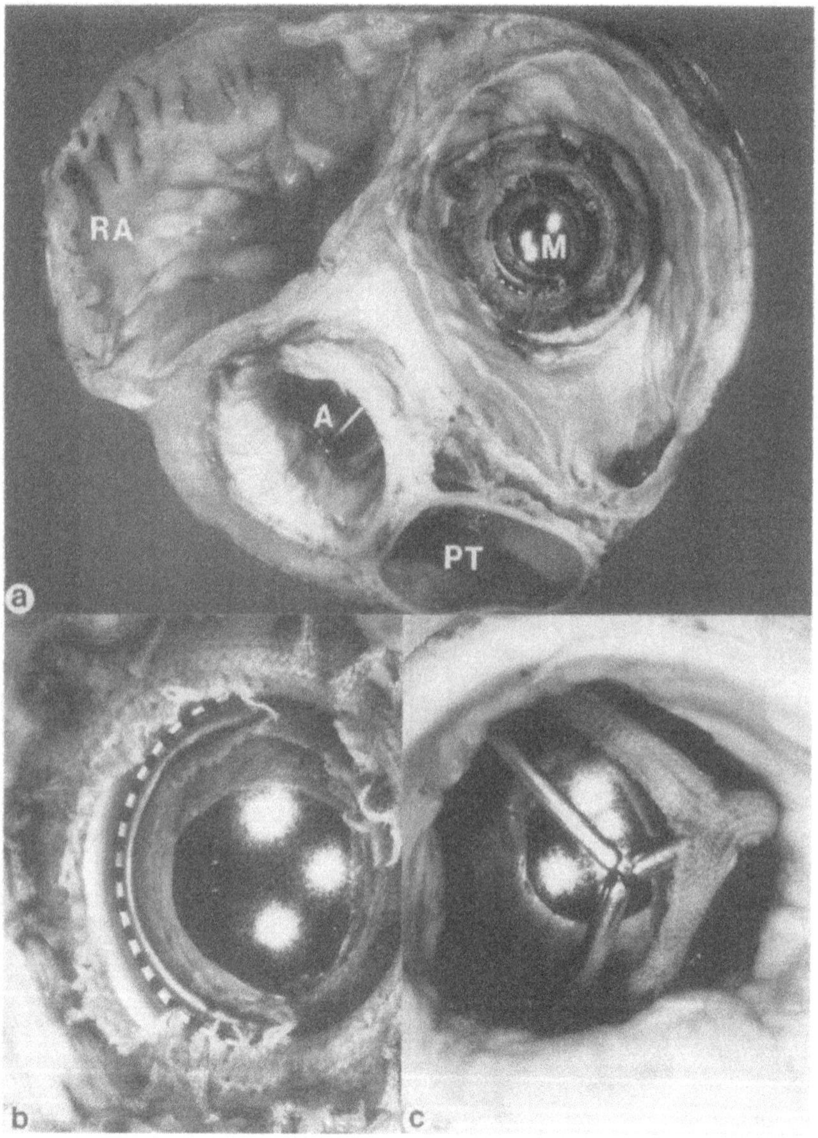

FIGURE 1. Photographs of the heart in the patient described. *a*, view of atria and great arteries from above showing the cloth-covered Starr-Edwards prostheses in the mitral (M) and aortic (A) valve positions. The cloth on the mitral prosthetic ring is frayed. PT = pulmonary trunk; RA = right atrium. *b*, close-up view of the mitral valve prosthesis from the left atrium with the torn cloth pulled away from the metallic ring. *c*, close-up view of the aortic valve prosthesis viewed from the aorta showing detachment of the cloth covering from each of the 3 struts due to wear of the cloth on the inside of the cage.

were usually not visible on gross inspection.

We recently studied a patient at necropsy who had multiple ventricular scars from cloth emboli from caged-ball prostheses. Such myocardial scars from this etiology have not been described previously.

A 58-year-old man underwent replacements of his stenotic mitral and aortic valves on January 23, 1970, and he died on November 1, 1988. Cloth-covered Starr-Edwards prostheses with metallic poppets, models 2310 and 6310, were implanted. Unilateral occlusion of a central retinal artery occurred at age 53 (13 years postoperatively); it resolved spontaneously and sight returned. A ventricular demand pacemaker was implanted at age 54 because of symptomatic bradycardia. Cardiac catheterization at that time disclosed a 10 mm Hg mean diastolic gradient between the pulmonary artery wedge and left ventricle, and no peak systolic gradient between the left ventricle (140/11 mm Hg) and aorta (140/85 mm Hg). The coronary arteries were normal by angiogram. On echocardiogram, the diameter of the left ventricular cavity was 55 mm in end-diastole and 38 mm in peak systole. Left ventricular fractional shortening was 31%. On evaluation 8 months before death, he was asymptomatic. Death resulted from injuries sustained when, as a pedestrian, he was struck by a truck traveling at a high speed.

Thirteen electrocardiograms recorded from July 16, 1969, to March 16, 1988, were reviewed. Each of the 3 recorded before double valve replacement showed atrial fibrillation, Q waves in leads V_1 through V_3 and total 12-lead QRS amplitudes of 234, 240 and 216 mm (10 mm = 1 mV).[8] The first 8 electrocardiograms recorded from 5 days to 14 years after the double valve replacement also showed Q waves in leads V_1 through V_3 and total 12-lead QRS amplitudes ranging from 129

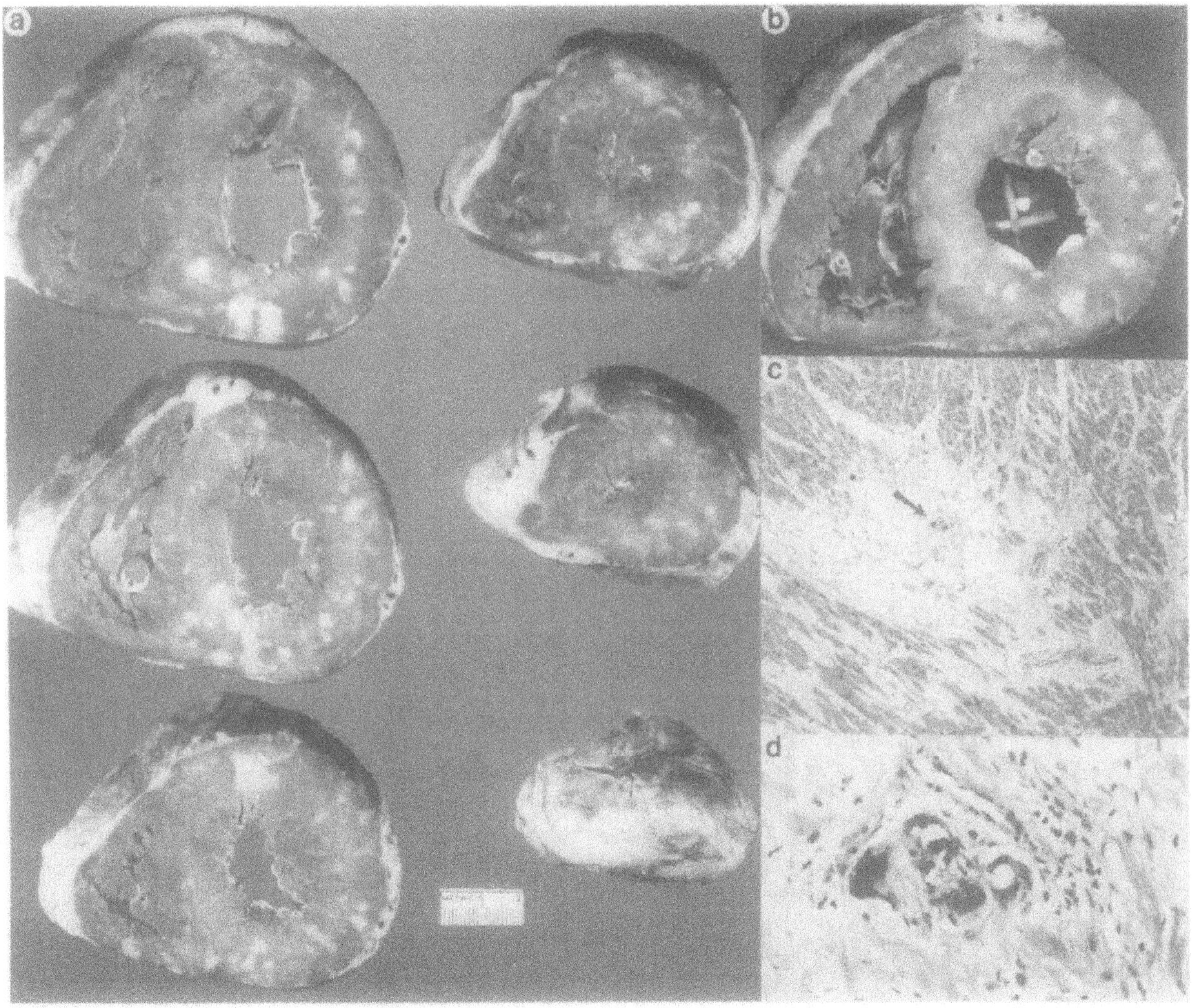

FIGURE 2. Ventricular myocardium in the patient described. *a*, views of the cardiac ventricles after transverse cutting showing numerous focal scars (*white*) in the walls of both ventricles. *b*, the most basal section showing the Starr-Edwards prosthetic valve in the mitral position. The cloth covering the struts of this valve is intact. *c*, photomicrograph of a portion of left ventricular myocardium showing a focal scar, in the center of which is basophilic staining, foreign body material (*arrow*) surrounded by multinucleated giant cells. *d*, higher power magnification of the embolized foreign-body material and associated giant cells seen in *c*. Hematoxylin and eosin stains, × 32 (*c*), × 250 (*d*).

to 179 mm (mean 164); atrial fibrillation was present in 5 and sinus rhythm in 3 of these 8 electrocardiograms. Two electrocardiograms recorded after the pacemaker was inserted showed total 12-lead QRS amplitudes of 199 and 213 mm, respectively.

At necropsy, the heart weighed 545 g. The epicardial coronary arteries were virtually devoid of atherosclerotic plaques. Cloth wear on both struts and rings was severe on both prostheses (Figure 1). There were numerous focal scars measuring 1 to 10 mm in the myocardial walls of both ventricles (Figure 2). Histologic examination revealed focal fibrosis and scattered basophilic staining, slightly refractile, foreign body material occluding small intramyocardial arteries, often surrounded by multinucleated giant cells (Figure 2). By polarized light this basophilic material was anisotropic and typical of cloth fragment. Histologic examination of the kidneys and brain disclosed similar foreign body material associated with multinucleated giant cells. The foreign body emboli in these organs was not associated with gross or microscopic scars. No foreign body material was found in lung, liver, spleen, pancreas or thyroid gland.

The extensive focal right and left ventricular wall scarring in this patient is presumed to have resulted from multiple cloth emboli dislodged from the cardiac valve prostheses. Despite these multiple emboli, there were no clinical or electrocardiographic consequences.

1. Niles NR, Sandilands JR. Pathology of heart valve replacement surgery: autopsies of 62 patients with Starr-Edwards prostheses. *Dis Chest 1969;56:373–382.*

2. Niles NR. Teflon embolism from Starr-Edwards valves. *J Thorac Cardiovasc Surg 1970;59:794–799.*

3. Boruchow IB, Ramsey HW, Wheat MW Jr. Complications following destruction of the cloth covering of a Starr-Edwards aortic valve prosthesis. *J Thorac Cardiovasc Surg 1971;62:290–293.*

4. Thomas CS Jr, Killen DA, Alford WC Jr, Burrus GR, Stoney WS. Cloth disruption in the Starr-Edwards composite mitral valve prosthesis. *Ann Thorac Surg 1973;15:434–438.*

5. Crawford FA, Sethi GK, Scott SM, Takaro T. Systemic emboli due to cloth wear in a Starr-Edwards Model 2320 aortic prosthesis. *Ann Thorac Surg 1973;16:614–619.*

6. Shah A, Dolgin M, Tice DA, Trehan N. Complications due to cloth wear in cloth-covered Starr-Edwards aortic and mitral valve prostheses and their management. *Am Heart J 1978;96:407–414.*

7. Huber S, Burckhardt D, Raeder EA, Follath F, Hasse J, Gradel E. Complications in patients with cloth-covered Starr-Edwards prostheses. *J Cardiovasc Surg 1980;21:19–24.*

8. Siegel RJ, Roberts WC. Electrocardiographic observations in severe aortic valve stenosis: correlative necropsy study to clinical, hemodynamic, and ECG variables demonstrating relation of 12-lead QRS amplitude to peak systolic transaortic pressure gradient. *Am Heart J 1982;103:210–221.*

Mitral Valve Replacement for Mitral Lipoma Associated with Severe Obesity

Allen L. Dollar, MD, Robert B. Wallace, MD, Kenneth M. Kent, MD, Michael W. Burkhart, MD, and William C. Roberts, MD

Adipose tissue is present in every mammalian heart. Its amount tends to increase with age. The most common location of fat in the heart is the subepicardium, particularly in the areas of the epicardial coronary arteries. Sometimes the subepicardial fat is so extensive that none of the myocardium covering the cardiac ventricles is visible. Occasionally the subepicardial fat is so extensive that it causes the heart to float in water.[1] Most patients with extensive subepicardial fat also have fat between clumps of myocardial cells in the right ventricular wall. Additionally, some patients have fat on the mural endocardium of right ventricle and, occasionally, left ventricle. Another common location of cardiac fat is the atrial septum. When fat deposits in the most cephalad portion of the atrial septum are large, the phrase "lipomatous hypertrophy of the atrial septum" has been applied.

From the Pathology Branch, National Heart, Lung, and Blood Institute, National Institutes of Health, Bethesda, Maryland 20892; the Departments of Surgery and Medicine (Cardiology), Georgetown University Medical Center, Washington, DC; and the Department of Medicine, City Hospital, Martinsburg, West Virginia. Manuscript received June 28, 1989; revised manuscript received and accepted August 24, 1989.

A rare location of cardiac fat is a cardiac valve. Although foam cells are commonly observed on the ventricular aspects of the mitral leaflets and on the aortic aspects of the aortic valve cusps, fatty tumorous deposits involving the mitral valve are extremely rare and no reports have described such tumors on a semilunar valve. At least 2 patients have been reported to have "lipomas" on 1 or more tricuspid valve leaflets.[2,3] At least 3 patients with either "lipomas" or "fibrolipomas" involving the mitral valve have been described.[4–6] All 3 previously reported patients with mitral lipomas had mitral regurgitation and each had mitral valve replacement. The present report describes another patient with a mitral lipoma excised at operation and briefly summarizes previously reported cases.

A 66-year-old obese (64 inches [163 cm] tall, 197 pounds [90 kg]) white woman, who had been well all her life, sought medical care after having 4 months of dyspnea (without chest pain) on climbing stairs or walking briskly. A grade 3/6 precordial murmur consistent with mitral regurgitation was heard. An echocardiogram (Figure 1) showed a 2-cm echo-dense mass "attached" to the posterior mitral leaflet and a smaller mass attached to a chorda tendinea arising from the posterior leaflet. The anterior leaflet was normal and both leaflets had good mobility. Mild mitral regurgitation was detected by pulsed Doppler examination. The other 3 cardiac valves were normal as were all 4 cardiac chamber sizes. Left ventricular contractility was normal. Chest radiograph (Figure 2) disclosed the cardiac silhouette to be enlarged and the subcutaneous tissues to be excessive. There were no symptoms or signs of infective endocarditis. At catheterization, the pressures (in mm Hg) were as follows: right atrial mean 9, A wave 15, V wave 12, right ventricle 45/12, pulmonary artery 50/25, and systemic artery 120/60. The cardiac index was 2.0 liters/min/m^2. Coronary angiograms showed normal epicardial coronary arteries. The systemic arterial saturation was 88% and the blood hematocrit was 33%. The mitral valve was excised and replaced with a Medtronic Hall prosthesis.

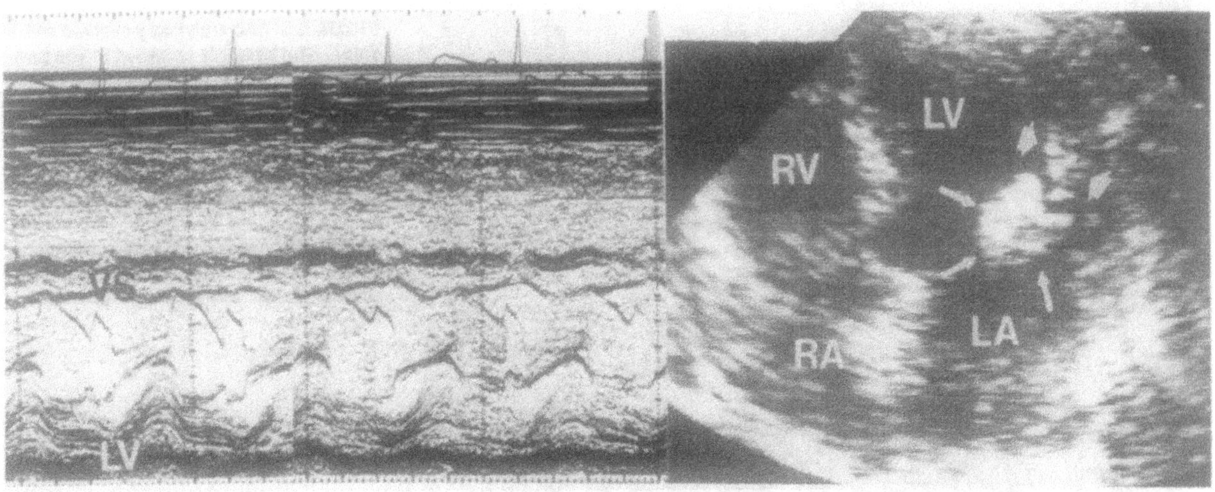

FIGURE 1. M-mode echocardiogram (*left*) showing the mitral valve leaflets (which do not appear thickened) and echo densities intermittently seen in the mitral orifice. LV = left ventricular wall; VS = ventricular septum. Apical 4-chamber (with aorta) 2-dimensional echocardiogram (*right*) showing a 2-cm echo-dense mass (*longer arrows*) attached to the posterior mitral leaflet and a smaller echo-dense mass (*shorter arrows*) associated with a chorda tendinea. LA = left atrial cavity; LV = left ventricular cavity; RA = right atrial cavity; RV = right ventricular cavity.

The posterior leaflet of the mitral valve (Figure 3) contained a lobular, yellow, firm mass measuring 2.2 × 1.7 × 0.5 cm. A second smaller mass, similar in composition, surrounded a chorda tendinea arising from the posterior leaflet. The posterior mitral leaflet together with the attached tumor weighed 2.0 g, and both leaflets with their attached chordae weighed 2.7 g. The posterior leaflet also was focally thickened by fibrous tissue and had outpouchings or "hoods." The anterior leaflet was normal. Microscopic examination of the mass (Figure 4) showed it to be a lipoma with well-differentiated adipose cells and a few fibrous septae.

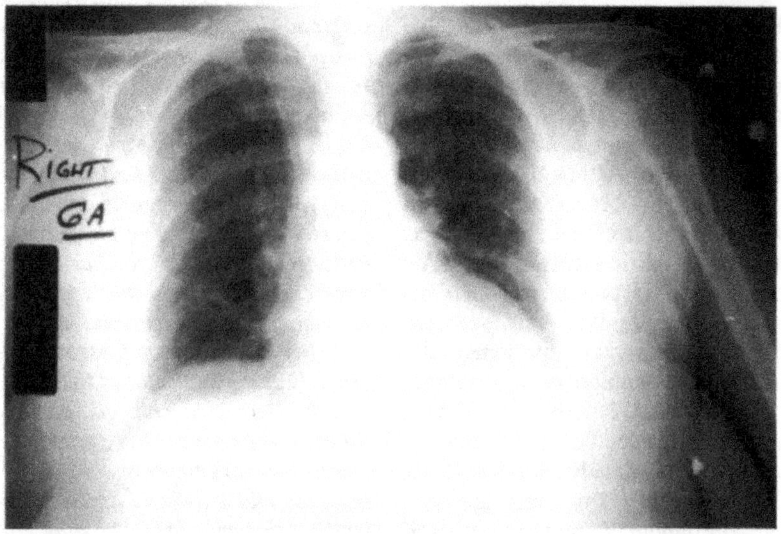

FIGURE 2. Chest x-ray showing an enlarged cardiac silhouette and markedly increased subcutaneous adipose tissue.

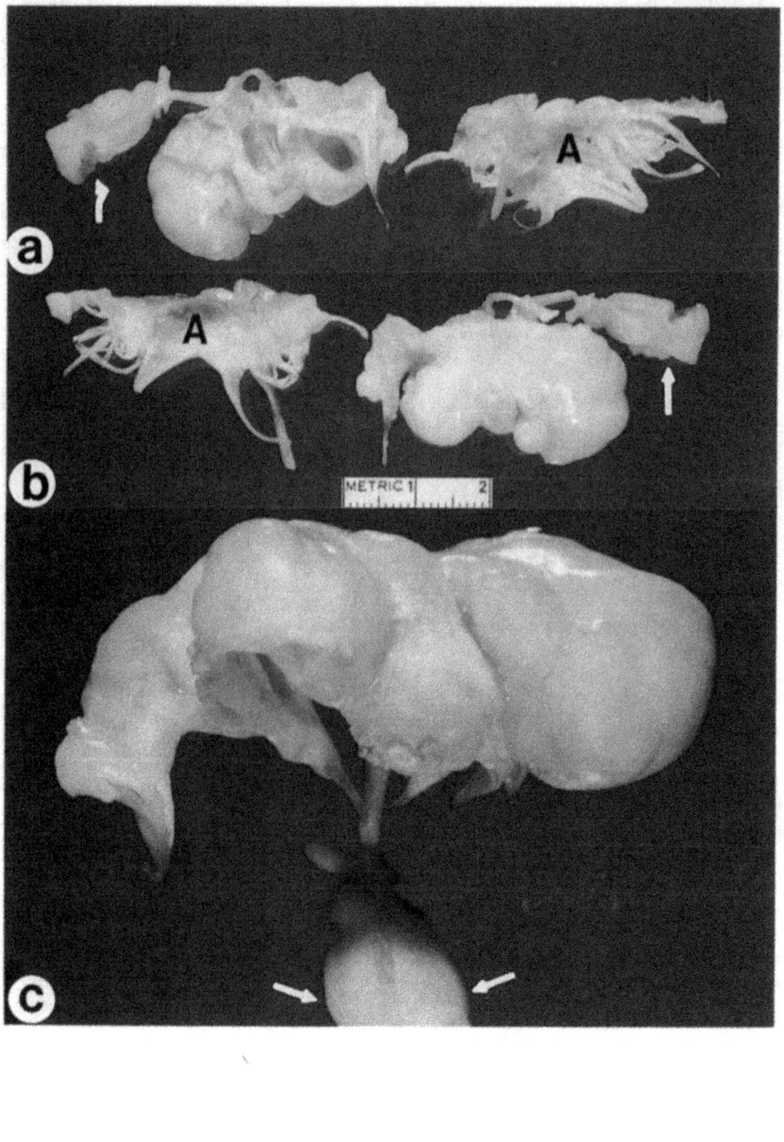

FIGURE 3. The surgically excised mitral valve. The tumor is confined to the posterior leaflet and an associated chorda tendinea (*arrows*). The underlying posterior mitral leaflet is thickened by fibrous tissue and contains out-pouchings or "hoods." The anterior (A) leaflet is normal. *a*, ventricular aspect. *b*, atrial aspect. *c*, close-up view of the atrial aspect of the posterior mitral leaflet and attached tumor. Small calcific deposits are present on the margins of the leaflet.

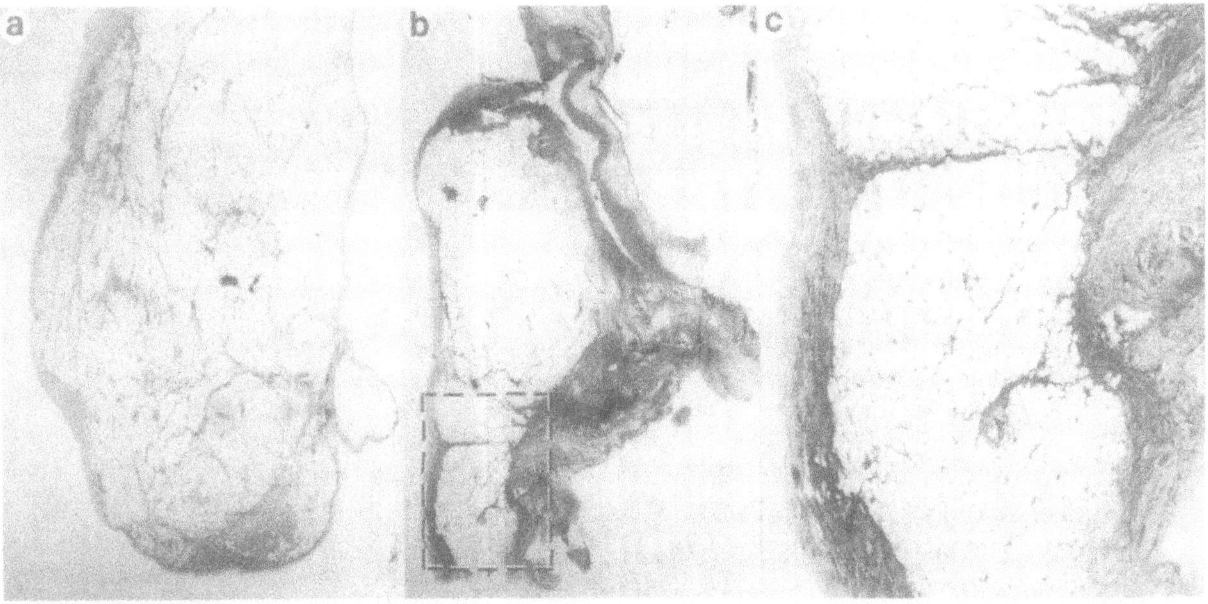

FIGURE 4. Photomicrographs of transverse sections of the tumor seen in Figure 3 showing a typical lipoma with mature adipose cells. The lipoma is *within* the leaflet, not attached to its surface. *a* and *b*, 2 different histologic sections of the tumor. *c*, higher-power magnification of the *area in brackets* shown in *b*. Hematoxylin and eosin stains; × 8 (*a,b*); × 32 (*c*).

The fatty tumors involving the mitral valve in the aforementioned patient and in each of the 3 previously reported patients were nonspecific echo-dense masses on echocardiogram. In 2 previously reported patients, a 12-year-old boy[4] and a 16-year-old girl,[5] the lipomas were limited to posterior mitral leaflet and to the posteromedial papillary muscle. In a previously reported 54-year-old man,[6] the lipoma involved both mitral leaflets and adjacent left ventricular myocardial wall. None of these 3 patients was obese. The 2 younger patients were asymptomatic but had precordial murmurs. The man had a dizzy episode that led to cardiac evaluation. Only 1 of the 3 previously reported patients had severe mitral regurgitation, and our patient had only mild regurgitation. In a previously reported patient with a mitral lipoma, the fatty nature of the tumor was revealed by computed tomography.[6]

1. Roberts WC, Roberts JD. The floating heart or the heart too fat to sink: analysis of 55 necropsy patients. *Am J Cardiol 1983;52:1286–1289.*
2. Verliac H, Morel L. Étude sur le lipome du coeur. *Arch Mal Coeur 1909;2:152–161.*
3. Esteves JM, Thompson DS, Levinson JP. Lipoma of the heart. *Arch Pathol 1964;77:638–642.*
4. Barberger-Gateau P, Paquet M, Desaulniers D, Chenard J. Fibrolipoma of the mitral valve in a child: clinical and echocardiographic features. *Circulation 1978;58:955–958.*
5. Behnam R, Williams G, Gerlis L, Walker D, Scott O. Lipoma of the mitral valve and papillary muscle. *Am J Cardiol 1983;51:1459–1460.*
6. Anderson DR, Gray MR. Mitral incompetence associated with lipoma infiltrating the mitral valve. *Br Heart J 1988;60:169–171.*

MORPHOLOGIC ABNORMALITIES IN EXPLANTED BIOPROSTHETIC HEART VALVES

VICTOR J. FERRANS, M.D., PH.D., STEPHEN L. HILBERT, PH.D., SHINSUKE FUJITA, M.D., PH.D., MICHAEL JONES, M.D., and WILLIAM C. ROBERTS, M.D.

A description of the normal and abnormal anatomic features of bioprosthetic (BP) heart valves is presented in this chapter, with emphasis on cuspal calcification and perforation, which are the major complications of their use. The following types of bioprosthetic (tissue) heart valves are considered: porcine aortic valvular bioprostheses, bovine and porcine parietal pericardial bioprosthetic valves, human dura mater valves, fascia lata valves, and human aortic homografts. Before describing the normal and abnormal features of these types of bioprosthetic valves, an outline is given of the techniques that are useful for their morphologic evaluation.

TECHNIQUES OF EXAMINATION

Systematic anatomic study should be made of the heart before the bioprosthetic valve itself is detached from its site of implantation. Certain important abnormalities can be detected only by *in situ* study of the implanted valve. Immediately after detachment from the heart, or after operative removal, a decision should be made as to whether it is necessary to obtain a microbiologic culture before the bioprosthetic valve is placed in a fixative solution. A mixture of 4% formaldehyde and 1% glutaraldehyde (McDowell-Trump solution)[1] is recommended when both light and electron microscopic studies are to be made of the same specimen, since it results in adequate fixation for electron microscopy without interfering with certain light microscopic stains such as the Masson, Movat, hematoxylin and eosin, and elastic fiber methods, all of which give poor results after fixation with glutaraldehyde alone. Visual inspection and gross photography of the inflow and outflow aspects of the bioprosthetic valve are followed by examination (and photography, as indicated by the findings) using a dissecting microscope at magnifications of 2× to 40×. Some features, such as small tears, thrombi, and calcific deposits, cannot be adequately observed by visual inspection without this magnification.

Radiographic examination is then performed using a Faxitron unit (Hewlett-Packard). It is important to use the proper exposure conditions to obtain adequate contrast of the calcific deposits and to distinguish them from soft tissue shadows. In radiographs of porcine bioprosthetic valves, calcific deposits in the basal regions of the cusps and in the aortic wall often appear superimposed and must be distinguished by taking radiographs after the individual cusps have been detached. Small, diffusely distributed calcific deposits may not be easily evident on radiographic study. Examination of von Kossa-stained sections is the most sensitive morphologic technique for detecting minimal calcification of cuspal tissue.

After the radiographic study is completed, the cusps are detached from the stent, radiographed again to further define the patterns of calcification, and cut for histologic study. Our usual practice is to obtain at least one section from the middle third of each cusp. This section is oriented from the base to the free edge. Sections from additional areas may be taken as needed. Additional cuts from the base to the free edge can be taken and processed for transmission and scanning electron microscopic study and for quantitative analysis of calcium and phosphorus content. For the latter, the sample consists of one half of each cusp, selected at random and submitted separately after careful dissection to remove the aortic wall from the base of the cusp. This large sample size is necessary to minimize variance in the quantitative data.[2, 3]

For histologic study, the sample is embedded in glycol methacrylate, after which 1-μm thick sections are cut with glass knives and stained with hematoxylin and eosin, alkaline toluidine blue, and the von Kossa method. Giemsa, Masson trichrome, and periodic acid–Schiff stains also can be made using these plastic sections; however, other connective tissue stains such as the Masson and Movat methods do not give satisfactory results. These tissues are not decalcified routinely. Paraffin embedding and histologic sectioning result in preparations of less satisfactory quality, owing to the hardness of the tissue.

The sample for transmission electron microscopy is subdivided into three pieces, which consist of the basal, middle, and distal thirds of the cusp. These pieces are washed with several changes of phosphate buffer, postfixed with osmium tetroxide in phosphate buffer, dehydrated, and embedded in epoxy resin. Flat embedding molds are used to orient the specimen so that the plane of sectioning includes both surfaces and the full thickness of the cusp. The 1-μm thick sections are cut and examined by light microscopy to select areas for ultrathin sectioning. Ultrathin sections are cut with a diamond knife, mounted on copper grids, and stained either with uranyl acetate and lead citrate or according to the Kajikawa method for the electron microscopic demonstration of elastic fibers.[4] For scanning electron microscopy, the sample is divided into two pieces in order to examine both cuspal surfaces. It is feasible to examine both surfaces of a single specimen.[5] The tissues are prepared by dehydration using the critical point drying method, followed by coating with carbon and gold-palladium.

ABNORMALITIES EVIDENT ON *IN SITU* EXAMINATION OF THE BIOPROSTHESIS

Abnormalities that are best (or only) diagnosed by *in situ* examination of the implanted bioprosthetic valve include perivalvular leak, obstruction to the left ventricular outflow tract or of a coronary ostium by a strut, entanglement of sutures, disproportion, abnormal angulation of the bioprosthesis, and compression of an anomalous left main or left circumflex coronary artery by the fixation rings of one or more bioprostheses.

Perivalvular Leak (Para-annular Prosthetic Ring Discontinuity)

A peribasilar leak may result from the use of too few sutures to secure the bioprosthesis and from inadequate placement or from pulling loose of sutures between the patient's tissues and the bioprosthetic sewing ring.[6] Peribasilar leaks (Fig. 17–1) tend to occur in instances in which the sutures are placed in tissues that are abnormal because of infection, extensive calcific deposits, or preexisting connective tissue disorders, such as Marfan's syndrome or valvular prolapse (floppy valves). However, they also can develop in patients who have papillary muscle dysfunction and normal perivalvular tissues.[6] Residual glutaraldehyde may remain in tissue valves after prolonged storage, even after careful preimplantation washing of the bioprosthesis,[7] and it has been suggested that it exerts toxic effects, including induction of necrosis of the host tissues of the valve ring, which are directly in contact with the sewing ring; such a necrosis could evolve into a perivalvular leak.

Abnormal Angulation

Angulation of a bioprosthetic valve can result from insertion and suturing of the valve away from the usual axis. This can take place when the annulus is distorted by calcification, infection, or dense scarring. Angulation also can result from partial detachment of sutures because of infection associated with a ring abscess.

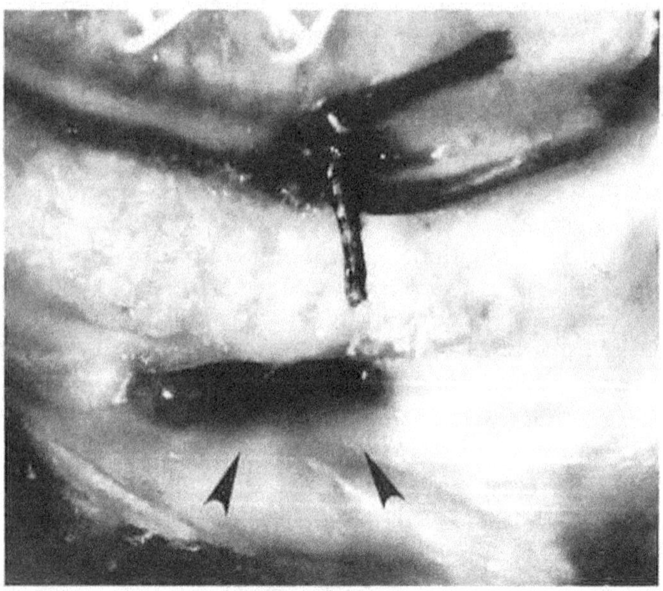

Figure 17–1. Peribasilar leak appears as dark space *(arrowheads)* just peripheral to sewing ring of bioprosthetic valve that had been implanted in a sheep for 20 weeks.

Disproportion and Hemodynamic Obstruction

Nearly all bioprosthetic valves present some degree of obstruction to forward flow and some degree (usually minimal) of regurgitant flow. The central flow pattern of bioprosthetic valves generally provides good hemodynamic function, but valves of small sizes may cause significant reduction in flow because the sewing ring and struts may occupy a larger fraction of the total orifice area of the bioprosthesis than is the case in larger-sized bioprostheses. Disproportion occurs when the substitute cardiac valve is too large for the ventricle or ascending aorta into which it is inserted.

Obstruction to a coronary ostium (Fig. 17–2) can result from malpositioning of the stent in a bioprosthesis implanted in the aortic position.[6] The left ventricular outflow tract may be obstructed (Fig. 17–3) by a strut of a bioprosthesis that has not been placed properly in the mitral position.[6, 8] Low profile bioprostheses are less likely to cause this complication. Compression of an anomalous left main or left circumflex coronary artery by mitral and aortic prosthetic rings is a rare complication of double valvular replacement.[6] Obstruction to flow through the central orifice of a bioprosthesis can result from progressive inward bending of polypropylene stents (Fig. 17–4).[9]

Ventricular Rupture and Ventricular Aneurysms

Ventricular rupture and ventricular aneurysms, both of which can be located at the level of the atrioventricular groove, at the site of excision of one or both papillary muscles, or midway between the mitral ring and the stumps of the papillary muscles, are major complications of mitral valvular replacement with any kind of prosthetic valve.[10] Both of these lesions can be caused by compression of the left ventricular wall by the struts of bioprosthetic valves at the time of valvular replacement (Fig. 17–5).[11]

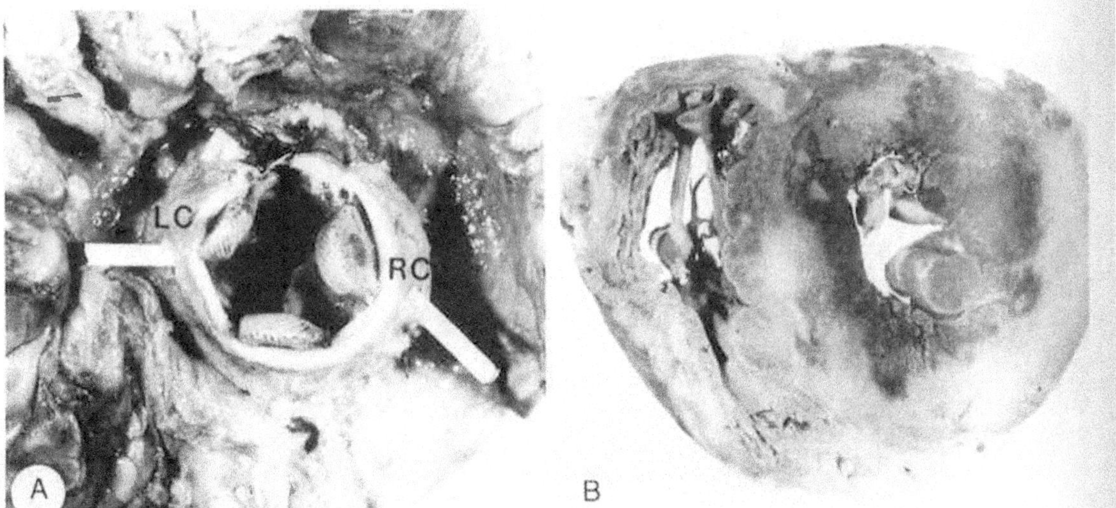

Figure 17–2. Coronary ostial occlusion by the struts of a 27-mm bioprosthetic valve in the aortic position in a 63-year-old woman who had had aortic stenosis. The patient died with pulmonary edema 36 hours after operation. *A.* View of the aortic prosthesis from above. A Teflon patch was used to attempt to widen the aorta. White sticks indicate the origins of the right and left coronary arteries (*RC* and *LC*). *B.* Section of ventricles showing extensive circumferential hemorrhagic necrosis.

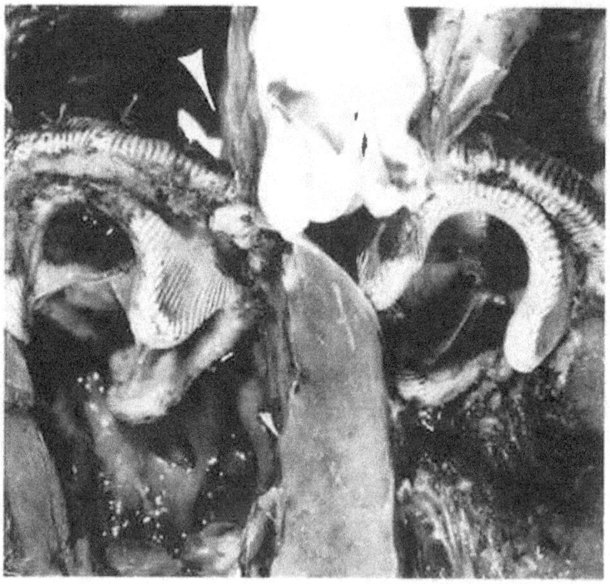

Figure 17–3. Partial obstruction to left ventricular outflow was produced by one strut of the mitral bioprosthetic valve in a woman who had mitral and tricuspid valve replacements who died 4 days later with a low cardiac output state. Prosthetic disproportion also occurred, as shown by the fact that the sewing rings of both prostheses appeared to indent the aorta *(arrowheads)* just above the valve.

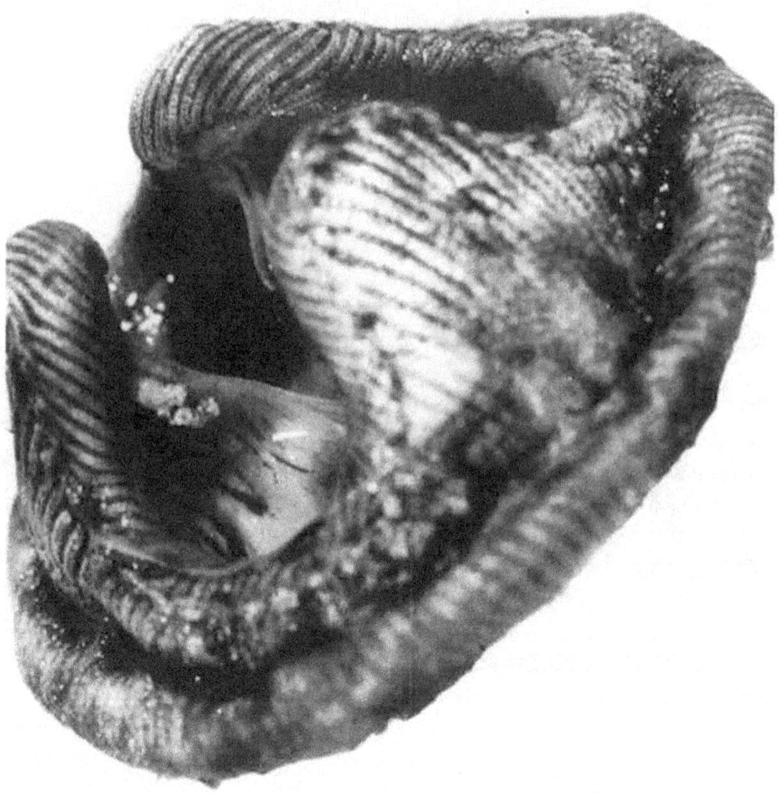

Figure 17–4. Marked inward bending of all three struts is evident in Hancock bioprosthetic valve that was removed 5.7 years after implantation in the mitral position.

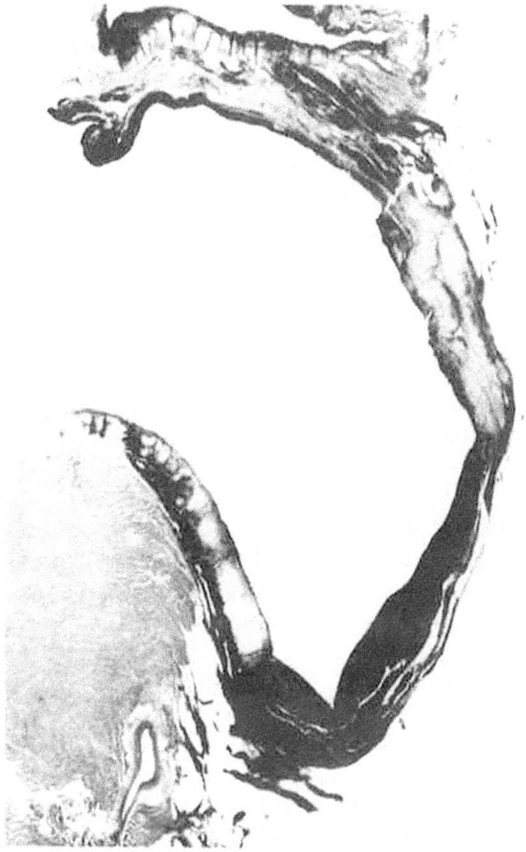

Figure 17–5. Low magnification view of histologic section through aneurysm that developed in left ventricular posterior wall of sheep that had a bovine pericardial bioprosthesis implanted in the mitral position. The wall of the aneurysm consists of collagenous and elastic tissue, and the circumflex coronary artery *(bottom left)* courses caudal to the aneurysm.

STRUCTURE OF UNIMPLANTED BIOPROSTHESES

Before describing the pathologic changes that develop in implanted bioprosthetic valves, it is convenient to review briefly the morphologic features of normal, unimplanted bioprostheses. Porcine bioprostheses, pericardial bioprostheses, fascia lata valves, and dura mater valves have all been configured as trileaflet valves, regardless of the valve position in which they are implanted. The only exceptions to this generalization are the pericardial unicusp or unileaflet valve[12] and the bicuspid pericardial valve;[13] neither has been used extensively. Most bioprostheses undergo preimplantation chemical treatment—porcine bioprostheses and pericardial bioprostheses with 0.25% to 0.6% glutaraldehyde and dura mater valves with glycerol. Homografts are sterilized, usually with antibiotics (several other methods were found to be less satisfactory), after which they may undergo cryopreservation but are not treated with aldehyde fixatives. Fascia lata valves were used without any chemical treatment. Some types of glutaraldehyde-treated bioprostheses are stored in dilute formaldehyde after processing, to improve sterility, because the antifungal and antibacterial action (especially against spores) of low concentrations of glutaraldehyde is poor.[14, 15] In general, the durability of unfixed or formalin-fixed porcine and pericardial bioprostheses is poor.[16–19] Anticalcification treatments have been devised to mitigate the problem of calcific deposits developing in bioprostheses. These include the preimplantation treatment of the bioprostheses with various chemical agents including surfactants (sodium dodecyl sulfate [T6 process], Tween 80 [PV2 process], Triton X-100 and lauroyl sarcosine), toluidine blue, and diphosphonates, which would be expected to mitigate the calcification of connective tissue in bioprostheses. The use of some of these processes (Triton X-100 and lauroyl sarcosine) has led to early bioprosthesis failure.[20] Clinical trials of valves prepared according to the T6 and PV2 processes are currently in progress. In the sheep model, both processes are effective in mitigating the calcification in porcine aortic valvular bioprostheses but not in pericardial BPs.[2, 3]

The stents on which the bioprosthetic tissue is mounted vary in structural design, flexibility, and composition (plastic and metal) from one manufacturer to another, and among different models of the same bioprosthesis, in which the stents may have been modified (e.g., to make them lower in profile); different stents may be used for the same type of valve according to whether it is to be used in the atrioventricular or the aortic valve position. Similarly, the techniques by which the tissues are attached to the stents vary, particularly among pericardial bioprostheses from different manufacturers (in efforts to minimize chances of cuspal disruption near the stent posts).

Porcine Aortic Valvular Bioprostheses

Glutaraldehyde-treated porcine bioprostheses are the most widely used type of bioprosthesis and consist of a porcine aortic valve and adjacent region of the aortic root. The porcine aortic valve (Fig. 17–6) is asymmetric. The right coronary cusp is larger than the other two cusps; its most basal region contains a layer of ventricular muscle cells that represent an extension of septal muscle and that impart a darker color and a firmer consistency to this region of the cusp (Fig. 17–6*B*). This muscle layer ("muscle shelf") sometimes is also found in the basal regions of the other two cusps. It can cause delayed and less complete opening of the right coronary cusp (compared with the other two cusps) of porcine bioprostheses, and it can become the site of calcific deposits involving the myocytes. For these reasons a "modified orifice valve" has been designed in which the right coronary cusp is removed and replaced by a cusp from another valve; this bioprosthesis has had very limited use. Other attempts have been made to eliminate part of this muscle shelf, either by curetting from the external surface before the valve is mounted on its stent or by tucking it into the sewing ring during mounting.

The porcine aortic valve[18] consists of three layers of tissue: the ventricularis, which faces the inflow side of the valve; the spongiosa, which occupies the central portion of the cusp; and the fibrosa, which faces the outflow surface of the valve (Fig. 17–6*A*). Both surfaces are completely covered by a single layer of endothelial cells. The tissue layers are better defined in the basal and middle thirds than in the distal third of the valve; the free edge may be thickened. The ventricularis contains collagen and elastic fibers. The latter are larger and more prominent than those in the other two layers and serve as a useful marker to identify the tissue layers of porcine bioprostheses. The spongiosa contains collagen, a few elastic fibers, and abundant amounts of proteoglycan material. The fibrosa has dense bundles of collagen as its main structural component. Much of this collagen is arranged parallel to the free edge. These collagen bundles form cords, which become thicker and more prominent as they course toward the commissures. These cords are responsible for the corrugated appearance of the outflow surface of the cusp (especially on scanning electron microscopic examination) and appear as focal thickenings of the fibrosa in the sections from the base to the free edge

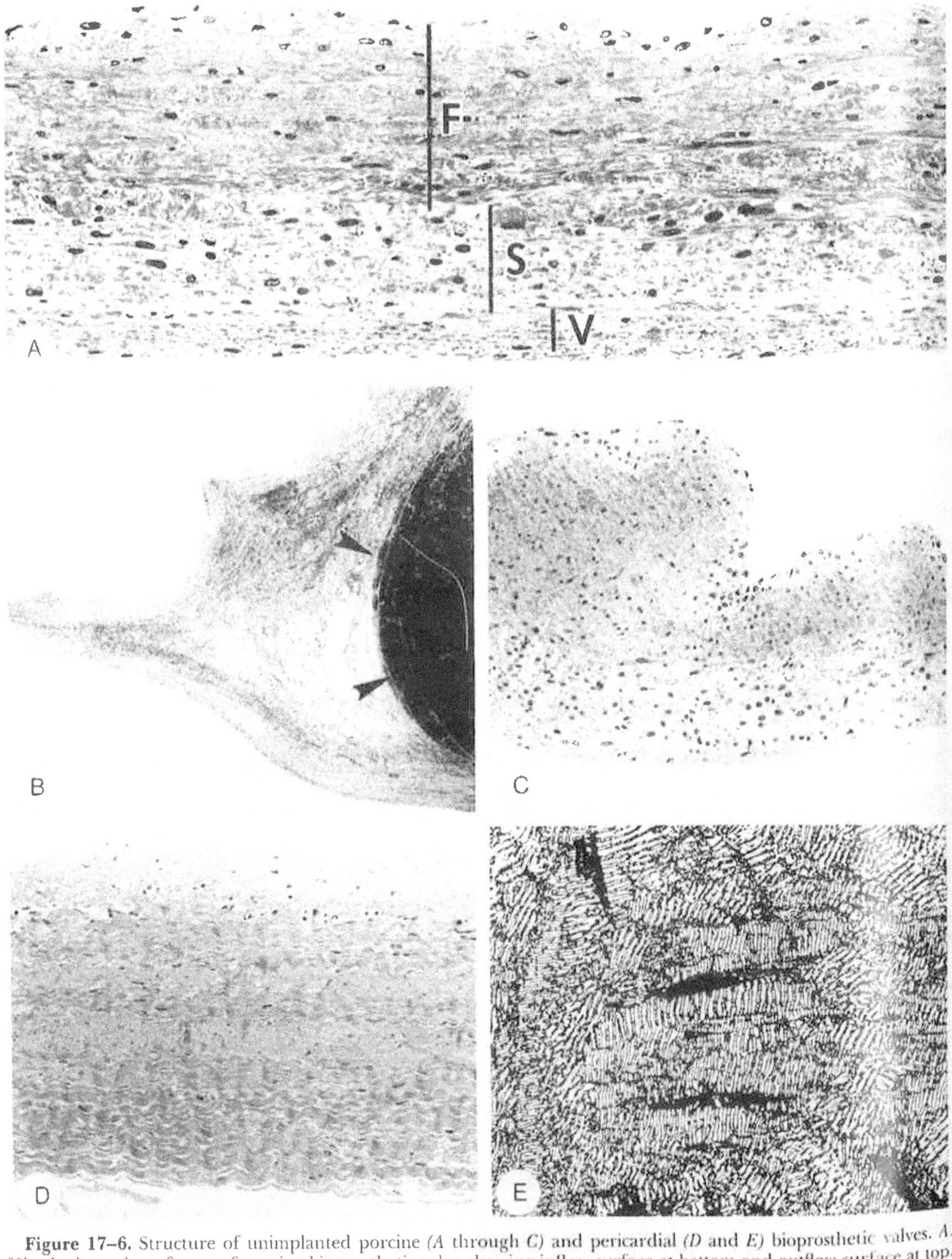

Figure 17–6. Structure of unimplanted porcine *(A* through *C)* and pericardial *(D* and *E)* bioprosthetic valves. *A*. Histologic section of cusp of porcine bioprosthetic valve showing inflow surface at bottom and outflow surface at top. Note the ventricularis *(V)*, the spongiosa *(S)*, and the fibrosa *(F)*. *B*. Basal portion of right coronary cusp showing the darkly stained muscle shelf *(arrowheads)*. *C*. Collagenous cords in cusp are sectioned transversely and appear as focal thickenings of the fibrosa (compare with *A*). *D*. Section of cusp of bovine pericardial bioprosthetic valve showing the inflow surface (the epipericardial layer) at bottom and the outflow surface (serosal layer) at top. The layers of connective tissue are poorly defined. *E*. Polarized light micrograph of section taken parallel to the surface of cusp of pericardial bioprosthetic valve showing multidirectional pattern of birefringence of collagen fibrils. (Hematoxylin and eosin: *A*, ×150; *C* through *E*, ×100 and toluidine blue: *B*, ×25)

of the cusps (Fig. 17–6*C*). Cellular elements in the porcine aortic valve consist of fibroblasts, myofibroblasts, and smooth muscle cells, which usually show poor ultrastructural preservation in commercially processed, unimplanted bioprostheses.[18] As a consequence of postmortem autolysis and preimplantation processing (chemical fixation, tissue handling), the structure of the native porcine valve undergoes several changes,[18] including partial or complete denudation of the endothelial cell layer on both surfaces, partial loss of the proteoglycan material from the spongiosa, loosening of the connective tissue bundles, and a reduction in basophilia and an increase in eosinophilia of all tissue components.

The thickness of the cusps and the waviness of the collagen fibers in porcine bioprostheses depend on the technique of fixation. Bioprostheses fixed by the standard method of fixation under pressure (70 to 80 mm Hg), to maintain the cusps in the fully closed position during the procedure, have thinner cusps, less prominent cords, and less wavy collagen than do bioprostheses fixed without pressure or under very low pressure (< 5 mm Hg). The latter technique has been proposed to minimize mechanical damage to collagen from the bending stresses to which the cusps are subjected, on the premise that such stresses are more evenly distributed in collagen that has a wavy (i.e., nonstretched) as opposed to a linear or stretched configuration.[21] Most porcine bioprostheses implanted up to the present time have been prepared by pressure fixation.

Pericardial Bioprostheses

Practically all pericardial bioprostheses are made of bovine parietal pericardium; the only exception appears to be the Polystan valves, which are made of porcine parietal pericardium and are used as parts of valved conduits that also have an inner lining of parietal pericardium.[22] The thickness of the cusps is greater in pericardial bioprostheses than in porcine bioprostheses. Parietal pericardium[23, 24] is composed of the serosal layer, which is formed by mesothelial cells; the fibrosa, which contains collagen, elastic fibers, nerves, blood vessels and lymphatics; and the epipericardial connective tissue, which has more loosely arranged collagen and elastic fibers (Fig. 17–6*D*). Thin, elongated fibroblasts are present in the pericardial fibrosa and epipericardial connective tissue layer, together with occasional adipose tissue cells, histiocytes, and mast cells. During preimplantation processing the mesothelial cell layer is partially or completely lost and the denuded serosal surface (i.e., that which faces the epicardial surface) appears smoother than the epipericardial surface. This difference is evident in histologic preparations but is particularly striking on scanning electron microscopic study, which reveals exposed basement membrane and collagen fibrils in the serosal surface and large, coarse bundles of collagen in the epipericardial surface. In pericardial bioprostheses, the serosal surface corresponds to the outflow surface of the valve and the rougher epipericardial surface corresponds to the inflow surface.[23, 24] The collagen fibrils in parietal pericardium (Fig. 17–6*E*) form relatively short bundles that are multidirectional and overlapping rather than highly oriented and well layered.[25]

Dura Mater Valves

Normal human dura mater is composed of two distinct layers: an outer or endosteal layer and an inner or meningeal layer.[26] The outer layer contains large bundles of collagenous fibers and constitutes about two thirds of the total thickness of the dura. About 50% of the bundles in this layer appear oriented in the same direction; the other 50% are multidirectional. The inner layer is thinner and has smaller bundles of collagen, many of which are arranged irregularly, often obliquely or at right angles to the main direction of orientation of the bundles in the outer layer. In some areas the two layers of the dura are closely apposed; in others they are separated by spaces of variable width. Blood vessels are present in some of these spaces. In both layers the collagen is wavy, elastic fibers are few and small, and proteoglycan content (judged by staining with alcian blue) is low. Cellular elements in dura mater are scarce and consist of elongated fibroblasts with spindle-shaped nuclei and scanty cytoplasm. On scanning electron microscopic examination, the endosteal layer shows a pattern of ridges and grooves that correspond to vascular elements. The meningeal surface is much flatter and smoother, and no cells are evident on this surface in dura mater valves. These valves have been used extensively in Latin America,[27–29] and in a clinical trial in England, they were frequently found to develop cuspal tears.[30, 31] Their use has decreased sharply in recent years.

Fascia Lata Valves

Fascia lata valves constructed of three cusps of autologous fascia lata mounted on a stent were used 20 years ago, but their use has been discontinued because of poor results, due to overgrowth of fibrous sheath of host origin and disintegration of cuspal connective tissue.[32–36] Fascia lata is composed of parallel arrays of collagen fibrils and a few associated fibroblasts; elastic fibers are few and small.[33]

Homografts

Human aortic valve homografts consist of a sleeve of tissue containing the aortic valve and a portion of ascending aorta; this sleeve is trimmed just below the cuspal attachments and is scalloped along its upper border into anchoring projections above the cuspal commissures. The cells in the graft have pale nuclei, but the collagen and elastic fibers are morphologically similar to those of normal aorta.[37–43]

POSTIMPLANTATION CHANGES IN BIOPROSTHESES

Many pathologic changes that occur in bioprostheses implanted as substitute cardiac valves are common to all types of these devices, reflecting three basic facts: (1) collagen is the most important structural element in these valves; (2) in bioprostheses there is no synthetic or renewal mechanism (such as that provided by the fibroblasts present in native valves) to replace the collagen that is gradually broken down, either because of proteolysis (although glutaraldehyde-treated collagen is very resistant to the effects of proteolytic enzymes) or because of the mechanical stresses to which the cusps are subjected; thus, the cumulative effect of this gradual breakdown can lead to the formation of cuspal tears and perforations; and (3) collagen in implanted bioprostheses tends to undergo a time-dependent process of focal calcification, which may result in stenosis and/or regurgitation and loss of mobility of the cusps.[18, 44–54]

Within a few days after implantation, bioprostheses become covered with a layer of fibrin, platelets, and a few erythrocytes; inflammatory cells usually are relatively few and consist mainly of macrophages and multinucleated giant cells; lymphocytes and plasma cells are scarce, as are neutrophils (Fig. 17–7*A* and *B*).[18] The presence of neutrophils in implanted bioprostheses is highly suggestive of infection. Plasma cells were relatively numerous in the bioprostheses of children who were considered to have an immunologic reaction to the bioprostheses;[55] such cases, however, are rare and there is little evidence to suggest that rejection or an immunologic reaction are of importance in the pathogenesis of calcification or other postimplantation changes.[56] Most leukocytes and macrophages remain confined to the surfaces, with little tendency to infiltrate the bioprosthetic tissue.[18] Clusters of

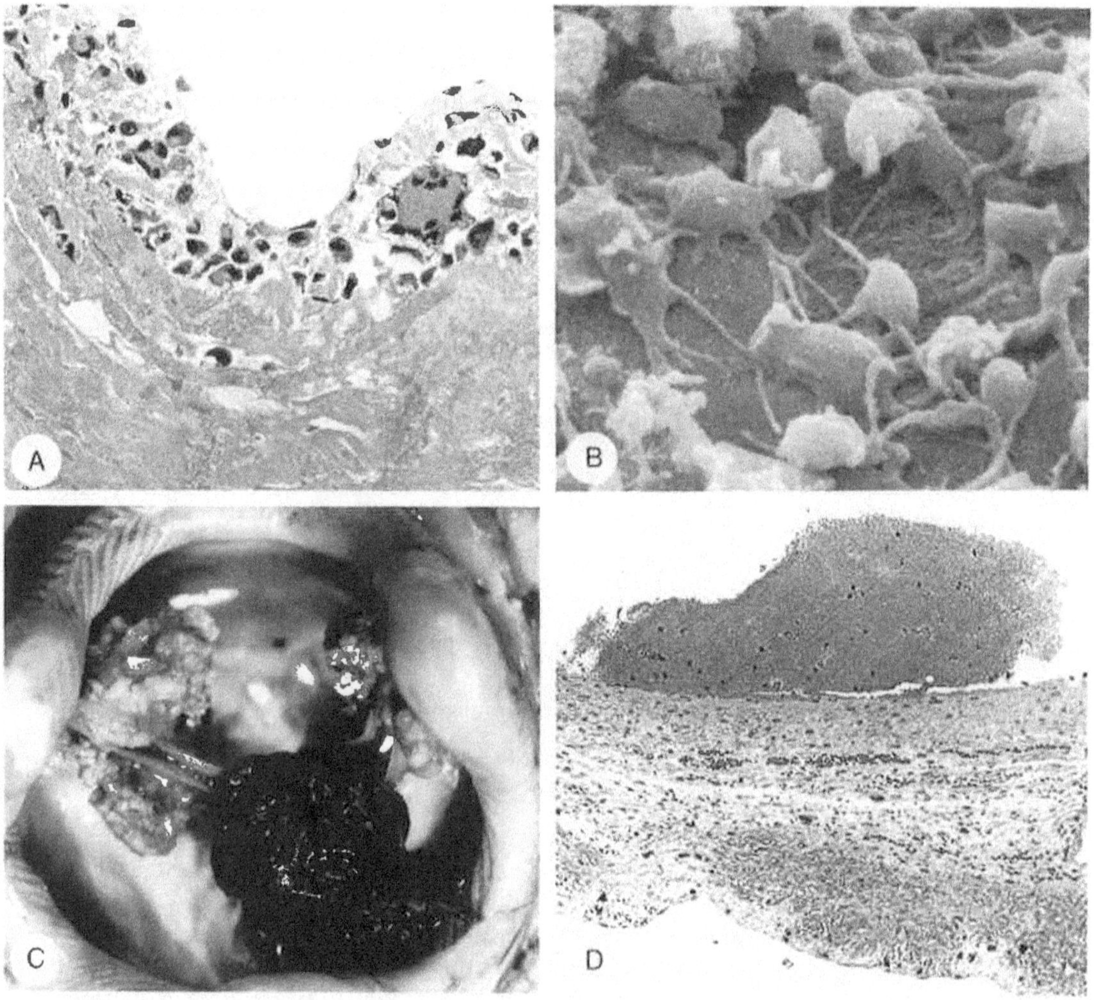

Figure 17–7. Cells *(A* and *B)* and thrombi *(C* and *D)* adherent to the surfaces of porcine bioprosthetic valves. *A*. Macrophages and multinucleated giant cells line the surface of a bioprosthetic valve implanted in a sheep for 20 weeks. *B*. Scanning electron micrograph (×2800) showing numerous platelets on the surface of a bioprosthetic valve removed because of dysfunction after being implanted for 76 months in the mitral position. *C*. A large thrombus and several calcific nodules, which are localized in the vicinity of the commissures, are present on outflow aspect of bioprosthetic valve that had been implanted for 5 years in the mitral position. *D*. Microthrombus is shown on the surface of bioprosthetic valve that had been implanted in a sheep for 20 weeks. (Hematoxylin and eosin: *A*, ×250; *D*, ×100)

lymphocytes, macrophages, and a few plasma cells are sometimes found in connective tissue of host origin at the junction between valve tissue and the sewing ring, particularly in the right coronary cusp of porcine bioprostheses. Multinucleated giant cells also may be numerous in these areas, where they may be associated with suture materials. In addition to the changes just described, plasma proteins penetrate into the substance of the bioprostheses because of the absence of an endothelial cell barrier, and the connective tissue structure becomes somewhat looser than in unimplanted bioprostheses. The surfaces of the implants may become gradually endothelialized, particularly in the basal regions of the cusps, and also may become covered with a fibrous sheath of host origin. This process may take from several months to several years.[57]

Aggregates of platelets also may develop on nonendothelialized regions of the surfaces, where they are in direct contact with collagen fibrils that form part of the surfaces.[18, 58, 59] This finding is not surprising in view of the tendency of collagen to induce platelet aggregation. This tendency is minimized by preimplantation treatment of bioprostheses with glutaraldehyde.[58] Activation, spreading and hyperactive responses of platelets, and circulating aggregates of platelets have been reported in some patients with bioprostheses, particularly in those with degenerated implants.[58] The clinical significance of these findings remains uncertain.

Thrombi in Bioprostheses and Embolic Phenomena

Although the lack of need for the use of anticoagulants is often cited as one of the advantageous features of bioprostheses, compared with mechanical heart valves, thrombi (Fig. 17–7*C* and *D*) and thromboembolic episodes do occur in patients with implanted bioprostheses, even in those receiving anticoagulants, but less frequently than in patients with mechanical valves.[29, 45–47, 50, 51, 54, 60–62] Thrombi in bioprosthetic valves may occur as early or late postimplantation phenomena. They tend to be localized on the outflow surfaces of the cusps and may be associated with calcific deposits.

Fatal coronary embolization was reported to have been caused by fragments of textile fibers from the packing material in a bioprosthesis.[63] Cotton fibers have been found to become adherent to the surfaces of pericardial bioprostheses, even after implantation.[23]

Bioprosthetic Infection

Infection of an implanted bioprosthesis (Fig. 17–8) continues to be a major complication of cardiac valvular replacement.[64–71] The overall incidence of infection is generally similar in patients with mechanical valves and in patients with bioprostheses.[69, 70]

The characteristics of infection differ in mechanical valves and in bioprostheses.[65–68] In mechanical valve prostheses, the infection involves the periprosthetic tissues, primarily at the site of attachment of the sewing ring to the tissue (valve ring abscess). Infection does not destroy mechanical valves, but it may cause them to malfunction and to become detached from the annulus. In contrast, infection of bioprostheses can involve the bioprosthetic cusps as well as fibrin, surface thrombi, or fibrous sheath of host origin. It also can involve the site of attachment of the sewing ring to host tissue. Thus, it can cause cuspal

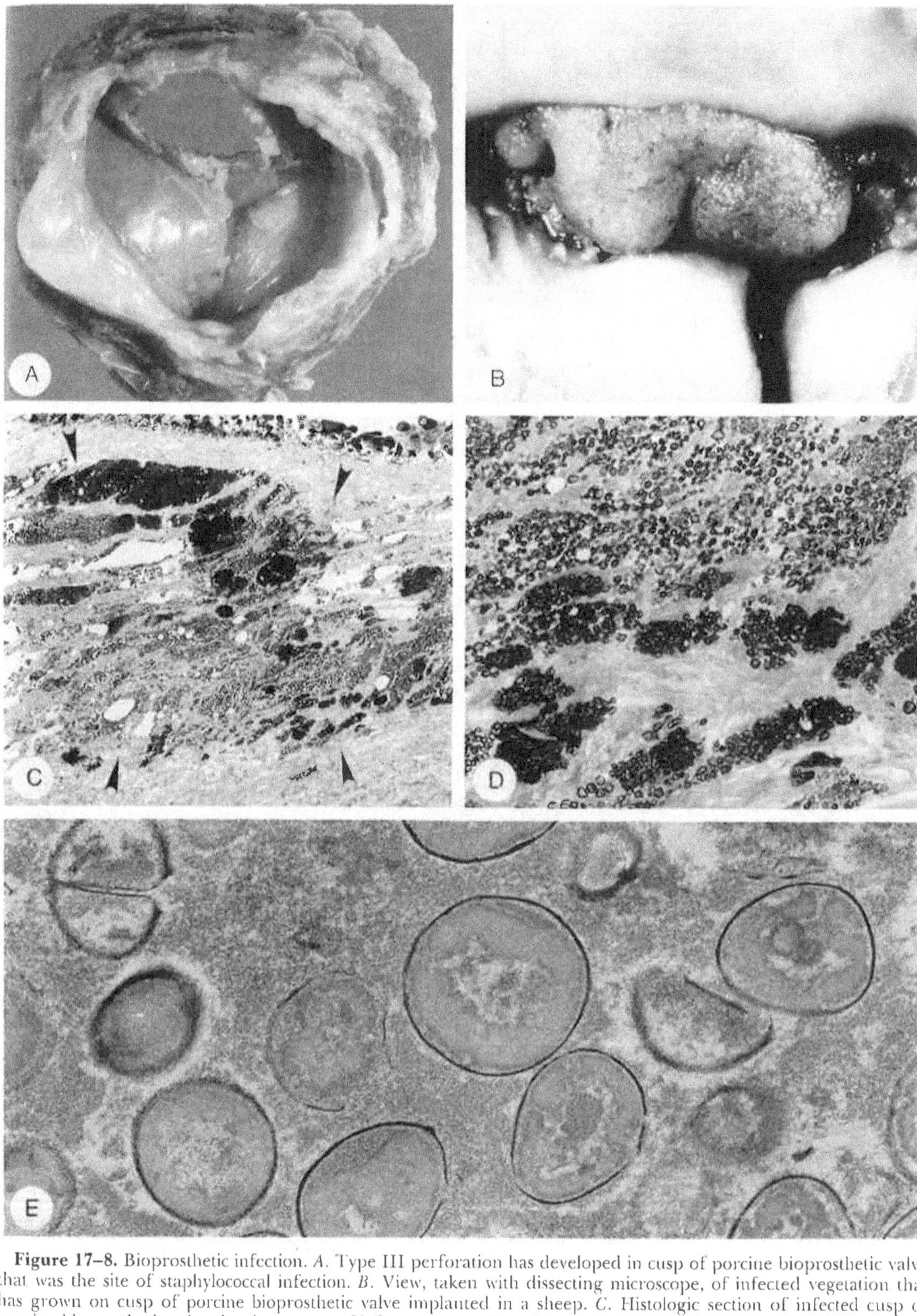

Figure 17–8. Bioprosthetic infection. *A.* Type III perforation has developed in cusp of porcine bioprosthetic valve that was the site of staphylococcal infection. *B.* View, taken with dissecting microscope, of infected vegetation that has grown on cusp of porcine bioprosthetic valve implanted in a sheep. *C.* Histologic section of infected cusp of porcine bioprosthetic valve showing masses of inflammatory cells and bacteria on the surface and within the spongiosa *(arrowheads)*. *D.* Higher magnification view of section shown in *C.* Note clusters of staphylococci. *E.* Electron micrograph showing numerous cocci in infected bioprosthetic valve. (Toluidine blue: *C,* ×100; *D,* ×800 and uranyl acetate and lead citrate: *E,* ×25,000)

perforations as well as ring abscesses;[67] nevertheless, these complications occur less frequently than in the case of infections of mechanical valves.

Cuspal perforations in infected bioprostheses occur more frequently in the aortic position than in the mitral position;[68] however, the possibility of infection must be considered in all cuspal perforations. Cuspal perforations associated with infection (Fig. 17–8*A*) tend to be of type III. In patients with multiple substitute cardiac valves, the one located the most downstream has the greatest propensity to infection.[65] Prosthetic valve infection is most common during the first few months after implantation but continues to represent a long-term risk.[69, 70] Early infections are more likely to be caused by staphylococci than are late infections. Staphylococci are extremely destructive to bioprosthetic and native tissues and continue to be the most common cause of infections involving either mechanical or bioprosthetic (Fig. 17–8*B* through *E*) valves. Numerous species of bacteria and fungi have been found to cause prosthetic valvular infection. Infections with *Mycobacterium chelonii* were reported in a group of patients with porcine bioprostheses,[14, 15] and one patient with Whipple's disease developed infection of a bioprosthesis with the organisms characteristically found in other tissues, such as intestine and native cardiac valves, of patients with this disease.[72]

Four stages of infection of bioprostheses are recognizable:[68] stage I, the initial stage, is characterized by localization of organisms only on thrombi adherent to the cuspal surfaces; stage II, by the presence of organisms on thrombotic material and on immediately subjacent cuspal collagen; stage III, by penetration of organisms into centrally located areas of cuspal tissue (i.e., the spongiosa of porcine bioprostheses and the middle third of the fibrosa in pericardial bioprostheses); and stage IV, by actual perforation of the cusp (Fig. 17–9).

In porcine bioprostheses, the loosely arranged spongiosa may provide a path by which infection can spread from the cusps toward the sewing ring (see Fig. 17–8*C*). Bacterial invasion of the spongiosa probably indicates that the bioprosthesis cannot be salvaged by therapy and eventually will be destroyed by the infection. Calcific deposits tend to develop in vegetations. It can be difficult to distinguish bacteria from calcific deposits on light microscopic study of vegetations in bioprostheses; in fact, the bacteria themselves can become calcified, and electron microscopic study can be helpful in their identification.[68, 71]

Cuspal Tears and Perforations

The connective tissue components of all bioprostheses are subjected to chemical and degradative processes that place certain limits on their durability. The most important of these processes seems to be the mechanical disruption of collagen fibrils, which occurs as a consequence of the flexing and bending that take place with each cycle of valvular opening and closure. The contribution of proteolytic enzymes in blood cells and plasma to this process of "collagen degeneration" is unclear. As mentioned previously, such a process is accentuated at certain sites in which mechanical stresses are high, thus causing focal breakdown of the connective tissue structure and giving rise to tears and perforations (Figs. 17–9 and 17–10). The collagen affected by these changes has a pale, hyaline appearance in histologic sections stained either with hematoxylin and eosin or with toluidine blue, and on transmission electron microscopic study the collagen fibrils are decreased in number, appear to be broken, with frayed tips, and are associated with large amounts of finely granular material.[18] Examination by polarized light microscopy shows changes that range from decrease and loss of the waviness (crimping) of

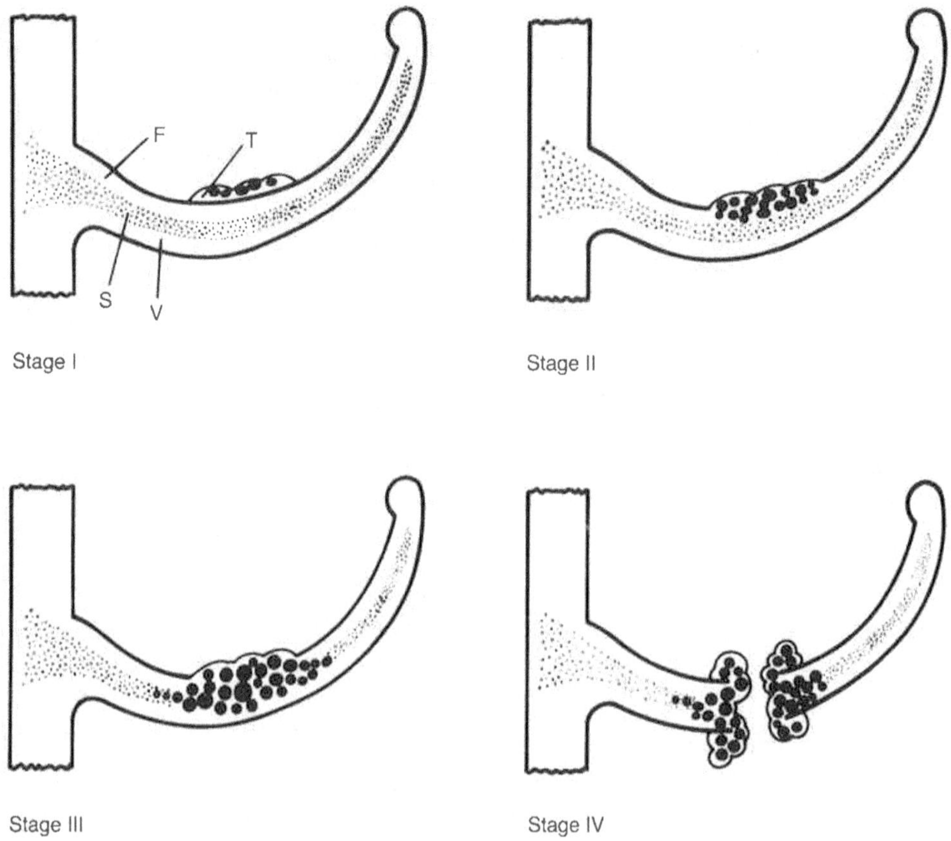

Figure 17–9. Stages of infection of bioprosthetic valves. Stage I is characterized by infection only in surface thrombi; stage II, by invasion of superficial layers of the cusp; stage III, by deeper invasion; and stage IV, by cuspal perforation.

collagen to a marked decrease in the birefringence of collagen in such areas.[25] For reasons that are not clear, collagen degradation is rapid in fascia lata valves[32–36] but slow in aortic homografts.[37–42]

Ishihara and associates have presented a system (Fig. 17–10) for the classification of cuspal lesions in bioprosthetic valves.[73] Type I lesions (Fig. 17–11*A* and *B*) are tears that involve the free edge of the cusp. Type II lesions (Fig. 17–11*C*) are linear perforations that extend along the base of the cusp, forming an arc parallel to the sewing ring. Type III lesions (see Fig. 17–8*A*) are large, round or oval defects that occupy the central portion of the cusp, often in association with severe cuspal destruction. Type IV lesions (Fig. 17–11*D*) are small and often multiple and appear as pinholes in the central regions of the cusps, usually in association with calcific deposits. These four lesions can be associated with "delamination" of the cuspal connective tissue (Fig. 17–11*E*), in which the normally compact collagen bundles are separated into loosely arranged, parallel layers.

Type I lesions are most frequent in the cusps of pericardial[74–78] and dura mater[30, 31] valves. They have been reported to be a relatively common complication in patients undergoing mitral valvular replacement with Ionescu-Shiley pericardial bioprostheses,[74–76] but they also have been encountered with other pericardial bioprostheses of more recent design.[77, 78] In both pericardial and dura mater valves, these lesions (flail cusp) tend to occur near the stent post rather than along the central region of the free edge. They have a similar preferential location in porcine bioprostheses. In pericardial bioprostheses, the attachment or alignment

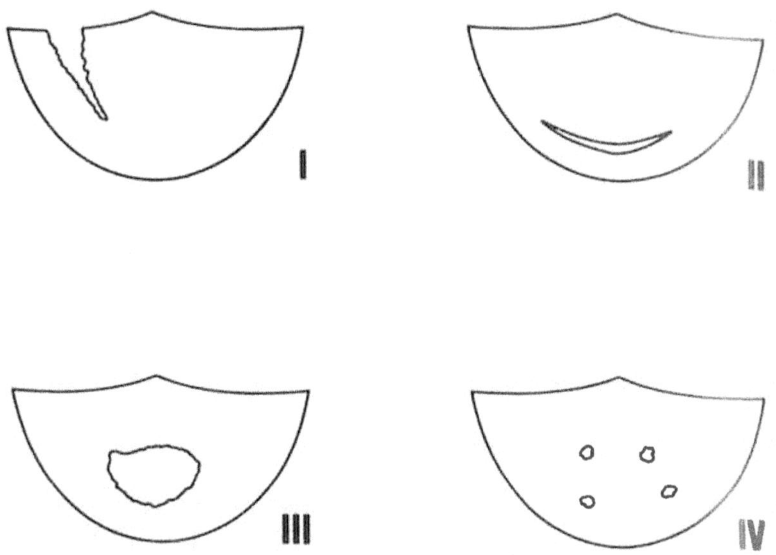

Figure 17–10. Classification of cuspal lesions in bioprosthetic valves. Type I lesions are tears that involve the free edge of the cusp. Type II are linear perforations along the base of the cusp. Type III lesions are large perforations in the center of the cusp. Type IV lesions are small, often multiple perforations that appear as pinholes and usually are associated with calcific deposits.

suture placed near the top of the post is believed to be of importance in the pathogenesis of these lesions.[79]

Ishihara and colleagues[73] have shown that breakage and degeneration of collagen fibrils occur along the edges of type I lesions (Fig. 17–11*F*). The lower frequency of occurrence of such lesions in porcine bioprostheses is explained by the fact that the cuspal free edges of these valves are reinforced by collagenous cords that run from one commissure to another; in contrast, the free edges of pericardial and dura mater valves are composed of sharply transected, multidirectional bundles of collagen without any reinforcing structures.[25]

Type II lesions are believed to be related to the phenomenon called "hinging," in which the cusps do not open with an even motion but tend to open by bending excessively at one localized site near the cuspal base. The cumulative effects of such a repeated hinging are believed to lead to separation of bundles of collagen and to the formation of a linear defect along the base of the cusp.[73] An extensive perforation involved the muscle shelf of the right coronary cusp of a porcine bioprosthesis.[80]

Type III lesions usually result from infection but also can be produced by the confluence of several type IV lesions. Type III lesions caused by infection have shown extensive destruction and necrosis of cuspal tissue at their edges. Type IV lesions usually occur in the vicinity of calcific deposits and are believed to result from mechanical forces acting on the collagen at the edges of such deposits.[73, 81] The importance of calcific deposits in the pathogenesis of cuspal tears and perforations has been emphasized by Stein and colleagues,[82] who studied 54 spontaneously degenerated bioprostheses and found calcification to be associated with tears and perforations of the cusps in 50% of all bioprostheses, in 56% of bioprostheses with torn cusps, and in 71% of bioprostheses with gross calcific deposits.

Comparisons of the extent of degeneration of bioprostheses in patients undergoing double valve replacements showed that bioprostheses in the mitral position undergo more rapid degeneration than those either in the aortic or the tricuspid position.[83, 84]

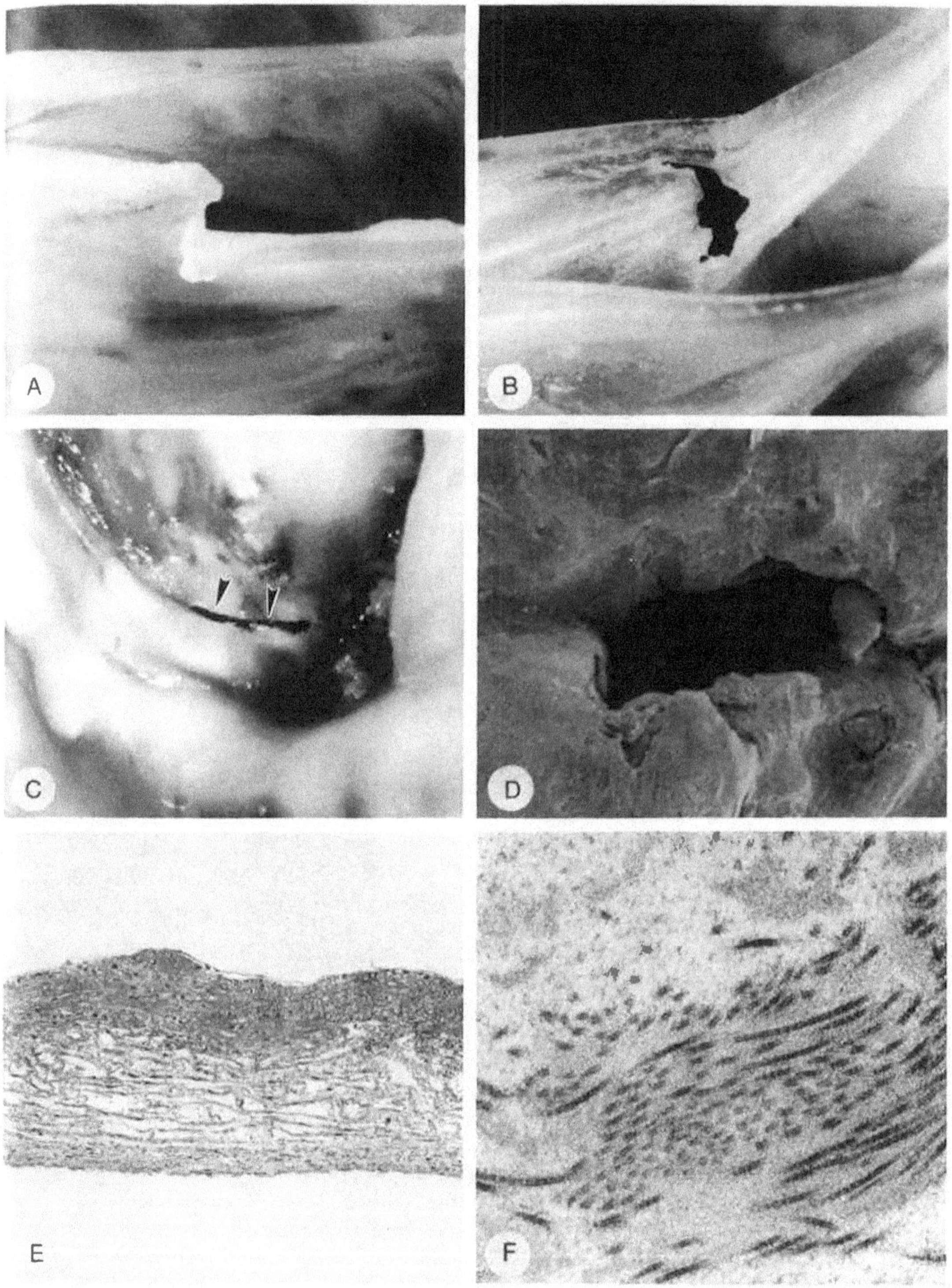

Figure 17–11. Cuspal tears and perforations. *A*. Type I lesion is a tear located near the commissure of a porcine bioprosthetic valve implanted in a sheep. *B*. Lesion has developed near the free edge (which appears very thin but not yet torn) in the region of a commissure of a porcine bioprosthetic valve implanted in a sheep. *C*. Type II lesion has developed in the shape of an arc along the basal portion of a cusp of a porcine bioprosthetic valve implanted in a sheep. *D*. Scanning electron micrograph (×50) of type IV lesion in a dura mater valve. *E*. Delamination of cusp of porcine bioprosthetic valve is characterized by separation of the connective tissue layers. Compare with histology of unimplanted valve in Figure 17–4. *F*. Electron micrograph of collagen fibrils undergoing disruption into finely granular material in bioprosthetic valve removed because of tear 76 months after implantation in the mitral position. (Hematoxylin and eosin: *E*, ×100 lead citrate and uranyl acetate: *F*, ×22,000)

Suture-induced Perforations

In addition to the four types of perforations described previously, suture-induced abrasions and perforations have been reported in bioprostheses implanted both in the mitral and in the aortic valve position, in instances in which the sutures anchoring the sewing ring had excessively long ends.[5] These long ends may make contact with the bioprosthetic cusps and eventually erode them, causing cuspal perforations (Figs. 17–12 and 17–13). These lesions have been produced by monofilament and by braided types of sutures, and they have been induced experimentally in sheep with bioprostheses.[5]

Fibrous Sheathing

Implanted bioprostheses gradually become partially or completely covered by a fibrous sheath of host origin.[57] This fibrous sheath appears to grow in from the region of the stent and spreads over both of the surfaces of cusps (Fig. 17–14). It is composed of fibrous connective tissue, and it is at least partially lined by

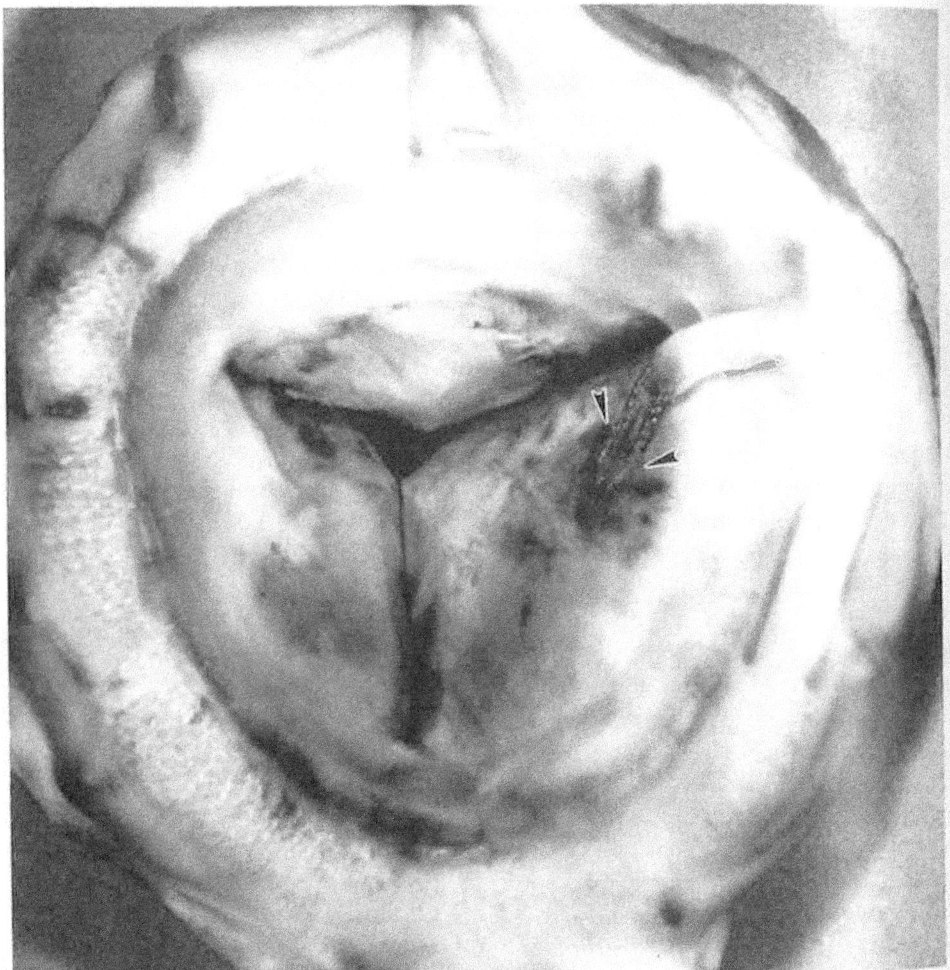

Figure 17–12. Inflow surface of bioprosthetic valve in which an excessively long suture end was left at the time of implantation. This end, partially covered by a fibrous sheath, is in contact with the inflow surface of one of the cusps and has produced a perforation (see Figure 17–13).

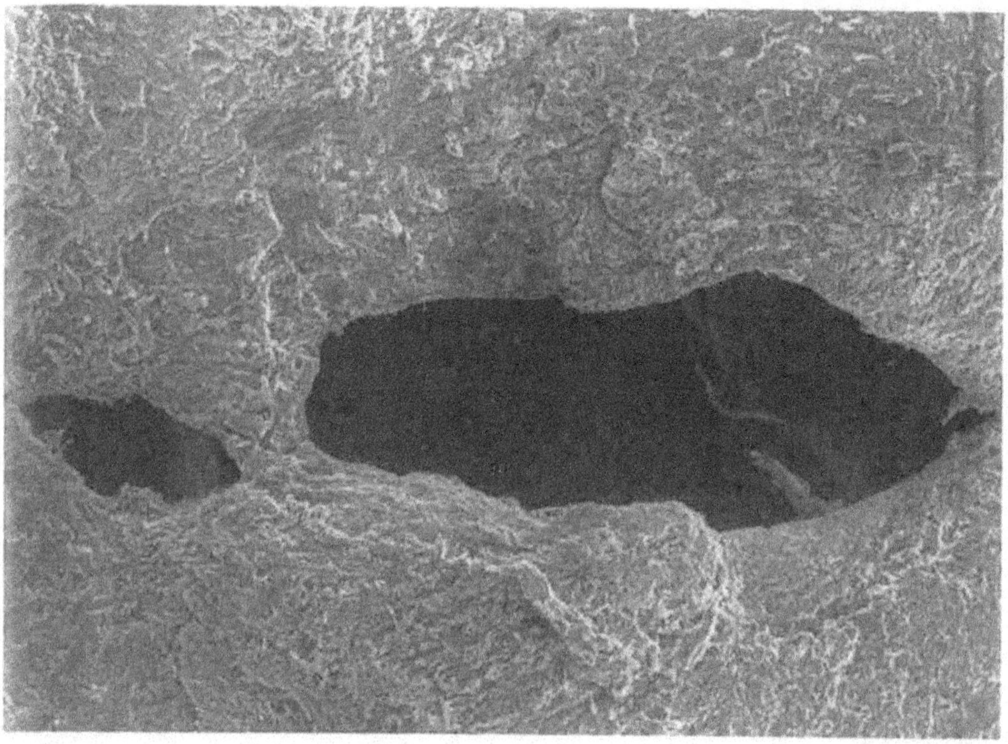

Figure 17–13. Scanning electron micrograph showing perforation produced by progressive erosion of the cuspal surface by the suture end. Note the fraying of the collagen at the surface. (×75)

endothelium. The fibrous tissue contains collagen and elastic fibers, and its distal end (i.e., that closest to the free edge of the cusp) often has the appearance of a partially organized thrombus. Actually, the fibrous sheath may develop as a consequence of the organization of small surface microthrombi (Fig. 17–14*B*). In bioprostheses in place for only a short time, the elastic fibers are few and small and most cells are elongated fibroblasts. In bioprostheses in place for longer periods, the elastic fibers are more numerous, the collagen is more dense, and the connective tissue cells are more differentiated in the direction of smooth muscle cells. The collagen in fibrous sheaths usually is easily distinguished from that in the bioprosthetic cusps because it is less eosinophilic; the nuclei of the host connective tissue cells are much more basophilic than those in the cusp itself (Fig. 17–14*C*). The thickness of the fibrous sheath can be equal to, or greater than, that of the cusp itself. In some instances metaplastic cartilage and even bone develop at the border between fibrous sheath and bioprosthetic cusp.[85]

Fibrous sheaths appear to have some protective effect in reinforcing the cuspal structure; however, in some instances they can grow excessively (Fig. 17–14*C*) and cause cuspal stiffening and even commissural fusion.[31, 44–47, 50–54, 57] Thus, they can produce significant cuspal stenosis. In sheep, fibrous sheathing can cover completely the cusps of pericardial valves, also producing subsequent retraction of cuspal tissue and bioprosthetic regurgitation.[3, 86] Similar fibrous sheathing occurs in dura mater valves,[28–31, 87] homografts,[37–42] and fascia lata valves.[31–36] Fibrous sheathing (sometimes referred to as "neointima") also is observed in valved right ventricle–pulmonary artery conduits, in which it can involve the bioprosthetic cusps, which become adherent to the inner wall of the conduit, causing both stenosis and regurgitation.[88]

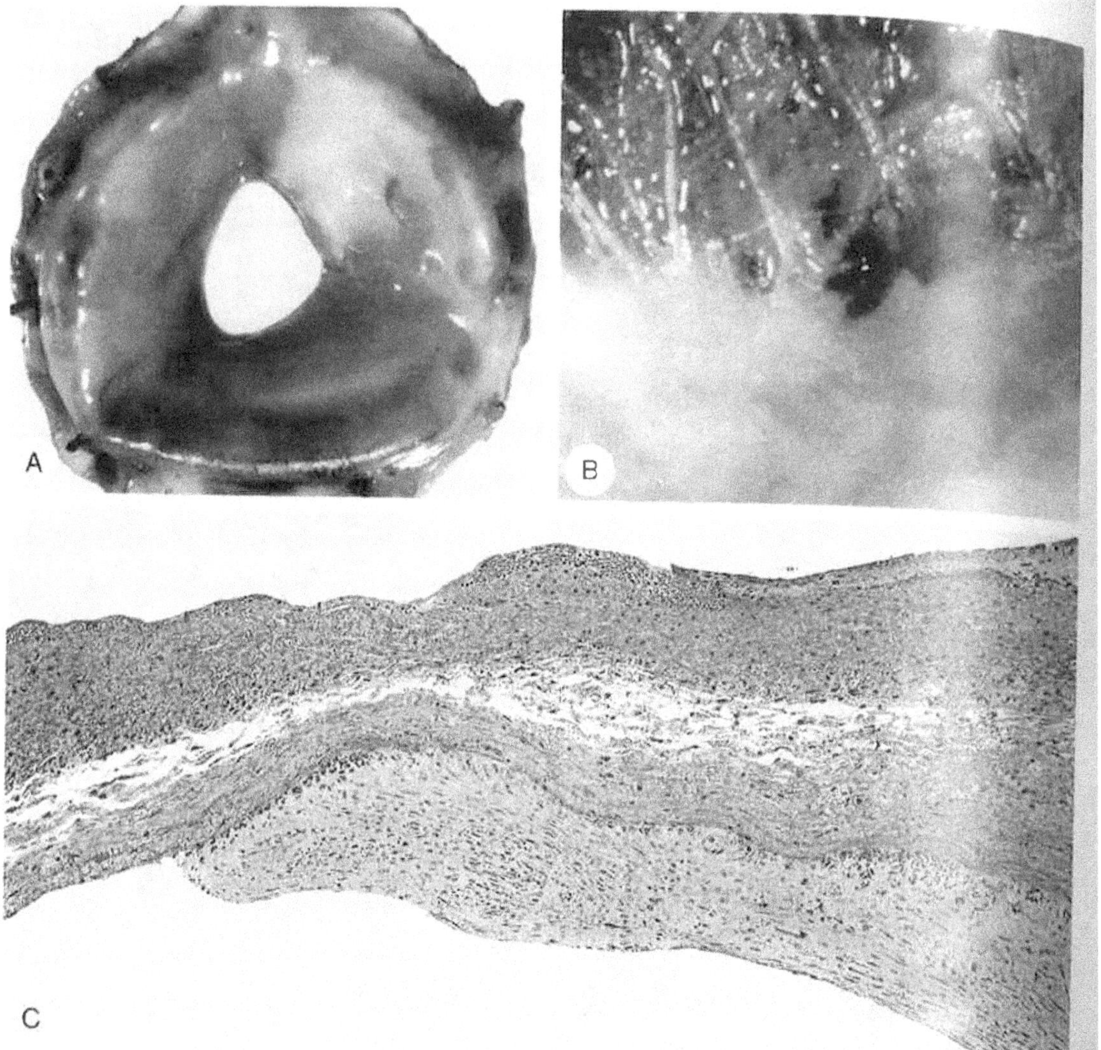

Figure 17–14. Fibrous sheathing in bioprosthetic valve. Histologic section of basal portion of cusp of porcine bioprosthetic valve showing fibrous sheath that has grown extensively on the inflow surface and to a much lesser extent *(upper right)* on the outflow surface. (Hematoxylin and eosin, × 100)

Calcification

Calcific deposits develop in most porcine bioprostheses implanted for 3 years or longer[18, 44–54] and can be the cause of stenosis because they can stiffen the cusps considerably and reduce their mobility. They also can be the cause of regurgitation because they often are associated with cuspal tears and perforations.

Calcific deposits affect the cusps of porcine bioprostheses,[2, 3, 18, 31, 44–54, 81, 82, 86] pericardial bioprostheses,[2, 3, 31, 47, 51, 54, 86] fascia lata valves,[33, 34] and dura mater valves (Fig. 17–15).[27–31, 89–91] Homografts tend to show much less cuspal calcification, although their aortic walls may become heavily calcified.[37–43] Bioprosthetic valves placed within right ventricular–pulmonary artery conduits also calcify.[88]

In all types of bioprostheses the most significant calcific deposits develop in association with collagen fibrils (intrinsic calcification) (Fig. 17–15*C* through *F*) and with organizing surface microthrombi (extrinsic calcification). They also can involve other structures, including the nuclei and the cytoplasm of cuspal connective tissue cells; porcine bioprostheses also may have calcific deposits in connective

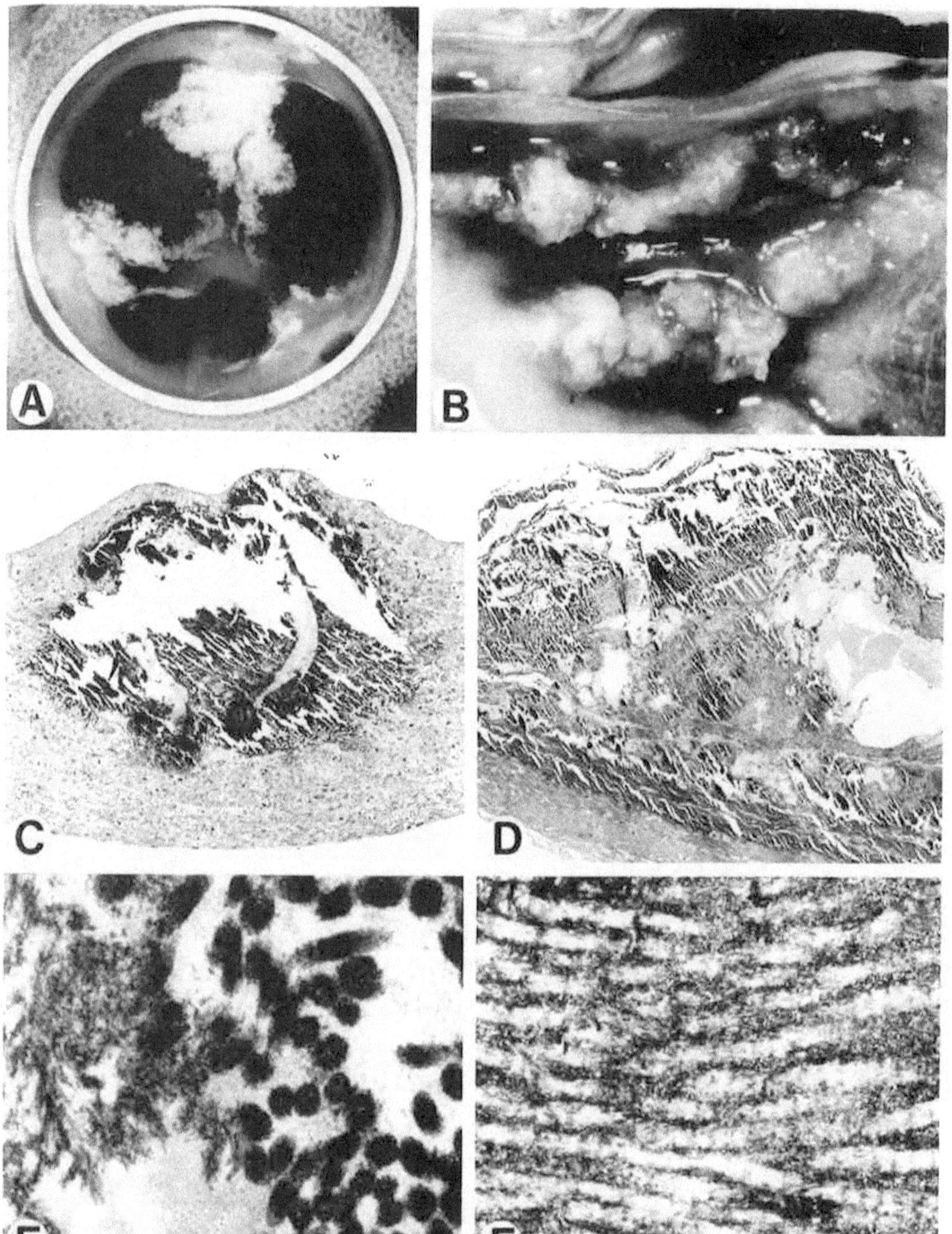

Figure 17–15. Calcific deposits on bioprosthetic valves. *A*. Radiograph of valve demonstrates multiple calcific nodules. *B*. Dissecting microscope view of multiple calcific deposits near a commissure of porcine bioprosthetic valve. *C*. Calcific deposits in porcine bioprosthetic valve implanted for 20 weeks in a sheep. *D*. Calcific deposits in pericardial bioprosthetic valve implanted for 20 weeks in a sheep. This region of the cusp is thickened and delaminated. *E* and *F*. Ultrastructure of calcific deposits associated with collagen. Deposits in *E* involve the entire thickness of the collagen fibrils, which have been sectioned transversely; deposits in *F* are confined to the interfibrillary spaces, so that the collagen fibrils appear lucent. (*B*, ×30; *C* and *D*, hematoxylin and eosin, ×150; *E* and *F*, uranyl acetate and lead citrate stain, ×54,000 and ×56, 000)

tissue cells in the aortic wall and in cardiac myocytes in the muscle shelf of the right coronary cusp.[3, 18] Calcific deposits usually are multiple; in porcine bioprostheses they tend to be concentrated near the commissures (Fig. 17–15*A* and *B*). The deposits associated with thrombi are raised and project above the cuspal surfaces. The collagen-associated deposits usually are most extensive in the spongiosa of porcine bioprostheses and in the middle third of the cusps of pericardial bioprostheses.

Electron microscopic examination (Fig. 17–15*E* and *F*) has revealed three patterns of association of calcific deposits with collagen fibrils: (1) deposits that involve the entire fibrils, (2) deposits confined to the surfaces of the fibrils, and (3) deposits that are mainly localized in the interfibrillary spaces.[18, 49] Analytical techniques have disclosed that the calcific deposits are composed of calcium hydroxyapatite.[92]

Factors known to predispose to the calcification of bioprostheses are young age of the patient, chronic renal disease, other causes of hyperparathyroidism, and bioprosthetic infection.[92] Both porcine and pericardial bioprostheses implanted in children may undergo rapid, clinically severe calcification within 3 years after implantation. There is considerable, unexplained variation in the extent to which calcific deposits develop in bioprostheses implanted in adults, in whom such deposits usually do not become clinically significant until 4 years or longer after implantation. Calcific deposits are the single most important cause of dysfunction of implanted bioprostheses in adults. The pathogenesis of calcific deposits is poorly understood.[92] Subcutaneous models of valve implantation have provided useful insights into this process.[93, 94]

Intracuspal Hematomas

Intracuspal hematomas are infrequent causes of stenosis of porcine aortic valvular bioprostheses. Intracuspal hematomas[95] are due to the penetration of red blood cells between the layers of the cusps, especially in the spongiosa, leading to an increase in cuspal thickness and stiffness (Fig. 17–16). The presence of blood imparts a characteristic dark color to the affected cusps. It has been suggested that the blood penetrates between the bioprosthetic cusps and the sewing ring.[95]

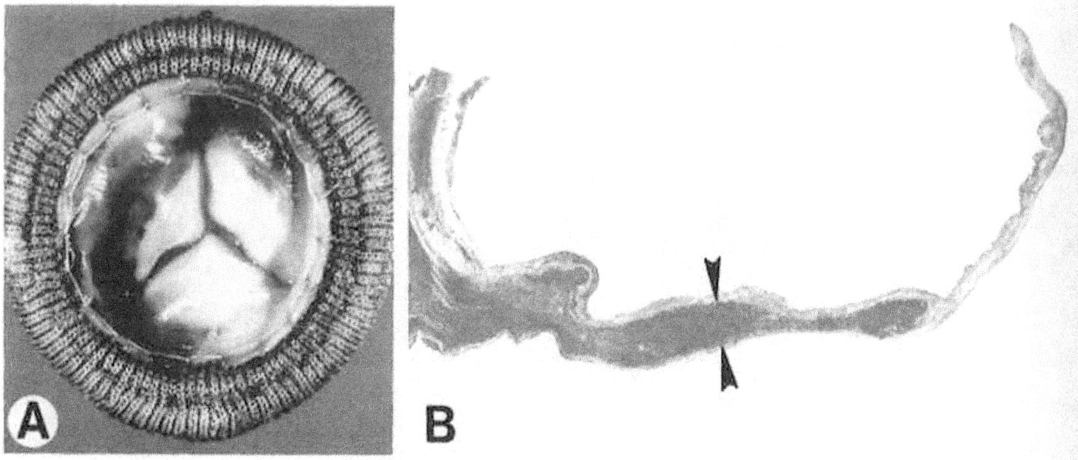

Figure 17–16. Intracuspal hematoma in a porcine bioprosthetic valve. *A*. View of the explanted bioprosthetic valve showing dark discoloration of basal regions of the cusps. *B*. Histologic examination shows penetration of blood *(arrowheads)* into spongiosa of the cusp, which has become thickened. (Hematoxylin and eosin, × 15)

Infiltration of Lipid Material and Amyloid

Infiltration of lipid material, presumably derived from blood plasma, has been reported to occur in extraordinary amounts in some implanted bioprostheses. Large crystals of cholesteryl esters have been demonstrated in some,[96, 97] and in others lipid infiltration has been very marked in areas adjacent to type I cuspal tears.[18] The true prevalence of such deposits is uncertain.

Goffin and co-workers[98] found microscopic deposits of amyloid in the sewing ring of one fascia lata valve and in cuspal tissue in 10 of 30 porcine bioprostheses. All amyloid-containing porcine bioprostheses had been in place for at least 33 months, and all except two showed dysfunction and/or severe degeneration of cuspal tissue. In the majority of the valves the amyloid deposits were permanganate sensitive and tryptophan positive. The pathogenesis and significance of these deposits are unknown.

REFERENCES

1. McDowell E: Fixation and processing. In Trump BF, Jones RT (eds): Diagnostic Electron Microscopy, vol 1, pp 113–139. New York, John Wiley & Sons, 1978
2. Jones M, Eidbo EE, Walters SM et al: Effects of two types of preimplantation proceses on calcification of bioprosthetic valves. In Bodnar E, Yacoub M (eds): Biologic and Bioprosthetic Valves. Proceedings of the Third International Symposium, pp 451–459. New York, Yorke Medical Books, 1985
3. Arbustini E, Jones M, Moses RD et al: Modification by the Hancock T6 process of calcification of bioprosthetic cardiac valves implanted in sheep. Am J Cardiol 53:1388, 1984
4. Kajikawa K, Yamaguchi T, Katsuda S, Miwa A: An improved elastic stain for elastic fibers using tannic acid. J Electron Microsc (Tokyo) 24:287, 1975
5. Jones M, Rodriguez ER, Eidbo EE, Ferrans VJ: Cuspal perforations caused by long suture ends in implanted bioprosthetic valves. J Thorac Cardiovasc Surg 90:557, 1985
6. Roberts WC, Ferrans VJ: Complications of replacement of either the mitral or aortic valve or both by either mechanical or bioprosthetic valves. In Cohn LH, Gallucci V (eds): Cardiac Bioprostheses, pp 331–345. New York, Yorke Medical Books, 1982
7. Gendler E, Gendler S, Nimni ME: Toxic reactions evoked by glutaraldehyde-fixed pericardium and cardiac valve tissue bioprostheses. J Biomed Mater Res 18:727, 1984
8. Roberts WC: Complications of cardiac valve replacement: Characteristic abnormalities of prostheses pertaining to any specific site. Am Heart J 103:113, 1982
9. Borken AM, McIntosh CL, Jones M et al: Inward stent-post bending of a porcine bioprosthesis in the mitral position: Cause of bioprosthetic dysfunction. J Thorac Cardiovasc Surg 83:105, 1982
10. Roberts WC, Isner JM, Virmani R: Left ventricular incision midway between the mitral anulus and the stumps of the papillary muscles during mitral valve excision with or without rupture or aneurysmal formation: Analysis of 10 necropsy patients. Am Heart J 104:1278, 1983
11. Jones M, Eidbo EE, Rodriguez ER et al: Ventricular aneurysms and other lesions produced by the struts of bioprosthetic valves implanted in sheep. J Thorac Cardiovasc Surg 95:729, 1988
12. Gabbay S, Frater RW: The unileaflet heart valve bioprosthesis: New concept. In Cohn LH, Gallucci V (eds): Cardiac Bioprostheses, pp 411–424. New York, Yorke Medical Books, 1982
13. Bodnar E, Bowden NL, Drury PJ et al: Bicuspid mitral bioprosthesis. Thorax 36:45, 1981
14. Center for Disease Control: Isolation of mycobacteria species from porcine heart valve prostheses. MMWR 26:42, 1977
15. Laskowski LF, Marr JJ, Spernoga JF et al: Fastidious mycobacteria grown from porcine prosthetic heart valve cultures. N Engl J Med 297:101, 1977
16. Buch WS, Kosek JC, Angell WW, Shumway NE: Deterioration of formalin-treated aortic valve heterografts. J Thorac Cardiovasc Surg 60:673, 1970
17. Dubiel WT, Johansson L, Willen R: Late changes in formalin-treated porcine aortic heterografts replacing human mitral valves. Scand J Thorac Cardiovasc Surg 9:16, 1975
18. Ferrans VJ, Spray TL, Billingham ME, Roberts WC: Structural changes in glutaraldehyde-treated porcine heterografts used as substitute cardiac valves: Transmission and scanning electron microscopic observations in 12 patients. Am J Cardiol 41:1159, 1978
19. Sade RM, Greene WB, Kurtz SM: Structural changes in a porcine xenograft after implantation for 105 months. Am J Cardiol 44:761, 1979
20. Jones M, Eidbo EE, Hilbert SL et al: Anticalcification treatments of bioprosthetic heart valves: *In vivo, in situ* studies in the sheep model. J Cardiac Surg 4:69, 1989

21. Broom ND, Thompson FJ: Influence of fixation conditions on the performance of glutaraldehyde-treated porcine aortic valves: Towards a more scientific basis. Thorax 34:166, 1979
22. Polystan Bioprostheses Information Bulletins BPA, BPB, BPC, BPD, BPE, BPF and BPI. Polystan A/S, Copenhagen, Denmark, 1980
23. Ishihara T, Ferrans VJ, Jones M et al: Structure of bovine parietal pericardium and of unimplanted Ionescu-Shiley pericardial valvular bioprostheses. J Thorac Cardiovasc Surg 81:747, 1981
24. Allen DJ, DiDio LJ, Zacharias A et al: Microscopic study of normal parietal pericardium and unimplanted Puig-Zerbini pericardial valvular heterografts. J Thorac Cardiovasc Surg 87:845, 1984
25. Hilbert SL, Ferrans VJ, Swanson WM: Optical methods for the nondestructive evaluation of collagen morphology in bioprosthetic heart valves. J Biomed Mat Res 20:1411, 1986
26. Allen DJ, DiDio LJA: Scanning and transmission electron microscopy of the encephalic meninges in dogs. J Submicrosc Cytol 9:1, 1977
27. Allen DJ, DiDio LJ, Highison GJ et al: Electron microscopic evaluation and x-ray microanalysis of prosthetic dural cardiac valves surgically recovered. Bull Assoc Anat 65:275, 1981
28. Nuno-Conceicao A, Puig LB, Verginelli G et al: Homologous dura mater cardiac valves: Structural aspects of eight implanted valves. J Thorac Cardiovasc Surg 70:499, 1975
29. Puig LB, Verginelli G, Iryia K et al: Homologous dura mater cardiac valves: Study of 533 surgical cases. J Thorac Cardiovasc Surg 69:722, 1975
30. Martelli V, Wain WH, Bodnar E, Ross DN: Mitral valve replacement with dura mater bioprosthesis. Artif Organs 4:163, 1980
31. Bodnar A, Ross DN: Mode of failure in 226 explanted biologic and bioprosthetic valves. In Cohn LH, Gallucci V (eds): Cardiac Bioprostheses, pp 401–407. New York, Yorke Medical Books, 1983
32. Willen R, Willen H, Dubiel WT, Johansson L: Composition of surface layers in unfixed autologous fascia lata heart valve grafts: A transmission electron microscopical study. Upsala J Med Sci 88:25, 1983
33. Silver MD, Trimble AS: Structure of autologous fascia lata heart valve prostheses. Arch Pathol 93:109, 1972
34. Olsen EG, Al-Janabi N, Salamao CS, Ross DN: Fascia lata valves: A clinicopathological study. Thorax 30:528, 1975
35. Willen R, Dubiel WT, Johansson L: Viability properties in autologous fascia lata heart valve grafts: A transmission electron microscopical study. Ann Thorac Surg 19:494, 1975
36. Willen R, Dubiel WT, Johansson L: Viability and surface properties of autologous fascia lata heart valve grafts: A radioautographic and scanning electron microscopical study. Ann Thorac Surg 18:597, 1974
37. Hudson REB: Pathology of the human aortic valve homograft. Br Heart J 28:291, 1966
38. Reichenbach DD, Mohri H, Merendino KA: Pathological changes in human aortic valve homografts. Circulation 39, 40(suppl I):I-47, 1969
39. Angell WW, Shumway NE, Kosek JC, Alto P: A five-year study of viable aortic valve homografts. J Thorac Cardiovasc Surg 64:329, 1972
40. Aparicio SR, Donnelly RJ, Dexter F, Watson DA: Light and electron microscopy studies on homograft and heterograft heart valves. J Pathol 115:147, 1975
41. Barratt-Boyes BG, Roche HG, Brandt PWT et al: Aortic homograft valve replacement: A long-term follow-up of an initial series of 101 patients. Circulation 40:763, 1969
42. Ross DN: Aortic valvar replacements. Br Heart J 33(suppl):39, 1971
43. Moodie DS, Mair DD, Fulton RE et al: Aortic homograft obstruction. J Thorac Cardiovasc Surg 72:553, 1976
44. Yarbrough JW, Roberts WC, Reis RL: Structural alterations in tissue cardiac valves implanted in patients and in calves. J Thorac Cardiovasc Surg 65:364, 1973
45. Spray TL, Roberts WC: Structural changes in porcine xenografts used as substitute cardiac valves: Gross and histologic observations in 51 glutaraldehyde-preserved Hancock valves in 41 patients. Am J Cardiol 40:319, 1977
46. Fishbein MC, Gissen SA, Collins JJ Jr et al: Pathologic findings after cardiac valve replacement with glutaraldehyde-fixed porcine valves. Am J Cardiol 40:331, 1977
47. Silver MD, Wilson GJ: Pathology of cardiovascular prostheses including coronary artery bypass and other vascular grafts. In Silver MD (ed): Cardiovascular Pathology, vol 2, pp 1225–1296. New York, Churchill Livingstone, 1983
48. Cipriano PR, Billingham ME, Oyer PE et al: Calcification of porcine prosthetic heart valves: A radiographic and light microscopic study. Circulation 66:1100, 1982
49. Ferrans VJ, Boyce SW, Billingham ME et al: Calcific deposits in porcine bioprostheses: Structure and pathogenesis. Am J Cardiol 46:721, 1980
50. Thiene G, Arbustini E, Bortolotti U et al: Pathologic substrates of porcine valve dysfunction. In Cohn LH, Gallucci V (eds): Cardiac Bioprostheses, pp 378–400. New York, Yorke Medical Books, 1982
51. Schoen FJ, Hobson CE: Anatomic analysis of removed prosthetic heart valves: Causes of failure in 33 mechanical valves and 58 bioprostheses, 1980 to 1983. Hum Pathol 16:549–559, 1985
52. Goffin YA, Deuvaert F, Wellens F et al: Normally and abnormally functioning left-sided porcine bioprosthetic valves after long-term implantation in patients: Distinct spectra of histologic and histochemical changes. J Am Coll Cardiol 4:324, 1984

53. Camilleri JP, Pornin B, Carpentier A: Structural changes of glutaraldehyde-treated porcine bioprosthetic valves. Arch Pathol Lab Med 106:490, 1982
54. Schoen FJ, Levy RJ: Bioprosthetic heart valve failure: Pathology and pathogenesis. Cardiol Clin 2(4):717, 1984
55. Rocchini AP, Weesner KM, Heidelberger K et al: Porcine xenograft valve failure in children: An immunologic response. Circulation 64(suppl II):II-162, 1981
56. Levy RJ, Schoen FJ, Howard SL: Mechanism of calcification of porcine bioprosthetic aortic valve cusps: Role of T-lymphocytes. Am J Cardiol 52:629, 1983
57. Ishihara T, Ferrans VJ, Jones M et al: Occurrence and significance of endothelial cells in implanted porcine bioprosthetic valves. Am J Cardiol 48:443, 1981
58. Magilligan DJ Jr, Oyama C, Klein S et al: Platelet adherence to bioprosthetic cardiac valves. Am J Cardiol 53:945, 1984
59. Dewanjee MK, Didisheim P, Kaye MP et al: Platelet deposition on and calcification of bovine pericardial valve. Eur Heart J 5(suppl D):1, 1984
60. Pumphrey CW, Fuster V, Chesebro JH: Systemic thromboembolism in valvular heart disease and prosthetic heart valves. Mod Concepts Cardiovasc Dis 51:131, 1982
61. Gonzalez-Lavin L, Tandon AP, Chi S et al: The risk of thromboembolism and hemorrhage following mitral valve replacement: A comparative analysis between the porcine xenograft valve and Ionescu-Shiley bovine pericardial valve. J Thorac Cardiovasc Surg 87:340, 1984
62. Selzer A: Present status of prosthetic cardiac valves. Arch Intern Med 143:1965, 1983
63. Tubbs RR, Picha GC, Levin HS et al: Cotton emboli (cellulose II polymorph, "rayon") of the coronary arteries. Hum Pathol 11:76, 1980
64. Magilligan DJ, Quinn EL, Davila JC: Bacteremia, endocarditis and the Hancock valve. Ann Thorac Surg 24:508, 1977
65. Arnett EN, Roberts WC: Prosthetic valve endocarditis: Clinicopathologic analysis of 22 necropsy patients with comparison of observations in 74 necropsy patients with active infective endocarditis involving natural left-sided valves. Am J Cardiol 38:281, 1976
66. Ferrans VJ, Boyce SW, Billingham ME et al: Infection of glutaraldehyde-preserved porcine valve heterografts. Am J Cardiol 43:1123, 1979
67. Bortolotti U, Thiene G, Milano A et al: Pathological study of infective endocarditis in Hancock porcine bioprostheses. J Thorac Cardiovasc Surg 81:934, 1981
68. Ferrans VJ, Ishihara T, Jones M et al: Pathogenesis and stages of bioprosthetic infection. In Cardiac Bioprostheses, pp 346–361. New York, Yorke Medical Books, 1982
69. Mundth ED, Hakki AH, Goel IP et al: Prosthetic valve endocarditis. Comparison of porcine heterograft and mechanical prosthetic valves. In Bodnar E, Yacoub M (eds): Biologic and Bioprosthetic Valves: Proceedings of the Third International Symposium, pp 537–549. New York, Yorke Medical Books, 1985
70. Jacobs ML, Buckley MJ, Austen WG et al: Early prosthetic valve endocarditis (PVE): Analysis of risk factors. In Bodnar E, Yacoub M (eds): Biologic and Bioprosthetic Valves: Proceedings of the Third International Symposium, pp 533–536. New York, Yorke Medical Books, 1985
71. Knight JP, Torell JA, Hunter RE: Bacterial associated porcine heterograft heart valve calcification. Am J Cardiol 53:370, 1984
72. Ratliff NB, McMahon JT, Naab JT, Cosgrove DM: Whipple's disease in the porcine leaflets of a Carpentier-Edwards prosthetic mitral valve. N Engl J Med 311:902, 1984
73. Ishihara T, Ferrans VJ, Boyce SW et al: Structure and classification of cuspal tears and perforations in porcine bioprosthetic cardiac valves implanted in patients. Am J Cardiol 48:665, 1981
74. Gabbay S, Bortolotti U, Wasserman F et al: Long-term follow-up of the Ionescu-Shiley mitral pericardial xenograft. J Thorac Cardiovasc Surg 88:758, 1984
75. Nistal F, Garcia-Satue E, Artinano E et al: Comparative study of primary tissue valve failure between Ionescu-Shiley pericardial and Hancock porcine valves in the aortic position. Am J Cardiol 57:161, 1986
76. Cooley DA, Ott DA, Reul GJ et al: Ionescu-Shiley pericardial bioprostheses: Clinical results in 2701 patients. In Bodnar E, Yacoub M (eds): Biologic and Bioprosthetic Valves: Proceedings of the Third International Symposium, pp 177–198. New York, Yorke Medical Books, 1985
77. Fournial G, Sauer M, Bernies M et al: Re-operation after Hancock pericardial valve replacement. In Bodnar E, Yacoub M (eds): Biologic and Bioprosthetic Valves: Proceedings of the Third International Symposium, pp 345–349. New York, Yorke Medical Books, 1985
78. Reece IJ, Fisher J, Sethia B et al: Early clinical results with 2 new pericardial bioprostheses. In Bodnar E, Yacoub M (eds): Biologic and Bioprosthetic Valves: Proceedings of the Third International Symposium, pp 749–757. New York, Yorke Medical Books, 1985
79. Wheatley DJ, Fisher J, Reece IJ et al: Primary tissue failure in pericardial heart valves. J Thorac Cardiovasc Surg 94:367, 1987
80. Valente M, Arbustini E, Bortolotti U et al: Perforation of muscle shelf of right coronary cusp causing acute regurgitation of porcine mitral xenograft. Am Heart J 108:180, 1984
81. Sabbah HN, Hamid MS, Stein PD: Estimation of mechanical stresses on closed cusps of porcine bioprosthetic valves: Effects of stiffening, focal calcium and focal thinning. Am J Cardiol 55:1091, 1985
82. Stein PD, Kemp SR, Riddle JM et al: Relation of calcification to torn leaflets of spontaneously degenerated porcine bioprosthetic valves. Ann Thorac Surg 40:175, 1985
83. Cohen SR, Silver MA, McIntosh CL, Roberts WC: Comparison of late (62 to 140 months)

degenerative changes in simultaneously implanted and explanted porcine (Hancock) bioprostheses in the tricuspid and mitral valve positions in six patients. Am J Cardiol 53:1599, 1984

84. Warnes CA, Scott ML, Silver MG et al: Comparison of late degenerative changes in porcine bioprostheses in the mitral and aortic valve position in the same patient. Am J Cardiol 51:965, 1983
85. Arbustini E, Jones M, Ferrans VJ: Formation of cartilage in bioprosthetic cardiac valves implanted in sheep: A morphologic study. Am J Cardiol 52:632, 1983
86. Barnhart GR, Jones M, Ishihara T et al: Bioprosthetic valvular failure. J Thorac Cardiovasc Surg 83:618, 1982
87. Allen DJ, Highison GJ, DiDio LH et al: Evidence of remodeling in dura mater cardiac valves. J Thorac Cardiovasc Surg 84:267, 1982
88. Ferrans VJ, Arbustini E, Eidbo EE, Jones M: Anatomic changes in right ventricular–pulmonary artery (RV-PA) conduits implanted in baboons. In Bodnar E, Yacoub M (eds): Biologic and Bioprosthetic Valves: Proceedings of the Third International Symposium, pp 316–328. New York, Yorke Medical Books, 1985
89. Harasaki H, Kiraly RJ, Jacobs GB et al: Bovine aortic and human dura mater valves: A comparative study in artificial hearts in calves. J Thorac Cardiovasc Surg 79:125, 1980
90. Harasaki H, Snow JL, Kiraly RJ, Nose Y: The dura mater valve: *In vitro* characteristics and pathological changes after implantation in calves. Artif Organs 3:176, 1979
91. Highison GJ, Allen DJ, DiDio LJ et al: A study of structural and chemical composition of surgically recovered defective dura mater cardiac valves using SEM, TEM, and x-ray analysis. Scan Electron Microsc 3:873, 1979
92. Dunn JM, Marmon L: Mechanisms of calcification of tissue valves. Cardiol Clin 3(3):385, 1985
93. Schoen FJ, Levy RJ, Nelson AC et al: Onset and progression of experimental bioprosthetic heart valve calcification. Lab Invest 52:523, 1985
94. Fishbein MC, Levy RJ, Ferrans VJ et al: Calcifications of cardiac valve bioprostheses: Biochemical, histologic, and ultrastructural observations in a subcutaneous implantation model system. J Thorac Cardiovasc Surg 83:602, 1982
95. Ishihara T, Ferrans VJ, Barnhart GR et al: Intracuspal hematomas in implanted porcine aortic valvular bioprostheses. J Thorac Cardiovasc Surg 83:399, 1982
96. Ferrans VJ, McManus B, Roberts WC: Cholesteryl ester crystals in a porcine aortic valvular bioprosthesis implanted for eight years. Chest 83:698, 1983
97. Arbustini E, Bortolotti U, Valente M et al: Cusp disruption by massive lipid infiltration: A rare cause of porcine valve dysfunction. J Thorac Cardiovasc Surg 84:738, 1982
98. Goffin YA, Gruys E, Sorenson GD, Wellens F: Amyloid deposits in bioprosthetic cardiac valves after long-term implantation in man: A new localization of amyloidosis. Am J Pathol 114:431, 1984

Extreme obstruction to left ventricular outflow by a bioprosthesis in the mitral valve position

William C. Roberts, MD, and Allen L. Dollar, MD.
Bethesda, Md.

Obstruction to left ventricular outflow is a recognized potential or real complication of mitral valve replacement.[1-13] It usually results from the use of a large-sized prosthesis or bioprosthesis in patients with relatively small-sized left ventricular cavities. As surgeons gained more experience in cardiac valve replacement and particularly when the use of smaller-framed prostheses became commonplace, left venticular outflow obstruction after mitral replacement became uncommon and is now rare. Recently we studied the heart of a patient who had extreme obstruction to left ventricular outflow after mitral replacement. Because this complication may be fatal and because it is preventable, a brief description of this patient is presented as a reminder of this unfortunate complication.

A 72-year-old woman, who was known for several years to have a precordial murmur, at age 70 developed atrial fibrillation and symptoms of congestive heart failure. Left ventricular angiography disclosed severe mitral valve prolapse, moderately severe mitral regurgitation, normal left ventricular systolic function, a normal-sized left ventricular cavity, and an enlarged left atrial cavity. She was electrically cardioverted to sinus rhythm and was treated with medication and her symptoms improved. At age 72, 6 months before death, exertional dyspnea worsened and nocturnal dyspnea appeared. Shortly before mitral replacement she was evaluated. She was 65 inches (163 cm) tall and weighed 110 pounds (50 kg). The blood pressure was 120/60 mm Hg, and the cardiac ventricular rate was 74 beats/min. A grade 3/6 holosystolic precordial murmur, consistent with mitral regurgitation, was present. The electrocardiogram showed atrial fibrillation and evidence

From the Pathology Branch, National, Heart, Lung, and Blood Institute, National Institutes of Health.
4/4/25888

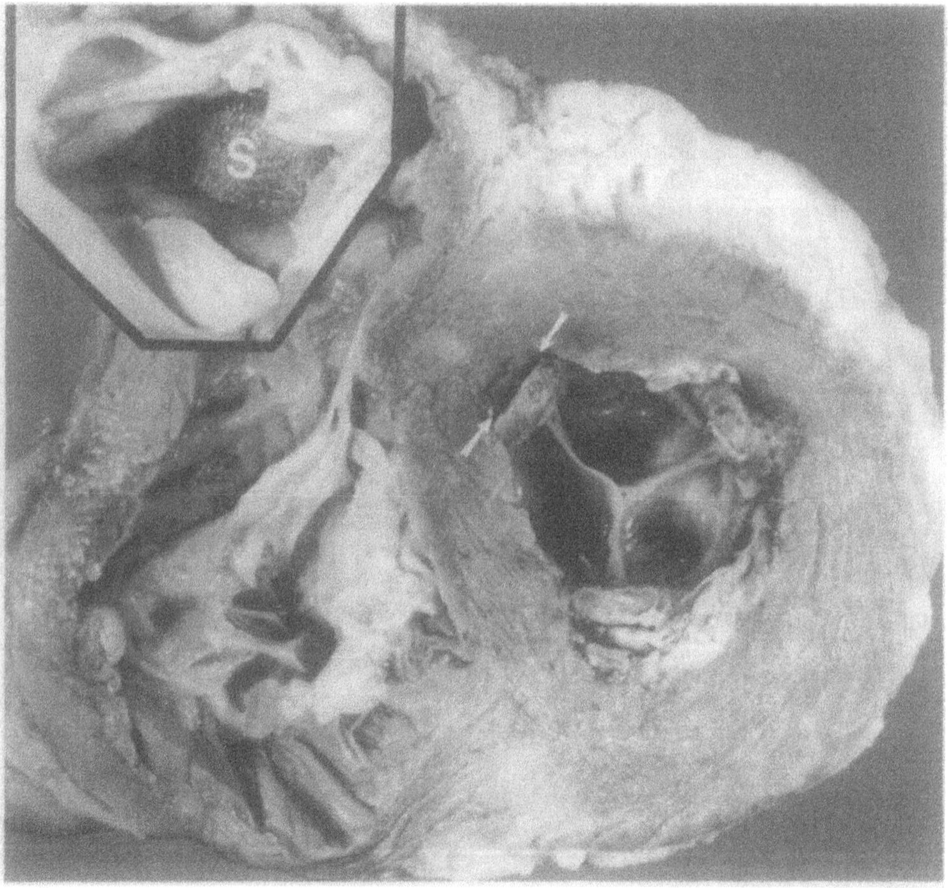

Fig. 1. Interior of the right and left ventricles, showing the bioprosthesis in the mitral valve position. Each of the three stents contacts left ventricular endocardium. *Arrows* indicate the minute area for left ventricular outflow. The insert *(upper left)* is a view of the obstructing stent(s) of the bioprosthesis in the mitral valve position from the aorta after the three aortic valve cusps had been excised.

of left ventricular hypertrophy. The chest radiograph showed an enlarged cardiac silhouette and evidence of chronic obstructive lung disease. At surgery, mitral valve repair was considered, but the valve leaflets were believed to be so abnormal that valve replacement was performed. The floppy mitral valve was excised and was replaced with a 29 mm Carpentier-Edwards bioprosthesis. The excised mitral valve was typical of mitral valve prolapse. The patient was weaned from cardiopulmonary bypass without difficulty; however, upon arrival in the recovery room, she was severely hypotensive and vasopressors were given. Nevertheless, the hypotension worsened, and 3 hours postoperatively, fatal cardiac arrest occurred. Initially, closed-chest cardiac massage was performed. When it was unsuccessful, the chest was opened, and the posterior wall of the left ventricle was found to have ruptured. The tear was repaired. The left ventricular cavity was distended and was difficult to empty by manual compression. (The ventricle likely ruptured as a result of external chest compressions on the distended, non-emptying left ventricle.) Further resuscitative efforts were unsuccessful. The heart weighed 425 gm. A 2.5 cm transverse tear in the posterior wall of the left ventricle had been closed with sutures. The ventricular cavities were of normal size. The bioprosthesis nearly occluded left ventricular outflow (Fig. 1). The three other cardiac valves were normal, no foci of myocardial necrosis or fibrosis were present, and the epicardial coronary arteries were normal.

In the above-described patient, the substitute cardiac valve inserted was too large (or the heart was too small), and the consequence was extreme obstruction to left ventricular outflow. Why was such a large-sized prosthesis inserted in this small-sized person? The hemodynamic mitral lesion before operation was pure regurgitation, i.e., no element of mitral stenosis, a lesion which when chronic usually results in dilatation of the left ventricular cavity. In the described patient, however, the left ventricular cavity was not dilated preoperatively (confirmed by left ventricular angiography). Although the heart was larger (425 gm) than normal in mass, it contained an excessive amount of fat, which probably accounted for the increased weight.

What precautions can a surgeon take to prevent this mechanical complication of mitral valve replacement? (1) He/she should utilize relatively small-sized prostheses in relatively small-sized persons irrespective of the type of hemodynamic lesion produced by the native valve to be replaced. (2) If the left ventricular cavity is of normal or near-normal size, the surgeon should err on the side of smaller-sized rather than larger-sized prostheses or bioprostheses. (3) The surgeon should be aware that any type of prosthesis or bioprosthesis is capable of producing left ventricular outflow obstruction, or specifically that a central flow substitute valve, as was inserted in the aforedescribed patient, does not prevent this complication. (4) If the prosthesis or bioprosthesis fills the entire "floor" of the left atrial cavity, it may be too large for the left ventricle, where the major portion of some substitute valves will reside. (5) Mechanical obstruction to left ventricular outflow (or inflow) may be suspected when a patient has a difficult time being weaned from cardiopulmonary bypass or develops severe hypotension shortly after weaning from bypass. (6) Intraoperatively, echocardiography is useful in diagnosing this complication.[13]

REFERENCES

1. Roberts WC, Morrow AG. Mechanisms of acute left atrial thrombosis after mitral valve replacement. Pathologic findings indicating obstruction to left atrial emptying. Am J Cardiol 1966;18:497-503.
2. Roberts WC, Morrow AG. Causes of early postoperative death following cardiac valve replacement. Clinico-pathologic correlation in 64 patients studied at necropsy. J Thorac Cardiovasc Surg 1967;54:422-37.
3. Roberts WC, Morrow AG. Anatomic studies of hearts containing caged-ball prosthetic valves. Johns Hopkins Med J 1967;121:271-95.
4. Shepard RL, Glancy DL, Stinson EB, Roberts WC. Hemodynamic confirmation of obstruction to left ventricular inflow by a caged-ball prosthetic mitral valve. Case report. J Thorac Cardiovasc Surg 1973;65:252-4.
5. Roberts WC, Bulkley BH, Morrow AG. Pathologic anatomy of cardiac valve replacement: a study of 224 necropsy patients. Prog Cardiovasc Dis 1973;15:539-87.
6. Seningen RP, Bulkley BH, Roberts WC. Prosthetic aortic stenosis. A method to prevent its occurrence by measurement of aortic size from preoperative aortogram. Circulation 1974;49:921-4.
7. Roberts WC, Hammer WJ. Cardiac pathology after valve replacement with a tilting-dics prosthesis (Björk-Shiley type). A study of 46 necropsy patients and 49 Björk-Shiley prostheses. Am J Cardiol 1976;37:1024-32.
8. Roberts WC. Complications of cardiac valve replacement: characteristic abnormalities of prostheses pertaining to any or specific site. AM HEART J 1982;103:113-22.
9. Rahimtoola SH. The problem of valve prosthesis–patient mismatch. Circulation 1978;58:20-4.
10. Pelikan PCD, Chew PH, Fortuin NJ, Yin FCP. Left ventricular outflow obstruction caused by a Starr-Edwards mitral prosthesis. Am J Cardiol 1983;52:552-3.
11. Currie PJ, Seward JB, Lam JB, Gersh BJ, Pluth JR. Left ventricular outflow tract obstruction related to a valve prosthesis: case caused by a low-profile mitral prosthesis. Mayo Clin Proc 1985;60:184-7.
12. Mihaileanu S, Marino JP, Chauvaud S, Perier P, Forman J, Vissoat J, Julien J, Dreyfus G, Abastado P, Carpentier A. Left ventricular outflow obstruction after mitral valve repair (Carpentier's technique). Circulation 1988;78:78-84.
13. Byrnes TJ, Cuillory WR, Hanley HG. Left ventricular outflow obstruction by a mitral valve prosthesis: Doppler ultrasound and cardiac catheterization findings. Cathet Cardiovasc Diagn 1989;17:34-8

Massive calcification of a porcine bioprosthesis in the aortic valve position and the role of calcium supplements

Heinrich G. Klues, MD, Lowell S. Statler, MD,
Robert B. Wallace, MD, and William C. Roberts, MD.
Washington, D.C., and Bethesda, Md.

The development of calcific deposits in porcine aortic valve cusps used in bioprostheses for cardiac valve replacement in humans is well recognized. Often the calcific deposits cause tearing of the porcine aortic valve cusps and the tearing may lead to severe valvular regurgitation. The calcific deposits on occasion may be large enough to decrease the mobility of the cusps and the immobility may lead to varying degrees of dysfunction. Bioprosthetic regurgitation, however, is a more common major complication of

From the Division of Cardiology, Department of Medicine, and the Department of Surgery, Georgetown University Medical Center; and the Pathology Branch, National Heart, Lung, and Blood Institute, National Institutes of Health.

Reprint requests: William C. Roberts, MD, Bldg. 10, Room 2N258, NHLBI-NIH, Bethesda, MD 20892.

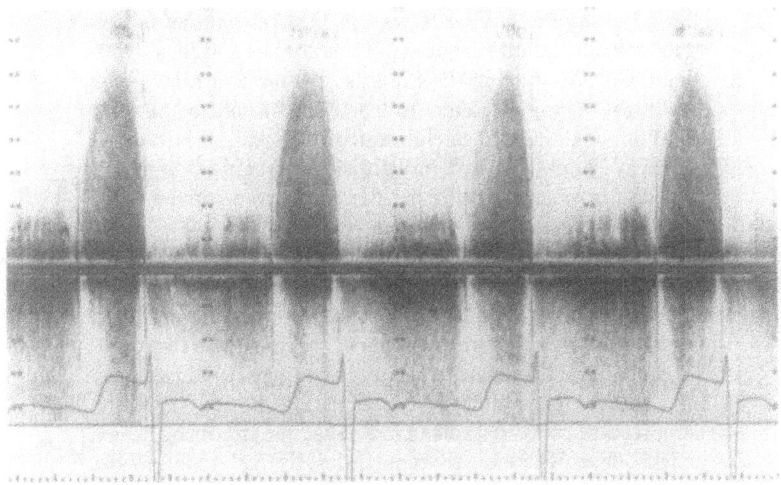

Fig. 1. Continuous-wave Doppler tracing obtained from the left ventricular apex demonstrating a 6 m/sec jet across the aortic valve, corresponding to a calculated peak systolic gradient of approximately 140 mm Hg between the left ventricle and aorta. The tracing also shows a mild aortic regurgitation jet.

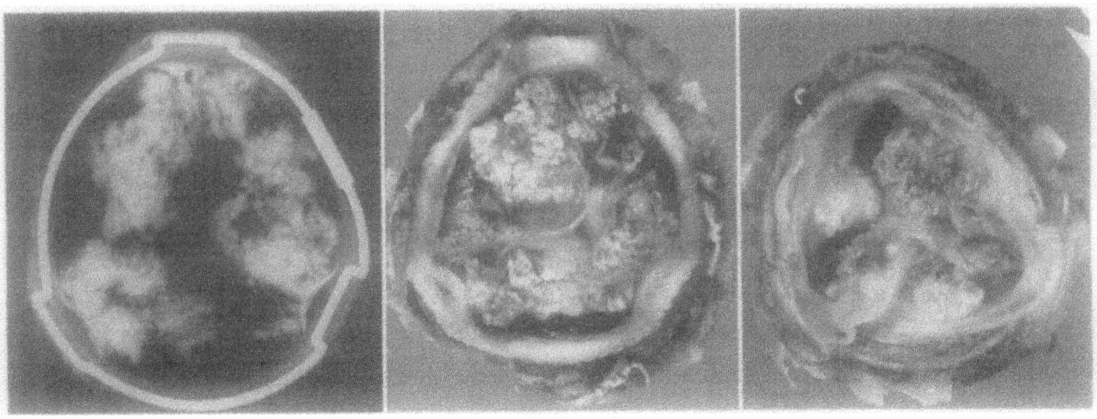

Fig. 2. Massively calcified bioprosthetic valve removed from the aortic valve position 126 months after implantation. **Left panel,** Radiograph; **center panel,** view from the aortic aspect; **right panel,** view from the ventricular aspect. It is extremely unusual to have calcific deposits on both ventricular and aortic aspects of the cusps; they are usually only found on the aortic aspects.

bioprosthetic replacement than is stenosis. In this report we describe massive calcific deposits with resulting extreme stenosis unassociated with significant regurgitation in a porcine bioprosthesis in the aortic valve position, and we discuss the possible relation of daily calcium supplements on the amount of bioprosthetic calcific deposits.

A 74-year-old woman had aortic valve replacement for a stenotic (47 mm Hg peak systolic pressure gradient between the left ventricle and the ascending aorta) congenitally bicuspid aortic valve stenosis in September 1978 when she was 64 years old. The native valve was replaced with a porcine bioprosthesis (Hancock 27 mm, Johnson & Johnson Cardiovascular, King of Prussia, Pa.). She was asymptomatic thereafter until January 1989, when while she was on a cruise, she noted dyspnea upon walking up stairs on the ship. Three days later, she was in acute pulmonary edema and was hospitalized. An echocardiogram (Fig. 1) disclosed a peak systolic pressure gradient between the left ventricle and the aorta of approximately 140 mm Hg. At cardiac catheterization, the bioprosthesis in the aortic valve position could not be crossed by the catheter despite repeated attempts. Five days after the onset of the dyspnea on the ship, the Hancock bioprosthesis in the aortic valve position was replaced with a Carpentier-Edwards bioprosthesis (29 mm, Baxter Healthcare Corp., Edwards Division, Santa Ana, Calif.). Eighteen months later (August 1990) she was asymptomatic and was working daily in her garden. The operatively excised Hancock bioprosthesis is shown in Fig. 2. Each cusp is heavily calcified, virtually immobile, and the deposits are present on both aortic and ventricular aspects of the cusps. No cusp is torn or perforated. Early postoperatively it was learned that this woman had been taking a calcium supplement daily for no specific medical indication for at least 20 years, including each of the 3769 days that the porcine bioprosthesis had been in the aortic valve position. Each Caltrate tablet (Lederle Laboratories, Pearl River, N.Y.) she took contained 1500 mg of calcium carbonate. Thus she took at least 5654 gm of Caltrate during the 3769 days. Each Caltrate tablet contains 600 mg of elemental calcium; therefore she took 2261 gm of elemental calcium during this 126-month postoperative period. Just before aortic valve replacement the blood urea nitrogen was 18 mg/dl and the creatinine was 1.0 mg/dl.

The unusual features of the patient described herein are the massive quantity of calcific deposits on the cusps of the porcine bioprosthesis, the degree of the pressure gradient across the bioprosthesis, the lack of tearing or perforations in the bioprosthetic cusps despite the huge calcific deposits, and the possibility that the taking of daily calcium supplements played a role in the development of the heavy calcific deposits. Search of reports describing late follow-up of patients having bioprostheses in the aortic valve position did not uncover any reported patients having a peak systolic pressure gradient >100 mm Hg across a bioprosthesis in the aortic valve position. Furthermore, we have not encountered any bioprostheses in any valve position previously having as extensive calcific deposits as were present in the bioprosthesis of the patient described herein. At least one other report has attempted to link heavy calcific deposits in a bioprosthesis to the taking of calcium supplements. Moront and Katz[1] described a 72-year-old woman who developed massive calcific deposits on a bioprosthesis in the mitral valve position in an 18-month period and the mean diastolic pressure gradient across the bioprosthesis was 19 mm Hg. This woman also took calcium carbonate supplements daily. It would appear from the study of the patient by Moront and Katz and from the study of the patient described herein that persons having bioprostheses should not take calcium supplements.

REFERENCE

1. Moront MG, Katz NM. Early degeneration of a porcine aortic valve bioprosthesis in the mitral valve position in an elderly woman and its association with long-term calcium carbonate therapy. Am J Cardiol 1987;59:1006-7.

Clinical and Anatomic Observations in Patients Having Mitral Valve Replacement for *Pure Mitral Regurgitation* and Simultaneous Tricuspid Valve Replacement

William C. Roberts, MD, and Erik A. Eways, BS

Among patients with chronic mitral valve dysfunction severe enough to warrant mitral valve replacement, associated tricuspid valve dysfunction is relatively common. Most patients having tricuspid valve replacement have simultaneous mitral valve replacement because of mitral stenosis (with or without associated mitral regurgitation). Among patients having simultaneous mitral and tricuspid valve replacement, relatively few have pure mitral regurgitation. This report describes certain clinical and morphologic findings in 17

From the Pathology Branch, National Heart, Lung, and Blood Institute, National Institutes of Health, Bethesda, Maryland 20892. Manuscript received April 25, 1991; revised manuscript received June 11, 1991, and accepted June 12.

TABLE I Clinical, Anatomic, and Hemodynamic Observations in 17 Patients with Mitral and Tricuspid Valve Replacement for Pure Mitral and Tricuspid Valve Regurgitation

Case	Surgical Number	Age (yr) at VR & Sex	Etiology of Valve Disease	Pressures (mm Hg) Right Atrium m	a	v	PAW or LA m	a	v	PA (s/d)	RV (s/d)	LV (s/d)	SA (s/d)	Interval VR → Death	Interval VR → Last Follow-Up
1	S78-38	41F	MVP	11	—	14	32	—	—	94/50	94/15	145/20	150/80	—	60 days
2	S75-5160	52M	MVP (RCT)	5	—	—	24	—	38	56/30	56/16	86/19	95/60	—	10 years
3	S79-37	65F	MVP	14	—	16	25	—	30	60/35	60/14	142/12	160/100	95 mos	—
4	S75-5056	66M	MVP	8	—	—	17	—	22	28/10	28/8	100/9	105/65	2 mos	—
5	S78-207	73M	MVP	14	—	18	35	—	65	50/27	50/10	120/13	120/79	2 mos	—
6	S83-126	27F	IE, healed (RCT)	16	21	20	30	30	50	75/40	75/20	110/22	110/80	68 mos	—
7	S75-5171	46F	IE, healed (RCT)	11	—	—	22	—	26	100/40	100/12	120/14	138/80	—	10 years
8	S79-128	63F	IE, healed	9	—	10	26	—	28	48/25	48/8	100/16	105/70	—	60 days
9	S83-145	60F	ASD with MVP	16	—	—	20	—	24	36/22	36/14	168/29	168/75	1 day	—
10	S77-149	64F	ASD with MVP	13	18	17	18	26	22	70/26	70/22	150/28	180/100	1 mo	—
11	S81-186	50M	HC with MVP	24	—	30	45	—	—	85/36	85/22	110/24	110/65	34 mos	—
12	S83-152	68M	HC with MVP	20	22	22	35	25	55	85/37	85/18	110/26	125/70	2 days	—
13	S81-8	70M	HC (IE → RCT)	14	—	24	38	—	55	85/35	85/12	120/14	120/60	28 days	—
14	S82-158	32M	HS	21	25	24	33	36	56	55/33	55/25	95/38	100/75	36 mos	—
15	S80-190	36M	HS	15	20	18	30	30	34	60/30	60/16	85/32	95/64	—	7 years
16	S78-142	45F	Rheumatic	19	—	22	26	—	36	50/30	50/6	125/14	125/70	—	10 years
17	S79-40	59M	Calcified PM*	18	—	22	30	—	55	85/30	85/18	160/22	170/90	—	60 days
Mean		54		15	21	20	30	29	40	66/32	66/14	121/21	128/75		

*Mitral leaflets and chordae tendineae were normal. Coronary arteries were angiographically normal.

a = a wave; ASD = atrial septal defect; HC = hypertrophic cardiomyopathy; HS = hypereosinophilic syndrome; IE = infective endocarditis; LA = left atrium; LV = left ventricle; m = mean; MVP = mitral valve prolapse; PA = pulmonary artery; PAW = pulmonary artery wedge; PM = papillary muscle; RCT = ruptured chordae tendineae; RV = right ventricle; SA = systemic artery; s/d = peak systole/end-diastole; v = v wave; VR = valve replacement.

patients having mitral replacement for severe, chronic, pure mitral regurgitation, and simultaneous tricuspid valve replacement for severe tricuspid valve dysfunction.

A total of 113 patients >20 years of age underwent simultaneous replacement of dysfunctioning native tricuspid and mitral valves at the Surgery Branch of the National Heart, Lung, and Blood Institute between September 1963 and December 1989. Of the 113 patients, the mitral valve was stenotic before valve replacement in 96 (85%) and purely regurgitant in 17 (15%). This report focuses exclusively on the latter 17 patients. Certain pertinent clinical and morphologic findings in them are listed in Table I and illustrated in Figures 1 to 5. Methods of diagnosis of both mitral and tricuspid regurgitation in the patients have been described elsewhere.[1,2] The 17 patients (8 (47%) women and 9 (53%) men, aged 27 to 73 years [mean 54]) underwent double valve replacement from 1975 to 1983. None of the 17 patients had clinical evidence of aortic valve dysfunction. Sixteen patients (94%) had pulmonary hypertension, including 8 (47%) with peak pulmonary arterial systolic pressure ≥70 mm Hg. All

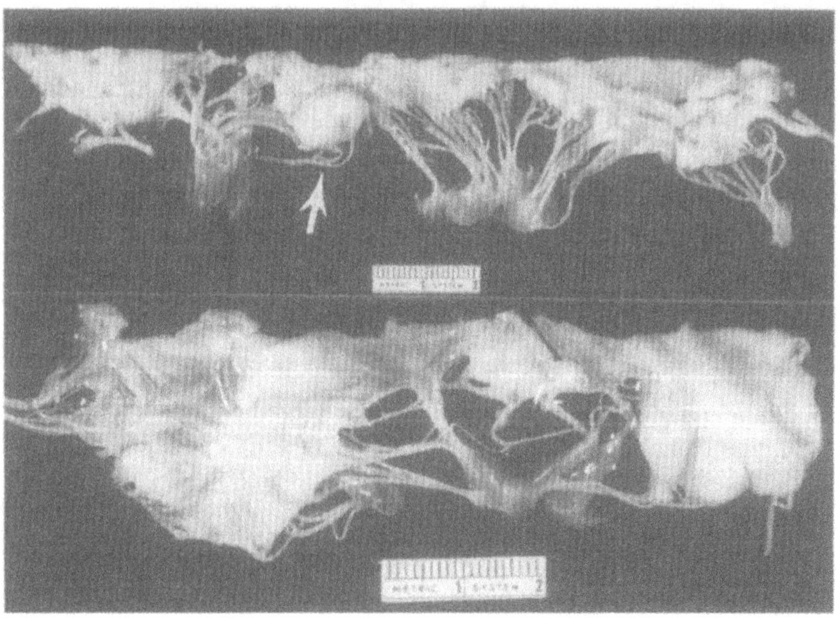

FIGURE 1. Case 4 (Table I). Opened mitral valve (*upper*) and tricuspid valve (*lower*). A portion of posterior mitral leaflet (*arrow*) is prolapsed. Tricuspid leaflets also show mild hooding.

had clinical evidence of severe tricuspid valve regurgitation and none had a pressure gradient between right atrium and right ventricle during ventricular diastole. Likewise, none had a pressure gradient between pulmonary arterial wedge position or left atrium and left ventricle during ventricular diastole.

The various etiologies of the mitral regurgitation are listed in Table I. Five patients had isolated mitral valve prolapse,[3,4] 2 had mitral valve prolapse associated with hypertrophic cardiomyopathy[5] and 2 had mitral valve prolapse associated with secundum type atrial septal defect. Infective endocarditis that

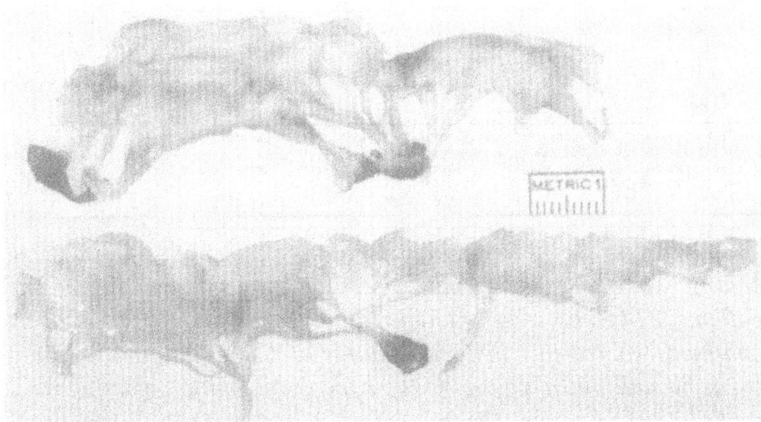

FIGURE 2. Case 9 (Table I). Opened mitral valve (*upper*) and tricuspid valve (*lower*) associated with atrial septal defect. Clinically, a portion of posterior mitral leaflet had prolapsed by left ventricular angiogram.

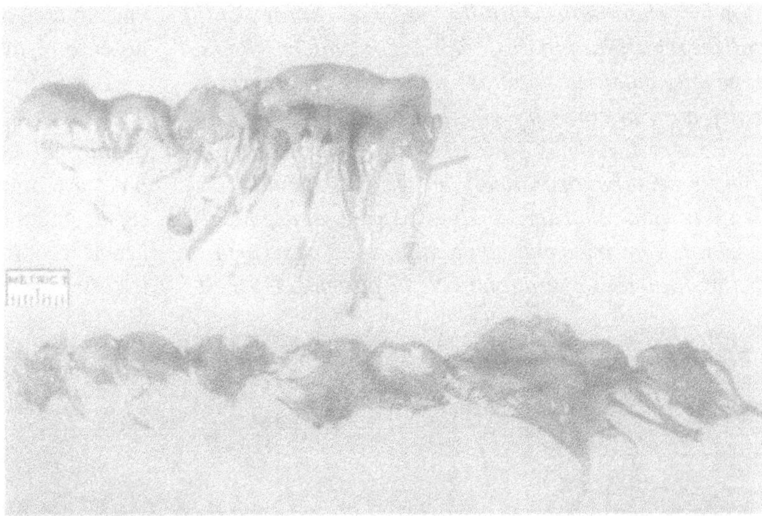

FIGURE 3. Case 12 (Table I). Opened mitral valve (*upper*) and tricuspid valve (*lower*). Mitral leaflets are thickened in a fashion typical of hypertrophic cardiomyopathy. Tricuspid valve leaflets are normal.

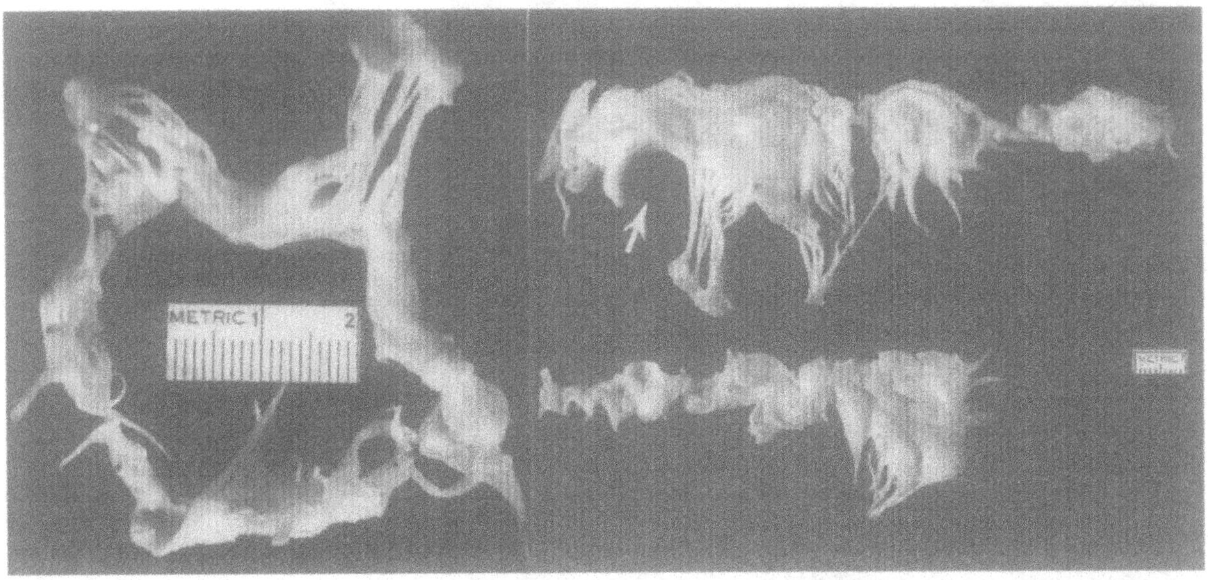

FIGURE 4. Case 13 (Table I). Intact mitral valve (*left*) showing a dilated anulus, opened mitral valve (*upper right*) showing an indentation (*arrow*) with loss of chordae tendineae in anterolateral half of anterior mitral leaflet, and opened normal tricuspid valve (*lower right*) in patient with hypertrophic cardiomyopathy associated with severe mitral and tricuspid valve regurgitation.

TABLE II Functional and Anatomic Status of the Tricuspid Valve in Patients Having Simultaneous Replacement of Both Mitral and Tricuspid Valves with Pure Mitral Regurgitation

Study	No. of Pts. with Pure MR	No. of Pts. with Pure TR	No. of Pts. with TS	Anatomic Status of Tricuspid Valve: Normal	Abnormal
Hauck et al (1988)	28	28	0	16 (57%)	12* (43%)
Roberts & Eways (1991)	17	17	0	15 (88%)	2† (12%)

*All 12 patients had "post-inflammatory" (rheumatic) heart disease of both the mitral and tricuspid valve leaflets.
†Both patients had hypereosinophilic syndrome with thrombi involving both mitral and tricuspid valve cusps.
MR = mitral regurgitation; TR = tricuspid regurgitation; TS = tricuspid stenosis.

healed[6] was the cause of mitral regurgitation in 4 patients, 1 of whom also had hypertrophic cardiomyopathy. Two patients had involvement of both the tricuspid and mitral valves by the hypereosinophilic syndrome.[7] In 1 patient, the cause of mitral regurgitation was rheumatic heart disease.[8] The etiology of the mitral regurgitation was unclear in 1 patient who had a heavily calcified papillary muscle but angiographically normal coronary arteries.

Except for the 2 patients with hypereosinophilic syndrome, the operatively excised tricuspid valve leaflets and chordae tendineae were anatomically normal. The tricuspid valve anuli were described as being dilated at operation in all 17 patients. Of the 17 patients, 5 died within 2 months of the double valve replacement and 4 others died from 34 to 95 months afterwards, 1 was known to be alive 7 years and 3 were known to be alive 10 years after valve replacement, and 3 were lost to follow-up within 2 months of the valve replacement operation.

Pure tricuspid valve regurgitation associated with pure mitral regurgitation in the absence of hypereosinophilic syndrome is usually associated with an anatomically normal tricuspid valve. Therefore, the tricuspid regurgitation in this setting appears to result from tricuspid anular dilation, which appears to be a consequence of right ventricular dilatation. The peak right ventricular systolic pressure averaged 66 mm Hg in the 17 patients and was <30 mm Hg in only 1 patient. The type of tricuspid valve dysfunction found in patients with pure mitral regurgitation is nearly always pure tricuspid regurgitation. Except in the patient with the carcinoid syndrome[9] or congenital cardiac anomalies, we have never encountered a patient with tricuspid valve stenosis in the absence of mitral valve stenosis.

It is difficult to compare the findings from this study with those reported previously. Hauck et al[10] examined operatively excised tricuspid valves in 28 patients who had pure mitral regurgitation with simultaneous mitral repair or replacement (Table II). From study of their article it is probable that all 28 of their patients had pure tricuspid valve regurgitation and that none of them had

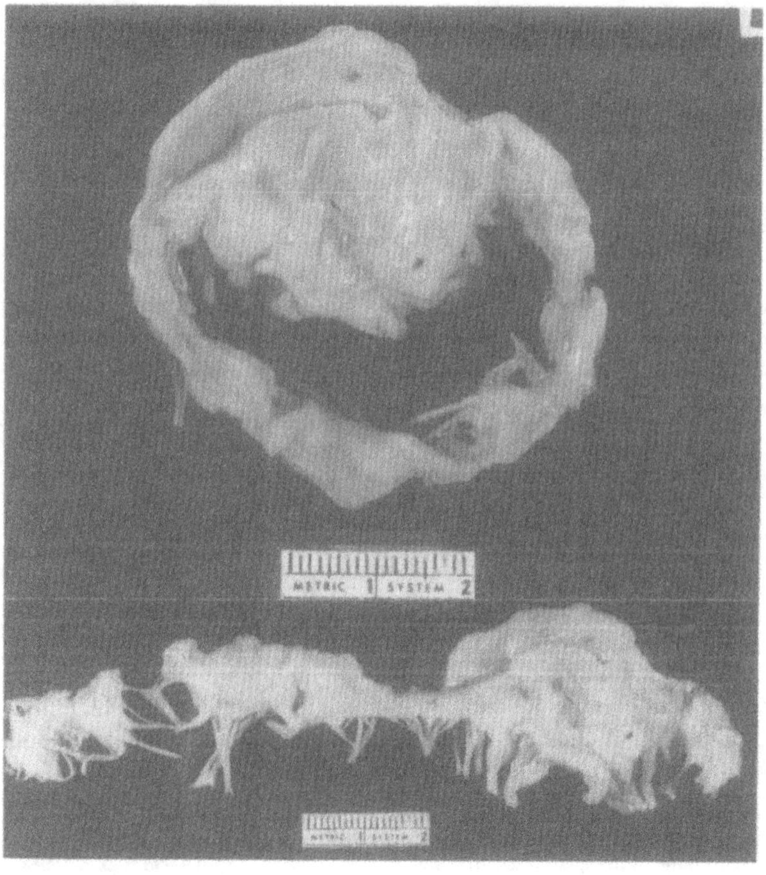

FIGURE 5. Case 16 (see Table I). Intact purely incompetent mitral valve (*upper*) and opened mitral valve (*lower*). Leaflets are diffusely fibrotic consistent with a rheumatic etiology. Tricuspid valve was anatomically normal.

stenotic tricuspid valves. Of their 28 patients, 16 (57%) had normal and 12 (43%) had diffusely fibrotic tricuspid valves. All of the latter 12 patients had postinflammatory (rheumatic) mitral and tricuspid valve disease. It is unclear whether some of the 28 patients reported by Hauck et al had associated aortic valve disease. The latter patients were excluded from our study. None of the 45 necropsy patients with pure tricuspid regurgitation reported by Waller et al[11] had pure mitral regurgitation.

Because in recent years there has been a tendency to perform anuloplasty for tricuspid regurgitation associated with left-sided valvular heart disease rather than tricuspid valve replacement, it is likely that right-sided valve replacement would not have been performed in most of the patients described herein were the operation performed today. Thus, the opportunity to examine the tricuspid valve in similar fashion in patients with pure, chronic mitral regurgitation will be less likely in the future.

In summary, the type of tricuspid valve dysfunction occurring in association with pure chronic mitral regurgitation is virtually always pure regurgitation, and the cause of the tricuspid valve regurgitation is usually dilatation of the tricuspid valve anulus.

1. Cohen SR, Sell JE, McIntosh CL, Clark RE. Tricuspid regurgitation in patients with acquired, chronic, pure mitral regurgitation. I. Prevalence, diagnosis, and comparison of preoperative clinical and hemodynamic features in patients with and without tricuspid regurgitation. *J Thorac Cardiovasc Surg* 1987;94:481–487.

2. Cohen SR, Sell JE, McIntosh CL, Clark RE. Tricuspid regurgitation in patients with acquired, chronic, pure mitral regurgitation. II. Nonoperative management, tricuspid valve annuloplasty, and tricuspid valve replacement. *J Thorac Cardiovasc Surg* 1987;94:488–497.

3. Roberts WC, McIntosh CL, Wallace RB. Mechanisms of severe mitral regurgitation in mitral valve prolapse determined from analysis of operatively excised valves. *Am Heart J* 1987;113:1316–1323.

4. Dollar AL, Roberts WC. Morphologic comparison of patients with mitral valve prolapse who died suddenly with patients who died from severe valvular dysfunction or other conditions. *J Am Coll Cardiol* 1991;17:921–931.

5. Roberts CS, Roberts WC. Morphologic features (of hypertrophic cardiomyopathy). *Prog Cardiol* 1989;2/2:3–32.

6. Roberts WC, Buchbinder NA. Healed left-sided infective endocarditis: a clinicopathologic study of 59 patients. *Am J Cardiol* 1977;40:876–888.

7. Harley JB, McIntosh CL, Kirklin JJW, Maron BJ, Gottdiener J, Roberts WC, Fauci AS. Atrioventricular valve replacement in the idiopathic hypereosinophilic syndrome. *Am J Med* 1982;73:77–81.

8. Roberts WC. Morphologic features of the normal and abnormal mitral valve. *Am J Cardiol* 1983;51:1005–1028.

9. Ross EM, Roberts WC. The carcinoid syndrome. Comparison of 21 necropsy subjects with carcinoid heart disease to 15 necropsy subjects without carcinoid heart disease. *Am J Med* 1985;79:339–354.

10. Hauck AJ, Freeman DP, Ackermann DM, Danielson GK, Edwards WD. Surgical pathology of the tricuspid valve. A study of 363 cases spanning 25 years. *Mayo Clin Proc* 1988;63:851–863.

11. Waller BF, Moriarty AT, Eble JN, Davey DM, Hawley DA, Pless JE. Etiology of pure tricuspid regurgitation based on anular circumference and leaflet area: analysis of 45 necropsy patients with clinical and morphologic evidence of pure tricuspid regurgitation. *J Am Coll Cardiol* 1986;7:1063–1074.

Clinical and Anatomic Observations in Patients Having Mitral Valve Replacement for *Mitral Stenosis* and Simultaneous Tricuspid Valve Replacement

Erik A. Eways, BS,* and William C. Roberts, MD

Certain clinical and morphologic findings are described in 67 patients (aged 23 to 76 years [mean 52]; 55 women [82%]) who had mitral valve replacement for mitral stenosis (with or without associated regurgitation), and simultaneous tricuspid valve replacement for pure tricuspid regurgitation (58 patients) or tricuspid stenosis (all with associated regurgitation; 9 patients). Of the 58 patients with pure tricuspid regurgitation, 21 had anatomically normal and 37 had anatomically abnormal (diffusely fibrotic leaflets) tricuspid valves. Among these 58 patients, no clinical or hemodynamic variable was useful before surgery in distinguishing the group without from that with anatomically abnormal tricuspid valves. All 9 patients with stenotic tricuspid valves had anatomically abnormal tricuspid valves. The latter group had a lower average right ventricular systolic pressure (tricuspid valve closing pressure) than those with pure tricuspid regurgitation, and none had severe pulmonary arterial hypertension (present in 20 [30%] of the 58 patients with pure tricuspid regurgitation).

(Am J Cardiol 1991;68:1367–1371)

From the Pathology Branch, National Heart, Lung, and Blood Institute, National Institutes of Health, Bethesda, Maryland. Manuscript received June 17, 1991; revised manuscript received July 12, 1991, and accepted July 15.

Address for reprints: William C. Roberts, MD, Building 10, Room 2N258, National Institutes of Health, 9000 Rockville Pike, Bethesda, Maryland 20892.

*Sophomore medical student, George Washington University School of Medicine and Health Sciences, Washington, D.C.

A significant percentage of patients with primary mitral valve disease have tricuspid valve dysfunction. Consequently, some patients undergoing mitral valve replacement or repair operations for primary mitral disease also have tricuspid valve replacement or other operative procedures performed on the right-sided atrioventricular valve. Among surgeons who perform many cardiac valve operations yearly, some rarely replace the tricuspid valve and others do so relatively frequently. If the tricuspid valve is stenotic, the decision is relatively easy; if it is purely regurgitant, the decision is more difficult. In the latter circumstance, the tricuspid valve leaflets may be anatomically abnormal, normal or virtually normal. In this report we focus on the frequency and type of structural abnormality of the tricuspid valve in patients having simultaneous replacement of both mitral and tricuspid valves for *mitral stenosis* and tricuspid valve dysfunction (either pure regurgitation or stenosis [with or without regurgitation]).

METHODS

Patients studied: In the Surgery Branch of the National Heart, Lung, and Blood Institute from September 1963 to December 1989, a total of 113 patients >20 years of age underwent simultaneous replacement of the native mitral and tricuspid valves without aortic valve replacement at any time. Of the 113 patients, 11 were excluded from further analysis because a peak systolic pressure gradient between the left ventricle and a systemic artery >10 mm Hg was present. Another 18 patients were excluded because either the operatively excised tricuspid and mitral valves were not available for reexamination or photographs of these operatively excised valves were unavailable. Of the remaining 84 patients, 67 had mitral stenosis and 17 had pure mitral regurgitation. This report focuses on the 67 patients with mitral stenosis. Thirty-two (48%) of the 67 patients previously had valvular commissurotomy operations: mitral valve only (28 patients), tricuspid valve only (2), and both mitral and tricuspid valve commissurotomy (2). None of the 67 patients had a previous anuloplasty procedure on either the tricuspid or mitral valve.

TABLE I Clinical, Hemodynamic and Anatomic Observations in 67 Patients Having Combined Mitral and Tricuspid Valve Replacement for Mitral and Tricuspid Valve Stenoses or Regurgitation, or Both

Group	Type of Valve Dysfunction	Valve Anatomically Abnormal	No. of Pts. (%)	Age (yrs) at VR Range (mean)	Women (%)	Men (%)	Pressures (mm Hg): Right Atrium Mean	Right Atrium V Wave	PAW or LA Mean	PAW or LA V Wave	RV (s/d) Average	LV (s/d) Average	RVSP ≤40 (%)	RVSP > 70 (%)	LVSP > 140 (%)	Dead After VR: ≤60 Days (%)	12 Mos	60 Mos	10 Yrs
1	MS,TR	MV	21 (31)	23–75 (54)	17 (81)	4 (19)	12	21	22	29	61/11	117/12	5 (24)	4 (19)	2 (10)	2/21 (10)	4/19	8/17	11/16
2	MS,TR	MV & TV	37 (55)	25–76 (54)	29 (78)	8 (22)	14	22	26	35	68/13	117/14	7 (19)	16 (43)	3 (8)	8/37 (22)	8/34	10/29	15/23
3	MS,TS	MV & TV	9 (14)	29–55 (40)	9 (100)	0 (0)	13	20	19	32	47/10	121/13	2 (22)	0 (0)	2 (22)	2/9 (22)	3/9	3/9	3/6
Totals or means			67 (100)	23–76 (52)	55 (82)	12 (18)	13	21	23	33	63/12	118/13	14 (21)	20 (30)	7 (10)	12/67 (18)	5/62 (24%)	21/55 (38%)	29/45 (64%)

LA = left atrium; LV = left ventricle; LVSP = left ventricular peak systolic pressure; MS = mitral stenosis (with or without mitral regurgitation); MV = mitral valve; PAW = pulmonary artery wedge; RV = right ventricle; RVSP = right ventricular peak systolic pressure; s/d = peak systole/end-diastole; TR = tricuspid regurgitation; TS = tricuspid stenosis; TV = tricuspid valve; VR = valve replacement.

Year of operation and surgeon: The 67 valve replacement operations were performed by 6 different surgeons during the following time periods: 1963 to 1965 (1 patient); 1966 to 1970 (13); 1971 to 1975 (20); 1976 to 1980 (16); 1981 to 1985 (10); and 1986 to 1989 (7).

Classifications and definitions: The clinical records of all 67 patients were reviewed. The operatively excised valves had all been examined and classified initially by WCR. Of the 134 operatively excised valves in the 67 patients, 62 were reexamined, and photographs of the other 72 were examined. The original description of the operatively excised valve by WCR was reviewed in all 67 patients.

The patients were divided into 3 groups on the basis of valvular function and structure (Table I). The leaflets in all stenotic valves (both mitral and tricuspid) were diffusely fibrotic, and the mitral leaflets were often focally calcified. Calcific deposits were absent in all stenotic tricuspid valves. Nonstenotic, purely regurgitant tricuspid valves considered anatomically abnormal were also diffusely fibrotic, but their orifices were nonstenotic. Tricuspid valves considered anatomically normal were free of diffuse leaflet or chordal thickening; some had small focal leaflet thickenings involving 1 or 2 leaflets. (These focal thickenings were considered consequences of increased right ventricular systolic or closing pressure on the leaflets.) All patients with mitral stenosis were considered to have rheumatic heart disease. Mitral and tricuspid stenoses were confirmed in all patients by cardiac catheterization before surgery. All 67 patients had right- and left-sided cardiac catheterization during the 6 weeks preceding simultaneous replacement of the native mitral and tricuspid valves.

RESULTS

Certain clinical, hemodynamic and morphologic findings in the 67 patients (55 women [82%]) are listed in Table I, and some valves are illustrated in Figures 1 to 5. Of the 67 patients, 9 (14%) had associated tricuspid valve stenosis (group 3) and, consequently, anatomically abnormal tricuspid valves; 58 (86%) had pure tricuspid valve regurgitation, 21 (31%) with anatomically normal (group 1) and 37 (55%) with anatomically abnormal tricuspid valves (group 2). No significant differences among the 3 groups were observed before surgery in mean right atrial pressure, average right atrial peak V wave, percentage of patients with peak right ventricular systolic pressure ≤40 mm Hg, peak left ventricular systolic pressure, percentage of patients with peak left ventricular systolic pressure >140 mm Hg, average peak systemic arterial systolic pressure, and mean and average V wave in the pulmonary artery wedge position or left atrium. Patients in group 3 (mitral and tricuspid stenoses) had lower average peak right ventricular systolic pressure and percentage of patients with right ventricular systolic pressures >70 mm Hg than those in the other 2 groups had.

DISCUSSION

The present study focuses on structural alterations in operatively excised tricuspid valves in patients having mitral valve replacement because of mitral stenosis. Pa-

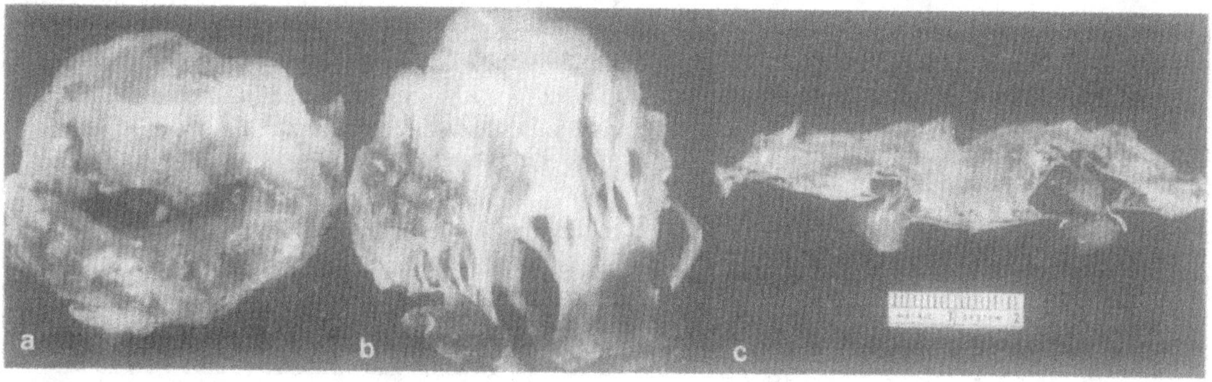

FIGURE 1. Operatively excised stenotic mitral valve *(a and b)*, and purely regurgitant and anatomically normal tricuspid valve *(c)* in 59-year-old woman (S74-5134). Mean diastolic gradient across mitral valve was 18 mm Hg. Right ventricular pressure was 50/7 mm Hg, and left ventricular pressure was 124/9 mm Hg.

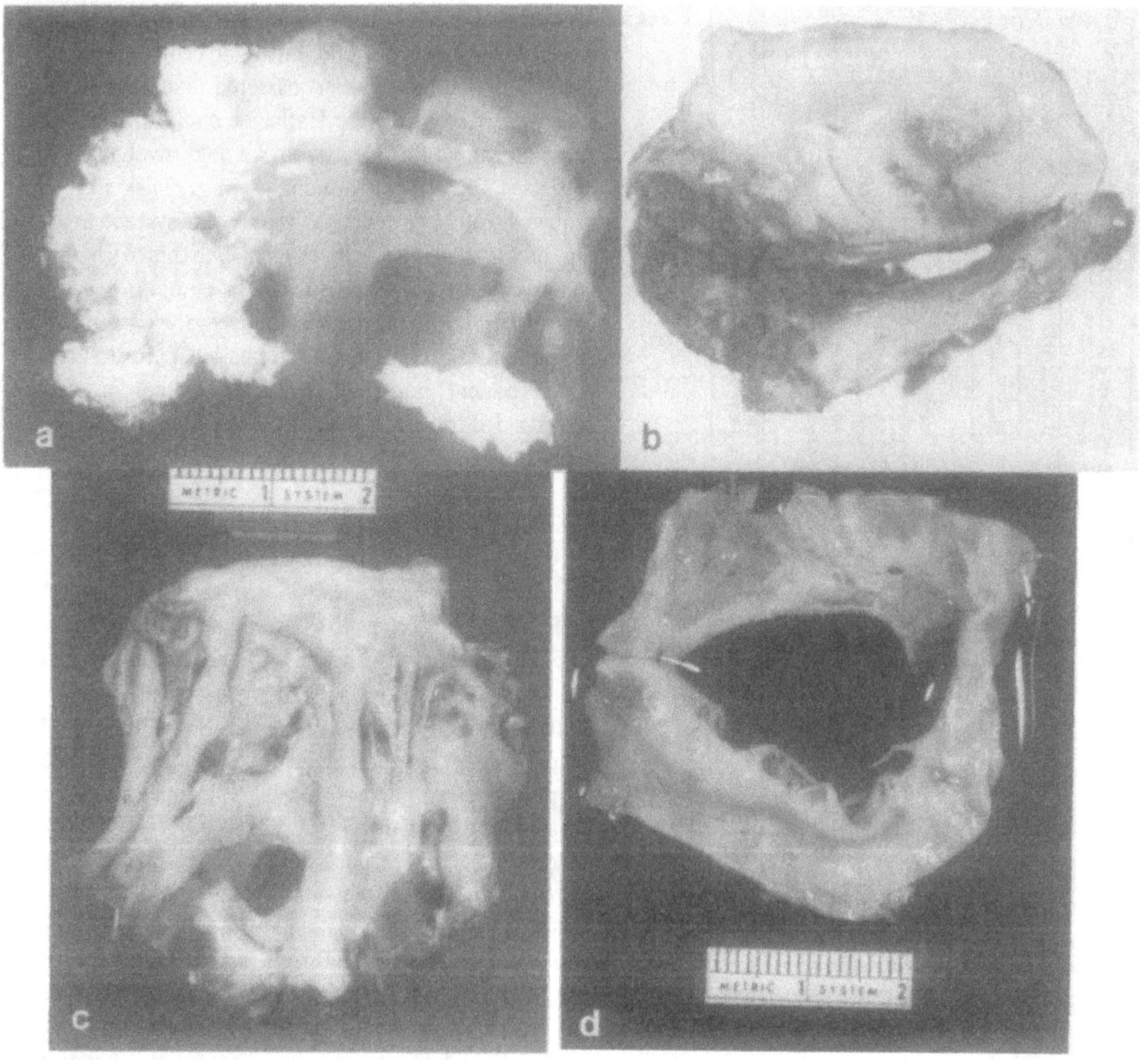

FIGURE 2. Operatively excised stenotic mitral valve *(a to c)* and purely regurgitant, diffusely fibrotic tricuspid valve *(d)* in 65-year-old man (S74-5046). Right ventricular pressure was 120/27 mm Hg, and left ventricular pressure was 100/25 mm Hg. The mitral valve is calcified.

tients whose indication for mitral valve replacement was pure mitral regurgitation were excluded from this study. Of the 67 patients having stenotic mitral valves replaced, the leaflets and chordae tendineae of all mitral valves were diffusely fibrotic with or without calcific deposits.[1,2] The operatively excised tricuspid valves in these patients were anatomically normal in 21 patients (31%) and anatomically abnormal (diffusely fibrotic) in 46 (69%). The tricuspid valves in the latter 46 patients were purely regurgitant in 37 (80%) and stenotic

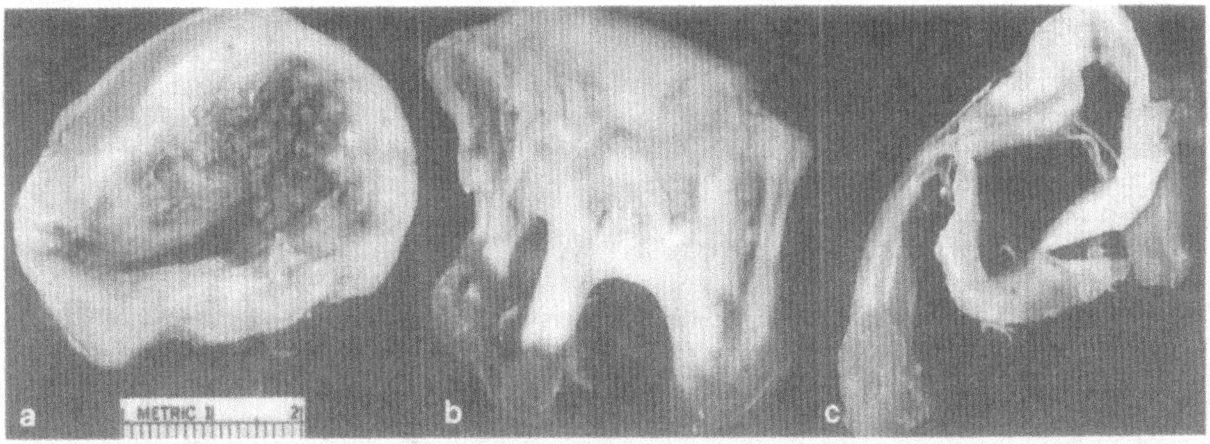

FIGURE 3. Operatively excised stenotic mitral valve *(a and b)* and diffusely fibrotic purely regurgitant tricuspid valve *(c)* in 54-year-old man (S68-2439). Right ventricular pressure was 65/10 mm Hg, and left ventricular pressure was 110/12 mm Hg.

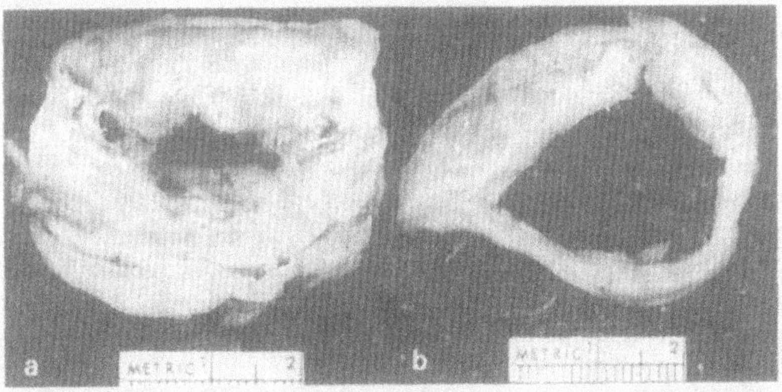

FIGURE 4. Operatively excised stenotic mitral valve *(a)* and diffusely fibrotic mildly stenotic tricuspid valve *(b)* in 55-year-old woman (S71-3034). Right ventricular pressure was 38/11 mm Hg, and left ventricular pressure was 148/14 mm Hg.

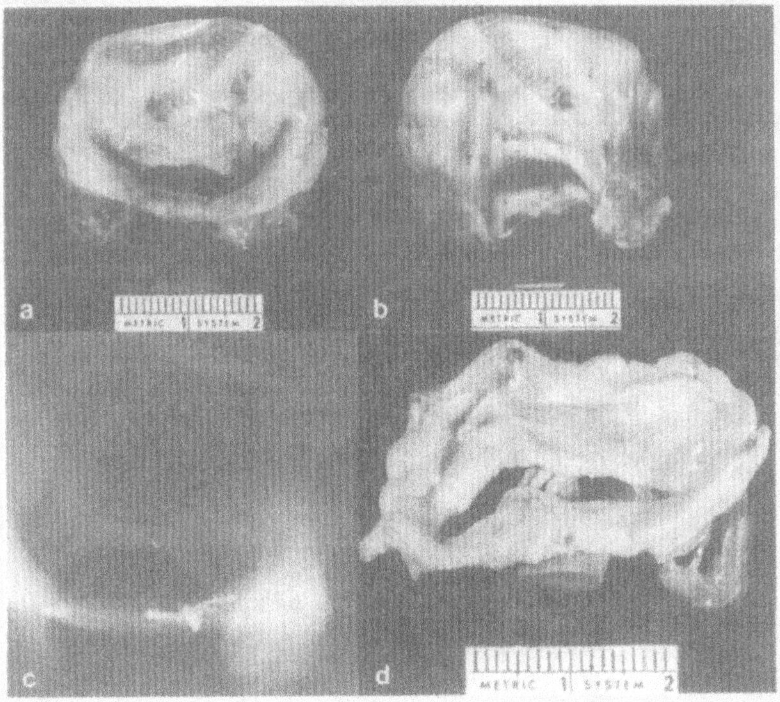

FIGURE 5. Operatively excised stenotic mitral valve *(a to c)* and stenotic tricuspid valve *(d)* in 29-year-old woman (S74-5057) whose right ventricular pressure was 45/15 mm Hg and whose left ventricular pressure was 110/18 mm Hg. Radiograph *(c)* shows only small deposit of calcium in 1 mitral leaflet.

(mean right atrial to right ventricular mean diastolic gradient ranged from 3 to 11 mm Hg [average = 6]) with or without associated regurgitation in 9 (20%).

When a cardiac valve (tricuspid or any other cardiac valve) is stenotic, the valve leaflets are diffusely fibrotic or extensively calcified (i.e., anatomically abnormal).[2,3] Among patients with mitral stenosis severe enough to warrant a mitral valve operation, associated tricuspid valve stenosis is infrequent (14% in the present study). This percentage, however, is much less if the analysis does not focus exclusively on patients having simultaneous replacement of both the mitral and tricuspid valves. In the study by Roberts[2] focusing on necropsy patients with fatal valvular heart disease (some of whom had had cardiac operations and some of whom had not), 434 (43%) of 1,010 patients ≥15 years of age had mitral stenosis with or without associated mitral regurgitation. Of the 434 patients, mitral stenosis was not associated with aortic valve dysfunction or tricuspid stenosis in 189 (44%); it was combined with aortic stenosis in 152 (35%), with pure aortic regurgitation in 65 (13%), with both aortic and tricuspid stenoses in 24 (6%) and with tricuspid stenosis alone in 4 (1%). Therefore, if the 176 patients with associated aortic stenosis (24 of whom also had tricuspid stenosis) and the 65 with pure aortic regurgitation were excluded from the necropsy study (as they were in the present study), only 4 (2%) of the remaining 193 patients with mitral stenosis had associated tricuspid valve stenosis.[2]

Among patients with mitral stenosis severe enough to warrant a mitral valve operation, a significant percentage of them will also have some degree of pure tricuspid regurgitation. Of the 67 patients with replaced stenotic mitral valves in the present study, 58 (86%) had purely regurgitant tricuspid valves and 9 (14%) had stenotic tricuspid valves. The 58 purely regurgitant tricuspid valves were anatomically abnormal in 37 patients (64%) and anatomically normal in 21 (36%). We found only 1 previously published report with which our observations could be meaningfully compared. Hauck et al[4] examined operatively excised tricuspid valves in 248 patients with mitral stenosis, and 163 (66%) of them had purely regurgitant tricuspid valves and 85 (34%) had stenotic tricuspid valves. Of the 163 patients with purely regurgitant tricuspid valves, the tricuspid leaflets and chordae tendineae were anatomically normal in 54 (22%) and diffusely fibrotic in 194 (78%). The patients reported by Hauck and associates and by us underwent valve replacement during similar time periods (1963 to 1989). Comparison of these 2 studies indicates that the patients with mitral stenosis undergoing replacement of both mitral and tricuspid valves at the Mayo Clinic (Hauck et al) had a higher frequency of associated tricuspid valve stenosis and, therefore, a lower frequency of pure tricuspid regurgitation than those having similar therapy at the National Institutes of Health (present study).

Tricuspid valve replacement is performed less frequently today than during the 1960s and 1970s when 50 patients (75%) described in the present study underwent valve replacement operations. Justifying tricuspid valve replacement in the presence of tricuspid valve stenosis is much easier than justifying tricuspid valve replacement in the presence of pure tricuspid valve regurgitation associated with mitral stenosis. When the tricuspid leaflets and chordae are anatomically normal, as they were in 21 (31%) of the 67 patients described herein, we believe that most surgeons today would rarely replace the tricuspid valve. When the tricuspid valve is purely regurgitant but the leaflets are diffusely fibrotic, the decision of replacement versus anuloplasty (with ring) is more difficult. Unfortunately, in the present study none of the clinical or hemodynamic variables analyzed (Table I) was useful in distinguishing before surgery patients with purely regurgitant anatomically normal tricuspid valves from those with purely regurgitant anatomically abnormal ones.

REFERENCES

1. Lachman AS, Roberts WC. Calcific deposits in stenotic mitral valves. Extent and relation to age, sex, degree of stenosis, cardiac rhythm, previous commissurotomy and left atrial body thrombus from study of 164 operatively-excised valves. *Circulation* 1978;57:808–815.

2. Roberts WC. Morphologic features of the normal and abnormal mitral valve. *Am J Cardiol* 1983;51:1005–1028.

3. Olson LJ, Subramanian R, Ackermann DM, Orszulak TA, Edwards WD. Surgical pathology of the mitral valve: a study of 712 cases spanning 21 years. *Mayo Clinic Proc* 1987;62:22–34.

4. Hauck AJ, Freeman DP, Ackermann DM, Danielson GK, Edwards WD. Surgical pathology of the tricuspid valve: a study of 363 cases spanning 25 years. *Mayo Clin Proc* 1988;63:851–863.

Pure Mitral Regurgitation Associated with a Malfunctioning Congenitally Bicuspid Aortic Valve Necessitating Combined Mitral and Aortic Valve Replacement

Daniel J. Fernicola, MD,* and William C. Roberts, MD†

Some patients with clinically significant aortic valve dysfunction have associated pure mitral regurgitation (no element of mitral stenosis), but usually the mitral regurgitation is of minimal or mild degree. On occasion, however, the degree of pure mitral regurgitation associated with clinically significant aortic valve dysfunction is considerable (i.e., severe enough to result in associated mitral valve repair or replacement at the time of aortic valve replacement). In the present study, we sought to determine the etiology of pure mitral regurgitation in a group of patients who had aortic valve replacement because of a dysfunctioning congenitally bicuspid aortic valve and simultaneous mitral valve replacement because of associated mitral regurgitation.

From the Pathology Branch, National Heart, Lung, and Blood Institute, National Institutes of Health, Bethesda, Maryland. Manuscript received January 4, 1994; revised manuscript received and accepted March 21, 1994.

*Division of Cardiology, Department of Medicine, Georgetown University, Washington, D.C. 20058.

†Baylor Cardiovascular Institute, Baylor University Medical Center, 3500 Gaston Avenue, Dallas, Texas 75246.

The surgical files of the Pathology Branch, National Heart, Lung, and Blood Institute, were reviewed to identify patients who had simultaneous replacement of both native mitral and aortic valves. A total of 115 cases were identified. Of them, 103 patients (90%) had 3-cuspid aortic valves, and 12 (10%) had congenitally bicuspid aortic valves. Of the latter 12 patients, 1 had associated congenital mitral stenosis and was therefore excluded from this study.[1] The other 11 patients with congenitally bicuspid aortic valves had associated pure mitral regurgitation. The 11 operatively excised congenitally bicuspid aortic valves and the simultaneously excised mitral valves were retrieved and reexamined. Certain clinical and cardiac morphologic features in each of the 11 patients are tabulated in Table I and illustrated in Figures 1 to 8.

All 11 patients were men, aged 25 to 77 years (mean 56). Four (cases 1 to 4, Table I) had pure aortic regurgitation and their mean age was younger than that of the 7 patients (cases 5 to 11, Table I) with some degree of aortic valve stenosis (with or without associated aortic regurgitation) (45 vs 63 years). Of the 7 patients with aortic stenosis, 6 had cardiac catheterization, and their

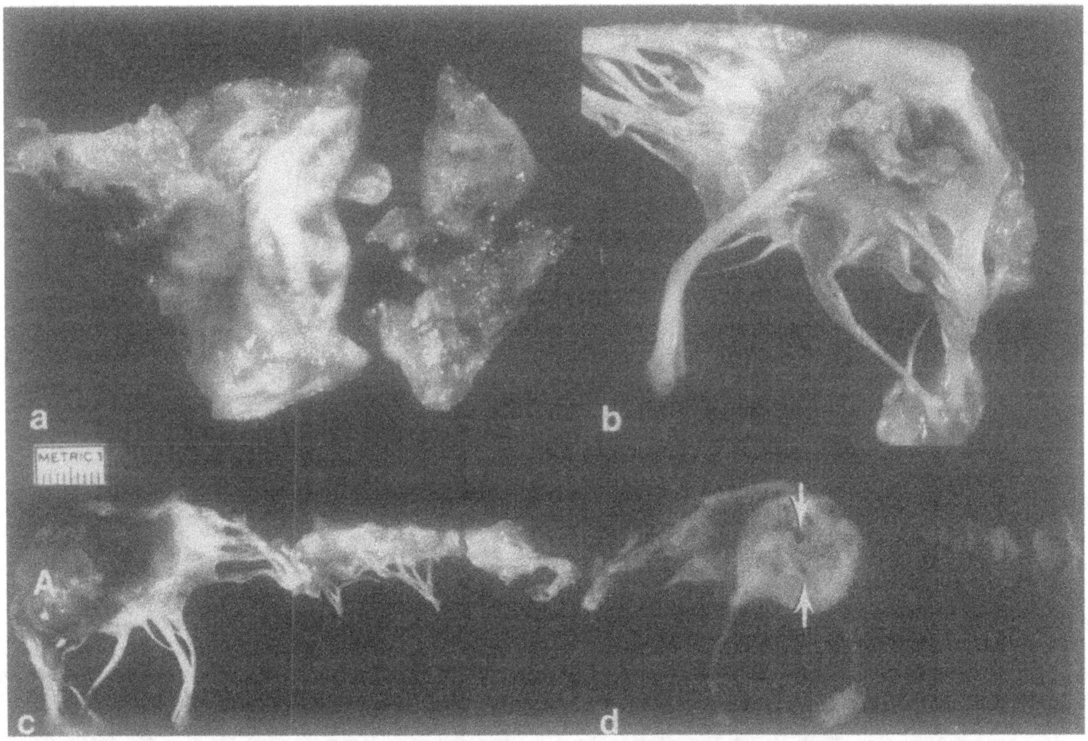

FIGURE 1. Patient 1. G. H. (GT #83-S-1910), a 25-year-old man, developed signs and symptoms of *Streptococcus bovis* endocarditis 4 months before valve replacement. Later he developed acute pulmonary edema due to severe aortic and mitral regurgitation. Both native left-sided cardiac valves were replaced with Carpentier-Edwards bioprostheses. *a*, excised aortic valve. Infective material is located on both cusps. *b*, ventricular aspect of anterior mitral leaflet. Infective material fills an aneurysm of the leaflet. *c*, opened mitral valve showing both leaflets. The large aneurysm (A) bulges toward the left atrium. *d*, radiograph of the mitral valve showing 2 perforations *(arrows)* in the aneurysm.

peak systolic pressure gradient ranged from 10 to 130 mm Hg (average 60). All 11 patients had pulmonary hypertension, with peak systolic pressures ranging from 37 to 90 mm Hg (average 64). Ten of the 11 patients had elevated mean pulmonary artery wedge pressures ranging from 24 to 35 mm Hg (average 29). The pulmonary artery V wave was >35 mm Hg in 7 of the 8 patients in whom this datum was available. The left ventricular angiogram in 8 patients indicated that the mitral regurgitation was 4+/4+ in 3, 3+/4+ in 3, and 2+/4+ in 2. In 4 patients with pure aortic regurgitation, aortic root angiogram indicated the regurgitation to be either 3+/4+ or 4+/4+. The left ventricular cavity was dilated, either by echocardiogram or left ventriculogram, in 9 of the 10 patients in whom either of these procedures

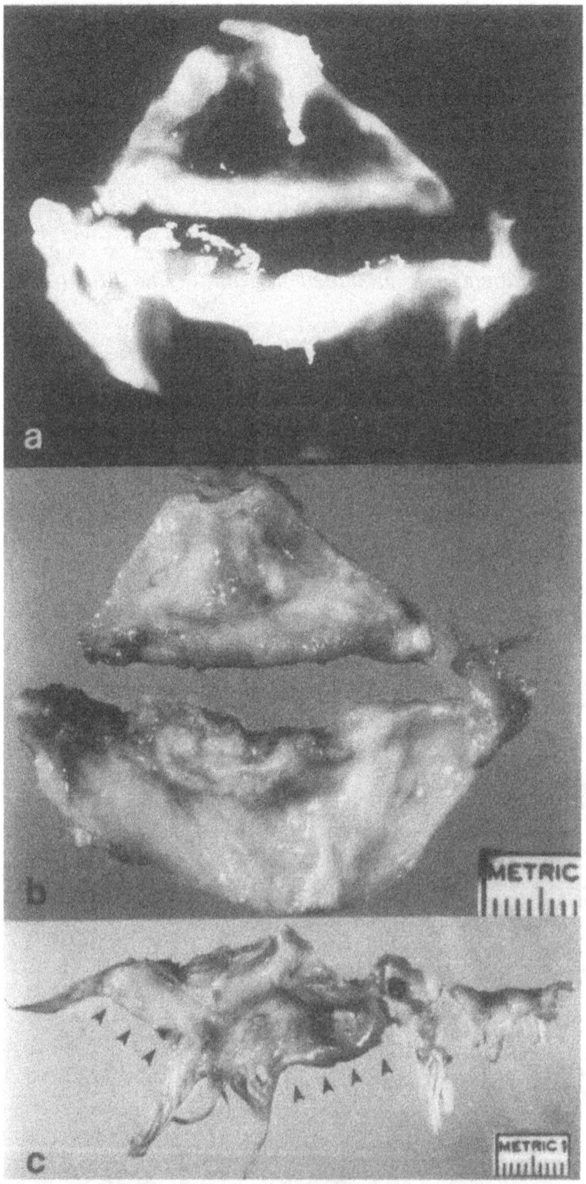

FIGURE 2. Patient 2. A. L. (NIH #S84-105), a 48-year-old man, had aortic regurgitation noted at age 38 years. He developed active infective endocarditis at age 44. A second episode of active infective endocarditis occurred 4 months before valve replacement. Within 3 months, the patient went from New York Heart Association functional class II to functional class IV. *a,* radiograph of the excised aortic valve showing small calcific deposits. *b,* excised aortic valve. The 2 cusps are of unequal size. *c,* excised mitral valve. Most chordae tendineae to the anterior mitral leaflet are ruptured (missing) *(arrowheads).*

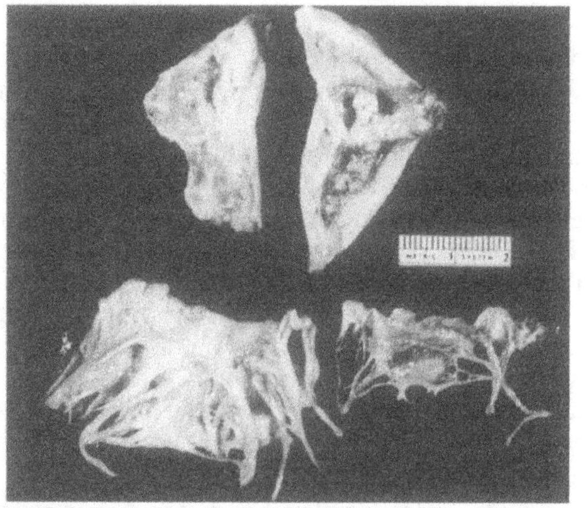

FIGURE 3. Patient 3. D. U. (NIH #S72-4111), a 51-year-old man, was first noted to have a precordial murmur at age 23 years. Symptoms began at age 50 years, approximately 1 year before valve replacement. The excised aortic valve *(top)* is diffusely thickened with a focal calcific deposit limited to the raphe. The excised mitral valve leaflets *(bottom)* are essentially normal.

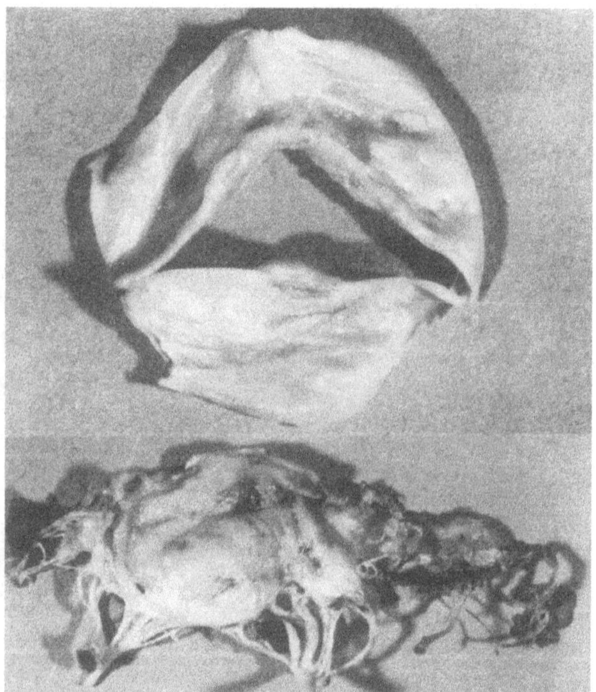

FIGURE 4. Patient 4. M. W. (NIH #S70-3100), a 55-year-old man, was noted to have a murmur of aortic regurgitation at the age of 47. The patient remained asymptomatic until 6 weeks before surgery when he developed acute pulmonary edema. The excised aortic valve *(top)* is mildly and diffusely fibrotic and purely regurgitant. The anterior leaflet of the mitral valve *(bottom)* is greatly thickened by fibrous tissue. The chordae tendineae to the anterior mitral leaflet are thickened by fibrous tissue and are very short. The commissure between the anterior and posterior leaflets is abnormal but not fused.

TABLE I Clinical and Morphologic Features of 11 Men with a Malfunctioning Bicuspid Aortic Valve and Associated Pure Mitral Regurgitation and Operative Excision of Both Valves

Case No.	Age at operation (years)	Interval (days) CC to VR	Pressures (mm Hg) RV (s/d)	PA (s/d)	PAW Mean	PAW V Wave	LV (s/d)	SA (s/d)	LV-SA psg	Angiogram MR (1+–4+)	AR (1+–4+)	No. CA >50%
1	25	1	—	50/20	25	—	120/30	120/60	0	2+	4+	—
2	48	30	50/12	45/24	29	41	100/35	110/45	0	3+	4+	0
3	51	4	80/10	80/35	30	65	125/22	125/55	0	3+	3+	—
4	55	21	65/10	65/25	25	65	120/24	120/55	0	4+	4+	—
5	52	30	56/10	55/30	30	36	120/25	110/65	10	2+**	2+	0
6	54	5	70/11	70/30	30	—	220/30	110/60	100	—	—	—
7	56	—	38/11	37/15	24	—	145/10	95/65	50	4+	0	0
8	58	4	—	70/25	35	45	—	118/50	—	—	—	1
9	71	14	90/4	90/40	35	38	210/20	90/60	130	—	—	0
10	71	—	80/15	80/25	10	16	140/16	100/70	40	4+	0	0
11	77	18	44/12	44/19	25	41	126/12	99/57	27	3+	—	3§§

Case No.	Cavity Size (mm) by Echocardiogram LV_s	LV_d	LA	Year of VR	Prosthesis in AV Position Type	Size	Prosthesis in MV Position Type	Size	Calcium (0–4+) AV	MV	BA-DM Length (cm) AML	PML	Etiology of MR IE	MVP	Ruptured MV CT
1	—		—	1983	CE	25	CE	29	0	0	1.4	0.7	+ (A)	0	0
2	51	75	45	1984	SE	24A*	SE	30M†	1+	0	2	—	+ (H)	0	+
3	—‡		—	1972	SE	27A§	SE	32M‖	1+	0	2	1.5	0	0	0
4	—‡		—	1970	SE	26A¶	SE	30M†	0	1+	2.5	1.0	+ (H)	0	0
5	60	65	53	1986	SE	24A*	SE	30M†	3+	1+	1.4	—	0††	0††	0††
6	—		33	1979	Ha	21	Ha	31	4+	0	2.2	1.7	0	0	0††
7	42	61	63	1989	SJM	21	SJM	29	2+	1+	1.8	—	+ (H)††	0††	0
8	62	69	56	1980	SE	24A*	SE	32M‖	3+	0	2.0	1.0	0	0	0
9	60	70	56	1983	Ha	21	Ha	29	4+	0	2.2	1.0	+ (H)	0	+
10	34	52	58	1991	MH	25	MH	31	3+	1+	2	2	0	+	+
11	—	58	40	1992	CE	23	CE	31	2+	1+	2	—	0	0	0

*Old terminology is 10A.
†Old terminology is 3M.
‡Left ventricle very large by left ventricular angiogram.
§Old terminology is 12A.
‖Old terminology is 4M.
¶Old terminology is 11A.
**No mitral regurgitation, however, by Doppler echocardiogram.
††Only the anterior mitral leaflet excised at operation.
§§Coronary artery bypass surgery performed at time of valve replacement.

A = active; AML = anterior mitral leaflet; AR = aortic regurgitation (by aortic root cineangiogram); AV = aortic valve; BA = basal attachment; CA = coronary artery; CC = cardiac catheterization; CE = Carpentier-Edwards bioprosthesis; CT = chordae tendineae; DM = distal margin; H = healed; Ha = Hancock bioprosthesis; IE = infective endocarditis; LA = left atrium; LV = left ventricle; LV_s = left ventricular (cavity size in systole); LV_d = left ventricular (cavity size in diastole); MH = Medtronic-Hall mechanical prosthesis; MR = mitral regurgitation (by left ventriculogram); MV = mitral valve; MVP = mitral valve prolapse; PA = pulmonary artery; PAW = pulmonary artery wedge; PML = posterior mitral leaflet; psg = peak systolic gradient; RV = right ventricle; SA = systemic artery; SE = Starr-Edwards mechanical prosthesis; s/d = peak systole/end-diastole; SJM = Saint Jude mechanical prosthesis; VR = valve replacement.

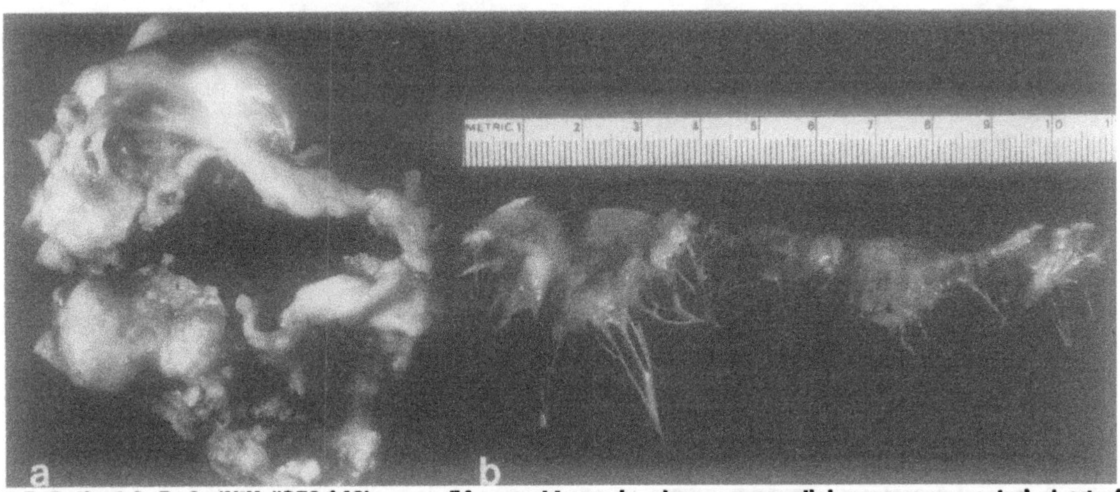

FIGURE 5. Patient 6. B. O. (NIH #S79-142) was a 54-year-old man in whom a precordial murmur was noted at age 43 years. At age 51, the peak systolic pressure gradient between left ventricle and aorta was 65 mm Hg. Over the next 2 years, congestive heart failure progressed. At the time of valve replacement, the peak systolic gradient across the aortic valve was 100 mm Hg. The patient died 12 days after operation from sepsis. *a*, excised heavily calcified aortic valve. *b*, opened mitral valve. Some segments of the posterior mitral leaflet are elongated.

was performed; the 1 patient (case 1, Table I) without cavity dilation had aortic regurgitation secondary to active infective endocarditis of short duration. The 1 patient who did not have either an echocardiogram or a left ventriculogram had an ejection fraction of 20%, and chest radiogram showed a large cardiac silhouette.

Infective endocarditis, either active (case 1) or healed (cases 2, 4, 7, and 9), was the etiology of the mitral regurgitation in 5 patients (45%). In 2 of the 4 patients with healed infective endocarditis, several chordae tendineae in each had ruptured (Figures 2 and 7). In the other 2 patients the diagnosis of infective endocarditis was made by a history of positive blood cultures. In 1 patient (case 4) the excised anterior mitral leaflet was diffusely thickened by fibrous tissue without calcific deposits, the attached chordae tendineae were thickened and short, and the posterior mitral leaflet was smaller than expected. The etiology of this distorted anatomy is uncertain, but infective endocarditis that healed and was not diagnosed clinically may have caused the local fibrous thickening. In 1 patient mitral valve prolapse was present and some chordae tendineae from the posterior mitral leaflet had ruptured. In 4 patients the excised mitral leaflets and chordae tendineae were anatomically normal, but the left ventricular cavities were very dilated.

In the 4 patients with purely regurgitant aortic valves, calcific deposits, determined by x-ray of the excised valves, were either absent or minute. In each of the 7 stenotic aortic valves, large calcific deposits were present. Of the 11 excised mitral valves, 5 had minute calcific deposits, confined to the annular region in 4.

Although most persons with a congenitally bicuspid aortic valve have a normally functioning mitral valve, the present study indicates that associated mitral regurgitation not only may occur, but also may be severe enough to warrant mitral valve replacement at the time of aortic valve replacement. It is well appreciated that the congenitally bicuspid aortic valve has a high propensity to be the site of infective endocarditis.[1–12] Furthermore, when active endocarditis of the aortic valve leads to aortic regurgitation, vegetations on the aortic valve may be dislodged retrogradely by the regurgitant jet and the vegetations may adhere to mitral chordae tendineae causing their rupture, or to the anterior mitral leaflet causing it to perforate or to become aneurysmal. The latter scenario appears to have been responsible for the mitral regurgitation in 5, and possibly 6, of the 11 patients in the present study.

Mitral valve prolapse without superimposed infective endocarditis was responsible for the mitral regurgitation

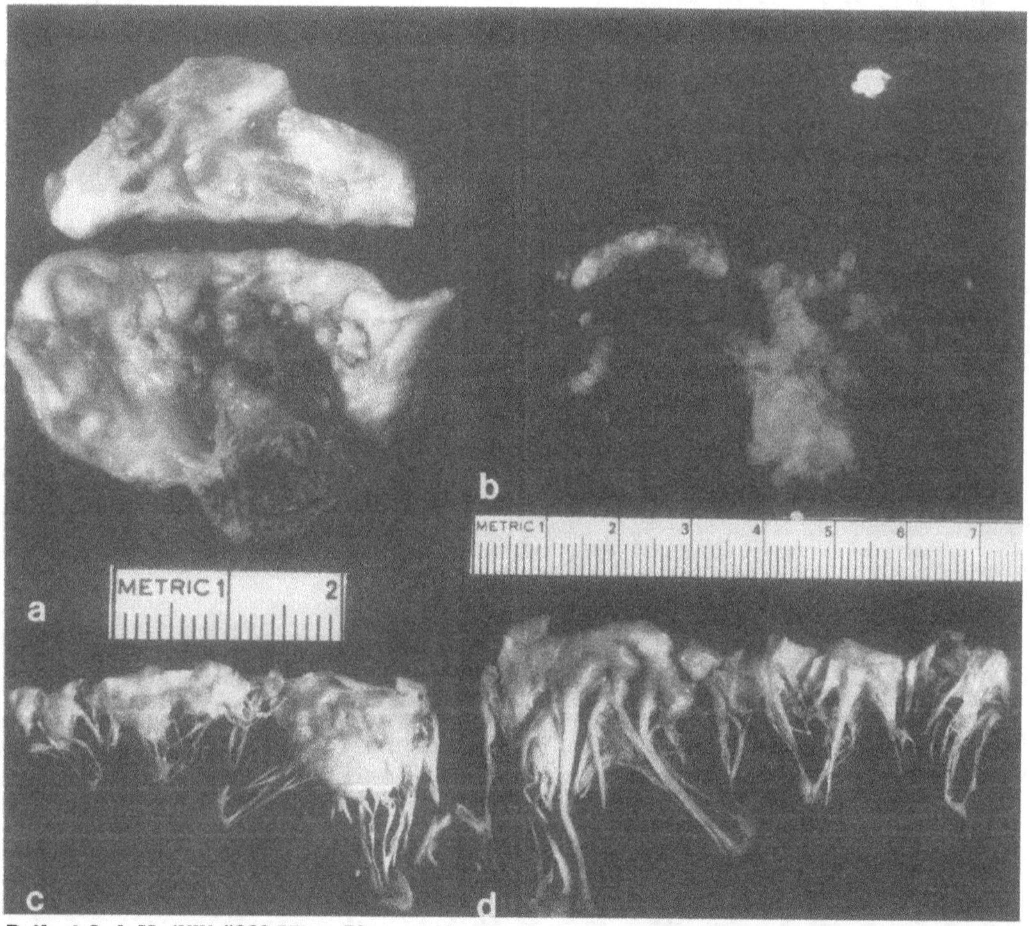

FIGURE 6. Patient 8. J. M. (NIH #S80-75), a 58-year-old man, had a precordial murmur since at least age 19 years. He remained asymptomatic until age 51 when he had an acute myocardial infarction. He developed acute pulmonary edema 2 weeks before valve replacement. *a*, excised aortic valve. *b*, radiograph of the aortic valve. The cusps are of different sizes and calcium is virtually limited to the largest cusp. *c and d*, excised mitral valve. Atrial *(c)* and ventricular *(d)* views of the excised mitral leaflets. Both leaflets are moderately thickened. Portions of the posterior leaflet are elongated.

in only 1 patient.[13–16] It is surprising that mitral valve prolapse (unassociated with infective endocarditis) is not seen more often in patients with congenitally bicuspid aortic valves, because mitral valve prolapse may occur in as many as 5% of the adult population, and the bicuspid aortic valve in as many as 1% of the population.[17] In 4 patients, the mitral leaflets and chordae tendineae were normal but the mitral annulae were quite dilated. Today, these latter 4 patients would probably have had mitral annuloplasty rather than replacement.

Although all 11 patients had pure mitral regurgitation, the type of aortic valve dysfunction was variable. Four patients had pure aortic regurgitation, in 3 due to superimposed infective endocarditis or at least worsened by the endocarditis, and in 1 patient due entirely to the bicuspid condition of the valve. Seven patients had stenotic aortic valves. Of the 4 purely regurgitant aortic valves, 3 had superimposed infective endocarditis; of the 7 stenotic aortic valves, 2 had superimposed infective endocarditis.

In summary, some patients with severely dysfunctioning congenitally bicuspid aortic valves develop pure mitral regurgitation severe enough to warrant mitral valve replacement or repair. The most common cause of the associated mitral regurgitation is leaflet and chordal damage from infective endocarditis.

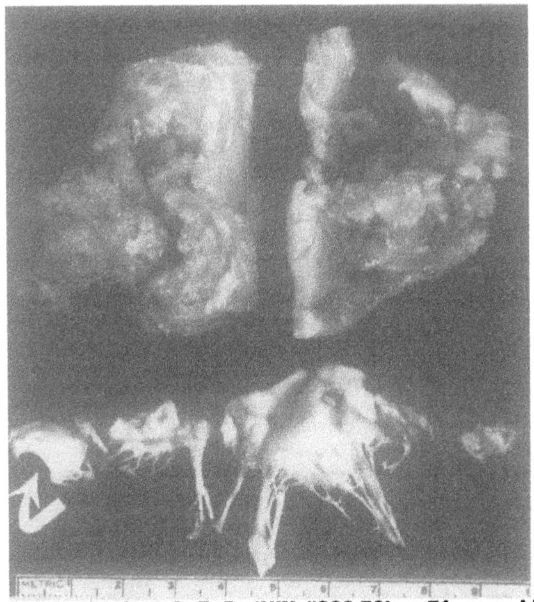

FIGURE 7. Patient 9. E. P. (NIH #S83-56), a 71-year-old man who developed congestive heart failure 9 months before valve replacement. Four months before valve replacement, he was treated with ampicillin for bronchitis. *Top,* excised aortic valve showing heavy calcific deposits. *Bottom,* excised mitral valve. A portion of posterior leaflet is indented *(arrow)* with missing chordae tendineae at this site. These latter findings are consistent with healed infective endocarditis.

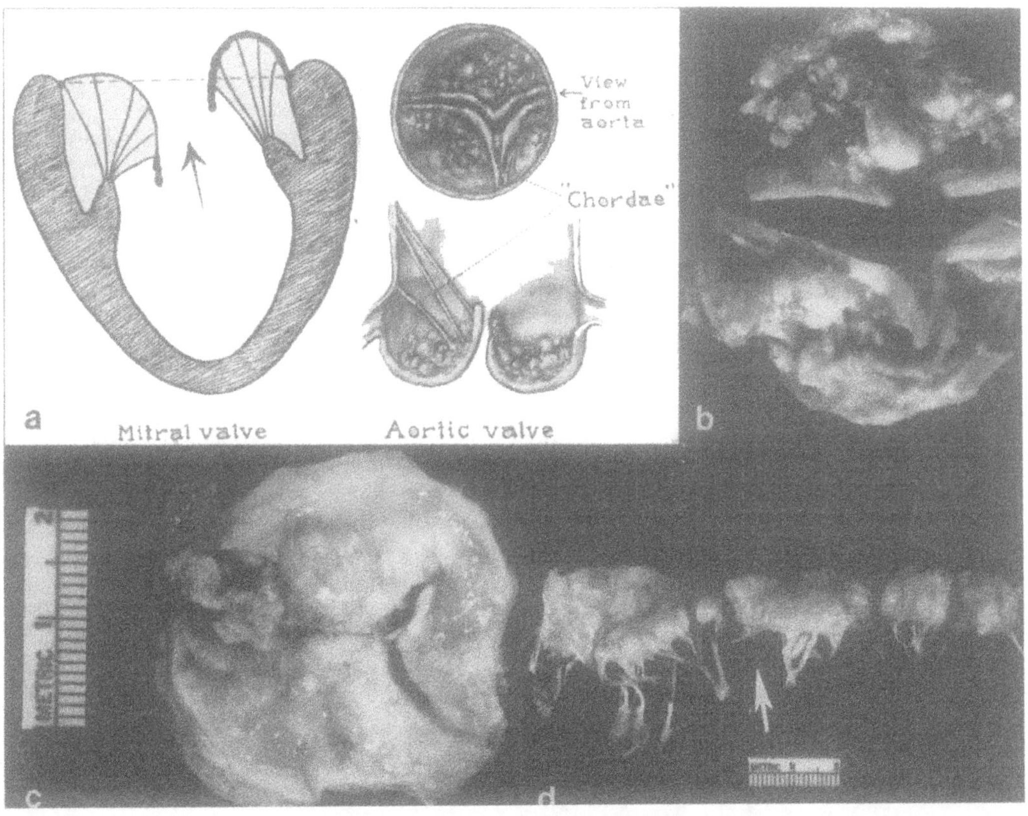

FIGURE 8. Patient 10. A. S. (GT #91S-6903), a 71-year-old man, developed acute pulmonary edema and severe mitral regurgitation 2 weeks before valve replacement. The patient had been in New York Heart Association functional class II before the development of severe mitral regurgitation. *a,* illustration of the mitral and aortic valves as they probably appeared in life. "Chordae" were present from the raphe of the aortic valve cusps to the wall of the aorta. *b,* excised aortic valve from the aortic aspect. *c,* aortic valve from the ventricular side. *d,* excised mitral valve showing "missing" chordae tendineae *(arrows).* An adjacent portion of posterior leaflet is hooded.

1. Roberts WC. The congenitally bicuspid aortic valve. A study of 85 autopsy cases. *Am J Cardiol* 1970;26:72–83.
2. Arnett EN, Roberts WC. Valve ring abscess in active infective endocarditis. Frequency, location, and clues to clinical diagnosis from the study of 95 necropsy patients. *Circulation* 1976;54:140–145.
3. Arnett EN, Roberts WC. Prosthetic valve endocarditis. Clinicopathologic analysis of 22 necropsy patients with comparison of observations in 74 necropsy patients with active infective endocarditis involving natural left-sided cardiac valves. *Am J Cardiol* 1976;38:281–292.
4. Arnett EN, Roberts WC. Active infective endocarditis: a clinicopathology analysis of 137 necropsy patients. *Curr Probl Cardiol* 1976;1:1–76.
5. Roberts WC, Buchbinger NA. Healed left-sided infective endocarditis: a clinicopathologic study of 59 patients. *Am J Cardiol* 1977:72:757–761.
6. Roberts WC, Morrow AG, McIntosh CL, Jones M, Epstein SE. Congenitally bicuspid aortic valve causing severe, pure aortic regurgitation without superimposed infective endocarditis. Analysis of 13 patients requiring aortic valve replacement. *Am J Cardiol* 1981;47:206–209.
7. Roberts WC, McIntosh CL, Wallace RB. Aortic valve perforation with calcific aortic valve stenosis and without infective endocarditis or significant aortic regurgitation. *Am J Cardiol* 1987;59:476–478.
8. Dressler FA, Roberts WC. Infective endocarditis in opiate addicts: analysis of 80 cases studied at necropsy. *Am J Cardiol* 1989;63:1240–1257.
9. Roberts WC. Living with a congenitally bicuspid aortic valve. *Am J Cardiol* 1989;64:1408–1409.
10. Brown PS Jr, Roberts CS, McIntosh CL, Roberts WC, Clark RE. Combined obstructive hypertrophic cardiomyopathy and stenotic congenitally bicuspid aortic valve. *Am J Cardiol* 1990;66:1273–1275.
11. Roberts WC. Morphologic aspects of cardiac valve dysfunction. *Am Heart J* 1992:123:1610–1632.
12. Roberts WC, Oluwole BO, Fernicola DJ. Comparison of active infective endocarditis involving a previously stenotic versus a previously nonstenotic aortic valve. *Am J Cardiol* 1993;71:1082–1088.
13. Rippe JM, Slors LJ, Angoff G, Alpert JS. Mitral valve prolapse in adults with congenital heart disease. *Am Heart J* 1979;97:561–573.
14. Chisholm JC. Mitral valve prolapse syndrome associated with congenital bicuspid aortic valve. *JAMA* 1981;73:921–923.
15. Roberts WC, McIntosh CL, Wallace RB. Mechanisms of severe mitral regurgitation in mitral valve prolapse determined from analysis of operatively excised valves. *Am Heart J* 1987;113:1316–1323.
16. Dollar AL, Roberts WC. Morphologic comparison of patients with mitral valve prolapse who died suddenly with patients who died from severe valvular dysfunction or other conditions. *J Am Coll Cardiol* 1991;17:921–931.
17. Roberts WC. The 2 most common congenital heart diseases. *Am J Cardiol* 1984;53:1198.

Severe late (16 years) dysfunction of a bioprosthesis in the mitral valve position without dysfunction of a bioprosthesis in the aortic valve position

Paul A. Grayburn, MD, Baron L. Hamman, MD, and William C. Roberts, MD

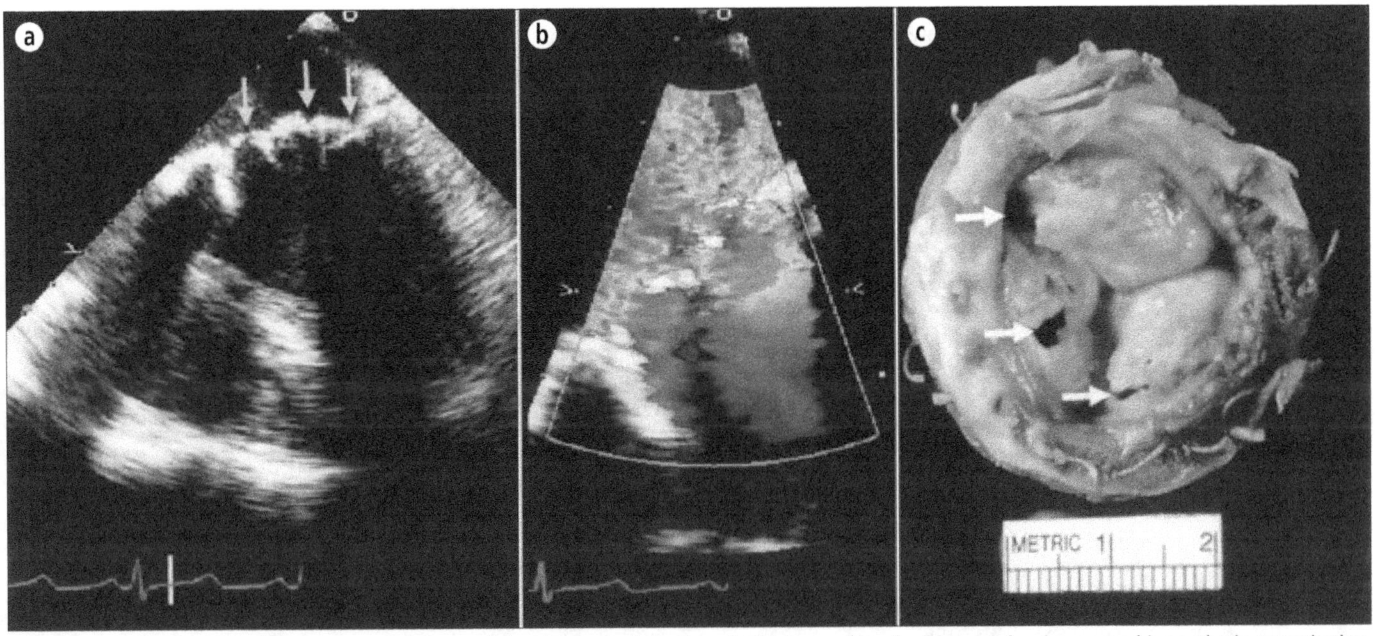

Figure. Echocardiographic and gross anatomic images of the bioprosthesis in the mitral valve position for 16 years showing severe bioprosthetic regurgitation. **(a)** A midesophageal 4-chamber view showing 3 distinct defects in the porcine cusps (arrows). **(b)** A magnified image in the same projection showing multiple color flow jets with severe mitral regurgitation through the cusps. There was no perivalvular leak. **(c)** The excised bioprosthesis with 3 perforations in the cusps (arrows). This is a classic example of structural porcine bioprosthetic deterioration.

A man who was born in 1939 underwent replacement of both mitral and aortic valves with porcine bioprostheses in 1987 (age 48). Thereafter, he was asymptomatic until 2003 (age 64), when he developed signs and symptoms of heart failure. Cardiac catheterization in late 2003 disclosed the following pressures in mm Hg: pulmonary artery, 70/31; right ventricle, 70/18; right atrial mean, 9; pulmonary artery wedge mean, 30, with v waves averaging 54; left ventricle, 108/25; and aorta, 104/65. Left ventricular angiography disclosed a normal-sized left ventricular cavity and severe mitral regurgitation. Aortic root angiogram disclosed trace aortic regurgitation. The preoperative echocardiogram and the operatively excised (late 2003) bioprosthesis, which had been in the mitral valve position, are shown in the *Figure*. Coronary angiography preoperatively showed insignificant coronary arterial narrowing.

This case demonstrates that when bioprostheses are placed in both mitral and aortic valve positions during the same operation, the bioprosthesis in the mitral valve tends to degenerate more rapidly than a similar bioprosthesis in the aortic valve (1). The likely reason is that the closing pressure exerted on the mitral bioprosthesis is the left ventricular systolic pressure, whereas the closing pressure exerted on the aortic prosthesis is the aorta's diastolic pressure, which in general is about a third lower than the left ventricular peak systolic pressure. In the present patient, the left ventricular peak systolic pressure was 108 mm Hg and the aorta's end-diastolic pressure was 65 mm Hg, a 40% difference.

1. Warnes CA, Scott ML, Silver GM, Smith CW, Ferrans VJ, Roberts WC. Comparison of late degenerative changes in porcine bioprostheses in the mitral and aortic valve position in the same patient. *Am J Cardiol* 1983;51:965–968.

From the Division of Cardiology, Department of Internal Medicine (Grayburn), Department of Cardiothoracic Surgery (Hamman), and Department of Pathology and the Baylor Heart and Vascular Institute (Roberts), Baylor University Medical Center, Dallas, Texas.

Corresponding author: Paul A. Grayburn, MD, Baylor Hamilton Heart and Vascular Hospital, 621 N. Hall Street, Dallas, Texas 75226 (e-mail: PaulGr@bhcs.com).

Severe Regurgitation Immediately After Replacement of a Dysfunctional Bioprosthesis in the Mitral Valve Position

Hassan Farooq, MD, Paul Grayburn, MD, and William Clifford Roberts, MD

Severe regurgitation immediately after replacement of a cardiac valve with a mechanical prosthesis or a bioprosthesis is a rare occurrence. Such, however, was the case in the patient described.

(Am J Cardiol 2005;95:703–704)

A 74-year-old woman, who was born in September 1929, had her purely regurgitant mitral valve replaced with a bioprosthesis in 1986, when she was 57 years old. Thereafter, she was asymptomatic until age 74, when exertional dyspnea appeared. Four months later, she entered the hospital. She was 57 inches tall and weighed 115 pounds (body mass index 25 kg/m^2). A grade 3/6 holosystolic murmur was heard over the cardiac apex, and it radiated into the left axilla. An echocardiogram disclosed a normal-sized left ventricle, a dilated right ventricle, and severe bioprosthetic regurgitation. At cardiac catheterization, the pressures in mm Hg were as follows: pulmonary artery wedge "a" wave, 33, V wave, 43, and mean, 28; right ventricle, 58/23, simultaneous left ventricle, 166/26, and aorta 162/92. Left ventricular angiography disclosed severe (4+/4+) bioprosthetic regurgitation.

• • •

Reoperation on April 14, 2004, disclosed that 1 of the 3 bioprosthetic cusps had prolapsed severely toward the left atrium, despite the absence of calcium in any of the bioprosthetic cusps. The dysfunctional bioprosthesis in the mitral position was replaced with another bioprosthesis (Carpentier-Edwards, 25 mm, Edwards Lifesciences, Irvine, California). At operation, the left atrium was opened by an incision parallel to the atrial septum just anterior to right superior pulmonary vein. After the excision of the initially inserted bioprosthesis and the insertion of the newer bioprosthesis, the patient apparently came off cardiopulmonary bypass, which lasted 68 minutes, without difficulty.

When entering the intensive care unit, the patient's blood pressure was 100/60 mm Hg, and her heart rate was 92 beats/min. Her extremities were cool, and the pedal pulses were barely palpable. Pulmonary artery pressure was 36/18 mm Hg. Later that day, the patient's blood pressure decreased to 60/30 mm Hg, and atrial fibrillation appeared. Sinus rhythm was restored by cardioversion (50 J) but without improvement in hemodynamics. On postoperative day 4, the patient again reverted to atrial fibrillation, but with amiodarone sinus rhythm returned. By day 8, she was still intubated, sinus tachycardia (110 beats/min) persisted, her respirations were rapid (25 breaths/min), and vasopressors were required to maintain adequate systemic arterial pressures. A repeat echocardiogram (Figure 1) showed severe bioprosthetic regurgitation, and a third cardiac operation was performed on postoperative day 9 (April 23, 2004). The left atrium was opened through the previous incision, and the bioprosthesis in the mitral position was excised. The orifice of the bioprosthesis was found to be in a fixed open position because of a single suture that had encircled 1 of the 3 stents, resulting in the tethering down of 2 cusps (Figure 1; see next page). After excision of the tethered bioprosthesis and replacement with another bioprosthesis, the patient came off cardiopulmonary bypass easily, and her postoperative course was relatively uneventful. She left the hospital on May 14, 2004.

• • •

In the early days of cardiac valve replacement, certain technical complications occurred fairly commonly simply because the procedure was new, and good techniques had to be developed. In recent years technical complications of cardiac valve replacement have been infrequent. The complication described in the present patient, namely, the tethering down of 2 bioprosthetic cusps by a suture tied down inadvertently on 1 bioprosthetic stent located on the ventricular aspect of the bioprosthesis, was originally described and reported in 1983.[1] The present case indicates that even 21 years later, this complication has not yet been completely eliminated. It is still a good idea before closing the left atrium after mitral replacement to ensure that each bioprosthetic cusp is freely mobile. Intraoperative transesophageal echocardiography should be used routinely to evaluate the valve before leaving the operating suite.

From the Baylor University Medical Center, Baylor Heart & Vascular Institute, Dallas, Texas. Dr. Roberts's address is: Baylor University Medical Center, Baylor Heart & Vascular Institute, 621 North Hall Street, Dallas, Texas 75226. E-mail: wc.roberts@baylorhealth.edu. Manuscript received and accepted October 29, 2004.

1. Silver MA, Oranburg PR, Roberts WC. Severe mitral regurgitation immediately after mitral valve replacement with a parietal pericardial bovine bioprosthesis. *Am J Cardiol* 1983;52:218–219.

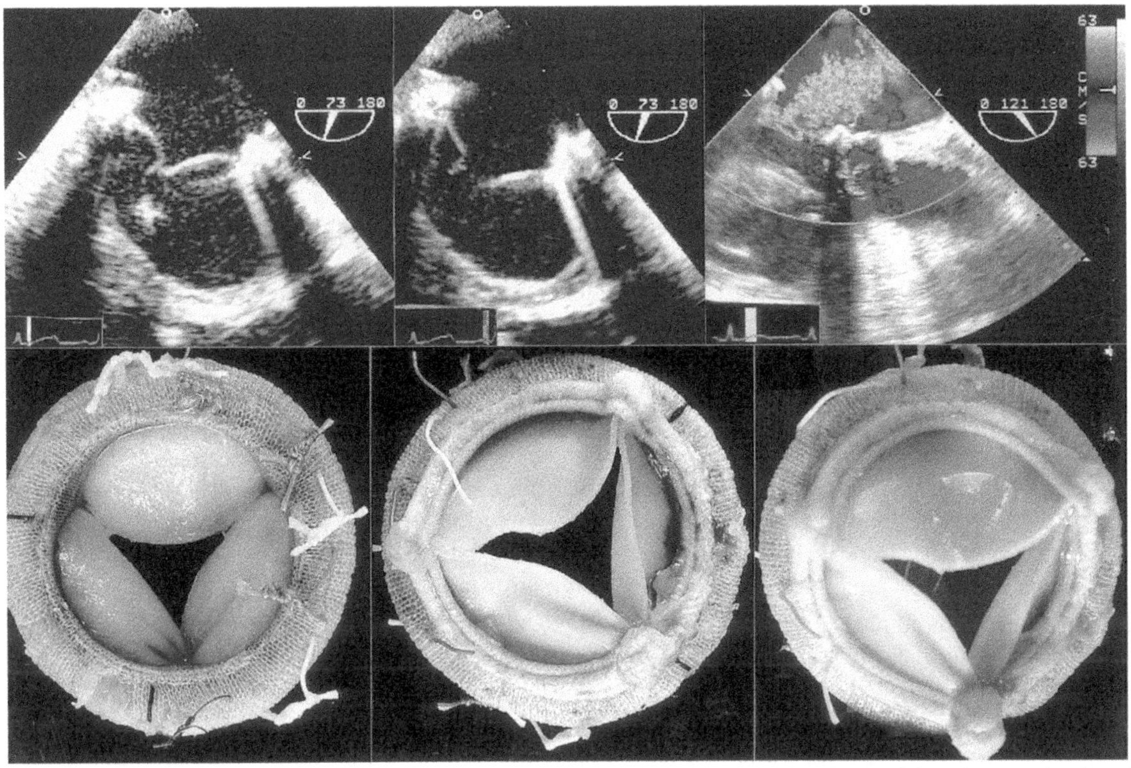

FIGURE 1. Transesophageal echocardiographic images *(top panels)* obtained in ventricular systole *(top left)* and ventricular diastole *(top middle)* showing marked restriction in the opening of 2 cusps. The *top right* shows mitral regurgitation by color Doppler flow mapping. The vena contracta of the mitral regurgitation jet measured 0.9 cm, a thickness consistent with severe mitral regurgitation. The *bottom panels* show the bioprosthetic valve as seen from the left atrial aspect *(bottom left)* and from the left ventricular aspect *(bottom middle and bottom right)*. A single suture encircled 1 of the 3 stents, tethering down 2 cusps and resulting in an opened, roughly triangular orifice in ventricular systole and diastole.

A Starr-Edwards Model 6120 Mechanical Prosthesis in the Mitral Valve Position for 38 Years

Mark A. Peterman, MD, Michael S. Donsky, MD, Gregory J. Matter, MD, and William Clifford Roberts, MD*

The Starr-Edwards caged-ball prosthesis for cardiac valve replacement was first successfully used in the mitral position in September 1960. Because of swelling of the silicone rubber poppet due to lipid infiltration, the processing of the silicone rubber was altered in 1965 in hopes of preventing poppet degeneration. We describe findings in a woman who had mitral valve replacement in 1965 utilizing the revised silicone rubber poppet; the prosthesis remained in place for 38 years.

• • •

A 78-year-old woman was admitted to Baylor University Medical Center in August 2003 in functional class IV heart failure. At age 38 (1963), she had had aortic valve replacement with a Starr-Edwards mechanical prosthesis and mitral valve commissurotomy. At age 40 (1965), she had repeat aortic valve replacement and mitral valve replacement, both with Starr-Edwards mechanical prostheses. She did well until age 63 (1988), when a third aortic valve replacement, this time with a St. Jude Medical prosthesis, and a tricuspid valve annuloplasty were performed. She also had chronic anemia, for which she had received several transfusions.

On admission, blood pressure was 110/63 mm Hg, and heart rate was 82 beats/min. Her body mass index was 23 kg/m^2. A grade 3/6 systolic murmur was heard at the left sternal border and a grade 2/6 diastolic murmur at the cardiac apex. Rales were heard at the bases of both lungs. The liver was large, and the lower legs were severely edematous. The hemoglobin was 9.5 g/dl, and the hemotocrit was 29.5%.

An echocardiogram disclosed that her mean transmitral diastolic gradient was 18 mm Hg; the left ventricular ejection fraction was about 50%. The aortic pressure was 150/59 mm Hg, and the pulmonary artery pressure, 75/20 mm Hg. Coronary arteriography showed no significant coronary narrowings.

The Starr-Edwards model 6120/30 mm (3M) mechanical valve, which had been in the mitral position for 38 years, was excised and a porcine bioprostheses was implanted via a right mini-thoracotomy approach. The patient recovered uneventfully and was discharged on the fifth postoperative day after reinitiation of warfarin therapy.

After photographing it, the excised Starr-Edwards prosthesis was sent to Edwards Lifesciences LLC (Irving, California), the laboratory that had originally produced the prosthesis. The prosthesis was disassembled to acquire the serial number of the valve, which confirmed it to be a model 6120. The poppet was deeply orange, swollen, and moved only when significant pressure was applied (Figure 1). A senior scientist at the manufacturer's laboratory determined that the prosthetic poppet weighted 7.4 g, a gain of 0.9 g from its original weight (14% increase). After cutting the poppet in half, the maximal diameter was 21.8 mm, an increase of 1.7 mm (8% increase) from its original diameter (Figure 2). Several cuts were present on the poppet's surface, each about 1 mm long, and light ware groovings, due to restricted motion/rotation, also were present on the poppet's surface. Additionally, micropores were evident on the poppet's surface on scanning electron microscopy (Figure 3). The maximal excursion of the poppet was about 0.5 cm. There was also host tissue overgrowth covering about 50% of the aortic aspect of the prosthetic ring (Figure 1). (This tissue overgrowth combined with the poppet swelling restricted poppet motion leading to both prosthetic stenosis and erythrocyte hemolysis. The latter resulted from high shear jetting backflow from incomplete seating of the poppets.) Other than a local burnish region on 1 of the 4 metallic struts, corresponding to the sliding contact of the poppet as opposed to the normal rolling contact, the cage and the other 3 metallic struts showed no evidence of wear.

• • •

The first successful mechanical prosthesis in the mitral valve position in humans was the Starr-Edwards Model 6000.[1] This model had a significant incidence of systemic embolization as well as ball variance[1] (occasionally lethal[2]). The model 6120 Starr-Edwards mitral valve prosthesis was introduced in 1965 with a reduction in the surface area of metallic components, and an improved barium-impregnated poppet.[1] This model had a far lower incidence of systemic embolization (3% vs 38%) compared with model 6000.[1] The next models (6300) were introduced in 1968 and added cloth covering to the stents. The modified cloth-covered series (model 6400 or track valve) was introduced in 1974 and discontinued in 1980, becauses results showed no advantage over the original 6120 model.

Although ball variance is usually discovered within 8 years of implantation, late ball variance has been described in early models in patients up to 20 years after implantation.[3] The longest interval

Departments of Internal Medicine (Cardiology Division), Cardiothoracic Surgery and Pathology, and the Baylor Heart & Vascular Institute, Baylor University Medical Center, Dallas, Texas. Manuscript received September 6, 2005; revised manuscript received and accepted October 11, 2005.

* Corresponding author: Tel: 214-820-7911; fax: 214-820-7533.

E-mail address: wc.roberts@BaylorHealth.edu (W.C. Roberts).

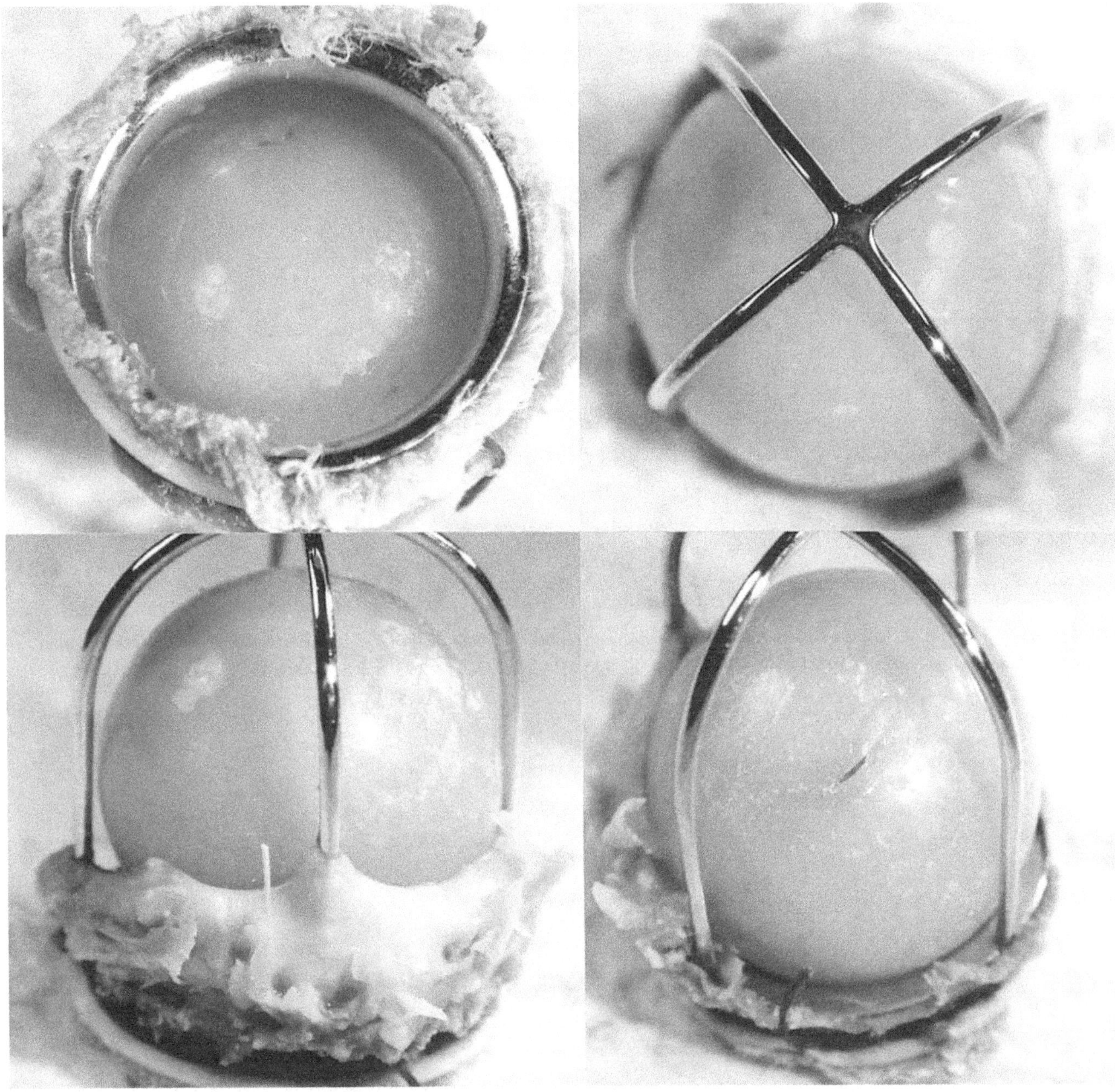

Figure 1. Views of the operatively excised model 6120 Starr-Edwards prosthesis that had been in place for 38 years.

previously reported from implantation to reoperation of a Starr-Edwards mitral prosthesis was 31 years in a cloth-covered model with a metal poppet.[4] To our knowledge, ball variance has not been reported in the model 6120 Starr-Edwards prosthesis. The present case is remarkable for the extremely late onset of prosthetic mitral valve stenosis and the occurrence of severe ball variance in a model 6120 Starr-Edwards mitral valve prosthesis.

1. Freimanis I and Starr A. The unnatural history of valvular heart disease. Late results with silastic ball valve prostheses. *J Cardiovasc Surg* 1984;25:191–198.
2. Roberts WC, Levinson GE, Morrow AG. Lethal ball variance in the Starr-Edwards prosthetic mitral valve. *Arch Intern Med* 1970;126:517–521.
3. Grunkemeier GL and Starr A. Late ball variance with model 1000 Starr-Edwards aortic valve prosthesis. Risk analysis and strategy of operative management. *J Thorac Cardiovasc Surg* 1986;91:918–923.
4. Goshima M, Shiono M, Yamamoto T, Inoue T, Hata M, Sezai A, Niino T, Nakamura T, Ye Z, Negishi N, Sezai Y. Reoperation for a Starr-Edwards ball valve prosthesis implanted in mitral position 31 years ago. *Jpn J Thorac Surg* 2003;56:535–540.

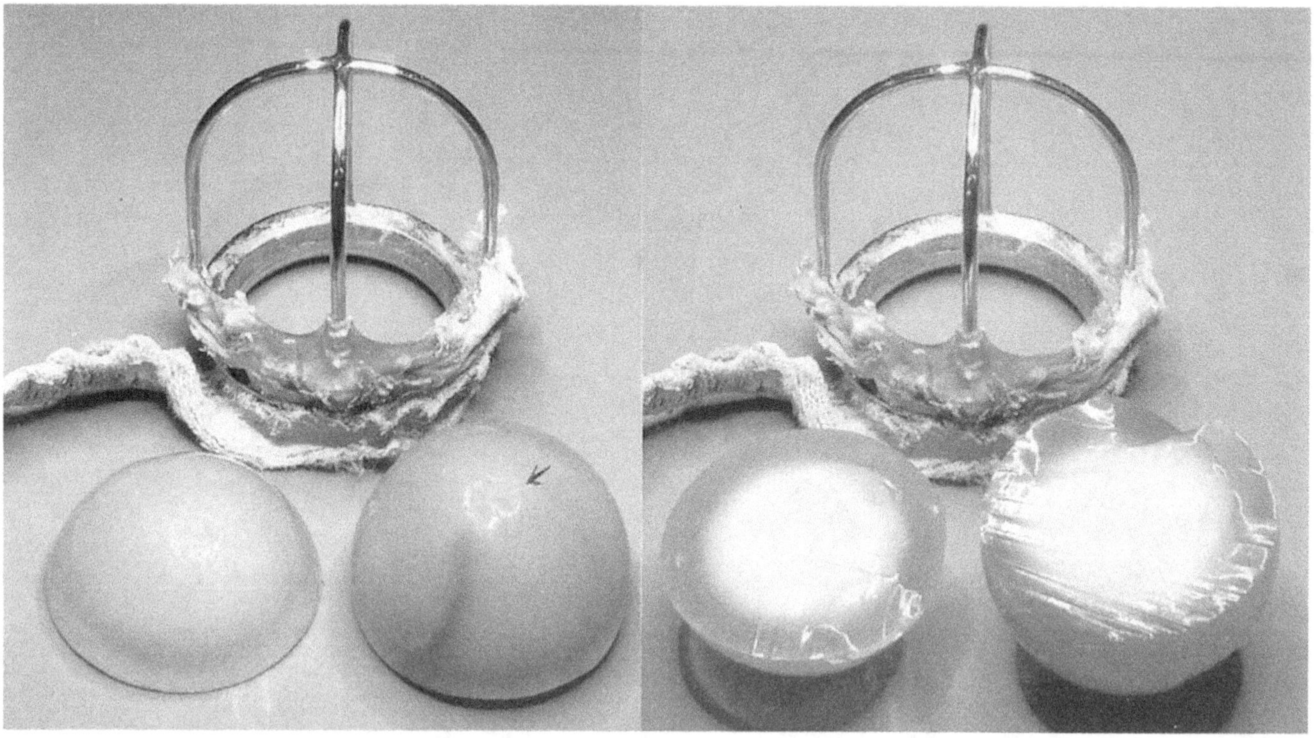

Figure 2. View of the poppet and age after incising the poppet in its mid-portion. The *arrow (left)* shows a region of elongated wear marks. The ball shows a demarcation of color probably corresponding to penetration of blood components, primarily lipids, by absorption *(right)*.

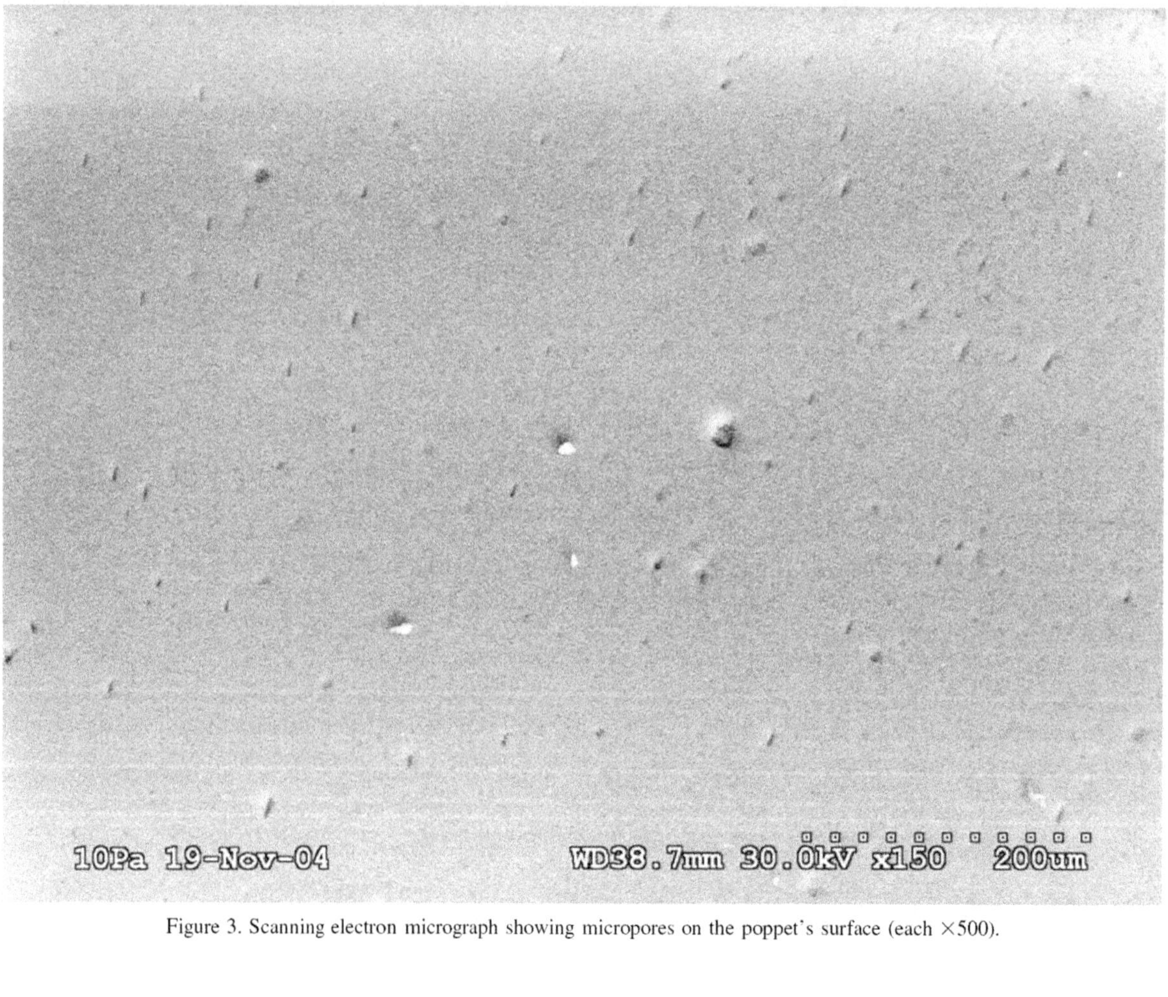

Figure 3. Scanning electron micrograph showing micropores on the poppet's surface (each ×500).

Comparison of the quantity of calcific deposits in bovine pericardial bioprostheses in the mitral and aortic valve positions in the same patient late after double-valve replacement

William Clifford Roberts, MD,[a,b,d] Carlos Ernesto Velasco, MD,[a] Jong Mi Ko, BA,[d] and Gregory John Matter, MD,[c] Dallas, Tex

Among patients undergoing cardiac valve replacement, the aortic valve is most commonly replaced, the mitral valve next, and, infrequently, both the mitral and aortic valves. When the latter situation occurs and when the substitute valves inserted are both bioprostheses, it is possible to compare the rates of degenerative change because one bioprosthesis serves as a control for the other. In 1983, Warnes and associates[1] reported on 5 patients with porcine bioprostheses in both the mitral and aortic valve positions from 18 to 107 months, and in each of the 4 patients in which the bioprosthesis was in place for greater than 18 months, the quantity of calcific deposits on the cusps of the bioprosthesis in the mitral valve position was much greater than that on the prosthesis in the aortic valve position. The present report was prompted by observing a patient who had a bovine parietal pericardial bioprosthesis in both the mitral and aortic positions explanted after they had been in place for 77 months; the quantity of calcium in the bioprosthesis in the aortic valve position was massive, and that in the bioprosthesis in the mitral position was minimal.

CLINICAL SUMMARY

A patient, who was born on March 25, 1949, had acute rheumatic fever in childhood and hypothyroidism since age 20 years. She was in her usual good health until April 2001 (age 52 years), when exertional dyspnea appeared, and it soon progressed to orthopnea, which prompted hospital admission. Echocardiographic and cardiac catheterization data are shown in Table 1. Electrocardiographic analysis disclosed sinus rhythm.

On May 22, 2001, both the mitral and aortic valves were replaced with Carpentier Edwards pericardial bovine bioprostheses treated with the XenoLogix tissue treatment process (Edwards LifeSciences, Irvine, Calif), which removes approximately 98% of phospholipids, which are calcium-binding sites. The excised anterior mitral leaflet weighed 0.77 g, and the 3-cuspid aortic valve weighed 0.74 g (Figure 1, *A* and *B*). Both valves were free of calcium.

The patient was thereafter well until April 2002, when a febrile illness developed. *Streptococcus sanguis* was cultured from the blood. She was treated with antibiotics, and her usual health returned. Vegetations were never observed on either bioprosthesis by means of echocardiographic analysis. Another echocardiogram in March 2003 disclosed stenosis of the bioprosthesis in the aortic valve position.

She continued to be well until August 2007, when exertional dyspnea recurred, and within 3 weeks, she was essentially bedridden. She was rehospitalized on September 24, 2007, and repeat cardiac catheterization (Table 1) and echocardiographic analysis showed mild bioprosthetic mitral regurgitation and nearly nonmovable bioprosthetic cusps in the aortic valve position. The bioprosthesis in the aortic valve position could not be crossed at cardiac

TABLE 1. Cardiac catheterization data in the patient presented

Variable	May 18, 2001 (before the first operation)	October 10, 2007 (before the second operation)
Pulmonary artery (mm Hg)	75/40	102/54
Right ventricle (mm Hg)	75/28	102/24
Right atrium (mm Hg)		
A wave	30	28
V wave	23	25
Mean	22	20
Pulmonary artery wedge (mm Hg)		
A wave	37	42
V wave	38	46
Mean	34	33
Left ventricle (mm Hg)	159/28	
Aorta (mm Hg)	165/95	130/82
Cardiac index ($L \cdot min^{-1} \cdot m^{-2}$)	1.8	2.0
Ejection fraction (%)	40	
Body weight (lbs)	156	138
Height (inches)	62	62

–, No information available.

From the Departments of Internal Medicine (Division of Cardiology),[a] Pathology,[b] and Cardiothoracic Surgery,[c] and the Baylor Heart and Vascular Institute,[d] Baylor University Medical Center, Dallas, Tex.

Received for publication Jan 29, 2009; accepted for publication Feb 8, 2009; available ahead of print March 27, 2009.

Address for reprints: William C. Roberts, MD, Baylor Heart and Vascular Institute, Baylor University Medical Center, 3500 Gaston Ave, Dallas, TX 75246 (E-mail: wc.roberts@baylorhealth.edu).

J Thorac Cardiovasc Surg 2009;138:1448-50
0022-5223/$36.00

doi:10.1016/j.jtcvs.2009.02.022

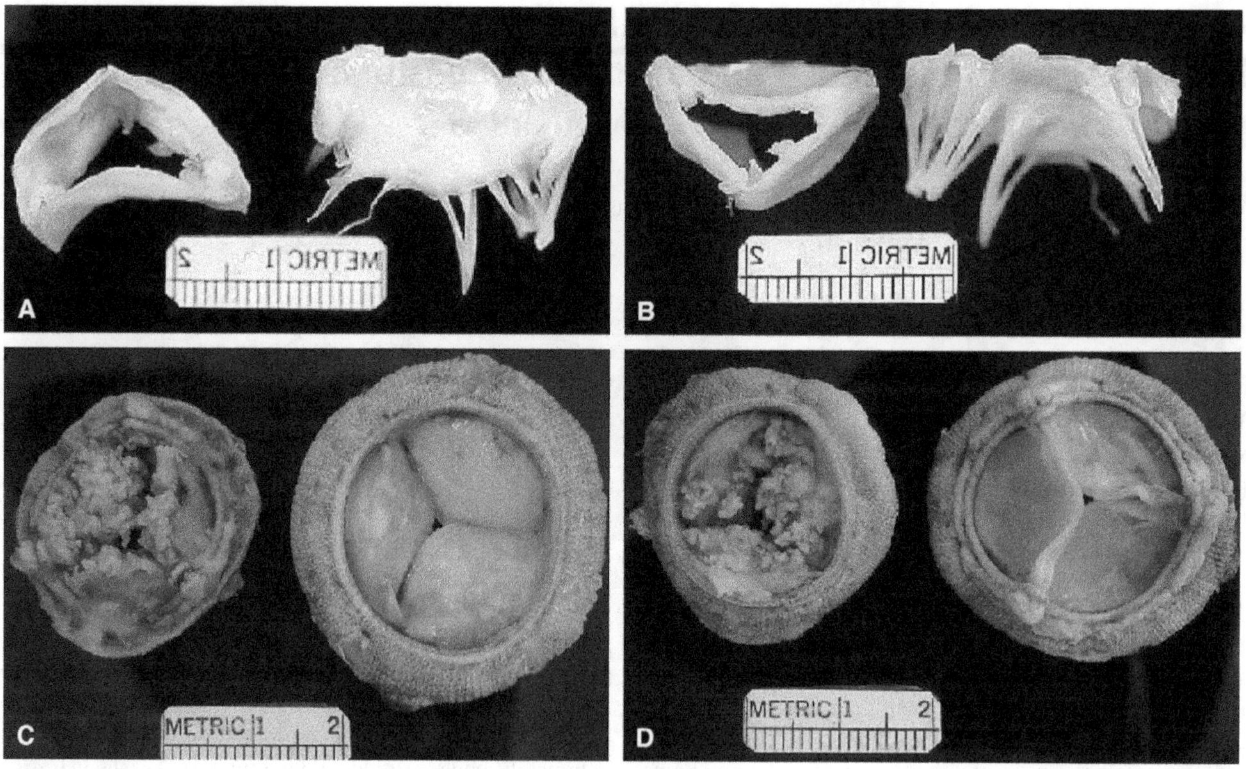

FIGURE 1. Native mitral and aortic valves (A and B) and bovine pericardial bioprostheses in the mitral and aortic valve positions (C and D) in the patient described. A, Anterior mitral leaflet from the atrial aspect and aortic valve from the ventricular aspect. B, Anterior mitral leaflet from the ventricular aspect and aortic valve from the aortic aspect. Both native valves are devoid of calcific deposits. C, Bioprosthesis in the mitral position from the atrial aspect and biopros thesis in the aortic position from the aortic aspect. D, Bioprosthesis in the mitral position from the ventricular aspect and bioprosthesis in the aortic position from the ventricular aspect. Heavy calcific deposits are present on both surfaces of the bioprosthesis in the aortic valve position.

catheterization. The coronary arteries were normal on angiographic analysis.

On October 12, 2007, both bioprostheses were replaced with mechanical prostheses, and a tricuspid valve annuloplasty was performed. At the time of the operation, a small paravalvular leak was seen in the mitral position. The bioprosthesis in the mitral position (no. 25) weighed 4.04 g, and the bioprosthesis in the aortic position (no. 21) weighed 3.86 g (Figure 1, *C* and *D*). Radiographs of the operatively excised bioprostheses showed huge calcific deposits in the aortic prosthesis and small deposits in the mitral prosthesis (Figure 2). Her postoperative course was relatively uneventful. As of November 2008, she is active, and her activities are not limited. By means of

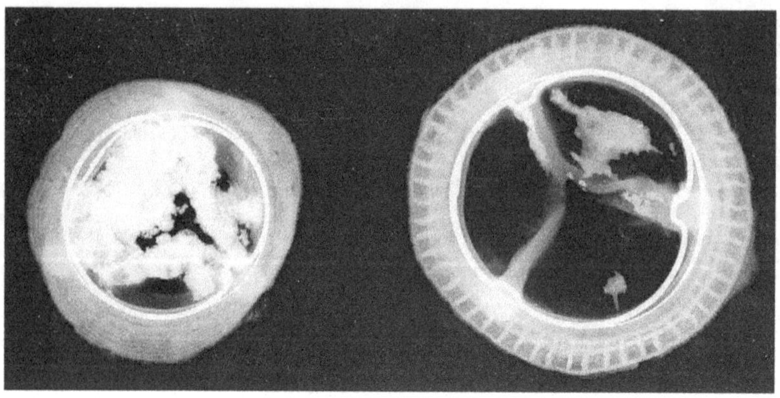

FIGURE 2. Radiograph of the bioprostheses excised from the aortic valve position *(left)* and the mitral valve position *(right)*. The calcific deposits are huge on the left and small on the right.

echocardiographic analysis, her pulmonary arterial systolic pressure had decreased to 34 mm Hg, and left ventricular ejection fraction had increased to 55%. There was only trace tricuspid valve regurgitation.

DISCUSSION

The patient described had parietal pericardial bovine bioprostheses in both the mitral and aortic valve positions for 77 months and during that period developed huge quantities of calcium on the cusps of the bioprosthesis in the aortic valve position and only small quantities of calcium on the cusps of the bioprosthesis in the mitral valve position. Because the closing pressure on the mitral bioprosthesis is usually about a third higher than that on the aortic bioprosthesis (peak left ventricular systolic pressure vs end-diastolic aortic pressure; normally approximately 120 vs 80 mm Hg), it might be expected that the degeneration of a bioprosthesis in the mitral position would be greater (more calcium and more tears) and more rapid than that of a bioprosthesis in the aortic position, but the opposite was the case in the patient described herein. Why might that be the case? Some possibilities include the following:

1. Parietal pericardial bovine bioprostheses are not the same as porcine aortic valve bioprostheses. The former are thicker and less flexible and possibly withstand the left ventricular peak systolic pressure and the aortic end-diastolic pressure more easily than the more delicate porcine aortic cusps.
2. The bovine bioprosthesis in the aortic position was defective and not properly prepared, whereas the one in the mitral position was not.
3. The febrile illness the patient had beginning 11 months after the initial cardiac operation could have been active infective endocarditis that affected the bioprosthesis in the aortic position but not the bioprosthesis in the mitral position.
4. Smaller bovine parietal pericardial bioprostheses calcify more rapidly and more extensively than do larger bovine pericardial bioprostheses.
5. The paravalvular leak in the mitral position and the absence of a leak in the aortic position provided a "bypass shunt," diminishing the effect of the full force of the peak left ventricular systolic pressure on the bioprosthetic cusps in the mitral position.

None of these 5 possibilities can be proved or disproved, but this report might stimulate careful follow-up of similar patients to determine whether this distribution of calcium in the 2 left-sided bioprostheses is a pattern or an exception.

Reference

1. Warnes CA, Scott ML, Silver GM, Smith CW, Ferrans VJ, Roberts WC. Comparison of late degenerative changes in porcine bioprostheses in the mitral and aortic valve position in the same patient. *Am J Cardiol*. 1983;51:965-8.

Combined mitral and aortic stenosis of rheumatic origin with double-valve replacement in an octogenarian

William Clifford Roberts [a,b,d,*], Jong Mi Ko [d], John Ryan Schumacher [a], Albert Carl Henry III [c]

[a] *Department of Internal Medicine, Division of Cardiology, Baylor University Medical Center, Dallas, TX, United States*
[b] *Department of Pathology, Baylor University Medical Center, Dallas, TX, United States*
[c] *Department of Cardiothoracic Surgery, Baylor University Medical Center, Dallas, TX, United States*
[d] *Baylor Heart and Vascular Institute, Baylor University Medical Center, Dallas, TX, United States*

Received 29 October 2008; accepted 1 November 2008
Available online 30 November 2008

Abstract

We describe double valve replacement for rheumatic mitral and aortic stenosis in an 83-year-old woman, a very uncommon event in an octogenarian.

Keywords: Mitral stenosis; Aortic stenosis; Rheumatic heart disease; Octogenarians; Double valve replacement

Replacement of both mitral and aortic valves in octogenarians is infrequent especially for combined mitral stenosis (MS) and aortic stenosis (AS) of rheumatic etiology. Such was the case, however, in the patient to be described herein.

An 81-year-old woman, who was born on 23 September 1925, had increasing dyspnea for several years became of what was believed to be "pulmonary fibrosis," worse in the lower lobes than the upper lobes. In December 2004, she was placed on home oxygen, and in January 2005, on continuous oxygen by nasal cannula. She had never smoked and had no history of acute rheumatic fever. Because of rather dramatic worsening of her dyspnea, she was hospitalized at Baylor University Medical Center on 1 May 2007. Her body mass index was 20 kg/m^2. Precordial examination disclosed an apical diastolic murmur and a basal ejection type systolic murmur. Electrocardiogram disclosed prolonged P–R interval and increased voltage compatible with left ventricular hypertrophy. Telemetric monitoring disclosed runs of atrial fibrillation.

Cardiac catheterization disclosed the following pressures in mm Hg: pulmonary artery wedge a-wave 21, v-wave 34, and mean 22; pulmonary artery, 68/26 (mean 39); left ventricle, 129/21 and aorta, 113/46; pulmonary arterial wedge — left ventricular mean diastolic gradient 8, and simultaneous left ventricular–aortic peak systolic gradient, 16. Cardiac index was 2.2 L/min/m^2. The calculated mitral valve area was 0.8 and the aortic valve area, 0.7 cm^2. Angiography disclosed insignificant coronary arterial narrowing.

On 4 May 2007, both left-sided cardiac valves (Fig. 1) were replaced with St. Jude Medical prostheses: mitral #29, and aortic #19. The postoperative course was relatively smooth. The pulmonary arterial pressure fell dramatically, and she was discharged to the Baylor Specialty Hospital on 14 May 2007 where she remained for 17 days.

Thereafter, she did well until about 1 January 2008, when she noted pedal edema which progressed to anasarca and a weight gain from 112 to 148 lb. She was rehospitalized on 4 February 2008. The blood hemoglobin was 9.8 g/L and the hematocrit, 30.3%. With diuretic therapy she lost 30 lb and returned home feeling much better. She was now in persistent atrial fibrillation. As of October 2008, she was doing well.

* Corresponding author. Department of Internal Medicine, Division of Cardiology, Baylor University Medical Center, Dallas, TX, United States.
E-mail address: wc.Roberts@baylorhealth.edu (W.C. Roberts).

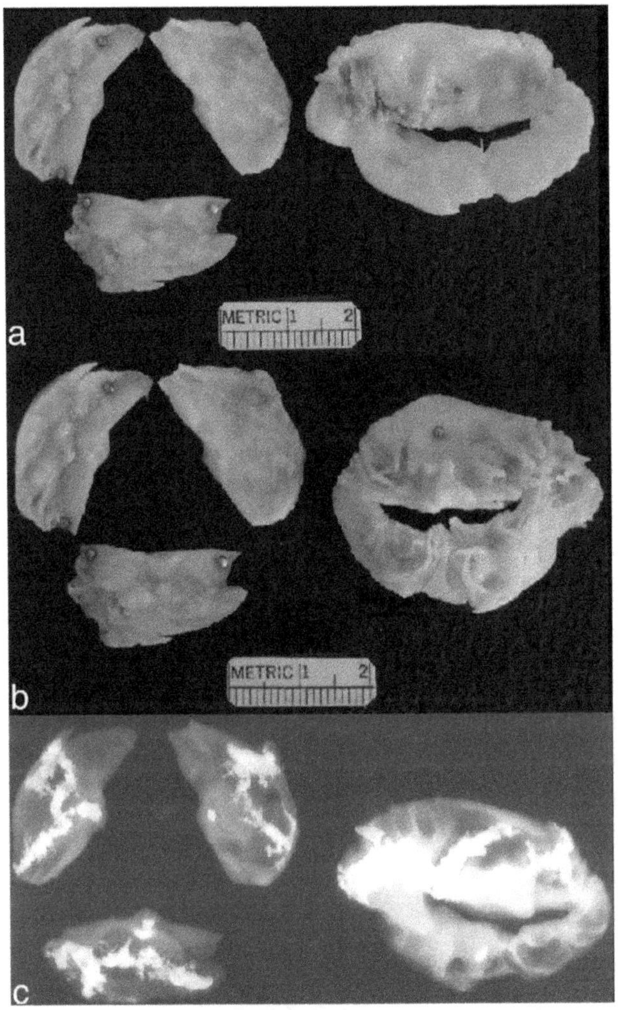

Fig. 1. Photographs of the operatively excised aortic valve (left) and mitral valve (right). The mitral valve is shown from the atrial aspect in a and from the ventricular aspect in b. Radiographs of each valve are shown in c.

Although now infrequent in the Western world, combined MS and AS of rheumatic origin was relatively common when acute rheumatic fever was far more prevalent. Roberts [1] collected 1010 cases at autopsy of valvular heart disease studied from approximately 1955 to 1980: isolated AS (with or without regurgitation) was the most frequent valve lesion (29%); isolated MS (with or without mitral regurgitation) was next (19%), and combined MS and AS was in third place (15%) (Table 1). None of the patients with combined MS and AS, however, was ≥80 years of age. In the last 3 decades, combined MS and AS of rheumatic etiology was infrequent in the Western world.

Combined MS and AS is particularly rare in octogenarians. Uricchio et al. [2] in 1959 reported 141 patients with combined MS and AS, all of whom had undergone both mitral and aortic commissurotomy: their ages ranged from 23 to 67 years. Katznelson et al. [3] studied 22 patients ranging in age from 23 to 61 years (mean 45); the average age of onset of symptoms of cardiac dysfunction was 40. Honey [4] studied 35 patients and their ages ranged from 24 to 54 years (mean 40). Reid et al. [5] studied 15 patients aged 26 to 48. Morrow et al. [6] studied 8 patients aged 20 to 48, all of whom had combined mitral and aortic valvulotomy. Zitnik et al. [7] studied 10 such patients who ranged in age from 34 to 55 (mean 42). Roberts and Sullivan [8] studied at necropsy 30 such patients who died within 60 days of double valve replacement for combined MS and AS: one was an octogenarian, aged 83, but the others were younger (mean age 57). Berman et al. [9] performed combined percutaneous mitral and aortic valvulotomy in 6 patients, aged 60 to 83. Thus, only 2 of the 267 patients in those studies with combined MS and AS were octogenarians.

Combined MS and AS is more common in women than in men. Of the 267 patients reported in the previously mentioned 8 studies [2–9], 171 (64%) were women.

Table 1
Functional and anatomic classification of valvular heart disease in 1010 necropsy patients aged >=15 years.[a]

Functional class	Patients	Anatomic class				
		AV	MV	MV-AV	TV-MV	TV-MV-AV
1. Aortic stenosis (AS)	292 (29%)	256 (88%)	0	35 (12%)	0	1 (0.3%)
2. Mitral stenosis (MS)	189 (19%)	0	117 (62%)	40 (21%)	13 (7%)	19 (10%)
3. MS+AS	152 (15%)	0	0	120 (79%)	0	32 (21%)
4. Aortic regurgitation (AR)[b]	119 (12%)	107 (90%)	0	10 (8%)	0	2 (2%)
5. Mitral regurgitation (MR)	97 (10%)	0	85 (88%)	8 (8%)	1 (1%)	3 (3%)
6. MS+AR	65 (6%)	0	52 (80%)	0	0	13 (20%)
7. MR+AR	45 (4%)	0	0	39 (87%)	0	6 (13%)
8. AS+MR	23 (2%)	0	0	21 (91%)	0	2 (9%)
9. Tricuspid stenosis+MS±AS	28 (3%)	0	0	0	4 (14%)	24 (86%)
Totals	1010 (100%)[c]	363 (36%)	254 (25%)	273 (27%)	18 (2%)	102 (10%)

AV = aortic valve; MV = mitral valve; TV = tricuspid valve.

Reproduced with permission from Elsevier and the author (Roberts WC. Am J Cardiol 1983;51:1005–1028).

[a] Excludes patients with mitral regurgitation secondary to coronary heart disease (papillary muscle dysfunction), carcinoid heart disease, hypertrophic cardiomyopathy, and those with infective endocarditis limited to 1 or both right-sided cardiac valves. Tricuspid valve regurgitation was present in many patients in most of the 9 functional groups. All patients were in functional class III or IV (New York Heart Association), and more than half had 1 or more cardiac operations.

[b] In many patients, the aortic valve cusps were normal or nearly normal and the regurgitation was the result of disease of the aorta (Marfan and Marfan-like syndrome, syphilis, systemic hypertension, healed aortic dissection).

[c] The hearts in all 1010 patients were examined and classified by WCR.

Several studies have examined cardiac hemodynamics in patients with combined MS and AS [2–9]. Although there are exceptions, the degree of AS when combined with MS is not as great (transvalvular peak systolic gradient) as in patients with isolated AS. Furthermore the MS, as emphasized by Zitnik et al. [7], can mask the presence of AS. If the AS is missed in this circumstance and mitral valve commissurotomy or replacement is performed and the downstream AS is neglected dire consequences can ensue. Obviously, it is best to diagnose both MS and AS preoperatively, but if one lesion is to be missed, it is far better to miss the upstream problem (MS) than the downstream problem (AS).

And finally, combined MS and AS can produce an operative challenge. First, the patients are most commonly women, some of whom, as in the present patient, are of small stature and, consequently, have relatively small hearts [8]. In combined MS and AS, neither the left ventricular cavity nor the ascending aorta is dilated, a circumstance which provides less space for either the mitral or the aortic mechanical prosthesis or bioprosthesis compared to the space provided in patients with isolated AS who often have congenitally bicuspid aortic valves and dilated ascending aortas.

Acknowledgment

The authors of this manuscript have certified that they comply with the Principles of Ethical Publishing in the International Journal of Cardiology [10].

References

[1] Roberts WC. Morphologic features of the normal and abnormal mitral valve. Am J Cardiol 1983;51:1005–28.
[2] Uricchio JF, Goldberg H, Sinha KP, Likoff W. Combined mitral and aortic stenosis: clinical and physiologic features and results of surgery. Am J Cardiol 1959;4:479–91.
[3] Katznelson G, Jreissaty RM, Levinson GE, Stein SW, Abelmann WH. Combined aortic and mitral stenosis. Am J Med 1960;29:242–56.
[4] Honey M. Clinical and haemodynamic observations on combined mitral and aortic stenosis. Brit Heart J 1961;23:545–55.
[5] Reid JM, Stevenson JG, Barclay RS, Welsh TM. Combined aortic and mitral stenosis. Brit Heart J 1962;24:509–15.
[6] Morrow AG, Awe WC, Braunwald E. Combined mitral and aortic stenosis. Brit Heart J 1962;24:606–12.
[7] Zitnik RS, Piemme TE, Messer RJ, Reed DP, Haynes FW, Dexter L. The masking of aortic stenosis by mitral stenosis. Am Heart J 1965;69:22–30.
[8] Roberts WC, Sullivan MF. Clinical and necropsy observations early after simultaneous replacement of the mitral and aortic valves. Am J Cardiol 1986;58:1067–84.
[9] Berman AD, Weinstein JS, Safian RD, Diver DJ, Grossman W, McKay RG. Combined aortic and mitral balloon valvuloplasty in patients with critical aortic and mitral valve stenosis: results in six cases. J Am Coll Cardiol 1988;11:1213–8.
[10] Coats AJ. Ethical authorship and publishing. Int J Cardiol 2009;131:149–50.

43.3-Year Durability of a Smeloff-Cutter Ball-Caged Mitral Valve

Stuart J. Head, BS, Jamie Ko, MD, Rajeev Singh, MD, William C. Roberts, MD, and Michael J. Mack, MD

Cardiopulmonary Research Science and Technology Institute, Dallas, Texas, Department of Cardio-Thoracic Surgery, Erasmus University Medical Center, Rotterdam, the Netherlands, Department of Pathology, The Baylor Health and Vascular Institute, Dallas, Department of Cardiology, The Diagnostic Clinic of Longview, Longview, and Heart Hospital Baylor Plano, Plano, Texas

Extended durability of mechanical heart valves has been documented for many years. We describe a case of a ball-caged mechanical valve implanted 43.3 years previous to developing valve dysfunction. The patient presented with both prosthetic valve stenosis and insufficiency. This Smeloff-Cutter valve (Cutter Laboratories, Berkeley, CA) in the mitral position was dysfunctional due to lipid absorption, which resulted in ball variance and concomitant pannus growth prevented optimal seating of the ball in its cage. This is the longest length of time in which a Smeloff-Cutter mechanical valve has been originally implanted.

(Ann Thorac Surg 2011;91:606–8)

In the early 1960s, heart valves were introduced for heart valve replacement, which resulted in the first mechanical valve prosthesis implantation of a Starr-Edwards valve (Edwards Lifesciences, Irvine, CA) in the mitral position in 1961 [1]. After this, newly developed ball-caged valves followed in quick succession, manufactured by a number of companies producing aortic and mitral valve prostheses. The Smeloff-Cutter valve (Cutter Laboratories, Berkeley, CA) was introduced in 1964, being the first "full-flow" valve, which was achieved by including an additional smaller cage on which the ball could rest during valve closure [2].

"Ball variance" is a previously documented cause of valve dysfunction [3], in which lipid absorption in the ball causes it to grow and form surface irregularities, increasing the risk of thromboembolic events and valve dysfunction. We report a case in which ball variance and pannus overgrowth caused a 43.3-year implanted Smeloff-Cutter ball-caged valve to fail. This case is the longest implantation time of this type of valve.

At age 13, mitral valve stenosis developed in the patient, due to rheumatic fever. Therefore, the patient underwent a valve replacement. Recently, the 56-year-old woman presented with New York Heart Association functional class IV symptoms of heart failure and

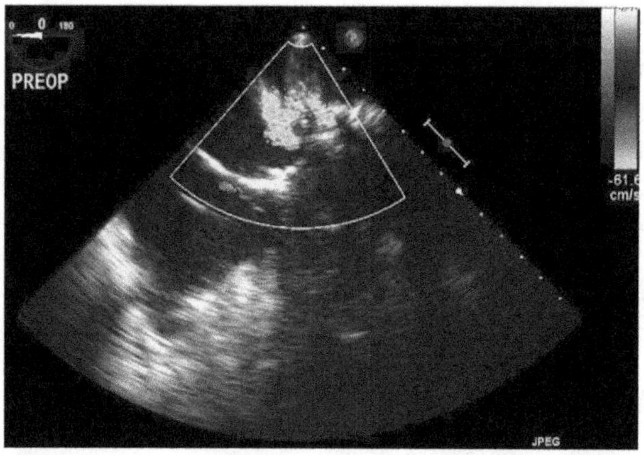

Fig 1. Preoperative echocardiogram showing both mitral stenosis and insufficiency.

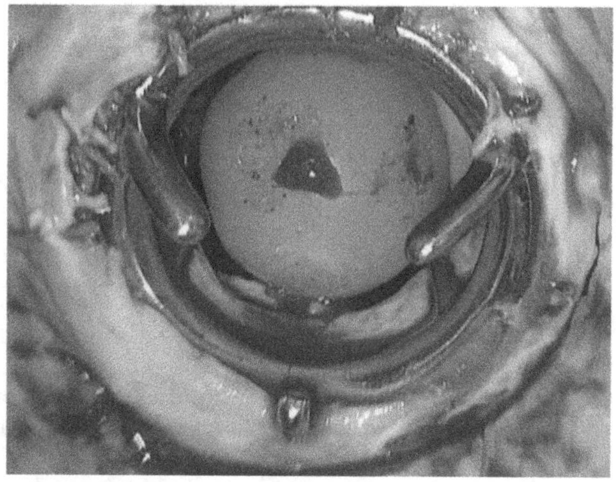

Fig 2. The 43.3-year-old Smeloff-Cutter valve in the mitral position. The valve was dysfunctional due to ball variance and pannus formation, both visible here. The ball shows signs of wear, having lost its perfect round shape and showing erosion.

palpitations as a result of long-standing persistent atrial fibrillation. Transthoracic and transesophageal echocardiography (Fig 1) revealed moderate to severe mitral valve regurgitation and severe mitral stenosis with a valve area of 0.7 cm^2 and a mean gradient of 15 mm Hg. There was decreased left ventricular function with an ejection fraction of 40%, systemic pulmonary hypertension, and severe tricuspid regurgitation.

The patient had been noncomplaint with warfarin therapy until suffering a stroke in 1988 after discontinuing therapy, which left her with a significant residual right hemipharesis. However, this event subsequently made her extremely diligent in taking the anticoagulant with good control and no further clinical events. For this reason, she opted for another mechanical valve.

At the time of the redo mitral valve replacement, a pre-cardiopulmonary bypass transesophageal echocardiographic finding consisted of the mitral valve prosthesis in a good position with severe mitral valve regurgitation. A 2.4 m/s maximum velocity was measured across the valve, calculating to a peak gradient of 23 mm Hg and a mean gradient of 9 mm Hg. The valve area was 2.3 cm^2 by pressure halftime and 0.7 cm^2 measured by continuity equation. Furthermore, a left ventricular ejection fraction of 40% was obtained. All measurements are consistent with preoperative findings.

The limited access procedure was performed exposing only the aorta and right atrium. A superior septal approach to the mitral valve was performed. Inspection of the valve revealed some erosion of the ball (Fig 2). Pannus formation built up around the valve prevented the ball to seat completely in its cage. There was an extensive amount of calcium built up both in the annulus and the ventricular muscle below the annulus. The 43.3-year-old valve was replaced with a 25-mm On-X bi-leaflet mechanical valve (On-X Life Technologies Inc, Austin, TX). After the valve was implanted, transesophageal echocardiography measured a maximum velocity across the valve of 1.3 m/s, with a peak-to-peak gradient of 7 mm Hg and a mean gradient of 3 mm Hg. By pressure half-time the valve area had improved to 3.5 cm^2. Concomitant tricuspid valve annuloplasty with a 26-mm tricuspid annulus ring and a full left-sided and right-sided Cryo maze procedure were performed. Her postoperative course was uneventful. She was discharged home on postoperative day 6. The patient is in New York Heart Association functional class I at her most recent follow-up at 6 weeks postoperatively.

Comment

Valve dysfunction after extended durability can be the result of a wide variety of causes, including lipid absorption into the ball and pannus formation, causing tissue impingement as the two most common. Absorption increases the size of the ball and causes it to lose its round shape [3]. This can cause denting, increasing the risk of complications, such as thrombus formation and hemolysis. Dysfunction occurs because ball vari-

Table 1. Valve Implantation Times ≥43 years

Valve Type	Position	Age at Surgery	Years in Position
Starr-Edwards	Aortic	19	46.3
Starr-Edwards [8]	Mitral	24	44
Starr-Edwards	Aortic	28	43.8
Starr-Edwards	Aortic and mitral	31	43.7
Smeloff-Cutter	Mitral	13	43.3
Starr-Edwards	Aortic	19	43.1
Starr-Edwards	Aortic	16	43.1
Starr-Edwards	Aortic	19	43

ance can make it impossible for the ball to move freely with regurgitation as a result, or can cause it to stick in the cage in the closed position. However, many causes of late valve dysfunction are not related to the design of the valve. Ozkokeli and colleagues [4] reported a case in which a 37-year implanted Starr-Edwards valve (Edwards Lifesciences) (model 1000-9A) developed acute prosthetic valve endocarditis, a complication unrelated to the implantation time. Also, indiscriminate to years of implantation, is the formation of tissue overgrowth. An article by Butany and colleagues [5] describes pannus growth in a DeBakey Surgitool (Travenol Laboratories Inc, Morton Grove, IL) mechanical aortic valve prosthesis implanted for 32 years. The valve itself did not show any signs of wear, but it became dysfunctional due to the excessive tissue. Schmitto and colleagues [6] reported a suboptimal but satisfactory working Starr-Edwards ball-caged valve at 39 years after initial implantation. However, a post-valvular ascending aortic aneurysm of 6.0 × 6.5 cm made it necessary to perform a Bentall procedure [6].

A few cases have been reported of patients with a mechanical aortic or mitral valve in place for more than 30 years in which the nonprosthetic valve in the systemic circulation was regurgitating, not the prosthesis [7]. In these cases, the prostheses were working satisfactory, but in many cases the decision was made to prophylactically replace the valve.

Reports of prolonged ball-caged valve durability are mostly Starr-Edwards valves, with survival of greater than 43 years in a number of cases (Table 1). In the literature, it is reported that Smeloff-Cutter valves have been explanted after as long as 37 years [7]. Until further results have been published, we believe that this case reports the longest implanted Smeloff-Cutter mechanical valve of 43.3 years.

References

1. Starr A, Edwards M. Mitral replacement: clinical experience with a ball-valve prosthesis. Ann Surg 1961;154:726–40.
2. Gott VL, Alejo DE, Cameron DE. Mechanical heart valves: 50 years of evolution. Ann Thorac Surg 2003;76:S2230–9.
3. Peterman MA, Donsky MS, Matter GJ, Roberts WC. A Starr-Edwards model 6120 mechanical prosthesis in the mitral valve position for 38 years. Am J Cardiol 2006;97:756–8.
4. Ozkokeli M, Ates M, Ekinci A, Akcar M. Thirty-seven-year durability of a Starr-Edwards aortic prosthesis. Tex Heart Inst J 2005;32:99–101.
5. Butany J, Naseemuddin A, Nair V, Feindel CM. DeBakey Surgitool mechanical heart valve prosthesis, explanted at 32 years. Cardiovasc Pathol 2004;13:345–6.
6. Schmitto JD, Ortmann P, Popov AF, et al. Bentall procedure 39 years after implantation of a Starr-Edwards aortic caged-ball-valve prosthesis. J Cardiothorac Surg 2010;5:12.
7. Si MS, Zapolanski A. A 37-year-old Smeloff-Cutter aortic valve. Ann Thorac Surg 2009;87:628–9.
8. Fernandez J, Farivar RS. Explantation of a 44-year-old Starr-Edwards mitral valve for delayed hemolysis. J Thorac Cardiovasc Surg 2010;140:e35–6.

Mitral Valve Replacement After Failed Mitral Ring Insertion With or Without Leaflet/Chordal Repair for Pure Mitral Regurgitation

William C. Roberts, MD[a,b,c,*], Meagan Moore[a,d], Jong Mi Ko, BA[a], and Baron L. Hamman, MD[e]

Mitral repair operations for correction of pure mitral regurgitation (MR) are generally quite successful. Occasionally, however, the reparative procedure incompletely corrects the MR or the MR recurs. From March 1993 to January 2016, twenty nine patients had mitral valve replacement after the initial mitral repair operation, and observations in them were analyzed. All 29 patients at the repair operation had an annular ring inserted and later (<1 year in 6 and >1 year in 21) mitral valve replacement. The cause of the MR before the repair operation appears to have been prolapse in 16 patients (55%), secondary (functional) in 12 (41%) (ischemic in 5), and infective endocarditis which healed in 1 (3%). At the replacement operation the excised anterior mitral leaflet was thickened in all 29 patients. Some degree of stenosis appeared to have been present in 16 of the 29 patients before the replacement operation, although only 10 had an echocardiographic or hemodynamic recording of a transvalvular gradient; at least 11 patients had restricted motion of the posterior mitral leaflet; 10, ring dehiscence; 2, severe hemolysis; and 2, left ventricular outflow obstruction. In conclusion, there are multiple reasons for valve replacement after earlier mitral repair. Uniformly, at the time of the replacement, the mitral leaflets were thickened by fibrous tissue. Measurement of the area enclosed by the 360° rings and study of the excised leaflet suggest that the ring itself may have contributed to the leaflet scarring and development of some transmitral stenosis.
(Am J Cardiol 2016;117:1790−1807)

Although the results of mitral valve repair operations performed in major medical centers by very experienced cardiac surgeons are usually excellent, an unfortunate consequence of mitral valve repair with ring insertion in a few patients is inadequate elimination of the mitral regurgitation (MR) or recurrence of mitral valve dysfunction after repair with ring insertion.[1−21] From 1994 through 2015 (23 years) 32 patients who earlier had had mitral valve repair with ring insertion underwent a second mitral valve operation. This report focuses on the 29 patients in whom the second operation was mitral valve replacement.

Methods

Since March 1993, all cardiac specimens excised at cardiac operations at Baylor University Medical Center (BUMC) have been described by one of us (WCR) and most have been photographed (mainly by JMK). During this 23-year period, 32 specimens of mitral annular rings with or without the anterior mitral leaflets were submitted to the surgical pathology laboratory of the Department of Pathology of BUMC. Three of them had a second mitral repair operation and they were eliminated from this study. The remaining 29 patients all had mitral valve replacement after the initial mitral repair operation and they form the basis of this study. After examining the operatively excised annular ring and anterior mitral leaflet and chordae, the clinical records were sought and examined. The interior of the complete rings was calculated by the formula for an ellipse, which is half the length of its major axis times half the length of its minor axis times *pi* (3.14).

The mitral valve replacement operations in the 29 patients were performed by 11 different surgeons: 10 by 1 surgeon; 6 by another; 4 by another; 2 by another, and 1 by each of 7 different surgeons. Of the mitral valve replacement surgeons, 10 had previously done the mitral valve repair operation.

The BUMC Institutional Review Board approved this study.

Results

Certain clinical and morphologic findings are tabulated for each of the 29 patients in Table 1. The ages of the patients at the time of the mitral valve repair operation ranged

[a]Baylor Heart and Vascular Institute; [b]Department of Internal Medicine (Division of Cardiology); [c]Department of Pathology, and [e]Department of Cardiothoracic Surgery, Baylor University Medical Center, Dallas, Texas; and [d]Second Year, Texas A&M University, College Station, Texas. Manuscript received March 2, 2016; revised manuscript received and accepted March 3, 2016.

This study was funded by the Baylor Health Care System Foundation through the Cardiovascular Research Review Committee and in cooperation with the Baylor Heart and Vascular Institute.

See page 1804 for disclosure information.

*Corresponding author: Tel: (+1) 214-820-7911; fax: (+1) 214-820-7533.

E-mail address: wc.roberts@baylorhealth.edu (W.C. Roberts).

Table 1
Certain clinical and morphologic findings in the 29 patients having mitral valve replacement after earlier mitral valve repair

Patient	Sex	Cause of MR	AF	SH	BMI (Kg/m²)	Age (yrs) at MV Repair and Ring Insertion	Age (yrs) at MVR and Ring Removal	Interval between Operations	MV Ring Size (mm) and type	MDG LA-LV (mmHg)	Explanted Ring Area (cm²)	Valve Type	CABG	AVR	Reason for MV Replacement						Figure Number
															MS	RD	Leaflet Repair Breakdown	H	Restricted PML	LVOTO	
1	Man	Prolapse	0	0	20	49	49	16 days	33 Duran		3.9	M	+	0	0	0	+	0	0	0	
2	Man	Prolapse	+	+	34	65	65	21 days	30 Edwards-physio II	5	3.9 (2.7[*])	M	0	0	+	0	0	0	+	+[†]	1
3	Man	Secondary (CAD)	0	+	28	58	58	53 days	–	12	3.3	M	+	0	+	0	0	0	0	0	2
4	Woman	Healed IE	0	+	43	68	68	63 days	28 miral flex	–	–	B	0	0	+	+	0	+	0	0	
5	Man	Secondary (CAD)	0	+	24	70	70[‡]	80 days	28 Carbomedics	4	–	B	+	0	+	+	0	0	0	0	3
6	Man	Prolapse	0	0	21	43	43	91 days	33 Duran	–	5.9	M	0	0	0	0	+	0	0	0	2
7	Man	Prolapse	0	+	27	69	69	161 days	33 Duran	–	–	M	+	0	0	0	0	+	0	0	5
8	Man	Prolapse	0	0	28	55	55	237 days	–	–	2.4	M	0	0	0	+	+	0	0	0	
9	Woman	Secondary (CAD)	0	+	29	57	58	1 year	–	–	2.3	M	+	0	0	0	+	0	0	0	6
10	Man	Secondary	0	+	36	62	63	1 year	38 ATS simulus semirigid	–	–	M	0	0	0	+	+	0	+	0	
11	Woman	Prolapse	0	+	44	30[†]	32	2 years	32 Carpentier Edwards	7	3.5	M	0	0	0	+	0	0	0	0	7
12	Woman	Secondary	0	+	22	45	47	2 years	26 Cosgrove-Edwards	–	0.3	M	0	+	+	+	0	0	+	0	
13	Man	Prolapse	0	+	"obese"	67	69	2 years	–	–	–	B	+	0	0	+	0	0	0	0	
14	Woman	Secondary[§]	0	+	29	63	66	4 years	26 Carpentier Edwards	–	2.4	M	0	0	+	+	0	0	+	0	8
15	Woman	Prolapse	+	+	35	57	61	4 years	30 Carpentier Edwards	8	3.2	M	0	0	+	0	0	0	+	0	9
16	Woman	Secondary	+	+	54	55	60	5 years	26 Carpentier Edwards	21	– (1.0[*])	B	0	+[¶]	+	0	0	0	+	0	10
17	Woman	Secondary (CAD)	+	+	25	62	67	5 years	–	52	0.3	B	+	0	+	0	0	0	0	+[†]	11
18	Woman	Secondary (CAD)	+	+	16	62	67[*]	5 years	–	–	3.1	B	+	0	+	0	0	0	+	0	12

(continued)

Table 1
(continued)

Patient	Sex	Cause of MR	AF	SH	BMI (Kg/m^2)	Age (yrs) at MV Repair and Ring Insertion	Age (yrs) at MVR and Ring Removal	Interval between Operations	MV Ring Size (mm) and type	MDG LA-LV (mmHg)	Explanted Ring Area (cm^2)	Valve Type	CABG	AVR	Reason for MV Replacement						Figure Number
															MS	RD	Leaflet Repair Breakdown	H	Restricted PML	LVOTO	
19	Woman	Secondary (CAD)	+	+	25	66	72	6 years	Duran	–	0.9	M	0	0	+	0	0	0	0	0	13
20	Man	Prolapse	0	0	29	66	74	8 years	Carpentier Edwards	–	–	M	+	0	0	0	+	0	0	0	14
21	Man	Prolapse	+	+	26	57	66	9 years	–	–	4.5	M	+	0	0	0	+[‖]	0	+	0	15
22	Woman	Secondary	0	+	34	29	39	10 years	–	13	3.9 (1.0*)	M	0	+	+	+	0	0	+	0	16
23	Man	Secondary	0	+	22	50	61	11 years	Carpentier Edwards	–	4.5	M	0	+	0	0	0	0	+	0	17
24	Man	Prolapse	0	+	32	53	64	11 years	30	–	6.4	M	+	+	0	+	+	0	+	0	18
25	Man	Prolapse	0	+	24	57	68	11 years	–	14	–	M	0	0	+	0	+	0	0	0	
26	Man	Prolapse	+	+	21	57	70	13 years	–	–	6.5	B	0	0	0	0	+	0	0	0	19
27	Woman	Prolapse	+	+	19	65	80	15 years	34 Carpentier Edwards	–	–	B	+	0	+	0	0	0	0	0	
28	Woman	Prolapse	0	+	27	21	43	22 years	–	–	–	M	0	0	+	0	0	0	0	0	
29	Man	Prolapse	+	+	28	47	71	24 years	–	12	3.4	B	0	0	+	0	0	0	+	0	20
Totals			8	18									12	5	16	10	10	2	12	2	

AF = atrial fibrillation; B = bioprosthesis; BMI = body mass index; CAD = coronary artery disease; CABG = coronary artery bypass grafting; EF = ejection fraction; H = hemolysis; IE = infective endocarditis; LA = left atrial; LV = left ventricular; M = mechanical prosthesis; MDG = mean diastolic gradient; MR = mitral regurgitation; MS = mitral stenosis; MV = mitral valve; MVR = mitral valve replacement; PML = posterior mitral leaflet; RD = ring dehisence; SH = systemic hypertension; – = not available.

* Area of ring calculated from echocardiogram.

† LV-aortic peak gradient at rest in case #2 was 46 mm Hg increasing to 85 mm Hg with Valsalva with severe systolic anterior motion of the anterior mitral leaflet. The LV-aortic peak systolic gradient at rest in case #17 was 41 mm Hg at rest.

‡ Left ventricular aneurysm also resected.

§ Previous acute lymphocytic leukemia treated by chemotherapy with subsequent dilated cardiomyopathy and 3+/4+ mitral regurgitation.

¶ Aortic valve dysfunction probably secondary to systemic lupus erythmatosis.

‖ An Alfiere stitch had dehised. Of the 13 patients in whom the MR was of functional or ischemic origin or secondary to cardiomyopathy or to infective endocarditis that had healed, only a ring was inserted in 12 (92%).

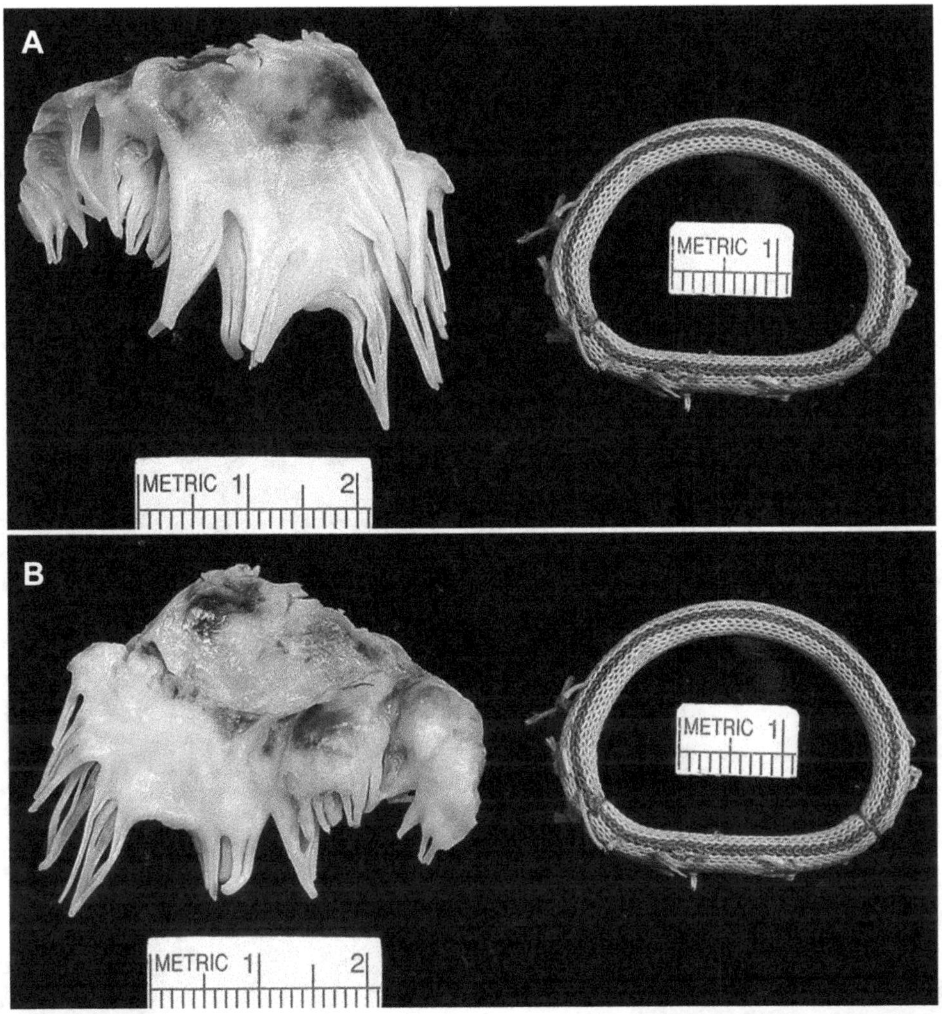

Figure 1. *Case #2.* Shown here is the anterior mitral leaflet *(A)*, ventricular aspect; *(B)*, atrial aspect and mitral ring which had been in place for 21 days before the mitral valve replacement. The ring (30 mm Edwards Physio II) pushed the anterior mitral leaflet into the left ventricular outflow tract causing severe outflow obstruction (left ventricular to aortic peak systolic gradient at rest 46 mm Hg rising to 88 m Hg with the Valsalva maneuver) and systolic anterior motion of the anterior mitral leaflet. The ring lying on about a third of the leaflet on its atrial aspect pushed the leaflet into the outflow tract causing the obstruction, complete heart block occurred at the replacement operation necessitating pacemaker implantation.

from 21 to 70 years (mean 55), and at mitral valve replacement operation, from 32 to 80 years (mean 61). The interval between the 2 operations was <1 year in 8 patients and between 1 and 24 years (mean 8) in the remaining 21 patients. The cause of the MR before the valve repair operation was prolapse in 16 patients (55%); secondary (functional) in 12 (41%), 5 of whom had coronary heart disease, and infective endocarditis, which had healed, in 1 (3%). Twelve patients (41%) had coronary artery bypass grafting, 11 at the time of the mitral repair: 6 (38%) of the 16 with mitral prolapse, and 5 (42%) of the 12 with secondary (functional) MR, and also in the 1 patient with healed infective endocarditis. Five patients had aortic valve replacement (for stenosis in 4) at the time of either the repair or replacement operation.

Examination of the operatively excised mitral leaflet (usually only the anterior one) in all 29 patients disclosed the leaflet to the thickened, at least focally, by fibrous tissue. The areas enclosed by the 360° annular rings (calculated in 19 patients) ranged from 2.4 to 6.4 cm^2 (mean 4.4 cm^2) in the 9 patients in whom the MR was the result of prolapse, and from 0.3 to 4.5 cm^2 (mean 2.3 cm^2) in the 9 patients with secondary MR. Either echocardiographic or hemodynamic mean left atrial to left ventricular diastolic gradients were measured in 5 of the 16 patients with prolapse and they ranged from 5 to 14 mm Hg (mean 9.2), and in 5 of the 12 patients with secondary MR, from 4 to 52 mm Hg (mean 20). In 2 patients (cases #2 and #22) the mitral area just before the replacement operation was measured by echocardiogram and also by measurement of the interior of the

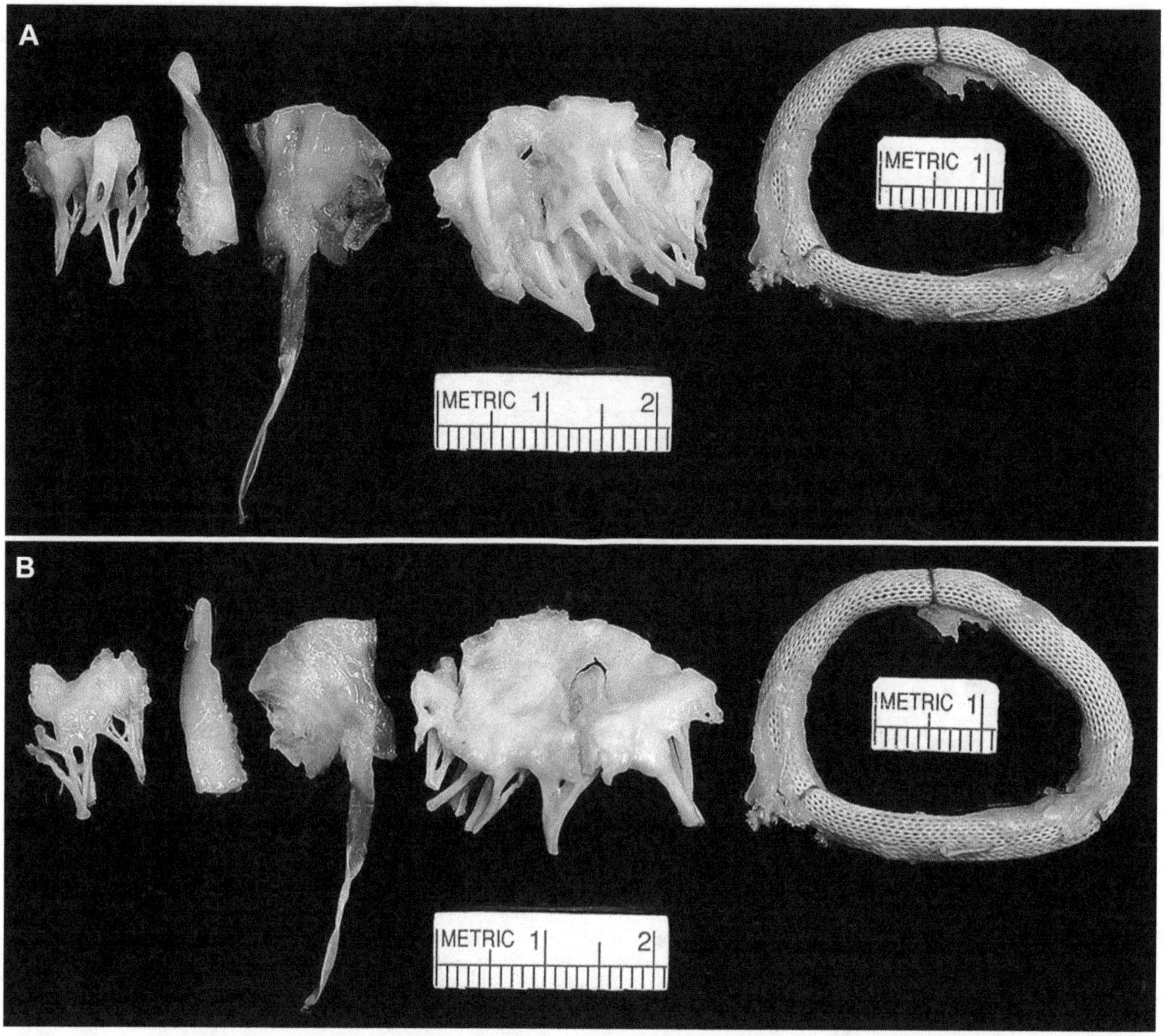

Figure 2. *Case #3*. Shown here are the mitral ring and the anterior mitral leaflet from the ventricular aspect (*A*) and from the atrial aspect (*B*). Fragments of posterior mitral leaflet, all of the anterior leaflet and the annular ring excised during mitral valve replacement 53 days after mitral valve repair procedure and coronary artery bypass grafting. The marginal portion of the anterior leaflet is thickened. After the initial repair procedure severe mitral regurgitation was present and it prompted the replacement operation. The reason for the mitral regurgitation after the repair procedure is not apparent from examination of the excised ring and leaflets, and the mechanism of the severe regurgitation was not mentioned in the operative note.

ring after its operative excision. In both cases the mitral area determined by echocardiogram was much smaller than that determined by morphologic measurement: 2.7 and 3.9 cm^2, respectively, in case #2, and 1.0 and 3.9 cm^2, respectively, in case #22.

Although MR, usually severe, was present immediately before the replacement operation in all 29 patients, some degree of mitral stenosis appeared to be present in 16 of the 29 patients, although confirmed physiologically in only 10 patients. The exact site of the stenosis was not easily determined from examination of the operatively excised leaflet and ring. Some rings appeared small: at least 2 had considerable "pannus" growing into the lumen of the ring, and the leaflets in all patients were thickened at the time of the replacement operation.

Morphologic features of the operatively excised mitral leaflets and/or rings are shown in Figures 1 to 20. A mechanical prosthesis was employed in 20 patients (69%) and a bioprosthesis in 9 patients (31%).

Discussion

Described herein is a heterogeneous group of patients who had a mitral annular ring inserted with or without leaflet/chordal repair for pure MR (no element of stenosis) and later underwent mitral valve replacement because of

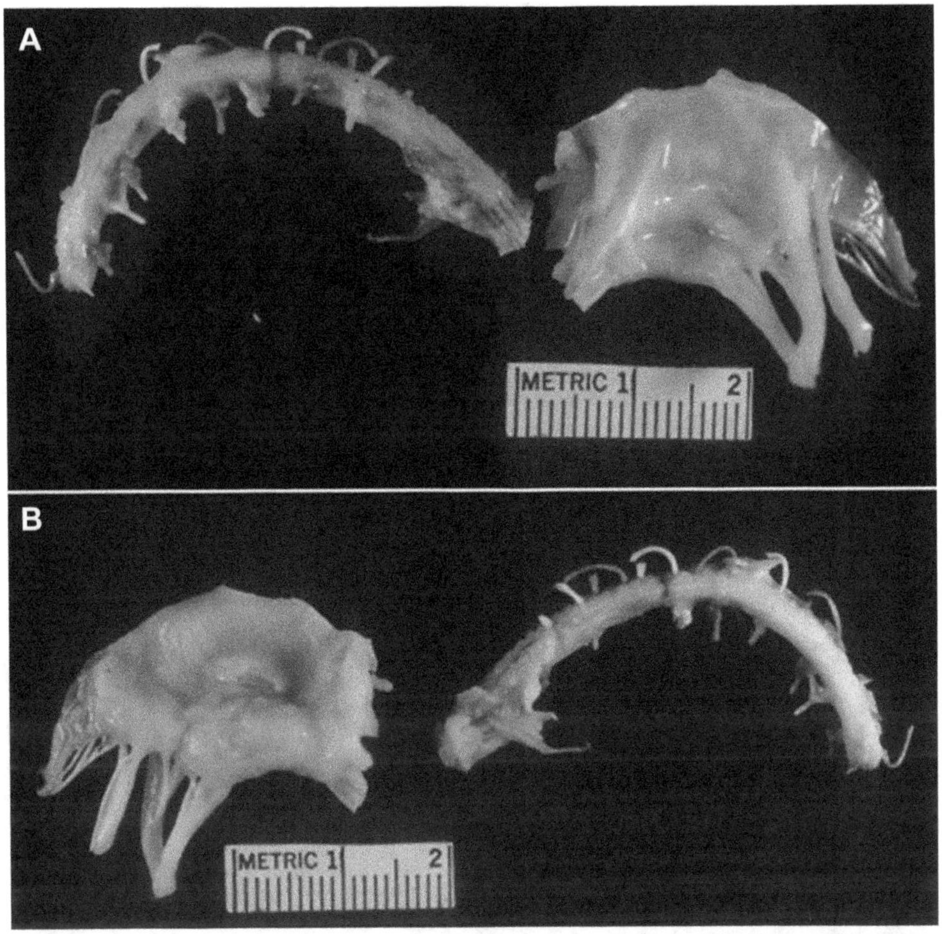

Figure 3. *Case #5.* Shown here is the anterior mitral leaflet from both the ventricular aspects *(A)* and atrial *(B)* plus the semicircular mitral ring, which has been opened up considerably. The margin of the anterior leaflet on the atrial aspect is thickened and several chordae from the anterolateral half of the anterior leaflet are thickened. The cause of the recurrence of mitral regurgitation, which at least initially was due to myocardial ischemia appears to have been partial ring dehiscence. One week after the repair operation for 4+/4+ mitral regurgitation, a 4 mm Hg mean gradient was present across the mitral valve. Only a ring was used for the repair.

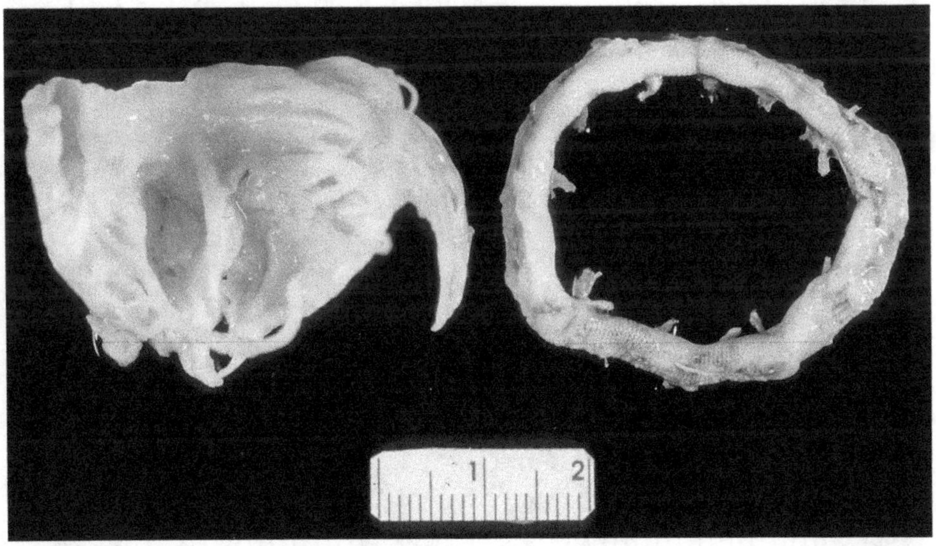

Figure 4. *Case #6.* Shown is the ventricular aspect of anterior mitral leaflet and the 360° ring which had been in place only 3 months. The distance from mitral annular region to distal margin of anterior mitral leaflet is elongated. The mitral annulus was found by the surgeon to be quite dilated. The 360° ring is mostly covered by fibrous tissue. Severe mitral regurgitation before the mitral replacement was attributed to both inadequate repair 91 days earlier and also to the annular dilatation. The interior area is 5.9 cm^2 suggesting that the mitral annulus had been quite dilated in this patient, both before the ring was inserted and probably afterwards.

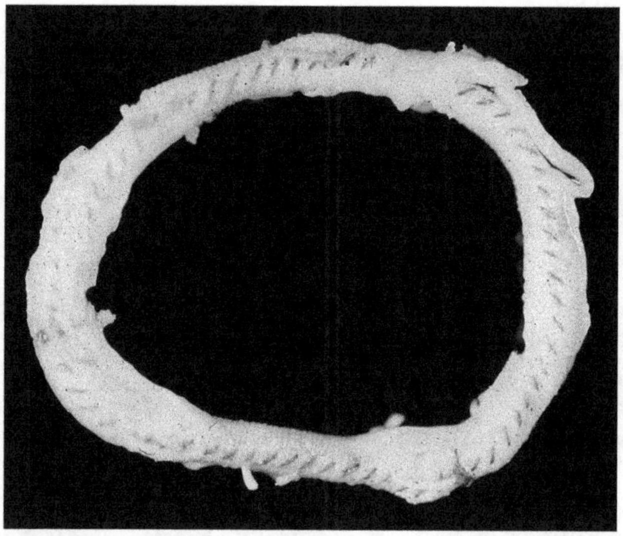

Figure 5. *Case #7*. Shown is the mitral ring which was excised 161 days after having been inserted. The ring apparently caused severe hemolysis which necessitated a blood transfusion at least once a week after the ring had been inserted. The ring is a 360° one and it is covered for the most part by fibrous tissue. The severe mitral regurgitation after valve repair was due to ring dehiscence plus prolapse of the anterior mitral leaflet.

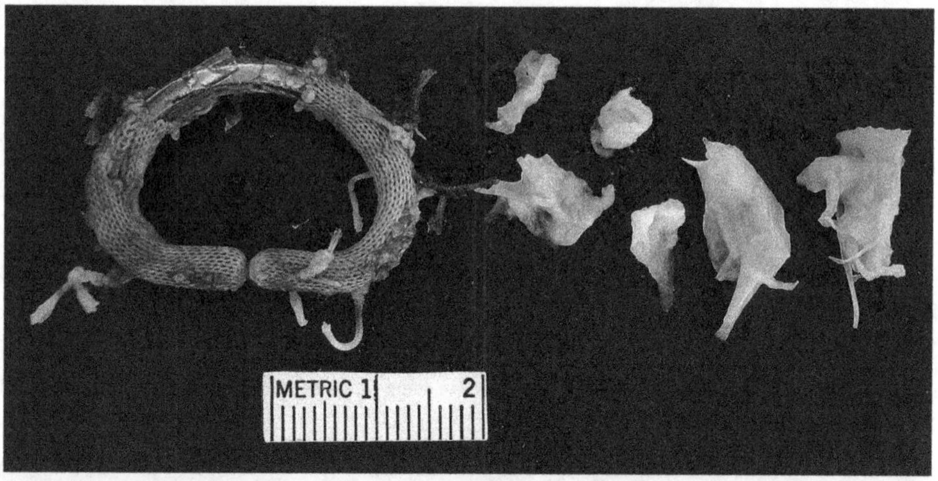

Figure 6. *Case #9*. Shown here are the operatively excised mitral ring and 6 fragments of the anterior mitral leaflet. The surgeon indicated that the previous mitral repair had failed and that was the reason for the recurrence of severe mitral regurgitation. The area enclosed by the mitral ring is 2.3 cm^2.

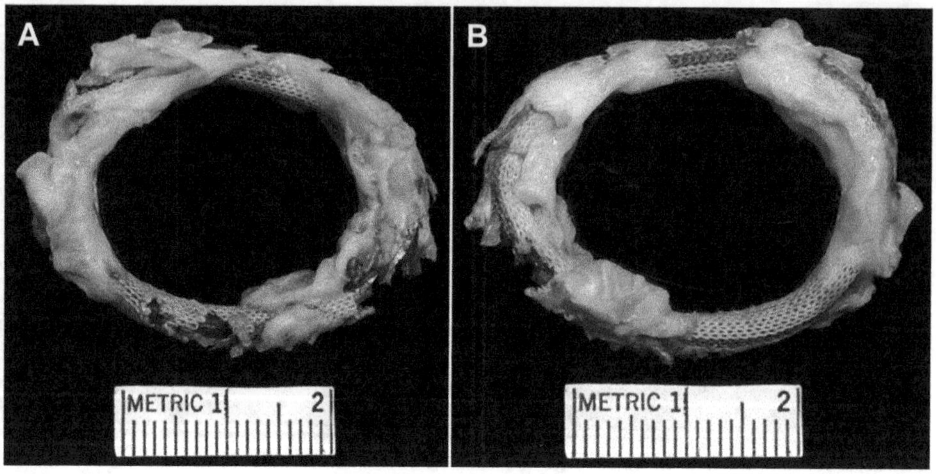

Figure 7. *Case #11*. This patient developed mitral stenosis (mean gradient between pulmonary artery wedge position and left ventricle, 7 mm Hg) after operative repair utilizing a 360° ring. The figures show the *top (A)* and *bottom (B)* aspects of the ring which is partially covered by white fibrous tissue. The orifice barely accepts the tip of my (WCR) index finger. Thus, this is acquired stenosis after "repair" of severe pure mitral regurgitation. The interior area of the ring measures is 3.5 cm^2.

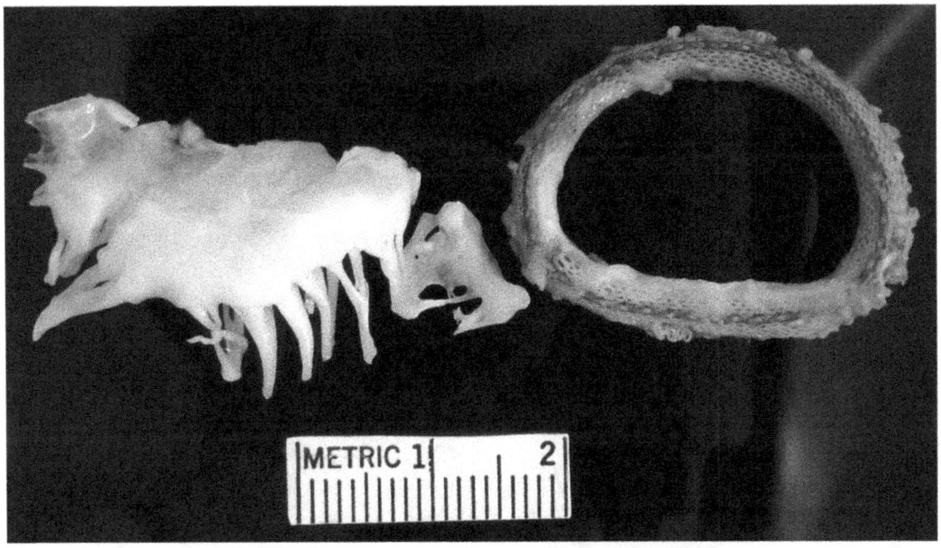

Figure 8. *Case #14.* Shown here is the operatively excised anterior mitral leaflet from its atrial aspect and the operatively excised ring. The area of the interior of the ring is 2.4 cm^2 suggesting that the ring had made the mitral orifice a bit stenotic. The mitral leaflet and several of its chords are thickened by fibrous tissue, an occurrence which could happen simply by the ring's being in the mitral annular position for 4 years as was the case in this patient. The distance from the margin of attachment to the central free margin was only 1.2 cm, suggesting that the mitral valve leaflets were quite small and further supporting the suggestion that the valve orifice was stenotic.

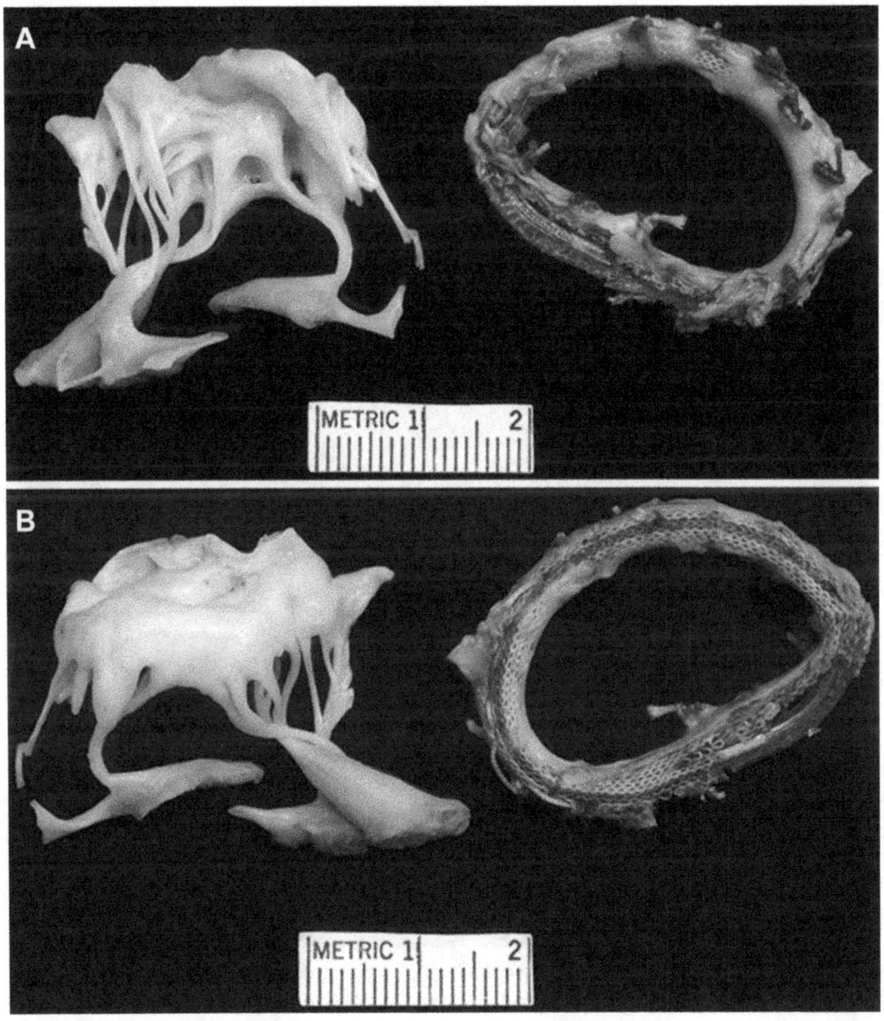

Figure 9. *Case #15.* Shown here is the anterior mitral leaflet with attached chords and papillary muscle and the mitral ring which had been in place for 4 years. *(A)* shows the mitral valve from the ventricular aspect and *(B)*, from the atrial aspect. The ring is shown from its view from left atrium in the *upper panel* and its attachment site in the *lower panel*. There was a mean diastolic gradient of 8 mm between pulmonary artery wedge position and left ventricle in this patient. The interior area of the ring is 3.2 cm^2.

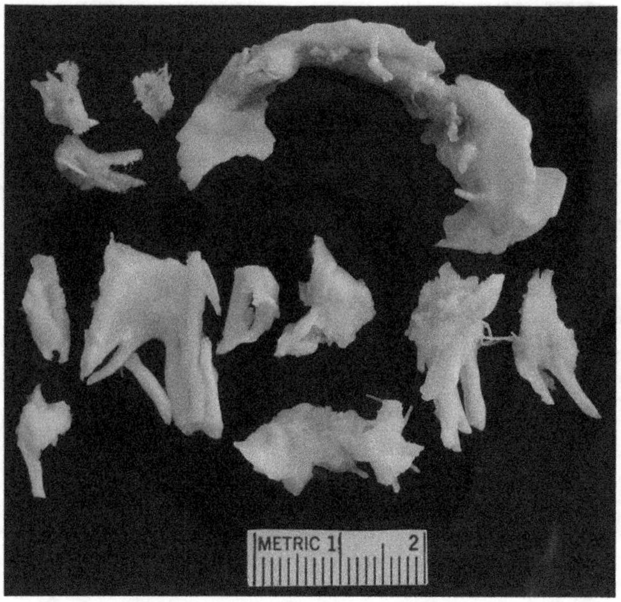

Figure 10. *Case #16*. Fragments of anterior and posterior mitral leaflets, which are diffusely fibrotic and focally calcified, and the severely fibrotic and small ring. The mitral ring had been inserted 5 years earlier for pure mitral regurgitation. An aortic valve replacement was also done at the time. The underlying etiology of the valve disease was considered systemic lupus erythematosis. Just before mitral valve replacement because of severe mitral stenosis (also mild mitral regurgitation) the mean pulmonary arterial wedge–left ventricular end-diastolic pressure was 21 mm Hg and the peak pulmonary arterial systolic pressure was 93 mm Hg. The body mass index was 54 Kg/m^2. The ring appears quite small. The mitral leaflets at the time of the repair operation were not described as being thickened.

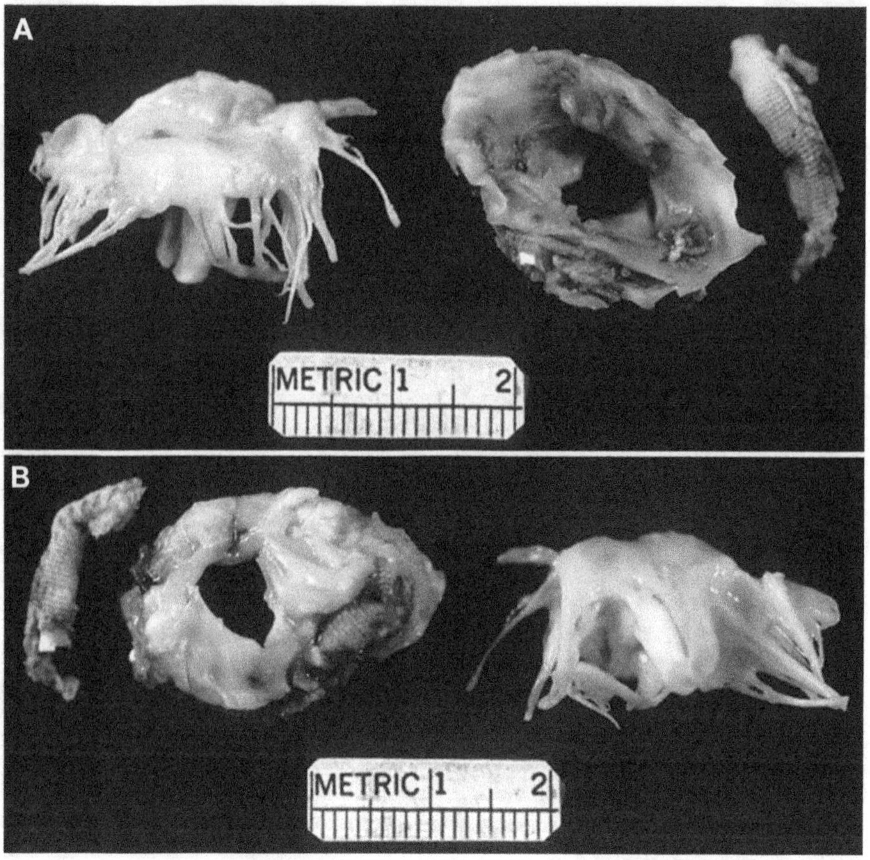

Figure 11. *Case #12*. Shown in *(A)* are the operatively excised anterior mitral leaflet (atrial aspect) and the mitral annular ring, which has been made severely stenotic by fibrous tissue covering much of the interior of the ring producing an extremely small orifice; *(B)* shows the ring as it would appear from the left atrium and the anterior mitral leaflet from its ventricular aspect. The orifice of the ring in the lower view is approximately 0.3 cm^2. Cardiac catheterization shortly before the mitral valve replacement yielded a left ventricular pressure of 124/11 and a simultaneous aortic pressure of 83/42. The pulmonary arterial wedge pressure A wave was 88, V wave 86, and mean 46 mm Hg. Thus, the mean diastolic gradient across the severely narrowed mitral ring was 52 mm Hg and the orifice area was 0.58 cm^2 and the index 0.34 cm/m^2. At the same time the cardiac index was 5.5 l/minute. The pulmonary arterial pressure was 114/41, and the right ventricular pressure, 114/14 mm Hg.

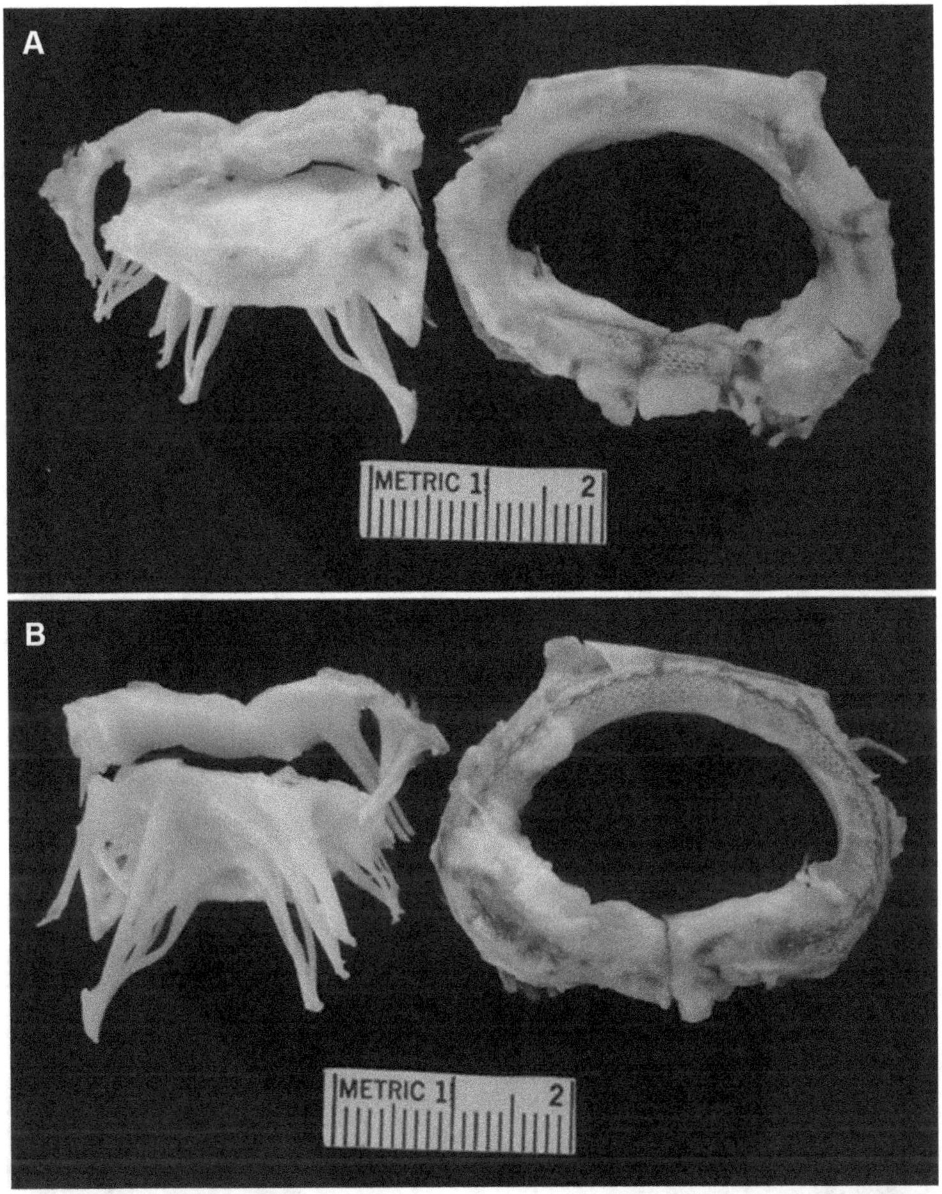

Figure 12. *Case #18.* Shown in *(A)* are the operatively excised anterior mitral leaflet from the atrial aspect and the previously inserted mitral ring from the atrial aspect; *(B)* shows the anterior mitral leaflet from the ventricular aspect and the ring which was adjacent to the left atrial wall. This patient also had a left ventricular aneurysm and severe coronary disease. The mitral regurgitation before the initial repair was considered ischemic in origin. The area of the interior of the mitral ring 3.1 cm^2.

continued or recurrent mitral valve dysfunction. Examination of the operatively excised mitral ring and anterior mitral leaflet at the time of mitral valve replacement disclosed the mitral leaflets in all 29 patients to be thickened, usually focally, by fibrous tissue. Examination of clinical notes, available echocardiographic findings, hemodynamic findings, and operative reports, and measurement of the area enclosed by the operatively-excised mitral ring suggest that possibly as many the 16 of the 29 (55%) patients had some degree of mitral stenosis before the mitral valve replacement operation. These findings at least raise the possibility that the mitral annular ring inserted at the "repair" operation was undersized in several of these patients. Fibrous tissue (pannus) within the area enclosed by the ring played the major role in at least 2 patients. The ring itself probably contributed to restriction of motion of the posterior mitral leaflet in 12 patients. The lesson of all this is that the insertion of a mitral annular ring is not a benign procedure and may in and of itself lead to leaflet fibrosis, to mitral stenosis, and to left ventricular outflow obstruction (if the ring is too large) (patients #2 and #17).[3]

Additional evidence for the occasional occurrence of mitral stenosis following mitral repair for MR comes from several recent reports.[17,19,20] Mesana and colleagues [17] studied 107 patients with severe MR from leaflet prolapse by stress echocardiography a mean of 4.3 years after mitral valve repair. The patients who had a complete ring—as did the patients in the present study—had a higher mean mitral

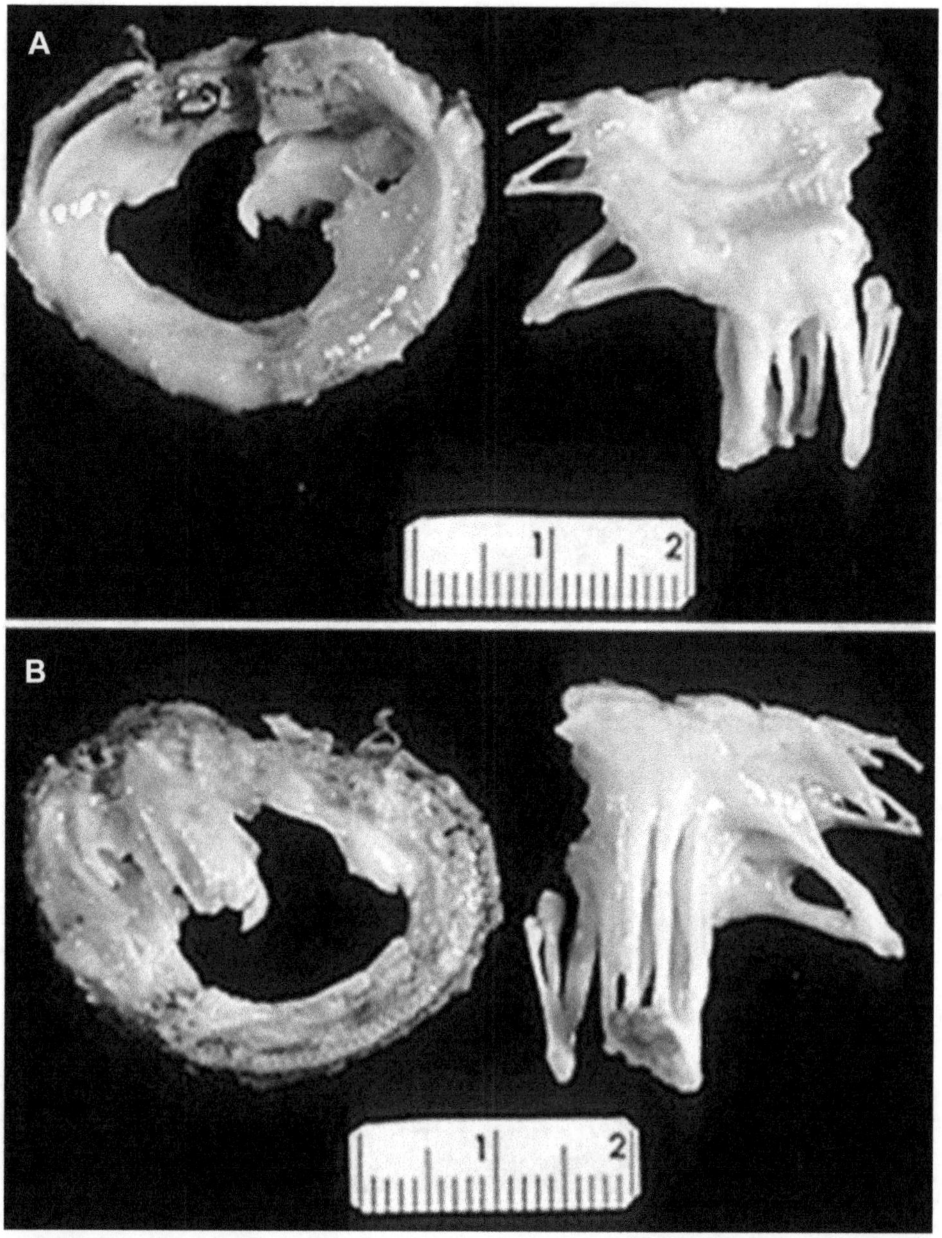

Figure 13. *Case #19*. Shown here are the mitral ring and the anterior mitral leaflet from the atrial aspect (*A*) and from the ventricular aspect (*B*). Mitral ring and a portion of anterior mitral leaflet in a 72-year-old woman with mitral regurgitation who underwent mitral valve replacement and ring excision 6 years after the initial mitral repair for sudden onset of mitral regurgitation. A portion of mitral leaflet is attached to the ring partially obliterating its orifice.

gradient after repair than those with a partial ring. These authors found a high degree of mitral stenosis after repair, particularly with the Duran ring. The mean mitral area at rest was 2.3 cm^2 in those patients with an incomplete ring ("band"), and 1.8 cm^2 in those with a complete ring. The mean mitral gradients were 3.8 and 5.8 mm Hg, respectively. Suh and colleagues [19] performed computed tomographic scans in patients who had mitral ring annuloplasty and found significant pannus "around the annuloplasty ring," leaflet thickening, and low mean mitral valve opening areas (2.5 ± 0.7 cm^2 [Carpentier-Edwards ring] and 2.2 ± 0.7 cm^2 [Duran ring]) (The normal mitral area in adults is 4 to 6 cm^2.). The annular area measured by computed tomography was 3.9 ± 0.5 cm^2 (C-E) and 3.9 ± 0.5 cm^2 (Duran ring). Of their 45 patients, 13 (29%) had transvalvular mitral gradients ≥5 mm Hg.

Some support of the above thesis is the recent examination at necropsy of the heart of a 70-year-old obese man who previously had undergone mitral valve repair for pure MR, percutaneous aortic valve implantation for aortic valve stenosis, and 2 previous coronary bypass grafting procedures. A new ring was inserted in the mitral valve annular region, and another ring in the tricuspid annular position (for tricuspid regurgitation), and during the 6-hour post-operative period he was in pulmonary edema. The area enclosed by the mitral ring measured 2.4 cm^2 and accepted only the tip of my (W.C.R.) index finger. The mitral ring was clearly undersized, something

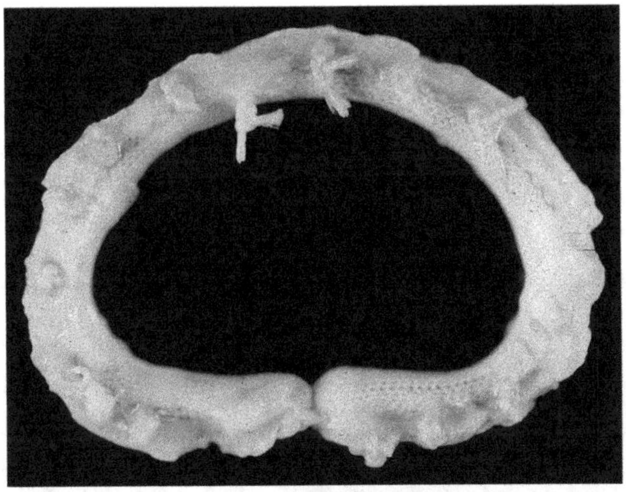

Figure 14. *Case #20*. Shown here is the atrial aspect of the mitral ring which is virtually completely covered by fibrous tissue. The ring had been in place for 8 years.

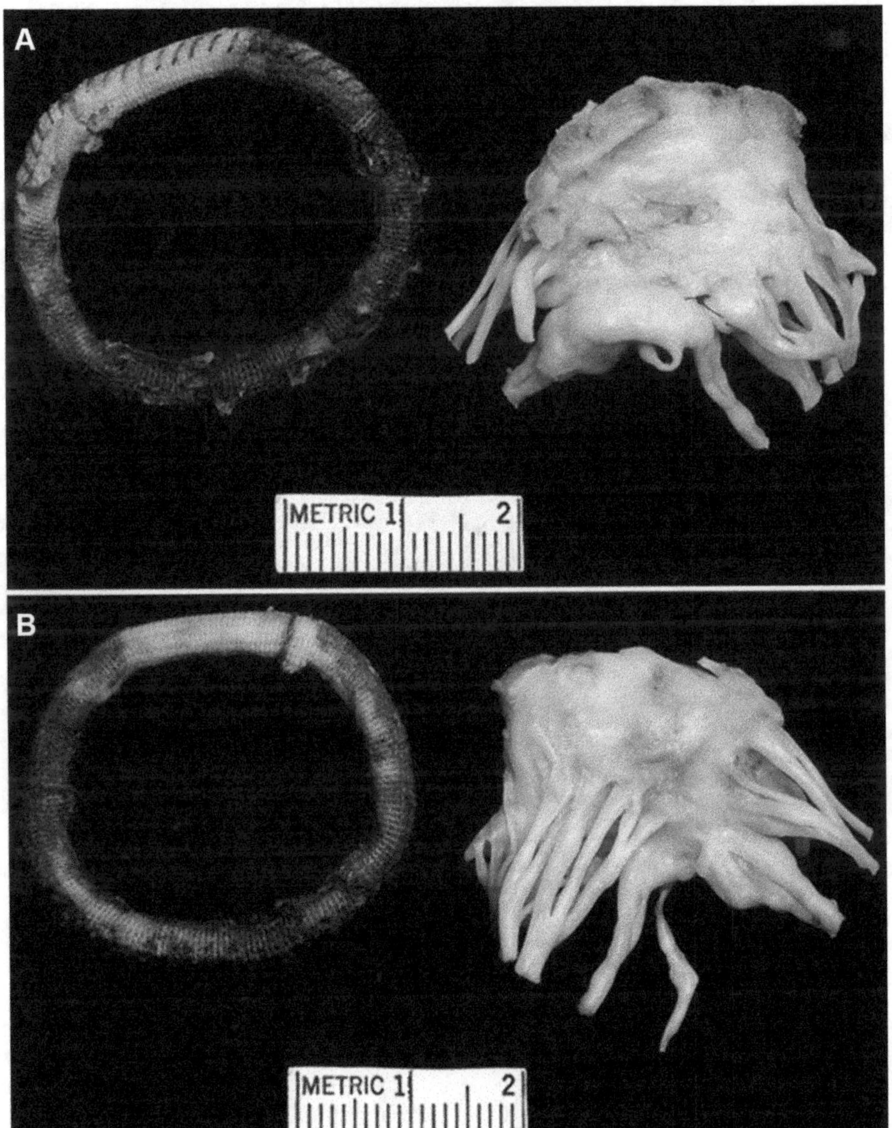

Figure 15. *Case #21*. Shown here are the mitral ring, which had been in place 9 years, and the anterior mitral leaflet from the atrial aspect *(A)* and from the ventricular aspect *(B)*. Green suture is present in the anterior mitral leaflet and was the result of an Alfieri stitch placed in both anterior and posterior leaflets 9 years earlier. Before the mitral replacement the posterior leaflet by echocardiogram was observed to be flail and at least one chord had ruptured. The area of the interior of the ring is 4.5 cm^2.

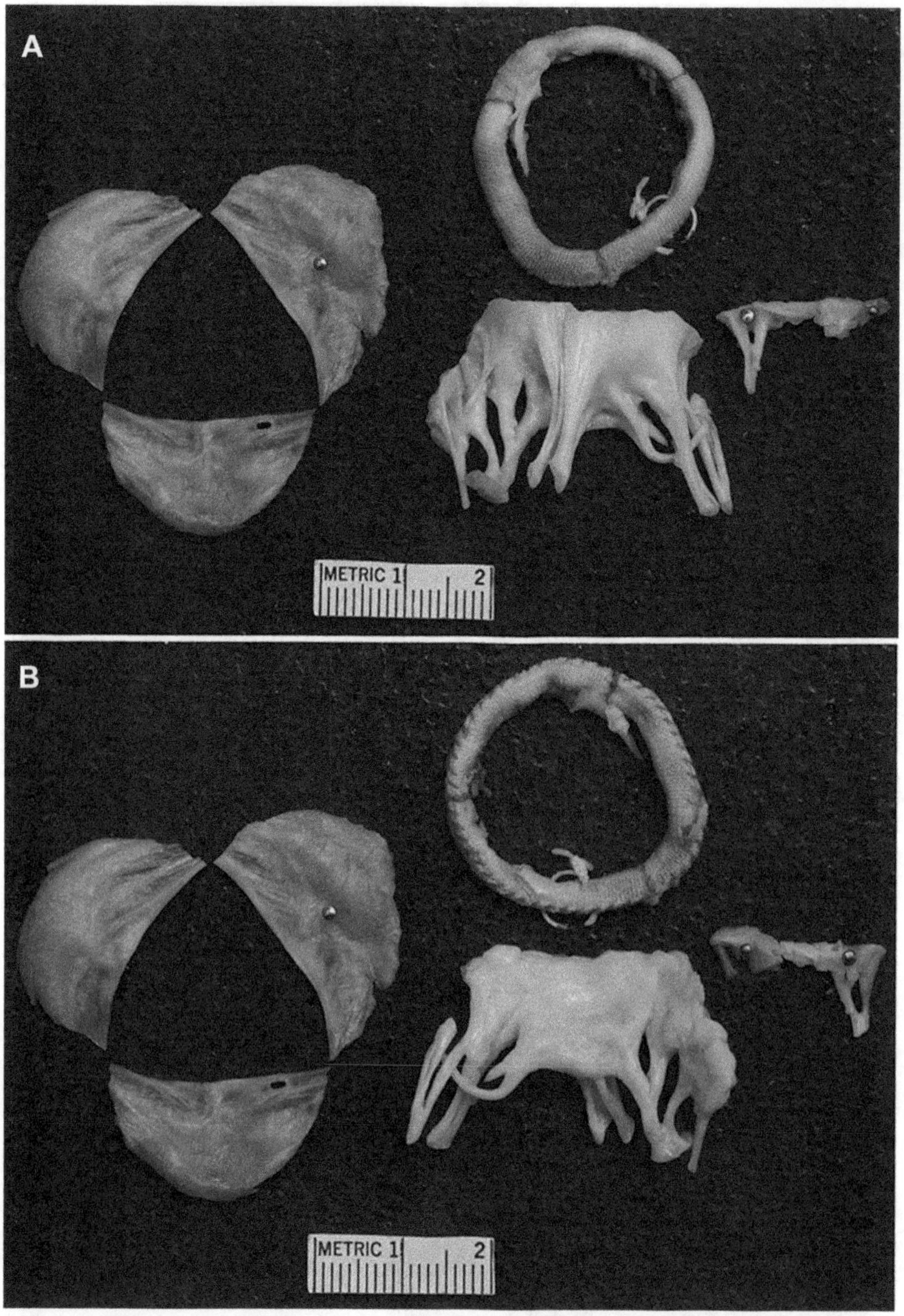

Figure 16. *Case #22.* Shown here is the operatively excised mitral ring (inserted 10 years earlier) and the anterior mitral leaflet from the left ventricular aspect *(A)* and atrial aspect *(right).* This patient had pure mitral regurgitation at the time of the repair operation and it recurred years later along with stenosis (mean diastolic pressure gradient between pulmonary wedge and left ventricular end-diastolic position of 13 mm Hg). Both anterior and posterior leaflets were thickened by fibrous tissue. This patient also had an aortic valve replacement at the time of the mitral replacement operation. The area enclosed by the ring was 3.9 cm^2 but by echocardiogram immediately before the replacement operation the mitral orifice area was 1.0 cm^2.

advocated in some quarters in some patients (Figure 21).[15,16]

Limitations of the present study include the lack of hemodynamic and/or echocardiographic data to confirm the presence of mitral stenosis in 6 of the 16 patients suspected of having morphologic evidence of stenosis. Possibly some of the "pannus" within the ring was "knocked off" during the excision process and thus that information was not available to us. Also, because the posterior mitral leaflet was usually not excised at the replacement operation we were entirely dependent on the description of that leaflet from the operative note and description of that leaflet was often absent in the operative note. Another limitation was non-availability of the operative note describing the

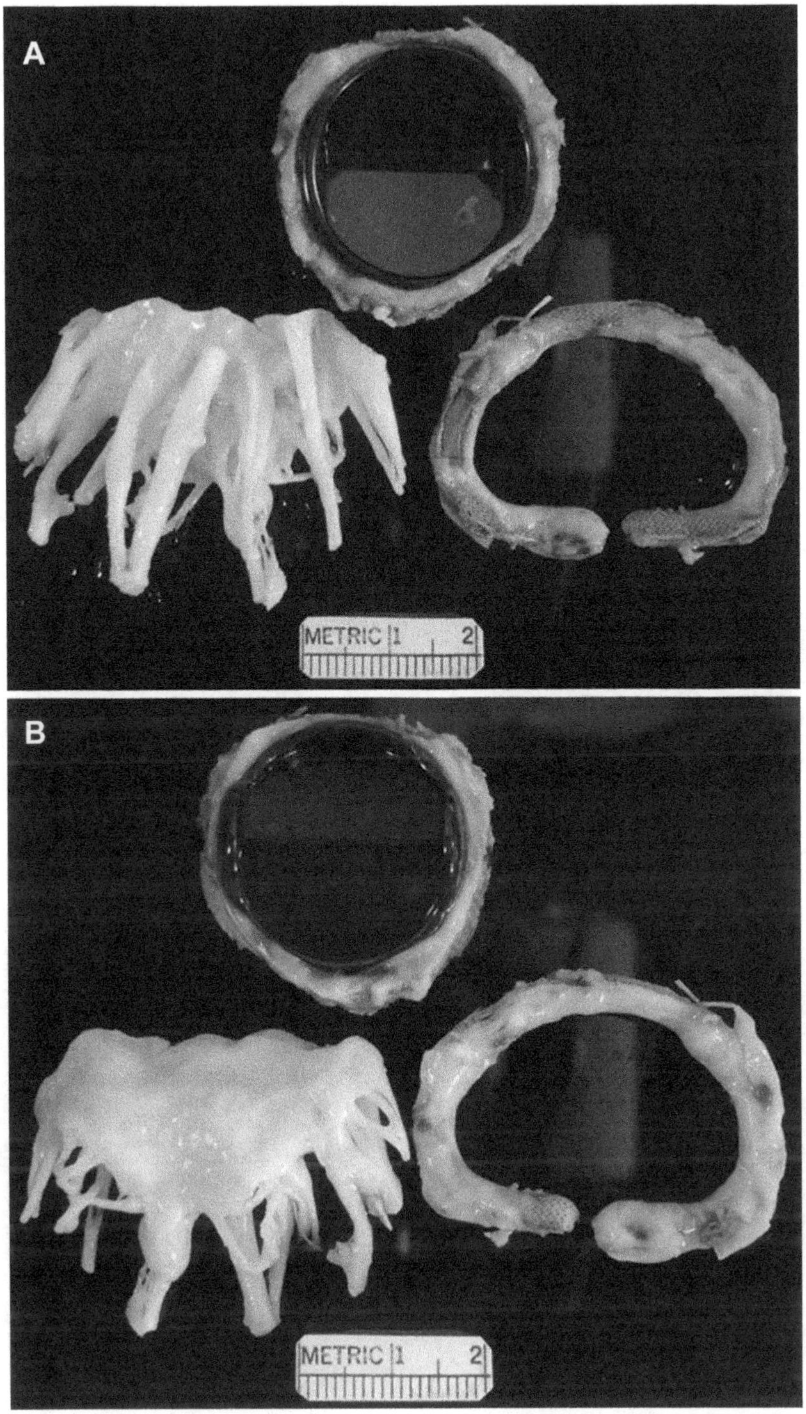

Figure 17. *Case #23*. Shown is the anterior mitral leaflet ventricular aspect *(A)* and atrial aspect *(B)*, mitral ring, and St. Jude Medical mechanical prosthesis which had been in the aortic valve position. The repair operation had occurred 11 years earlier. The mitral leaflets appear to have thickened by fibrous tissue between the 2 operations. Unfortunately, at cardiac catheterization just before the replacement operation a left ventricular pressure was not recorded so whether a pressure gradient was present across the mitral ring or leaflets is uncertain.

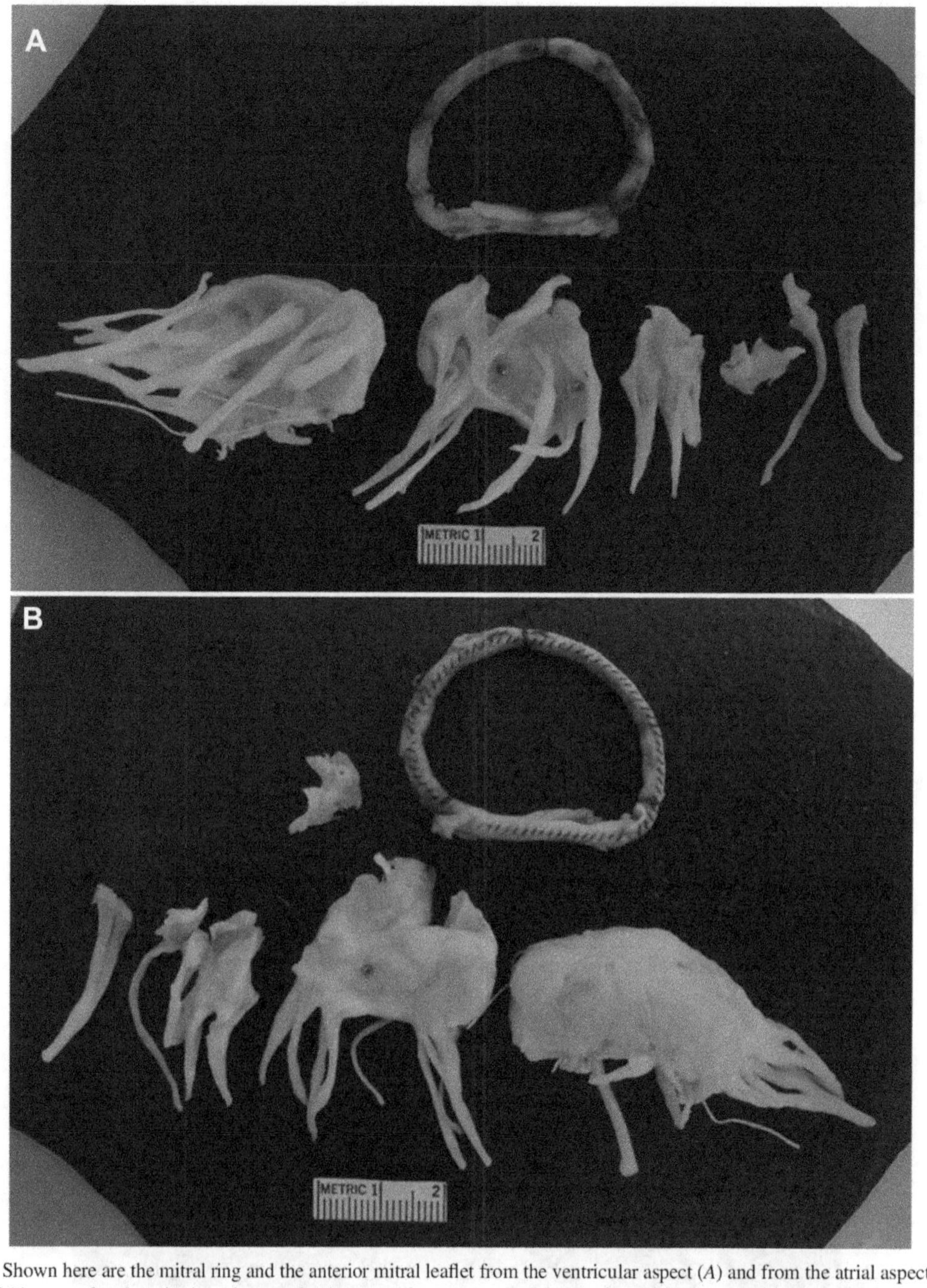

Figure 18. *Case #24*. Shown here are the mitral ring and the anterior mitral leaflet from the ventricular aspect (*A*) and from the atrial aspect (*B*). Mitral ring and mitral leaflets excised 11 years after the mitral repair operation because of severe post-repair mitral regurgitation secondary to mitral valve prolapse. The mitral ring had partially dehisced. A left ventricular pressure was not recorded just prior to the mitral valve replacement operation. A large parabasil disruption had occurred at the site of the earlier aortic valve replacement (St. Jude Medical mechanical prosthesis) and was responsible for prosthesis regurgitation.

findings at the time of the repair procedure (sometimes performed >20 years earlier). A positive feature of the present study is that it is the first to illustrate and measure the areas enclosed by the mitral rings inserted to eliminate the MR.

There are no other reported studies to which to compare the present findings. Although the immediate postoperative echocardiogram after repair may not have shown any degree of stenosis, late echocardiographic observations are relatively infrequent and thus some degree of stenosis may be more common than previously realized. It is likely that the degree of mitral dysfunction after repair may change with time.

Disclosures

The authors have no conflicts of interest to disclose.

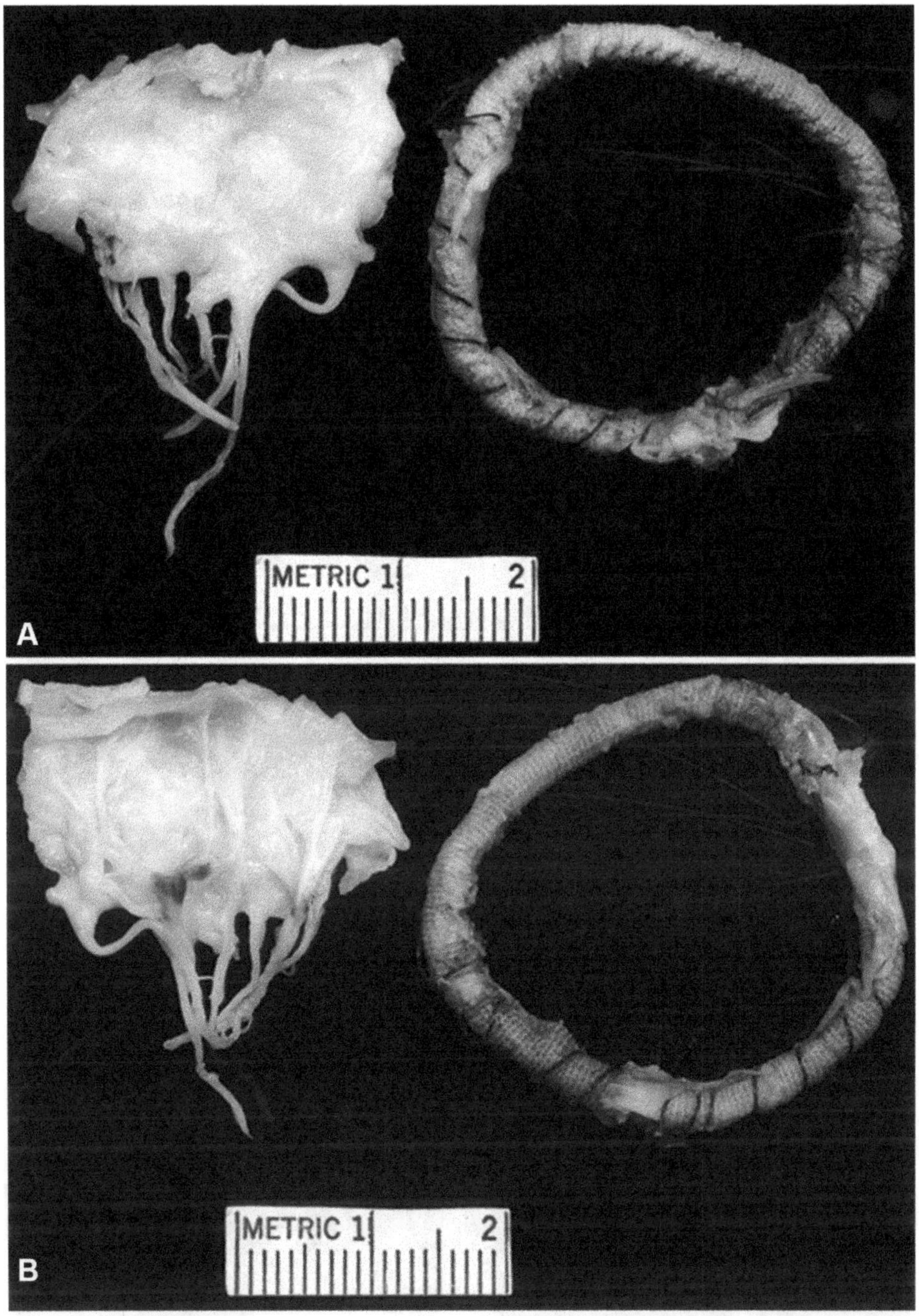

Figure 19. *Case #26*. Shown here is a portion of posterior mitral leaflet which was said to be flail by the operating surgeon and it was "swinging in the breeze." *(A)* shows the atrial aspect and *(B)*, the ventricular aspect. The ring was intact at operation. The area of the interior of the ring is 6.5 cm^2. The mitral leaflet is typical of mitral valve prolapse.

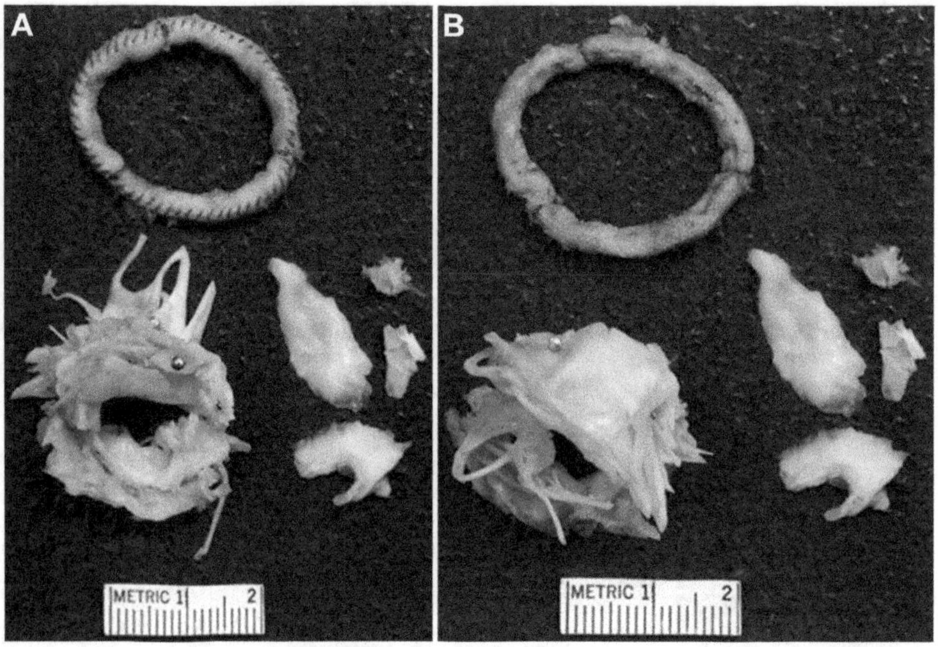

Figure 20. *Case #29*. The mitral valve from the atrial aspect *(A)* and a few fragments excised separately plus the mitral annular ring; *(B)* shows the anterior mitral leaflet and a portion of posterior leaflet from the ventricular aspect. In *(A)*, the mitral annular region is discernable where the ring had been placed and it appears that the ring squeezed the mitral leaflets, so to speak such that the orifice is quite stenotic. Before the mitral repair operation the mitral valve was purely regurgitant. The area of the interior of the mitral ring is 3.4 cm^2. Immediately before mitral valve replacement the mean diastolic gradient between pulmonary artery wedge position and left ventricle was 12 mm Hg.

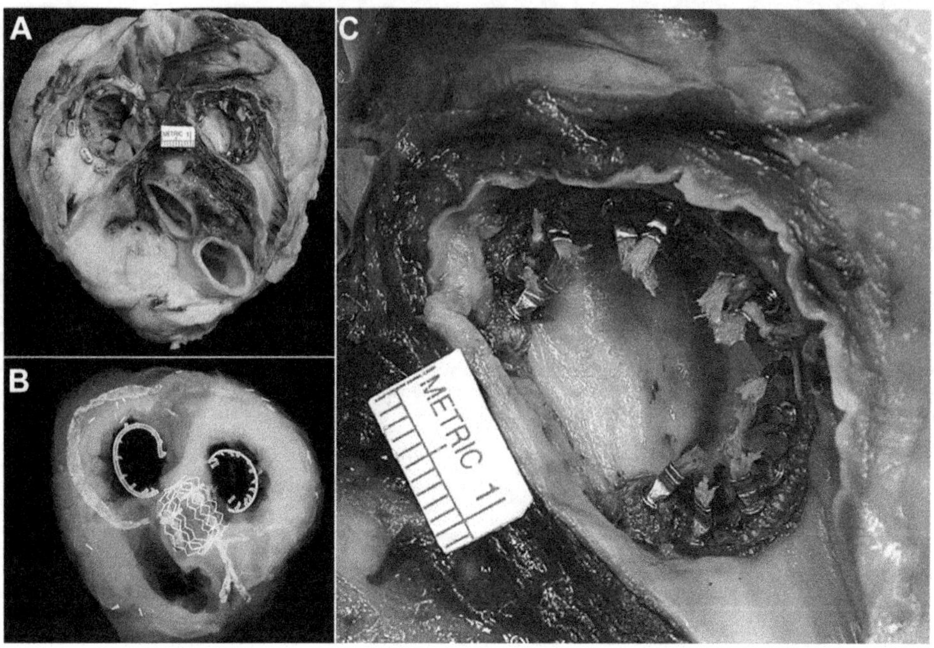

Figure 21. Photograph *(A)* and radiograph *(B)* of the rings placed in the tricuspid valve and mitral valve positions and a close-up of the mitral ring *(C)* in the 70-year old man who was in pulmonary edema for his terminal 6 hours after the ring insertion. The ring in the tricuspid valve position of course is much larger than the one in the mitral valve position. The area of the ring in the mitral position is approximately 2.4 cm^2. The orifice is covered in this view by anterior mitral leaflet *(C)*. The mitral ring appears to be considerably undersized. This ring also hinders free movement of the anterior mitral leaflet. The coronary arteries are heavily calcified and the bioprosthesis had earlier been inserted into the aortic valve position by the percutaneous route.

1. Marwick TH, Stewart WJ, Currie PJ, Cosgrove DM. Mechanisms of failure of mitral valve repair: an echocardiographic study. *Am Heart J* 1991;122:149–156.
2. David TE, Armstrong S, Sun Z, Daniel L. Late results of mitral valve repair for mitral regurgitation due to degenerative disease. *Ann Thorac Surg* 1993;56:4–7.
3. Lee KS, Stewart WJ, Lever HM, Underwood PL, Cosgrove DM. Mechanism of outflow tract obstruction causing failed mitral valve repair. Anterior displacement of leaflet coaptation. *Circulation* 1993;88:II24–II29.
4. Enriquez-Sarano M, Tajik AJ, Schaff HV, Orszulak TA, Bailey KR, Frye RL. Echocardiographic prediction of survival after surgical correction of organic mitral regurgitation. *Circulation* 1994;90: 830–837.
5. Cerfolio RJ, Orszulak TA, Pluth JR, Harmsen WS, Schaff HV, Mitchell RS, Duran CG, Kafrouni G. Reoperation after valve repair for mitral regurgitation: early and intermediate results. *J Thorac Cardiovasc Surg* 1996;111:1177–1184.
6. Gillinov AM, Cosgrove DM, Lytle BW, Taylor PC, Stewart RW, McCarthy PM, Smedira NG, Muehrcke DD, Apperson-Hansen C, Loop FD, David TE, Carpentier AF, Cohn LH. Reoperation for failure of mitral valve repair. *J Thorac Cardiovasc Surg* 1997;113:467–475.
7. Braunberger E, Deloche A, Berrebi A, Abdallah F, Celestin JA, Meimoun P, Chatellier G, Chauvaud S, Fabiani JN, Carpentier A. Very long-term results (more than 20 years) of valve repair with Carpentier's techniques in nonrheumatic mitral valve insufficiency. *Circulation* 2001;104:I8–I11.
8. David TE, Ivanov J, Armstrong S, Christie D, Rakowski H. A comparison of outcomes of mitral valve repair for degenerative disease with posterior, anterior, and bileaflet prolapse. *J Thorac Cardiovasc Surg* 2005;130:1242–1249.
9. Shekar PS, Couper GS, Cohn LH. Mitral valve re-repair. *J Heart Valve Dis* 2005;14:583–587.
10. Adams DH, Anyanwu A. Pitfalls and limitations in measuring and interpreting the outcomes of mitral valve repair. *J Thorac Cardiovasc Surg* 2006;131:523–529.
11. Dumont E, Gillinov AM, Blackstone EH, Sabik JF, Svensson LG, Mihaljevic T, Houghtaling PL, Lytle BW. Reoperation after mitral valve repair for degenerative disease. *Ann Thorac Surg* 2007;84: 444–450.
12. DiBardino DJ, ElBardissi AW, McClure RS, Razo-Vasquez OA, Kelly NE, Cohn LH. Four decades of experience with mitral valve repair: analysis of differential indications, technical evolution, and long-term outcome. *J Thorac Cardiovasc Surg* 2010;139:76–84.
13. Wong RHL, Lee APW, Ng CSH, Wan IYP, Wan S, Underwood MJ. Mitral valve repair: past, present, and future. *Asian Cardiovasc Thorac Ann* 2010;18:586–595.
14. Kwon MH, Lee LS, Cevasco M, Couper GS, Shekar PS, Cohn LH, Chen FY. Recurrence of mitral regurgitation after partial versus complete mitral valve ring annuloplasty for functional mitral regurgitation. *J Thorac Cardiovasc Surg* 2013;146:616–622.
15. Asgar AW, Mack MJ, Stone GW. Secondary mitral regurgitation in heart failure: pathophysiology, prognosis, and therapeutic considerations. *J Am Coll Cardiol* 2015;65:1231–1248.
16. Asgar AW, Mack MJ, Stone GW. Reply: secondary mitral regurgitation. *J Am Coll Cardiol* 2015;66:1947.
17. Mesana TG, Lam BK, Chan V, Chen K, Ruel M, Chan K. Clinical evaluation of functional mitral stenosis after mitral valve repair for degenerative disease: potential affect on surgical strategy. *J Thorac Cardiovasc Surg* 2013;146:1418–1423.
18. Kron IL, Hung J, Overbey JR, Bouchard D, Gelijns AC, Moskowitz AJ, Voisine P, O'Gara PT, Argenziano M, Michler RE, Gillinov M, Puskas JD, Gammie JS, Mack MJ, Smith PK, Sai-Sudhakar C, Gardner TJ, Ailawadi G, Zeng X, O'Sullivan K, Parides MK, Swayze R, Thourani V, Rose EA, Perrault LP, Acker MA; CTSN Investigators. Predicting recurrent mitral regurgitation after mitral valve repair for severe ischemic mitral regurgitation. *J Thorac Cardiovasc Surg* 2015;149:752–761.
19. Suh YJ, Chang BC, Im DJ, Kim YJ, Hong YJ, Hong GR, Kim YJ. Assessment of mitral annuloplasty ring by cardiac computed tomography: correlation with echocardiographic parameters and comparison between two different ring types. *J Thorac Cardiovasc Surg* 2015;150: 1082–1090.
20. Chan V, Mesana TG. Functional mitral stenosis after mitral valve repair is a true anatomic problem that originates from the time of surgery. *J Thorac Cardiovasc Surg* 2015;150:1091–1092.
21. Suri RM, Clavel M-A, Schaff HV, Michelena HI, Huebner M, Nishimura RA, Enriquez-Sarano M. Effect of recurrent mitral regurgitation following degenerative mitral valve repair: long-term analysis of competing outcomes. *J Am Coll Cardiol* 2016;67:488–498.

Smeloff-Cutter Mechanical Prosthesis in the Aortic Position for 49 Years

Robin A. Chalkley, MD[a,b,c], Chong W. Kim, MD[a,b,c], James W. Choi, MD[a,b,c], William C. Roberts, MD[a,b,c], and Jeffrey M. Schussler, MD[a,b,c,*]

We describe a 76-year-old male physician who at age 27 underwent replacement of his stenotic aortic valve with a Smeloff-Cutter mechanical prosthesis which functioned normally for 49 years. He died of a noncardiac condition. A normally functioning substitute cardiac valve for this length of time has not been previously reported (1). © 2019 Published by Elsevier Inc. (Am J Cardiol 2019;124:457–459)

Smeloff-Cutter valve first design began production in 1964; a second design was implemented in 1966 and was produced until the end of 1989 at which time the Smeloff-Cutter valve was no longer manufactured.[2] It was one of the first commercially available prosthetic heart valves and the first with double cage design.[2] The double cage design was intended to reduce the risk of thromboembolism secondary to the "self-washing" effect.[3] The Smeloff-Cutter was a popular ball-in-cage valve and had 72,000 valves implanted.[4] It was mostly used in aortic position.[4] Smeloff-Cutter valve durability was comparable to the more popular Starr-Edwards valve and had 25 year survival of 31%.[5] Longest reported implanted Smeloff-Cutter valve was 43 years reported in publications.[1] We recently encountered a physician who had the Smeloff-Cutter valve implanted for 49 years in the aortic position without any complications secondary to the Smeloff-Cutter valve and who died of noncardiac causes. A description of Smeloff-Cutter valve implanted for this length of time has not been previously described.

Case Description

This 76-year-old man underwent replacement of his stenotic aortic valve for congenital bicuspid aortic stenosis at age 27 years by Dr. Denton A. Cooley. During the 49 years that followed, he took warfarin intermittently; he did not take warfarin for approximately a decade because of recurrent gastrointestinal bleeding. No episodes occurred that suggested prosthetic thrombosis or systemic embolism. Later in life, he developed coronary artery disease for which he received 3 drug-eluting stents for unstable angina, and heart failure due to ischemic cardiomyopathy for which he received an implantable cardioverter defibrillator. Weeks before his death, echocardiogram revealed a peak left ventricular outflow velocity of 2.18 m/sec, an aortic valve velocity time integral of 44.2 cm, an aortic valve peak transvalvular gradient of 19 mm Hg and an aortic valve area of 2.9cm^2. His mechanical valve type was identified while he was living using a radiographic guide developed by Mehlman and Resnekov[6] and confirmed at necropsy to be a Smeloff-Cutter type cage in ball. The patient died from chronic renal failure.

The patient was originally from South Korea where he graduated from Seoul National Medical School. He eventually came to the United States where he practiced internal medicine for 40 years. He was strongly desirous that his mechanical prosthesis be examined after his death. The excised poppet of the prosthesis was discolored but its surface was smooth and devoid of indentions and cracks. The poppet moved normally in its cage.

Comments

The Smeloff-Cutter valve was first produced in 1964.[2] It was the first substitute valve to have a double cage in which

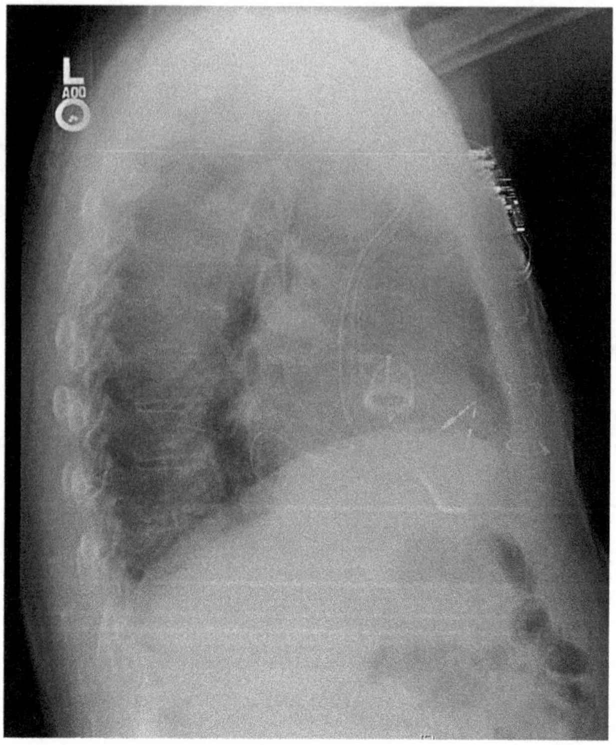

Figure 1. Lateral chest radiograph the distinctive double cage design.

[a]Baylor Scott & White Heart and Vascular Hospital, Dallas, Texas; [b]Baylor University Medical Center, Dallas, Texas; and [c]Texas A&M College of Medicine, Dallas, Texas. Manuscript received February 15, 2019; revised manuscript received and accepted May 6, 2019.

See page 459 for disclosure information.

*Corresponding author: Tel: 469-800-7400; fax: 469-800-7401.

E-mail address: Jeffrey.Schussler@BSWHealth.org (J.M. Schussler).

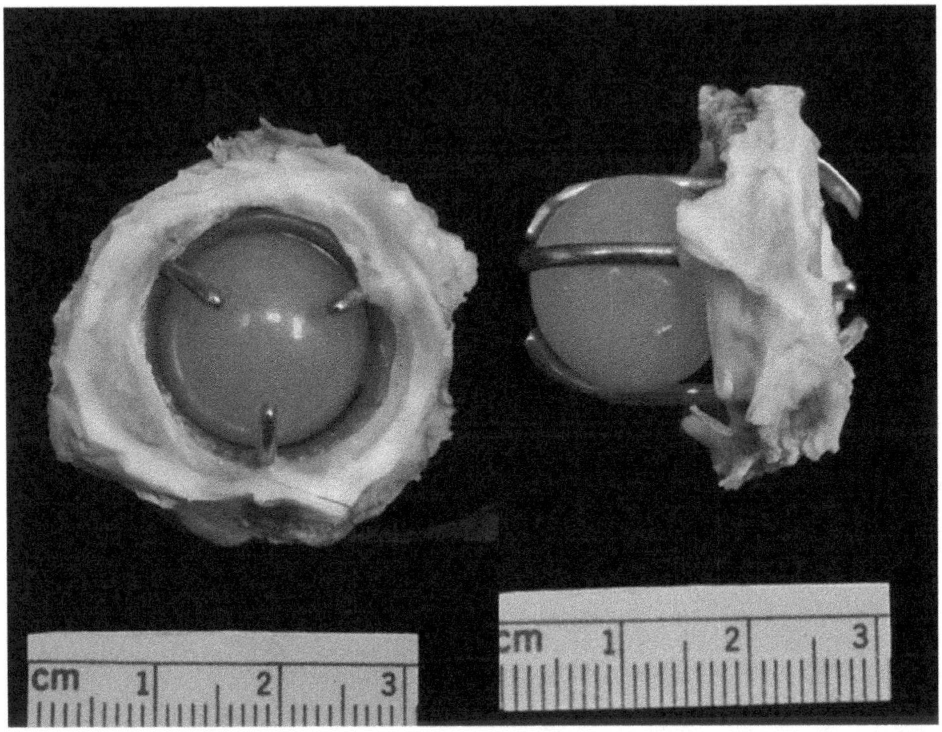

Figure 2. Smeloff-Cutter valve post mortem, note the ball discoloration from lipid absorption.

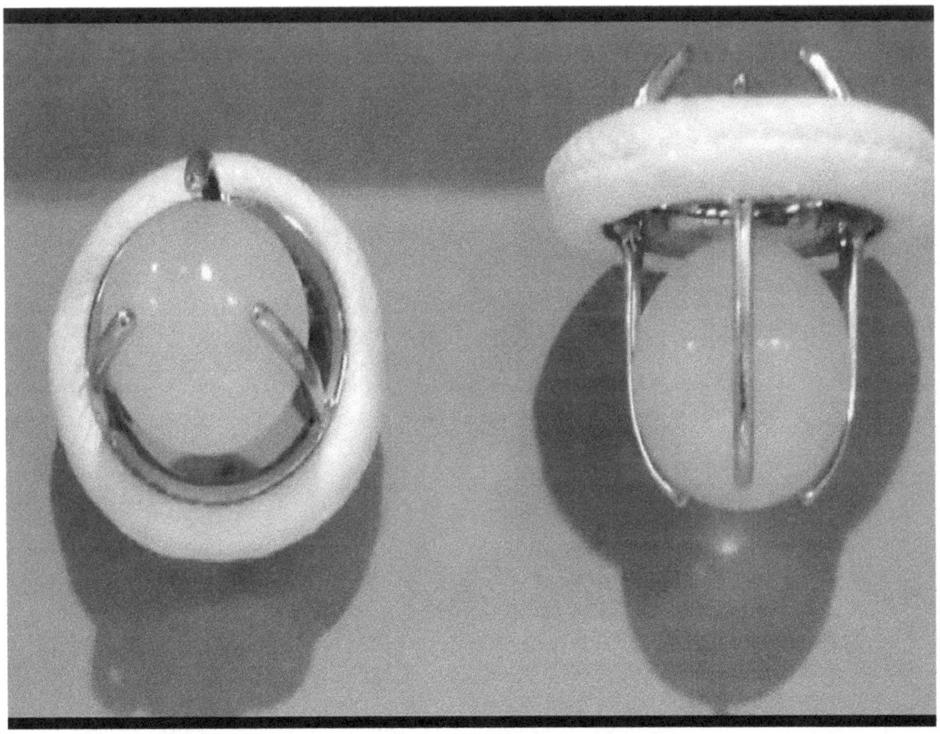

Figure 3. New Smeloff-Cutter valve.

the silicone rubber ball moved.[2] It also had a "self-washing" effect thought to reduce the risk of thrombosis.[3] This first design (produced from 1964 to 1966) was plagued with poppet malfunction. The poppet absorbed lipids which caused it to swell, a situation that could lead to immobility of the poppet in the cage.[1,2] The second iteration (produced from 1966 to 1989) included changes to the silicon rubber processing (as it did for many other ball and cage valves

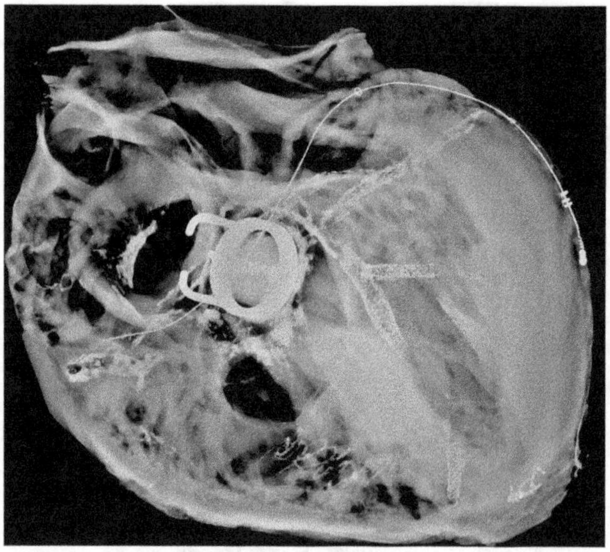

Figure 4. Post mortem radiograph of the heart.

including the more popular Starr-Edwards valve) and the cage was changed slightly.[2] In the newer version, the housing was titanium and the ball was silicone rubber.[2] The incidence of thromboembolism in patients with this valve in the aortic position without anticoagulation was 1% per patient year.[3] Of the 72,000 valves implanted (the Starr-Edwards poppet-in-cage 250,000 has been implanted).[4] The 10, 20, and 25 year survival postvalve implantation was 69%, 47%, and 31%, respectively.[5] The 10, 20, and 25 actuarial freedom rate of valve complication, reoperations or death was 73%, 47%, and 20% respectively.[5] These rates are similar to Starr-Edwards valve.[5] That our patient suffered no complications with his mechanical prosthesis is testament to the durability of the design of the Smeloff-Cutter valve, particularly in the aortic position (Figures 1–4).

Disclosures

The authors have no conflicts of interest to disclose.

1. Head SJ, Ko J, Singh R, Roberts WC, Mack MJ. 43.3-year durability of a Smeloff-Cutter ball-caged mitral valve. *Annal Thora Surg* 2011;91: 606–608.
2. Gott VL, Alejo DE, Cameron DE. Mechanical heart valves: 50 years of evolution. *Annal Thora Surg* 2003;76:S2230–S2239.
3. Gometza B, Duran CM. Ball valve (Smeloff-Cutter) aortic valve replacement without anticoagulation. *Annal Thor Surg* 1995;60: 1312–1316.
4. Belenkie I, Carr M, Schlant R, Nutter D, Symbas P. Malfunction of a cutter-Smeloff mitral ball valve prosthesis: diagnosis by phonocardiography and echocardiography. *Am. Heart J* 1973;86:399–403.
5. Godje O, Fischlein T, Adelhard K, Mair H, Reichart B. 25 years follow-up of patients after replacement of the aortic valve with a Smeloff-cutter prosthesis. *Thora Card Surg* 1996;44:234–238.
6. Mehlman DJ, Resnekov L. A guide to the radiographic identification of prosthetic heart valves. *Circulation* 1978;57:613–623.

www.ingramcontent.com/pod-product-compliance
Lightning Source LLC
LaVergne TN
LVHW062134200926
848484LV00007B/1814